CARDIAC NURSING

SANDRA L. UNDERHILL R.N., M.N.

Assistant Professor, Department of Physiological Nursing
University of Washington, Seattle, Washington

SUSAN L. WOODS R.N., M.N.

Associate Professor, Department of Physiological Nursing
University of Washington, Seattle, Washington

ERIKA SEIBERLER SIVARAJAN R.N., M.A.

Co-Director, Cardiac Rehabilitation, Center for Health Enhancement, Education and Research
Center for Health Sciences; and Assistant Clinical Professor, School of Nursing
University of California at Los Angeles, Los Angeles, California
Formerly, Research Assistant Professor, Department of Physiological Nursing
University of Washington, Seattle, Washington

CAROL JEAN HALPENNY R.N., M.A.

Doctoral Student, School of Nursing; Formerly, Assistant Professor
Department of Physiological Nursing, University of Washington, Seattle, Washington

With 32 additional contributors

J. B. LIPPINCOTT COMPANY Philadelphia · Toronto

CARDIAC NURSING

Library of Congress Cataloging in Publication Data
Main entry under title:

Cardiac Nursing.

  Bibliography
  Includes index.
  1. Cardiovascular disease nursing. I. Underhill, Sandra L.
[DNLM: 1. Cardiovascular diseases—Nursing.
WY 152.5 C2672]
RC674.C3   616.1   81-5973
ISBN 0-397-54275-5   AACR2

The authors and publisher have exerted every effort to ensure
that drug selection and dosage set forth in this text are in accord
with current recommendations and practice at the time of
publication. However, in view of ongoing research, changes in
government regulations, and the constant flow of information
relating to drug therapy and drug reactions, the reader is urged
to check the package insert for each drug for any change in
indications and dosage and for added warnings and precautions.
This is particularly important when the recommended agent is a
new or infrequently employed drug.

Printed in the United States of America

*To our families and friends
for their enduring support*

CONTENTS

CONTRIBUTORS

Eleanor F. Bond, R.N., M.A.
Doctoral Student
Department of Physiology and Biophysics
University of Washington
Seattle, Washington

Mary Boozer, R.N., M.N.
Associate Professor
Department of Physiological Nursing
University of Washington
Seattle, Washington

Jenille Bradly, R.N.
Coordinator of Medical Subspecialty Clinics
U.S. Public Health Service Hospital
Seattle, Washington

Lora E. Burke, R.N., M.N.
Director, Cardiac Rehabilitation
St. Vincent Medical Center
Los Angeles, California

Dianne J. Christopherson, R.N., M.N.
Assistant Director of Staff Development
St. Joseph's Mercy Hospital
Ann Arbor, Michigan

Marie J. Cowan, R.N., Ph.D.
Assistant Professor
School of Nursing, Department of Physiological
Nursing
and School of Medicine, Departments of Pathology
and Medicine, Division of Cardiology
University of Washington
Seattle, Washington

Ruth F. Craven, R.N., M.N.
Assistant Professor
Department of Physiological Nursing
University of Washington
Seattle, Washington

Paul S. Fardy, Ph.D.
Director, Department of Cardiac Rehabilitation
St. Catherine Hospital
East Chicago, Indiana

Linda Ann Felthous, B.S. in Pharm., R.Ph.
Drug Information and Education Coordinator
Group Health Cooperative of Puget Sound
Seattle, Washington

B. Lynn Grose, R.N., M.N.
Educational Coordinator
Critical Care Unit
Harborview Medical Center
Clinical Assistant Professor
Department of Physiological Nursing
University of Washington
Seattle, Washington

Margaret Hall, R.N., M.D.
Resident
University of Washington
Seattle, Washington

Janet B. Haskin, B.S.N., R.N.
Supervisory Clinical Nurse, CCU
U.S. Public Health Service Hospital
Seattle, Washington

Rose Homan, R.N., M.A., D.D.S.
Formerly, Assistant Professor
Department of Physiological Nursing
University of Washington
Seattle, Washington

Patricia A. Hong, R.N., M.A.
Captain, U.S. Air Force Nurse Corps
Anchorage, Alaska
Formerly, Instructor
Department of Physiological Nursing
University of Washington
Seattle, Washington

Jon S. Huseby, M.D.
Respiratory Disease Specialist
The Polyclinic
Clinical Assistant Professor
Department of Physiological Nursing
University of Washington
Seattle, Washington

Kathleen A. Kominski, R.N., M.N.
Staff Nurse, Coronary Care Unit
U.S. Public Health Service Hospital
Seattle, Washington

Debra Laurent-Bopp, R.N., M.N.
Cardiovascular Clinical Nurse Specialist
Virginia Mason Hospital
Clinical Assistant
Department of Physiological Nursing
University of Washington
Seattle, Washington

Kathryn A. Lee, R.N., M.N.
Research Associate
Department of Physiological Nursing
University of Washington
Seattle, Washington

Katherine M. Newton, R.N., M.A.
Lecturer
Department of Physiological Nursing
University of Washington
Seattle, Washington

Nancy A. Niles, R.N., M.A.
Clinical Nurse Specialist, Critical Care Units
U.S. Public Health Service Hospital

Clinical Instructor
Department of Physiological Nursing
University of Washington
Seattle, Washington
Thomas A. Preston, M.D.
Director of Cardiology
U.S. Public Health Service Hospital
Seattle, Washington
Wanda Roberts, R.N., M.N.
Assistant Professor
Department of Physiological Nursing
Educational Coordinator of Burn Center
Harborview Medical Center
University of Washington
Seattle, Washington
Joanne Schnaidt Rokosky, R.N., M.N.
Assistant Professor
Department of Physiological Nursing
University of Washington
Seattle, Washington
Sarah J. Sanford, R.N., M.A.
Critical Care Medical-Surgical Nursing Administrator
Overlake Hospital
Bellevue, Washington
Clinical Assistant Professor
Department of Physiological Nursing
University of Washington
Seattle, Washington
Cynthia C. Scalzi, R.N., M.N.
Research Associate, School of Nursing
Doctoral Candidate, School of Public Health
University of California at Los Angeles
Los Angeles, California
Joan Shaver, R.N., Ph.D.
Assistant Professor
Department of Physiological Nursing
University of Washington
Seattle, Washington

Brenda J. Siewicki, R.N., M.N.
Nurse Consultant
Medicus Company
Evanston, Illinois
Formerly, Teacher—Practitioner
School of Nursing
Rush Presbyterian St. Luke's University
Chicago, Illinois
Sandra D. Solack, R.N., M.S.N.
Predoctoral Student
Department of Physiology and Biophysics
University of Washington
Seattle, Washington
Gene Trobaugh, M.D.
Assistant Professor
Department of Cardiology
Harborview Medical Center
and School of Medicine
University of Washington
Seattle, Washington
Martha Tyler, R.N., M.N.
Assistant Professor
Department of Physiological Nursing
Adjunct Assistant Professor of Medicine
Division of Respiratory Diseases
Harborview Medical Center
University of Washington
Seattle, Washington
Robert E. Wills, M.D.
Clinical Assistant Professor
Formerly, Assistant Professor of Medicine
Department of Physiological Nursing
University of Washington
Seattle, Washington
Karen S. Wulff, R.N., M.N.
Cardiovascular Clinical Specialist
University Hospital
Clinical Instructor
Department of Physiological Nursing
University of Washington
Seattle, Washington

PREFACE

Nurses are accountable for their practice. The scope of all nursing practice has expanded because of increased professional expectations, advanced technology, and greater demands by health-care consumers. Because coronary artery disease is the number one health problem in the United States and other Western industrialized nations, a great deal of medical and nursing research and public education have been focused on heart disease. As a result, the scope of the subspecialty of cardiac nursing has grown to an even greater extent than the scope of general medical–surgical nursing.

All patients have the right to receive safe, competent, individualized nursing care. A sample of this philosophy can be seen in the Patient's Bill of Rights in Chapter 45. Key features of nursing responsibility are coordination and continuity of patient care. The responsibility of patients and families is to participate actively in the care.

Cardiac nurses are primarily concerned with the recognition and management of the problems, both physiological and psychological, of patients with coronary artery disease; however, they must also be prepared to care for cardiac patients with other types of cardiovascular disease. The knowledge base of the cardiac nurse is expanding to include an appreciation of coronary artery disease as being a continuum, of which the patient's hospitalization experience is only a small part.

The priorities of cardiac nursing interventions are based on Maslow's hierarchy of needs: physiological, safety, love and belonging, esteem, and self-actualization.[1] Life-threatening needs, such as control of lethal arrhythmias, must be met before the nurse can assist the cardiac patient with meeting other needs. It is essential that the cardiac nurse be clinically competent, first, to meet these life-threatening needs, and second, to assist the patient and family affected by coronary artery disease to function optimally.

Nursing is organized around the nursing process: assessment, planning, implementation, and evaluation. *Cardiac Nursing* is based on the *Standards of Cardiovascular Nursing Practice,*[2] which were defined jointly by the American Heart Association Executive Committee of the Council of Cardiovascular Nursing and the American Nurses' Association Executive Committee on the Division of Medical–Surgical Nursing Practice:

Standards of Cardiovascular Nursing Practice

Cardiovascular nursing practice is defined as the nursing care of individuals who have a known or predicted alteration in cardiovascular physiologic function. In planning nursing interventions, nurses who engage in cardiovascular nursing practice must take into account related physiological, social and behavioral problems resulting from or affecting the individual's response and/or adjustment to the cardiovascular alteration. The practice of cardiovascular nursing is carried out in those settings which deliver primary, acute and long term care.

1. Maslow AH: Motivation and Personality. New York, Harper and Row, 1954
2. Standards of Cardiovascular Nursing Practice. Kansas City, American Nurses' Association, 1975. Reproduced with permission.

The scope of cardiovascular nursing practice encompasses those nursing activities which assist the individual to modify his life style and environment so that he can attain optimum cardiac function and acceptable quality of life in congruence with life goals.

STANDARD I
The collection of data about the health status of the individual is systematic and continuous. These data are recorded, retrieved, and communicated to appropriate persons.
Data are obtained by interview, physical examination, review of records and reports, and consultation.
Priority of data collection is determined by the immediate health care problems of the individual.

STANDARD II
Nursing diagnosis is derived from health status data. Nursing diagnosis is a concise statement and the end product of the assessment phase identifying the individual's presenting problems, strengths and limitations and methods of adapting to the current situation.

STANDARD III
Goals for nursing care are formulated. A goal is the end state toward which nursing action is directed.

STANDARD IV
The plan for nursing care prescribes nursing actions to achieve the goals.
The plan for nursing care describes a systematic method to meet the goals. The plan is initiated following nursing diagnosis.

STANDARD V
The plan for nursing care is implemented. The plan must be implemented to achieve the goals.

STANDARD VI
The plan for nursing care is evaluated. Individual's response is compared with observable outcomes which are specified in the goals.

STANDARD VII
Reassessment of the individual, reconsideration of nursing diagnosis, setting of new goals, and revision of the plan for nursing care are a continuous process. The steps of the nursing process are taken concurrently and recurrently.

In order to meet these standards of cardiovascular nursing and to develop critical-thinking and decision-making skills, we believe the cardiac nurse must have a current and sound scientific as well as clinical base.

Cardiac Nursing was written to provide the cardiac nurse with a comprehensive book that approaches the care of the cardiac patient from a nursing standpoint and incorporates our philosophy of patient care. In order to meet these objectives, we selected nurses as the primary contributors. The thrust of *Cardiac Nursing* is the care of patients with coronary artery disease and their related cardiovascular problems.

Because the work of the four authors was shared equally, the sequence in which the authors are listed is the result of random selection.

Sandra L. Underhill, R.N., M.N.
Susan L. Woods, R.N., M.N.
Erika Seiberler Sivarajan, R.N., M.A.
Carol Jean Halpenny, R.N., M.A.

ACKNOWLEDGMENTS

We thank Louise W. "Susie" Mansfield, Professor of Nursing, Emeritus, University of Washington, for her inspiration, support, and guidance in the preparation of this book. Her critical review was invaluable.

We are grateful to Alison Ross, Editor in the School of Nursing, University of Washington, for her interest, encouragement, and editorial expertise.

We thank Diana Intenzo, Editor at JB Lippincott Company, for the production of this book.

We appreciate the support and encouragement that Maxine Patrick, Chairman of our Department, gave us during the writing of this book, and we appreciate the faculty and staff of many departments within the University of Washington and School of Nursing who provided us with many valuable resources.

We are grateful to the many persons who reviewed chapters.

We also wish to thank Mary Whitacre, Ruth Haze, Madhavi Rajaguru, Debbie Browne-Palalay, and Mary Kristensen for their assistance in typing the manuscript.

CARDIAC NURSING

CARDIOVASCULAR ANATOMY AND PHYSIOLOGY

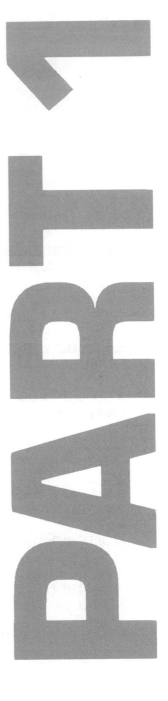

Functional Cardiac Anatomy

CAROL JEAN HALPENNY, R.N., M.A.

The section on the Coronary Circulation was written by
ELEANOR F. BOND, R.N., M.A.

The function of the heart is intimately related to its structural characteristics. Knowledge of cardiac anatomy is essential for understanding cardiac physiology.

GENERAL DESCRIPTION

Position of the Heart in the Thorax

The heart is situated in the middle mediastinum (Fig. 1-1). It lies in the space between the two pleural sacs and is encased in its own serous membrane, the pericardium. Two-thirds of the heart extends to the left of the body's vertical midline.

The long axis of the heart is directed obliquely leftward, downward, and forward.[5] Any factor that changes the shape of the thorax changes the position of the heart and thus modifies the directional axis. Respiratory alterations in the level of the diaphragm or expansion of the rib cage change the cardiac axis. For example, with a deep inspiration, the heart descends and rotates to the right.[26] Factors that may cause axis variations in normal individuals include age, weight, pregnancy, body shape, and the shape of the thorax. A tall, thin person usually has a more vertical heart, whereas a short obese person usually has a more horizontal heart. Pathologic conditions of the heart, lungs, abdominal organs, and other structures also influence the direction of the cardiac axis.

Consideration of the anterior, posterior, inferior, right, and left surfaces of the heart provides a basis for understanding the location of cardiac structures and for understanding the location of myocardial infarctions or other pathologic conditions.[26] The anterior, or sternocostal, cardiac surface is formed by the right ventricle and parts of the right atrium and the left ventricle (Fig. 1-1). The left atrium is behind the ascending aorta and pulmonary trunk when the heart is viewed from the front. Thus the right heart (right atrium and ventricle) lies anteriorly and to the right of the left heart (left atrium and ventricle) in the frontal plane.

The small portion of the lower left ventricle that extends anteriorly forms a blunt tip that is composed of the apical part of the interventricular septum and the left ventricular free wall. Because of the forward tilt of the heart, the movement of this apex portion of the left ventricle during cardiac contraction forms the "point of maximal impulse" that can be observed in normal persons in the fourth or fifth intercostal space at the midclavicular line, six or seven centimeters (cm) from midline. The sternum, costal cartilages of the third to sixth ribs, part of the lungs, and the thymus (in children) overlie the arterior cardiac surface.

The inferior or diaphragmatic surface of the heart, comprised chiefly of the left ventricle, lies almost horizontally on the upper surface of the diaphragm.[26] A portion of the inferior cardiac surface is formed by the right ventricle.

The lateral wall of the left ventricle forms the left heart border; this portion of the left ventricle articulates with the left lung and sometimes is referred to as the pulmonary surface. The right atrium forms the lateral right heart border and thus is close to the right lung.

The base of the heart, comprised of the left atrium and small sections of the right atrium and ventricle, is directed backward and forms the posterior surface of the heart (Fig. 1-2).[26] The thoracic aorta, esophagus, and vertebrae are posterior to the heart (Fig. 1-3).

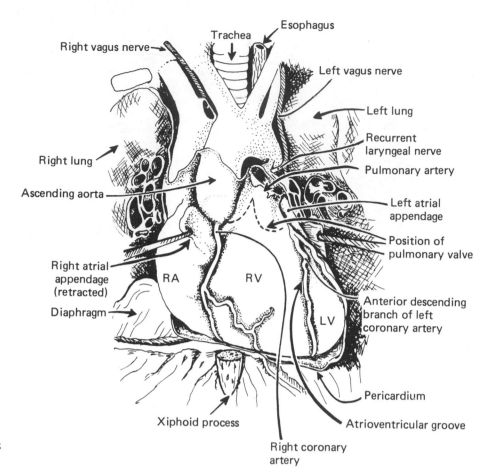

Fig. 1-1. Anterior view of the heart. The anterior thoracic wall has been removed. The lungs have been retracted. The anterior fibrous and parietal layers of the serous pericardium have been resected; free cut edges of the pericardium are shown. *RA* = right atrium; *RV* = right ventricle; *LV* = left ventricle.

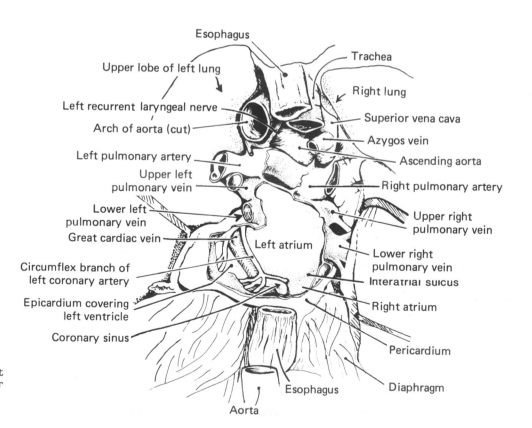

Fig. 1-2. Posterior view of the heart. The lower lobe of the left lung, the esophagus, and the fibrous pericardium have been removed. The left upper lobe and the right lung have been retracted. The epicardium has been removed in the region of the atrioventricular sulcus to expose the left ventricle and the coronary vessels lying in the sulcus. The left ventricle may be seen from the back when the upper lobe of the left lung is retracted and the lower lobe is removed. *LA-* left atrium.

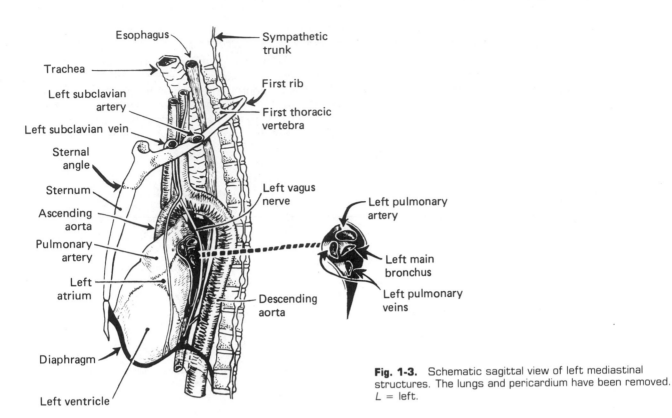

Esophagus

Trachea

Left subclavian artery

Left subclavian vein

Sternal angle

Sternum

Ascending aorta

Pulmonary artery

Left atrium

Diaphragm

Left ventricle

Sympathetic trunk

First rib

First thoracic vertebra

Left vagus nerve

Descending aorta

Left pulmonary artery

Left main bronchus

Left pulmonary veins

Fig. 1-3. Schematic sagittal view of left mediastinal structures. The lungs and pericardium have been removed. *L* = left.

Fig. 1-4. Schematic view of the fibrous skeleton, illustrating the attachment of the cardiac valves and chambers. The four annuli and their extensions lie in different planes, so it is impossible to depict them accurately on a plane surface. *T* = tricuspid valve, *M* = mitral valve, *A* = aortic valve, *P* = pulmonic valve. (Adapted from Rushmer RF: Cardiovascular Dynamics, p 77. Philadelphia, WB Saunders, 1976)

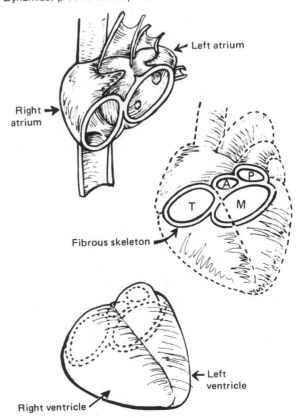

Left atrium

Right atrium

Fibrous skeleton

Right ventricle

Left ventricle

The coronary, or atrioventricular, sulcus (groove) is the external landmark denoting the separation of the atria from the ventricles. It encircles the heart obliquely and contains the coronary blood vessels and epicardial fat. It is interrupted by the aorta and pulmonary artery anteriorly. The right and left ventricles are separated on the external heart surface by the anterior and posterior interventricular sulci. The crux of the heart is the point on the external posterior heart surface where the posterior interventricular sulcus intersects with the coronary sulcus externally and where the interatrial septum joins the interventricular septum internally.

Size

The normal adult male heart weighs approximately 300 to 350 grams (g), with a normal upper limit of 400 g. The female heart weighs approximately 250 to 300 g.[15] Tables have been derived to indicate normal ranges of heart size for various ages and body weights.[25]

The average heart is approximately 12 cm long from its base at the beginning root of the aorta to the left ventricular apex, 9 cm wide transversely at the widest part, and 6 cm in anteroposterior diameter.[2,15,27] However, heart size and weight are obviously influenced by age, body weight and build, frequency of physical exercise, and heart disease.

CARDIAC STRUCTURES

Fibrous Skeleton

Four adjacent rings of dense fibrous connective tissue, the annuli fibrosi, and the extensions that arise from them provide the central supporting structure of the heart (Fig. 1-4).[17,26] The four cardiac valves extend from the rings of the fibrous skeleton. The annuli are attached together and connected by a central fibrous core. The fibrous skeleton divides the atria from the ventricles by providing the site of attachment for much of the atrial and ventricular cardiac muscle. Each annulus and valve has a different orientation, but the skeleton is generally oriented obliquely within the mediastinum.

Chambers

The four cardiac chambers are composed of two atria and two ventricles (Fig. 1-5). Approximate wall thicknesses of the chambers are as follows:[21]

right atrium	2 millimeters (mm)
right ventricle	3–5 mm
left atrium	3 mm
left ventricle	13–15 mm

The wall thickness of each cardiac chamber reflects the degree of high-pressure work done by the chamber.

The two atria serve functionally as reservoirs and conduits for blood that is being funneled into the ventricles. The left ventricle is two to three times as thick as the right ventricle because the left ventricle pumps blood into the high-pressure systemic system, whereas the right ventricle pumps blood into the low-pressure pulmonary system.

The interatrial septum between right and left atria extends obliquely forward from right to left. The interatrial septum includes the fossa ovalis. During fetal life an orifice at this site, the foramen ovale, permits passage of blood from right to left atrium. The foramen usually closes shortly after birth. The lower portion of the interatrial septum is formed by the lower medial right atrial wall on one side and the aortic outflow tract of the left ventricular wall on the other side. An extension of the fibrous skeleton downward between the right atrium and left ventricle forms the upper or membranous part of the interventricular septum. The lower muscular portion of the interventricular septum extends from this membranous septum.

The Right Heart. The posterior and septal walls of the right atrium are smooth, whereas the lateral wall and the right atrial appendage (auricle) have parallel muscular ridges, termed pectinate muscles.[20] The right auricle extends over the aortic root.[20]

The inferior wall of the right atrium and part of the superior wall of the right ventricle are formed by the tricuspid valve. The anterior and inferior walls of the right ventricle are lined by muscle bundles, the trabeculae carneae cordis, which form a rough-walled inflow tract for blood. One muscle group, the moderator band, extends from the lower interventricular septum to the anterior right ventricular papillary muscle.

Another thick muscle bundle, the christa supraventricularis, extends from the septal wall to the anterolateral wall of the right ventricle. The christa supraventricularis helps to divide the right ventricle into an inflow and outflow tract. The smooth-walled outflow tract, also called the infundibulum, extends to the pulmonary artery (see Fig. 1-5).

The concave free wall of the right ventricle is attached to the slightly convex septal wall. The internal right ventricular cavity is cresent shaped or triangle shaped. The right ventricle also forms a cresent laterally around the left ventricle. Right ventricular contraction causes the right ventricular free wall to move toward the interventricular septum. This bellowslike action is effective in ejecting large and variable volumes into a low-pressure system (Fig. 1-6).[17]

Venous blood enters the right atrium from the upper and lower posterior part of the atrium through the superior and inferior venae cavae. Most of the venous drainage from the heart itself enters the right atrium by way of the coronary sinus, which is located between the entrance of the inferior vena cava into the right atrium and the tricuspid valve. Blood flows medially and anteriorly from the right atrium through the tricuspid orifice into the right ventricle.[17,20]

Blood enters the right ventricle in an almost horizontal but slightly leftward, anterior, and inferior direction. It is ejected superiorly and posteriorly through the pulmonary valve (Fig. 1-7).

The Left Heart. Four pulmonary veins return blood from the lungs to openings in the posterolateral wall of the left atrium (see Fig. 1-6). The left atrium is a cuboidal structure that lies between the aortic root and the esophagus. The left

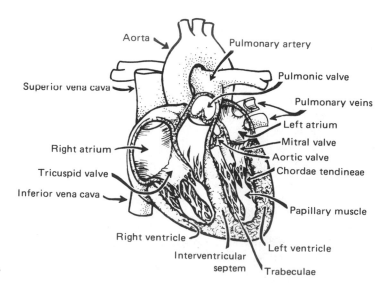

Fig. 1-5. Schematic illustration of cardiac structures.

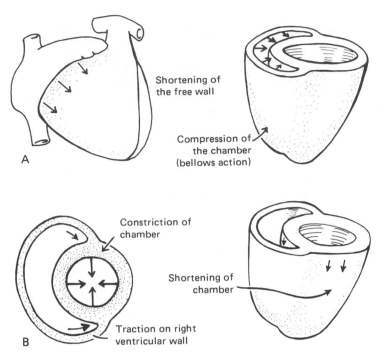

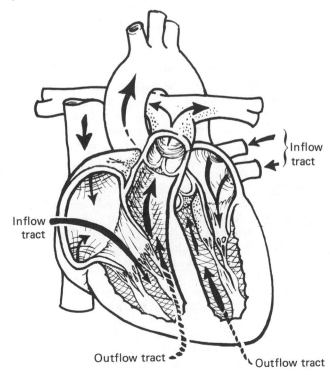

Fig. 1-6. Right and left ventricular contraction. **(A)** Right ventricular contraction. Right ventricular ejection of blood is accomplished primarily by shortening and movement of the free wall toward the interventricular septum. Note the crescent shape of the right ventricle. **(B)** Blood is ejected from the left ventricle primarily by a reduction in the diameter of the chamber. There is some ventricular shortening. (Adapted from Rushmer R: Cardiovascular Dynamics, p 92. Philadelphia, WB Saunders, 1976)

atrial appendage, or auricle, extends along the border of the pulmonary artery. The walls of the left atrium are smooth except for pectinate muscle bundles in the atrial appendage.

The left ventricle is oval shaped. The left ventricular free wall forms a large portion of the left ventricle. The interventricular septum is shaped like a triangle with the base at the aortic area. Anatomically and functionally the septum between the right and left ventricles is more an integral part of the left ventricle than of the right ventricle. The muscular

Fig. 1-7. Blood flow through cardiac chambers and valves.

septum forms the interomedial wall of the left ventricle. The upper septum is smooth walled. The lower septum and free walls of the left ventricle are ridged with trabeculae carneae muscle bundles, so the interior surface of the entire ventricle is rough.

Blood is directed obliquely forward out of the left atrium and enters the left ventricle in an anterior, leftward, inferior direction. Blood flows outward from the apex toward the aorta in a superior and rightward direction (Fig. 1-7). The left ventricular inflow tract is formed by the mitral valve and attachments. The outflow tract is formed by the anterior surface of the anterior mitral valve cusp, the intraventricular septum, and the left ventricular free wall.[20,26] Blood is ejected from the left ventricle mainly by circumferential contraction of the muscular wall, that is, by decreasing the diameter of the cylinder. There is some longitudinal shortening.[17] The ventricular cavity has a small surface area in relation to the volume contained, but high pressures can be developed because of the amount of ventricular muscle, the shape of the cavity, and the way the muscles contract.

Thus blood flows from posterior orifices into both ventricles in a leftward direction and is ejected superiorly toward the center of the heart. The right ventricular tract is more tubular, with outflow oriented at approximately a 60-degree angle to inflow. The left ventricular tract is more conical, with outflow oriented at approximately a 90-degree angle to inflow (Fig. 1-7).[11,20]

Valves

Atrioventricular Valves. The atrioventricular (mitral and tricuspid) valve complexes function as a unit. These complexes are composed of six components: atria, annuli fibrosi, valves, chordae tendineae, papillary muscles, and ventricular walls (see Fig. 1-5).

The mitral and tricuspid valve leaflets or cusps attach to the valve rings of the fibrous skeleton; the site of attachment is termed the commissure. The valves are composed of fibrous connective tissue and are covered by endothelium. The chordae tendineae are fibrous cords that are attached to the free margins and ventricular surfaces of the valve leaflets. The papillary muscles are muscle bundles that are oriented parallel to the ventricular walls and extend from the walls to the chordae tendineae (see Fig. 1-5). The chordae tendineae provide many cross connections from one papillary muscle to two valve leaflets or from trabeculae carne in the ventricular wall directly to valves.

The tricuspid orifice is larger in diameter than the mitral orifice. Three fingers can be admitted through the tricuspid valve compared to two fingers through the mitral valve. The combined surface area of the atrioventricular valve cusps is larger than the surface area of the valvular orifice, so the cusps resemble curtainlike flaps that overlap.

In each ventricle the number of major papillary muscles usually corresponds to the number of atrioventricular cusps. There are three tricuspid cusps: the anterior, the inferior (posterior), and the septal. There are two principal right ventricular papillary muscles, the anterior and inferior, and a smaller set of accessory papillary muscles attached to the ventricular septum.[26]

The arrangement of the two triangular mitral valve cusps has been compared to a bishop's hat, or mitre. The larger anterior cusp extends from the medial posterior septum to the anterior papillary muscle and the anterolateral ventricular wall (diagonally leftward). The ventricular surface of the anterior mitral valve leaflet forms the upper part of the aortic outflow tract.[20] Thus, disease of the aortic valve can affect the mitral valve, or mitral disease may affect aortic function (see Chap. 48). The posterior cusp is less mobile.[20]

The atrioventricular valves open and close passively in response to pressure changes and fluid movements.[14] During diastole the valves open because the pressure in the ventricles is lower than that in the atria. The open valve resembles a funnel, which helps to promote blood flow into the ventricles (see Fig. 1-7). Toward the end of diastole, movement of blood in a circular motion behind the cusps helps to close the valve.[14] During systole the increased ventricular pressures would force the valve cusps to pass into the atria if the papillary muscles did not contract and pull the overlapping edges of the cusps together and downward.[17]

Semilunar valves. The two semilunar (aortic and pulmonic) valves are each composed of three cup-shaped cusps of approximately equal size that arise from the fibrous skeleton. They are thicker than the atrioventricular valves. The cusps are attached to the outflow tract only at the base and therefore do not have the supporting structures that the atrioventricular valves have (see Fig. 1-5). The valve cusps are convex from above, with thickened nodules at the center of the free margins. The cusps are composed of fibrous connective tissue and lined with endothelium; the endothelial lining on the nonventricular side of the valves closely resembles and merges with that of the intima of the arteries beyond the valves. The aortic cusps are thicker than the pulmonic.

The pulmonic valve cusps are usually termed right anterior, left anterior, and posterior. The aortic cusps are most clearly named from the coronary arteries that leave the aorta immediately behind the aortic valve; that is right coronary, left coronary, and noncoronary; however, other names may be used.[26] There is a pouch or sinus of Valsalva behind (above) each semilunar cusp. In the closed position the two semilunar valves are approximately at right angles to each other. The pulmonic valve is above the aortic valve.[26]

The semilunar valve cusps do not overlap each other. During systole the cusps are thrust upward as blood flows from an area of greater pressure in the ventricle to an area of lesser pressure in the aorta or the pulmonary artery. During diastole the cusps drop back passively and backflow is prevented because of the cusps' fibrous strength, their close approximation, and their shape.

CARDIAC TISSUE

The major portion of the heart wall is composed of cardiac muscle tissue, the myocardium. This muscular layer is covered internally and externally by thin layers of endocardium and epicardium, respectively.

Endocardium

The endocardium is composed of a layer of endothelial cells and a few layers of connective tissue and elastic fibers. It is in continuation with the tunica intima of the blood vessels.[2]

Epicardium

The epicardium is the visceral or heart layer of the serous pericardium. Branches of the coronary blood vessels, nerves, and fat are enclosed in the epicardium and the superficial layers of the myocardium.

The epicardium completely encloses the external surface of the heart and extends several centimeters along each great vessel, encircling the aorta and pulmonary artery together. It merges with the tunica adventia of the great vessels, at which point it doubles back upon itself as the parietal pericardium. This continuous membrane thus forms the pericardial sac and encloses a potential space, the pericardial cavity (see Fig. 1-1). The fibrous pericardium extends beyond the serous pericardium and is attached by ligaments and loose connections to the sternum, diaphragm, and structures in the posterior mediastinum.

The pericardial cavity is usually filled with 10 to 30 milliliters (ml) of thin, clear serous fluid.[15,20] It is capable of containing approximately 300 ml without creating serious interference with cardiac function and may contain up to a liter of fluid in disease. Sudden filling of the pericardial sac with fluid drastically hampers filling of the ventricles. During slow accumulations of fluid, the heart may be able to make compensatory adaptations.

The main function of the pericardium and its fluid is to lubricate the moving surfaces of the heart. The pericardium also helps to retard ventricular dilation, helps to hold the heart in position, and forms a barrier to the spread of infections and neoplasia. The pericardium has many similarities with pleural and peritoneal serous membranes, so that inflammation of all three membranes may occur with certain systemic conditions such as rheumatoid arthritis.

Myocardium

The largest portion of the cardiac chamber wall is composed of cardiac muscle tissue, or myocardium, which is firmly anchored to the fibrous skeleton (see Fig. 1-4). The thin-walled atria are composed of two major muscle systems, one that surrounds both of the atria and another that is arranged at right angles to the first and that is separate for each atrium.

Ventricular muscle fibers have been found to spiral downward on the epicardial ventricular wall, pass through the wall, spiral up on the endocardial surface, cross the upper part of the ventricle, and go back down through the wall (Fig. 1-8). Such a vortex arrangement of nested figure of eights is functionally efficient for ventricular contraction.[21] The fibers form a fanlike arrangement of interconnecting muscle fibers when dissected horizontally through the ventricular wall.[22] The orientation of these fibers gradually rotates through the thickness of the wall, so that at the endocardial surface the fibers are circumferentially oriented, whereas at the epicardial surface the fibers are oriented more perpendicularly (Fig. 1-9). This arrangement allows for the circumferential generation of tension throughout the ventricular wall.[22]

Conduction System

Nodal and Purkinje cells generate and conduct electrical impulses to myocardial cells, which are then stimulated to contact (see Chaps. 2 and 3). The anatomic arrangement of cardiac conducting tissue influences the timing and sequencing of atrial and ventricular contraction.[3]

The sinus node lies close to the epicardial surface of the heart just above the tricuspid valve near the anterior entrance of the superior vena cava into the right atrium. The node is approximately 3 to 20 mm long, 3 to 5 mm wide, and 1 to 2 mm thick.[9,19] The sinus nodal artery courses very close to the node, as do autonomic nerves and ganglia.

There is controversy regarding whether or not there are tracts of specialized conducting tissue in the right atrium and whether such tracts have functional significance. Bach-

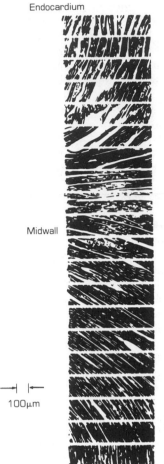

Endocardium

Midwall

←| |←
100μm

Epicardium

Fig. 1-9. Changing ventricular muscle fiber angles at different depths. Reconstructed from a series of microphotographs. (Streeter D, Jr: Circ Res 24:342, 1969. By permission of the American Heart Association, Inc.)

mann originally described an interatrial myocardial bundle conducting impulses from the right atrium to the left atrium.[1] James presented evidence for three internodal pathways from the sinus node to the atrioventricular node.[7,10] There is controversy regarding physiologic support for this theory in terms of specialized paths of depolarization (see Chap. 3).[11,19]

The atrioventricular (AV) node lies subendocardially in the right atrial wall close to the septal leaflet of the tricuspid valve and the ostium of the coronary sinus. The mitral valve

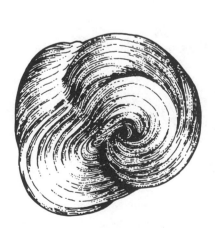
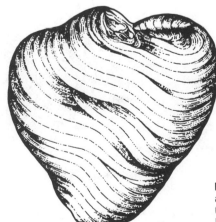

Fig. 1-8. Schematic view of spiral arrangement of ventricular muscle fibers. (Katz A: Physiology of the Heart, p 4. New York, Raven Press, 1977)

is close on the other side of the interatrial septum (Fig. 1-10).[6] In the adult, the node is 3 to 8 mm long, 2 to 4 mm wide, and 1 mm thick, with considerable variation.[12,19,23] Specialized conducting fibers are irregularly interspersed with normal myocardial fibers in the AV nodal region, which leads to difficulties in identifying the boundaries of the node.

The specialized conducting fibers from the AV node converge into a shaft termed the atrioventricular bundle, the common bundle, or the bundle of His. The His bundle passes from the lower right atrial wall anteriorly and laterally through the membranous septum, which is part of the fibrous skeleton. Thus the His bundle provides the only muscular connection between the atria and the ventricles. This section of the bundle is sometimes termed the penetrating portion.

Accessory tracts have been described that join the atria and ventricles through connections outside the main AV node and His bundle (Kent bundles). Tracts from the His bundle to the upper interventricular septum (the paraspecific fibers of Mahaim) have been documented.[24]

The common bundle usually divides into two branches in the region of the crest of the muscular interventricular septum (Fig. 1-10). This section of the bundle is sometimes termed the branching portion. The common bundle is approximately 10 mm long and 2 mm wide.[12] Pathologic problems of the central fibrous body or of the tricuspid, mitral, or aortic valves may affect the AV node or common bundle. Any dysfunction of this portion of the conducting system may affect the coordinated functioning of the atria and ventricles (see Chaps. 3, 17, and 26).

The right bundle branch (RBB) is usually a well-defined single slender group of fibers approximately 45 to 50 mm long and 1 mm thick that arises as a continuation of the common bundle.[12,16,23] Initially it courses downward along the right side of the interventricular septum. It continues through the moderator band of muscular tissue near the right ventricular apex and then to the base of the anterior papillary muscle.[19] If a small segment of the bundle is damaged, the entire distal distribution is affected, owing to the right bundle's thinness, length, and relative lack of arborization.

A widely accepted description of the left bundle branch (LBB) is that it arises almost perpendicularly from the His bundle as the common left bundle branch.[16] This common left bundle, approximately 10 mm long and 4 to 10 mm wide, then divides into two discrete divisions (Fig. 1-10). The left anterior fascicle, or left anterior bundle branch (LABB), is approximately 25 mm long and 3 mm wide.[16] The LABB courses over the left ventricular surface to the anterior papillary muscle and the base of the left ventricle, crossing the aortic outflow tract. This anterior fascicle usually arises directly from the common bundle close to the origin of the right bundle and after the origin of the posterior fascicle. Aortic valve dysfunction as well as myocardial infarction can affect this bundle (see Chaps. 17, 26, and 48).

The large thick left posterior fascicle or left posterior bundle branch (LPBB) arises either from the first portion of the common left bundle or directly from the His bundle. The left posterior fascicle goes inferiorly and posteriorly across the left ventricular inflow tract to the base of the posterior papillary muscle, then spreads diffusely through the posterior inferior left ventricular free wall. It is approximately 20 mm long and 6 mm wide.[16] This fascicle often seems to be the least vulnerable segment of the ventricular conducting system because of its diffuseness, its location in a relatively protected nonturbulent portion of the ventricle and its dual blood supply. There is physiologic evidence for the trifascicular configuration of the bundle branches, because many conduction defects involving partial bundle branch block may be explained on the basis of this model (see Chap. 26).[16]

Other investigators have identified three rather than two fascicular divisions of the left bundle branch or have found that the common left bundle fans out diffusely along the septum and the free ventricular wall.[13] Many individual

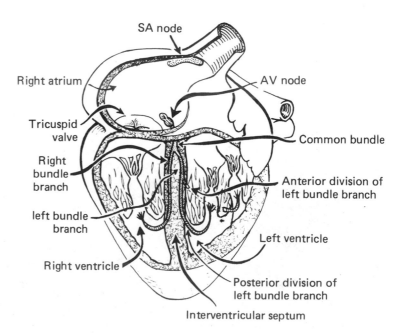

Fig. 1-10. Schematic illustration of human cardiac conducting system. Cardiac structures are labeled on the right and conducting tissue is labeled on the left. (After Katz A: Physiology of the Heart, p 5. New York, Raven Press, 1977)

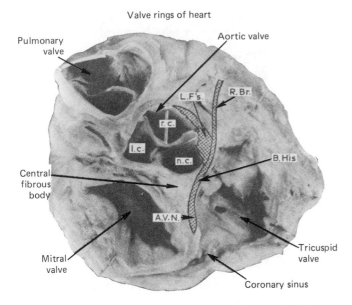

Valve rings of heart

Pulmonary valve

Aortic valve

L.F's.

R. Br.

r.c.

l.c.

n.c.

B. His

Central fibrous body

A.V.N.

Mitral valve

Tricuspid valve

Coronary sinus

Fig. 1-11. Relationship of the atrioventricular conducting system to cardiac valves. Viewed from above. *A.V.N.* = atrioventricular node. Note the proximity of the A.V.N. to the aortic, mitral, and tricuspid valves and the proximity of the valves to each other. *L.F.* = left ventricular conducting fibers, *R. Br.* = right (bundle) branch, *B. His* = bundle of His, *r.c.*, *l.c.*, and *n.c.* = right, left, and noncoronary cusps of the aortic valve. (Hudson R: Br Heart J 29:652, 1967)

variations in left bundle branch configuration have been found in human autopsy dissections, with no definite prevalence of two discrete fascicular divisions (Fig. 1-11).[13]

Purkinje fibers form a complex network of conducting fibers that provide a continuation of the bundle branches, coursing down toward the ventricular apex and then up toward the fibrous rings. They spread over the subendocardial surfaces of both ventricles and then spread from the endocardium throughout the myocardium, thus spreading from inside outward.

CORONARY CIRCULATION

The heart is continuously active. It must receive oxygen and metabolic substrates and have carbon dioxide and other wastes removed in order to maintain aerobic metabolism and contractile activity (see Chap. 2).

Coronary Arteries

The major coronary arteries in man are the right coronary artery and the left coronary artery, sometimes called the left main coronary artery. These arteries branch from the aorta in the region of the sinus of Valsalva (Figs. 1-12, 1-13). They extend over the epicardial surface of the heart and branch several times, the branches usually coming off the parent artery at right angles.[8,9] The arteries plunge inward through the myocardial wall and undergo further branching. Partly because the branches to the epicardial layers exit first, the blood supply to the endocardial (internal) myocardium is more easily compromised than is the blood supply to the epicardial (outer) myocardium. The arteries continue branching and eventually become arterioles, then capillaries.

There is much individual variation in the pattern of coronary artery branching. Table 1-1 indicates the major cardiac structures and their usual arterial supply, with common variations that may occur. For example, it illustrates that a cardiac structure such as the AV node may be supplied by either the right or the left coronary artery. Figures 1-12, 1-13, and 1-14 illustrate the major anatomic features of the coronary circulation.

The left main coronary artery arises from the aorta in the ostium behind the left cusp of the aortic valve. This artery passes between the left atrial appendage and the pulmonary artery and then typically divides into two major branches, the left anterior descending artery and the left circumflex artery.

The left anterior descending artery (LAD) supplies portions of the left and right ventricular myocardium and much of the intraventricular septum. The LAD often appears to

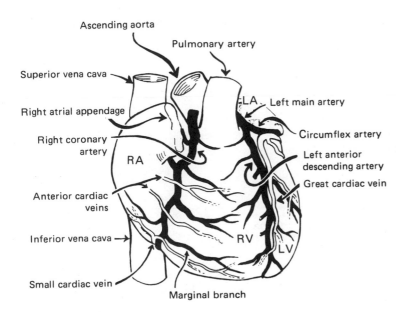

Ascending aorta

Pulmonary artery

Superior vena cava

LA — Left main artery

Right atrial appendage

Circumflex artery

Right coronary artery

RA

Left anterior descending artery

Great cardiac vein

Anterior cardiac veins

Inferior vena cava

RV

LV

Small cardiac vein

Marginal branch

Fig. 1-12. Principal arteries and veins on the anterior surface of the heart. Part of the right atrial appendage has been resected. The left coronary artery arises from the left coronary aortic sinus behind the pulmonary trunk. *RA* = right atrium, *RV* = right ventricle, *LA* = left atrium, *LV* = left ventricle.

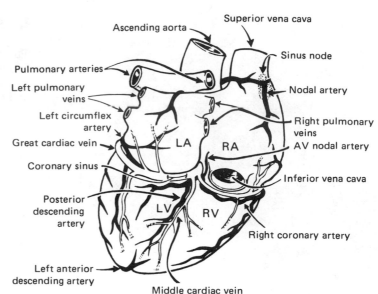

Fig. 1-13. Principal arteries and veins on the inferior-posterior surfaces of the heart. This schematic drawing illustrates the heart tilted upward at a nonphysiologic angle; normally, little of the inferior cardiac surface is visible posteriorly. The sulci are not depicted; the coronary sinus courses in the atrioventricular sulcus; the middle cardiac vein and the posterior descending artery course in the interventricular sulcus. The crux region is represented by the junction of these sulci with each other and with the shallow interatrial sulcus. The right coronary artery is shown to cross the crux and to supply the atrioventricular node. The artery to the sinus node is depicted as arising from the right coronary artery. *RA* = right atrium, *RV* = right ventricle, *LA* = left atrium, *LV* = left ventricle.

be a direct continuation of the left main coronary artery. The LAD courses down the anterior interventricular sulcus to the ventricular apex, where it may terminate or ascend upward in the posterior interventricular groove. It may give off several anterior septal branches.

The left circumflex artery supplies blood to parts of the left atrium and left ventricle. In 45% of autopsied human hearts, it supplies the major perfusion of the sinus node; in 10% of autopsied hearts, it supplies the AV node.[8] It courses in the groove between the left atrium and left ventricle to the left margin of the heart and sometimes extends posteriorly. The left circumflex gives off an obtuse marginal artery

TABLE 1-1 AREA SUPPLIED BY COMMON ARTERIES

Structure	Usual Arterial Supply	Common Variants
Right atrium	Sinus node artery, branch of RCA (55%)*	Sinus node artery, branch of L circumflex (45%)
Left atrium	Major L circumflex†	Sinus node artery, branch of L circumflex (45%)
Right ventricle		
Anterior	Major RCA Minor LAD	
Posterior	Major RCA; posterior descending branch of RCA	Posterior descending may branch from L circumflex (10%)
	Minor LAD (ascending portion)	LAD terminates at apex (40%)
Left ventricle		
Posterior (diaphragmatic)	Major L circumflex, posterior descending branch of RCA	Posterior descending may branch from L circumflex (10%)
	Minor LAD (ascending portion)	LAD terminates at apex (40%)
Anterior	LCA; L circumflex and LAD	
Apex	Major LAD	
Intraventricular septum	Major septal branches of LAD	
	Minor posterior descending branch of RCA and AV nodal branch of RCA	Minor posterior descending may branch from L circumflex and AV nodal may branch from L circumflex
LV papillary muscles		
Anterior	Diagonal branch of LAD; other branches of LAD, other branches of L circumflex	Diagonal may branch from circumflex
Posterior	RCA and L circumflex	RCA and LAD
Sinus node	Nodal artery from RCA (55%)	Nodal artery from L circumflex (45%)
AV node	RCA (90%)	L circumflex (10%)
Bundle of His	RCA (90%)	L circumflex (10%)
Right bundle	Major LAD septal branches Minor AV nodal artery	
Left anterior bundle	Major LAD septal branches Minor AV nodal artery	
Left posterior bundle	LAD septal branches and AV nodal artery	

* Percentages in parentheses denote frequency of occurrence in autopsy studies.
† Major and minor refer to degree of predominance of an artery in perfusing a structure.
RCA = right coronary artery
LAD = left anterior descending artery
L = left
(Data from James TN: Anatomy of the Coronary Arteries. New York, Paul B. Hoeber, 1961; James TN: Anatomy of the coronary arteries and veins. In Hurst JW (ed): The Heart, 4th ed, pp 32—47, New York, McGraw-Hill, 1978)

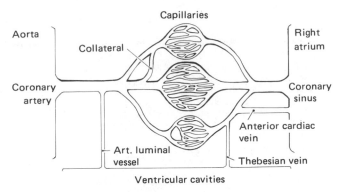

Fig. 1-14. Schematic model of coronary circulation. As in other circulatory beds, the coronary circulation is comprised of arteries, capillaries, and veins. Some veins drain directly into the ventricles. Collateral channels may link arterial vessels. Art. = arterial. (Adapted from Ruch TC, Patton HD: Physiology and Biophysics II, p 249. Philadelphia, WB Saunders Co., 1975)

that travels to the apex. A smaller left diagonal artery may branch from the LAD or the left circumflex artery and extend downward over the left ventricle.

The right coronary artery supplies the right atrium, right ventricle, and a portion of the posterior and inferior surfaces of the left ventricle. It supplies the AV node and bundle of His in 90% of hearts and the sinus node in 55% of hearts in some documented autopsy series.[8] It originates behind the right aortic cusp and passes behind the pulmonary artery, coursing in the right atrioventricular groove laterally to the right margin of the heart and then posteriorly. Its three major branches are the conus branch, supplying the upper part of the right ventricle, the right marginal branch, which passes over the right ventricle to the apex of the heart, and the posterior descending branch, which lies in the posterior interventricular sulcus. The posterior descending branch arborizes further into the posterior septal branches to the intraventricular septum.

Collateral Circulation

Collateral arteries are interarterial vessels that can connect two branches of a single coronary artery or connect branches of the right coronary artery with branches of the left. In the human heart, collaterals are found through the full thickness of the myocardium, with the highest density near the endocardial surface.[4] Vasoactive drugs that dilate or constrict other coronary arteries apparently do not directly affect collateral diameter.[18] Collaterals are present normally; however they greatly enlarge in diseases such as coronary atherosclerosis that involve gradual narrowing of proximal coronary arteries (see Chap. 11). Compensatory collateral development is also seen with chronic anemia or chronic hypoxemia.

Coronary Capillaries

Blood passes from the arteries into arterioles, then into capillaries, where exchange of oxygen and other materials takes place (see Chap. 5). The heart has a dense capillary network with approximately 3300 capillaries per square millimeter (cap/mm^2) or approximately one capillary per muscle fiber.[28] Blood flow through the capillaries is regulated according to cardiac metabolic needs (see Chap. 2).

Myocardial cells increase in size with hypertrophy of the heart muscle. The capillary network, however, does not appear to proliferate.[28] The same capillaries must now perfuse a larger mass of tissue. The distance over which materials must diffuse is increased. Thus, with hypertrophy, the coronary circulation must perfuse a larger mass of tissue while at the same time the efficiency of exchange has decreased.

Coronary Veins

Most of the venous drainage of the heart is through epicardial veins. The large veins course close to the coronary arteries. Two veins sometimes accompany an artery.[8] The major veins feed into the great cardiac vein, which runs alongside the circumflex artery, becomes the coronary sinus, and then empties into the right atrium (see Fig. 1-13). An incompetent (incompletely shut) semilunar valve, the valve of Vieussens, marks the junction between the great cardiac vein and the coronary sinus; a similar structure, the Thebesian valve, is also incompetent and is found at the entry of the coronary sinus into the right atrium.[17] Venous blood from the right ventricular muscle is drained to a large extent by two to four anterior cardiac veins that empty directly into the right atrium, bypassing the coronary sinus (see Fig. 1-12).

Some veins empty directly into the ventricles; these are known as Thebesian veins (see Fig. 1-14). They are more common on the right side of the heart, where the pressure gradient is favorable for such flow. Only a small amount of venous blood is returned directly to the left ventricle. When blood is returned to the left ventricle it constitutes a component of physiologic shunt, or unoxygenated blood entering the systemic circulation. Many collateral channels are found in the venous drainage system.

Lymph Drainage

Cardiac contraction assists lymphatic drainage outward through an abundant system of lymphatic vessels in the myocardium to lymph nodes in the anterior mediastinum that empty into the superior vena cava.[2] Cardiac lymphatic obstruction rarely occurs.

CARDIAC NERVES

Sensory nervous fibers from ventricular walls, coronary blood vessels, the pericardium, and other tissues transmit impulses through the cardiac nerves to the central nervous system. The motor fibers from the central nervous system to the heart are autonomic; sympathetic stimulation accelerates firing of the sinus node, enhances conduction through the atrioventricular node, and increases the force of cardiac contraction, whereas parasympathetic stimulation slows the heart rate, slows conduction through the atrioventricular node, and may decrease ventricular contractile force. The nervous innervation of the heart is described more fully in Chapter 6.

REFERENCES

The selections marked with an asterisk (*) are helpful for further reading.

1. Bachmann G: The inter-auricular time interval. Am J Physiol 41:309–314, 1916
2. Bloom W, Fawcett DW: A Textbook of Histology, 10th ed, pp 416–419. Philadelphia, WB Saunders, 1975*
3. Fozzard HA: Conduction of the action potential. In Berne RM (ed): Handbook of Physiology, Sec 2: The Cardiovascular System, Vol I, The Heart, pp 335–356. Bethesda, Md, American Physiological Society, 1979
4. Fulton WFM: The Coronary Arteries. Springfield, Ill, Charles C Thomas, 1965*
5. Gardner E, Gray DJ, O'Rahilly R: Anatomy, 4th ed, p 291. Philadelphia, WB Saunders, 1975
6. Hudson REB: Surgical pathology of the conducting system of the heart. Br Heart J 29:646–670, 1967
7. James TN: Anatomy of the conduction system of the heart. In Hurst JW (ed): The Heart, 4th ed, pp 47–57. New York, McGraw-Hill, 1978
8. James TN: Anatomy of the Coronary Arteries. New York, Paul B Hoeber, 1961*
9. James TN: Anatomy of the coronary arteries and veins. In Hurst JW (ed): The Heart, 4th ed, pp 32–47. New York: McGraw-Hill, 1978
10. James TN: The connecting pathways between the sinus node and AV node and between the right and the left atrium in the human heart. Am Heart J 66(4):498–508, 1963
11. Katz AM: Physiology of the Heart, pp 1–24. New York, Raven Press, 1977*
12. MacLean WA, Waldo AL, James TN: Formation and conduction of the cardiac electrical impulse. In Yu PN, Goodwin JF (eds): Progress in Cardiology. Philadelphia, Lea & Febiger, 1974
13. Massing GK, James TN: Anatomical configuration of the His bundle and bundle branches in the human heart. Circulation 53(4):609–621, 1976
14. Parmley WW, Talbot L: Heart as a pump. In Berne RM (ed): Handbook of Physiology, Sec 2: The Cardiovascular System, Vol 1, The Heart, pp 449–457. Bethesda, Md, American Physiological Society, 1979*
15. Robbins S, Cotran RS: Pathologic Basis of Disease, 2nd ed, pp 643–645. Philadelphia, WB Saunders, 1979*
16. Rosenbaum MB, Elizari MV, Lazzari JO: The Hemiblocks. Oldsmar, Fla, Tampa Tracings, 1971
17. Rushmer RF: Cardiovascular Dynamics, pp 89–98; pp 411–418. Philadelphia, WB Saunders, 1976*
18. Schaper W: The Collateral Circulation of the Heart. New York, American Elsevier, 1971
19. Scher AM, Spach MS: Cardiac depolarization and repolarization and the electrocardiogram. In Berne RM (ed): Handbook of Physiology, Sec 2: The Cardiovascular System, Vol I, The Heart, pp 357–392. Bethesda, Md, American Physiological Society, 1979
20. Silverman ME, Schlant RC: Anatomy of the normal heart and blood vessels. In Hurst JW (ed): The Heart, 4th ed, pp 19–32. New York, McGraw-Hill, 1978
21. Streeter DD, Jr: Gross morphology and fiber geometry of the heart. In Berne RM (ed): Handbook of Physiology, Sec 2: The Cardiovascular System, Vol I, The Heart, pp 61–112. Bethesda, Md, American Physiological Society, 1979
22. Streeter DD, Jr, Spotnitz HM, Patel DP et al: Fiber orientation in the canine left ventricle during diastole and systole. Circ Res 24(3):339–347, 1969
23. Titus JL, Daugherty GW, Edwards JE: Anatomy of the normal human atrioventricular conduction system. Am J Anat 113(3):407–415, 1963
24. Truex RC: Structural basis of atrial and ventricular conduction. Cardiovasc Clin 6(1):1–24, 1974
25. Ungerleider HE, Clark CP: A study of the transverse diameter of the heart silhouette with prediction table based on the teleoroentgenogram. Am Heart J 17(1):92–102, 1939
26. Walmsley R, Watson H: Clinical Anatomy of the Heart. New York, Churchill Livingston, 1978*
27. Warwick R, Williams PL: Gray's Anatomy, 35th ed, p 599. Philadelphia, WB Saunders, 1973
28. Wearn JT: Morphological and functional alterations of the coronary circulation. Harvey Lect 35:243–270, 1940*

ADDITIONAL READING

Berne RM, Rubio R: Coronary circulation. In Berne RM (ed): Handbook of Physiology, Sec 2: Circulation, Vol I, The Heart, pp 873–952. Bethesda, Md, American Physiological Society, 1979

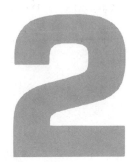

Physiology of the Heart
ELEANOR F. BOND, R.N., M.A.

The section on Myocardial Metabolism was written by
SANDRA SOLACK, R.N., M.S.N.
and
CAROL JEAN HALPENNY, R.N., M.A.

MOLECULAR BASIS FOR MYOCARDIAL FUNCTION

Structure of the Myocardial Cells

In shape, myocardial cells are long, narrow, and often branching. A limiting membrane, the sarcolemma, surrounds each cell. A portion of the sarcolemma is modified to form a special type of cell-to-cell junction, the intercalated disc. The major cellular components are the contractile elements or myofibrils, the mitochondria, the transverse tubules, and the sarcoplasmic reticulum. Cells usually have one nucleus and a small amount of cytoplasm called sarcoplasm (Fig. 2-1).

The *sarcolemma* is a thin sheath of phospholipid and protein that separates the cell contents from the extracellular space, maintaining differences of ionic concentration and electrical charge. Electrical currents flowing across the sarcolemma initiate contraction.

The *intercalated discs* are at right angles to the long axis of the cell. These discs form a physical barrier between cells; they offer much less resistance to the spread of electrical current than does the remainder of the sarcolemma. Impulses pass easily and rapidly across these junctions. Because of these junctions, the heart functions as a syncytium of coordinated cells, although anatomically the cells are discrete units.

The *myofibrils* are long rodlike structures that run the length of the cell. They contain the contractile proteins, which convert chemical energy into mechanical energy and thus are responsible for the generation of tension (see definition of tension in glossary) and the muscle shortening

that occurs during contraction. It is the highly organized alignment of these contractile proteins that gives the myocardial cell its striated (striped) appearance.

Mitochondria are small rod-shaped membranous structures. They are the sites of the breakdown and resynthesis of high-energy substrates; the relative abundance of these organelles in cardiac muscle reflects the high level of biochemical activity in cardiac cells.

Transverse tubules (t-tubules) are membrane-surrounded tubes that form from invaginations of the sarcolemma. The t-tubule membrane is a continuation of the surface membrane, and the channels formed are in direct contact with the extracellular fluid.

The *sarcoplasmic reticulum* (SR) is an extensive self-contained internal membrane system. Both the t-tubule and the SR participate in excitation–contraction coupling, that is, in the linking of electrical depolarization of the surface membrane to the mechanical activity of the contractile protein filaments.

The *nucleus* contains the genetic material of the cell. One of its major roles is to direct the synthesis of the new protein components of the cell.

Types of Myocardial Cells

Various types of cardiac muscle cells have been identified on the basis of anatomic characteristics. In general, myocardial cells have either a mechanical or an electrical function.

Working myocardial cells generate the contractile force of the heart. These cells have a markedly striated appearance because of the orderly arrays of the abundant contractile

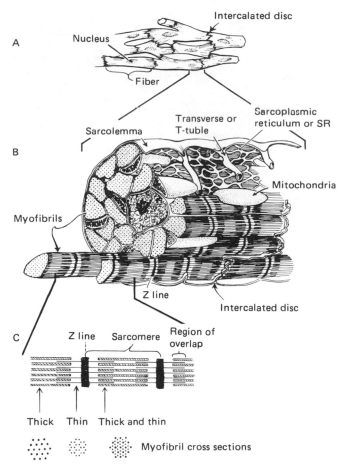

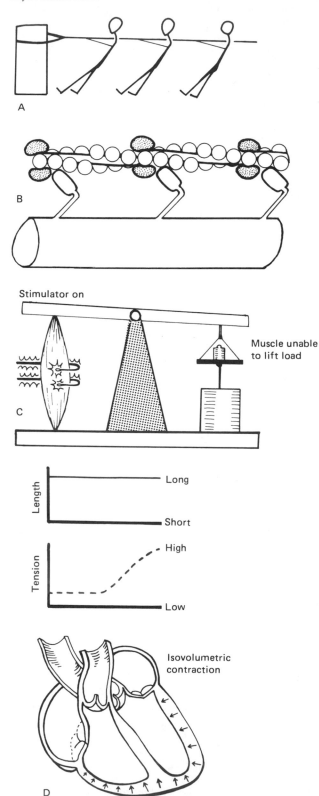

Fig. 2-1. The microscopic structure of working myocardial cells. (**A**) Working myocardial cells as seen under the light microscope. Note the branching network of fibers and intercalated discs. (**B**) Schematic illustration of the internal structure of the working myocardial cell. Note the striated appearance of the myofibrils, the intimate association of the sarcoplasmic reticulum with the myofibrils, the presence of t-tubules, and the large number of mitochondria. (**C**) Structure of the sarcomere, illustrating alignment of thick and thin filaments. Cross sections taken at three different positions along the sarcomere illustrate a region with only thick filaments, a region with only thin filaments, and a region of overlap where the thick and the thin filaments interdigitate. (Adapted from Braunwald E, Ross J, Sonnenblick E: Mechanisms of Contraction of the Normal and Failing Heart, 2nd ed, p 3. Boston, Little, Brown & Co, 1976)

Fig. 2-2. Isometric contraction. (**A**) In an isometric contraction, force is generated while muscles are held at a constant length. Schematically, this is analogous to the stick men pulling a load they cannot dislodge: A large force is generated but no movement takes place. (**B**) At the molecular level, myosin heads attach to actin and pull, but filaments do not slide significantly past one another. (**C**) An experimental preparation producing isometric contraction consists of a muscle mounted on a lever with a very large load as counterweight. The muscle generates a force when stimulated, but the load is so great that the muscle cannot lift it. (**D**) In the heart, ventricular contraction is primarily isometric prior to the opening of the semilunar valves: Tension increases but no major shortening takes place. (**A** and **B** adapted from Katz AM: Physiology of the Heart, p 118. New York, Raven Press, 1977)

protein filaments. Working myocardial cells make up the bulk of the walls of both atrial and both ventricular chambers.

Nodal cells are specialized for pacemaker function. They are found in clusters in the sinus node and in the atrioventricular node. These cells contain few contractile filaments, little SR, and no t-tubules. They are the smallest of the myocardial cells.

Purkinje cells are specialized for rapid conduction of electrical impulses, especially through the thick ventricular wall. The large size, elongated shape, and sparse contractile proteins reflect this specialization. These cells are found in the common His bundle and in the left and right bundle branches, as well as in a diffuse network throughout the ventricles. Purkinje cell cytoplasm is rich in glycogen granules, which may contribute to these cells' resistance to damage during periods of anoxia.

A secondary function of the Purkinje cells is to serve as a potential pacemaker locus. In the absence of an overriding impulse from the sinus node, Purkinje cells can initiate a cardiac impulse (see Chap. 3).

In areas where one cell type makes contact with another cell type, there is often an area of gradual transition in which the cells are intermediate in appearance.

Overview of Contraction

As seen in Figure 2-1, the myofibril is composed of a series of repeating units, sarcomeres. The *sarcomere* is the basic functional as well as structural unit of the myofibril. Dark-staining Z lines are seen at each end of the sarcomere. Attached to the Z line are the thin filaments. The center of the sarcomere is composed of the dark-appearing thick filaments. Interdigitating thin and thick filaments overlap to a variable extent. The amount of this overlap is altered during shortening, when the proteins of the thick and thin filaments interact and the filaments slide past one another.

The individual thick and thin filaments do not themselves change in length; the sarcomere (and the muscle as a whole) shortens. If shortening of the sarcomere (or the muscle cell) is prevented, the interaction of thick and thin filaments is manifested as tension generation. When a stimulated muscle is allowed to shorten, tension generated by the muscle is not increased and the contraction is said to be *isotonic*. If, on the other hand, the muscle is held at a fixed length, tension increases, and the contraction is said to be *isometric* (Figs. 2-2, 2-3). In the heart, early systolic contraction is primarily isometric: Tension increases and muscle length remains fairly constant. Later in systole, the contraction is primarily isotonic: The heart muscle shortens and the blood is expelled into the aorta. Little additional tension (see definition in the glossary) is developed (see Chap. 4).

Molecular Basis for Contraction

The *thin filaments* are composed primarily of bead-shaped molecules of the protein actin arranged in an intercoiled double-stranded chain. Two other proteins, troponin and tropomyosin, are located on the thin filaments at periodic intervals (Fig. 2-4).

The *thick filaments* are composed primarily of the protein myosin. The myosin molecule consists of a long rodlike tail with two "heads" protruding at one end. In the thick filament, the rodlike portions of a number of myosin mole-

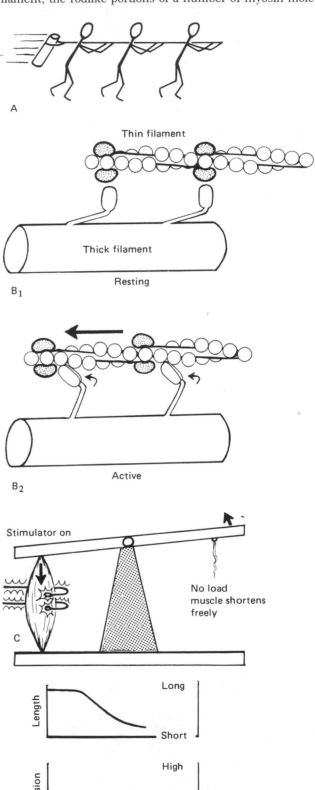

Fig. 2-3. Isotonic contraction. **(A)** In an isotonic contraction, muscles shorten freely, and little tension is developed. Schematically this is analogous to the stick men running with a very small load. Little force is generated but movement takes place. **(B)** At the molecular level, myosin heads attach briefly to actin and pull the thin filament, then release in a cyclic fashion. The sarcomere shortens. **(C)** An experimental preparation producing isotonic contraction consists of a muscle mounted on a lever without significant counterload. The stimulated muscle shortens freely, not increasing its tension. (**A** and **B** adapted from Katz AM: Physiology of the Heart, pp 87, 112. New York, Raven Press, 1977)

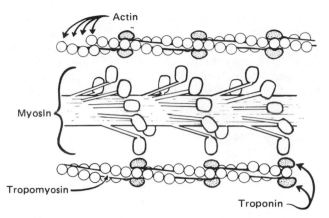

Fig. 2-4. The organization of the contractile proteins. The thick filament is composed primarily of myosin molecules. The long "tails" of the myosin are parallel and form the backbone of the thick filament; the heads protrude at regular intervals. The thin filaments consist of actin, troponin, and tropomyosin. Beadlike actin molecules form two intertwining chains with tropomyosin and troponin attached at regular intervals.

cules are arranged end to end, and the globular heads protrude in spiraling arrangements from the two ends of the myosin rod (Fig. 2-4).

The myosin head functions as an enzyme that breaks down the high-energy molecule, adenosine triphosphate (ATP). When myosin interacts with actin, the rate of turnover of ATP is greatly increased. The chemical energy released from ATP is converted to the mechanical energy of contraction.

According to the *crossbridge theory* of muscle contraction, a bond or crossbridge forms, linking the thick and thin filaments. It is thought that the protuberant myosin head

contains the actin binding site and forms the crossbridge. This crossbridge is capable of binding, flexing, releasing, and binding again, thus pulling the thin filament toward the center of the sarcomere in an isotonic contraction. If the muscle is held at a fixed length and is unable to shorten (an isometric contraction), tension is generated by the pulling of the crossbridge.

When the muscle is relaxed during diastole, the interaction of myosin and actin is inhibited by tropomyosin and troponin. Electrical signals across the cell membrane trigger the release of calcium ion (Ca^{2+}) into the sarcoplasm from within the SR and from extracellular fluid by way of the sarcolemma and t-tubule membranes. This increase in intracellular Ca^{2+} concentration is in turn a trigger for contraction. Ca^{2+} binds troponin; tropomyosin rotates in a manner such that resting inhibition to crossbridge formation is removed. Crossbridges form (Fig. 2-5).

Molecular Basis for Relaxation

Following contraction, Ca^{2+} must be removed from the sarcoplasm. Troponin releases its bound Ca^{2+}; tropomyosin returns to the position in which actin and myosin interaction was blocked. The cell relaxes again (Fig. 2-5).

Removal of Ca^{2+} is essential in this sequence. Two mechanisms are involved in this process. The SR pumps Ca^{2+} into its core. This is an active process and requires chemical energy from ATP breakdown. The cell membrane also actively pumps Ca^{2+} into the extracellular fluid.

The ATP required for the removal of Ca^{2+} from the cell and for the cycling of crossbridges may be depleted, for example, in myocardial ischemia. When this happens, crossbridges form and are not broken. The muscle is stiff.

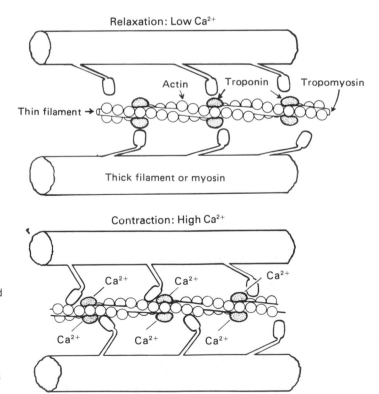

Fig. 2-5. Molecular interactions during relaxation and contraction proposed by the crossbridge theory of muscle contraction. During relaxation, when Ca^{2+} concentration is low, no crossbridges form. When intracellular Ca^{2+} concentration rises, as it does following the membrane action potential, troponin combines with Ca^{2+}, and the tropomyosin—troponin system changes in such a way as to allow attachment and pulling by crossbridges.

MECHANICAL PROPERTIES OF THE MYOCARDIUM

The heart is a pump. Its function is to add energy to the flowing blood, thus propelling it through the systemic and pulmonary circulations. The performance of the heart as a pump can be described in terms of the cardiac output (*CO*). This is the volume of blood pumped by one ventricle in one minute. It is equal to the stroke volume (*SV*), or volume of blood pumped with each beat, times the number of cardiac contractions (heart rate; *HR*) in one minute (*CO* = *SV* × *HR*). Typical normal values in a 70-kg man at rest of 68 beats per minute and 80-ml stroke volume produce a cardiac output of 5440 ml or 5.4 liters per minute.

The stroke volume is determined by the degree of ventricular filling during diastole, or preload, the pressure against which the ventricle must pump, or afterload, and the contractile state of the myocardim. In the remainder of this section these factors are discussed in more detail, and the manner in which they interact to influence the mechanical function of the heart is described.

Preload and Afterload

Preload. Preload refers to the distending force stretching the ventricular muscle immediately prior to electrical excitation and contraction. Figure 2-6 further defines preload and illustrates the role of preload in the contraction of a simple muscle preparation and in the heart. Left ventricular end-diastolic pressure is the left ventricular preload. In the absence of pathologic changes in the mitral valve, left atrial pressure and pulmonary capillary wedge pressure are useful indices of left ventricular preload (see Chap. 21).

Afterload. A related term often used to describe cardiac mechanical function is afterload. This is the force opposing ventricular ejection. In the absence of pathologic changes in the aortic valve, aortic pressure constitutes the afterload of the left ventricle. Figure 2-7 illustrates the role of afterload in a simple muscle preparation and in the heart. (See The Role of Afterload.)

The Role of Preload

The Length–Tension Relationship. Early in this century, Starling observed that, within limits, an increase in the volume of the left ventricle at the end of diastole resulted in the generation of increased active pressure and increased volume pumped during the ensuing contraction. Beyond a certain volume this mechanism was no longer operational; increased end-diastolic volume resulted instead in decreased pressure developed and a decreased volume of blood ejected.[12] This property is known as Starling's law of the heart or the length–tension relationship of cardiac muscle (or sometimes, the Frank-Starling law of the heart). It is commonly illustrated in a graph (Fig. 2-8). Although the increment in active pressure generated is related to volume of the ventricle and consequently to the length of the ventricular muscle fibers, it is common to use preload (*i.e.,* filling pressure) as an index of ventricular volume (see Compliance below).

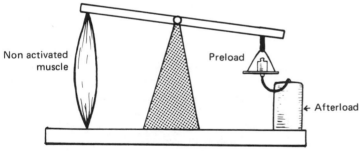

Non activated muscle

Preload

← Afterload

A

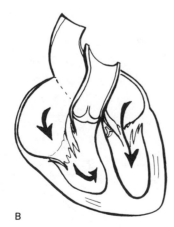

B

Preload = load stretching the resting ventricle to its end–diastolic volume

Fig. 2-6. Preload. (**A**) In the isolated muscle preparation, preload is the load stretching the resting muscle. Thus preload determines the resting length of the muscle. (**B**) In the heart, the ventricular preload is determined by the volume of blood stretching the resting ventricles.

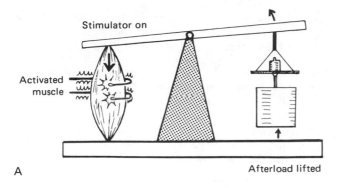

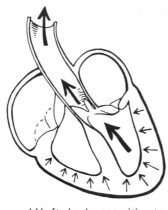

LV afterload = opposition to
LV ejection offered by
aortic pressure

B

Fig. 2-7. Afterload. **(A)** In the isolated muscle preraration, afterload is the force opposing shortening. The muscle must generate enough tension to lift the afterload before it can shorten. **(B)** In the heart, the aortic pressure constitutes the left ventricular (LV) afterload. The heart must generate a pressure slightly greater than the aortic pressure before the myocardium can undergo significant shortening.

The length–tension mechanism is a functional one. It is thought to contribute to maintaining overall matching between left and right ventricular output.[14] For instance, if a person reclines after being in a standing position (or elevates his legs when in a reclining position), the volume of blood returning to the heart transiently increases. The right ventricle is stretched and increases its force of contraction, pumping a larger stroke volume to the lungs and generating higher pressures. Pulmonary vascular pressures rise. This raises the left ventricular filling pressure or preload. Left ventricular filling volume increases. The left ventricle generates increased active pressure and pumps a larger stroke volume, and arterial vascular pressures rise (see Chap. 6).

Some forms of therapy are designed to take advantage of the length–tension characteristics of the heart. Examples of this are leg raising and intravascular volume expansion in the shock patient. These therapies both increase central blood volume and improve cardiac contractile force. Indices of central blood volume (*e.g.*, central venous pressure or, more ideally, pulmonary capillary wedge pressure, left atrial, or left ventricular end-diastolic pressure) are used to monitor ventricular filling or stretch at end diastole and hence indicate position on the Starling curve (see Chap. 21).

The mechanical function of the heart is not characterized by a single curve describing the length–tension relationship but rather by a number of curves (Fig. 2-8). Positive inotropic factors, that is, factors that increase the contractility of the heart, such as sympathetic stimulation, cause the heart to operate on a higher length–tension curve so that a higher tension is generated at the same left ventricular end-diastolic volume.

In heart failure, the heart may be characterized by a lower length–tension curve (Chap. 27). Heart failure is not characterized by movement onto the descending limb of the normal length–tension curve. This would be disastrous: A vicious cycle would develop wherein increased dilatation of the heart would reduce the contractile force, less blood would be pumped, and still greater dilatation would occur. It is unlikely that this happens in the intact heart, even when diseased.

The crossbridge theory of muscle contraction partly accounts for the length–tension relationship of cardiac muscle (Fig. 2-9). Tension generated by muscle is proportional to the number of crossbridges formed. At short lengths, thin filaments overlap one another and interfere with crossbridge formation. Maximum tension development occurs in the range of muscle lengths at which the myosin crossbridge regions maximally overlap the thin filaments without the thin filaments themselves overlapping one another. If the muscle is stretched still further, the region of crossbridge overlap is diminished; less tension is developed.[3]

Other factors also contribute to the shape of the Starling curve. For instance, when the heart is stretched, more cells may be brought into parallel with the axis of shortening and be able to contribute more effectively to the total development of force within the ventricle.[5]

Compliance. Starling's law of the heart relates end-diastolic length, rather than end-diastolic pressure, to the strength of contraction. End-diastolic length and pressure are, however, related. Compliance is the term used to describe that relationship. Compliance (C) is the change in volume (ΔV) that results for a given change in pressure (ΔP). ($C = \Delta V/\Delta P$) Stiffness (S) is the inverse of compliance ($S = \Delta P/\Delta V$). Increased stiffness is the same as decreased compliance.

Fig. 2-8. The length–tension relationship of the heart. End-diastolic volume determines the end-diastolic length of the ventricular muscle fibers and is proportional to tension generated during systole as well as to cardiac output, stroke volume, and stroke work. A change in cardiac contractility causes the heart to perform on a different length–tension curve.

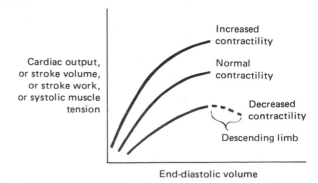

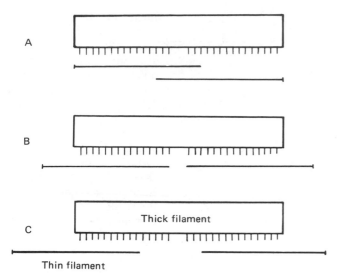

Fig. 2-9. Schematic view of variations in overlap between the thick and thin filaments that account for the length–tension relationship of cardiac muscle. (**A**) Sarcomere on ascending limb of length–tension curve. The thin filaments begin overlapping, interfering with attachment by crossbridges. (**B**) Sarcomere with maximum effective overlap of thin and thick filaments and hence at the peak of the length–tension curve. (**C**) Sarcomere stretched beyond maximum overlap and hence on the descending limb of the length–tension curve. As the actin chains are pulled further out, fewer actin sites are available for crossbridge attachment. (**A** and **B** adapted from Katz AM: Physiology of the Heart, 1977, pp 129, 130. New York, Raven Press, 1977)

Compliance of the heart is determined by the inherent properties of the muscle tissue as well as by the chamber geometry. The state of the pericardium can also influence the cardiac pressure–volume relationship. Figure 2-10, curve 1, illustrates a normal relationship between pressure and volume at end diastole in the left ventricle. Compliance changes with volume. As the ventricular volume increases, compliance decreases: It takes larger increments in filling pressure to achieve a given increment in volume.

A number of clinical states alter compliance. The tissue itself becomes stiffer with hypoxia, ischemia, and scarring, for example, following a myocardial infarction (curve 2, Fig. 2-10).[9] Infiltrative myocardial diseases such as amyloidosis increase muscle stiffness. Pericardial constriction, for example, with pericarditis or tamponade, can cause increased stiffness. Hypertrophy can increase chamber stiffness. Whenever the left ventricle operates at a greater end-diastolic volume, stiffness is invariably increased. This might be seen, for example, with valvular incompetence (either aortic or sometimes mitral) or with saline or colloid overloads, for example, due to excess iatrogenic infusion or renal failure.

Implications for Patient Care. It is important to consider left ventricular compliance in patient care. In monitoring preload, the nurse commonly measures indices of left ventricular end-diastolic *pressure*. Yet, therapeutic goals are related to achieving an end-diastolic *volume* change that will take advantage of the length–tension relationship of the heart to maintain or increase cardiac output. The pressure change is important, too, because elevated left ventricular filling pressures result in pulmonary congestion and edema.

For example, the first few days following a myocardial infarction are generally characterized by an increase in myocardial stiffness (Fig. 2-10).[4] The same end-diastolic volume may be accompanied by such a markedly increased end-diastolic pressure that signs of left ventricular failure such as rales appear (see Chap. 27). In this case, inotropic agents (which increase the force of contraction) would be of little or no benefit. However, unloading therapies that could decrease the end-diastolic volume could eliminate the damaging elevation in end-diastolic pressures. Furthermore, lowered ventricular pressures throughout diastole may improve coronary arterial filling. Better perfusion can improve tissue oxygenation and further diminish stiffness (see Chaps. 27 and 36 and Fig. 27-6).

The Role of Afterload

The Force–Velocity Relationship. The heart's ability to contract is influenced by the amount of active pressure above the preload it must generate. With a smaller afterload (*i.e.,* low aortic pressure), the heart is able to contract more rapidly. Against very large afterload (*i.e.,* high aortic pressure), contraction is much slower. This is often referred to as the force–velocity of shortening or simply the force–velocity relationship (Fig. 2-11). Changes in the initial muscle length or changes in contractility can alter the force–velocity relationship.

An intuitive understanding of the force–velocity relationship can be gained by reviewing the stick-figure cartoons of Figure 2-11. The lighter the load, the faster A, B, and C can run; the heavier the load, the slower they can move. If the load they are pulling is the Rock of Gibraltar, they will be unable to move it at all.

At the molecular level, the rate of cycling of crossbridges might be equated with the speed of shortening. Generation

Fig. 2-10. The stiffness of the left ventricle. Stiffness is the slope of the pressure–volume relationship. Curve 1 represents normal stiffness; curve 2 represents an increase in stiffness such as that which might occur following a myocardial infarction. In both cases, increases in volume result in increased pressure and an increased increment in pressure for a given increment in volume. Compliance is the inverse of stiffness. (Adapted from Forrester JS, Diamond GA: In Corday E, Swan HJC (eds): Myocardial Infarction, p 147. Baltimore, Williams & Wilkins, 1973)

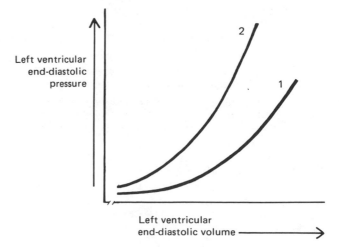

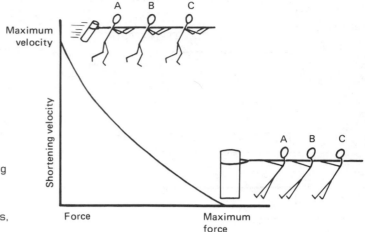

Fig. 2-11. Approximation of the force–velocity of shortening relationship of cardiac muscle. Velocity of shortening is maximal with extremely light afterload. Shortening is impossible with large afterloads. (Adapted from Katz AM: Physiology of the Heart, pp 87, 126. New York, Raven Press, 1977)

of tension might be equated with attachment and pulling by the crossbridges. The amount of tension the muscle can generate is determined by the number of crossbridges the muscle is able to form. This is determined in part by the preload, or the amount of diastolic stretch placed on the muscle. Once a critical pressure is reached—that of the afterload—the muscle shortens. The speed of that shortening that might be equated with the speed of cycling of crossbridges is determined in part by the pressure of the afterload.

The Effect of Afterload on the Volume Ejected by the Ventricle. In addition to influencing the speed of shortening, afterload is related to extent of shortening.[8] Increases in aortic pressure, at a constant end-diastolic pressure, result in decreased volume pumped by the left ventricle. When pumping against decreased aortic pressure, the left ventricle pumps a larger volume.

Implications for Patient Care. It is important to consider the force–velocity relationship in myocardial performance. Vasopressors that increase the systemic vascular resistance increase the afterload. Because of the inverse nature of the force–velocity relationship, the development of greater force is accompanied by a slower velocity of shortening. There may be a concomitant fall in stroke volume and cardiac output.

Contractility of Cardiac Muscle

Contractility describes the heart's ability to contract: It describes the ability of the heart muscle to shorten, develop tension, or both. Altered contractility is a change in the ability of the heart to contract independent of variations induced by altering either preload or afterload (Figs. 2-8, 2-12). In Figure 2-8, when the ordinate is "systolic muscle tension," the curves other than "normal" represent alterations in contractility.

Contractility is a property intrinsic in the muscle. Its physiologic basis is not yet understood. Although contractility is difficult to define or measure, it is a property of critical importance, for abnormalities in contractility are a major problem in the failing heart, and many therapies are designed to enhance contractility.

It is important to note that contractility is not equivalent to cardiac performance, which can be influenced by valvular function and circulating blood volume as well as by myocardial contractility.

Factors that affect the contractility of the heart are called inotropic agents. Positive inotropic agents increase contractility. These include sympathetic stimulation, excess thyroid hormone, epinephrine, norepinephrine, dopamine or isoproterenol infusion, and calcium salt infusion. Negative inotropic agents decrease contractility; these include myocardial hypoxia, anoxia or ischemia, barbiturates, alcohol, procaine amide and quinidine, propranolol, and possibly lidocaine.

Cardiac Reserve

The interaction of the mechanical properties of the heart can be illustrated by considering the reserve capacity of the heart. Cardiac reserve refers to the ability of the heart to increase its output. In the normal healthy person, the reserve capacity is used to meet demands for increased blood flow, such as during exercise. Normal cardiac output is 5.5 liters of blood per minute in a healthy 70-kg male. Utilization of

Fig. 2-12. Positive and negative inotropic effects on tension development or myocardial shortening. An increase in myocardial contractility enhances the amount of tension developed, the rate of shortening, or both, without an increase in initial cardiac muscle length. A decrease in myocardial contractility reduces the amount of tension developed, the rate of shortening, or both, without a decrease in initial cardiac muscle length. (Adapted from Katz AM: Physiology of the Heart, p 166. New York, Raven Press, 1977)

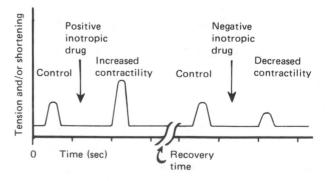

cardiac reserve could typically increase cardiac output with activity to 18 liters per minute. Heart disease often limits the total possible output, and the patient may have to rely on reserve capacity simply to maintain a normal cardiac output at rest. The two components of cardiac reserve are increases in heart rate and stroke volume.

Increases in heart rate increase the cardiac output. However, at rates higher than about 180 beats per minute, diastole is so shortened that diastolic filling is reduced. Stroke volume is then diminished as predicted by the Starling relationship. Furthermore, the coronary arteries are perfused during diastole, and fast heart rates diminish coronary blood flow. This in turn may result in ischemia, which in turn diminishes myocardial compliance and contractility. The stiff ventricle requires greater filling pressures to expand it to the same diastolic volume and may well operate at a smaller volume, further diminishing stroke volume, again as defined by the Starling relationship. Beyond a certain point, increasing the heart rate will so decrease the volume pumped per beat that cardiac output will fall.

During diastole the heart can fill to a larger volume than usual, thereby increasing its stroke volume as defined by the Starling relationship. This is sometimes called the diastolic cardiac reserve. Increases in diastolic volume are accompanied by increases in end-diastolic pressure. Left ventricular end-diastolic pressures beyond about 20 to 25 mm Hg typically result in pulmonary congestion and edema (see Chap. 27). The more dilated the ventricle, the more oxygen it requires (see below); this may be a limiting problem in the patient with coronary artery disease.

The heart is capable of ejecting a larger portion of its volume than it normally does, that is, it can contract to a smaller end-systolic volume. This is sometimes called the systolic reserve; it comes into play when the afterload is decreased (force–velocity relationship) or contractility increased. Increases in the velocity of contraction or contractility also make extra demands on the heart in terms of oxygen requirements and may be intolerable for the patient with coronary artery disease.

Factors involved in mechanical performance interact continuously. For example, an increase in afterload may result in a decrease in the stroke volume ejected. This in turn will result in a larger volume of blood in the heart at the end of systole. The addition of an unchanged amount of blood during the subsequent diastole will increase the end-diastolic volume. The ensuing contraction will be more forceful and stroke volume increased owing to the Starling effect.

In hemorrhage, the filling pressure may diminish. However, the afterload may also decrease. This tends to raise the stroke volume. Adrenergic outflow also contributes to increased stroke volume. The cardiac output may increase despite lowered filling pressures.

This section has discussed means by which the heart can increase its output. Just as a budget deficit can be corrected either by increasing income or by carefully managing spending, the cardiovascular system can meet demands for increased perfusion both by increasing output and by more efficiently using its present output. It can, for instance, shift blood flow to more active regions and extract more oxygen from the blood (Chap. 6).

Patient Assessment

Assessment of the patient includes the evalution of numerous indices of overall pump performance:

- Urine output, mental status, skin color, and temperature are indices of the adequacy of cardiac output to various organs and tissues.
- Cardiac output may be measured directly.
- Blood pressure is the product of cardiac output and systemic vascular resistance.

These observations measure end products of many complicated interacting variables that together compose the reserve capacity of the cardiovascular system. In making these assessments, we should not only ask whether blood flow and pressure are adequate but also probe more deeply:

- How much of the patient's reserve capacity must be used to maintain his level of functioning?
- Is he already tachycardiac, with a dilated left ventricle?
- Is his heart already receiving a high level of endogenous catecholaminergic outflow?
- How much of his reserve capacity is left? Of that which is left, how much can be used in planning the patient's care?

MYOCARDIAL METABOLISM

The heart, like other muscle tissue in the body, depends on the breakdown of adenosine triphosphate (ATP) to adenosine diphosphate (ADP) and inorganic phosphate (P_i) to liberate the energy required for many biologic processes:

$$ATP + H_2O \xrightleftharpoons{Mg^{2+} \, + \, ATPase} ADP + P_i + H^+ + 7.5 \, kcal \; energy$$

This reaction is spontaneous in an aqueous environment but proceeds slowly. Therefore, the cell uses selective enzymes to speed ATP hydrolysis (breakdown in water). These catalysts also couple the release of energy with specific activities such as muscle contraction and relaxation, electrical excitation, membrane transport, and biosynthesis of large molecules.

When a person is at rest, the myocardium uses some of the available ATP to synthesize a high-energy storage compound—creatine phosphate (CP). This process is catalyzed by creatine phosphokinase (CPK):

$$ATP + Creatine \xrightleftharpoons{CPK} CP + ADP$$

Because the myocardium is continuously active, CP stores are limited. A reverse of the storage reaction occurs when energy requirements increase. This reversal provides an immediate, though limited, source of ATP. Normally, however, ATP must be continuously synthesized to maintain myocardial function.

The hydrolysis and storage of ATP are simple biochemical processes. In contrast, the formation of ATP occurs in a series of efficient, but complex, enzyme-dependent reactions (Fig. 2-13). The bulk of myocardial ATP is synthesized in an aerobic environment. The presence of large amounts of mitochondria, the sites of aerobic synthesis of ATP, in the

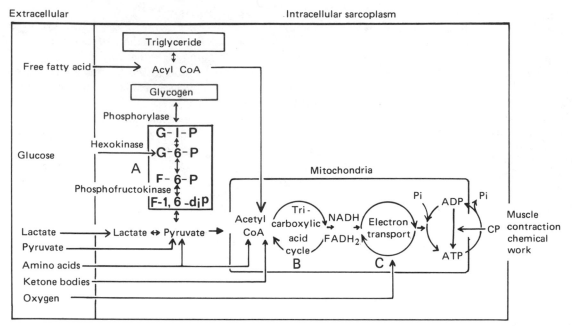

Fig. 2-13. Summary of energy-producing processes in the myocardial cell. Glycolysis (**A**) and substrate simplification occur in the sarcoplasm. The tricarboxylic acid cycle (**B**) and oxidative phosphorylation (**C**) take place in the mitochondria. A total of 36 moles ATP are formed for each mole of glucose metabolized in the presence of oxygen. Under anaerobic conditions, acetyl CoA production slows, anaerobic glycolysis proceeds, and pyruvate is metabolized to lactate. A net gain of 2 moles ATP for 1 mole glucose occurs. (Adapted from Hurst JW: The Heart, 4th ed, p 108. New York, McGraw-Hill, 1978)

myocardial cell attest to the need for oxygen as an energy substrate. The myocardium contains more mitochondria than does any other type of muscle cell.[15]

An important feature of overall ATP synthesis is its close link to energy demand. A number of control points closely couple the intermediate steps in ATP production to facilitate its use by the cell. The links in the chain responsible for the synthesis of ATP include substrate simplification, the tricarboxylic acid (TCA) cycle, and oxidative phosphorylation.

Substrate Simplification

Simplified dietary substances—glucose, free fatty acids (FFA), and amino acids—provide the fuel needed for energy production. These foodstuffs are initially oxidized through different pathways. (Oxidation is defined as the addition of oxygen or the loss of electrons with or without the loss of a hydrogen atom from a molecule.) However, all dietary substrates eventually converge into a common metabolic pathway, the tricarboxylic acid (TCA) cycle. This is accomplished by producing an intermediate, acetyl coenzyme A (CoA), which readily enters that cycle. The nutrients used by the myocardium are determined by their arterial concentration, availability of oxygen, cellular metabolism and storage, hormonal factors, and total energy requirements.[10]

Free fatty acids are the preferred myocardial fuel, particularly when the individual is in the fasting state. They enter the cell through the plasma membrane by passive diffusion. Plasma and myocardial triglycerides and lipoproteins are simplified by an enzyme, lipoprotein lipase, to FFA. The activity of this catalyst is regulated by hormones, one of which is epinephrine.[5] Once in the cell, FFA are simplified and combine with CoA to form acyl CoA. The fatty acyl CoA

enters the mitochondria if ATP is present. It is then broken down into acetyl CoA for entry into the TCA cycle. This breakdown step is absolutely dependent on oxygen.[11]

Glucose or its storage form, glycogen, can serve as an additional substrate for energy metabolism. Whereas glucose contributes only 15% to myocardial ATP synthesis in the fasting individual, its role increases to nearly 50% in the postprandial state.[11] Glucose enters the cell by carrier-mediated diffusion. Its transport is accelerated by epinephrine, insulin, or hypoxia and is inhibited by FFA oxidation.[5]

The initial step in the breakdown of glucose to form energy is called glycolysis. Each molecule of glucose undergoes several chemical reactions resulting in the net gain of 2 molecules ATP and the formation of 2 pyruvate molecules. The fate of pyruvate depends on the state of cellular oxygenation. In aerobic conditions, pyruvate is converted into acetyl CoA, which can be oxidized to carbon dioxide (CO_2) and water (H_2O) in the TCA cycle. When the cell is hypoxic, pyruvate is converted into lactate. This conversion results in less ATP formed, but it allows glycolysis to proceed in the absence of oxygen (see Table 11-1). It is a mechanism vital for the survival of the ischemic myocardium, because it is the only way in which ATP can be synthesized under anaerobic conditions (see Chap. 11).[2]

Amino acids play a minor role in energy metabolism of the heart. In starvation, however, amino acid intermediates may enter the TCA cycle at various points.[14]

The TCA Cycle

The production of acetyl CoA from fats, carbohydrates, and proteins occurs only in the oxygenated cell. It enables the TCA cycle to proceed in the direction of ATP synthesis.

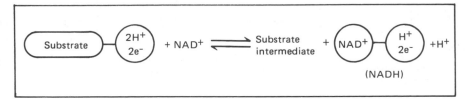

Fig. 2-14. Electron transfer to energy cofactors.

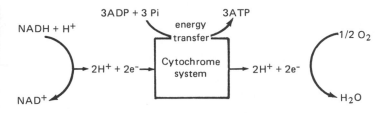

Fig. 2-15. The oxidation of NADH is coupled to ATP synthesis in the mitochondrial cytochrome chain. $FADH_2$ (not shown) is also oxidized in the same system. (Adapted from Vander AJ, Sherman JH, Luciano DS: Human Physiology, p 81. New York, McGraw-Hill, 1980)

Although a small amount of ATP is produced in the cycle, its major role is to link the breakdown of acetyl CoA to the synthesis of ATP that occurs in the cytochrome chain of the mitochondria. As acetyl CoA combines with the TCA cycle intermediates, CO_2 and H_2O are formed and electric charges are transferred to cofactors, nicotinamide adenine dinucleotide (NAD) and flavin adenine dinucleotide (FAD). They act as vehicles for the transfer of energy from one form (electric charge) to another (ATP) (Fig. 2-14).[16]

Oxidative Phosphorylation

The final step in aerobic ATP synthesis occurs in the cytochrome chain located in the inner membrane of the mitochondria. A cytochrome is a molecule that can accept or donate electric charges. The energy cofactors (NAD, FAD) used in the TCA cycle pass electric charges through the chain. This process releases a sufficient amount of energy so that an inorganic phosphate can be added to ADP to form ATP (Fig. 2-15). The final transfer of charge from a cytochrome to oxygen to form water occurs at the end of the chain.

The production of ATP through the cytochrome chain is called oxidative phosphorylation. Oxidative phosphorylation is the coupling of oxidation of a substance with phospho-

rylation (adding P_i) of another molecule. In this case, cytochrome pairs undergo oxidation and reduction while ADP is phosphorylated. The major metabolic pathways for energy production are summarized in Table 2-1 and Figure 2-16.

PHYSIOLOGY OF THE CORONARY CIRCULATION

Under normal conditions at rest, the heart extracts a large amount of oxygen from the blood perfusing it: The difference in oxygen content between the arterial and coronary sinus blood is approximately 11.4 ml O_2/100 ml blood (see Chap 6).[13] It is difficult to extract much more oxygen than this, yet the oxygen requirement of the heart may increase many fold. This additional oxygen can only be supplied by increasing the coronary blood flow. Coronary blood flow increases proportionately to myocardial metabolism and oxygen consumption.

Determinants of Myocardial Oxygen Consumption (MV̇O₂)

Some oxygen is used in the "housekeeping" activities of the heart cells. This refers to those activities that are independent of contraction and includes such functions as maintenance of the proper ionic environment and repair or replacement of intracellular proteins. The amount of oxygen used in these functions is relatively small and stable.

Each contraction of the heart involves movements of ions across the cell membranes. By removing Ca^{2+} from the fluid bathing the heart cells, the heart can be excited without actively developing tension. Such experiments have shown that the cost of electrical depolarization and repolarization is small.[7] It is possible that cycling of pumps that maintain Na^+ and K^+ concentrations is responsible for this oxygen requirement (see Chap. 3).

In addition to these two fairly constant and low requirements for oxygen, there are factors related to activity and the state of the heart that determine how much oxygen the heart will need. These constitute the major determinants of myocardial oxygen consumption (MV̇O₂) and include intramyocardial tension, heart rate, shortening, and contractile state.

TABLE 2-1. ATP Yield from Complete Oxidation of Glucose

Reaction Sequence	ATP Yield Per Glucose
	Molecules
Glycolysis	
Glucose → 2 pyruvate Occurs in cytoplasm Uses 2 NAD+	2
2 Pyruvate → 2 acetyl CoA	
Occurs in mitochondria Uses 2 NAD+	
TCA cycle	
Occurs in mitochondria Uses 6 NAD+ and 2 FAD	2
Oxidative phosphorylation	
Occurs in mitochondria Uses 10 NADH and 2 FADH₂	32
TOTAL	36

Oxidation of FFA produces more ATP than does oxidation of glucose; the number of molecules ATP produced by oxidation of FFA depends on the specific fatty acid utilized. (Adapted from Biochemistry 2nd ed. by Lubert Stryer. W.H. Freeman and Company. Copyright © 1981.)

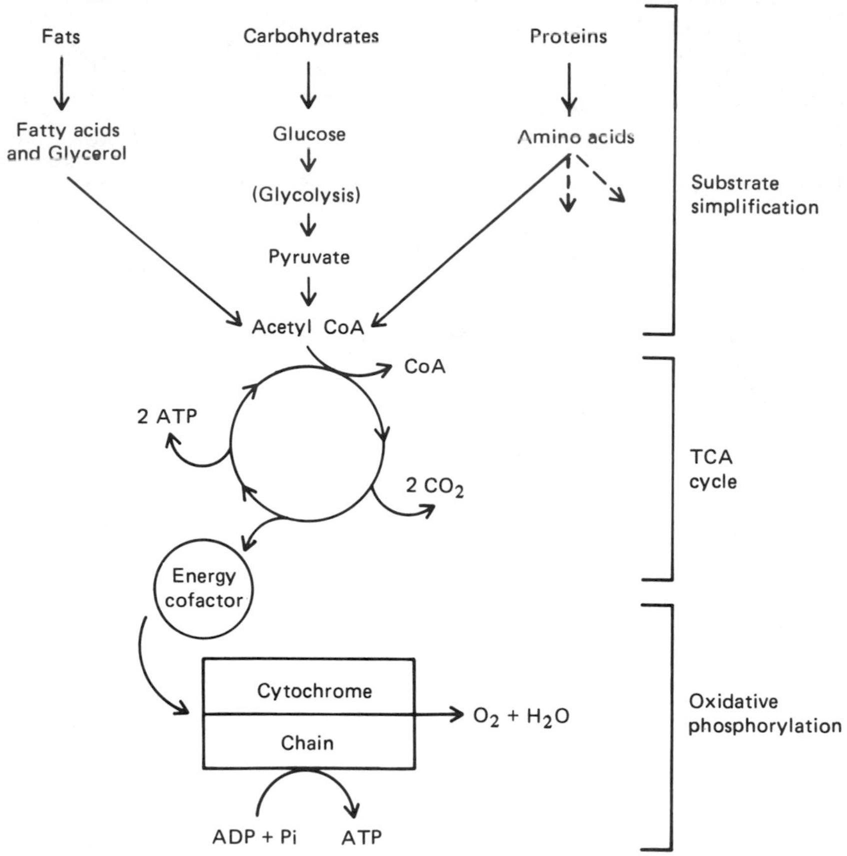

Fats

Carbohydrates

Proteins

Fatty acids
and Glycerol

Glucose

Amino acids

(Glycolysis)

Substrate
simplification

Pyruvate

Acetyl CoA

CoA

2 ATP

2 CO_2

TCA
cycle

Energy
cofactor

Cytochrome

O_2 + H_2O

Oxidative
phosphorylation

Chain

ADP + Pi   ATP

Fig. 2-16. Synthesis of energy in the aerobic cell. Adenosine triphosphate (ATP) is the major form of energy used by the myocardial cell. It is formed when free fatty acids, amino acids, and glucose are degraded by a variety of metabolic pathways. Glucose goes through three major metabolic processes when it is oxidized to carbon dioxide (CO_2) and water (H_2O). Its initial breakdown into two pyruvate molecules occurs in glycolysis. The pyruvate is converted to acetyl coenzyme A (CoA) when oxygen is present. Acetyl CoA is formed in the mitochondria and is oxidized to CO_2 and water by the tricarboxcylic acid (TCA) cycle. ATP is formed and energy cofactors are reduced. (Reduction is the process by which electrons or a hydrogen atom are added to a substance.) The cofactors then use the cytochrome chain to produce more ATP. (Adapted from Stryer L: Biochemistry, 2nd ed. p 272. San Francisco, WH Freeman & Co, 1981)

Tension. *The law of Laplace* is used to calculate intramyocardial tension. This law states

$$T \propto \frac{P \cdot R}{Th}$$

where T = intramyocardial wall tension, P = internal pressure within the ventricular cavity, R = radius of the ventricular cavity, Th = thickness of the ventricular wall, and $\propto$ = proportional to. An increase in the afterload of the left ventricle (*i.e.*, aortic pressure) causes the left ventricle to develop more pressure during the systolic period, thereby increasing intramyocardial tension and oxygen consumption. A rise in the preload or filling pressures of the left ventricle increases tension, because both internal pressure and the radius of the ventricular cavity are increased, and the thickness decreased. Again oxygen consumption is increased.

Clinical Implications. It is useful to consider the Laplace relationship when evaluating oxygen demand in clinical states. For example, *hypertrophy of ventricular muscle* results in an increase in the thickness of the ventricular wall. This is advantageous in that wall tension is lower for the same left ventricular cavity size (the same end-diastolic volume); hence oxygen consumption is decreased. However, development of hypertrophy is a two-edged sword. At the same time that wall tension is decreased, the mass of tissue requiring oxygen is increased; the net result may well be a greater demand by the heart for oxygen. Furthermore, because hypertrophy tends to increase the size of the muscle cells without increasing the tissue capillarity,[17] diffusional

distances are increased. The supply of oxygen to the interior of the fiber may be significantly impaired.

With *cardiac dilation*, the radius of the left ventricle is increased. A larger end-diastolic volume is associated with higher end-diastolic pressure and increased pressure generation during systole according to the Starling law. The Laplace relationship predicts that both factors lead to increased intramyocardial wall tension. The stretching out of the heart wall is associated with decreased wall thickness, further increasing intramyocardial wall tension. The increase in oxygen demand can be significant.

Heart Rate. It is not surprising that increased heart rate (at the same preload and afterload) increases the myocardial oxygen consumption. Each beat represents the generation of tension by the myocardium.

Shortening. In an *isotonic twitch*, there is a component of the oxygen consumption that is proportional to the amount of shortening by a muscle, that is, there is a metabolic cost that is related to shortening. This is sometimes called the Fenn effect and is a characteristic of cardiac as well as of skeletal muscle. In cardiac muscle, a contraction with a large amount of shortening is one that expels a large stroke volume.

Contractile State. *Contractility* correlates with the amount of oxygen consumed by the heart. Postive inotropic factors increase the oxygen consumption of the heart. Negative inotropic agents decrease oxygen consumption.

Pressure Versus Volume Work. Work done by the heart is proportional to the pressure generated times the volume pumped. (Stroke work = (mean arterial pressure-left atrial pressure) × stroke volume.) Pressure generated is a component of the intramyocardial tension as described by the Laplace relationship and thus contributes to the overall $M\dot{V}O_2$. The size of the stroke volume is related to the amount of myocardial shortening, and thus it, too, contributes to the $M\dot{V}O_2$. Although equal amounts of work can be obtained by altering pressure or volume, the cost in terms of $M\dot{V}O_2$ is much greater for high-pressure work than it is for high-volume work. Thus cardiac work is poorly correlated with $M\dot{V}O_2$.

Indices of $M\dot{V}O_2$. There is no single readily available indicator of the oxygen requirements of the myocardium. Ideally such an indicator would take into account all major determinants of the $M\dot{V}O_2$. The pressure–rate product and the tension–time index are two commonly used methods of estimation that have been validated.[6] Each takes into account one of the major determinants of the $M\dot{V}O_2$, the heart rate. Another major determinant, tension, is also considered in these indices. However, what is actually measured is pressure. For pressure to be an indicator of tension, the other factors in the Laplace equation, that is, radius of the ventricular cavity and thickness of the ventricular wall, must be constant.

The pressure–rate product is calculated by multiplying the heart rate times either systolic or mean arterial pressure and dividing by 100.

The tension–time index might more appropriately be called the pressure–time index. It is calculated by multiplying the area under the left ventricular pressure curve times the heart rate.

Control of Coronary Blood Flow

Flow of blood in the coronary circulation is, as in all vascular beds, proportional to the perfusion pressure and inversely proportional to the resistance of the bed. Resistance in the coronary bed is altered by compression on it during systole and by metabolic, neural, and hormonal factors. Coronary artery disease can impose significant resistance.

The pressure difference that drives the perfusion of the heart is the gradient between aortic pressure and the pressure in the right atrium into which most of the coronary blood flows (Chap. 5). However, the coronary circulation is autoregulated. This means that changes in the perfusion pressure over the range of approximately 60 to 180 mm Hg make little change in the amount of blood flowing to the heart if the other factors influencing perfusion are held constant. Because the heart develops its own perfusion pressure, a fall in aortic pressure can reduce coronary perfusion, which in turn may further decrease cardiac function and pressure development. A cycle of deterioration may result.

During systole, the tension in the myocardial wall is high. This compresses the coronary arteries and prevents perfusion. Thus, the heart has the unique property of receiving most of its blood flow during diastole (Fig. 2-17). Rapid

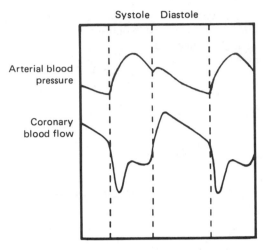

Fig. 2-17. Effect of systolic compression on coronary blood flow. Note the decrease in flow during systole, and the increase during diastole. (Folkow B, Neil E: Circulation, p 421. Oxford, Oxford University Press, 1971)

heart rates decrease the time spent in diastole and may impinge on coronary perfusion.

Intramyocardial tension tends to be highest in the subendocardial regions of the left ventricle. Thus myocardial oxygen consumption is probably highest in this region; yet systolic compression is also greatest here. This in part explains why this area has an increased incidence of infarction. In transmural infarctions (*i.e.*, ones that involve the full thickness of the left ventricular wall) the area of involvement is typically greater on the subendocardial surface than on the subepicardial surface (Chap. 12). A factor that also contributes to this pattern of involvement in infarction is the pattern of coronary artery distribution. Because arteries enter the myocardium on the epicardial surface and plunge inward through the wall, the most easily compromised distal segments of the coronary arteries perfuse the endocardium.

The coronary arteries are innervated by alpha sympathetic and by parasympathetic fibers. The direct effects of neural outflow are the same in the coronary bed as in other systemic beds. Alpha adrenergic stimulation (or norepinephrine) constricts arteries, and parasympathetic (vagal) stimulation dilates them. Pharmacologic doses of the beta adrenergic drug isoproterenol dilate the coronary artery bed. However, often the direct effect of neural outflow on the coronary bed is masked because the autonomic nervous sytem also affects myocardial metabolism and contractility, and the effect of these latter factors often predominates.

Local metabolic conditions are the predominant determinants of coronary perfusion (see Chap. 5). Increased metabolism or hypoxia leads to vasodilation and increases myocardial blood flow. The mechanism that mediates this effect is unknown. One hypothesis suggests that adenosine is released from myocardial tissue in proportion to the amount of oxygen being consumed and that perfusion correlates with the amount of adenosine released.[1] This hypothesis is as yet unproved.

With atherosclerosis, significant resistance can develop in the coronary arteries. Lesions that occupy more than two-thirds of the vessel's cross-sectional area may impinge significantly on flow at rest. Such lesions can prevent the increases in flow necessary when myocardial oxygen demand increases.

REFERENCES

1. Berne RM, Rubio R: Coronary circulation. In Berne RM (ed): Handbook of Physiology, Sec 2: The Cardiovascular System, Vol 1, The Heart, pp 873–952. Bethesda, Md, American Physiological Society, 1979
2. Davies RE: Biochemical processes in cardiac function. In Braunwald E (ed): The Myocardium: Failure and Infarction, pp 29–35. New York, HP Publishing, 1974
3. Gordon AM, Huxley AF, Julian FJ: The variation in isometric tension with sarcomere length in vertebrate muscle fibres. J Physiol (Lond) 184:170–192, 1966
4. Hood WB, Jr, Bianco JA, Humar R et al: Experimental myocardial infarction: Compliance in the healing phase. J Clin Invest 49:1316–1323, 1970
5. Katz AM: Physiology of the Heart, pp 1–227. New York, Raven Press, 1977
6. Kitamura K, Jorgensen CR, Gobel FL et al: Hemodynamic correlates of myocardial oxygen consumption during upright exercise. J Appl Physiol 32:516–522, 1972
7. Klocke FJ, Braunwald E, Ross J, Jr: Oxygen cost of electrical activation of the heart. Circ Res 18:357–365, 1966
8. Levy MN, Imperial ES, Zieske H, Jr: Ventricular response to increased outflow resistance in absence of elevated intraventricular end-diastolic pressure. Circ Res 12:107–117, 1963
9. Lewis BS, Gotsman MS: Current concepts of left ventricular relaxation and compliance. Am Heart J 99:101–112, 1980
10. Oliver MF: The metabolic response to a heart attack. Heart Lung 4(1):57–60, 1975
11. Oliver MF: Metabolism of the normal and ischemic myocardium. In Dickinson CJ, Marks J (eds): Developments in Cardiovascular Medicine, pp 145–164. Baltimore, University Park Press, 1978
12. Patterson SW, Per HP, Starling EH: The regulation of the heart beat. J Physiol (Lond) 48:465–513, 1914
13. Regan TJ, Frank MJ, Lehan PH et al: Myocardial blood flow and oxygen uptake during acute red blood cell volume increments. Circ Res 13:172–181, 1963
14. Schlant RC: Normal physiology of the cardiovascular system; Metabolism of the heart. In Hurst JW (ed): The Heart, 4th ed, pp 71–100; pp 107–113. New York, McGraw-Hill, 1978
15. Shepherd JT, Vanhoulte PM: The Human Cardiovascular System, pp 46–47. New York, Raven Press, 1979
16. Stryer L: Biochemistry, 2nd ed, pp 235–332, pp 539–556. San Francisco, WH Freeman, 1981
17. Wearn JT: Morphological and functional alterations of the coronary circulation. Harvey Lect 35:243–270, 1940

ADDITIONAL READING

Myocardial Mechanics

Carlson D, Wilkie DR: Muscle Physiology. Englewood Cliffs, NJ, Prentice-Hall, 1974

Forrester JS, Diamond GA: Clinical applications of left ventricular pressures. In Corday E, Swan HJC (eds): Myocardial Infarction. Baltimore, Williams & Wilkins, 1973

Kones RJ: Myocardial mechanics: Evaluation of the heart as muscle and determinants of ventricular performance. In Cardiogenic Shock: Mechanism and Management, pp 39–78. Mt Kisco, NY, Futura, 1974

Schlant RC: Normal physiology of the cardiovascular system. In Hurst JW (ed): The Heart, 4th ed, pp 71–100. New York, McGraw-Hill, 1978

Weber KT, Janicki JS: The heart as a muscle–pump system and the concept of heart failure. Am Heart J 98:371–384, 1979

Myocardial Metabolism

Oliver MF: Metabolism of the normal and ischemic myocardium. In Dickinson CJ, Marks J (eds): Developments in Cardiovascular Medicine, pp 145–168. Baltimore, University Park Press, 1978

Oxygen Consumption and Coronary Blood Flow

Braunwald E: Control of myocardial oxygen consumption. Am J Cardiol 27:416–432, 1971

Braunwald E, Sobel BE: Coronary blood flow and myocardial ischemia. In Braunwald E (ed): Heart Disease, Vol 2, pp 1279–1308. Philadelphia, WB Saunders, 1980

Feigl EO: The coronary circulation. In Ruch TC, Patton HD (eds): Physiology and Biophysics, Vol II, 20th ed, pp 247–261. Philadelphia, WB Saunders, 1974

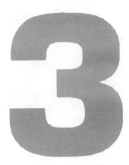

Cardiac Electrophysiology

CAROL JEAN HALPENNY, R.N., M.A.

The heart's intrinsic ability to generate an electrical impulse, propagate the impulse through the heart, and then sustain a relatively lengthy cardiac muscle contraction differentiates it from other body organs that function only in response to external nervous control. A lengthy cardiac muscle contraction is functionally efficient in terms of ejecting blood from the cardiac chambers (see Chap. 2).

CARDIAC ACTION POTENTIAL

Cardiac electrical activity is generated by the movement (flux) of ions (charged particles) across the myocardial cell membrane. The change in cardiac intracellular voltage over time is termed the cardiac action potential. Action potential diagrams represent recorded electrical changes within a single cell; the characteristics of individual human cardiac cells vary somewhat from the following generalized descriptions.

Effect of Ionic Movement on Cell Membrane Potential

Electrical (voltage) differences across the cell membrane are usually referred to in terms of the intracellular voltage, with an extracellular voltage of zero as a reference. The measured membrane potential difference (usually shortened to "membrane potential") for a resting Purkinje cell is approximately -90 millivolts (mV); this means that the voltage measured by a microelectrode inserted into the cell is 90 mV less than that measured by a microelectrode outside the cell (Fig. 3-1).[14]

The total net movement of ions across the cell wall determines the membrane potential of the cell at any specific point in time. The number of ions moving across the wall is small in terms of the total number within and outside the cell. Cardiac intracellular ionic composition differs greatly from that of the extracellular fluid surrounding the cells. Table 3-1 illustrates the approximate intra- and extracellular concentrations of the major ions involved in cardiac electrical activity.

Fig. 3-1. Schematic illustration of how intracellular electrical changes are recorded. When the tip of one microelectrode penetrates a cell, the oscilloscope trace shifts from the reference 0 potential and records the intracellular negative resting potential. (Vassale M: Cardiac Physiology for the Clinician, p 2. New York, Academic Press, 1976)

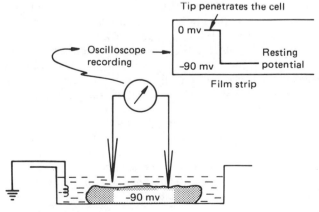

TABLE 3-1 INTRACELLULAR AND EXTRACELLULAR ION CONCENTRATIONS IN CARDIAC MUSCLE

Ion	Extracellular Concentration	Intracellular Concentration*	Ratio of Extracellular to Intracellular Concentration	E_i
Na^+	145 mM	15 mM	9.7	+60 mV
K^+	4 mM	150 mM	0.027	−94 mV
Cl^-	120 mM	5 mM	24	−83 mV
Ca^{2+}	2 mM	10^{-7} M	2×10^4	+129 mV

Na^+ = sodium; K^+ = potassium; Cl^- = chloride and Ca^{2+} = calcium. E_i = equilibrium potential; mM = millimole per kilogram; mV = millivolt; M = mole.

Values given are approximations and differ slightly in different published tables. Table values may be given in mM per liter or per kilogram body water (see Chap. 9). Most of the intracellular calcium is bound to proteins or sequestered in the sarcoplasmic reticulum; thus, total intracellular calcium content is approximately 2 mM/kg. Actual free sodium concentration may approach 1 mM, because some intracellular sodium may be sequestered in the sarcoplasmic reticulum.

Chloride appears to be passively distributed across the cell membrane according to the resting cell-membrane potential (electrical potential difference across the cell membrane), so that during the resting phase of the action potential, the net efflux of chloride equals the net influx of chloride.

(Sperelakis N: Origin of the cardiac resting potential. In Berne RM (ed): Handbook of Physiology, Sec 2, The Cardiovascular System, Vol I, The Heart, p 193. Bethesda, Md, American Physiological Society, 1979)

Ionic Movement Across Cell Membranes

Ions move across the cardiac cellular membrane in response to both passive and active forces. The cardiac membrane must be permeable to a specific ion for that ion to move passively across the membrane. This selective permeability makes it easier or more difficult for each ion to move across the membrane and thus limits ionic diffusion. The passive diffusion of ions is influenced principally by differences in electrical charge and chemical concentration on each side of the membrane. Active forces, usually using energy, move ions across the membrane in a direction that is opposite to the forces operating passively.

Potassium. Potassium is the major intracellular positive ion (cation) (Table 3-1). The membrane potential of the resting Purkinje cell is determined primarily by potassium movement across the cell membrane.[5,19]

Because potassium has an intracellular concentration of approximately 150 millimole/liter (mM/liter) and an extracellular concentration of 3 to 4 mM/liter, there is a chemical concentration difference (chemical gradient) promoting the movement of potassium out of the cell (Fig. 3-2). Potassium moves through the semipermeable cell membrane from the intracellular region of greater potassium concentration to the extracellular region of lesser potassium concentration.

The cell becomes more negative as potassium moves outward. The electrical difference (electrical gradient) between the inside and the outside of the cell increases. Potassium is then influenced by the electrical difference to move back into the cell; that is, because potassium is a positive ion, it is drawn by the accumulation of increased negative charge in the cell to move back into the cell.

The point at which there is an equilibration between the concentration forces promoting potassium efflux (outward movement) and the electrical forces promoting potassium influx (inward movement) is termed the *equilibrium potential* for potassium; the forces promoting influx are equal and opposite to the forces promoting efflux. Small amounts of potassium continuously move back and forth across the membrane, but the concentration gradients for potassium remain stable and net movement is zero.

The equilibrium potential for potassium is approximately −95 mV.[27] Each ion has a different equilibrium potential,

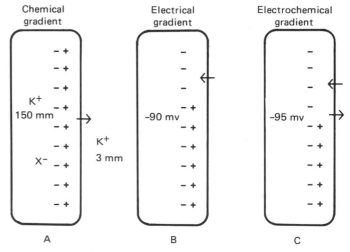

Fig. 3-2. Development of potassium equilibrium potential. **(A)** The cell is assumed to have no intracellular electrical potential gradient because positive potassium (K^+) ions are matched by negative protein (X) charges. A chemical gradient directed outward favors the outflow of K^+. **(B)** An electrical difference promotes the inward movement of potassium. **(C)** Potassium equilibrium is established when the inside of the cell has become sufficiently negative to oppose any further net potassium outflow. Note that the equilibrium potential for potassium (−95 mV) is slightly more negative than the resting Purkinje cell (−90 mV) (see text). *mM* = millimoles, *mV* = millivolts. (Adapted from Vassale M: Cardiac Physiology for the Clinician, p 4. New York, Academic Press, 1976)

which depends on its specific chemical and electrical gradients (Table 3-1). The Nernst equation mathematically defines the equilibrium potential for any ion. (The Nernst equation can be found in the Glossary.)

Because the membrane potential for potassium is −95 mV and the resting Purkinje membrane potential is approximately −90 mV, it is apparent that the resting cell membrane is permeable to potassium. However, the resting membrane potential is also influenced to some extent by the movement of other positive ions, principally sodium.[21]

Sodium. The equilibrium potential for sodium at an extracellular concentration of 150 mM/liter and an intracellular concentration of 15 to 30 mM/liter is +40 to +60 mV.[10,14,21] A resting cell membrane potential of −90 mV should

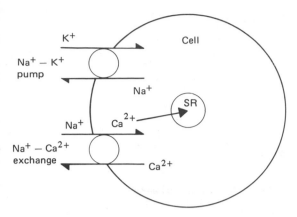

Fig. 3-3. Schematic view of active ion movements. See text for description. Calcium (Ca^{2+}) is sequestered in the sarcoplasmic reticulum SR and participates in cardiac contraction (see Chap. 2). (Adapted from Noble D: The Initiation of Heartbeat, published by Oxford University Press, 2nd edition, p 18. © Oxford University Press, 1979)

promote the passive influx of sodium. Although in Purkinje cells there is a small amount of inward sodium movement under resting conditions, the resting cell membrane is relatively impermeable to sodium, and there is not a large influx of sodium.

Movement of sodium out of the cell requires energy because it occurs against the sodium equilibrium potential. The cell has a pumping mechanism located in the cell membrane that moves sodium ions out of the cell and potassium ions into the cell; this mechanism is referred to as the *sodium–potassium pump*.[21,24] The energy for this pump is provided by adenosine triphosphate (ATP) and requires magnesium and the enzyme sodium-potassium-ATPase. This pump helps to reestablish the resting concentrations of intracellular and extracellular sodium and potassium after cardiac depolarization. The ratio of sodium ions pumped out to potassium ions pumped in varies from 3 Na^+ :3 K^+ to 3 Na^+:2 K^+ depending upon the situation.[10] A ratio of 3:2 helps to make the cell more negative.[14,28]

Calcium. There is evidence for a cellular exchange mechanism that couples the efflux of one calcium ion with the influx of two sodium ions by indirectly using energy from the electrochemical gradient for sodium. (Fig. 3-3).[14,21,24] The relationships and ratios of transmembrane ion exchanges may be reversed or changed in the calcium–sodium exchange reaction.[21] There are probably other active transport mechanisms for sodium, calcium, and potassium.[14]

Phases of the Action Potential

The changes in cardiac intracellular voltage that lead to the creation of the cardiac impulse are described below. Processes in cardiac muscle seem to be more complex than those in skeletal muscle, perhaps because multiple mechanisms are necessary to maintain the cardiac functions essential to life.[10] Although recognizing the complexities of cardiac impulse generation and conduction during the following discussion, there are some simple essential points regarding the electrical activity of cardiac cells to remember (Fig. 3-4):

1. Depolarization means that the interior of the cell becomes less negative. Repolarization means the return of membrane potential toward the original negative voltage after depolarization. Electrophysiologists often refer to a movement of the original membrane potential toward zero as being a decrease in potential, whereas a movement toward greater negativity is termed an increase in potential. To avoid confusion, the terms increased or decreased potential are not used in this text but instead voltage changes are referred to either as being more negative or less negative or as moving from the original position toward or away from zero.

2. Cardiac cells depolarize rapidly. They remain partly depolarized during a relatively long plateau period before repolarization. This plateau period differentiates cardiac muscle from skeletal muscle or nerve tissue. Cardiac muscles thus have time to contract and relax and are incapable of developing tetanic contractions (see Chap. 2).

3. The selective membrane permeability for specific ions varies during different phases of the action potential. These increased permeabilities are referred to as separate ionic "channels" through which specific ions diffuse into or out of cardiac cells more readily.[7,16,28] This ionic movement through the channels is referred to as being controlled by "gates" in the membrane that open and shut in response to changes in time and voltage.

4. Myocardial cells have two basic functions: to conduct electrical impulses and to contract. There are electrophysiologic differences among different types of cardiac cells.[2,3,16] Purkinje cells have been studied more intensively than other cardiac cells, so the Purkinje cell is used as a prototype for describing the time periods and events of the cardiac action potential. Differences between Purkinje cells and other cardiac cells are mentioned later.

Phase Zero. Rapid depolarization of the Purkinje cell is represented by the rapid upstroke labeled 0 in Figure 3-4. Intracellular voltage is altered approximately from -90 mV to $+20$ mV within milliseconds (msec), with a maximum velocity of depolarization of 600 to 800 mV/msec.[2,3]

This rapid voltage change is caused by the membrane suddenly becoming more permeable to sodium, that is, a "rapid sodium channel" opens and permits the rapid inward movement of sodium. This channel seems to be voltage

Fig. 3-4. Cardiac action potential. See text for description. (Katz A: Physiology of the Heart, p 230. New York, Raven Press, 1977)

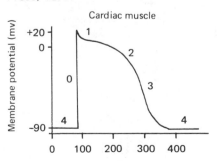

dependent; it opens and closes when the intracellular voltage is at certain levels. Recovery (ability to function again) of the channel seems to be voltage and time dependent; it also takes a fixed amount of time to recover.

During rapid depolarization, potassium movement out of the cell is decreased. Calcium moves into the cell during the latter part of phase 0.[3,25]

Phase 1. In Purkinje fibers there is a rapid early repolarization from +20 mV to 0 mV or −20 mV. This rapid repolarization seems to be caused by a rapid partial closing of the fast sodium channel, so that sodium influx decreases.[2,7,28] At the same time there also seems to be an inward flow of chloride.[2,28] Because chloride is negative, this makes the cell more negative.[7]

Plateau (Phase 2). The membrane potential remains between 0 mV and −20 mV for over 100 msec. The plateau is due to a balance between the effects of small inward and outward electrical flows (currents) that result from several ionic fluxes.[28]

A slow inward movement of calcium occurs during the late part of phase 0 and continues through phase 2; this "slow inward current" helps to maintain the plateau.[28] Movement through this "slow channel" is voltage and time dependent. Sodium may also move inward through the calcium slow channel or another slow channel.[3,14,16,25]

Phase 3 is a period of rapid repolarization. The relatively neutral (0 mV) membrane potential that was maintained during the plateau period rapidly becomes more negative. An increase in potassium efflux appears to be the major factor responsible for returning the membrane potential to resting values of approximately −90 mV.[2,6,7,14,29]

Phase 4. Figure 3-4 depicts a Purkinje cell that maintains an unchanging resting membrane potential of −90 mV

Fig. 3-5. Major ionic movements during a Purkinje cell action potential. *Arrows* indicate approximate times when the indicated ion movement influences membrane potential. The arrows point in the direction of the effect, upward for depolarization and downward for repolarization. (Modified from Fozzard H and Gibbons WR: Cardiol 31:182–192, 1973)

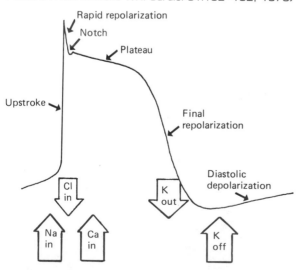

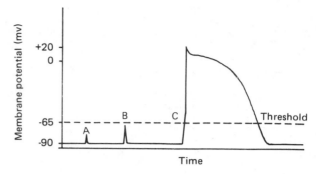

Fig. 3-6. Initiation of an action potential when the membrane potential is depolarized to threshold. Small depolarizing stimuli (**A** and **B**) that fail to reach threshold (*dashed line*) are unable to initiate an action potential. When depolarization reaches threshold (**C**), a regenerative action potential is produced. Once the latter begins, further depolarization becomes independent of the initial stimulus. (Katz A: Physiology of the Heart, p 236. New York, Raven Press, 1977)

during the resting phase (phase 4) of the action potential. The sodium–potassium–ATPase pump helps to maintain resting sodium and potassium intracellular concentrations. Figure 3-5 summarizes some of the major ionic movements occurring during a single episode of cell depolarization and repolarization.

Threshold Potential

Depolarization does not occur again until the membrane potential reaches a voltage level termed the threshold potential. In Purkinje cells the threshold potential is approximately −60 or −65 mV.[13,27] The cell must be depolarized to this point either by an electrical stimulus from a neighboring cell or by spontaneous depolarization. When this voltage is reached, the rapid sodium channels open and complete rapid depolarization results (Fig. 3-6.)

Although once threshold is reached the cell will completely depolarize, the amplitude of the action potential can be decreased if the distance between the resting potential and the threshold potential is less than usual.[2] Stimuli that do not depolarize a cell to threshold are not effective in initiating action potentials. However, such stimuli can have an effect on ionic movements; in pathophysiologic situations these stimuli may influence cardiac arrhythmias (see Chap. 26).

Refractory Period. The period of time following depolarization during which it is difficult or impossible to reexcite the cell is termed the refractory period (Fig. 3-7). Refractoriness reflects the effects on depolarization of time and voltage requirements for the opening and closing of ionic channels.

The effective refractory period is the time when no action potential can be initiated by an external electrical stimulus. This period is determined by the time needed for the reopening of channels permitting sodium and calcium influx. The effective refractory period extends from phase 0 through the middle of phase 3.

During the relative refractory period only stimuli greater than those that normally depolarize the cell to threshold can initiate an action potential. The relative refractory period

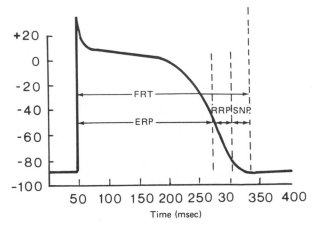

Fig. 3-7. Excitability during the cardiac action potential. The effective refractory period (*ERP*), during which electrical stimuli of any strength are unable to initiate a propagated action potential, is followed by the relative refractory period (*RRP*), during which only stimuli greater than those that normally reach threshold can cause a propagated action potential. This is followed by the supernormal period (*SNP*), during which stimuli slightly less than those which normally reach threshold can cause a propagated action potential. The action potentials generated during the RRP and SNP usually propagate slowly. Full recovery time (*FRT*) is the interval following depolarization after which threshold returns to normal and stimulation produces a normally propagated action potential. (Adapted from Katz A: Physiology of the Heart, p 248. New York, Raven Press, 1977)

occurs during the latter part of repolarization. Under certain conditions, a stimulus that is weaker than usual may initiate an action potential during the last part of phase 3 and the beginning of phase 4; this is termed the supernormal period (Chap. 26).

The entire period between depolarization and complete repolarization is termed the *full recovery time*. Under normal conditions cardiac cells are not depolarized until they have had time to recover fully from the previous depolarization.

• The upper limits of normal heart rate responses and the time allowed for ventricular filling depend upon normal cardiac electrical refractoriness.

Cells with longer action potential durations have longer refractory periods under normal conditions.

• Abnormal refractory periods resulting from pathophysiologic situations may create cardiac arrhythmias (see Chap. 26).

Automatic Cells

Any cell that has been shown to be capable of spontaneous depolarization under physiologic conditions has been termed an automatic cell.[3,9] Cells of the cardiac conduction system are automatic. Myocardial cells in the atria and ventricles do not spontaneously depolarize under physiologic conditions.[3,9]

When Purkinje cells are not depolarized to threshold by an electrical impulse from a neighboring cell, the Purkinje membrane potential has been shown to become less negative

over time during phase 4 (Fig. 3-8). A time-dependent decrease in the outward movement of potassium coupled with a slow inward movement of sodium appears to be the major mechanism responsible for this spontaneous depolarization to threshold (Fig. 3-9).[2,14,27,28]

Thus, in spontaneously depolarizing cells, the membrane potential does not remain stable or "resting" during phase 4. The membrane potential during phase 4 is frequently termed the "diastolic" potential, because it coincides with the diastolic phase of the cardiac cycle. The voltage level of maximum negative repolarization is termed maximum diastolic repolarization.

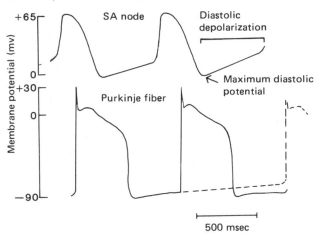

Fig. 3-8. Action potentials of sinus node cells and Purkinje cells. Purkinje-cell action potentials are usually elicited by propagated impulses. If Purkinje cells are not discharged by impulses from the sinus node or elsewhere, the Purkinje diastolic depolarization progresses enough to attain threshold. (After Vassale M: Cardiac Physiology for the Clinician, p 35. New York, Academic Press, 1976)

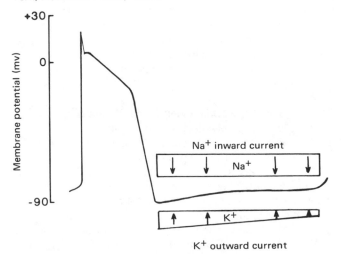

Fig. 3-9. Schematic representation of the ionic movements during diastolic depolarization in Purkinje fibers. Outward movement of potassium decreases as a function of time. Inward sodium movement makes the cell become more positive. (Vassale M: Cardiac Physiology for the Clinician, p 44. New York, Academic Press, 1976)

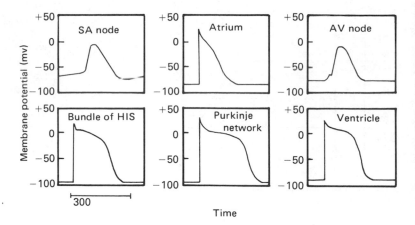

Fig. 3-10. Characteristic action potentials in different regions of the heart. See text for description. (Katz A: Physiology of the Heart, p 251. New York, Raven Press, 1977)

Electrical Characteristics of Other Cardiac Cells

Sinus Node Cells. The rate of spontaneous depolarization during phase 4 and maximum negative repolarization voltage levels are different in sinus node cells compared to Purkinje cells (Fig. 3-10). Cells in the sinus node spontaneously depolarize to threshold more rapidly than do other cardiac cells under normal conditions. Inward movement of calcium appears to be an important mechanism for sinus node diastolic depolarization as well as for a decrease in the outward movement of potassium.[2,3,14,27,28]

Maximum sinus node repolarization voltage levels are approximately −60 mV.[14] There is a less abrupt transition from the rate of depolarization before and after reaching threshold in sinus node cells than in Purkinje cells.

During the rapid depolarization phase (phase 0), the maximum rate of sinus node depolarization and the magnitude of depolarization (approximately to 0 mV) are less than that of Purkinje cells. Sinus node cells do not seem to have rapid sodium channels, but slow channel calcium and sodium influx have been shown to be responsible for sinus node depolarization.[10,16]

There is no definite sinus node plateau phase (phases 1 and 2). The total sinus node action potential duration is slightly less than that of Purkinje cells.

Atrial Myocardial Cells. Atrial myocardial cells undergo rapid depolarization. These cells have essentially no plateau period, but repolarization is slower than in Purkinje cells. The total action potential duration of atrial cells is shorter than that of Purkinje cells. Atrial cells do not spontaneously depolarize.[10]

Cells in the Atrioventricular Node. In general, spontaneously depolarizing cells of the atrioventricular node show similarities to sinus node cells in terms of rate of depolarization and of maximum repolarization voltage (Fig. 3-10). These characteristics indicate that atrioventricular conducting cells probably do not have fast sodium channels but depolarize because of the movement of calcium and sodium through slow channels.[3] Figure 3-11 illustrates the different electrophysiologic characteristics of cells termed atrionodal (A-N), nodal (N) and nodal-His (N-H); these action poten-

tials were recorded from the upper, middle, and lower junctional areas.[15]

Other investigators have contended that the electrophysiologic properties of A-N, N, and N-H cells are not correlated with definite anatomic areas.[8] It has also been claimed that only cells in the upper and lower atrioventricular junctional regions spontaneously depolarize and that cells within the atrioventricular node itself do not spontaneously depolarize.[3,9]

Cells in the Bundle of His and Purkinje System. The electrophysiologic characteristics of His bundle cells closely resemble those of Purkinje cells in the distal conducting system. However, the duration of the His bundle action potential is slightly less than that of cells in the Purkinje network. The most rapid period of depolarization and the longest period of repolarization occur in Purkinje cells at the distal end of the conducting system (Fig. 3-10).

Ventricular Myocardial Cells. Ventricular myocardial cells are similar to Purkinje cells except that the total action potential duration is slightly shorter. These cells do not spontaneously depolarize under normal conditions.[9]

SPREAD OF THE CARDIAC IMPULSE

The spread of the electric impulse through the heart reflects the electrical characteristics of the different myocardial cells described previously and the anatomic characteristics of the conducting system that were described in Chapter 1. When one segment of the membrane of a cardiac cell is depolarized,

Fig. 3-11. Schematic action potentials from atrial (**A**), atrionodal (**A–N**), nodal (**N**), nodal–HIS (**N–H**), and His bundle (**H**) cells. See text for discussion. (Myerburg R, Lazzara R: Cardiovasc Clin 5:2–19, 1973)

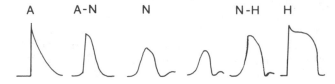

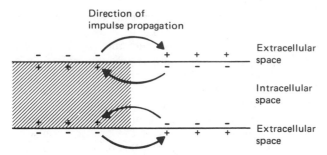

Fig. 3-12. Cable properties of a strand of cardiac muscle transmitting a propagated impulses from left to right. Current flow between the depolarized tissue (*shaded, left*) and resting tissue (*unshaded, right*) is indicated by arrows. Current flows away from the depolarized tissue along the outside of the cell, and the circuit is completed when current flows toward the depolarized region inside the cell. (Katz A: Physiology of the Heart, p 298 New York, Raven Press, 1977)

the entire cell is rapidly depolarized.[14] An electrical circuit is established along the cell (fiber), then current flows from depolarized cells to adjacent resting cells that are capable of excitation. (Fig. 3-12; see Chap. 26).[14,27] A wave of depolarization is propagated that spreads longitudinally from cell to cell across intercalated discs.[5,26] Because the cells have a branching arrangement, the impulse may pass in a zigzag fashion from one cell to another across the intercalated discs.[26] Resistance to current flow is less across the gap junctions at the ends of the cells than along the sides of the cell membranes, so the impulse does not readily spread laterally across adjacent cell membranes.[5,22]

The direction of the impulse spread is also determined by the refractory period of cardiac tissue adjacent to a depolarized fiber. As the impulse spreads through the heart it normally depolarizes tissue in front of it that has recovered and is excitable but cannot depolarize tissue behind it because that tissue is still refractory. Because the cardiac impulse spreads rapidly through the atria, slowly through the atrioventricular junction, and then rapidly through the ventricles, both atria contract almost synchronously, there is time for the ventricles to receive blood from the contracting atria, and then both ventricles contract almost synchronously (see Chap. 4).

Atrial Conduction

Because sinus nodal cells normally depolarize more rapidly than other cardiac automatic cells during phase 4, the sinus node normally initiates the electrical impulse that is conducted to other areas of the myocardium (see Fig. 3-8).[3,6,18] This impulse depolarizes all other cells of the conducting system before those cells have time to depolarize to threshold.

The electrical impulse seems to spread outward in relatively concentric circles from the sinus node through the atria, moving from the upper right atrium to the lower left atrium.[18,20] Conduction velocity (speed with which the impulse spreads) through the atria is approximately 1 meter/ second (m/sec) (Table 3-2).[18] Conduction velocities are not equal through the atria; for example, conduction velocity is more rapid by way of Bachman's tissue bundle into the left atrium than in other areas of the interatrial septum. There do not seem to be specialized pathways from the sinus node

to the atrioventricular node in which conduction is more rapid than in surrounding atrial tissue (Chap. 1).[3,18,20,26,27] Atrial repolarization seems to spread in the same direction as depolarization.[18,20]

Junctional Conduction

The cardiac impulse is not conducted through the connective tissue of the cardiac skeleton, so the atrioventricular junction cardiac muscle tissue provides the only pathway for electrical conduction from the atria to the ventricles (see Chap. 1). Conduction velocity through the atrioventricular node is approximately 50 mm/sec (0.05 m/sec), although in some areas it has been found to be as slow as 0.02 m/sec.[18,20] Not only does this slowing of the cardiac impulse at the atrioventricular junction prevent the atria and ventricles from contracting at the same time; it also protects the ventricles from abnormally fast heart rates that can be generated in the atria under abnormal situations (see Chap. 26).

The initial normal slowing of conduction through the atrioventricular junction and later increase in the strength and speed of conduction have been correlated by some but not all investigators with electrophysiologic differences in A-N, N, and N-H cells.[11,12,20] Other mechanisms that have been postulated to be responsible for the slowing of conduction through the junction are the small size of the junctional conducting cells and the amounts of connective tissue interspersed among conducting cells.[20] The property of a propagating impulse becoming successively weaker is termed *decremental conduction*. Extreme decremental conduction leads to atrioventricular blocks (see Chap. 26).

Although anatomic evidence in adults for accessory connections between the atria and ventricles by way of specific Kent fiber bundles outside the main bundle of His has been questioned, there is electrophysiologic support for such accessory pathways.[17,20] Preexcitation syndromes, such as the Wolff-Parkinson-White syndrome, have been explained on the basis of these pathways (see Chaps. 17 and 26).[20]

Ventricular Conduction

Cells in the His–Purkinje system have the most rapid conduction velocities in the heart, approximately 2 to 4 m/ sec.[18,23] The large size of the Purkinje fibers provides less

TABLE 3-2 NORMAL CARDIAC ACTIVATION SEQUENCE

Normal Sequence of Activation	Conduction Velocity (M/sec)	Time for Impulse to Traverse Structure (sec)	Rate of automatic discharge (per minute)
SA node		~0.15	60–100
Atrial Myocardium	1.0–1.2		None
AV node	0.02–0.05		See text
AV bundle	1.2–2.0	~0.08	40–55
Bundle branches	2.0–4.0		25–40
Purkinje network			
Ventricular myocardium	0.3–1.0	~0.08	None

(Adapted from Katz AM: *Physiology of the Heart*, pp 229–264; pp 355–370. New York, Raven Press, 1977)
~ = approximately.

resistance to current flow than that of smaller fibers. Cells with rapid sodium channels have more rapid rates (steeper slopes of phase 0) and greater ampltitudes of depolarization than cells that have only slow calcium channels.[14,25,27] These two factors help to explain Purkinje cells' rapid conduction velocities.

Although the cardiac impulse spreads from the common His bundle through the bundle branches and Purkinje fiber system in a sequential manner, three general phases of ventricular activation may be described for discussion purposes: septal depolarization, apex depolarization, and basal depolarization (Fig. 3-13) (see Chap. 17).

The middle to the basal ventricular septum has been found to be the first part of the ventricles to be activated (Fig. 3-13A).[20] The major wave of septal depolarization is from left to right, although the septum is activated from both the right and the left bundle branches.[18]

The extensive ventricular ramifications of the conduction system facilitate the rapid spread of the impulse over the ventricular walls toward the ventricular apices (Fig. 3-13B). Activation spreads from the endocardium toward the epicardium.[18,20]

Purkinje fibers are sparsely distributed in the basal (upper) sections of the ventricles, particularly in the right ventricle.[12,20] The basal and posterior portions of both ventricles are the last to be activated (Fig. 3-13C).

Although Purkinje fibers conduct the cardiac impulse more rapidly than any other cardiac cells, Purkinje cells in the distal terminations of the conducting system have longer action potential durations and refractory periods than do ventricular muscle fibers. Because conduction is slower in cells with longer action potential durations and refractory periods, the conduction velocity of the cardiac impulse is slowed at the point where Purkinje fibers connect with myocardial fibers (Fig. 3-14).[13] Theoretically, the distal Purkinje fibers then function like a "gate," the length of the refractory period in distal Purkinje fibers normally controlling the rate at which ventricular muscle fibers depolarize, and excitation–contraction coupling and the rate of cardiac contraction therefore may be controlled by this gating mechanism. The clinical importance of this gating mechanism has been questioned.[20]

Ventricular repolarization proceeds from the epicardium to the endocardium and seems to spread from the ventricular bases to the apices.[1,20] Thus, ventricular repolarization generally proceeds in a direction that is opposite to the direction of depolarization, and all portions of the ventricle recover at approximately the same time. Chapter 17 discusses the

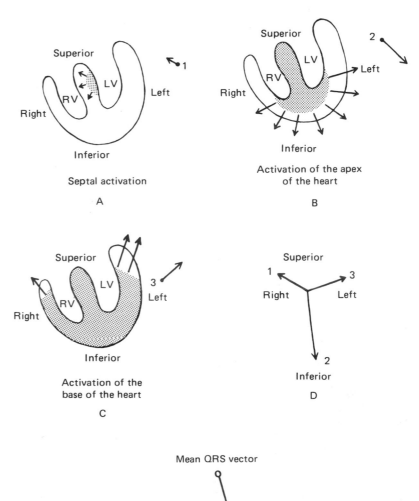

Fig. 3-13. Schematic representation of normal sequence of ventricular depolarization. **(A)** Septal depolarization is directed to the right, anteriorly, and superiorly (beginning of the QRS complex). **(B)** Depolarization of the apex of the heart involves both ventricles and is directed to the left, posteriorly, and inferiorly (midportion of the QRS complex). **(C)** Depolarization of the base of the heart involves both ventricles and is directed to the left, posteriorly and superiorly (terminal portion of the QRS complex). The impulse terminates in the left ventricle and septum. **(D)** The sequence of ventricular activation. **(E)** The sum of these three vectors—the mean QRS complex vector. See text and Chapter 17. *RV* = right ventricle, *LV* = left ventricle. (Adapted from Katz A: Physiology of the Heart, p 275–277. New York, Raven Press, 1977)

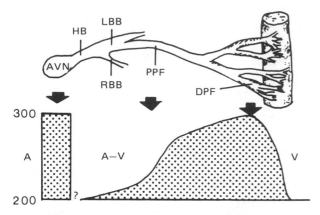

Fig. 3-14. Schematic representation of refractory periods in the atrioventricular conducting system. The shaded areas represent refractory periods. The diagram at the top represents the A-V node (*AVN*), bundle of His (*HB*), bundle branches (*RBB, LBB*), and a tract of conducting tissue from the bundle branch to ventricular muscle, subdivided into proximal (*PPF*) and distal (*DPF*) Purkinje fibers. The *shaded areas* at the bottom represent refractory periods along the length of the conducting system. Maximum local refractory periods occur at the AVN (*first arrow*) and a few millimeters proximal to the junctions of Purkinje fibers with ventricular muscle cells. The '?' symbol at the level of the His bundle and the most proximal bundle branches indicates the current limitation of knowledge of local functional properties in this region. (Myerburg RJ, Gelband H, Castellanos A et al: In Wellens HJJ, Lie KJ, Janse MJ (eds): The Conduction System of the Heart, p 353. Philadelphia, Lea & Febiger, 1976)

relationship of the electrocardiogram to the spread of the cardiac impulse (see Fig. 3-13D, E).

FACTORS MODIFYING ELECTROPHYSIOLOGIC FUNCTION

General Effects of Alterations

Factors that alter cardiac cell depolarization and repolarization do so by affecting the rates of change (slopes), the magnitudes of voltage changes or the time intervals of the phases of the cardiac action potential. Such changes affect cardiac impulse generation, impulse conduction, or both of these; normally occurring examples of the following summarized factors have been previously mentioned.

Impulse generation, or automaticity, is influenced by a cardiac cell's level of maximum diastolic repolarization, threshold level, and rate of spontaneous depolarization to threshold (slope of phase 4) (see Fig. 34-1). If maximum diastolic repolarization becomes more negative, if threshold becomes less negative, or if the slope of phase 4 becomes less steep, the rate at which the entire cell is depolarized can become slower (see Chaps. 26, 34).

Cardiac impulse conduction velocity is influenced by the slope of phase 0, the amplitude of phase 0, the distance from resting potential to threshold level, action potential and refractory period durations, and resistance to current flow. If the rate or amplitude of phase 0 is decreased, the distance from resting potential to threshold level is increased, action potential or refractory periods are lengthened, or resistance

to current flow is increased, the rate of conduction can become slower. For example, cells with rapid sodium channels have greater amplitudes and more rapid rates of depolarization than cells that have only slow calcium channels, so Purkinje cells have faster conduction velocities than do junctional cells.[14,25]

Cardiac impulse generation or conduction or both can be altered by the effects on cardiac cells of changes in the ratio of extra to intracellular ionic concentrations, acid–base changes, sympathetic and parasympathetic stimulation, myocardial stretch, cooling, ischemia and heart rate changes (Chaps. 26, 34, and 35). These factors often affect different cardiac cells in different ways; the following section discusses selected examples of these alterations.

Alterations in Extracellular Ionic Concentrations

In clinical situations, alterations in the ratio of extracellular to intracellular concentrations of one ion can directly or indirectly affect the concentrations of other ions, often influencing several ionic channels simultaneously and affecting the behavior of active membrane exchange mechanisms. Conversely, the sodium–potassium–ATPase pump and other active mechanisms can help to correct imbalances, for example by exchanging three instead of two potassium ions for three sodium ions.[21]

Increased Extracellular Potassium. When the concentration of extracellular potassium increases, the chemical gradient for potassium efflux decreases. In general, less potassium then moves out of the cell, the resting membrane potential becomes less negative, and as a result, the membrane potential moves closer to threshold potential.[2]

Increases in extracellular potassium increase the refractory period of the fast sodium channel.[2] Because this inactivates the rapid sodium channels, the velocity and amplitude of depolarization and conduction velocity are decreased in cells such as Purkinje fibers that have rapid sodium channels.[29] The cell becomes less and less capable of being depolarized. The plateau duration is increased but the rate of repolarization also is increased in Purkinje fibers with increases in extracellular potassium; thus the action potential duration is decreased. The slope of phase 4 is decreased in Purkinje fibers, so automaticity is decreased.[2] Eventually intraventricular conduction is depressed.[4] Sinus node cells are less responsive to extracellular potassium increases than are most other myocardial cells (Fig. 3-15A) (see Chaps. 17 and 26).[2,9]

Decreased Extracellular Potassium. When the concentration of extracellular potassium decreases, the membrane potential becomes more negative, thus moving the membrane potential further from threshold.[4] This makes it more difficult for the cell to be excited. However, this effect may be counteracted by the increases in the slope of phase 4 in both Purkinje and sinus node cells that can occur with decreases in extracellular potassium.[4,9,28] This increase in automaticity may be strong enough to cause the cell to reach threshold.[2] The action potential duration is lengthened and

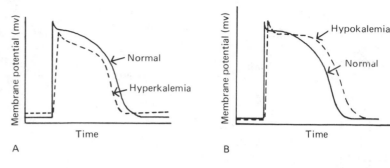

Fig. 3-15. Electrophysiologic effects of increased (**A**) or decreased (**B**) levels of extracellular potassium. See text for discussion. (Katz A: Physiology of the Heart, pp 356, 358. New York, Raven Press, 1977)

normal repolarization is lengthened (Fig. 3-15B).[2] Decremental conduction through the atrioventricular junction may lead to atrioventricular block (see Chaps. 17 and 26).[4,10]

Increased and Decreased Extracellular Sodium. Increases and decreases in extracellular sodium usually have little clinical significance because the cell membrane is not particularly permeable to sodium and because the changes in serum sodium levels necessary to alter the action potential are usually not seen clinically. Alterations in extracellular sodium primarily affect the amplitude and rate of rise of the phase 0, particularly in cells with rapid sodium channels.[3,4] The observation that alterations in extracellular sodium had few effects on sinus node cells led to the discovery that these cells apparently have no fast sodium channels; however, depolarization of sinus node cells is inhibited by the complete absence of sodium.[2,3] Theoretically, changes in extracellular sodium should affect the sodium influx during phase 4 that contributes to automaticity. However, sinus node diastolic depolarization (phase 4) is relatively insensitive to changes in extracellular sodium.[2]

Increased and Decreased Extracellular Calcium. Alterations in extracellular calcium have the greatest effects on the slow inward calcium channel, although sodium and potassium movements are affected also.[5,9] Alterations in extracellular calcium affect cardiac contraction as well as the cardiac action potential (see Chap. 2).[2]

In sinus node cells, increases in extracellular calcium levels (up to 4–7 mM/liter) increase the rate of rise and amplitude of phase 0 and also increase the rate of diastolic depolarization.[3,9] A more positive plateau is maintained with increased extracellular calcium, and the action potential duration usually is shortened (Fig. 3-16A).[3,10]

Decreases in extracellular calcium decrease the slow inward current; however, because sodium can also move through this (these) channel(s), the effect of decreased calcium is not as much as would otherwise be predicted.[16]

The plateau level is more negative, and the action potential duration usually is lengthened.[2] There can be a decrease in the rate of rise and amplitude of phase 0 (Fig. 3-16B).[10] Decremental conduction may occur with clinical levels of hypocalcemia (see Chap. 26).[4,10]

Adrenergic and Cholinergic Effects

Catecholamines. Catecholamines generally have similar effects whether they are secreted by sympathetic nerve endings, are endogenous hormones, or are adrenergic drugs; however, there are specific differences in the effects of different adrenergic substances (Chap. 35). The catecholamines have multiple effects and probably work through affecting cyclic adenosine monophosphate (C-AMP).[2] Catecholamines increase the rate of diastolic depolarization (slope of phase 4) in both Purkinje cells and the sinus node. The increased rate of firing of the sinus node appears to be the most important mechanism by which adrenergic effects increase heart rate (Fig. 3-17). Repolarization becomes faster and the action potential duration is shortened.[14] The amplitude and rate of rise of phase 0 is increased in junctional cells, which increases conduction velocity through the atrioventricular node.[2]

Acetylcholine. Cholinergic effects are stronger on sinus node cells, atrial muscle, and atrioventricular junctional cells than on His–Purkinje tissue or ventricular muscle. The rate of diastolic depolarization (slope of phase 4) is decreased in sinus node cells as a result of vagal (cholinergic) activity (Fig. 3-18).[2,10] The maximum diastolic potential usually becomes more negative. These effects slow heart rate. There is a decreased rate of rise and amplitude of phase 0 and a decreased action potential duration in cells of the atrioventricular node; this has a powerful effect on slowing conduction through the atrioventricular node.[2,14]

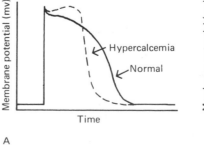
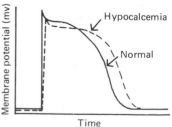

Fig. 3-16. Electrophysiologic effects of increased (**A**) or decreased (**B**) levels of extracellular calcium. (Katz A: Physiology of the Heart, pp 360, 361. New York, Raven Press, 1977)

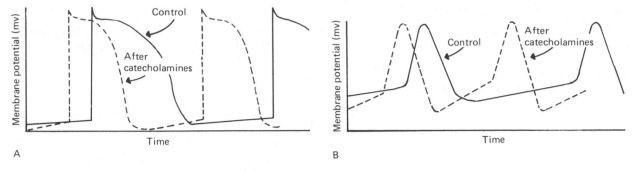

Fig. 3-17. Electrophysiologic effects of catecholamines on Purkinje cells (**A**) and sinus node cells (**B**). See text for discussion. (Katz A: Physiology of the Heart, pp 366, 367. New York, Raven Press, 1977)

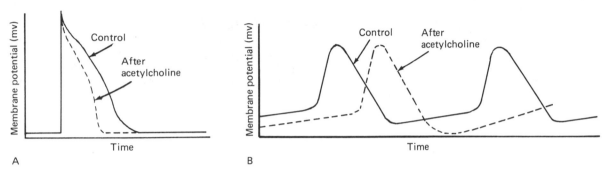

Fig. 3-18. Electrophysiologic effects of acetylcholine (vagal stimulation) on atrial muscle (**A**) and sinus node cell (**B**). (Katz A: Physiology of the Heart, pp 362, 363. New York, Raven Press, 1977)

Interval Duration

The action potential duration is related to the length of the preceding diastolic interval. When heart rate increases and the interval between successive cardiac impulses decreases, repolarization is faster in most cardiac cells and there is a shorter action potential duration. At slower heart rates, the action potential duration lengthens.[2,14]

Other Effects

In experimental situations, the effects of *warming the heart* are somewhat similar to adrenergic effects; for example, diastolic depolarization is increased in automatic fibers. *Cooling* the heart depresses spontaneous depolarization in automatic cells. Repolarization is delayed and conduction is decreased.[9] Arrhythmias may occur during cooling; this is clinically relevant for the cardiac surgical patient who has been subjected to hypothermia (see Chap. 24).

Stretching cardiac fibers increases the rate of diastolic depolarization and makes the maximum diastolic potential less negative in automatic fibers. Myocardial fiber stretch may cause arrhythmias during heart failure (Chap. 27).

Acidosis slows repolarization and prolongs the action potential duration in Purkinje fibers.[2] The sodium–potassium–ATPase pump is inhibited with acidosis.[21] *Alkalosis* shortens the action potential duration and increases diastolic depolarization.[2] The effects of *ischemia* on the action potential are discussed in Chapter 11.

REFERENCES

The selections marked with an asterisk (*) are helpful for further reading.

1. Burgess MJ: The sequence of normal ventricular recovery. Am Heart J 84(5):660–669, 1972
2. Carmeliet E, Vereecke J: Electrogenesis of the action potential and automaticity. In Berne RM (ed): Handbook of Physiology, Sec 2, The Cardiovascular System, Vol I, The Heart, pp 269–334. Bethesda, Md, American Physiological Society, 1979
3. Cranefield PF: The Conduction of the Cardiac Impulse, pp 1–153. Mt Kisco, NY, Futura, 1975
4. Fisch C: Relation of electrolyte disturbances to cardiac arrhythmias. Circulation 47(2):408–419, 1973
5. Fozzard HA: Conduction of the action potential. In Berne RM (ed): Handbook of Physiology, Sec 2: The Cardiovascular System, Vol I, The Heart, pp 335–356. Bethesda, Md, American Physiological Society, 1979
6. Fozzard HA, Das Gupta DS: Electrophysiology and the electrocardiogram. Mod Concepts Cardiovasc Dis 44(6):29–34, 1975*
7. Fozzard HA, Gibbons WR: Action potential and contraction of heart muscle. Am J Cardiol 31(2):182–192, 1973*
8. Hecht HH, Kossmann CE: Atrioventricular and interventricular conduction. Am J Cardiol 31(2):232–244, 1973
9. Hoffman BF, Cranefield PF: The physiological basis of cardiac arrhythmias. Am J Med 37(5):670–684, 1964
10. Katz AM: Physiology of the Heart, pp 229–264; pp 355–370. New York, Raven Press, 1977*
11. Mendez C, Moe GH: Atrioventricular transmission. In Mello WC (ed): Electrical Phenomena in the Heart, pp 263–291. New York, Academic Press, 1972*
12. Myerburg RJ, Gelband H, Castellanos A et al: Electrophysiology of endocardial intraventricular conduction. In Wellens HJJ, Lie

KJ, Janse MJ (eds): The Conduction System of the Heart, pp 336–359. Philadelphia, Lea & Febiger, 1976

13. Myerburg RJ, Lazzara R: Electrophysiologic basis of cardiac arrhythmias and conduction disturbances. Cardiovasc Clin 5:2–19, 1973
14. Noble D: The Initiation of the Heartbeat, 2nd ed. Oxford, Clarendon Press, 1979*
15. Paes de Carvalho A, de Almelda DF: Spread of activity through the atrioventricular node. Circ Res 8:801, 1960
16. Reuter H: Properties of two inward membrane currents in the heart. Annu Rev Physiol 41(1128):413–424, 1979
17. Roberts NK: The Cardiac Conducting System and the His Bundle Electrogram, pp 1–28. New York, Appleton-Century-Crofts, 1975
18. Scher AM: Electrocardiogram. In Ruch TC, Patton HD (eds): Physiology and Biophysics II, pp 65–101. Philadelphia, WB Saunders, 1974
19. Scher AM, Kerrick WG: Electrical characteristics of the cardiac cell. In Ruch TC, Patton HD (eds): Physiology and Biophysics II, pp 49–64. Philadelphia, WB Saunders, 1974*
20. Scher AM, Spach MS: Cardiac depolarization and repolarization and the electrocardiogram. In Berne RM (ed): Handbook of Physiology, Sec 2, The Cardiovascular System, Vol 1, The Heart, pp 357–392. Bethesda, Md, American Physiological Society, 1979
21. Sperelakis N: Origin of the cardiac resting potential. In Berne RM (ed): Handbook of Physiology, Sec 2 The Cardiovascular System, Vol I, The Heart, pp 187–236. Bethesda, Md, American Physiological Society, 1979
22. Sperelakis N: Propagation mechanisms in the heart. Annu Rev Physiol 41(1230):441–457, 1979
23. Surawicz B: The input of cellular electrophysiology into the practice of clinical electrocardiology. Mod Concepts Cardiovasc Dis 44(8):41–46, 1975
24. Sweadner KJ, Goldin SM: Active transport of sodium and potassium ions. N Engl J Med 302(14):777–783, 1980
25. Trautwein W: Membrane currents in cardiac muscle fibers. Physiol Rev 54(4):793–835, 1973
26. Truex RC: Structural basis of atrial and ventricular conduction. Cardiovasc Clin 6(1):1–24, 1974*
27. Vassale M: Cardiac Physiology for the Clinician, pp 1–59. New York, Academic Press, 1976*
28. Vassale M: Electrogenesis of the plateau and pacemaker potential. Annu Rev Physiol 41(1229):425–440, 1979
29. Weidmann S: Heart: Electrophysiology. Annu Rev Physiol 36(1108):155–169, 1974

ADDITIONAL READING

Marriott HJL, Myerburg RJ: Recognition and treatment of cardiac arrhythmias and conduction disturbances. In Hurst JW (ed): The Heart, 4th ed, pp 637–641. New York, McGraw-Hill, 1978

Smith J, Kampine JP: Circulatory Physiology: The Essentials, pp 76–84. Baltimore, Williams & Wilkins, 1980

4

The Cardiac Cycle
CAROL JEAN HALPENNY, R.N., M.A.

Every ventricular contraction that propels blood to the body or lungs is the result of the sequential activation of cardiac chambers through the coordinated functioning of the electrical and mechanical factors that were discussed separately in Chapters 2 and 3. Figure 4-1, the cardiac cycle, illustrates the coordinated sequence of cardiac events that must be understood in order to understand and assess normal or abnormal cardiac functioning.

For the sake of simplicity, the description of events occurring during the cardiac cycle will begin with events in the left heart. Figure 4-1 should be referred to frequently in order to obtain an understanding of what is occurring concurrently with respect to atrial, ventricular, and aortic pressures, ventricular volumes, valvular activity, heart sounds, and electrical activity.

There are some general points about pressures and timing to remember during the following discussion. Blood flows from a chamber with a greater pressure to one with a lesser pressure (Chap. 5). When valves are open between two chambers, pressures in both chambers change until eventually they are approximately equal. When valves between two chambers are closed, the pressures in the chambers change relatively independently of each other. Table 19-3 indicates pressures in the cardiac chambers.

Ventricular systole and diastole divide the cardiac cycle into two major phases. The cardiac cycle can be further subdivided into several different mechanical periods occurring during systole and diastole.[17] Because the cardiac cycle is continuous, the description of these periods can begin at any point.

SEQUENCE OF LEFT VENTRICULAR CARDIAC EVENTS

Ventricular Systole

Isovolumic Ventricular Contraction. (Period a, Fig. 4-1.) Ventricular contraction follows the ventricular depolarization that is reflected by the electrocardiographic R wave (Chap. 17). Ventricular pressure increases rapidly.

At the onset of this period, pressures in the atrium and ventricle are approximately equal, but atrial pressure decreases with atrial muscle relaxation and repolarization. The mitral valve closes when pressure in the ventricle is higher than in the atrium (Chap. 1).[13] The aortic valve remains closed until left ventricular pressure becomes greater than aortic pressure. Bulging of the cardiac valves due to abrupt ventricular pressure increases may cause slight increases in atrial and aortic pressure during this period.[7]

During this brief time when both mitral and aortic valves are closed, there are no actual changes in ventricular volume because no blood is flowing into or out of the ventricle. The ventricle changes its shape during this period. The apparent increase in ventricular volume recorded on the ventricular volume curve in Figure 4-1 occurs because ventricular volumes are calculated from ventricular circumference.[13]

This period has been termed the isometric phase of ventricular contraction because tension is increasing rapidly while the muscle fibers are not shortening very much until they have overcome the afterload of aortic pressure (see

Chap. 2).[16] However, muscle contraction is not completely isometric because the ventricles do change dimensions.[13,16]

Rapid Ventricular Ejection. (Period b, Fig. 4-1.) Ventricular muscle contraction continues and the aortic valve opens when left ventricular pressure exceeds aortic pressure, at

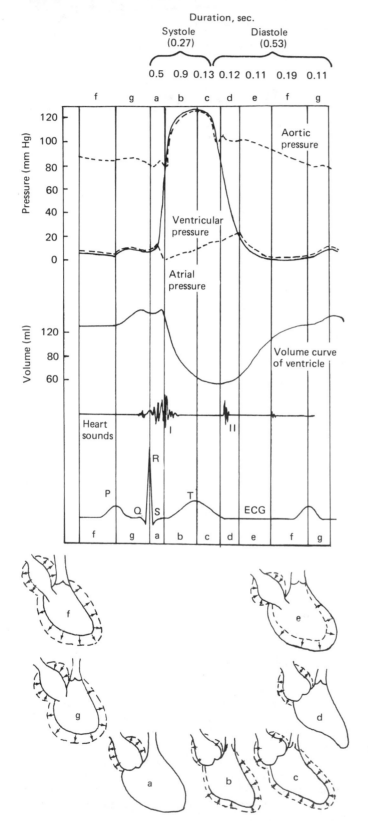

TABLE 4-1   DURATION OF CARDIAC CYCLE PERIODS

	Seconds
Isometric contraction	.05
Maximum ejection	.09
Reduced ejection	.13
TOTAL SYSTOLE	.27
Protodiastole	.04
Isometric relaxation	.08
Rapid inflow	.11
Diastasis	.19
Atrial systole	.11
TOTAL DIASTOLE	.53

(Heart rate approximately 75 beats per minute)
(Scher AM: Mechanical events of the cardiac cycle. In Ruch TC, Patton, HD (eds): Physiology and Biophysics II, pp 102–116. Philadelphia, WB Saunders, 1974)

approximately 80 mm Hg. The aorta and left ventricle are essentially a common cavity at this time. Ventricular pressure continues to rise rapidly during the initial part of this period, then rises less rapidly during the latter part of the period to an approximate maximum of 120 mm Hg.

Ventricular volume decreases rapidly; two-thirds of the stroke volume is ejected during this rapid ejection period of 0.09 sec (Table 4-1). Aortic flow reaches its peak velocity during the period of rapidly increasing ventricular pressure and before the point of maximum ventricular pressure. Aortic pressure may actually slightly exceed ventricular pressure during the latter part of rapid ventricular ejection, but blood continues to flow into the aorta because of the forward momentum of the blood (see Chap. 5).[13]

The left atrium is relaxed at this time. Atrial pressure slowly begins to rise as blood from the lungs accumulates in the atrium. Ventricular repolarization begins.

Reduced Ventricular Ejection. (Period c, Fig. 4-1.) Pressure in the ventricles begins to decrease about 0.13 sec before the end of ventricular contraction. During this time, ventricular muscle fibers are no longer contracting as forcefully as during the previous period, because the fibers have reached a shorter length and are contracting isotonically.[13] This period of reduced ventricular ejection comprises approximately the latter two-thirds of the total ejection period (Table 4-1).[12] Ventricular and aortic pressures begin decreasing. Blood continues to flow from the left ventricle into the aorta because of the momentum of forward blood flow.[2,14] Ventricular volume continues to fall, although at a slower rate than during rapid ejection.

Fig. 4-1. The cardiac cycle, illustrating the changes in aortic, ventricular, and left atrial pressures, and in left ventricular volume, in relation to the phonocardiogram and the electrocardiogram during the cardiac cycle. The duration of each phase at a heart rate of approximately 75 beats per minute is indicated at the top of the figure. a = isovolumetric ventricular contraction, b = rapid ventricular ejection, c = slow ventricular ejection, d = isovolumetric relaxation, e = rapid ventricular filling, f = diastasis, g = atrial contraction. I = first heart sound, II = second heart sound. Insets: Changes in the configuration of the left atrium, mitral valve, left ventricle, and aortic valve during various phases of the cycle. (Adapted from Shepherd JT, Vanhoutte PM: The Human Cardiovascular System, p 68. Raven Press, 1979)

Atrial pressure and volume continue to increase. Ventricular repolarization is usually complete by this time, as indicated by the end of the T wave.

Ventricular Diastole

Protodiastole. (Initial part of period d, Fig. 4-1.) As ventricular muscle relaxation begins, there is a brief period termed the protodiastolic period before ventricular pressure becomes lower than aortic pressure. During this time a slight transient decrease in atrial pressure may occur, reflecting the effect of ventricular relaxation. The aortic valve closes when the ventricular pressure has decreased below aortic pressure. The second heart sound occurs.

Isovolumic Ventricular Relaxation. (Latter part of period d, Fig. 4-1.) Ventricular pressure decreases rapidly as the ventricle relaxes. During this period when all the cardiac valves are closed there is no change in ventricular volume. Atrial pressure continues to increase as the atrium continues to receive pulmonary venous blood.

Rapid Ventricular Filling. (Period e, Fig. 4-1.) The atrioventricular (mitral) valve opens when ventricular pressure becomes lower than atrial pressure. The ventricle fills rapidly with blood that has been accumulating in the atrium, but ventricular pressure continues to decrease during this period because ventricular relaxation continues. Most of the blood that had been sequestered in the atrium during systole has been emptied into the ventricle by the time the ventricle has reached maximum diastolic size. Atrial pressure decreases as the atria empty, but remains very slightly greater than ventricular pressure throughout this period.

Late Diastole (Diastasis). (Period f, Fig. 4-1.) The mitral valve remains open and pressures in the atrium and ventricle have equilibrated between the time following rapid ventricular filling and the beginning of atrial contraction. Blood from the lungs continues to enter the left ventricle passively, so ventricular volume and pressure slowly increase. Coronary artery blood flow usually is maximal during this time (Chap. 2). The beginning of atrial depolarization is illustrated by the upstroke of the electrocardiographic P wave (Fig. 4-1; see Chap. 17).

Atrial Contraction. (Period g, Fig. 4-1.) Atrial contraction follows atrial depolarization. Contraction results in a slight increase in left atrial pressure. Ventricular volume is increased as the atrium forces most of its remaining blood into the ventricles. Approximately 20% of the total end-diastolic ventricular volume is comprised of blood that has been ejected from the atrium during atrial contraction. The contribution of atrial contraction to total ventricular volume normally varies between 15% and 25%, depending upon venous return and heart rate; it is less at faster heart rates.[5,13] This atrial contribution to ventricular volume may be lost when the atria and ventricles are electrically and mechanically dissociated, such as during atrial fibrillation or complete heart block (Chap. 26).

Toward the end of this period, the ventricles begin to depolarize. Diastole ends with the onset of ventricular contraction, and the cardiac cycle is repeated.

RIGHT VENTRICULAR CARDIAC CYCLE

The sequence of events in the right ventricle during the cardiac cycle is exactly the same as in the left ventricle. The timing of the events in the two ventricles is slightly different. Right ventricular and pulmonary artery pressures are much lower than left ventricular and aortic pressures (see Table 19-3). Right atrial pressures are usually slightly less than left atrial pressures.[3]

Several factors lead to differences in the timing of events between the right and left heart. Contraction of the left ventricle begins before contraction of the right ventricle.[3,14] Left ventricular isovolumetric contraction and relaxation last longer than right ventricular isovolumetric contraction and relaxation because the left ventricle must develop more contractile force to overcome higher systemic pressures.[14] Right ventricular ejection begins before and lasts longer than left ventricular ejection, because pressures in the pulmonary artery are less than in the aorta.[3,14] Thus, right ventricular filling and ejection periods are longer than left ventricular periods.

CARDIAC VALVULAR EVENTS AND NORMAL HEART SOUNDS

Valvular Events

The differences in timing of right and left ventricular events lead to differences in timing of right and left valvular events. The atrioventricular valves close at the onset of ventricular systole. The mitral valve normally closes before the tricuspid valve because left ventricular contraction begins before right ventricular contraction.

The aortic and pulmonic valves open when ventricular pressures exceed arterial pressures. The pulmonic valve opens before the aortic valve because right ventricular isovolumetric contraction is shorter than left ventricular isovolumetric contraction.

The aortic and pulmonic valves close when ventricular pressures become less than arterial pressures. The aortic valve closes before the pulmonic valve because the right ventricular ejection period is longer than the left.[13,14] During inspiration, the time between closure of the aortic and pulmonic valve is increased because the increased right ventricular stroke volume leads to a longer right ventricular ejection time (see Chaps. 5, 14).

The atrioventricular valves open during diastole when ventricular pressures are less than atrial pressures. The tricuspid valve opens before the mitral valve because of the more rapid isovolumetric right ventricular relaxation.

Normal Heart Sounds

The specific mechanisms that are responsible for heart sounds are disputed. Sudden accelerations and decelerations of blood, turbulent blood flow, and the movements of valves, heart walls and blood vessels may all contribute to the production of vibrations audible at the body surface as sounds.[4,8,10 – 15]

First Heart Sound. Closure of the atrioventricular valves and oscillations in the movement of blood in the ventricles are associated with vibrations of the entire valvular apparatus and of atrial and ventricular walls. This creates the early components of the first heart sound.[6,8,12,15] Later components of the first heart sound may be due to tricuspid valve closure or to the acceleration of blood ejected into the aorta.[8,11,12,15]

Second Heart Sound. The second heart sound actually seems to begin before semilunar valve closure.[4,11] The mechanisms responsible for the second heart sound seem to include arterial blood flow decelerations due to ventricular relaxation, closure of the semilunar valves, blood vessel wall vibrations, and valvular vibrations. The closure of the pulmonic valve after the aortic valve leads to a two-component sound that is accentuated during inspiration.[6,8,13] Other heart sounds that do not usually occur in adults over 30 years old are discussed in Chapters 14 and 48.

CLINICAL APPLICATIONS OF CARDIAC EVENTS

Systolic Events

The stroke volume (SV) ejected by the ventricle, 60 to 130 ml/min/meter^2 body surface area (m^2 BSA), is illustrated by the ventricular volume downstroke of Figure 4-1; it is the difference between the ventricular end-diastolic volume and end-systolic volume (see Table 19-3). The SV times the number of cardiac cycles per minute (heart rate) equals the cardiac output. Approximately 24 to 36 ml/m^2 BSA remains in the ventricle at the end of systole (see Table 19-3). The ejection fraction (EF) is the percentage of total ventricular volume that is ejected during each contraction, that is, stroke volume divided by end-diastolic volume. The EF is a frequently used index of ventricular function; it normally is greater than 50% and usually is approximately 65% (see Chap. 19).

The maximum rate of left ventricular force development and rise of left ventricular pressure over time (peak dP/dt) occurs during isovolumic ventricular contraction.[1,18] Peak dP/dt is an important clinical measure of ventricular contractility (see Chap. 2).[1]

Specific phases of the left ventricular systolic time intervals can be measured and used to diagnose ventricular dysfunction. Total electromechanical systole (Q-S$_2$), the preejection period (PEP), and left ventricular ejection time (LVET) are derived from simultaneous noninvasive electrocardiogram, phonocardiogram, and carotid artery pulse tracing recordings (see Chap. 20).[1] The tension time index was mentioned in Chapter 2. These time intervals vary with heart rate.[18] They provide useful diagnostic and prognostic information about impairment of myocardial function in persons with cardiac disese.[9]

Diastolic Events

Diastole comprises a greater portion of the cardiac cycle (approximately 65%) than does systole (approximately 35%) at normal heart rates (see Table 4-1). At faster heart rates

both systole and diastole are shortened, diastole proportionally more so than systole. For example, at a heart rate of 180 beats per minute, diastole comprises approximately 40% and systole approximately 60% of the cardiac cycle.[5] Chapter 2 discusses the importance of this diastolic shortening at faster heart rates in terms of the decreased amount of time available for ventricular and coronary artery filling, which may lead to impaired myocardial functioning.

REFERENCES

The selections marked with an asterisk (*) are helpful for further reading.

1. Ahmed SS, Levinson GE, Schwartz CJ et al: Systolic time intervals as measures of the contractile state of the left ventricular myocardium in man. Circulation 46(3):559–571, 1972
2. Berne RN, Levy MN: Cardiovascular Physiology, 3rd ed, p 85. St Louis, CV Mosby, 1977*
3. Braunwald E, Fishman AP, Cournand A: Time relationship of dynamic events in the cardiac chambers, pulmonary artery and aorta in man. Circ Res 4(1):100–106, 1956
4. Chandraratna PA, Lopez JM, Cohen LS: Echocardiographic observations on the mechanism of production of the second heart sound. Circulation 51(2):292–296, 1975
5. Folkow B, Neil E: Circulation, pp 156–161. New York, Oxford University Press, 1971
6. Hurst JW, Schlant RC: Principles of auscultation. In Hurst JW (ed): The Heart, 4th ed, pp 226–227. New York, McGraw-Hill, 1978
7. Katz AN: Physiology of the Heart, pp 20–23. New York, Raven Press, 1977*
8. Leatham A: The first and second heart sounds. In Hurst JW (ed): The Heart, 4th ed, pp 237–254. New York, McGraw-Hill, 1978
9. Lewis RP, Boudoulas H, Welch TG et al: Usefulness of systolic time intervals in coronary artery disease. Am J Cardiol 37(5):787–796, 1976
10. Luisada AA, MacCanon DMF: Functional basis of heart sounds. Am J Cardiol 16(5):631–633, 1965
11. Piemme TE: Relationship of heart sounds to acceleration of blood flow. Circ Res 18(3):303–315, 1966
12. Rushmer RF: Cardiovascular Dynamics, 4th ed, pp 88–91; pp 411–430. Philadelphia, WB Saunders, 1976*
13. Scher AM: Mechanical events of the cardiac cycle. In Ruch TC, Patton HD (eds): Physiology and Biophysics II, pp 102–116. Philadelphia, WB Saunders, 1974*
14. Schlant RC: Sequential phases of the cardiac cycle. In Hurst JW (ed): The Heart, 4th ed, pp 73–74. New York, McGraw-Hill, 1978
15. Waider W, Craig E: First heart sound and ejection sounds. Am J Cardiol 35(3):346–356, 1975
16. Wiggers CJ: Circulatory Dynamics, pp 53–60. New York, Grune & Stratton, 1952*
17. Wiggers CJ: Studies on the consecutive phases of the cardiac cycle. Am J Physiol 56(3):415–459, 1921
18. Yang SS, Bentivoglio LG, Maranhao V et al: From Cardiac Catheterization Data to Hemodynamic Parameters, 2nd ed, pp 257–264. Philadelphia, FA Davis, 1978

ADDITIONAL READING

Delman AJ: Hemodynamic correlates of cardiovascular sounds. Annu Rev Med 18:139–158, 1967
Kones RJ: Cardiogenic Shock, pp 131–134. Mt Kisco, NY, Futura, 1974
Smith JJ, Kampine JP: Circulatory Physiology: The Essentials, pp 39–46. Baltimore, Williams & Wilkins, 1980
Weissler AM: Systolic time intervals. N Engl J Med 296(6):321–324, 1977

5

Systemic and Pulmonary Circulations
CAROL JEAN HALPENNY, R.N., M.A.

A single-celled organism can exchange material directly with the outside environment, but a multicelled organism with many different tissues and organs needs a transport system to bring the outside environment into proximity with all body cells. The peripheral vascular system supplies metabolic substrates such as oxygen and glucose to the tissues, removes metabolic end products such as carbon dioxide, maintains the normal fluid volume and distribution of electrolytes in the tissues, transports hormones and immunologic substances, and helps regulate internal temperature through heat exchange at the body surface. These exchange activities occur in the capillaries. Arteries function as a distribution system to transport blood to the capillaries, and veins function as a collecting system to carry blood back to the heart.

Ventricular contraction supplies the driving force for the movement of blood through these transport systems. The two divisions of the circulatory system, the left heart and systemic circulation and the right heart and pulmonary circulation, are serially connected in a closed system. Overviews of some structural and functional characteristics of the circulatory system are illustrated in Figures 5-1 and 5-2.

The term peripheral vascular system may be used to refer either to the systemic circulation or to both systemic and pulmonary circulations. In this chapter the term peripheral vascular system denotes circulation through all vascular beds.

Blood flow to each area of the body is governed by physical laws that describe fluid movement in a tube and is affected by the relationships between blood vessel characteristics and the specific cardiovascular regulatory mech- anisms that are operating at one particular point in time. This chapter is a discussion of the first two of these factors and Chapter 6 considers regulatory mechanisms.

PHYSICAL FACTORS THAT AFFECT BLOOD FLOW AND VELOCITY

Definition of Flow

Flow (F or Q) is the volume (amount) of fluid movement per unit of time. In clinical practice this is usually expressed as liters or milliliters/minute (ml/min); sometimes flow is expressed as cubic centimeters/second (cm^3/sec). The car- diac output (CO) is the total flow through the systemic or pulmonary circulation per minute.

Determinants of Flow

Nonturbulent flow in a tube or in one segment of a horizontal blood vessel is determined by the pressure (P) difference between the inflow and outflow ends of that segment (*in* minus *out*) or ΔP (change in pressure) divided by the resistance (R) to flow provided by that segment. Thus, $F = \Delta P/R$. These relationships are illustrated in Figures 5-3 and 5-4. (See Poiseuille's and Ohm's laws in the Glossary.)

Pressure Difference. Pressure is force per unit area; in a liquid system, it is the force exerted on the liquid per unit area. Gravitational forces affect pressure and must be con-

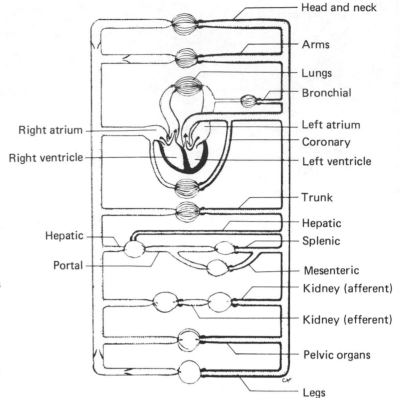

Fig. 5-1. Schematic diagram of the parallel and series arrangement of the vessels composing the circulatory system. The capillary beds are represented by thin lines connecting the arteries on the right with the veins on the left. The crescent-shaped thickenings proximal to the capillary beds represent the arterioles. (Berne RM, Levy MN: Cardiovascular Physiology, 3rd ed. St. Louis, The CV Mosby Co., 1977; redrawn from Green HD: In Glasser O (ed): Medical Physics, Vol. 1. Chicago, Year Book Medical Publishers, 1944)

sidered in nonhorizontal situations (Chap. 6). Pressure is expressed as mm Hg, cm H_2O, dynes per square centimeter (dyn/cm²), torr, or kilopascals. One mm Hg = 1.36 cm H_2O = 1 torr = 1333 dyn/cm² (see Table 21-1).

Flow is directly proportional to inflow minus outflow pressure differences, because fluid moves from a region of greater pressure to a region of lesser pressure. It is important to remember that it is the pressure difference or gradient and not just the upstream pressure that provides the impetus for flow.

Resistance. Resistance is the opposition to force, and hemodynamic resistance is the opposition provided by the blood vessels to blood flow, that is, the several factors that collectively constitute the resistance to blood flow are in opposition to the driving force for flow provided by a pressure difference.[11] In clinical practice, resistance is derived from pressure and flow measurements because resistance is difficult to measure. Because pressure = dyn/cm², flow = cm³/sec, and $R = \Delta P/F$ (by transposing the equation $F = \Delta P/R$), the units of resistance are dyn/sec/cm⁻⁵.

Peripheral resistance units (PRU), expressed as PRU or as mm Hg/ml of flow/min, may be used to compare the resistances of different vascular beds.[3,11,29] PRUs often are expressed per 100 grams of tissue.

Vascular resistance is proportional to a constant $(8/\pi)$, the viscosity of the blood (η), and the length of the vessel (l), and is inversely proportional to the fourth power of the radius (r^4).[16,29] Thus, $R = 8\eta l/\pi r^4$ (Fig. 5-3).

Blood vessel radius is the principal factor determining resistance in the vascular system. Because resistance is inversely proportional to the fourth power of the radius,

small changes in the radius lead to large changes in resistance.[28]

In considering viscosity, thick fluid provides a greater resistance and flows less easily than does thin fluid. The relative viscosity of blood is slightly different in the capillaries than in larger blood vessels, but blood viscosity in the body as a whole does not change under normal conditions. Thus, viscosity changes usually do not play an important role in blood flow.[7] A large change in the hematocrit, however, may alter blood viscosity. Under conditions of polycythemia, the advantage of a greater blood oxygen-carrying capacity due to increased amounts of hemoglobin may be counteracted by decreased flow at the capillary level secondary to the increased blood viscosity.[28]

Flow is less in longer tubes, because increased tube length increases resistance. Because blood vessel length is relatively fixed, this factor is not of primary importance in altering blood flow.

The arterioles and precapillary sphincters are the major sites of changes in radius and thus in resistance in the vascular system. Therefore the arterial system is frequently called the "resistance system." Capacitance is the inverse of resistance. The venous system is in general a low-resistance system, so it is frequently termed the "capacitance system."

In the systemic circulation, blood flows from the aorta [mean arterial pressure (MAP) 100 mm Hg] to the right atrium [mean right atrial pressure (RAP) 0–6 mm Hg] (see Table 19-3). In the pulmonary circulation, blood flows from the pulmonary artery (mean pressure 15 mm Hg) to the left atrium (mean pressure 1–10 mm Hg) (see Table 19-3).

Total resistance in the systemic circulation is termed

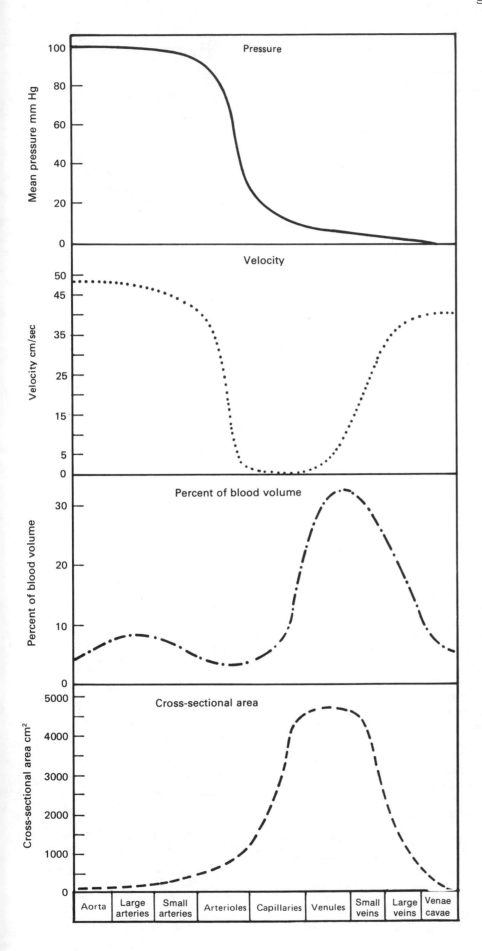

Fig. 5-2. Pressure, velocity of flow, cross-sectional area, and capacity of the systemic blood vessels. Note the major pressure drop at the arterioles, the minimal velocity of flow in the capillaries, and the large cross-sectional area and blood volume capacity of the venous system. (Adapted from Berne RM, Levy MN: Cardiovascular Physiology, 3rd ed. St. Louis, The CV Mosby Co, 1977)

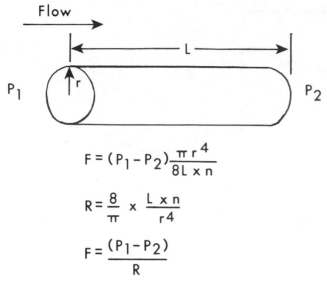

$$F = (P_1 - P_2)\frac{\pi r^4}{8L \times n}$$

$$R = \frac{8}{\pi} \times \frac{L \times n}{r^4}$$

$$F = \frac{(P_1 - P_2)}{R}$$

Fig. 5-3. Relations between pressure, flow, and resistance. F = flow (ml/min); P = pressure (mm Hg); R = resistance (dyn/sec/cm^{-5}); L = length (mm); r = radius (mm); n = viscosity; $\pi/8$ is the proportionality constant. Although these relationships were derived from Poiseuille's work with fluids flowing in a nonpulsatile manner through rigid tubes, the importance of alterations in diameter as the key determinant of the resistance to flow in blood vessels is illustrated (see text). (Adapted from Shepherd JT, Vanhoutte PM: The Human Cardiovascular System: Facts and Concepts, p 8. New York, Raven Press, 1979)

systemic vascular resistance (SVR), and ranges from 770 to 1500 dyn/sec/cm^{-5} (see Table 19-3). Substituting clinical entities in the previous equation $F = \Delta P/R$, $CO = (MAP - RAP)/SVR$; that is, the difference between aortic and right atrial pressure divided by the systemic vascular resistance determines the overall blood flow to the body. The relationship CO = blood pressure $(BP)/SVR$ is often used in clinical practice; this is a less exact interpretation of the equation $F = \Delta P/R$, because blood pressure by itself does not directly connote a change in pressure.

Resistance in the lungs is termed pulmonary vascular resistance (PVR) and ranges from 20 to 120 dyn/sec/cm^{-5} (average 100 dyn/sec/cm^{-5}) (see Table 19-3).[23] Peripheral vascular resistance was formerly abbreviated PVR. Because peripheral vascular resistance usually connotes systemic vascular resistance and not a combination of systemic and pulmonary resistances, the term peripheral vascular resistance is increasingly being replaced by the more precise terms systemic and pulmonary resistance.

An additional factor that affects resistance in a total system is whether blood vessels are arranged in series or in parallel. Total resistance is additive when blood vessels are arranged in series; total resistance is less than the resistance in any individual tube in a parallel arrangement. Blood flow to and from the individual vascular beds is serially arranged through the aorta and large veins. The capillaries and most of the individual vascular beds of the body are arranged in parallel, thus decreasing total resistance. The arrangement of the vascular beds in parallel also provides a situation in which resistance in one area may be selectively increased; for example, by closure of precapillary sphincters (see below). Although this does not immediately and directly

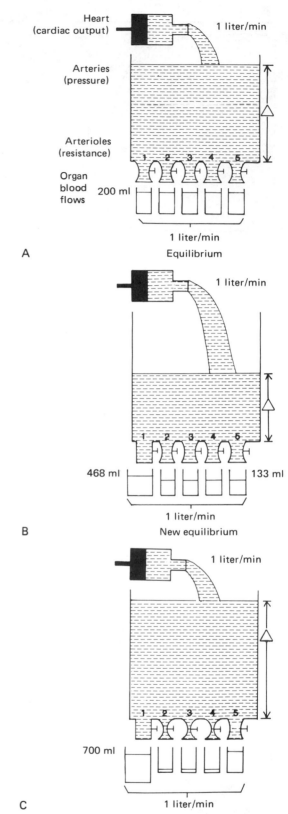

Fig. 5-4. Schematic representation of relations between pressure, flow, and resistance. (**A**) Equilibrium. (**B**) Dilation of one arterial bed with unchanged resistances in the other arterial beds. Flow to the dilated bed is increased and the change in pressure is decreased. (**C**) Dilation of one arterial bed and constriction of some other arterial beds so that total resistance remains constant. (After Vander AJ, Sherman JH, Luciano DS: Human Physiology, p 300. New York, McGraw-Hill, 1980)

affect flow to other areas, the body attempts to maintain blood pressure and flow relatively constant by subsequent compensatory changes (Fig. 5-4; Chap. 6).

Velocity

Velocity is the rate of fluid movement per unit of time and is expressed as cm/sec. Volume flow is expressed as cm³/sec. Velocity varies inversely with the total cross-sectional area. Because the capillaries have a combined cross-sectional area approximately one thousand times that of the aorta, flow is much slower in the capillaries where nutrient and waste product exchange take place (see Fig. 5-2).

Streamlined Versus Turbulent Flow

In most blood vessels, blood flows in layers of molecules that move parallel to each other in longitudinal streams, with the layers in the center of the vessel moving slightly faster than those layers adjacent to the vessel walls; this is called laminar (layered) flow. Laminar flow is silent.

Under certain conditions, flow ceases to be streamlined and becomes turbulent, with eddies and swirls. Turbulent flow may occur with high-flow velocities, with vessel constrictions or bifurcations, with increased tube diameter, or with lowered blood viscosity.[11,29] Under normal conditions, turbulent flow only occurs in the ventricles and in the ascending aorta during rapid systolic ejection.[13] Increases in turbulent ventricular flow may give rise to the third and fourth heart sounds and to palpable precordial thrills. Turbulent flow due to peripheral blood vessel constriction (atherosclerotic plaques) or dilation (aneurysms) can be auscultated as a bruit or palpated as a thrill (see Chaps. 14 and 48).

THE SYSTEMIC CIRCULATION

Flow, pressure, and resistance are intimately related; in order to maintain equilibrium or homeostasis, a change in one factor must be compensated for by changes in one or both of the other factors. Discussion of these changes in the body necessitates a consideration of the structural and functional characteristics of the systemic and pulmonary circulations. The systemic circulation will be used as a prototype for both circulations because the general characteristics of both systems are similar; differences between the two systems are noted in the discussion of the pulmonary circulation.

Structural Characteristics

The structure of blood-vessel walls in different parts of the peripheral vascular system is appropriately related to the function of each part of the system. For example, most arteries have thicker walls than most veins (Figs. 5-5 and 5-6). The arterial walls are composed of three layers: the tunica intima, which is the most internal; the tunica media, the thickest layer; and the tunica adventitia.[14] The intima is composed of an endothelial lining and an internal elastic membrane. The media contains smooth muscle and elastic

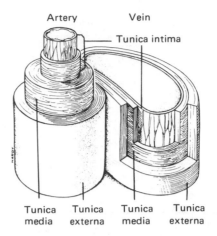

Fig. 5-5. Schematic presentation of tissue layers of blood vessel walls. (Chaffee EE: Basic Physiology and Anatomy, 4th ed, p 332. Philadelphia, JB Lippincott, 1980)

tissue. The adventitia consists of collagenous and elastic tissue; it merges with the loose connective tissues around each blood vessel (Fig. 5-5).[14,31] The large arteries have a considerable amount of elastic tissue. The arterial walls become progressively thicker, more muscular, and less elastic as the arteries get smaller (Fig. 5-6).[2,8,31]

Arterioles have an endothelial layer and one continuous layer of smooth muscle and range in size from 20 to 50 micrometers (μm) (Fig. 5-6). Some vascular beds have metarterioles (10–15 μm) connecting the arterioles to the arterial capillaries. The metarterioles have a single noncontinuous layer of smooth muscle. Capillaries branch from arterioles and metarterioles. Immediately before the capillary there is often a band or cushion of vascular smooth muscle cells termed the precapillary sphincter.[32]

Capillaries have a single layer of endothelium surrounded on the outer side by a basement membrane.[32] Most arterial capillaries are slightly smaller (outside diameter 5 μm) than venous capillaries (8 μm). There is no smooth muscle in the walls of true capillaries. Venous capillaries extend to nonmuscular venules, which have elastic tissue, then to muscular venules (Fig. 5-7).

Veins are more numerous than arteries, have a large diameter, and have thinner walls (Fig. 5-6). The elastic venous walls are sparsely covered with smooth muscle. The three muscle layers of the veins are often indistinct.[4] Superficial veins form a rich anastomosis with deeper veins.

Medium-sized veins (diameter > 1 mm) in the extremities and neck have valves, which are paired semilunar membranes of thin connective tissue. The valves are oriented in the direction of blood flow and prevent the retrograde flow of venous blood.[11] There is a sinus at the intersection of the vein wall and the valve; the wall of the vein is thinner in this region. (See Chapter 53 for a discussion of varicose veins.) The intrathoracic, intra-abdominal, and intracerebral veins usually have no valves.

The adventitia of arteries and veins is supplied with sensory and autonomic nerves.[31] The resistance vessels, particularly the arterioles, and the splanchnic and cutaneous veins, are densely innervated (Chap. 6).[28] Nerves do not always extend to metarterioles and precapillary sphincters and do not innervate capillaries.[31,32] Thus, external control

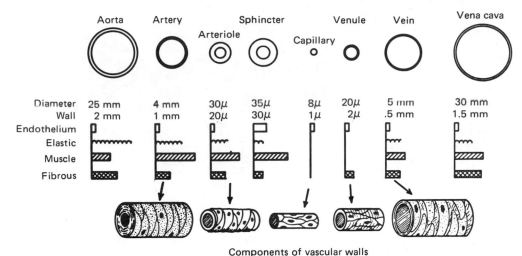

Components of vascular walls

Fig. 5-6. Components of blood vessel walls. The relative amounts of elastic and fibrous tissues are greatest in the aorta. Smaller arterial vessels have more prominent smooth muscle. This illustration is not drawn to scale because of the extent of diameter differences between arteries and the venae cavae and the capillaries. (Rushmer RF: Cardiovascular Dynamics, p 135. Philadelphia, WB Saunders, 1976)

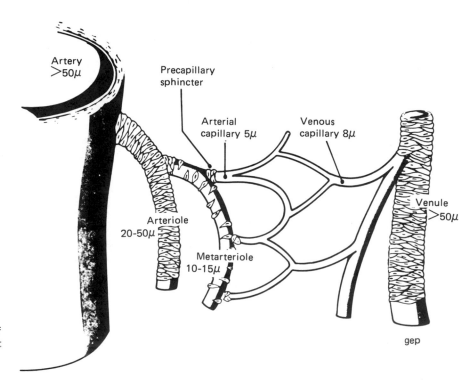

Fig. 5-7. Schematic representation of the capillary bed. (Ruch TC, Patton HD: Physiology and Biophysics II, p 130. Philadelphia, WB Saunders, 1974)

through nervous stimulation can be exerted on arterioles, whereas the metarterioles and precapillary sphincters seem to be under local control.

Functional Characteristics of the Arterial System

Arterial Pressures. The pressure drop between the aorta and the capillaries provides the impetus for blood flow through the arterial system. Adenosine triphosphate (ATP) provides the energy for mechanical ventricular contraction. The energy of ventricular contraction is transmitted to the aorta in the form of potential energy and kinetic energy, which provides the force for forward blood flow.[6]

Systolic arterial pressure is generated by ventricular contraction. The peak systolic pressure is mainly determined by the left ventricular stroke volume, the peak rate of ejection, and the distensibility of the aortic walls (Fig. 5-8; see Chap. 2).[27]

During systole, the elastic walls of the aorta and large arteries stretch as more blood enters than is capable of immediately running off. Thus, much of the stroke volume is retained by the distensible aorta. During diastole there is passive elastic recoil of the arterial walls. This recoil imparts

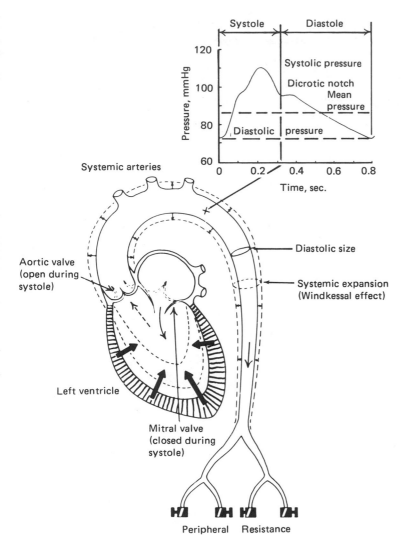

Fig. 5-8. Changes in aortic pressure during the cardiac cycle and the dampening role of the aorta and large arteries on the pulsatile flow from the heart during systole (sometimes termed the Windkessel effect.) (Shepherd JT, Vanhoutte PM: The Human Cardiovascular System: Facts and Concepts, p 78. New York, Raven Press, 1979)

energy to the stored blood, which is ejected out of the aorta into the peripheral arteries. The elastic recoil transforms pulsatile flow into more continuous flow into the smaller vessels (Fig. 5-8).[11,13,28]

The pressure in the arteries continues to decrease during diastole until the next ventricular contraction. Minimal diastolic pressure is determined by the systolic pressure, the arterial elastic recoil, the arterial peripheral resistance, and the length of diastole. These factors affect the magnitude and the rate of the diastolic pressure drop.[27,28,29]

Pulse pressure is the difference between systolic and diastolic pressure. It is affected by the determinants of systolic and diastolic pressure, particularly stroke volume and the elasticity of the arteries.[28]

Mean arterial pressure is the average pressure during a cardiac cycle. Arterial pressure during systole is greater than mean arterial pressure, and arterial pressure during diastole is less than mean arterial pressure. Thus, an accurate mean arterial pressure is determined by the magnitude and amount of time during which the pressure is greater than mean pressure and the magnitude and amount of time during which the pressure is less than mean pressure. Mean arterial pressure is most accurately computed by using intra-arterial pressure measurement and dividing the area under the

arterial pressure curve by the time of one cardiac cycle.[3,27] Because at normal heart rates systole occupies approximately one-third of the cardiac cycle, mean pressure can be approximated by adding the diastolic pressure to one-third of the pulse pressure.[3,27]

Mean arterial pressure is obviously dependent upon the cardiac output and the peripheral resistance. Stroke volume and heart rate determine cardiac output, whereas the elasticity of the arteries and the amount of precapillary vasoconstriction affect peripheral resistance. Therefore, all these factors affect arterial pressure.[3]

The Arterial Pressure Waves. The pressure contour in the aorta is illustrated in Figures 4-1 and 5-8. There is a sharp upstroke reflecting the pressure increase during the rapid ejection phase of ventricular systole and a slower rise during later systole (see Chap. 4). The aortic downstroke corresponding to a decrease in pressure during decreased ventricular ejection and ventricular relaxation is interrupted by a sharp notch denoting blood rebound following aortic valve closure. There is a slower decline in aortic pressure during the rest of ventricular diastole.

Pressure waves in the arterial system undergo changes as pressure is transmitted down the arterial tree. Systolic

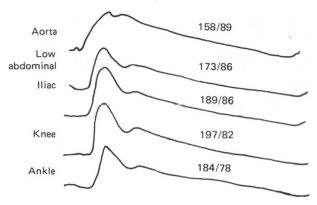

Aorta — 158/89
Low abdominal — 173/86
Iliac — 189/86
Knee — 197/82
Ankle — 184/78

Fig. 5-9. Changes in the arterial pressure wave from the aortic arch to the ankle. (Remington JW, O'Brien LJ: Am J Physiol, 218:437–447, 1970)

pressures increase slightly, so that systolic pressure is up to 20 or more mm Hg higher in the brachial and femoral arteries than in the aorta (Fig. 5-9). Systole becomes shorter and the pressure decrease following systole is faster, creating a narrower and more sharply elevated wave. Diastolic pressures decrease slightly. Consequently the pulse pressure is greater and the mean pressure is lower in the large arteries than in the aorta.[24,25] These changes appear to be due in some part to reflected waves from peripheral vessels that have less elasticity than the aorta.[13,24,25]

The arteries become less elastic with advancing age. With less ability to store potential energy and develop diastolic recoil, the arteries are less helpful in maintaining the forward blood flow. Thus, ventricular work is increased.[17] Larger arteries may remain somewhat distensible because they increase in diameter, but smaller arteries become less distensible because of decreased elasticity. There is often an increase in systolic pressure. Pulse pressure increases. If the aorta does become less distensible, the decreased aortic recoil will cause the diastolic pressure to fall more rapidly and there will be a decreased diastolic pressure as well as an increased systolic pressure (Chap. 47).[29]

Arterial Resistances. The normal overall pressure drop from the aorta to the terminal arteries is relatively small, approximately 25 mm Hg. The greatest pressure drop in the vascular system occurs at the arterioles, where vascular smooth muscle constriction provides most of the vascular resistance (Fig. 5-2). Alterations in the diameter of the precapillary sphincters control capillary blood flow and also control the pressures within the capillaries and veins. Thus, these resistance vessels have important effects on arterial blood pressure, on capillary exchange, and on venous function.

Arterial Volumes. The arterial system is a high-pressure, high-resistance, low-volume system. In such a system the blood vessels are not very compliant, so that increases in volume are accompanied by pressure increases of a similar relative magnitude.

Arterial Velocities. Mean velocity of flow in the aorta is approximately 40 cm/sec. The aorta has the most rapid flow velocity of any section of the peripheral vascular system (Fig. 5-2).[27]

Functional Characteristics of the Capillary System

Flow Through the Capillaries. Thin-walled capillaries can withstand relatively high pressures without rupturing because of their small lumens, an example of the law of Laplace (P — *tension/radius*, see the Glossary). In the human aorta, tension at normal pressures is approximately 20,000 dyn/cm, whereas in the capillaries it is approximately 17 dyn/cm, or 12,000 times less than in the aorta.[3,13,27]

Pressure differences between the arterial end of the capillary bed (approximately 32 mm Hg) and the venous end (approximately 15 mm Hg) provide the impetus for flow through the capillaries.[32] The velocity of blood flow in the capillaries, 0.3 to 0.5 mm/sec, is slow, because the total cross-sectional area is large.[13] This slow flow provides the setting for many substances to diffuse out of the blood vessel into the interstitial tissue and for substances to move from the interstitium into the blood vessel.

Characteristics of Capillary Membranes. Materials are exchanged between the interstitium and all body cells. Endothelial permeability and pressure differences and concentration gradients between the blood vessel and the surrounding interstitium determine the nature and rate of the exchange of materials between the blood and the interstitium.

Capillary endothelial membranes vary from continuous to fenestrated to discontinuous (Fig. 5-10). Continuous vascular endothelium is the least permeable and is found in nervous, muscular, subcutaneous, connective, and pulmo-

Fig. 5-10. Schematic illustration of transport pathways in the capillary endothelium. **(A)** Transport through the endothelial cell. **(B)** Pinocytosis. **(C)** Intercellular junctions. **(D)** Intercellular fenestrations. **(E)** Tight junctions in the brain. **(F)** Large gaps found in sinusoids of the liver and spleen. (Shepherd JT, Vanhoutte PM: The Human Cardiovascular System: Facts and Concepts, p 20. New York, Raven Press, 1979)

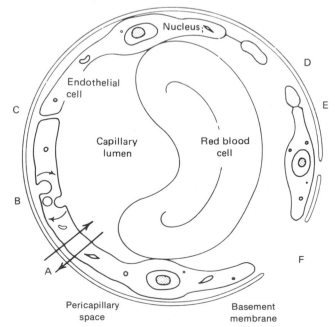

nary tissue (Fig. 5-10). Nervous tissue has extremely tight junctions between capillary endothelial cells, so few substances can penetrate between cells; this creates a blood–brain barrier. Fenestrated vascular endothelium has pores and is found in glands, the kidney, and the intestine. Discontinuous endothelium is the most permeable and is found in the liver, spleen, and bone marrow (Fig. 5-10).[18,32]

Most solutes travel across the capillary membrane by diffusion along concentration gradients (Chap. 9). The capillary endothelium permits only lipid-soluble substances to pass easily through the wall, so lipid-soluble substances such as oxygen, carbon dioxide, anesthetic agents, and alcohol diffuse relatively rapidly and freely through the capillary wall (Fig. 5-10). It appears that most lipid-insoluble substances cross vascular epithelial cells through pores that are in cells or pass through clefts between cells (Fig. 5-10). The size of the pore limits the movement of larger substances. The size of the molecules that easily penetrate capillary membranes varies in different vascular beds.[10] In general, molecules larger in diameter than 40 Å or with a molecular weight greater than 60,000 do not easily penetrate the vessel wall.[3,32]

Water and water-soluble materials such as electrolytes appear to diffuse through the endothelium principally through intercellular clefts.[32] The rate at which water moves across the capillary membrane is often used as a measure of capillary exchange rates and is expressed as the capillary filtration coefficient (CFC) of a specific vascular bed.[3]

The capillaries offer little restriction to diffusion for small molecules. The rate of blood flow and the size of the capillary bed provide the most important limitations to net movement of small molecules across the vessel wall.[3]

Albumin (diameter 30–35 Å) is the smallest of the plasma proteins and is able to cross the capillary wall more readily than the globulins or fibrinogen.[13] Nevertheless, there is some movement of globulins across the vessel wall; this is necessary because globulins participate in humoral immunity. The movement of the larger plasma proteins through the vessel walls seems to be due to pinocytosis or to transport by way of vesicles within the endothelial cells (Fig. 5-10).[32] Small amounts of larger cellular elements seem able to penetrate directly through the endothelial cell or to pass through endothelial clefts.[32] The mechanisms of transcapillary solute and fluid transport continue to receive intensive investigation.[10]

Capillary Filtration and Reabsorption. The amount and direction of fluid movement across the capillary wall is governed by capillary permeability, which remains unchanged under normal conditions, and by the equilibrium between four forces: blood vessel and interstitial hydrostatic pressures, and blood vessel and interstitial oncotic pressures.

The capillary hydrostatic (blood) pressure tends to force fluid into the tissues, more so at the arterial end of the capillary where capillary hydrostatic pressure (approximately 32 mm Hg) is higher, than at the venous end (approximately 15 mm Hg) (Table 5-1). Interstitial (tissue) hydrostatic pressure tends to force fluid into the blood vessel. It is difficult to measure interstitial hydrostatic pressure, and there is controversy regarding the values for this pressure, but it approximates atmospheric pressure or is close to 0 to 2 mm Hg (with atmospheric pressure considered to be 0 mm Hg).[28,32]

The plasma proteins exert an attraction promoting the movement of fluid into the capillary (plasma colloid osmotic, or oncotic, pressure, Chap. 9); this oncotic pressure is approximately 25 mm Hg at the arterial end of the capillary and is slightly higher at the venous end, because there is less fluid in the capillary at the venous end. Because there is only a small amount of protein in the tissues, the tissue colloid osmotic pressure is relatively slight, approximately 10 mm Hg.[32]

Because tissue hydrostatic and colloid pressures are both low, it is primarily the net balance between the capillary hydrostatic pressure promoting outward movement and the capillary colloid osmotic pressures promoting inward movement that determines fluid movement. At the arterial end of the capillary the net balance promotes outward fluid movement. When the capillary colloid osmotic pressure exceeds the capillary hydrostatic pressure toward the venous end of the capillary, flow reverses and there is fluid movement into the capillary (Fig. 5-11).

Although it is helpful to think of fluid going out of the capillary at the arterial end and coming back into the capillary at the venous end, it should be remembered that the filtration–reabsorption process actually occurs throughout the capillary. It is the balance of these four forces that governs the direction of net flow.

The original hypothesis regarding capillary tissue fluid balance (the Starling-Landis hypothesis) considered that the only relevant factors affecting capillary filtration and reabsorption were capillary hydrostatic and oncotic pressures, because it was assumed that tissue hydrostatic and oncotic pressures were negligible and that the two pressures balanced each other.[10,20] Some measurements indicate that tissue oncotic pressures are higher than were previously estimated, so that the balance of pressures promoting net fluid movement out of the capillary may actually be greater than the balance of pressures promoting net fluid movement back into the capillary (Table 5-1).[32] However, there also appears to be a greater permeability and surface area available for absorption at the venous end of the capillary than at the arterial end.[32] Because the balance of forces promoting net inward fluid movement is greater than the balance of forces promoting net outward fluid movement in the venous portion of the capillary, this factor promotes greater reabsorption. Thus, the greater tissue oncotic pressures promoting net outward movement may be balanced by the effect of promoting a net inward movement where there is a larger available surface area for reabsorption. Thus the original concept of a balance between the forces promoting filtration and the forces promoting reabsorption seems appropriate, although the relationships may not be as simple as originally conceived.[32] Another major factor that compensates for net filtration of fluid out of capillaries is removal of the tissue fluid and materials such as protein by the lymphatic system.[33]

Alterations in Capillary Filtration and Reabsorption. The capillaries are not capable of altering their own diameter because they have no smooth muscle and are not innervated. An increase in arterial resistance proximal to the capillary

TABLE 5-1 APPROXIMATE VALUES FOR PRESSURES PROMOTING CAPILLARY FILTRATION AND REABSORPTION

Original Starling-Landis hypothesis:

ARTERIAL END		VENOUS END	
Capillary hydrostatic pressure	32 mm Hg	Capillary hydrostatic pressure	15 mm Hg
Tissue hydrostatic pressure	− negligible	Tissue hydrostatic pressure	− negligible
Promoting capillary outflow	32 mm Hg	Promoting capillary outflow	15 mm Hg
Capillary oncotic pressure	25 mm Hg	Capillary oncotic pressure	25 mm Hg
Tissue oncotic pressure	− negligible	Tissue oncotic pressure	− negligible
Promoting capillary inflow	25 mm Hg	Promoting capillary inflow	25 mm Hg
Net pressure gradient for fluid flow	32 mm Hg	Net pressure gradient for fluid flow	15 mm Hg
	− 25 mm Hg		− 25 mm Hg
	7 mm Hg (promotes capillary outflow)		− 10 mm Hg (promotes capillary inflow)

Revised hypothesis:*

ARTERIAL END		VENOUS END	
Capillary hydrostatic pressure	32 mm Hg	Capillary hydrostatic pressure	15 mm Hg
Tissue hydrostatic pressure	− 2 mm Hg	Tissue hydrostatic pressure	− 2 mm Hg
Promoting capillary outflow	30 mm Hg	Promoting capillary outflow	13 mm Hg
Capillary oncotic pressure	25 mm Hg	Capillary oncotic pressure	25 mm Hg
Tissue oncotic pressure	− 10 mm Hg	Tissue oncotic pressure	− 10 mm Hg
Promoting capillary inflow	15 mm Hg	Promoting capillary inflow	15 mm Hg
Net pressure gradient for fluid flow	30 mm Hg	Net pressure gradient for fluid flow	13 mm Hg
	− 15 mm Hg		− 15 mm Hg
	15 mm Hg (promotes capillary outflow)		− 2 mm Hg (promotes capillary inflow)

*(Data from Wiederhielm CA: The capillaries, veins, and lymphatics. In Ruch TC, Patton HD (eds): Physiology and Biophysics II, pp. 129–145. Philadelphia, WB Saunders, 1974)

decreases capillary hydrostatic pressure because arterial pressure increases are prevented from being transferred to the capillary bed by constriction of the precapillary sphincters[3] (Fig. 5-11C). An increase in venous resistance distal to the capillary bed increases capillary hydrostatic pressures.

However, precapillary vasoconstriction and vasodilation affect the number of open versus closed capillaries and affect the amount of fluid entering the capillaries, which in turn affects the amount available for filtration. Under normal steady-state conditions, all factors except precapillary resistance are relatively constant, so it is principally changes in precapillary resistance that determine changes in fluid movement across the capillary walls.[3] Figure 5-11 illustrates the decreased filtration that results from precapillary vasoconstriction.

Figure 5-11 also illustrates the leaking of proteins into the interstitial fluid in conditions such as inflammation, when the capillary becomes more permeable. It further illustrates the effect of hypoproteinemia; both hypoproteinemia and inflammation as well as increased venous pressure can lead to edema. Usually no edema occurs until venous pressure increases or plasma oncotic pressure decreases are greater than 10 mm Hg.[32]

Local Regulation of Systemic Vascular Beds

The metarterioles and precapillary sphincters have been found by some investigators to demonstrate an alternating vasoconstriction and vasodilation termed vasomotion.[13,32] This vasomotion seems related to intrinsic factors that influence local blood flow, so the capillary vascular bed is autoregulated. Autoregulation in the peripheral vasculature is the ability to maintain constant local capillary flow in the face of varying perfusion pressures (Fig. 5-12). Local factors not under neural or hormonal control cause constriction or dilation of the precapillary sphincters.[11,13,27] Local autoregulation may work in concert with neurohormonal control of arterioles or may oppose this centrally mediated regulation (see Chap. 6).

Three different factors have been postulated to be responsible for autoregulation.[11] The chemical theory of autoregulation is based on findings that chemical factors related to actively metabolizing tissue may cause constriction or dilation of precapillary sphincters. Decreased tissue or arterial levels of oxygen, increased carbon dioxide levels, or increased levels of hydrogen ion concentration (decreased

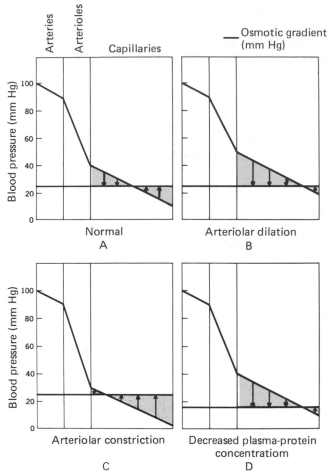

Fig. 5-11. Schematic illustration of capillary filtration and reabsorption. *Arrows* going down indicate filtration out of the capillary; *arrows* going up illustrate filtration into the capillary. The *shaded* areas denote the relative magnitudes of the fluid movements. Elevated venous pressure (not shown) would create increased capillary hydrostatic pressure, force fluid into the tissue, and resemble the situation in **B**. (Vander AJ, Sherman JH, Luciano DS: Human Physiology, 2nd ed, p 295. New York, McGraw-Hill, 1980)

pH) have been shown to cause vasodilation. Tissues that do not have enough oxygen, have too much carbon dioxide, or are acidotic obviously need to increase their blood flow. The prostaglandins are a group of phospholipids that have been found in almost every tissue. Prostaglandin E(PGE) and other prostaglandins have been demonstrated to be potent renal and coronary vasodilators.[30] Local vasodilation or constriction has also been demonstrated with alterations in the levels of calcium, potassium, magnesium, adenosine, cyclic adenosine monophosphate (C-AMP), hyperosmolality, and other substances.[1,5,13,19,30]

The effects of intravascular pressures may provide the stimulus for constriction or dilation of the precapillary sphincters. According to this myogenic theory of autoregulation, increased pressures stretch vascular smooth muscle. The muscle responds by vasoconstriction.[13]

It has been suggested that increases in local tissue pressure in confined tissues leads to capillary venoconstriction and then to increased resistance to blood flow. This is termed the tissue–pressure hypothesis of autoregulation.[11]

Different mechanisms seem to contribute to autoregulation in different vascular beds (see Chap. 6).[30]

Functional Characteristics of the Venous System

The venous system serves as a conduit to transport blood back to the heart. The veins also serve as a low-pressure reservoir that has the capacity to contain a variable and large volume of blood.

Venous Pressures. The pressure difference between the venules (10 mm Hg) and the right atrium (0–5 mm Hg), approximately 5 to 10 mm Hg in the recumbent position, provides the driving force for returning blood to the heart. Skeletal muscle contractions in the extremities help to propel venous blood toward the heart. Backward flow is prevented by the valves. This is particularly important during standing and exercise (see Chaps. 6 and 7). Valves also promote the one-way flow of blood from superficial to deep veins.

The pressure difference promoting flow from the venules to the right atrium is altered by alterations in intrathoracic and intra-abdominal pressures and by cardiac events. Central venous pressures are approximately atmospheric (0 mm Hg), reflecting the subatmospheric (−3 to −4 mm Hg) pressures in the thoracic cavity.[6,13,27]

Intrathoracic pressures become more negative (−7 to −8 mm Hg) during inspiration. Intra-abdominal pressures increase during inspiration and so the blood is propelled toward the heart.[3,27,28] Right ventricular stroke volume is increased, and eventually left ventricular stroke volume is increased. However, during deep inspiration, left atrial filling and consequently left ventricular stroke volume may transiently decrease. The increased blood in the lungs resulting from the increased right ventricular stroke volume is then transmitted to the left atrium with a subsequent expiration.[13,23] The results of some investigations have indicated that the fall in left ventricular stroke volume with inspiration

Fig. 5-12. Schematic representation of autoregulation. The blood flow remains relatively constant between mean blood pressures of 60 to 190 mm Hg. (Ruch TC, Patton HD: Physiology and Biophysics II, p 122. Philadelphia, WB Saunders, 1974)

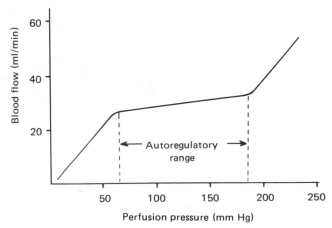

appears to be due to more complex factors than simple pooling of blood in the lungs.[26]

If the respiratory and intra-abdominal muscles contract to produce a forced expiration against a closed glottis (Valsalva maneuver), the intrathoracic pressure increases drastically to 40 mm Hg or more. This collapses the venae cavae. Blood that was contained in the venae cavae is forced into the right atrium, but further flow of blood through the venae cavae is stopped.[27]

Positive-pressure breathing also increases intrathoracic pressure and decreases venous return to the right heart. Some investigations have indicated that neural or hormonal mechanisms rather than increased intrathoracic pressures may be responsible for the decreased cardiac output that accompanies positive end expiratory pressure breathing.[22] There are indications that in some situations positive-pressure breathing may lead to vaso- and venoconstriction that partly compensates for the decreased venous return.

Atrial and ventricular pressure and shape changes appear to affect venous return. Rapid systolic ejection helps to push the ventricles downward, elongate the atria, and promote the flow of blood into the atria. Atrial relaxation during systole may help increase atrial inflow. During diastole, ventricular relaxation helps to promote venous return, although atrial contraction during late diastole decreases atrial inflow.[13]

Right atrial pressure changes are reflected backward into the venae cavae and the subclavian and jugular veins. Figure 21-10 illustrates these changes.

Venous Volumes. The veins contain approximately 75% of the total systemic blood volume, whereas the arteries contain 20% and the capillaries, 5%.[27,32] It is a common misconception that capillaries are the most numerous type of blood vessels; actually venules have been found to be more numerous than capillaries.[32]

The thin walls of the veins are flattened and their cross sections are elliptical when empty. As they fill with blood, they passively change to a circular shape. Because of this passive accommodation to volume increases, the veins are capable of receiving large volumes of fluid with only small increases in pressure, that is, they are quite compliant. For example, a six-fold increase in volume can lead to only a 10-mm Hg increase in venous pressure.[32]

The larger veins, particularly in the splanchnic circulations, skin, and muscle are capable, by venoconstriction, of mobilizing a large volume of the blood that is effectively "stored" in the venous system. Thus, changes in the caliber of veins lead to volume changes whereas changes in the caliber of the arterial vessels lead to pressure changes.

Venous blood flow velocities are slower than those in the arterial system because of the greater area in the venous system. Velocity of flow in the venae cavae (10 cm/sec) is approximately one-quarter that in the aorta.

Lymphatic System

Approximately 20 liters of fluid and other substances are filtered per day by the capillaries (excluding the kidneys) and 16 to 18 liters are reabsorbed. Two-to-four liters per day of fluid, plasma proteins, and some other substances are removed from the interstitial tissues by the lymphatic system.[28,32]

Lymphatic capillaries are usually blind terminal sacs with a discontinuous basement membrane and endothelium similar to that of the vascular capillaries.[33] The terminal lymphatics seem to be in free communication with the interstitial space.[32] Large lymphatic vessels have valves and some smooth muscle.

The lymphatic channels travel back to the heart close to the veins. Arteries, veins, and lymphatics usually are enclosed together in fibrous sheaths.

Peripheral lymphatic pressures seem to be similar to tissue pressures, 1 to 2 mm Hg. In larger lymphatics, the pressures are 5 to 10 mm Hg. The forces promoting the movement of lymph from the tissues toward and into the subclavian veins seem to include active contraction of lymph walls and passive wall compression by skeletal muscle.[27,28,32] Although the larger lymphatic vessels are supplied by nerves, nervous stimulation seems to have little effect on lymph flow.[32]

Besides removing fluid and protein from tissue spaces, the lymphatic system is influential in the removal of foreign particles from tissue spaces and serous cavities. Lymphatic channels empty into lymph nodes that are 1 to 25 mm in diameter. Bacteria and blood cells are phagocytized by fixed macrophages and other reticuloendothelial cells in the lymph nodes.

Lymph nodes are involved in the formation of some antibodies (see Chap. 8). In the alimentary tract, the lymphatics participate in the absorption of chylomicrons (fat particles). Lymph tissue is also present in the spleen, tonsils, genitourinary tract, respiratory tract, bone marrow, vermiform appendix, and the thymus.

THE PULMONARY CIRCULATION

The pulmonary circulation is in series with the systemic circulation and receives the same cardiac output, approximately 5 to 6 liters/min at rest for an adult 70-kg male. The primary function of the pulmonary circulation is to expose the blood to alveolar air so that oxygen can be taken up by the blood and carbon dioxide excreted. Carbon dioxide removal effects body acid-base balance (Chap. 9). Lung capillary endothelial cells also produce, remove, modify, or inactivate certain bioactive substances such as prostaglandins, angiotensin, bradykinin, and norepinephrine.[28]

Structural Characteristics

The walls of the pulmonary arteries are approximately 30% as thick as the walls of the aorta. Pulmonary arteries contain much less smooth muscle than do systemic arteries of comparable size. Pulmonary veins contain little smooth muscle.[21] Both pulmonary arteries and pulmonary veins are supplied with sympathetic constrictor nerves. The capillaries (diameter 7–9 μm) form networks surrounding each alveolus. The pulmonary capillary bed is approximately one-fortieth the size of the systemic capillary bed.[21]

Functional Characteristics

Low-pressure, Low-Resistance, High-Flow System. Pulmonary artery mean pressure is approximately 15 mm Hg, or one-seventh that of mean systemic arterial pressures. Mean left atrial pressure is approximately 5 mm Hg (see Table 19-3).[21] Thus, the total driving pressure for flow from the pulmonary artery to the left atrium is approximately 10 mm Hg versus approximately 90 to 95 mm Hg for the systemic circulation.

Pulmonary capillary pressures are approximately 10 mm Hg, whereas capillary oncotic pressure is the same as in the systemic circulation, 25 mm Hg. Thus, the capillary hydrostatic pressure does not provide a gradient for fluid flow out of the capillary; this prevents fluid from entering the alveoli under normal circumstances.

Because they have less smooth muscle, pulmonary vessels have less ability to alter vessel diameter than systemic vessels. The pulmonary blood vessels are quite compliant. Consequently, the pulmonary system is a low-resistance system. Pulmonary vascular resistance is seven to eight times less than systemic resistance.

No other single organ receives the entire output of one ventricle. Consequently the lungs have high blood flows.

Pulmonary blood volume is increased with exercise, the supine position, and systemic vasoconstriction. Pulmonary blood volume is decreased with positive-pressure breathing, the upright position, systemic vasodilation, and decreases in cardiac output.

Blood Reservoir. As in the systemic circulation, there is a large volume of blood sequestered in the pulmonary veins that can be mobilized by pulmonary venoconstriction.[13] When this occurs, the left heart transiently increases its output over that of the right heart.

Effects of Lung Pressures. Because the alveolar air spaces surround collapsible capillaries, intrapleural and alveolar pressures affect pulmonary capillary pressures. Pulmonary blood flow reflects this influence during respiration and in the upright position (see above and Chap. 6).

Perfusion—Ventilation Matching

Pulmonary precapillary vasomotor and bronchiolar responses serve to match pulmonary capillary perfusion to alveolar ventilation. Unlike in the systemic circulation where hypoxemia, decreased pH, or increased amounts of carbon dioxide cause local vasodilation, in the pulmonary vascular system any of these conditions may cause pulmonary arteriolar vasoconstriction. However, the precapillary blood vessels are immediately adjacent to respiratory bronchioles that sense the partial pressure of oxygen in the air passages. In regions that are well ventilated there is little vasoconstriction in response to deoxygenated blood. In poorly ventilated areas where the amount of alveolar oxygen is less than normal, such as when a bronchus is obstructed, vasoconstriction occurs and blood is shunted to other lung areas.[13] When blood flow to a certain lung area is reduced, this decreases the alveolar carbon dioxide concentration in the alveolus. The bronchial smooth muscle responds to the decreased

alveolar carbon dioxide levels by constricting, thus shifting ventilation away from a poorly perfused area.[9]

If the mismatch is of significant magnitude, these compensatory mechanisms are not adequate to prevent inequalities in ventilation and perfusion. Hypoxemia results if compensation is not adequate (Chap. 51).

Alveolar—Capillary Transfer of Oxygen and Carbon Dioxide

Each gas in a mixture of gases behaves as if it alone occupied the total volume and exerts a partial pressure that is independent of the other gases present. Gases equilibrate across the alveolar—capillary membranes by simple passive diffusion, moving from the area of their greater partial pressure to the region of their lesser partial pressure.

The partial pressure of oxygen in pulmonary arterial blood (which is venous blood from the body) is approximately 40 mm Hg whereas pulmonary alveolar partial pressures of oxygen are approximately 100 mm Hg, so oxygen moves into the blood. The partial pressure of systemic arterial oxygen is slightly less than 100 mm Hg, however, because blood from pulmonary veins is mixed with some deoxygenated blood from bronchial veins and from Thebesian veins draining cardiac muscle tissue (Chap. 1).

Carbon dioxide is removed in the pulmonary capillary. The partial pressure of carbon dioxide in pulmonary arterial blood (systemic venous blood) is 46 mm Hg and that of blood leaving the lung (which becomes systemic arterial blood) is 40 mm Hg.

Transport of Oxygen and Carbon Dioxide

Oxygen. At the normal systemic arterial oxygen partial pressure (PaO_2) of approximately 97 mm Hg, each 100 ml of blood contains approximately 19.7 ml of oxygen. Approximately 0.3 ml of this oxygen is in physical solution and 19.4 ml is carried within the red blood cells, chemically bound to hemoglobin (Hb). Thus, most of the total oxygen normally carried by the blood is bound to hemoglobin, in a relationship that is described by the oxygen—hemoglobin dissociation curve (Fig. 5-13).

Hemoglobin is a protein of four subunits of porphyrin and iron. Each of the four units can bind one molecule of oxygen. Thus four molecules of oxygen are carried by one molecule of hemoglobin when the hemoglobin is completely (100%) saturated. Oxygenation of the first heme unit in the hemoglobin molecule increases the affinity of the unit for oxygen, that is the affinity of the last heme unit for oxygen is much greater than the affinity of the first unit for oxygen.

Thus, it is easier for oxygen to combine with hemoglobin when the hemoglobin is already partially saturated with oxygen. This is the situation that occurs in the lung, so that at a normal PaO_2 of 95 to 97 mm Hg, the hemoglobin is 97% saturated. The flat shape of the upper portion of the curve in Figure 5-13 means that at a PaO_2 of 80 or 90 mm Hg, oxygen transport by hemoglobin cannot be greatly increased by increasing the concentration of oxygen in the lung.

It is less difficult for oxygen to be given up by hemoglobin if the hemoglobin is only partially saturated with oxygen. As

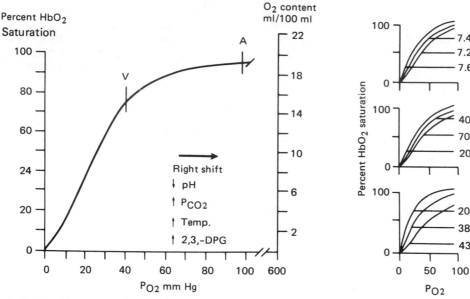

Fig. 5-13. The oxygen–hemoglobin dissociation curve illustrates the relationship between the partial pressure of oxygen (PO_2) and the percentage of oxyhemoglobin (HbO_2) saturation. (**A**) indicates the situation in the lungs and (**V**) indicates the situation in venous blood returning from the tissues; see text for discussion. The small insets on the right indicate the effects of pH, PCO_2, and temperature. (Smith JJ, Kampine JP: *Circulatory Physiology—the Essentials*, p 9. Baltimore, Williams & Wilkins, 1980)

oxygenated blood is transported to the tissues and begins to give up oxygen, it becomes increasingly easy for the oxygen to be released by hemoglobin, that is, the downward slope of the curve in Figure 5-13 becomes increasingly steep.[12] The point where the curve changes from flat to steep (approximately PaO_2 60 mm Hg) is important because at this point any further decrease in the oxygen partial pressure results in a big decrease in hemoglobin oxygen saturation and consequently in tissue oxygenation.

Deoxygenated blood returning to the lungs with a PaO_2 of 40 mm Hg has a hemoglobin saturation of approximately 75% and an oxygen content of approximately 15 ml/100 ml blood. Thus, under normal conditions, there is a reserve of oxygen available for cells that increase their activity (Chap. 6).

Several factors alter the affinity of hemoglobin for oxygen. An increased temperature or a decreased pH causes hemoglobin to require a higher PaO_2 to bind a given amount of oxygen. These relationships can be expressed by other curves that can be drawn to the right of the "normal" curve in Figure 5-13. Hemoglobin appears to lose oxygen more easily in the tissues under these conditions. This is helpful in situations of active metabolism such as exercise. Conversely, under conditions of alkalosis or decreased temperature, hemoglobin appears to lose oxygen less easily in the tissues than normally.

The concentration of 2,3 diphosphoglycerate (2,3-DPG), a product of glycolysis present in red blood cells, also affects the hemoglobin–oxygen affinity. Increases in red cell 2,3-DPG occur at high altitudes and with anemia and seem to facilitate the delivery of oxygen to the tissues. Banked blood that is stored with acid–citrate–dextrose solution has decreased amounts of 2,3-DPG and consequently has a decreased ability to release oxygen to the tissues.

Shifts in the oxygen–hemoglobin dissociation curve affect events in the tissues more than in the lungs, because the relationships in the lungs are described in the flat upper position of the curve.[12] A frequently used index of right and left shifts of the dissociation curve is the P_{50}, which is the PaO_2 at which hemoglobin is 50% saturated. A P_{50} that is higher than normal means a lower than normal affinity for oxygen.

Carbon Dioxide. Carbon dioxide is carried in the blood by three mechanisms. Approximately 6% of the total is carried in physical solution, 4% to 5% combines with hemoglobin, and most of it combines with hydrogen to form bicarbonate (see Chap. 9).

REFERENCES

The selections marked with an asterisk (*) are helpful for further reading.

1. Altura BT, Altura BM: Factors affecting vascular responsiveness. In Kaley G, Altura BM (eds): Microcirculation, Vol. II, pp. 547–615. Baltimore, University Park Press, 1978
2. Bader H: The anatomy and physiology of the vascular wall. In Hamilton WF, Dow P (eds): Handbook of Physiology, Sec 2: Circulation, Vol II, pp. 865–887. Washington, DC, American Physiological Society, 1962
3. Berne RM, Levy, MN: Cardiovascular Physiology, 3rd ed., pp. 53–74; pp. 99–136. St Louis, CV Mosby, 1977*
4. Bloom W, Fawcett DW: A Textbook of Histology, 10th ed., pp. 386–412. Philadelphia, WB Saunders, 1975
5. Bohr DF, Greenberg S, Bonaccorsi A: Mechanisms of action of vasoactive agents. In Kaley G, Altura BM (eds): Microcirculation, Vol II, pp. 311–348. Baltimore, University Park Press, 1978

6. Burch GE: A Primer of Venous Pressure. Springfield, Ill, Charles C Thomas, 1972

7. Burton AC: Physical principles of circulatory phenomena: The physical equilibria of the heart and blood vessels. In Hamilton WF, Dow P (eds): Handbook of Physiology, Sec 2: Circulation, Vol I, pp 85–106. Washington, DC, American Physiological Society, 1962

8. Burton AC: Relation of structure to function of the tissues of the wall of blood vessels. Physiol Rev 34(4):619–642, 1954

9. Comroe JH: Physiology of Respiration, pp 160–166. Chicago, Year Book, 1965

10. Crone C, Christensen O: Transcapillary transport of small solutes and water. In Guyton AC, Young DB (eds): International Review of Physiology III, Vol. 18 pp 149–213. Baltimore, University Park Press, 1979

11. Feigl EO: Physics of the cardiovascular system; The arterial system. In Ruch TC, Patton HD (eds): Physiology and Biophysics II, pp. 10–22; 117–128. Philadelphia, WB Saunders, 1974

12. Finch CA, and Lenfant C: Oxygen transport in man. N Engl J Med 286(8):407–415, 1972

13. Folkow B, Neil E: Circulation, pp 3–145. London, Oxford University Press, 1971

14. Goss CM: Gray's Anatomy, pp 765–769. Philadelphia, Lea & Febiger, 1959

15. Green JF: Determinants of systemic blood flow. In Guyton AC, Young DB (eds): International Review of Physiology III Vol. 18 pp 33–65. Baltimore, University Park Press, 1979

16. Green JF: Mechanical Concepts in Cardiovascular and Pulmonary Physiology, pp 3–63. Philadelphia, Lea & Febiger, 1977*

17. Henry JP, Meehan JP: The Circulation: An Integrative Physiologic Study. Chicago, Year Book, 1971

18. Johnson PC: Peripheral Circulation, pp 1–11. New York, John Wiley & Sons, 1978

19. Kaley G: Microcirculatory–endocrine interactions: Role of prostaglandins. In Kaley G, Altura BM (eds): Microcirculation, Vol II, pp. 503–529. Baltimore, University Park Press, 1978

20. Landis EM, Pappenheimer JR: Exchange of substances through the capillary walls. In Hamilton WF, Dow P (eds): Handbook of Physiology, Sec 2: Circulation, Vol II, pp 961–1034. Washington, DC, American Physiological Society, 1963

21. Lenfant C: Pulmonary circulation. In Ruch TC, Patton HD (eds): Physiology and Biophysics II, pp 277–284. Philadelphia, WB Saunders, 1974

22. Liebman PR, Patten MT, Manny J et al: The mechanism of depressed cardiac output on positive end-expiratory pressure (PEEP). Surgery 83(5):594–598, 1978

23. Milnor WR: Pulmonary hemodynamics. In Bergel DH (ed): Cardiovascular Fluid Dynamics, Vol 2, pp 299–340. London, Academic Press, 1972

24. O'Rourke MF: The arterial pulse in health and disease. Am Heart J, 82(5):687–702, 1971

25. Remington JW, O'Brien LJ: Construction of aortic flow pulse from pressure pulse. Am J Physiol 218(2):437–447, 1970

26. Robotham JL, Lixfield W, Holland L et al: Effects of respiration on cardiac performance. J Appl Physiol 44(5):703–709, 1978

27. Rushmer RF: Cardiovascular Dynamics, 4th ed, pp 1–75. Philadelphia, WB Saunders, 1976*

28. Shepherd JT, Vanhoutte PM: The Human Cardiovascular System: Facts and Concepts, pp 1–106. New York, Raven Press, 1979*

29. Smith JJ, Kampine JP: Circulatory Physiology: The Essentials, a, pp 1–20; b, pp 53–72; c, pp 129–161. Baltimore, Williams & Wilkins, 1980*

30. Sparks HV, Belloni FL: The peripheral circulation: Local regulation. Annu Rev Physiol 40(1186):67–92, 1978

31. Stehbens WE: Anatomy and structure of blood vessels. In Hemodynamics and the Blood Vessel Wall, pp 3–74. Springfield, Ill, Charles C Thomas, 1979

32. Wiederhielm CA: The capillaries, veins, and lymphatics. In Ruch TC, Patton HD (eds): Physiology and Biophysics II, pp 129–145. Philadelphia, WB Saunders, 1974

33. Zweifach BW, Silberberg A: The interstitial–lymphatic flow system. In Guyton AC, Young DB (eds): International Review of Physiology III, Vol. 18 pp 215–260. Baltimore, University Park Press, 1979

ADDITIONAL READING

Crouch JE: Functional Human Anatomy, 3rd ed., pp 427–462; 463–469. Philadelphia, Lea & Febiger, 1978

Ganong WF: Review of Medical Physiology, 9th ed, pp 443–456. Los Altos, Calif, Lange, 1979

Scharf SM, Ingram RH: Influence of abdominal pressure and sympathetic vasoconstriction on the cardiovascular response to positive end-expiratory pressure. Am Rev Respir Dis 116:661–670, 1977

Schwartz CJ, Werthessen NT, Wolf S: Structure and Function of the Circulation, Vol. 1, pp 537–630; 729–803. New York, Plenum Press, 1980

Vander AJ, Sherman JH, Luciano DS: Human Physiology, 2nd ed, pp 280–300. New York, McGraw-Hill, 1980

West JB: Respiratory Physiology: The Essentials, 2nd ed. pp 32–78. Baltimore, Williams & Wilkins, 1979

West JB(ed): Pulmonary Gas Exchange, Vol. I. New York, Academic Press, 1980

6

Regulation of Cardiac Output and Blood Pressure

CAROL JEAN HALPENNY, R.N., M.A.

Life is dependent on the integrated functioning of the cardiovascular system. Tissue blood supply needs are continuously changing even at rest; blood flow to different regions of the body must continuously be altered to meet these needs. Sensors in the tissue respond to changes in pressure, blood gas composition, and other factors and either transmit this information to the central nervous system, initiate local responses, or both.

The focus of this chapter is summarized in Figure 6-1, which illustrates the major factors and relationships that influence cardiac output and blood pressure. Local or intrinsic peripheral vascular regulation functions to maintain flow to an area in proportion to that area's needs through local changes in vascular resistance and perfusion pressure (see Chap. 5). Local autoregulation may override central nervous system influences. The heart has intrinsic mechanisms that respond to local conditions; for example, the strength of ventricular contraction is increased in response to increases in diastolic volume (see Chap. 2).

The central nervous system coordinates cardiac output, blood pressure, and vascular resistance responses to maintain cardiovascular equilibrium and to provide for the integrated functioning of the organism as a whole. Because cardiac output equals perfusion pressure divided by vascular resistance (see Chap. 5), alterations in one of these factors must be compensated for by coordinated alterations in one or both of the other factors in order to adjust appropriately to changing situations. Cardiac output is dependent upon venous return; changes in arterial resistance affect the distribution of the cardiac output to the tissues, whereas changes in venous capacitance affect the volume of blood in the central circulation.[20]

CENTRAL NERVOUS SYSTEM INTEGRATION

Sensory or afferent fibers from the blood vessels, the heart, the lungs, and other tissue transmit impulses from stretch receptors, chemoreceptors, and other types of receptors to the brain stem, hypothalamus, and other areas of the brain where cardiovascular reflex responses are mediated. Motor or efferent fibers act on cardiac and vascular smooth muscle cells to influence heart rate, myocardial contractility, arterial resistance, and venous capacitance.

The motor section of the nervous system is composed of the involuntary or autonomic system and the voluntary, somatic, or skeletal muscle motor system. The autonomic nervous system, the motor section of the nervous system primarily concerned with the maintenance of essential body functions, has two major anatomic subdivisions: sympathetic or adrengeric nerves that usually secrete norepinephrine from terminal nerve endings, and parasympathetic or cholinergic nerves that secrete acetylcholine from terminal nerve endings. Both subdivisions of the autonomic nervous system consist of at least two nerves in series: preganglionic fibers that exit from the brain or spinal cord and, using acetylcholine as the neurotransmitter, make synaptic connections in ganglia outside the central nervous system with postganglionic fibers. Besides their effects on the heart and vascular smooth muscle, autonomic nerves have numerous effects on smooth muscle of the gastrointestinal, genitourinary, and respiratory tracts, the eye, and other organs (Table 6-1, Fig. 6-2). Afferent and efferent nerves often travel together in nerve plexuses that accompany arteries and veins. Neurotransmitters secreted by nerve endings or

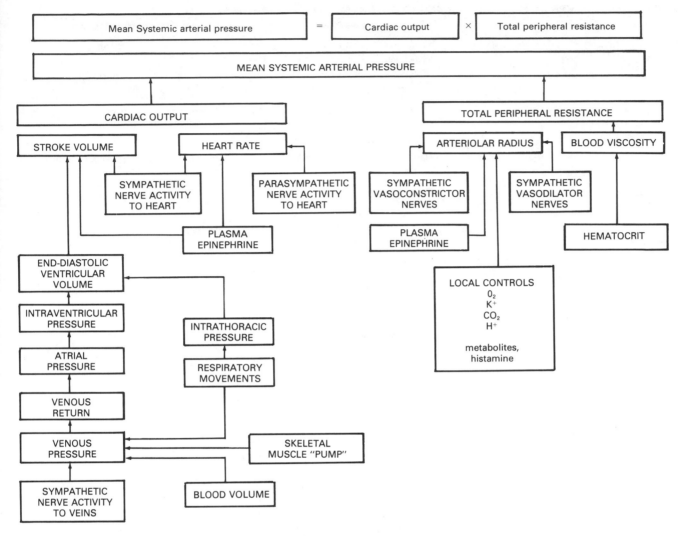

| Mean Systemic arterial pressure | = | Cardiac output | × | Total peripheral resistance |

Fig. 6-1. Summary of effector mechanisms and efferent pathways that regulate systemic arterial pressure. (Vander A, Sherman JH, Luciano DS: Human Physiology, 3rd ed, pp 304, 305. New York, McGraw-Hill, 1980)

glands interact with effector cells to convey information from nerves to other nerves, muscles, and glands.

Peripheral sensory information received in the brain stem and other centers is relayed throughout the brain by complex networks of interneurons that eventually excite or inhibit autonomic outflow with a resultant effect on cardiovascular functioning. Although it is useful to simplify the discussion of these interactions by considering specific responses to be limited to certain groups of cell bodies and nerve fiber tracts, research continues to demonstrate further interactions between cardiovascular responses that were formerly considered to be specific and discrete.[27] Chemical neurotransmitters that participate in exciting or inhibiting receptors of succeeding interneurons in the brain and spinal cord include norepinephrine, epinephrine, dopamine, 5-hydroxytryptamine (serontonin), and acetylcholine.[43]

The solitary tract nucleus in the brain stem is the major site of reception of afferent impulses from arterial and cardiac stretch receptors; most chemoreceptor impulses also appear to terminate here (Fig. 6-3).[26,27] Impulses are relayed from the solitary tract nucleus to parasympathetic and sympathetic brain-stem outflow areas, the hypothalamus, and other areas of the brain.[26]

Cells in and adjacent to the ambiguous nucleus in the medullary area of the brain stem are collectively termed the vagal nucleus and are major sites for parasympathetic outflow. Because parasympathetic excitation has a generally depressant cardiac effect, this area has been referred to as the cardioinhibitory area.[27,43]

The paramedian nucleus and adjacent areas in the brain-stem reticular formation are major areas for sympathetic outflow; this area is sometimes termed the vasomotor center (Fig. 6-3). In the past this area has been referred to as the cardioexcitatory center; however, that term is inexact because inhibitory as well as excitatory effects on sympathetic activity are initiated here.[43]

The hypothalamus receives and sends information relating to cardiovascular function to and from the brain stem, the thalamus, the cerebral cortex, and other areas. The hypothalamus participates in temperature regulation, the secretion of antidiuretic hormone, and exercise and emotional responses.

TABLE 6-1 RESPONSES OF EFFECTOR ORGANS TO AUTONOMIC NERVE IMPULSES

EFFECTOR ORGAN	RECEPTOR TYPE*	Adrenergic Impulses RESPONSE	Cholinergic Impulses RESPONSE
Eye	α	Mydriasis	Miosis
Heart	β	↑ Heart rate, automaticity ↑ Conduction velocity ↑ Contractility	↓ Heart rate, automaticity ↓ Conduction velocity ↓ Contractility
Vascular smooth muscle	α	Arterial and venous vasoconstriction	Vasodilation in coronary and skeletal muscle arteries
	β	Vasodilation in coronary, skeletal muscle, and hepatic arteries	
Lung	β	Bronchial muscle relaxation	Bronchial muscle contraction, bronchial glandular secretion

Stomach
  Sphincters
  Motility
	
	α
	β
		
		Contraction
		Decreased
			
			Relaxation
			Increased

Intestine
  Sphincters
  Motility & tone
  Secretion
	
	α, β
		
		Contraction
		Decreased
			
			Relaxation (usually)
			Increased
			Stimulation

Urinary bladder
  Detrusor muscle (bladder emptying)
  Sphincter
	
	β
	
	α
		
		Relaxation (usually)
		
		Contraction
			
			Contraction
			
			Relaxation

Skin
  Pilomotor muscles
  Sweat glands
	
	α
	α
		
		Contraction
		Palmar secretion
			
			Generalized secretion

Liver	α, β	Glycogenolysis, gluconeogenesis	

* Beta adrenergic receptor sites in the heart have been classified as β_1 receptors; in most other tissues, they have been identified as β_2 receptors.

(Adapted from Goodman AG, Goodman LS, Gilman A: The Pharmacological Basis of Therapeutics, 6th ed. pp 60–61. New York, Macmillan, 1980)

Cerebellar participation in cardiovascular reflexes has been demonstrated.[27] The cerebellum also coordinates input from the vestibular apparatus of the ear that is involved in spatial orientation reflexes; the response to spatial changes often involves cardiovascular changes.[27,43]

The cerebral cortex participates in cardiovascular functioning through complex pathways. Cerebral cortical perception of sensations such as pain can initiate responses that eventually affect blood pressure, heart rate, or cardiac contractility. Stimulation of certain areas of the motor cortex has resulted in decreases in blood pressure and heart rate; the clinical relevance of these effects is being investigated in relation to the use of relaxation techniques or biofeedback for volitional control of cardiovascular function (see Chaps. 22 and 47).[27]

EFFERENT NERVOUS ACTIVITY

Adrenergic (Sympathetic) Nerves

Axons of interneurons from sympathetic brain-stem areas travel by way of the bulbospinal tract in the intermediolateral column of the spinal cord to preganglionic fibers whose cell bodies are located in the anterior horns of the thoracolumbar segments of the spinal cord (Fig. 6-3). These interneurons from the brain stem to the spinal cord appear to excite or inhibit preganglionic sympathetic nerves and thus modulate the adrenergic outflow from the spinal cord.[27,43] Most sympathetic ganglia lie in a chain close to the spinal cord, so usually sympathetic preganglionic fibers are short and postganglionic fibers are long (Fig. 6-2).

Distribution. Adrenergic fibers to the heart arise mainly from the second, third, and fourth thoracic segments of the spinal cord.[30,36] Most of these fibers connect with postganglionic fibers in the stellate ganglion. Most postganglionic adrenergic nerves to the heart travel by way of the superior, middle, and inferior cardiac nerves; however, several cardiac nerves with variable locations have been identified.[29,30,36] Fibers from the right sympathetic ganglia appear to innervate the sinus node, the right atrium, and the anterior ventricular walls, whereas fibers from the left sympathetic ganglia innervate the atrioventricular node and the posterior and inferior left ventricles.[36]

Postganglionic adrenergic nerves are distributed widely to most blood vessels (Fig. 6-3). The most dense distribution is to areas that are the most responsive to neurohumoral control, such as the arterioles of the splanchnic (gastrointestinal, spleen, and liver) circulation and skeletal muscle, the afferent arterioles of the kidney, and the splanchnic and cutaneous veins.[1,25,43]

Alpha and Beta Adrenergic Effects. The differential response to specific blocking agents of adrenergic receptor sites on effector cells has led to the classification of alpha (α) and beta (β) adrenergic receptors, although no anatomic basis for these different responses has yet been demonstrated (see Table 6-1).[14] Increased α-adrenergic activity in vascular smooth muscle cells results in vasoconstriction of most resistance vessels and in splanchnic and cutaneous veno-

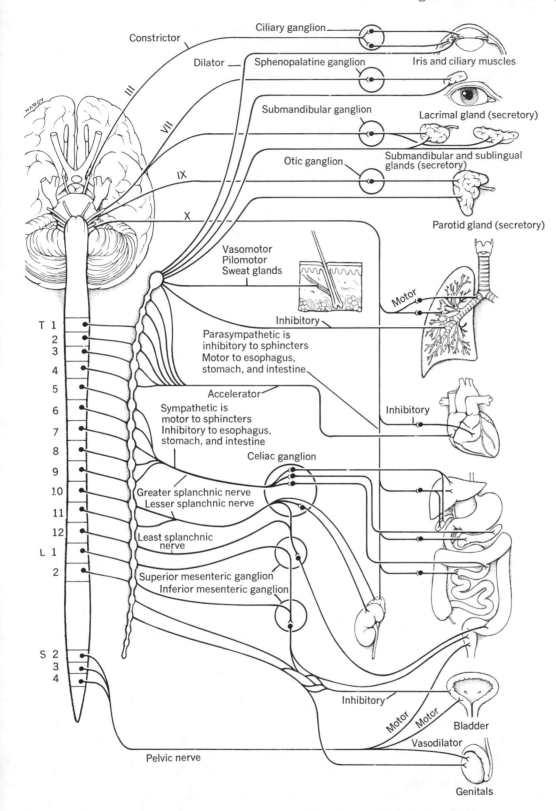

Fig. 6-2. The autonomic nervous system. Parasympathetic (craniosacral) fibers have long preganglionic fibers that synapse with short postganglionic fibers in ganglia located close to the innervated organs. Sympathetic (thoracolumbar) fibers have relatively short preganglionic fibers that synapse with long postganglionic fibers in the paravertebral and other ganglia. (Rodman MJ, Smith DW: Pharmacology and Drug Therapy in Nursing, 2nd ed, p 318. Philadelphia, JB Lippincott, 1979)

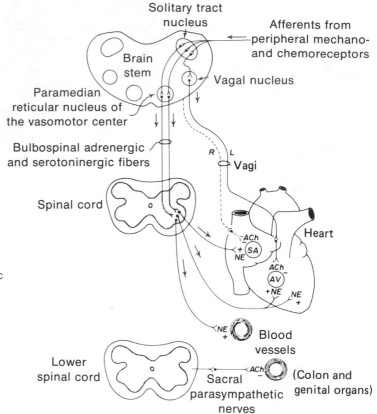

Fig. 6-3. Major origins and distributions of the adrenergic and cholinergic nerves to the cardiovascular system (see text for details). Not shown are vagal fibers that innervate blood vessels and nerve fibers that originate in higher centers, relay in the hypothalamus, travel with sympathetic (adrenergic) nerves, innervate skeletal muscle arterial vessels, and release acetylcholine under the influence of strong emotion. *ACh* = acetylcholine, *NE* = norepinephrine, *SA* = sinus node, *AV* = atrioventricular node. (Shepherd JT, Vanhoutte PM: *The Human Cardiovascular System: Facts and Concepts*, p 124. New York, Raven Press, 1979)

constriction. Under normal conditions a low level of continuous α-adrenergic activity in conjunction with local factors maintains tonic vaso- and venoconstriction in tissues such as skeletal muscle and the abdominal organs; dilation occurs when there is inhibition of α-mediated tonic constriction in these areas.[1,14]

Beta adrenergic effects have been subdivided into beta$_1$ (β$_1$) and beta$_2$ (β$_2$) responses. β$_1$ responses have major effects on the heart, causing more rapid firing of the sinus node, increased velocity of conduction throughout the conducting system, and an increase in myocardial contractility. β$_2$ receptors cause bronchial smooth muscle dilation and have other noncardiac effects (see Table 6-1).[28] β$_2$ receptors have been shown to cause vasodilation in some vascular smooth muscle cells, such as skeletal muscle, cardiac muscle, and hepatic arterioles.[14,24]

Peripheral Neurohumoral Transmitters. Norepinephrine, epinephrine, and dopamine are among the catechol-containing group of sympathomimetic amines that are collectively termed catecholamines (see Chap. 35). Most of the norepinephrine present in the plasma is synthesized from dopamine and stored in vesicles near adrenergic nerve endings. Norepinephrine activates adrenergic receptors on effector cells when released from the nerve endings. Norepinephrine has α and β$_1$ effects. Norepinephrine appears to promote the influx of calcium into myocardial and vascular smooth muscle cells and to increase the release of intracellular calcium stores, which in turn promotes muscle contraction (see Chap. 2).[3,45] Increased calcium influx appears to be one mechanism by which norepinephrine enhances

sinus node firing (see Chap. 3). Part of the released norepinephrine is taken up and stored again by the adrenergic nerve endings and part of it is degraded by enzymatic reactions.

At least some of the cardiac effects of norepinephrine and other catecholamines seem to be due to activation of an enzyme that converts cytoplasmic ATP to cyclic 3′, 5′-adenosine monophosphase (C-AMP). The cyclic AMP then mediates inotropic β-adrenergic activity.[45]

The adrenal medulla in a certain sense functions like a postganglionic sympathetic nerve, because it secretes epinephrine and norepinephrine when activated by acetylcholine from preganglionic sympathetic nerve endings. Epinephrine constitutes 80% of the adrenal medullary catecholamine secretion, whereas norepinephrine constitutes 20%.[43] Epinephrine has mainly α and β$_1$ properties; however, epinephrine in low concentrations can also activate β$_2$ receptors, resulting in vasodilation of skeletal muscle and other arterioles.[43] Epinephrine also increases cellular metabolism, which secondarily stimulates blood flow. Epinephrine is not usually present in the plasma in large amounts except when adrenal medullary catecholamine secretion is increased under stress situations such as during strong emotion, exercise, or hypoglycemia. Circulating epinephrine is mainly destroyed in the liver.[43]

Cholinergic Nerves

Distribution. Most preganglionic cholinergic fibers exit from the medulla by way of the vagus (tenth cranial) nerve or from sacral segments of the spinal cord (see Fig. 6-2).

Parasympathetic ganglia generally lie close to innervated organs, so most preganglionic fibers are long and postganglionic fibers are short. Cardiac branches of the vagus nerve supply the heart with preganglionic parasympathetic fibers. There is a dense supply of vagal fibers to the sinus node, the atrioventricular node, and the ventricular conducting system; consequently, there are many parasympathetic ganglia in the region of the sinus and atrioventricular nodes (Fig. 6-3). Vagal fibers also innervate both atria and to a lesser extent both ventricles.[30,36] Right vagal fibers seem to have more effect on the sinus node and left vagal fibers more effect on the atrioventricular node and ventricular conduction system, but there is overlap.[30]

Branches of the vagus nerve also supply cholingeric fibers to the arteries of the brain, the heart, the tongue, the gastrointestinal system, and the lungs. Sacral fibers supply cholinergic innervation to the arteries of the colon and the genitalia and to veins of erectile tissue.

Effects. Increased vagal activity slows the heart rate and slows conduction through the atrioventricular node and the ventricular conducting system. Cholinergic activity increases the potassium permeability of myocardial conducting tissue leading to increased potassium efflux (see Chap. 3).[30,43] The parasympathetic system seems to be dominant in the control of normal heart rate.[4] It was formerly thought that cholinergic fibers had no effect on ventricular contractility, but increasing evidence seems to indicate that some reduction in ventricular contractile force occurs during cholinergic stimulation.[36]

Cholinergically mediated vasodilation has been demonstrated in coronary, cerebral, and pulmonary arteries; the functional significance of these effects is not yet entirely clear.[10,14] Increased parasympathetic activity to the erectile tissue of the penis and clitoris causes arteriolar vasodilation and venous constriction, creating vascular congestion.[43]

Release of polypeptide kinins appears to be partly responsible for the vasodilation and increased capillary permeability seen during parasympathetic cholinergically stimulated glandular secretion in salivary glands. Acetylcholine is inactivated by the enzyme acetylcholinesterase.

Sympathetic Cholinergic Nerves. There are cholinergic nerves that arise in the cerebral cortex, form synaptic connections in the hypothalamus, bypass the brain-stem cardiovascular centers, form synaptic connections again in the sympathetic ganglia, and travel with sympathetic nerves to skeletal muscle arterioles. These fibers seem to be excited by emotional stress or by the anticipation of exercise; they appear to secrete acetylcholine and to cause vasodilation. Although these fibers have been shown to cause significant vasodilation during exercise in animals, the extent of their effect on skeletal muscle vasodilation in humans continues to be debated.[1,37,43] Sweat glands are supplied by sympathetic nerves but secrete acetylcholine from postganglionic terminals.[2]

PERIPHERAL SENSORS AND CARDIOVASCULAR REFLEXES

Arterial Baroreceptor Reflex

Specialized nerve tissue in the wall of both internal carotid arteries at the point where the internal carotids bifurcate from the common carotids and in the wall of the aortic arch is sensitive to stretch. This tissue increases its rate of discharge when it is stretched by blood pressure elevations. Because these nerve cells respond to mechanical factors, they are frequently referred to as aortic and carotid mechanoreceptors; because the stretch is caused by pressure

Fig. 6-4. Outline of the arterial baroreceptor reflex response. When the blood pressure changes, stretch receptors principally in the carotid sinus alter their rate of discharge to the medulla. The medullary centers alter the frequencies of vagal and sympathetic nerve impulses, which in turn affects heart rate, peripheral resistance, and, to some extent, stroke volume. The blood pressure is ultimately maintained within a "normal" range. *Dotted lines* indicate neural connections. (Ruch TC, Patton HD: *Physiology and Biophysics II*, p 150. Philadelphia, WB Saunders, 1974)

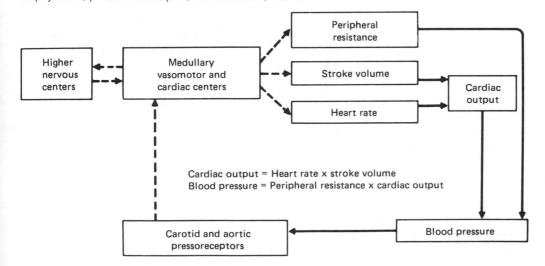

Cardiac output = Heart rate x stroke volume
Blood pressure = Peripheral resistance x cardiac output

changes, the receptors are often referred to as baroreceptors or pressoreceptors. The increased nerve activity is transmitted over the glossopharyngeal (ninth cranial) nerve from the carotid and over the vagus (tenth cranial) nerve from the aorta to the cardiovascular areas in the brain stem, where it initiates an increase in parasympathetic activity and a decrease in sympathetic activity. Consequently, the heart rate and vaso- and venoconstriction are decreased. This combined response thus decreases both cardiac output and peripheral resistance, working in a coordinated way to return the blood pressure to its previous levels (Fig. 6-4).[40] There is controversy regarding whether decreases in myocardial contractility are as influential in this reflex response as previously believed.[1,4,13] The parasympathetic heart rate response occurs in 3 to 4 seconds; it is more rapid and more influential in the situation of increased pressure than is the sympathetic response, which occurs in approximately 20 seconds.[40]

When the baroreceptors sense a decreased blood pressure, sympathetic responses result in an accelerated heart rate and adrenergically mediated vaso- and venoconstriction.[1,40] The arterial baroreceptors seem to be relatively more effective in compensating for a fall in arterial pressure than a rise in pressure.[26]

Although the arterial baroreceptors respond to changes in both the mean blood pressure and the pulse pressure between approximately 70 and 180 mm Hg, the receptors are most responsive during periods of changing blood pressure.[8,13,43] The aortic receptors seem to be relatively inactive within the ranges of normal pressure; they respond to higher pressures.[13,35]

Within 3 to 4 days of continued high blood pressures, the baroreceptors show adaptation, that is, they are "reset" to respond from a higher mean pressure baseline.[8,13] Because the arterial baroreceptors are not particularly responsive at very low or very high pressures and because they show adaptation to continued high pressure, the receptors are unable to compensate for extreme situations such as profound shock or sustained hypertension. However, they are extremely important in the minute-to-minute maintenance of cardiovascular stability during normal activities.[13]

Cardiac and Respiratory Mechanoreceptor Responses

There are stretch receptors located in the right atrium close to the entrances of the venae cavae, in the left atrium close to the entrances of the pulmonary veins, and throughout all cardiac chambers that are connected to brain-stem cardiovascular areas by afferent nerves that accompany the vagal nerve. The receptors at the venoatrial junctions respond to central or pulmonary venous volume changes, so these receptors are variously referred to as volume, low-pressure, or stretch receptors. A sympathetically mediated increase in heart rate and other responses similar to arterial baroreceptors responses follow mechanical distention of venoatrial receptors.[6,31,33,47]

Vagal afferent stretch receptors from ventricular muscle have been shown in experimental situations to initiate reflex slowing of the heart rate and a fall in blood pressure.[1] Afferent fibers throughout the heart, which travel with sympathetic nerves to the spinal cord, seem to convey pain and other sensations.[6,12] There are stretch receptors in the lungs that affect cardiovascular functioning.[1,25,33,41]

Renal Effects of Arterial and Cardiac Mechanoreceptor Activity

Antidiuretic Hormone Release. Renal diuresis seems to accompany distention of venoatrial mechanoreceptors.[6] Results from several investigations have indicated that moderate distention of atrial stretch receptors, such as occurs with increases in central venous volume, inhibits the release of antidiuretic hormone (ADH) by the posterior pituitary, which in turn by the action of ADH on the renal collecting duct promotes diuresis (see Chap. 9).[1,6,31,42] The arterial baroreceptors have also been shown to influence ADH release and to interact with the cardiac receptors.[42] The central nervous system links between atrial stretch receptors and the hypothalamus have not been clearly identified, so the existence of a relationship between the atrial mechanoreceptors and ADH release has been challenged.[6,31]

Renin Release. Decreased arterial and cardiac baroreceptor firing in response to lowered blood pressure has been shown to increase the transmission of impulses from sympathetic brain-stem areas to the kidney. This causes vasoconstriction of the afferent renal arteriole, leading to a decrease in renal blood flow, which in turn promotes renin release by the renal juxtaglomerular cells. A direct effect of adrenergic activity in promoting renin release has also been demonstrated.[9,11,46] Increased renin secretion initiates the renin–angiotensin–aldosterone response in which sodium is retained by the kidney, with a resultant increase in water retention (see Chap. 9).

Cardiovascular Effects of ADH and Angiotensin. The primary effects of baroreceptor-mediated ADH and renin release are on renal volume regulation; blood volume changes then affect cardiovascular function. Vasopressin (ADH) is a potent vasoconstrictor, but in the concentrations normally present in the plasma it exerts minimal direct effects on blood pressure.[19]

The concentration of angiotensin II normally present in the blood is small, and it was formerly considered to have little direct effect on vasoconstriction.[34] However, it is increasingly apparent that angiotensin affects blood pressure in several ways, for example, by enhancing the effects of epinephrine on vascular smooth muscle cells and by increasing blood pressure through direct effects on the brain.[16,43] The effects of angiotensin seem to become influential in situations of volume depletion and congestive heart failure.[22]

Chemoreceptor Responses

The carotid and aortic bodies are groups of nerve receptors close to the arterial stretch receptors that are sensitive to chemical stimuli. There are also chemoreceptor centers in the medullary area of the brain stem. Increases in plasma carbon dioxide or hydrogen ion concentrations or decreases in oxygen content sensed by the chemoreceptors initiate reflex increases in respiratory rate and depth. The cardiovascular responses to chemoreceptor stimulation are complex, reflecting interactions between peripheral and central chemoreceptors, respiratory responses, and baroreceptor responses.[7] The cardiac chemoreceptor responses may be important in severe hemorrhage accompanied by hypotension and hypoxia.

Vagally mediated bradycardia and decreased myocardial contractility occur when the cardiac effects of the chemoreceptor reflex can be observed without superimposed respiratory effects.[7,15,40] This occurs during the diving reflex, in which the head is submerged under water and there are no respirations. In this situation, cardiac depression is helpful in protecting the myocardium, because hypoxia cannot be alleviated by increased respirations.[7,15,40]

Other Cardiovascular Reflex Responses

Sensory input from the vestibular apparatus in the semicircular ear canals, from the abdominal organs, from muscles, joints, and elsewehere affect cardiovascular responses. Spinal cord reflex arcs affecting cardiovascular function are usually influenced by input from higher centers. When this input is cut off, for example by spinal cord transsection, sensory input from a distended bladder, muscle spasms, or pain can lead to reflex vasoconstriction in areas below the level of the cord lesion.[27] Cardiovascular responses to emotional stress are discussed in Chapter 11.

Temperature Regulation Responses

Cardiovascular function is affected during the reflexes initiated in response to central or peripheral temperature changes. When the cells of the hypothalamus sense an increase in body core temperature reflected in the blood perfusing the hypothalamus, hypothalamic reflex input to cardiovascular outflow centers in the brain stem initiates dilation of cutaneous arterioles and veins and the opening of direct arteriovenous channels between small skin arteries and veins. Blood is shunted to the skin, where heat is then lost by radiation, conduction, and, with sweating, by convection.[38] The opposite effects occur in response to cold, with vasoconstriction and constriction of arteriovenous anastomoses.

CARDIOVASCULAR RESERVE

Cardiac and Cardiovascular Reserve

At rest and during daily activities, an individual uses only a small amount of his cardiovascular functional capacity. The difference between the amount of oxygen used at rest and during maximal physical stress illustrates the reserve capacity of the cardiovascular system (see Chap.7). An individual's maximal achievable cardiac output determines his cardiac reserve capability and is achieved by increasing heart rate, stroke volume, or both, by intrinsic and neurohumoral mechanisms (Fig. 6-5) (see Chap. 2). In addition to increasing cardiac output, the body can redistribute blood flow to rapidly metabolizing tissue and extract more oxygen

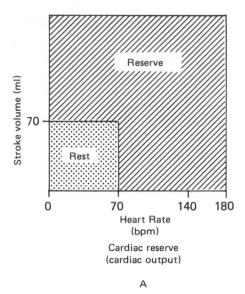

A

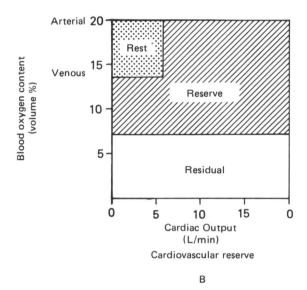

B

Fig. 6-5. Cardiac and cardiovascular reserve. **(A)** Cardiac reserve. Cardiac output can be increased by increasing stroke volume or heart rate, or both. **(B)** Cardiovascular reserve. Oxygen delivery to the tissues is determined by the product of the arteriovenous oxygen difference and the cardiac output. Residual oxygen remains in the mixed venous blood even at maximal levels of oxygen transport. (Rushmer RF: Cardiovascular Dynamics, p 270. Philadelphia, WB Saunders, 1976)

from the blood; collectively these mechanisms constitute the cardiovascular reserve capacity (Fig. 6-5) (see also Table 7-1).

Blood-flow redistribution involves the interaction of local and neurohumoral factors. Neural responses are faster than intrinsic vasomotor responses.[21] In situations of moderate physical stress, such as moderate hemorrhage, neural control is able to divert blood flow to vital areas such as the heart and brain. Under extreme physical stress, such as irreversible shock or maximal exercise in a hot environment, intrinsic local controls may override integrative neural controls.

TABLE 6-2 REGIONAL BLOOD FLOW AND OXYGEN UPTAKE AT REST

Tissue	Blood Flow* ml/min	Blood Flow* ml/min/100g	% Total CO	Oxygen Uptake ml/min/100g	A-VO$_2$ Difference ml/100 ml
Myocardium	250 (1200)	80 (400)	5	8	10
Brain	750 (1500)	55	14	3	6
Kidney	1200 (1500)	400 (500)	22	5	1.3
Skeletal muscle	900 (18000)	3 (60)	20	0.2	5
Skin	200 (3000)	10 (180)	6	0.2	2.5
Liver	1500 (3000)	60 (150) ⎱	23	2	6
GI Tract	1000 (5000)	35 (250) ⎰			
WHOLE BODY AVERAGE	5500	8.6	100	0.4	5

* Approximate values for a 70-kg resting male. Numbers in parentheses are approximate maximal flows.
(Slightly modified from Bard P (ed): Medical Physiology, 11th ed. St. Louis, CV Mosby, 1961)

Regional Circulations

Table 6-2 and Figure 6-6 illustrate regional blood flows at rest and during vasodilation. Neural control usually predominates at rest in regional circulations that have wide ranges of metabolism and blood flow. For example, the splanchnic (gastrointestinal) circulation has metabolic fluctuations during digestion, muscle blood flow reflects muscle activity levels, and temperature regulation affects skin blood flow.[32,37,38] Oxygen extraction from the blood perfusing these areas can be altered in response to local needs and changes in blood flow (Chap.7).

The splanchnic, muscle, and skin curculations also have in common an ability to augment central blood volume by mobilization of blood reposing in venous reservoirs. Active venous constriction in the splanchnic area is a major mechanism for providing an autotransfusion of blood into the central circulation. Also, when the venous perfusion pressure is decreased by arteriolar vasoconstriction, the veins passively collapse and venous blood is displaced from them.

Skeletal muscle has the greatest potential range of blood flow of any of the organ circulations; at rest about 15% of total cardiac output goes to muscle, but during exercise the muscle may receive 85% of the cardiac output.[37] Muscle

exhibits more evidence of dual control than does any other vascular bed. At rest, muscle blood flow is predominantly under extrinsic neural control, whereas during exercise local tissue hypoxia or the accumulation of carbon dioxide and lactic acid stimulates local vasodilation.

Skin blood flow also demonstrates dual control in response to temperature changes. Changes in body core temperature intiate reflex responses (above). The cutaneous circulation also responds to local changes; skin blood flow increases in response to elevated skin temperatures and decreases with local cooling within the ranges of cold usually encountered by humans.[38,44] When core temperature and skin temperature change in the same direction (i.e., central and skin heating), the skin blood flow increases are additive, whereas when core temperature and skin temperature change in the opposite direction, the local effects of temperature changes are counteracted by responses to the internal body temperature changes.[38]

Vascular autoregulation due to local control usually predominates in the heart, brain, and kidneys. A constant blood supply to the heart and brain and ultimately to the kidney is necessary for survival. Because the coronary arteries have achieved near-maximal oxygen extraction under resting conditions, increases in coronary blood flow provide the major mechanism by which the oxygen supply to working myocardial muscle can be increased when myocardial oxygen needs are increased (see Chap. 2).

Brain blood flow and oxygen extraction remain relatively constant, even under conditions of extreme stress such as maximal exercise. The arterial carbon dioxide tension seems to be the most important controlling factor for cerebral blood flow, although concurrent changes in hydrogen-ion concentration (pH) have been implicated as equally or more important.[10] An increased PCO$_2$ or decreased pH leads to cerebrovascular vasodilation. A severely decreased PO$_2$ also can lead to vasodilation.

The kidneys receive approximately 25% of the cardiac output at rest, which facilitates fluid, electrolyte, and acid–base regulation (Chap. 9). Under normal conditions, the kidney has a low arteriovenous oxygen difference, because renal blood flow is much greater than renal metabolic needs (see Table 6-2). Renal autoregulation may be overriden by sympathetically mediated vasoconstriction of the afferent renal arterioles. Thus, during physical stress, a large portion of the cardiac output can be diverted away from the kidneys into the central circulation.

Fig. 6-6. Blood flow at rest and during maximum vasodilation: Approximate values for a 70-kg man with a mean arterial perfusion pressure of 100 mm Hg. The *hatched* portions of the bars indicate the blood flow at rest, and the maximum flow is shown by the *total height* of the bars. (Mellander S, Johansson B: Pharmacolog Rev 20:132, 1968)

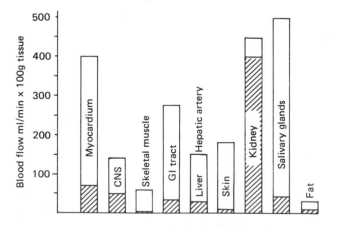

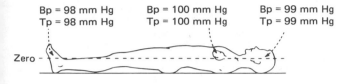

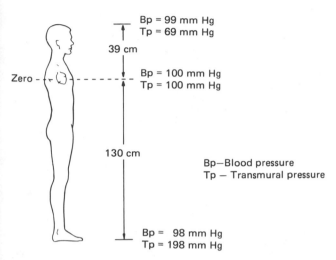

Fig. 6-7. Pressure effects of upright posture. In a closed system, the pressure due to gravitational force counterbalances the pressure change due to gravity. However, the transmural pressure (the force exerted across blood vessel walls) is altered by the height of the column of blood above it. Thus, when an individual is lying down, the transmural pressure equals the blood pressure, but when the individual is standing the transmural pressure above the heart is less and below the heart is greater than the transmural pressure at heart level. (Ruch TC, Patton HD: Physiology and Biophysics II, p 12. Philadelphia, WB Saunders, 1974)

INTEGRATED RESPONSES— POSTURAL CHANGE

Responses to postural change illustrate cardiovascular integration. Pressure in upright fluid columns such as the blood vessels in the standing position equals the height of the fluid column, the density of the blood, and a gravitational constant. When an individual assumes upright posture, the arteriovenous pressure difference is not changed, but transmural arterial and venous pressures are increased in areas below heart level and decreased in areas above heart level (Fig. 6-7). Thus, when pressures are measured in nonsupine positions, they should be reported with reference to heart level (see Chap. 21).

Approximately 500 ml of blood from the heart and lungs is displaced to the legs during standing, with a resulting decrease in venous filling; cardiac output is decreased by 15% to 30% and stroke volume is decreased by 40% to 50%.[18,39] Within 10 to 15 seconds, cardiac and carotid sinus baroreceptor responses compensate for the decreased cardiac output and blood pressure by initiating an increase in heart rate and in systemic vasoconstriciton. The arterial blood pressure is maintained at near resting supine values; however, stroke volume and cardiac output during quiet standing remain less than during supine rest. Renal blood flow decreases and renin secretion increases during upright posture.[46] There is some reduction in splanchnic blood flow.

During prolonged quiet standing, capillary transmural pressures are increased in the legs and the dependent veins are distended; this leads to increased fluid movement from the capillaries into the interstitial tissue.[18,23] Fainting from loss of blood due to this dependent edema can be prevented by moving the legs, which promotes venous return and, by decreasing venous pressures, decreases the capillary pressures that led to the edema (see Chap. 5).[39]

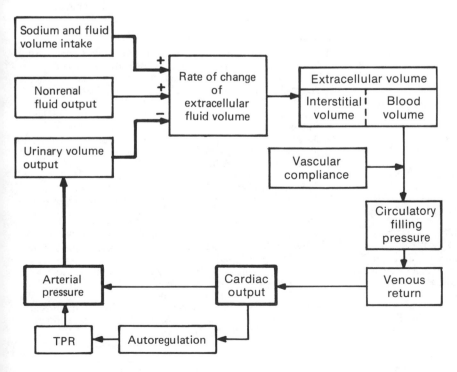

Fig. 6-8. Relationships between arterial pressure and body fluid volume. *TPR =* total peripheral resistance. (Onesti G, Brest AN (eds): Hypertension: Mechanisms, Diagnosis and Treatment, p 8. Philadelphia, FA Davis, 1978)

Blood flow in the lungs is affected by gravitational changes because the pulmonary vessels are compliant and are surrounded by air spaces. Alveolar and tissue hydrostatic pressures are greater than venous pressures in the upper areas of the lung in the upright position. Blood flow in these upper areas becomes a function of arterial and alveolar pressures instead of a function of arterial and venous pressures, so blood flow to the lung bases is greater than to the lung apices when the thorax is upright.[43] There is also a decrease in blood flow to the uppermost lung in the lateral recumbent position.

LONG-TERM VOLUME REGULATION OF CARDIAC OUTPUT AND BLOOD PRESSURE

Most of the neurohumoral and local factors that control cardiac output and blood pressure are concerned with the distributional flow of a certain blood volume. The amount of blood volume in the central circulation, that is, the venous return, may be altered by altering blood flow distribution or by altering amounts of blood sequestered in the veins, but total volume is not substantially altered.

Regulation of total body fluid volume by the kidney is thought by many investigators to have a major long-term effect on cardiac output and blood pressure (Figs. 6-8 and 9-5).[5,8,17,21] Renal fluid volume control is influenced by the amount and composition of the circulating blood volume and by arterial pressure. Although this has only been discussed in relation to baroreceptor responses, cardiovascular–volume–sodium interactions are numerous and complex. Cardiovascular-renal and pressure-volume balance are reciprocally related. Continued investigation of these relationships is particularly relevant to understanding the mechanisms involved in congestive heart failure and hypertension (see Chaps. 2, 5, 9, 27 and 47).

REFERENCES

The selections marked with an asterisk (*) are helpful for further reading.

1. Abboud FM, Heistad DD, Mark AL et al: Reflex control of the peripheral circulation. Prog Cardiovasc Dis 18(5):371–403, 1976
2. Barr ML: The Human Nervous System, 3rd ed, pp 283–290. Hagerstown, Md, Harper & Row, 1979
3. Bohr DF: Vascular smooth muscle. In Johnson PC (ed): Peripheral Circulation, pp 13–43. New York, John Wiley & Sons, 1979
4. Braunwald E: Regulation of the circulation. N Engl J Med 290(20):1124–1129, 1974; 290(25):1420–1425, 1974
5. Braunwald E, Ross J: Control of cardiac performance. In Berne RM (ed): Handbook of Physiology, Sec 2: The Cardiovascular System, Vol 1, The Heart, pp 533–580. Bethesda, Md, American Physiological Society, 1979
6. Brown AM: Cardiac reflexes. In Berne RM (ed): Handbook of Physiology, Sec 2: The Cardiovascular System, Vol 1, The Heart, pp 677–689. Bethesda, Md, American Physiological Society, 1979
7. Coleridge JCG, Coleridge HM: Chemoreflex regulation of the heart. In Berne RM (ed): Handbook of Physiology, Sec 2: The Cardiovascular System, Vol 1, The Heart, pp 653–676. Bethesda, Md, American Physiological Society, 1979
8. Cowley AW: Perspectives on the physiology of hypertension. In Onesti G, Brest AN (eds): Hypertension: Mechanisms, Diagnosis and Treatment, pp 1–21. Philadelphia, FA Davis, 1978
9. Cunningham S, Feigl EO, Scher AM: Carotid sinus reflex influence on plasma renin activity. Am J Physiol 234(6):H670–H678, 1978
10. D'Alecy, LG: The cerebral circulation. In Ruch TC, Patton HD (eds): Physiology and Biophysics II, pp 262–276. Philadelphia, WB Saunders, 1974
11. Donald DE: Studies on the release of renin by direct and reflex activation of renal sympathetic nerves. Physiologist 22:39–42, 1979
12. Donald DE, Shepherd JT: Reflexes from the heart and lungs: Physiological curiosities or important regulatory mechanisms. Cardiovasc Res 12(8):449–469, 1978
13. Downing SE: Baroreceptor regulation of the heart. In Berne RM (ed): Handbook of Physiology, Sec 2: The Circulation, Vol 1, The Heart, pp 621–652. Bethesda, Md, American Physiological Society, 1979
14. Feigl EO: The arterial system. In Ruch TC, Patton HD (eds): Physiology and Biophysics II, pp 117–128. Philadelphia, WB Saunders, 1974
15. Folkow B, Neil E: Circulation, pp 265–363. London, Oxford University Press, 1971
16. Ganong WF, Rudolph CD, Zimmerman H: Neuroendocrine components in the regulation of blood pressure and renin secretion. Hypertension 1(3):207–218, 1979
17. Gauer OH, Henry JP: Neurohumoral control of plasma volume. In Guyton AC, Cowley AW (eds): Int Rev Physiol II, Vol. 9, pp 145–190. Baltimore, University Park Press, 1976
18. Gauer OH, Thron HL: Postural changes in the circulation. In Hamilton WF, Dow P (eds): Handbook of Physiology, Sec 2: Circulation, Vol III, pp 2409–2438. Washington, DC, American Physiological Society, 1965
19. Goodman, AG, Goodman LS, Gilman A: The Pharmacological Basis of Therapeutics, 6th ed, pp 647–656; and 916–925. New York, Macmillan, 1980
20. Green JF: Determinants of systemic blood flow. In Guyton AC, Young DB (eds): Int Rev Physiol III, Vol 18, pp 33–65. Baltimore, University Park Press, 1979
21. Guyton AC, Cowley AW, Young DB et al: Integration and control of circulatory function. In Guyton AC, Cowley AW (eds): Int Rev Physiol II, Vol 9, pp 341–385. Baltimore, University Park Press, 1976
22. Haber E: The role of renin in normal and pathological cardiovascular homeostasis. Circulation 54(6):849–861, 1976*
23. Hainsworth R, Linden RJ: Reflex control of vascular capacitance. In Guyton AC, Young DB (eds): Int Rev Phys III, Vol 18, pp 67–124. Baltimore, University Park Press, 1979
24. Hanson KM: Liver. In Johnson PC (ed): Peripheral Circulation, pp 285–314. New York, John Wiley & Sons, 1979
25. Johnson PC: Principles of peripheral circulatory control. In Johnson PC (ed): Peripheral Circulation, pp 111–139. New York, John Wiley & Sons, 1978
26. Kirchheim HR: Systemic arterial baroreceptor reflexes. Physiol Rev 56(1):100–176, 1976*
27. Korner PI: Central nervous control of autonomic cardiovascular function. In Berne RM (ed): Handbook of Physiology, Sec 2: The Cardiovascular System, Vol I, The Heart, pp 691–739. Bethesda, Md, American Physiological Society, 1979
28. Lefkowitz RJ: Selectivity in beta-adrenergic responses. Circulation 49(5):783–786, 1974
29. Levy MN: Complexity of the neural regulation of the cardiovascular system. Fed Proc 31(4):1197–1198, 1972
30. Levy MN, Martin PJ: Neural control of the heart. In Berne RM (ed): Handbook of Physiology, Sec 2: The Cardiovascular System, Vol 1, The Heart, pp 581–620. Bethesda, Md, American Physiological Society, 1979
31. Linden RJ: Reflexes from the heart. Prog Cardiovasc Dis 18(3):201–221, 1975

32. Lundgren O: The alimentary canal. In Johnson PC (ed): Peripheral Circulation, pp 255–283. New York, John Wiley & Sons, 1978

33. Mancia G, Lorenz RR, Shepherd JT: Reflex control of circulation by heart and lungs. In Guyton AC, Cowley AW (eds): Int Rev Phys II, Vol 9, pp 111–144. Baltimore, University Park Press, 1976

34. Mellander S, Johansson B: Control of resistance, exchange and capacitance functions in the peripheral circulation. Pharmacol Rev 20(3):117–196, 1968

35. Oberg B: Overall cardiovascular regulation. Annu Rev Physiol 38(1159):537–570, 1976

36. Randall RC: Neural Regulation of the Heart. New York, Oxford University Press, 1977

37. Rowell LB: Circulation to skeletal muscle. In Ruch TC, Patton HD (eds): Physiology and Biophysics II, pp 200–214. Philadelphia, WB Saunders, 1974

38. Rowell LB: The cutaneous circulation. In Ruch TC, Patton HD (eds): Physiology and Biophysics II, pp 185–199. Philadelphia, WB Saunders, 1974

39. Rushmer RF: Cardiovascular Dynamics, 4th ed, pp 105–132; pp 186–195; pp 217–239. Philadelphia, WB Saunders, 1976*

40. Scher AM: Control of arterial blood pressure. In Ruch TC, Patton HD (eds): Physiology and Biophysics II, pp 146–169. Philadelphia, WB Saunders, 1974*

41. Scher AM: Control of cardiac output. In Ruch TC, Patton HD (eds): Physiology and Biophysics II, pp 170–184. Philadelphia, WB Saunders, 1974*

42. Share L, Claybaugh JR: Regulation of body fluids. Annu Rev Physiol 34(1079):235–260, 1972*

43. Shepherd JT, Vanhoutte PM: The Human Cardiovascular System: Facts and Concepts, pp 107–193. New York, Raven Press, 1979*

44. Sparks HV: Skin and muscle. In Johnson PC (ed): Peripheral Circulation, pp 193–230. New York, John Wiley & Sons, 1978

45. Stull JT, Mayer SE: Biochemical mechanisms of adrenergic and cholinergic regulation of myocardial contractility. In Berne RM (ed): Handbook of Physiology, Sec 2: The Cardiovascular System, Vol I, The Heart, pp 741–774. Bethesda, Md, American Physiological Society, 1979

46. Zanchetti A, Stella A: Neural control of renin release. Clin Sci Mol Med 48:215s–223s, 1975

47. Zoller RP, Mark AL, Abboud FM et al: The role of low pressure baroreceptors in reflex vasoconstrictor responses in man. J Clin Invest 51:2967–2972, 1972

ADDITIONAL READING

Ganong WF: Review of Medical Physiology, 9th ed, pp 457–495. Los Altos, Calif, Lange, 1979

Guyton AC, Coleman TG, Granger HJ: Circulation: Overall regulation. Ann Rev Physiol 34(1072):13–46, 1972

Sancho J, Re R, Burton J et al: The role of the renin–angiotensin–aldosterone system in cardiovascular homeostasis in normal human subjects. Circulation 53(3):400–405, 1976

Smith JJ, Kampine JP: Circulatory Physiology: The Essentials, a, pp 114–120; b, pp 141–213; c, pp 235–253. Baltimore, Williams & Wilkins, 1980

Vander AJ, Sherman JH, Luciano DS: Human Physiology, 3rd ed, pp 300–314. New York, McGraw-Hill, 1980

7

Normal Physiologic Responses to Exercise

PAUL S. FARDY, Ph.D.

and

CAROL JEAN HALPENNY, R.N., M.A.

A single muscle contraction is anaerobic, that is, no oxygen is required; however, without oxygen, exercise causes muscle fatigue within 1 or 2 minutes because exercising skeletal muscles require oxygen to resynthesize energy-providing phosphates. The use of oxygen to provide energy for muscle contraction is dependent upon the integration of several physiologic mechanisms: pulmonary ventilation, diffusion of oxygen from the lungs into the blood, the oxygen-carrying capacity of the blood, cardiac output, diffusion of oxygen into cells, and use of oxygen by the mitochondria.

Exercising muscles require an increased blood flow to supply oxygen and nutrients and also to remove metabolic waste products. There is controversy regarding whether maximal physical activity is limited more by the ability of the cardiovascular system to supply oxygen to working muscle, by the functional capacities of the respiratory system, or by the metabolic capabilities of skeletal muscle.[2,22] An individual's ability to do physical work appears to be determined primarily by the functional capabilities of his cardiovascular system.[22]

ACUTE PHYSIOLOGIC ADJUSTMENTS TO EXERCISE

Oxygen Uptake

The oxygen uptake of a specific organ of the body such as skeletal or cardiac muscle is determined by the blood supply to that tissue and by the amount of oxygen removed from the blood perfusing that organ (see Chap. 6). Maximum oxygen uptake represents the greatest amount of oxygen that can be used by the entire body per minute and is determined by the maximum cardiac output and the maximum arteriovenous oxygen difference. Maximum oxygen uptake is the most reproducible measure of maximum physical work capacity available; it is the single best indicator of cardiovascular function.[3,4] The difference between oxygen uptake at rest and during maximum exercise illustrates the reserve capacities of the cardiovascular system (Chap. 6). (The term "maximum" usually denotes the physiologic work capacity limit possible for humans, whereas the term "maximal" usually denotes a person's work capacity limit.)

Oxygen uptake increases linearly with increasing levels of activity and then often plateaus briefly (for approximately 1 minute) at the point of exhaustion beyond which an individual can no longer continue exercising when the physical workload is increased further (Fig. 7-1). Maximum oxygen uptake is approximately 3 to 3.5 liters/minute (liters/min) in normal adult males, an increase of twelve times resting values.[3,16] Maximum oxygen uptake varies with body weight and mass, particularly during upright exercise, so it is most commonly adjusted for body weight and ranges from 20 to 40 ml/(kg min) for sedentary adult males.[7] A sedentary person is one who does not exercise vigorously enough to perspire at least one time per week.

Cardiac Output

Cardiac output increases linearly with increasing levels of exercise. It approximates four times resting values at maximal exercise (maxima of 20 + liters/min) and is augmented

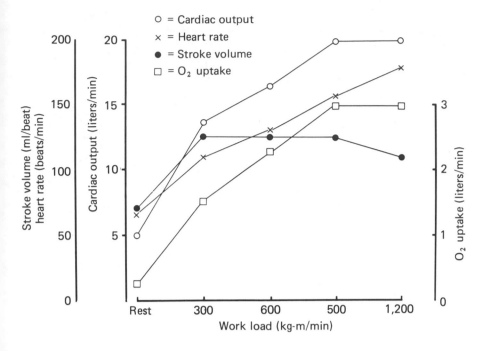

Fig. 7-1. Changes in heart rate, stroke volume, cardiac output, and oxygen uptake with increasing workloads (measured with bicycle exercise as kg-m/min). (Vander AJ, Sherman JH, Luciano DS: Human Physiology, p 362. New York, McGraw-Hill, 1980)

both by increasing heart rate and by increasing stroke volume.

Heart Rate

Heart rate increases abruptly with the onset of activity in sedentary adults, then increases more slowly but progressively to maximum levels of approximately three times resting values (age-adjusted maxima of 180 to 200 beats per minute) during maximal activity.[8] This heart rate response results from increased sympathetic and decreased vagal stimulation.

Stroke Volume

In the normal sedentary adult, stroke volume increases rapidly at the beginning of exercise and usually plateaus at near maximal values before less than half of maximal exercise capacity is reached. Average maximal stroke volumes of 140 to 150 ml for upright sedentary adult males are approximately two times resting values.[24] Blood that has been redistributed to skeletal and cardiac muscle from other areas is returned to the heart, causing an increase in diastolic filling (preload), which results in an increased stroke volume (Starling effect). Increased myocardial contractility resulting from sympathetic stimulation also helps to increase stroke volume.

Increases in Arteriovenous Oxygen Difference

The amount of oxygen extracted from the blood is increased in both exercising muscle and nonexercising areas. During rest, an average of 5 to 7 ml oxygen (O_2)/100 ml systemic blood is extracted, whereas during exercise 15 ml oxygen or more is extracted.[3,24]

Redistribution of Blood Flow

Blood is shunted from nonexercising arterial beds and from venous storage areas to cardiac muscle and exercising skeletal muscles (Table 7-1). Skeletal muscle blood flow is increased approximately 18 times over resting values at maximal exercise.[8] Increased sympathetic vasomotor outflow to regional vascular beds increases arteriolar renal, splanchnic and nonexercising muscle vasoconstriction, and constriction of the splanchnic and other veins. Also, the veins passively collapse when the venous perfusion pressure is decreased by arteriolar vasoconstriction (Chap. 6). Muscle pumping action helps to return blood to the heart.

Increases in coronary blood flow provide the major means by which oxygen supply to working myocardial muscle is increased, because the coronary arteries have achieved near maximal vasodilation and oxygen extraction under resting conditions (see Chaps. 2 and 6). Increases in myocardial contractility, wall tension, and heart rate contribute to the increased demands for myocardial oxygen (see Chap. 2). The derived product of heart rate times systolic blood pressure/100 has been shown to correlate with myocardial oxygen consumption (see Chap. 18).

TABLE 7-1 REDISTRIBUTION OF BLOOD FLOW AT REST AND DURING HEAVY WORK

Major Organs	Resting Conditions (%)	Strenuous Exercise (%)
Lungs	100	100
Liver	20–25	3.5
Heart	4–5	4–5
Kidneys	20	2–4
Bone	3–5	1
Brain	15	3–4
Skin and muscles	20–25	85

(Åstrand PO, Rohdal K: Textbook of Work Physiology, pp 11–34; pp 143–205. New York, McGraw-Hill, 1977)

Blood flow to the brain changes little during exercise. Blood flow to the skin reflects the opposing factors of the need for vasodilation to dissipate the temperature increases that result from increased metabolism and the need for vasoconstriction to shunt blood to exercising muscle. Skin arterioles constrict at the beginning of exercise, relax as central body temperature increases, but remain relatively constricted at maximal exercise.[21,22] Exercise in a hot environment can lead to collapse from an inability to maintain stroke volume and blood pressure as the cutaneous blood vessels dilate.[22]

Total systemic vascular resistance decreases to approximately 2.7 times resting values. Pulmonary vascular resistance is approximately two times less than resting values.[8]

Respiration

Pulmonary minute ventilation ($\dot{V}_E$) refers to the amount of air that is moved in and out of the lungs per minute. At rest, $\dot{V}_E$ is approximately 5 to 10 liters/min[29] and can increase with exercise to 100 to 150 liters/min.[3] Pulmonary ventilation is closely related to oxygen uptake at moderate levels of work, although the relationship is altered at near maximal activity. Pulmonary ventilation can be increased beyond that achieved at maximal work capacity.[2]

Because hemoglobin is almost fully saturated with oxygen when a person is at rest, the arterial partial pressure of oxygen remains relatively constant at maximal exercise.[29] The increased temperature and levels of carbon dioxide and decreased pH that occur during exercise cause hemoglobin to give up oxygen more readily at the tissue level than at rest. There is a "shift to the right" of the oxyhemoglobin dissociation curve.[3]

Coordination of Responses

Exercise responses represent a combination of local and central nervous system responses. Local autoregulation controls blood flow to exercising muscle, the heart, the brain, and to some extent the skin (see Chaps. 5 and 6). The afferent inputs to the central nervous system that initiate the coordinated responses to exercise have not been completely identified.[22] It is possible that chemical and other receptors in skeletal muscle and joints participate in the initial reaction to exercise.[3,22,24] Emotional responses may also be involved, because skeletal muscle vasodilation due to sympathetic cholinergic stimulation from the hypothalamus may actually precede activity (see Chap. 6).

Baroreceptors modify cardiovascular responses during exercise, and carotid chemoreceptors participate in respiratory responses (see Chap. 6).[22,29] The hypothalamus and higher brain centers are also involved in coordinating exercise responses.[3] There is coordination of nervous system output to skeletal muscles as well as autonomic output to the cardiovascular, respiratory, and other systems.

Skeletal Muscle Structure and the Contractile Process

Muscle fibers are elongated, cylindrical cells arranged in parallel and grouped together into bundles (fasciculi) that make up the muscle. The muscle fiber is made up of a series of contiguous units known as sarcomeres. The sarcomere possesses even smaller protein filaments, actin and myosin, which also run in parallel. Actin and myosin form crossbridges and slide past each other when stimulated (see Chap. 2). The sliding causes a shortening in the sarcomere units and eventually leads to a change in the length of the muscle fiber and the muscle itself.

The functional unit (motor unit) that permits skeletal muscular excitation consists of a number of muscle fibers and a single motor nerve fiber that supplies the neural stimulus. The neural impulse is transmitted along the nerve fiber until it meets the muscle fiber at the myoneural junction. The impulse is then transmitted to the muscle fiber by the chemical transmitter acetylcholine. The impulse travels along the muscle fiber to the sarcomere and initiates the contraction of the muscle (see Chap. 2).

Interest has increased during the last decade in the study of the types of muscle fibers and the type of contraction for which they are responsible. With the development and improvement of biopsy and histochemical techniques, it has become possible to classify two principal muscle fiber types according to their enzymatic activity, as slow-twitch and fast-twitch fibers. Slow-twitch fibers have oxidative enzymes and are responsible for oxidative activity, that is, aerobic exercise, whereas fast-twitch fibers have glycolytic enzymes and are responsible for glycolytic activity, that is, anaerobic work.[13,26,27] The amount of each type of muscle fiber characterizes the potential for endurance or power activity. Endurance athletes, for example, possess a higher percentage of slow-twitch fibers in their muscles whereas there are greater amounts of fast-twitch fibers present in the muscles of power athletes.

Energetics of Muscle Contraction. The energy provided for muscle contraction is derived either from aerobic (oxidative) or anaerobic (glycolytic) metabolic pathways. The immediate supply of energy at the onset of activity is anaerobic, as a result of the breakdown of high-energy adenosine triphosphate bonds (ATP) to adenosine diphosphate (ADP) and phosphate, which is facilitated by the action of the enzyme ATPase (see Chap. 2). Intramuscular supplies of creatine phosphate (CP) combine with ADP to resynthesize ATP (Chap. 2), but the total amount of creatine phosphate available to provide energy for contraction is extremely small and is quickly depleted. The maintenance of a continued supply of ATP for exercising muscle depends upon the delivery of adequate amounts of oxygen and metabolic substrates. Glucose in the blood, glycogen from muscle stores, and free fatty acids (FFA) from adipose tissue are the principal substrates available as energy fuels. Proteins rarely provide metabolic substrates for activity except under conditions of starvation. When protein is used as the principal source of energy, muscle tissue is degraded and muscular weakness ensues.

The food substrate or combination of substrates serving as fuel for energy is a factor in the potential intensity and duration of physical effort. At rest, approximately equal amounts of fats and carbohydrates (glycogen or glucose) are metabolized. During low-level and moderate exercise there is a greater dependence upon free fatty acids; as the intensity of work increases, there is a gradual shift to

TABLE 7-2 CHANGES IN RESPIRATORY QUOTIENT (RQ) DURING EXERCISE

Treadmill Workload (METS)	Heart Rate bpm	$\overset{\bullet}{V}O_2$ (ml/kg min)	RQ
2	81	10.4	0.74
4	94	15.8	0.80
6	112	22.2	0.88
8	132	28.7	0.94
10	153	36.5	1.00

1 MET = Basal O_2 requirement of the body at rest, approximately 3.5 ml/(kg min)

(Fardy PS: Exercise physiology for cardiac rehabilitation. In Fardy PS, Bennett JL, Reitz NL, Williams MA: Cardiac Rehabilitation: Implications for the Nurse and Other Health Professionals. St. Louis, CV Mosby, 1980)

carbohydrates as the main supplier of energy. The respiratory exchange ratio or exchange quotient (RQ) is the ratio of carbon dioxide to oxygen used. The RQ depends upon the energy substrate used and is 1.0 for carbohydrates and approximates 0.7 for fats. The RQ at rest is approximately 0.8 and increases to 1.0 with strenuous activity (Table 7-2).

Efficiency of Energy Conservation. The energy produced from metabolism of substrates is transformed into energy available for muscular contraction (Chap. 2; Fig. 2-16). Complete aerobic oxidation of 1 mole of glucose provides 36 to 38 moles of ATP and 686 kcal energy.[3] Because 7 kcal of energy per mole ATP is used in the process of muscle contraction and the remainder is dissipated as heat, the efficiency of energy conservation is approximately 38 × 7/686 × 100 = 38%. When glycogen is used as the substrate, an additional mole of ATP is formed.[3] However, these figures are likely to be underestimates. Under intracellular conditions of energy supply, the reversible ATP ↔ ADP and phosphate reaction probably involves a change in the energy level that is higher than 7 kcal/mole. It may be as high as 10 to 16 kcal, which gives an efficiency of the conservation of ATP energy as high as 55% to 87%, whereas the mechanical efficiency of physical work, as estimated from the ratio of mechanical work to oxygen use, is at most 20% to 25%.[3]

When the supply of oxygen is insufficient to meet the demand for oxygen imposed by the tissue cells of contracting muscles, anaerobic metabolism becomes the principal provider of energy. As explained in Chapter 2, glucose generates more ATP per gram mole aerobically than anaerobically. Conservation of energy is also less with anaerobic metabolic processes, that is, 27% for glucose and 38% for glycogen.

Because circulatory functions do not adjust immediately to physical exertion, ATP and CP are quickly depleted with the onset of exercise. Until aerobic metabolism resumes (approximately 1 minute), anaerobic metabolism is the principal source of energy. The maximal amount of energy supplied with anaerobic metabolism is approximately 30 kcal. Efforts extending beyond 1 minute derive a much greater contribution from aerobic metabolism, with a direct relationship existing between the duration of work and the relative contribution of aerobic and anaerobic metabolism. (Table 7-3).[12]

The buildup of lactic acid, the principal by-product of anaerobic metabolism, may be a contributing factor in the development of muscle fatigue. The toxic effect of increased lactate is underdetermined. Increased acidity results in lowered blood and muscle pH and may limit work performance by inhibiting glycolysis. Lactic acid may impede the contractile process by interfering with the interaction of the myosin and actin filaments.[12]

POPULATION DIFFERENCES IN EXERCISE RESPONSES

The maximal levels of exercise that can be achieved and maximal achievable oxygen uptakes differ among populations grouped according to physical activity level, age, sex, and cardiovascular–respiratory health. Any given level of exercise requires approximately the same oxygen uptake by any individual when skill is not a factor, but performing a given amount of physical work requires a greater percentage of maximal exercise capacity from some groups of people than from other groups (Chap. 43).[2] For example, a certain level of exercise can be accomplished by a physically conditioned young person without using any of the cardiac reserve, that is, with a minimal increase in heart rate and no change in stroke volume, whereas an older sedentary person will have to use a considerable portion of the cardiovascular reserve to accomplish the same exercise.

The percentage decrease in blood flow to nonessential areas appears to be much the same across population groups.[23] For example, the relative percentage of decrease in blood flow to the splanchnic area at 50% of maximal exercise is similar in sedentary and trained individuals.

Physical Conditioning

Athletes have a greater physical work capacity than do sedentary individuals. The conditioned person's oxygen uptakes and augmented stroke volumes are greater. Physical conditioning must be of a certain duration, frequency, and intensity before cardiovascular and muscular changes occur

TABLE 7-3 RELATIVE CONTRIBUTION OF ANAEROBIC AND AEROBIC METABOLISM TO TOTAL ENERGY OUTPUT DURING MAXIMAL EXERCISE OF DIFFERENT DURATION

Work Time at Maximal Exercise	Energy Source (kcal) ANAEROBIC	AEROBIC	TOTAL	Relative Contribution (%) ANAEROBIC	AEROBIC
10 seconds	20	4	24	83	17
1 minute	30	20	50	60	40
2 minutes	30	45	75	40	60
5 minutes	30	120	150	20	80
10 minutes	25	245	270	9	91
30 minutes	20	675	695	3	97
1 hour	15	1200	1215	1	99

(Adapted from Gollnick PD, Hermansen L: Biochemical adaptation to exercise: Anaerobic metabolism. In Wilmore JH (ed): Exercise and Sport Science Reviews, Vol 1, pp 1—43. New York, Academic Press, 1974)

TABLE 7-4 CARDIOVASCULAR ADAPTATION TO LONG-TERM AEROBIC TRAINING

Variable	At Rest	Standard-Submaximal Work	Maximal Effort
Oxygen uptake	No change	No change	Increased
Heart rate	Decreased	Decreased	No change
Stroke volume	Increased	Increased	Increased
Systolic blood pressure	Decreased	Decreased	No change
Diastolic blood pressure	Decreased	Decreased	No change
Pressure rate product	Decreased	Decreased	No change
Arterial-venous O$_2$ difference	No change	No change	Increased

(Fardy PS: Training for aerobic power. In Burke E (ed): Toward Understanding of Human Performance. Ithaca NY: Mouvement, 1977)

(Chap. 42).[10] Genetic endowment is the dominant factor affecting maximal aerobic power. In most cases, regular training can only increase maximal oxygen uptake by 10% to 20%[1,3] Habitual activity, particularly during pubesence and prepubescence, can exert considerable influence upon aerobic power. Maximal oxygen uptakes for trained individuals are 40 to 60 ml/(kg min) and for highly trained athletes, 60 to 80 ml/(kg min).

Resting heart rate is normally in the range of 60 to 80 beats per minute (bpm). Endurance athletes often have rates between 40 and 50 bpm, and rates as low as 30 bpm have been observed (Table 7-4). The magnitude of the increase, that is, the change from rest to maximal heart rate, is greater in more highly trained individuals because of the resting and submaximal bradycardia that results from training (Table 7-4). The better conditioned person has a greater cardiac rate reserve. In spite of the greater range of athletes' heart rates, their maximal heart rates do not appear to be any higher than those of less highly trained individuals.[5]

Stroke volume has been found by some investigators to be increased with training because of the development of increased left ventricular contractility (Table 7-4).[28] Because heart rate at rest and during submaximal exertion is lower with training, there is more time per beat for ventricular emptying and filling. As predicted by the Frank-Starling principle, increased filling time and subsequent ventricular stretch also enhance stroke volume. Lower heart rates provide a longer period for coronary arterial blood flow during diastole (see Chaps. 2 and 4).

Cardiac output at rest and during submaximal effort after training remains relatively unchanged because of the increase in stroke volume.[29] Because training does not affect maximal heart rates, the increased cardiac output achievable during maximal effort is attributed solely to an augmented stroke volume (Table 7-4).

Myocardial oxygen consumption decreases at standard workloads with training, reflecting increased myocardial efficiency. In contrast, maximal myocardial oxygen consumption increases with training, which indicates enhanced myocardial potential.

Pulmonary ventilation is as high as 200 liters/min in highly conditioned persons. The difference between arterial and venous saturation of oxygen increases with long-term training as a result of increased oxygen uptake at the cellular level.[5]

Trained athletes use more fatty acids and less carbohydrates than do sedentary individuals at a standard level of exercise.[11] There is an advantage to this during prolonged activity because there are approximately forty times greater stores of fat in the body than carbohydrates.[3,14]

The long-term consequences of regular physical training on muscle tissue consist in biochemical and morphologic alterations.[13] Skeletal muscles have been observed to undergo an increase in aerobic potential as a result of augmented muscle myoglobin and oxidative enzyme activity. The ability to increase the capacity for prolonged strenuous work is also significantly enhanced by an increased metabolism of fat and a concomitant sparing of glycogen. These adaptive activities are also influenced to a large degree by various structural changes in the muscle. Muscle hypertrophy (increased fiber size), possible increases in the number of muscle fibers, greater intramuscular capillarization, and increases in the size and possibly in the number of mitochondria are other long-term adaptive responses of exercise that can enhance aerobic capacity.

The potential usefulness of slow-twitch and fast-twitch muscle fiber classification is intriguing. The capability of classifying athletes according to the muscle metabolic potential (endurance versus power) to which they are genetically predisposed is exciting although sobering. The ability to estimate and predict performance potential may appear useful and desirable, but the biopsy technique does not take into account those intangible items of motivation, desire, hard work, and skill that make maximum athletic abilities a difficult end point to predict. It may be possible to alter muscle fiber types with systematic training.[27]

Age

Maximal oxygen uptake and work capacity appear to decrease with increasing age after young adulthood.[1,6,9,15] Maximal heart rate is equal to 220 minus age in years and decreases at an approximate rate of one beat per year (Table 7-5). Individuals who exercise regularly have less of a

TABLE 7-5 RELATIONSHIP OF AGE AND MAXIMAL HEART RATE

Age	Average Max Hr
20	200
25	195
30	190
35	185
40	180
45	175
50	170
55	165
60	160
65	155

(From Fardy PS: Exercise physiology for cardiac rehabilitation. In Fardy PS, Bennett JL, Reitz NL, Williams MA: Cardiac Rehabilitation: Implications for the Nurse and Other Health Professionals. St. Louis, CV Mosby, 1980)

decrease in maximal work capacity than do sedentary older people.[9,15]

Sex

Females appear to have lower work capacities than age- and activity-matched males. This may be because of the males' greater proportion of lean body mass or higher hematocrit.[4]

Cardiac Disease

Maximal exercise capacity is usually reduced in persons with cardiovascular impairment; exercise responses correlate to some extent with the amount of cardiac impairment (see Chap. 18). Maximal heart rate may be reduced slightly, but the inability to increase stroke volume is the major factor that limits exercise capacity in persons who have cardiac impairment.[7,17] Greater increases in heart rate occur at lower work loads to compensate for the reduced stroke volume.

Persons with coronary heart disease already have near-maximal coronary vasodilation. Further increases in myocardial oxygen requirements that cannot be met by increased coronary blood flow result in inadequate tissue oxygenation. The ischemic myocardium is unable to increase contractility in proportion to the increased work demand (see Chap. 42).

DIFFERENCES IN TYPES OF PHYSICAL ACTIVITY

Static and Dynamic Exercise

Static or isometric exercise such as a sustained hand grip involves sustained muscle tension at a constant muscle length (see Chap. 2). Blood flow is mechanically impeded during strong sustained isometric muscle contractions, and there is no dilation of muscle arterioles, so the increased cardiac output required for the exercise is accomplished with some increase in heart rate but with much greater increases in systolic and diastolic blood pressures than occur with a comparable level of isotonic exercise.[18,20] This increases myocardial afterload, increases myocardial pressure work, and thus increases myocardial oxygen consumption. Dynamic exercise such as walking involves rhythmic isotonic muscle contraction and muscle relaxation, which is much less stressful on the heart. Most exercises and activities in man involve both isometric and isotonic components; it is the proportion of isometric to isotonic work that determines the amount of myocardial pressure work.

Supine and Upright Exercise

The highest possible oxygen uptake in the supine flat position is less than the maximal oxygen uptake in the upright position.[22,25] Although stroke volume and cardiac output are greater in the supine position than in the upright stationary position, leg movement in the upright position benefits from an increased driving force for tissue perfusion (see Chaps. 6 and 30).

Arm and Leg Exercise

Maximal arm work results in peak oxygen uptakes approximately 70% of maximal oxygen uptake during upright leg exercise.[22] Arm exercises frequently involve substantial isometric work, such as during lifting activities.

Peak oxygen uptake during cycling is less than the maximal oxygen uptake achieved during running on an incline, apparently because of the restriction to blood flow that occurs during cycling.[2,16,19] Arterial mean pressure, heart rate, pressure rate product, peripheral vascular resistance, and pulmonary ventilation have been found to be higher with bicycle exercise, leading some investigators to believe that bicycle exercise places a slightly greater hemodynamic stress on an individual than does treadmill exercise.[19]

Individuals rarely achieve maximal work capacities except during test conditions. However, knowledge of the responses involved in exercise is useful for evaluating individual responses to any physical activity (see Chaps. 18 and 42).

REFERENCES

The selections marked with an asterisk (*) are helpful for further reading.

1. Åstrand PO: Physical performance as a function of age. JAMA 205:105–109, 1968
2. Åstrand PO: Quantification of exercise capability and evaluation of physical capacity in man. Prog Cardiovasc Dis 19(1):51–67, 1976*
3. Åstrand PO, Rohdal K: Textbook of Work Physiology, pp 11–34; pp 143–205. New York, McGraw-Hill, 1977*
4. Balke B, Ware RW: An experimental study of "physical fitness" of Air Force personnel. U.S. Armed Forces Med J 10:675–688, 1959
5. Barnard RJ: Long-term effects of exercise and cardiac function. In Wilmore JH (ed): Exercise and Sport Science Reviews, Vol 3, pp 113–133. New York, Academic Press, 1975
6. Bruce RA, Fisher LD, Cooper MN et al: Separation of effects of cardiovascular disease and age on ventricular function with maximal exercise. Am J Cardiol 34:35–41, 1974
7. Bruce RA, Gey GO, Cooper MN et al: Seattle heart watch: Initial clinical, circulatory and electrocardiographic responses to maximal exercise. Am J Cardiol 33:459–469, 1974
8. Buskirk ER: Cardiovascular adaptation to physical effort in healthy men. In Naughton JP, Hellerstein HK, Mohler IC (eds): Exercise Testing and Exercise Training in Health and Disease, pp 23–31. New York, Academic Press, 1973
9. Dehn MM, Bruce RA: Longitudinal variations in maximal oxygen uptake with age and activity. J Appl Physiol 33(6):42–44, 1972
10. Fardy PS: Training for aerobic power. In Burke E (ed): Toward Understanding of Human Performance. Ithaca, NY, Mouvement, 1977
11. Gollnick PD: Free fatty acid turnover and the availability of substrates as a limiting factor in prolonged exercise. In The Marathon: Physiological, Medical, Epidemiological and Psychological Studies. Vol 301, pp 64–71. Ann NY Acad Sci, 1977
12. Gollnick PD, Hermansen L: Biochemical adaptation to exercise: Anaerobic metabolism. In Wilmore JH (ed): Exercise and Sport Science Reviews. Vol 1, pp 1–43. New York, Academic Press, 1974
13. Gollnick PD, Sembrowich WL: Adaptations in human skeletal muscle as a result of training. In Amsterdam EA, Wilmore JH, DeMaria AN (eds): Exercise in Cardiovascular Health and Disease, pp 70–94. New York, Yorke, 1977

14. Holloszy JO: Biochemical adaptives to exercise: Aerobic metabolism. In Wilmore JH (ed): Exercise and Sport Science Reviews, Vol 1, pp 45–71. New York, Academic Press, 1974

15. Kanstrup I, Ekblom B: Influence of age and physical activity on central hemodynamics and lung function in active adults. J Appl Physiol 45(5):709–717, 1978

16. Lange-Anderson K: The determinants of physical performance capacity in health and disease. In Naughton JP, Hellerstein HK, Mohler IC (eds): Exercise Testing and Exercise Training in Health and Disease, pp 33–44. New York, Academic Press, 1973

17. McDonough JR, Danielson RA, Wills RE et al: Maximal cardiac output during exercise in patients with coronary artery disease. Am J Cardiol 33:23–29, 1974

18. Mitchell JH, Wildenthal K: Static (isometric) exercise and the heart: Physiological and clinical considerations. Annu Rev Med 25(7119):369–381, 1974

19. Niederberger M, Bruce RA, Kusumi F et al: Disparities in ventilatory and circulatory responses to bicycle and treadmill exercise. Brit Heart J 36(4):377–382, 1974

20. Nutter DO, Schland RC, Hurst JW: Isometric exercise and the cardiovascular system. Mod Concepts Cardiovasc Dis 41(3):1115, 11–15, 1972*

21. Roberts MF, Wenger CB: Control of skin blood flow during exercise: Thermal and nonthermal factors. J Appl Physiol 46(4): 780–796, 1979

22. Rowell LB: Human cardiovascular adjustments of exercise and thermal stress. Physiol Rev 51(1):75–159, 1974

23. Rowell LB: The splanchnic circulation. In Ruch TC, Patton HD (eds): Physiology and Biophysics II, pp 215–233. Philadelphia, WB Saunders, 1974

24. Rulli V: Normal cardiovascular/pulmonary responses to exercise. In James WE, Amsterdam EA (eds): Coronary Heart Disease, Exercise Testing and Cardiac Rehabilitation, pp 81–93. New York, Stratton Intercontinental, 1977*

25. Saltin B: The interplay between peripheral and central factors in the adaptive response to exercise and training. In The Marathon: Physiological, Medical, Epidemiological, and Psychological Studies. Vol 301, pp 224–231, Ann NY Acad Sci, 1977

26. Saltin B: Metabolic fundamentals in exercise. Med Sci Sports 5:137–146, 1973*

27. Saltin B, Henriksson J, Nygaard E, Andersen P: Fiber types and metabolic potentials of skeletal muscles in sedentary man and endurance runners. In The Marathon: Physiological, Medical, Epidemiological, and Psychological Studies. Vol 301, pp 3–29. Ann NY Acad Sci, 1977

28. Scheuer J, Stezowski SW: The effect of physical training on the mechanical and metabolic response of the rat heart to hypoxia. Circ Res 30:418–429, 1972

29. Wasserman K, Whipp BJ: Exercise physiology in health and disease. Am Rev Respir Dis 112:219–249, 1975*

ADDITIONAL READING

Smith JJ, Kampine JP: Circulatory Physiology: The Essentials, pp 213–233. Baltimore, Williams & Wilkins, 1980

Wilmore JH: Acute and chronic physiological responses to exercise. In Amsterdam EA, Wilmore JH, DeMaria AN (eds): Exercise in Cardiovascular Health and Disease. New York, Yorke, 1977

8

Normal Hematopoiesis and Coagulation

JOANNE SCHNAIDT ROKOSKY, R.N., M.N.

Each cellular constituent of the blood assists the body in maintaining homeostasis despite changing environmental stimuli: Erythrocytes carry oxygen, leukocytes and lymphocytes protect against foreign invasion, and platelets participate in blood clotting. In addition, the plasma serves as a transport medium for hormones and for end products of cellular metabolism. Because of these vital functions, a significant blood loss has devastating consequences for all body tissues. Protection against such blood losses and potential exsanguination from minor injuries is achieved by a complex series of events leading to hemostasis. This system is balanced by an equally complex mechanism of fibrinolysis in which formed clots are dissolved. Knowledge of these normal processes is important as a basis for understanding the many alterations that may occur as a result of disease states or drug administration.

HEMATOPOIETIC CELLS

Hematopoietic cells are produced in the bone marrow through successive mitoses and differentiations of stem cells. Stem cells are primitive, undifferentiated cells capable of dividing to produce identical daughter cells. Some of their progeny mature into one or more adult cell types, whereas others maintain the stem-cell pool. The most primitive stem cells are believed to be pluripotential, that is, to have the capacity to differentiate into either lymphoid or myeloid (erythrocytes, granulocytes, monocytes, platelets) lines. More specialized stem cells differentiate exclusively into either lymphoid or myeloid cells. These specialized stem cells are called restricted cell lines (Fig. 8-1).[4,10,17]

Erythrocytes

The rate of bone marrow stem cell differentiation into erythrocytes is primarily controlled by erythropoietin. The bulk of this hormone is produced by the kidney, although small amounts are also produced by extrarenal tissue, such as the Kupffer cells of the liver.[8]

In the bone marrow, the immature red blood cell progressively loses its nucleus and changes its shape. The mature red cell is a biconcave disc that provides an ideal surface for diffusion. The prime purpose of erythrocytes is to serve as a vehicle for oxyen transport from the pulmonary alveoli to the systemic tissues. Oxygen diffuses into the alveolar capillary, then into the erythrocyte, where it is carried on each of four heme binding sites on the hemoglobin portion of the cell (see Chap. 5). In addition, hydrogen is buffered in red cells, thus providing an instantaneous means of compensating for cellular acid production (see Chap. 9).

Leukocytes

White cells, all of which defend against injury and foreign invasion, can be separated into two groups: phagocytic cells and immune cells. Phagocytic cells are classified according to their different morphologies, as polymorphonuclear leukocytes and monocytes. Immune cells include T and B lymphocytes.

The *polymorphonuclear leukocytes,* also called granulocytes because of their abundant cytoplasmic granules, include neutrophils, basophils, and eosinophils (see Fig. 8-1). *Neutrophils* are small, short-lived, rapidly mobile cells that emigrate from the blood and initiate phagocytosis within an hour of the onset of an inflammatory reaction. Their half-

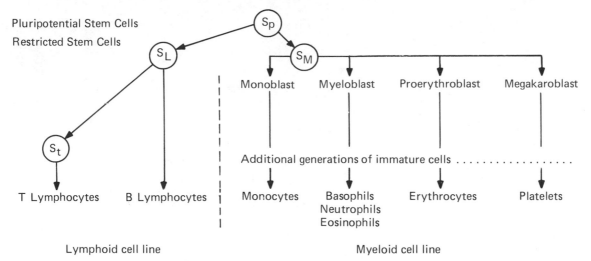

Pluripotential Stem Cells

Restricted Stem Cells

Lymphoid cell line

Myeloid cell line

Fig. 8-1. Hematopoietic cellular differentiation. Formation of blood cells originates within the bone marrow from stem-cell division. Those stem cells that are capable of forming all hematopoietic cells are called pluripotential stem cells and are designated S_p. Other stem cells also exist that produce selected hematopoietic cells. All are referred to as restricted stem cells. The cells designated S_m differentiate into myeloid cells. Stem cells that differentiate exclusively into lymphoid cells include those designated S_l and S_t. (Adapted from Phillips RA, Jones EV, Miller RG: In Golde DW et al (eds): ICN-UCLA Symposia on Molecular and Cellular Biology, X, 1978 and Ganong WF, Review of Medical Physiology, p 397. Los Altos, Lange Medical Publications, 1979)

life is approximately 7 hours. Huge numbers of neutrophils are produced daily.[4] *Eosinophils* and *basophils* also enter inflammatory reactions, but the function and importance of each is poorly understood. Increases in the number of eosinophils correlate with allergic diseases, and they may phagocytize antigen–antibody complexes. Basophils, also known as mast cells, contain heparin and histamine.[4] Their function remains elusive, although attachment of antibody to mast cells is known to occur in some immunologic disorders.

A fourth phagocytic white cell, *the monocyte,* is large and contains a single nucleus and relatively few cytoplasmic granules. Its value is its nonspecific phagocytic activity and its ability to survive adverse environmental conditions. Monocytes that have emigrated from blood to tissues are also known as macrophages or histiocytes. The influx of monocytes from the blood into an acute inflammatory focus occurs later than neutrophil entry and is also characteristic of chronic inflammatory conditions. Additional macrophages are permanently "fixed" in one location, for example those of the lung (alveolar macrophages) and liver (Kupffer cells).

Regulation of leukocyte production is believed to occur in a manner similar to the regulation of erythrocytes by erythropoietin. A glycoprotein substance that increases granulocyte production from committed precursor cells has been isolated from human urine. The primary source of this substance, termed colony-stimulating factor (CSF), is believed to be the monocyte.[10,18]

Lymphocytes are either T lymphocytes, involved with cell-mediated immunity, or B lymphocytes, which produce the antibodies leading to humoral immunity. As with the other cells already described, stem-cell differentiation occurs in the bone marrow. However, the lymphocytes produced in this manner are incapable of participating in immune reactions. Instead, the cells enter the circulating blood and

migrate to other lymphoid organs where they further mature to become competent immune cells. Under the influence of the thymus, T lymphocytes mature into cells ready to participate in cell-mediated immune reactions. Cell-mediated activities are of particular importance in graft rejection and in defense against fungal and viral infections. B lymphocytes mature into cells that respond to stimulation from foreign protein by differentiating into plasma cells. The plasma cells in turn mature and produce the specific antibodies that inactivate or destroy foreign protein.[19]

The activities of phagocytic and immune cells overlap in numerous mutually beneficial ways. For example, immune cells often participate in chronic inflammatory reactions. Conversely, engulfment of foreign protein by phagocytic cells is a preparatory step leading to antibody production.

Platelets

Huge numbers of platelets are formed within the bone marrow from their precursor cell, the megakaryocyte.[6] Their production is regulated by thrombopoietin, another humoral stimulator that functions in a manner similar to erythropoietin. Thrombopoietin increases both the number of megakaryocytes and the rate and quantity of platelet production by megakaryocytes.[13] The primary functions of platelets include the formation of a cellular plug that temporarily arrests bleeding and the contribution of substances to the subsequent coagulation process.

HEMOSTASIS

The arrest of bleeding, called hemostasis, is a fundamental protective mechanism. The adaptive necessity of blood clotting to prevent exsanguination from the minor injuries

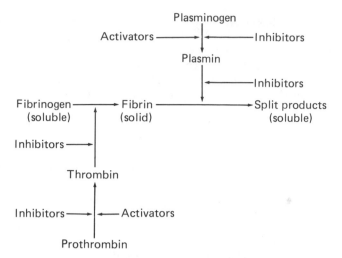

Fig. 8-2. The hemostatic balance. Under normal circumstances, coagulation and fibrinolysis are balanced so that neither unnecessary clotting nor excessive clot breakdown occurs. Both coagulation and fibrinolysis are complex processes with numerous activators and inhibitors. (Adapted from Astrup T, Thorsen S: Med Clin North Am 56:154, 1972)

we encounter in daily life is obvious. Likewise, eventual reestablishment of vascular patency is essential to preserve the normal blood supply to tissues. Hemostasis is thus part of a continuum involving clot formation and breakdown (Fig. 8-2).

The process of hemostasis involves three time-sequenced phases: the vascular phase, the platelet phase, and the coagulation phase (Fig. 8-3). Vessel type and size determine

whether one or all three phases are required to arrest bleeding.

Vascular Phase

The vascular phase refers to several instantaneous compensatory responses that occur when a vessel is severed. The initial vascular reaction to injury is constriction of vascular smooth muscle that limits blood loss.[16] Blood loss is also reduced by the apposition of surrounding tissues and by the pressure of interstitial fluid, the increase of which is due to escape of blood from the vessel into the interstitium. Although the vascular phase is usually insufficient to stop bleeding by itself, it can arrest venular or capillary bleeding or seal puncture wounds of larger vessels.[3,15]

Platelet Phase

The platelet phase refers to the formation of a soft mass of aggregated platelets that provides a temporary patch over the injured, bleeding vessel. Almost immediately after vascular injury, platelets begin to adhere to the exposed subendothelial collagen of the vessel wall. The activator of this phenomenon is unknown, but it has been theorized that erythrocytes may release a platelet-activating agent that initiates platelet adherence to the exposed collagen.[5] Adherent platelets release adenosine diphosphate (ADP), which causes platelets to change from their normal shape into a more rounded form with pseudopods. Although doubt has been raised about the significance of this shape change *in vivo*, the formation of these projections is generally believed

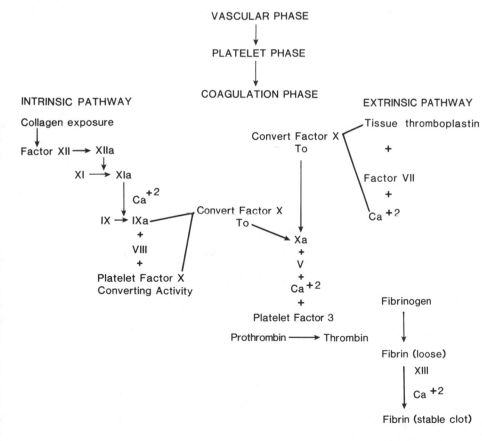

Fig. 8-3. Hemostasis. Hemostasis includes three phases: Vasoconstriction occurs in a severed vessel during the vascular phase; the platelet phase involves the formation of a soft mass of platelets over the site of vascular injury; and the coagulation phase refers to the formation of the more stable fibrin clot. Coagulation can be initiated by damage to the vessel endothelium, a process called the *intrinsic pathway*. Clotting can also be initiated by the release of substances from damaged cells outside the vessel, that is, by the *extrinsic pathway*. Regardless of the mechanism initiating clotting, Factor X is eventually activated and a fibrin clot formed.

to enhance platelet adhesion and subsequent aggregation.[6,15,20]

Most ADP is released from the dense granules contained within platelets themselves.[20] Collagen and thrombin are among the substances known to induce granule release.[15] The mechanism by which ADP causes aggregation is unclear, although it is postulated to involve actomyosin and calcium. The process is believed to be similar to the one leading to skeletal muscle contraction.[6,21] Aggregation is at first reversible but becomes permanent as more ADP is released. Throughout this process, various short-lived compounds are formed that further affect platelet aggregation and release. For example, prostaglandin E_2 enhances platelet aggregation, whereas prostaglandin E_1 inhibits it.[7]

Coagulation Phase

The final phase is coagulation or the formation of a fibrin blood clot. Although the subject of continued study, the coagulation process is most commonly viewed as a series of enzymatic reactions in which clotting factors are sequentially activated. Twelve different substances have been officially designated as clotting factors by the International Committee on Blood Clotting Factors (Table 8-1). The elucidation of additional factors has led to revisions shown under the heading Contemporary Version. This Contemporary Version is not yet officially recognized by the International Committee.

As studied in the laboratory, the coagulation process can be initiated by two different pathways: rapidly through the "extrinsic mechanism" and more slowly and complexly by the "intrinsic mechanism." Although these two mechanisms interact and are probably less clearcut when they occur within the body, differentiation between them is helpful for understanding pathologic mechanisms, medication actions, and coagulation tests. Both extrinsic and intrinsic mechanisms eventually lead to the activation of Factor X, with the remaining steps of the coagulation sequence being identical.

The extrinsic pathway involves the combination of Tissue Factor (Factor III) with Factor VII and ionized calcium, which together convert Factor X to its activated form, Factor Xa.[11] Tissue factor, also called tissue thromboplastin, is known to be a lipoprotein complex and is found in several subtypes throughout the body, including brain, lung, and placental tissue.[2] Although the ability of these tissue extracts to influence clotting has been recognized for over 100 years, the precise mechanisms by which this occurs remain unclear. Coagulation initiated by the extrinsic pathway occurs in approximately 10 to 15 seconds and is examined in the laboratory by the prothrombin time (see Chap. 15).[12]

Because the intrinsic pathway involves a greater number of factors, 30 to 60 seconds are required for coagulation to occur.[12] In the laboratory, intrinsic activation can be initiated by contact of blood with a negatively charged surface such as glass. Intrinsic activation is commonly analyzed by tests such as whole blood clotting time (Lee-White), recalcification time, and partial thromboplastin time (see Chap. 15). Exposure to subendothelial collagen is believed to be the major means by which Factor XII is activated in vivo. Once activated, Factor XII then stimulates the activation of Factor XI. Subsequently, activated Factor XI, together with ionized calcium, causes activation of Factor IX. In turn, Factor IX combines with Factor VIII and calcium to convert Factor X to Factor Xa, the activated form. A platelet substance, known as Factor X-converting activity, assists in the interaction of calcium and Factors IXa and VIII for the activation of Factor X.[20] From here, the coagulation process proceeds in an identical manner regardless of whether initiation was extrinsic or intrinsic.

This final common sequence involves the combination of Factors Xa, V, and calcium into a complex that converts prothrombin to thrombin. The process is accelerated by platelet Factor 3, a lipoprotein complex on or near the surface of the platelet membrane. This surface is exposed during the process of platelet aggregation.[6,7,20] The formed thrombin subsequently converts fibrinogen to fibrin, a loose web of fibers that is capable of stopping the bleeding in small and medium-sized arteries and veins. Over the next 1 to 2 hours, the fibrin clot is stabilized and thickened by the actions of Factors XIII and calcium. In the laboratory,

TABLE 8-1 THE COAGULATION PROTEINS

Official Number	Synonym	Contemporary Version
I	Fibrinogen	I (Fribrinogen)
II	Prothrombin	II (Prothrombin)
III	Tissue thromboplastin	III (Tissue Factor)
IV	Calcium	IV (Calcium)
V	Labile Factor	V (Labile Factor)
		VI: PF₃ (Platelet coagulant activities)
		VI: PF₄
VII	Stable Factor	VII (Stable Factor)
VIII	Antihemophilic Factor	VIII: AHF (Antihemophilic Factor)
		VIII: VWF (von Willebrand Factor)
		VIII: RAq (Related-Antigen)
IX	Christmas Factor	IX (Christmas Factor)
X	Stuart-Prower Factor	X (Stuart-Prower Factor)
XI	Plasma Thromboplastin (Antecedent)	XI (Plasma Thromboplastin Antecedent)
XII	Hageman Factor	XII: HF (Hageman Factor)
		XII: PK (Prekallikrein, Fletcher)
		XII: HMWK (High Molecular Weight Kininogen)
XIII	Fibrin Stabilizing Factor	XIII: Fibrin Stabilizing Factor

The Roman numerals and synonyms designating each clotting factor accepted by the International Committee on Blood Clotting Factors are located in the left-hand columns. Note the absence of Factor VI. The version in the right-hand column incorporates more recently recognized clotting factors but is not officially recognized.
(Green D: General considerations of coagulation proteins. Ann Clin Lab Sci 8(2):95–105, 1978)

platelets can be shown to express the fluid trapped in the clot and further compress the fibrin mass. The significance of this phenomenon, known as clot retraction, remains unknown.[16]

Intrinsic activation is probably most important for normal hemostasis.[9,11,20] However, both pathways are known to interact *in vivo* and in all probability synergize each other's activities. For example, thrombin produced by the extrinsic pathway has been shown to accelerate intrinsic coagulation by activating Factors V and VIII.[12] Conversely, a fragment of Factor XII from the intrinsic pathway is known to convert Factor VII to a more active form, thus accelerating extrinsic coagulation.[9]

Coagulation is modulated by various inhibitors. The most important inhibitor is antithrombin III, which forms complexes with and thus inhibits the action of Factors VII, IXa, XIa, and thrombin. In addition to several other molecular inhibitors, rapid blood flow and clearance of clotting factors by the liver help to maintain coagulation within physiologically beneficial limits.[11]

FIBRINOLYSIS

Of the numerous mechanisms known to result in fibrinolysis, most investigators consider the process mediated by plasmin to be of greatest significance.[14] Plasmin is found only in minute quantities in plasma, but its precursor, plasminogen, is normally abundant. Plasminogen is a betaglobulin with a molecular weight of approximately 90,000 and is believed to be synthesized by the liver.[1,12] Whether or not fibrinolysis occurs is controlled by the complex interplay of some substances that can activate plasminogen and others that keep it inactive. Under normal circumstances, the balance is in favor of those substances that prevent activation.

Activators of plasminogen are found in various tissues, blood, and urine. Particularly high levels of activator are found in healing tissues. The activation process involves cleavage of a bond on the plasminogen molecule that converts it to plasmin, a trypsinlike enzyme that can break down fibrin and other proteins.[1] The plasminogen inhibitors that usually prevent this activation are also present in blood and in various tissues.[1]

The mechanism by which formed clots are lysed remains controversial. However, the most commonly accepted theory is that plasminogen is incorporated into the fibrin clot as it polymerizes and becomes firm. Subsequent activation occurs in this localized region by the later diffusion of activators that convert the plasminogen to plasmin.[12,14] Fragments of the fibrin clot, known as fibrin split products, are then phagocytized and enter the lymphatic drainage system. Some of the larger fragments are themselves capable of inhibiting either platelet plug or fibrin clot formation.[12]

ABNORMAL HEMOSTASIS AND COAGULATION

Hemostatic Failure

Numerous defects in the hemostatic system are possible, including ineffective or insufficient platelets to form a platelet plug, deficient clotting factors, or bleeding from vessels too large for the hemostatic mechanisms to control. Furthermore, many drugs inhibit hemostasis (see Chap. 38). This phenomenon may be either the intended drug action or a side effect. In either event, knowledge of these pharmacologic activities is important for patient care and for patient teaching.

Inappropriate Coagulation

Excessive or inappropriate coagulation is also of great clinical significance. Venous thrombosis involves the interacting conditions of stasis, vascular damage, and hypercoagulability (Chap. 28). Its most common life-threatening complication, pulmonary embolism, is a major cause of mortality in hospitalized patients (Chap. 28). Patients with multisystem disease may also develop disseminated intravascular coagulation, a complex syndrome in which thrombosis and hemorrhage occur concomitantly. Recognition of patients likely to have or to develop any of these conditions is a nursing responsiblity.

REFERENCES

The selections marked with an asterisk (*) are helpful for further reading.

1. Astrup T, Thorsen S: The physiology of fibrinolysis. Med Clin North Am 56(1):153–162, 1972
2. Bennett B, Ratnoff OD: The normal coagulation mechanism. Med Clin North Am 56(1):95–104, 1972
3. Bithell TC, Wintrobe MM: Bleeding. In Wintrobe MM, Thorn, GW, Adams RD et al (eds): Harrison's Principles of Internal Medicine, 7th ed, pp 300–309. New York, McGraw-Hill, 1974
4. Boggs DR, Winkelstein A: White Cell Manual, 3rd ed. Seattle, University of Washington, 1975*
5. Born GVR: Fluid–mechanical and biochemical interactions in haemostasis. Br Med Bull 33(3):193–197, 1977
6. Crawford N, Taylor DG: Biochemical aspects of platelet behaviour associated with surface membrane reactivity. Br Med Bull 33(3):199–206, 1977
7. Deykin D: Emerging concepts of platelet function. N Engl J Med 290(3):144–151, 1974
8. Erslev AJ, Kansu E, Caro J: The biogenesis and metabolism of erythropoietin. In Golde DW et al (eds): Hematopoietic Cell Differentiation. ICN-UCLA Symposia on Molecular and Cellular Biology, Vol 10, 1978
9. Esnouf MP: Biochemistry of blood coagulation. Br Med Bull 33(3):213–218, 1977
10. Golde DW, Cline MJ: Regulation of granulopoiesis. N Engl J Med 291(26):1388–1395, 1974
11. Green D: General considerations of coagulation proteins. Ann Clin Lab Sci 8(2):95–105, 1978
12. Harker LA: Hemostasis Manual, 2nd ed. Philadelphia, FA Davis, 1974*
13. Harker LA: Platelet production. N Engl J Med 282(9):492–494, 1970
14. Kernoff PBA, McNicol GP: Normal and abnormal fibrinolysis. Br Med Bull 33(3):239–244, 1977
15. Mustard JF, Packham MA: Normal and abnormal hemostasis. Br Med Bull 33(3):187–192, 1977
16. Nossel HL: Bleeding. In Isselbacher KJ, Adams RD, Braunwald E et al (eds): Harrison's Principles of Internal Medicine, 9th ed, pp 272–279. New York, McGraw-Hill, 1980
17. Phillips RA, Jones EV, Miller RG: Differentiative potential of hematopoietic stem cells. In Golde DW et al (eds): Hemato-

poietic Cell Differentiation. ICN-UCLA Symposia on Molecular and Cellular Biology, Vol 10, 1978

18. Robinson WA: Leukopoiesis. In Froelich ED (ed): Pathophysiology: Altered Regulatory Mechanisms in Disease, 2nd ed, pp 597–607. Philadelphia, JB Lippincott, 1976

19. Sell S: Immunology, Immunopathology and Immunity, 2nd ed. Hagerstown, Md, Harper & Row, 1975

20. Sixma JJ, Wester J: The hemostatic plug. Semin Hematol 14(3):265–299, 1977

21. Weiss HJ: Platelet physiology and abnormalities of platelet function, Part I. N Engl J Med 293(11):531–541, 1975

ADDITIONAL READING

Cooper MO, Lawton AR: The development of the immune system. Sci Am 231(5):59–72, 1974

Ganong WF: Review of Medical Physiology, 9th ed. Los Altos, Calif, Lange, 1979 (Helpful for review of stem cells and concise summary of clotting)

Nysather JO, Katz AE, Lenth JL: The immune system: Its development and functions. Am J Nurs 76(10):1614–1618, 1976

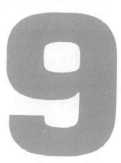

Fluid and Electrolyte Balance

JOANNE SCHNAIDT ROKOSKY, R.N., M.N.

and

JOAN SHAVER, R.N., Ph.D.

Energy metabolism involves numerous complex chemical reactions, all of which take place in a fluid environment inside the cell. The ingredients for cellular metabolism are acquired from the external environment outside the body or are produced by specialized cells within the body. From either source, they gain access to the blood, which flows to all tissue beds and delivers metabolic substrates and modulators to the cells. From the blood these substances are admitted preferentially to the interior of the cells, generally in accordance with cellular needs. By-products of cell function leave the cell, move through the fluid surrounding the cells, and also enter the blood. Blood flow delivers the by-products to tissues that either reorganize their structure for reuse or excrete them into the external environment.

A person continually makes exchanges with the environment external to the body. The exchanges consist of ordered forms of energy, such as chemicals (food, water, oxygen, carbon dioxide) and sensations (sound, light, heat). This flow of information from the external environment to the cell and back again takes place entirely through fluid mediums. Therefore, the extracellular environment is dynamically active and highly regulated both in terms of volume and composition (Fig. 9-1). The aim of this chapter is to review the state of normal fluid environments, dynamic exchange between them, how they are maintained, and the potential for altering the normal state.

BASIC CONCEPTS OF BODY FLUID ENVIRONMENTS

The human body can be viewed as having two fluid-filled chambers: an extracellular compartment and an intracellular compartment. The solutions in each contain numerous dissolved substances. Dissolved substances are called solutes, and the fluid in which they are dissolved is the solvent. In the human body, the solvent is water. The solutes are both organic, such as glucose, amino acids, and fatty acids, and inorganic, such as sodium, phosphate, and sulfate.

The Importance of Water

Cellular metabolism involves many complex chemical reactions between molecules. Water dissolves substances, so they can interact chemically. When molecules are dissolved in water, water facilitates dissociation, that is, the breakdown of loosely associated molecules into individual atoms or groups of atoms. Particles that contain atoms with incomplete orbital electrons are called ions. Substances capable of dissociating into ions are called electrolytes. The particles may be negatively charged (anions) or positively charged (cations), and they may have single or multiple charges. Important positively charged ions include sodium, potassium, hydrogen, magnesium, and calcium. Important negatively charged ions include chloride, bicarbonate, sulfate, phosphate, organic acids, and protein.[8] Ions constitute a large proportion of the total solutes present in body fluids. Although concentrations of these ions vary between the intracellular and extracellular compartments, the total numbers of ions are roughly equal.

Measurement of the Fluid Environment

Solute Concentration. The amount of any one solute dissolved in solvent is usually referred to as the concentration of that species of molecule. The concentration of solute in solution is expressed as the number of moles of the solute dissolved in one liter of water at some specified temperature. A mole is the weight in grams of a substance in an amount

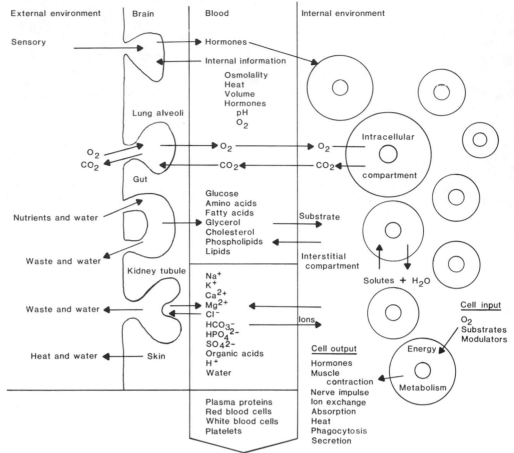

Fig. 9-1. Schemata of exchange of oxygen, nutrients, and waste with the environment; compartmentalization of body fluids and composition of blood. (Clark AL, Affonso R: *Childbearing: A Nursing Perspective*, 2nd ed. p 153. Philadelphia, FA Davis 1979)

equal to its molecular weight (gram molecular weight = GMW). Molecular weight is determined by summing the atomic weights of all elements specified in the formula for that molecule.[13] Atomic weights for major constituents of body fluids are listed in Table 9-1. Because the concentrations of substances dissolved in body fluids are rather small, they usually are expressed in 1/1000 of a mole or millimoles (mM). One mole of a nondissociable substance has the same number of molecules present as one mole of any other substance that does not dissociate.[13] For example, one mole of sodium (molecular weight = 23) has the same number of molecules as one mole of chloride (molecular weight = 35.5).

Concentrations of some solutes in body fluids are expressed clinically as weight (mg) per 100 milliliters (equal to 1 deciliter) volume. For example, a glucose concentration in serum is expressed as 120 mg/dl.

Electrolytes in solution are usually expressed as equivalents (Eq) or milliequivalents (mEq) because they chemically combine with each other in proportion to their ionic valence rather than in proportion to weight. One equivalent of an ion is that amount that can replace or combine with one gram of hydrogen. Clinically, electrolytes are usually expressed in mEq/liter, that is, as 1/1000 equivalent.[8] One mEq of an ion is that amount that can replace or combine with one milligram of hydrogen. Multivalent ions have greater chemical combining ability than do univalent ions. Therefore, if one millimole of calcium (Ca^{2+}) is added to solution, it can react with two millimoles of chloride (Cl^-).

TABLE 9-1   ATOMIC AND MOLECULAR WEIGHTS OF PHYSIOLOGICALLY IMPORTANT SUBSTANCES

Subtance	Symbol or Formula	Atomic or Molecular Weight
Calcium ion	Ca^{2+}	40.1
Carbon	C	12.0
Chloride ion	Cl^-	35.5
Hydrogen ion	H^+	1.0
Magnesium ion	Mg^{2+}	24.3
Nitrogen	N	14.0
Oxygen	O	16.0
Phosphorus	P	31.0
Potassium ion	K^+	39.1
Sodium ion	Na^+	23.0
Sulfur	S	32.1
Ammonia	NH_3	17.0
Ammonium ion	NH_4^+	18.0
Bicarbonate ion	HCO_3^-	61.0
Carbon dioxide	CO_2	44.0
Glucose	$C_6H_{12}O_6$	180.0
Phosphate ion	PO_4^{3-}	95.0
Sulfate ion	SO_4^{2-}	96.1
Urea	NH_2CONH_2	60.0
Water	H_2O	18.0

(Rose BD: Clinical Physiology of Acid–Base and Electrolyte Disorders, p 4. Copyright © 1977, McGraw-Hill. Used with the permission of the McGraw-Hill Book Company)

It follows that the addition of one millimole of a univalent ion is equal to adding one milliequivalent of that ion. The number of milliequivalents of a univalent ion can be determined by dividing the weight in milligrams by the atomic number. For example, 230 mg of sodium divided by the atomic weight (23) equals 10 mEq. For a multivalent ion, the milligrams must be multiplied by the valence prior to division by the atomic weight. For example, 40 mg of calcium is multiplied by its valence (2), then divided by the atomic weight, which equals 40. Thus 40 mg of calcium equals 2 mEq.[8]

Total Solute in Relation to Solvent (Osmolarity). The total number of dissolved particles per unit volume (in liters) or unit weight (in kilograms) of solvent is measured and expressed as the osmolarity or osmolality, respectively, of the solution. This property refers to overall degree of concentration or of dilution of the solution. The osmolality depends only on the number of dissolved particles rather than on their mass, electrical charge, or chemical formula. The number of particles is expressed as osmoles or milliosmoles, the latter referring to 1/1000 osmole.

If a substance is put into solution and the molecules do not dissociate, the number of particles added in milliosmoles is the same as the particles measured in millimoles. An example of such a substance is glucose. Although one millimole of a multivalent ion like calcium provides twice as many chemical equivalents (*i.e.*, 2 mEq), it does not dissociate into any more particles than a univalent ion; therefore, one millimole of calcium adds one milliosmole to the solution. However, when a substance such as sodium chloride that dissolves into two particles is added to the solution, one millimole adds two milliosmoles to the solution.

The osmolality of solutions affects movement of fluid between body-fluid compartments. Under conditions in which fluid volumes of differing osmolality are separated by a membrane that is permeable to water but not to the solute, osmotic forces are generated. In an effort to equalize its own concentration on either side of the membrane, water moves to the compartment that has more solute present. This process is called osmosis and the driving force is osmotic pressure, expressed in millimeters of mercury. Net flux of water to the more solute-concentrated side occurs until osmolality on both sides is equal.

The osmotic pressure is defined as the magnitude of the hydrostatic pressure required to oppose net water flux across the membrane. The measurement of osmolality of a solution is based on the change in certain physical properties of a solution that vary with the number of particles present in a volume of solvent. These are referred to as the colligative properties of the solution and include an increase in the boiling point, a decrease in the freezing point, and a decrease in the vapor pressure, all of which occur with increased concentration of solutes in solvent. Clinically, osmolality can also be determined by summing the positively and negatively charged ions. Because sodium ions account for most of the positive charges in the extracellular fluid, serum osmolality can be approximated by doubling the serum sodium value.

The extracellular and intracellular compartments of the body are bounded by biologic membranes that are freely permeable to water and that are relatively impermeable to many solutes. Normally, all body fluids have an equal osmolality of about 285 mOm/kg of water, so that net flux of water does not occur and the volume of the spaces remains fairly constant. However, an alteration in the osmolality of the extracellular fluid in relation to the intracellular fluid causes net flux of water between these compartments. Water moves into or out of cells, so that cell volume changes. When the extracellular fluid becomes lower in osmolality than normal, more water enters the cells than leaves, causing them to swell. When the extracellular fluid becomes higher in osmolality than normal, more water leaves the cell than enters and the cell volume shrinks.

THE CELLULAR ENVIRONMENT

Body-Fluid Spaces and Their Volume

Water is the most prominent constituent of the body, which underscores the importance of maintaining fluid balance for health. Water accounts for 45% to 60% of body weight[8] but varies somewhat from person to person, depending on size, body build, sex, and age. Fat tissue contains much less water than does lean muscle tissue, so women and, particularly, obese people have a smaller body water content proportional to their weight. Infants have a larger water content because of their undeveloped lean muscle tissue.

For people in a normal water-balanced state, total body water in liters can be estimated by dividing the body weight in pounds by four. This is based on the following calculation:

$$1 \text{ liter of water weighs } 1 \text{ kg} = 2.2 \text{ lbs}$$

If body water is 55% of body weight, then body water equals

$$\frac{\text{(body weight in pounds)}}{2.2} \times 0.55 \text{ (body water in liters)} = \frac{1}{4}$$

$$\text{Example: Weight} = \frac{160 \text{ lbs}}{4}; \text{ body water} = 40 \text{ liters.}$$

If a person is obese, the calculated body water is reduced by 10%. If the person is lean, 10% is added to the calculation.[2,15]

Although there is continual movement of water and solutes between compartments, the body strives to keep the proportions of solute and water the same in all compartments, so the volume of fluid contained in each one remains constant. That is, the extracellular and intracellular fluid volumes are regulated around a constant normal level.

The largest volume of water is inside cells where slightly over half of the total body water is localized. A little less than half of the total body water is outside the cells and occupies several spaces (Fig. 9-2). Only part of the water external to cells is available for exchange with the environment. Because not all extracellular water is exchangeable, the distribution of body water is often approximated as two-thirds intracellular and one-third extracellular.

The extracellular fluid that is located within the vascular compartment totals roughly 5 liters. Substrates for and modulators of cellular metabolism are absorbed or secreted into the blood and dissolved in the plasma portion, whose total volume is about 3 liters.[8] The remainder of the blood volume largely consists of white blood cells, red blood cells,

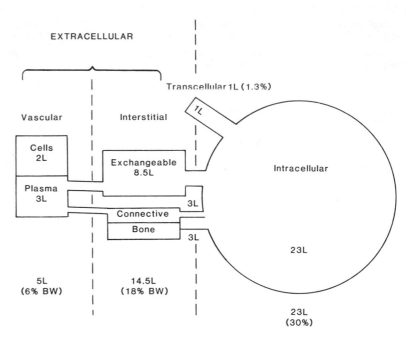

Fig. 9-2. Relative volume of fluid in body compartments. Of the total extracellular fluid, only 14.5 liters is exchangeable.

Total Body Water = 43.5L = 55–60% Body Weight

B.W. = Body Weight

and platelets. The ratio of red blood cell volume to plasma volume is expressed as the hematocrit. The normal hematocrit is about 45% for men and 40% for women, although there is a range of normal. The addition of extracellular water to the plasma decreases the hematocrit; removal of plasma fluid causes it to increase.

Another portion of extracellular fluid is the interstitial fluid, which is outside the blood vessels and bathes the cells. The volume of this space is roughly 8.5 liters.[8] Although this fluid used to be envisioned as a dynamically exchanging but free-floating pool, part of it is now known to be in a gel-like state.[8] Its structure is due to a large quantity of complex molecules called mucopolysaccharides.

Interstitial fluid exchanges with intracellular fluid, blood, and lymph. The lymphatic system actively propels fluid through its channels. When interstitial fluid pressure is normal, lymph flow is minimal. If excess fluid accumulates in the interstitial space and pressure in that space increases, lymph flow can increase by ten to fifty times to remove excess fluid (see Chap. 5). Extracellular water is also present within dense connective tissue and bone, but this fluid is not readily exchangeable. These relatively inaccessible fluids amount to about 6 liters.[8]

Some fluid is present in the body as transcellular fluid. These fluids include saliva, cerebrospinal fluid, sweat, the fluids of the gastrointestinal tract, and other secretions from epithelial cells (Table 9-2).[13] The ionic composition of these liquids differs from that of plasma and interstitial fluid.[13] In general, they are hypotonic compared with plasma. The transcellular volume is estimated as 1 liter at any one time, because much of the secreted fluid is reabsorbed.[8,13] In sum, extracellular fluid volume comprises about 19 liters but only 14.5 liters of this is dynamically interactive.[8]

Compared with total extracellular fluid volume, the volume of water inside cells is considerably larger. Intracellular

TABLE 9-2 MEAN ELECTROLYTE CONTENT OF THE TRANSCELLULAR FLUIDS

Fluid	Na^+ mEq/L	K^+ mEq/L	Cl^- mEq/L	HCO_3^- mEq/L
Saliva	33	20	34	0
Gastric juice*	60	9	84	0
Bile	149	5	101	45
Pancreatic juice	141	5	77	92
Ileal fluid	129	11	116	29
Cecal fluid	80	21	48	22
Cerebrospinal fluid	141	3	127	23
Sweat	45	5	58	0

* The Cl^- concentration exceeds the $Na^+ + K^+$ concentration by 15 mEq/L in gastric juice. This largely represents the secretion of H^+ by the parietal cells.

(Rose BD: Clinical Physiology of Acid–Base and Electrolyte Disorders, p 22. Copyright © 1977, McGraw-Hill. Used with the permission of the McGraw-Hill Book Company)

fluid cannot be measured directly but is deduced from measurements of fluid outside cells and measurements of total body water to be roughly 23 liters.[8] The total body fluid volume is 42 to 44 liters.

Body-Fluid Compartment Composition

The cell is a discrete entity bounded by a plasma membrane. Movement of most substances back and forth across the plasma membrane is highly controlled by specific enzyme systems embedded in the membrane, allowing the intracellular environment to be regulated by selective transmembrane transport. Such highly selective transport creates an electrical charge and an ion distribution differential across the membrane that is essential to normal cell metabolism. Therefore, the extracellular and intracellular compartments have very different compositions with respect to ion concentrations. The intracellular fluid is high in potassium, magnesium, phosphate, and protein but low in sodium and chloride. In contrast, extracellular fluid is mainly a salt solution with sodium electrically balanced by chloride and some bicarbonate (Table 9-3).

The plasma membrane is not freely permeable to ions, although small amounts continually leak into and out of cells. To preserve the ion distribution across the cell membrane, sodium must be extruded from the cell and potassium must be returned to the cell against their respective concentration gradients. The mechanism that pumps sodium out of the cell in exchange for potassium entering the cell is an enzyme complex called the Na^+–K^+ ATPase, which uses energy from the breakdown of adenosine triphosphate (ATP). This transport system is crucial to maintaining the ion differences between intracellular and extracellular milieux. Interference with production of ATP, the enzyme complex utilizing ATP, or availability of ion substrates impairs the cell's ability to maintain a normal electrochemical distribution and ultimately jeopardizes its own integrity.

Osmolality is approximately equal between the vascular and interstitial spaces. Exchange between these spaces takes place across the capillary membrane, which is composed of very thin endothelial cells. The capillaries are leaky because small gaps form where the endothelial cells join each other. These spaces are small enough to restrict cellular and large protein components of blood but allow flow of plasma water and crystalloid solutes through them under pressure. Hydrostatic pressure within the arterial capillary tends to force fluid out of the vasculature through the spaces. Diffusion of water and solute across the endothelial cells also occurs.

The plasma proteins that are too large to pass through the capillary wall exert an osmotic force tending to oppose water flow out of the vasculature. The osmotic pressure due to impermeable plasma proteins is called oncotic pressure. Net flux of fluid out of the capillary at the arterial end and net reabsorption of fluid into the capillary at the venous end

are determined by the balance between hydrostatic pressure tending to force fluid out of the capillary and oncotic pressure tending to keep fluid in. Similar forces of smaller magnitude operate in opposite directions from the interstitial space (see Chap. 5).

Solutes in plasma such as proteins and lipids normally constitute about 7% of the plasma volume. If either proteins or lipids are significantly altered in concentration, an apparent change is produced in the concentration of the ions per volume of total plasma. For example, hyperlipidemia or hyperproteinemia renders ion concentrations artificially low. This change reflects the change in total plasma volume, not an alteration of plasma water. In Table 9-3, the serum ion concentrations are expressed per liter of serum (column 1) and per liter of serum water (column 2). Laboratory measurements are usually expressed in liters of total serum.

THE CONCEPT OF BALANCE

To be healthy, a person must maintain a state of balance with regard to the fluid environments. That is, there must be internal balance whereby the proportions of water and solutes are normally distributed among the various body-fluid compartments. Likewise, there must be external balance whereby any substance that has entered plus any that is produced within the body must equal the amount degraded or leaving the body.[18] It is possible to create illness by altering intake, production, distribution, or excretion of solute and water.

External Balance

Water and ions usually enter the body by ingestion. Balance requires that water intake be matched with output (Fig. 9-3). If body water is lacking, drinking behavior is effected through thirst, for which there are centers located in the hypothalamus. Thirst is affected not only by lack of water but also by a host of factors not directly related to the need for water such as feeding behavior, nature of the diet, and climatic conditions. At least 70% of total water intake is closely associated with meals, and high-protein diets induce a larger turnover of water than do diets high in carbohydrates or fats. People drink greater amounts of water in a warm environment, irrespective of water loss. Normal feeding, drinking, and temperature regulation all require proper hypothalamic brain center functioning. The major ions are ingested with food but, like water intake, ion intake is not entirely related to body needs or controlled by appetite.

Balanced intake and output of ions and water depend mainly on regulation of their excretion. Water is lost from the skin primarily to eliminate heat. Loss of water through the skin without sweat formation is called insensible loss. This form of loss increases with increased metabolic rates as in fever and includes that lost from expiration of air out of the lungs.

Normally about 2500 ml of water are produced or consumed daily: 1200 ml as ingested liquid, 1000 ml in ingested food, and 300 ml produced from oxidative metabolism. To maintain balance, 2500 ml of water are also excreted daily:

TABLE 9-3 CONCENTRATION OF ELECTROLYTES IN SERUM, SERUM WATER, AND INTRACELLULAR WATER

Electrolyte		Serum mEq/L	Serum Water mEq/L	Intracellular Water mEq/kg
Cations				
Sodium		142	152.7	±10
Potassium		4	4.3	156
Calcium		5	5.4	3.3
Magnesium		2	2.2	26
	Total	153	164.6	195.3
Anions				
Chloride		102	109.7	±2
Bicarbonate		26	28	±8
Phosphate		2	2.2	95
Sulfate		1	1.1	20
Organic acids		6	6.5	
Protein		16	17.6	55
	Total	153	165.1	180

(Adapted from Hays RM: Dynamics of body water and electrolytes. In Maxwell MH, Kleeman CR (eds): Clinical Disorders of Fluid and Electrolyte Metabolism, 3rd ed., p 13. Copyright © 1980, McGraw-Hill. Used with the permission of McGraw-Hill Book Company)

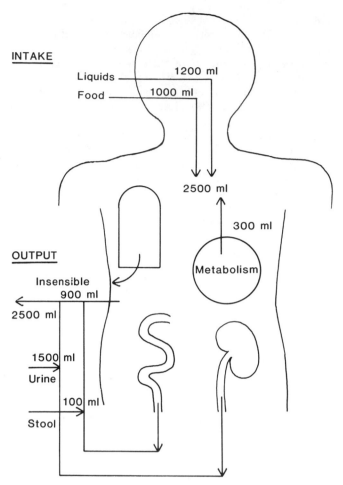

INTAKE

Liquids —— 1200 ml

Food —— 1000 ml

2500 ml

300 ml

Metabolism

OUTPUT

Insensible
900 ml

2500 ml

1500 ml

Urine

100 ml

Stool

Fig. 9-3. Approximate water intake and loss in 24 hours. Total intake, including water from liquids, solid food, and metabolism, equals 2500 cc. Total output, including that from urine, stool, and insensible loss, equals 2500 cc.

1500 ml as urine, 100 ml in stool, and 900 ml as insensible loss. Intake of sodium is about 155 mEq per day with output of about 140 mEq of sodium in urine and 5.0 mEq per day through the stool and insensible loss.[16,18]

Internal Balance

The volume of the extracellular and intracellular body fluid compartments remains constant if the distribution of solute and water remains constant in the two spaces. The osmolality of the extracellular compartment is caused almost entirely (97%) by sodium and its attendant anions. Therefore, the amount of sodium is a major determinant of extracellular volume. The amount of extracellular sodium is regulated by the kidney, which retains sodium when a deficit is imminent and excretes sodium to prevent abnormal accumulation. As the kidney retains or excretes sodium, water is retained or lost with it in order to preserve osmolality balance. As a result, retention or excretion of sodium leads to an increase or decrease in extracellular volume.

Regulation of Extracellular Fluid Volume

Sodium excretion depends upon the difference between glomerular filtration rate (GFR) and tubular reabsorption. Under normal circumstances, 99% of filtered sodium is reabsorbed. Variations in sodium reabsorption are largely affected by the hormone aldosterone. However, other factors also operate, including hydrostatic pressure changes, increases in blood flow to the medullary area of the kidney, sympathetic nervous system activity within the kidney and, possibly, a natriuretic hormone that remains unidentified.[11]

Reabsorption of sodium is known to occur in all areas of the nephron. After being filtered by the glomerulus, the first opportunity for sodium reabsorption is in the proximal tubule, where 50% to 75% of filtered sodium is reabsorbed. A balance exists between the amount of sodium filtered and the amount reabsorbed, so, as the filtered load increases, sodium reabsorption by the proximal tubule proportionately increases as well (Fig. 9-4). This reabsorption is isotonic, that is, sodium and water are reabsorbed in proportions identical to plasma. Both active and passive sodium reabsorption is believed to occur and is coupled to the reabsorption of bicarbonate, glucose, chloride, and amino acids. The descending limb of the loop of Henle is impermeable to sodium, but sodium passively follows as chloride is actively reabsorbed in the ascending limb. In the distal convoluted tubule, sodium reabsorption is active and controlled by aldosterone as described below. Additional active reabsorption occurs in the cortical collecting tubule and medullary collecting duct.[11]

Although it is well established that renal management of sodium occurs in response to changes in extracellular fluid volume, the specific means by which such changes are relayed to the kidney remain subject to investigation. When extracellular fluid volume decreases, aldosterone is secreted and increases sodium reabsorption by the distal tubule. Several inputs to the kidney are believed to signal the kidney that a diminished effective circulatory volume is present. These include decreased afferent arteriolar pressure, decreased sodium load to the macula densa (specialized cells composing the first portion of the distal tubule), and increased renal sympathetic nervous system input.[20] Such information provokes the kidney to release the hormone renin, which splits angiotensin I from angiotensinogen. Another ensyme splits angiotensin I into angiotensin II, which has several actions including vasoconstriction, augmented sympathetic nervous system outflow, thirst stimulation, and stimulated aldosterone secretion. The aldosterone secreted from the adrenal cortex acts on the distal convoluted tubule where it increases the reabsorption of sodium and urinary excretion of potassium. Water passively follows the sodium, which is reabsorbed into the circulating blood (Fig. 9-5).

Regulation of Osmolality

Man shares with other mammals the capacity to alter renal water excretion as a means of regulating body osmolality. Changes in renal water handling accompanied by the sensation of thirst serve to replace body water and maintain the normal osmolality of 285 to 290 mOm.[19]

The principal control of osmolality is by antidiuretic hormone, ADH, a hormone synthesized by the hypothalamus but stored in and released from the posterior pituitary. Changes in osmolality are sensed by osmoreceptors, cells located in several areas within the hypothalamus. When body water is displaced, body fluids become hyperosmolar

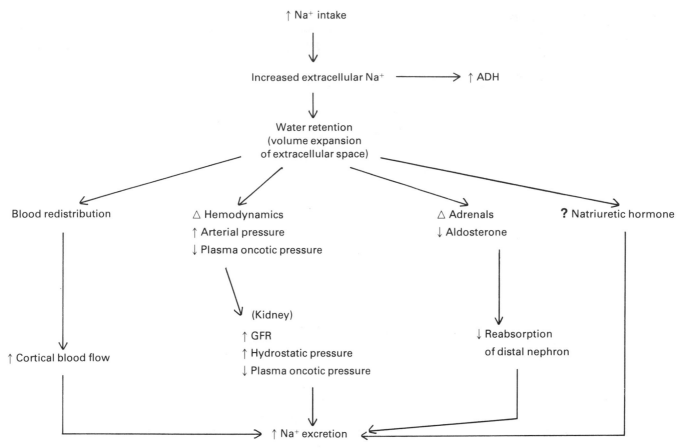

Fig. 9-4. Mechanisms of kidney function acting to correct for a sodium addition to the extracellular fluid. Multiple factors that operate to maintain extracellular volume include a rise in blood pressure causing increased renal blood flow, flow redistribution, and decreased aldosterone release. The existence of a natriuretic hormone is postulated. ECF = extracellular fluid, ECS = extracellular space, GFR = Glomerular filtration rate.

Fig. 9-5. Mechanisms influencing renal augmentation of extracellular fluid volume. Distal tubular reabsorption of sodium is augmented by aldosterone while the concurrent increased water permeability of the tubule occurs through the action of antidiuretic hormone (ADH).

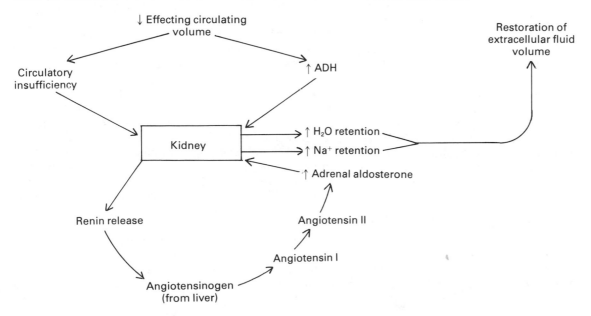

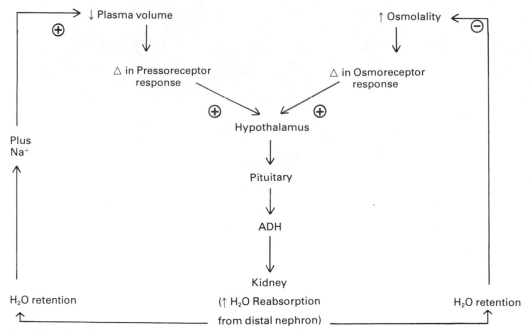

Fig. 9-6. Synchronous plasma volume and osmolality states turning on ADH induced water retention. The major stimulus for ADH secretion is increased serum osmolality. A secondary stimulus is a severe decrease in extracellular volume.

and cells, including the osmoreceptor neurons, shrink. Probably as a result of changed electrical activity,[19] these neurons stimulate the release of ADH. Conversely, if body water is increased over normal, body fluids decrease in osmolality and cells swell. The osmoreceptor cells also swell leading to inhibition of ADH secretion.

ADH exerts its effects upon the collecting ducts and the terminal portions of the distal convoluted tubule. Under the influence of ADH, the walls of these structures become permeable to water. The water diffuses through these walls into the adjacent interstitium and thence back into the blood. When ADH is decreased, the walls of the collecting duct remain impermeable to water, and the water flows down the collecting duct and is excreted in the urine.

ADH secretion and resultant urine volume can be altered by pain, fear, and a variety of other factors. An important secondary stimulus for ADH secretion is a decrease in extracellular volume. Decreases in extracellular volume are relayed by the baroreceptors located in the carotid sinus, aortic arch, and other areas to the hypothalamus and lead to increased antidiuretic hormone secretion. When plasma volume decreases along with an increase in osmolality, ADH release responds to synchronized messages (Fig. 9-6). However, if fluid volume and osmolality both decrease, one output is stimulatory to ADH whereas the other is inhibitory. The outcome will be in response to the strength of the inputs.

EXTRACELLULAR FLUID IMBALANCES

The foregoing mechanisms normally maintain constancy of the internal milieu despite changing environmental conditions. However, disruption of either fluid volume or osmo-

lality is possible when external balance is severely changed or when the mechanisms for maintaining internal balance are impaired. Although volume and osmolality can be altered simultaneously, it is conceptually easier to consider these problems separately first.

Losses and Gains of Extracellular Fluid

Terminology referring to changes in extracellular fluid volume includes saline excess and deficit, extracellular fluid excess and deficit, isotonic expansion and contraction, and hyper and hypovolemia. All these terms refer to either a gain or loss of isotonic fluid from the extracellular space. Such gains or losses occur in proportion to the distribution of extracellular fluid, so approximately one-third goes to the intravascular space and two-thirds to the interstitium.

Extracellular Volume Deficit. Loss of extracellular fluid volume occurs whenever losses of isotonic fluid exceed renal reabsorption or exogenous replacement. The most classic cause is hemorrhage. Excessive renal excretion of sodium and water may also result in an extracellular volume deficit; for example, after administration of potent diuretics or as a result of adrenal cortical insufficiency leading to impaired aldosterone secretion.[7]

The key indication of extracellular volume deficit is a history of saline loss because the kidney ordinarily reabsorbs sodium so well that inadequate sodium intake is rare.[17] The clinical picture of extracellular volume deficit depends upon the severity and rapidity of isotonic volume loss. The most sensitive manifestations are those of inadequate vascular volume, such as a postural drop in blood pressure (Chap. 14), tachycardia, and collapsed neck veins. Eventually, these signs culminate in the picture of hypovolemic shock. Monitoring indications of inadequate fluid volume provides data both about the severity of the initiating cause and the adequacy of fluid replacement.

An extracellular volume deficit is treated by replacement of isotonic fluids. Replacement fluid ideally is identical to the fluid lost, for example, blood loss is replaced by blood. Isotonic intravenous solutions include 0.9% (normal) saline, Ringer's solution, and lactated Ringer's. Table 9-4 shows the tonicity of various parenteral fluids.

Extracellular Volume Excess. An excess of extracellular volume occurs whenever gains of isotonic fluid exceed the renal excretion ability. Such an excess is possible iatrogenically, as when excessive isotonic solutions are infused intravenously. More commonly, an excess of extracellular volume reflects impairment of circulating blood flow to the kidneys so that sodium and water retention ensues. Such a sequence may occur with left ventricular failure (Chap. 27), advanced cirrhosis of the liver, and renal failure.

Manifestations of increased extracellular volume are both vascular and interstitial. Vascular changes include increased blood pressure, bounding pulse, and those parameters reflecting ventricular overload (see Chaps. 14 and 21). An excess of interstitial fluid is noted as edema. Considerable increases in extracellular volume may occur before detectable edema results. For example, a supine patient may accumulate 4 to 8 liters of fluid without edema.[17] When severe enough, the volume overload exceeds left ventricular capacity and pulmonary edema results. Because each liter

of water weighs 1 kg, increases in extracellular volume result in weight gain as well.

In contrast to the preceding clinical indications of extracellular gain or loss of fluid, laboratory signs are less helpful. Because hematocrit measures the proportion of red cell volume to plasma volume, a gain or loss of extracellular fluid may result in a decreased or increased hematocrit, respectively. If the extracellular volume excess develops slowly, hematocrit may not change.[17] Obviously, interpretation of hematocrit decreases must be made with consideration of possible blood loss. Because the extracellular osmolality is unchanged, the serum sodium value remains normal.

Treatment of extracellular volume excess depends upon the severity. Manifestations of pulmonary edema obviously require massive diuresis and measures to decrease venous return. In milder situations, sodium restriction with or without administration of a diuretic may suffice.

A special instance of extracellular volume excess is third-space sequestration of fluids. Although classified as an extracellular volume excess, this problem is unique in that the accumulated fluid does not circulate. As a result, the vascular space may have a normal, decreased, or increased volume. The classic third-space accumulation is ascites, a peritoneal sequestration of fluid as a result of advanced cirrhosis. In addition, third-space accumulations may result from severe burns, peritonitis, intestinal obstruction, and other causes.[7] Two key points should be remembered in relation to third-space fluid accumulation: This fluid may

TABLE 9-4 COMPOSITION OF COMMONLY USED INTRAVENOUS SOLUTIONS

Solution	Solute	Concentrations g/100 ml	Tonic Concentration					Mosmols Contributed by Glucose*	Mosmols Contributed by Electrolytes†
			$[Na^+]$	$[K^+]$	$[Ca^{2+}]$	$[Cl^-]$	$[HCO_3^-]$		
Dextrose in water									
5.0%	Glucose	5.0						278	
10.0%	Glucose	10.0						556	
Saline									
Hypotonic (0.45%, half-normal)	NaCl	0.45	77			77			154
Isotonic (0.9%, normal)	NaCl	0.90	154			154			308
Hypertonic	NaCl	3.0	513			513			1026
		5.0	855			855			1710
Dextrose in saline									
5% in 0.22%	Glucose	5.0						278	
	NaCl	0.22	38.5			38.5			77
5% in 0.45%	Glucose	5.0						278	
	NaCl	0.45	77			77			154
5% in 0.9%	Glucose	5.0						278	
	NaCl	0.90	154			154			308
Alkalinizing solutions									
Hypertonic sodium bicarbonate (0.6 *M*)	$NaHCO_3$	5.0	595				595		1190
Hypertonic sodium bicarbonate (0.9 *M*)	$NaHCO_3$	7.5	893				893		1176
Polyionic solutions									
Ringer's	NaCl	0.86							
	KCl	0.03	147	4	5	156			309
	$CaCl_2$	0.03							
Lactated Ringer's	NaCl	0.60							
	KCl	0.03							
	$CaCl_2$	0.02	130	4	3	109	28		274
	Na lactate	0.31							

* Once administered, glucose is rapidly metabolized and therefore makes no long-term contribution to tonicity.
† Primary contribution to tonicity; solutions approximating 285 mosmols/liter are considered isotonic.
(Adapted from Rose BD: Clinical Physiology of Acid–Base Disorders, p 243. Copyright © 1977, McGraw-Hill. Used with the permission of McGraw-Hill Book Company)

eventually be mobilized to the circulation and lead to a vascular excess, and the vascular status must be assessed before therapy is instigated.

Osmolality Imbalances

In contrast to isotonic disturbances of extracellular volume, which affect only the extracellular fluid compartment, changes in osmolality also affect the intracellular compartment. Whenever the osmolality of extracellular fluid is changed, water shifts between the extracellular and intracellular compartments. As a result of this passive water movement, osmolality is again equalized between the two compartments. However, it remains increased or decreased in relation to normal serum osmolality.

The major clinical manifestations of changes in osmolality thus result from water movement into or out of the cells. As a result of this fluid shift, the cells either swell or shrink. Changes in the volume of central nervous system cells are manifested as changes in neurologic function. As a result, the primary clinical manifestations of osmolality imbalances are neurologic changes ranging from mental confusion to seizures.

The major laboratory sign of osmolality disturbance used in the clinical setting is an abnormal serum sodium value. Because sodium is the major cation of extracellular fluid, doubling the serum sodium value gives an approximate value for the total number of positively and negatively charged ions. That is, the serum sodium is doubled to estimate serum osmolality.[17] A decreased osmolality is defined as a serum sodium under 130 mEq per liter, whereas increased osmolality refers to a serum sodium greater than 145 mEq per liter.[17]

Significant elevations in the glucose or fat content of blood distort the serum osmolality as determined by the preceding method. In the case of hyperglycemia, osmolality is corrected by adding 2 mEq/liter to the sodium value for each 100 mg/dl glucose elevation over normal. For example, if the blood glucose is 1100 mg/dl, the serum sodium must be increased by 20 mEq. Thus, a serum sodium value of 130 mEq/liter would be corrected to 150, then multiplied by two to produce an osmolality of 300 mOsm. In the case of hyperlipidemia, the serum sodium value would have to be adjusted upward by the same percentage as the fat content is elevated.[17]

Decreases and increases in serum osmolality are often referred to by other names, many of which are confusing. These names all refer to an alteration in the ratio of water to particles in the extracellular fluid, that is, to a change in osmolality. Commonly used synonyms for increased osmolality include water deficit, dehydration, and hypernatremia. Synonyms for decreased osmolality are water excess, water intoxication, and hyponatremia.

Increased Serum Osmolality (Water Deficit, Hypernatremia, Dehydration). An increase in serum osmolality occurs whenever losses of electrolyte-free water exceed ADH-mediated water reabsorption in the collecting duct. Often this imbalance occurs when there is neurologic impairment, so thirst is either not sensed or appropriately responded to.

Increased serum osmolality may result from the administration of high-protein tube feedings to patients with impaired consciousness. The high protein and electrolyte content creates a significant osmolar load, which obligates large urine volumes for excretion of the metabolic end products. If adequate water is not provided, increased serum osmolality eventually results. Persons with impaired concentrating abilities, including the elderly, are at particularly great risk.[6] Prophylaxis involves the choice of tube feedings with moderate protein content, dilution with or provision of additional water, and monitoring of sodium values.

Serum osmolality can also be elevated in response to deficient ADH. Alcohol ingestion causes a temporary inhibition of ADH secretion[7] and results in the common phenomenon of diuresis while imbibing. More prolonged and possibly permanent deficiencies in ADH secretion can follow head injuries involving the hypothalamus or can be idiopathic in origin.[13] Impairment of ADH secretion, regardless of cause, is called diabetes insipidus and is managed by ADH replacement.

An increased serum osmolality causes an increase in the serum sodium value beyond the normal range. Replacement of electrolyte-free water, either orally by tap water or intravenously by injection of 5% dextrose in water, reduces the osmolality to normal. The dextrose in the infusion allows parenteral infusion without bursting or crenation of red cells but is metabolized almost immediately, leaving "free water" to hydrate the individual.

Decreased Serum Osmolality (Water Excess, Hyponatremia, Water Intoxication). The converse situation, a decrease in serum osmolality, occurs when excessive electrolyte-free water is retained. Usually, impaired excretion of free water by the kidney is a prerequisite. A decrease in osmolality occurs with end-stage renal failure, with tumor involvement of the hypothalamus, and also with nonhypothalamic tumors that secrete ADH. ADH secretion is often temporarily increased by pain, by some drugs, and early in the postoperative period.[13]

Excessive antidiuretic hormone secretion, by lowering the serum osmolality below normal, causes water to move from the extracellular to the intracellular compartment in order to equalize osmolality between the compartments. The result is cell swelling. Again, the major clinical manifestations are neurologic dysfunctions. The most important laboratory indication is a decrease in serum sodium that reflects a greater proportion of free water in the vascular space. Treatment involves restriction of electrolyte-free water until the kidneys are able to excrete the excess water. Rapid changes in osmolality may precipitate seizures. For that reason as well as the risk of inducing a volume excess, hypertonic solutions are used only in emergency situations.[17]

Combined Volume and Osmolality Changes

In many instances both extracellular volume and osmolality are disordered. These disturbances are combinations of the problems already discussed and, as such, are recognized and managed separately. For example, if an extracellular volume deficit and an increased serum osmolality coexist, the volume deficit is diagnosed by clinical indications of inadequate vascular volume and corrected by replacement of isotonic fluids. The increased osmolality is meanwhile diagnosed by an increase in the serum sodium concentration accompanied by clinical indications of altered sensorium when severe. That problem is treated by administration of electrolyte-free water.

Extracellular Volume Deficit Plus Increased Osmolality. This combination of problems most often results from loss of transcellular fluids, in particular the loss of gastrointestinal fluids and large quantities of sweat. Although classified as extracellular fluids, these fluids are different in that they are hypotonic compared with plasma (see Table 9-2). As a result, simultaneous losses occur in isotonic fluid, leading to extracellular volume deficit, and in free water, leading to an increased serum osmolality. Therefore, manifestations develop of both extracellular deficit, such as postural blood pressure drop, and increased osmolality, as evidenced by the increase in serum sodium.

Because two different problems have occurred, each is treated separately. The extracellular deficit is treated by replacement of isotonic fluids, the increased osmolality, by replacement of electrolyte-free water. A common pattern clinically for patients undergoing nasogastric suction is intravenous replacement with alternating isotonic fluids, such as lactated Ringer's, and hydrating fluids, such as 5% dextrose in water. Another method is continuous infusion of half-strength saline, that is, 5% dextrose in 0.45% saline. If losses are extreme, exact determination of electrolyte content of gastrointestinal losses may prove necessary.

Extracellular Volume Deficit Plus Decreased Osmolality. When an extracellular volume deficit is treated only with electrolyte-free water, the simultaneous development of a volume deficit and decreased serum osmolality may occur. An extreme example is treatment of hypovolemic shock exclusively with 5% dextrose in water. More commonly, these two problems result when transcellular losses are replaced only with water. As described before, these fluids are electrolyte-containing, albeit in lower concentrations than plasma. Correct replacement requires administration of both isotonic solutions and electrolyte-free water.

Persons liable to lose transcellular fluids need to be taught appropriate replacement. For example, individuals with vomiting and diarrhea should drink sodium-containing fluids such as boullion. Because sensible perspiration contains sodium in amounts ranging from 30 to 70 mEq per liter,[7] people undergoing strenuous physical exertion also require electrolyte replacement. The beverage Gatorade provides 21 mEq sodium per liter.[7]

Water retention leading to a decreased serum osmolality may also be a physiologic compensation for a volume deficit. When extracellular volume is severely compromised, baroreceptor stimulation leads to ADH release in an attempt to increase the amount of circulating fluids.[13,19]

Regardless of cause, a coexisting decrease in extracellular volume and osmolality necessitates simultaneous replacement of isotonic fluid and restriction of free water. The effect of free-water restriction is monitored by following serum sodium values. Adequacy of isotonic replacement is determined by monitoring postural blood pressure and other indicators of circulating blood volume.

Extracellular Volume Excess Plus Decreased Osmolality. This combination usually represents severe physiologic dysfunction, so that the kidneys inappropriately reabsorb electrolyte-free water despite an extracellular volume excess. Although the exact mechanisms remain elusive, the situation is recognized as representing an end-stage event of many chronic disease states such as heart failure or cirrhosis.[12,17] Part of this sequence may involve third-space sequestration of fluid so that circulating blood volume is diminished. As a result, ADH secretion increases and excessive free water is reabsorbed.[13] Inappropriate water retention cannot develop without concomitant water ingestion. Therefore, ingestion of electrolyte-free water must be limited.[13] The excessive extracellular volume is simultaneously managed by sodium restriction and, when appropriate, by the administration of diuretics.

Extracellular Volume Excess Plus Increased Osmolality. This combination results from overly aggressive free water restriction in the situation just described. The possibility of over-restriction underscores the need for frequent monitoring of serum sodium values to estimate serum osmolality.

POTASSIUM BALANCE

The major intracellular cation, potassium, helps to regulate many cell functions, including protein and glycogen synthesis.[13] The intracellular potassium concentration is 150 to 160 mEq/liter and accounts for approximately 98% of the total body content. In contrast, extracellular potassium averages 4.0 to 5.0 mEq/liter or only 2% of the total.[13] Both the absolute amount of potassium and the ratio of intracellular to extracellular potassium are important.

External balance of potassium occurs when intake is equivalent to renal and extrarenal excretion. Daily intake in the diet is 1 to 1.5 mEq/kg body weight per day.[14] More than 90% of ingested potassium is excreted in the urine. Urinary excretion can vary from 5 mEq/day or less under conditions of body deficit, up to several hundred milliequivalents per liter per day. Extrarenal excretion is mainly through the feces in amount of 7 to 15 mEq per day. Small amounts are lost in sweat.[14] Most of the potassium filtered at the glomerulus is reabsorbed in the proximal tubule and loop of Henle. The distal tubule and collecting ducts regulate potassium balance. When the diet is deficient in potassium, reabsorption continues throughout the distal tubule and collecting duct. When dietary intake is in excess of body needs, potassium is secreted into the distal nephron and is excreted in the urine (Fig. 9-7).[13]

Potassium excretion by the kidney is basically determined by the potassium level inside distal nephron cells and by aldosterone action. An increased concentration of potassium inside cells enhances the gradient for potassium movement into the lumen of the tubule. In addition, aldosterone promotes potassium secretion at the same time as it augments sodium reabsorption. Aldosterone secretion can result from a response by the renin–angiotensin system to a decreased plasma volume or from a direct response of the adrenal cortex cells to the potassium concentration of the

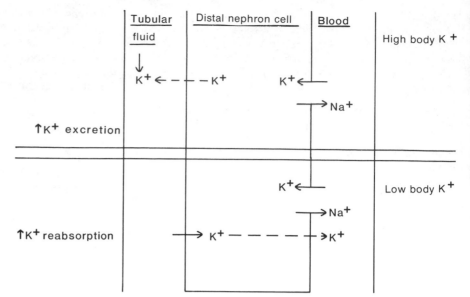

Fig. 9-7. Potassium transport in distal nephron under conditions of K+ load and K+ deficit. When excess potassium is ingested, potassium is secreted into the distal tubule and excreted in the urine. In conditions of potassium deficit, potassium is instead reabsorbed.

fluid surrounding them. In the latter case, an increased extracellular potassium concentration raises the level of the cellular potassium, which then stimulates aldosterone secretion.[14]

Although external balance is maintained by the kidney, internal balance can be altered by shifts of potassium between the cellular and extracellular compartments. In the case of a total potassium deficiency, the plasma potassium concentration tends to drop, which leads to a higher than normal efflux of potassium out of cells. The opposite flux of potassium occurs when there is a surfeit of total body potassium.

Shifts of potassium between compartments can also occur without total body potassium deficit or excess. Most commonly, the hydrogen ion concentration of plasma influences internal balance. When extracellular [H+] increases, potassium moves out of cells in exchange for hydrogen movement in. The opposite exchange occurs with a [H+] decrease.

Because the quantity of extracellular potassium is minute compared with that inside the cells, small variations in extracellular potassium can markedly alter the extracellular to intracellular ratio.[13] The result of a changed ratio is an increase or decrease in the resting membrane potential of the cell and an effect on action potential generation (see Chap. 3). Alterations in neuromuscular transmission can occur throughout the body, although cardiac muscle is particularly vulnerable. Either a decrease (hypokalemia) or an increase (hyperkalemia) in the extracellular potassium concentration is thus important, whether or not the intracellular potassium concentration has been altered.

Hypokalemia

Etiology. Hypokalemia can follow severe vomiting or diarrhea, excessive loss through the kidney (as in diuretic therapy), excessive or profound diaphoresis. In these instances cellular potassium is depleted. Hypokalemia can also result from the increased shift of potassium into cells that accompanies alkalosis or hyperinsulinism.[13] In these instances, total body potassium is usually normal.

Cardiac Manifestations. The increased resting membrane potential in the myocardial conduction system leads to prolonged repolarization (see Chap. 3) and produces a flat, broad T wave, enlarged U wave, and ST-segment depression on the electrocardiogram.[9] A wide variety of arrhythmias may occur as hypokalemia worsens, culminating in ventricular fibrillation.[9,13] Refer to Chapter 17 for a complete description of the electrocardiographic changes found in hypokalemia. In addition, hypokalemia increases the risk of digitalis toxicity with its attendant arrhythmias (see Chap. 34).

Effects of hypokalemia on contractility are unclear. Experimental evidence from animal studies associates acute hypokalemia with increased contractility but chronic severe hypokalemia with decreased contractility. The clinical relevance of these findings is unknown.[9]

Systemic Manifestations. Hypokalemia renders the cell membrane's resting potential more negative than normal, so that the cell has difficulty reaching threshold and cannot generate action potentials. As a result, muscles become weak and even paralyzed. The muscles of the feet and legs are usually impaired first, but the weakness progresses to the muscles of the hands and arms and gastrointestinal tract and eventually culminates in respiratory failure. Although these symptoms are generally associated with a plasma level of potassium under 2.5 mEq liter, individual variation occurs, depending on the serum calcium value and on the rate of hypokalemia development.[13]

Another effect of hypokalemia is impaired glucose tolerance, which is due at least in part to decreased insulin release.[14] Many other systemic effects are possible, including impaired urine concentration and other changes in renal function, alterations in sensorium, and rhabdomyolysis.[13]

Treatment. Mild hypokalemia can be treated by oral replacement with potassium-rich foods or various pharmacologic preparations of potassium chloride. Intravenous replacement is required for treatment of severe potassium depletion as well as for prophylaxis in patients receiving nothing by mouth who are likely to develop potassium loss. Maximal intravenous replacement of potassium diluted in a glucose solution is usually limited to 10 to 20 mEq/hour.[13]

Hyperkalemia

Etiology. A plasma potassium concentration above 5.0 mEq/liter can result from increased intake or decreased excretion of potassium or a shift of potassium from cells to the extracellular fluid. High oral intake of potassium rarely leads to hyperkalemia without a coexisting defect in excretion. Impaired renal elimination of potassium can be due to acute or chronic renal failure, decreased aldosterone secretion, or counteraction of aldosterone by potassium-sparing diuretics.[13] As previously described, cellular compensation for acidosis temporarily creates hyperkalemia until the pH is returned to normal. Additional situations causing potassium shifts from the intracellular to extracellular fluid include insulin deficiency, extreme tissue catabolism, and massive digitalis overdose. The last situation results from digitalis inhibition of the Na^+–K^+ ATPase pump such that potassium diffuses out of cells.[13]

Cardiac Manifestations. Initially, hyperkalemia enhances cell membrane permeability so that potassium moves out of the cells more rapidly and the rate of repolarization is increased (see Chap. 3). Electrocardiographic manifestations at this stage, usually when the serum potassium is about 6 mEq/liter, include peaked T waves and a shortened QT interval (Chap. 17). When the serum potassium reaches 7 or 8 mEq/liter, depolarization is delayed as evidenced by widened QRS intervals proceeding to sine waves. Ventricular fibrillation or asystole then follows.[13]

Systemic Manifestations. Hyperkalemia also changes the cell's resting membrane potential. In this case, the membrane potential moves closer to threshold potential, so that the initial action potential is enhanced but subsequent repolarization is impaired. As is the case for hypokalemia, the outcome for skeletal muscles is weakness beginning in the legs. Cranial nerves and respiratory muscles are ordinarily not affected.[13]

Treatment. As is true for hypokalemia, chronic elevations of potassium are usually better tolerated than are sudden rises.[13] However, whenever the serum potassium rises over 8 mEq/liter, emergency treatment is required to move potassium into the cells. This shift can be accomplished by administration of insulin, usually given with glucose, or by administration of bicarbonate. Intravenous calcium protects the heart by making the threshold potential less negative than normal and hence counteracting the abnormally shortened distance between the resting and threshold potentials.[13] Actual elimination of excess potassium from the body can be achieved by dialysis or by the use of the cation exchange resin, sodium polystyrene sulfonate (Kayexalate).[13]

ACID–BASE BALANCE
Hydrogen Ion and Acidity

An acid is commonly defined as a substance that donates a proton H^+ in chemical reactions, and a base is defined as an acceptor of H^+. Acids that dissociate freely into hydrogen ion and anion base are called strong acids, whereas acids that dissociate minimally in comparison are called weak acids.[4] In solution, weak acids reach an equilibrium where the tendency for molecules to dissociate is balanced with the tendency to reassociate.

Acidity is commonly measured as the hydrogen ion concentration $[H^+]$ in blood and is expressed as the negative logarithm of $[H^+]$, which is called pH. The pH of arterial plasma is normally maintained between 7.35 and 7.45. The state that occurs when plasma pH drops below 7.35 is called acidemia and the process by which pH is lowered, acidosis. Conversely, alkalemia is the state that occurs when serum pH is greater than 7.45, and alkalosis refers to a process with the potential to increase pH.

Buffering

Body fluids contain a number of substances acting as weak acids and conjugate bases. When a strong acid or base is added to body fluids, the change in $[H^+]$ is less than the amount of hydrogen added. This occurs when the hydrogen complexes with bases so they do not contribute to acidity. This process is called buffering, and the acid–base pairs are called buffers.

The body has several buffer systems that accept H^+ as they are admitted into the extracellular fluid, so the acidity of body fluids does not change significantly. These include hemoglobin and other proteins, which are negatively charged at body pH and therefore accept hydrogen, inorganic phosphate, and organic phosphate groups. However, the major buffer of extracellular fluid is carbonic acid (H_2CO_3) and its conjugate base, bicarbonate (HCO_3^-).

Carbon dioxide dissolved in plasma water combines with water to form carbonic acid. The chemical reaction is reversible and inside certain cells is accelerated by the enzyme, carbonic anhydrase. The amount of carbon dioxide gas dissolved in fluid is proportional to the partial pressure of that gas in contact with the fluid. Therefore, the determinant of the concentration of carbonic acid in plasma is the partial pressure of carbon dioxide ($PaCO_2$) in the blood. Carbonic acid has two hydrogen atoms, but one hydrogen bond is sufficiently weak to dissociate into a hydrogen ion and a bicarbonate ion, as expressed in the following equation:

$$\text{Dissolved } CO_2 + H_2O \rightleftarrows H_2CO_3 \rightleftarrows H^+ + HCO_3^-$$

These reactions form the basis for deriving the equation to calculate pH as follows:[1,5]

$$[H^+]\,[HCO_3^-] = K(H_2CO_3)$$
$$[H^+] = \frac{K(H_2CO_3)}{(HCO_3^-)}$$
$$K = \text{dissociation constant at body temperature}$$
$$\log [H^+] = \log K + \log \frac{(H_2CO_3)}{(HCO_3^-)}$$
$$-\log H = -\log K - \log \frac{(H_2CO_3)}{(HCO_3^-)}$$
$$pH = pK + \log \frac{(HCO_3^-)}{(H_2CO_3)}$$

In practice, H_2CO_3 is replaced by $PaCO_2$ since the concentration of H_2CO_3 is very low and its measurement difficult:

$$pH = 6.1 + \log \frac{(HCO_3^-) mEq/liter}{PaCO_2 \; mm \; Hg}$$

Substitution of normal values for HCO_3^- and $PaCO_2$ shows how a normal pH of 7.4 is obtained. Note that the pH value does not change as long as the 20:1 ratio of HCO_3^- to $PaCO_2$ is maintained:

$$pH = 6.1 + \log \frac{24}{(0.03 \times 40)}$$
$$pH = 6.1 + \log \frac{24 \; mEq/liter}{1.2 \; mEq/liter}$$
$$pH = 6.1 + \log 20$$
$$pH = 6.1 + 1.30$$
$$pH = 7.4$$

Regulation of Acid–Base Balance

Changes in plasma acidity can occur either through an effect on $PaCO_2$ or by an effect on bicarbonate concentration. These variables can be altered independently, and an understanding of the physiologic factors influencing them is a prerequisite to comprehending acid–base assessment.

Plasma Bicarbonate Concentration. The regulation of bicarbonate concentration is a secondary effect of the mechanisms that regulate extracellular hydrogen ion concentration. When HCO_3^- is consumed, restoration of the bicarbonate pool depends on the kidney's ability to effect net hydrogen ion secretion. Net secretion of hydrogen is associated with regeneration by the kidney of HCO_3^-, which is returned to the extracellular pool.

Bicarbonate ions are freely filtered at the glomerulus but are reabsorbed by an indirect mechanism (Fig. 9-8). Sodium ions that electrically balance the HCO_3^- in tubular fluid enter the kidney tubule cell in exchange for hydrogen ions

Fig. 9-8. Reabsorption of filtered bicarbonate. Hydrogen ion is secreted into the tubular lumen in exchange for sodium entry into renal tubular cells. The H^+ combines with HCO_3^- to form H_2CO_3, which converts to H_2O and CO_2. The CO_2 readily enters the cell. Inside the cell CO_2 and H_2O form H_2CO_3, which again breaks down to H^+ and HCO_3^-. The HCO_3^- is reabsorbed. The H^+ is secreted into the tubular lumen to start the cycle again. O = active transport pump.

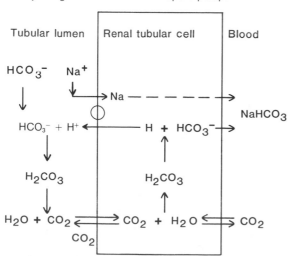

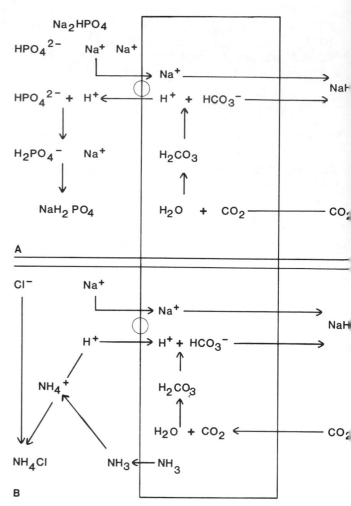

Fig. 9-9. Execretion of hydrogen and addition of new bicarbonate to plasma by reaction of secreted hydrogen. The top portion of the diagram (**A**) shows the sequence for H^+ combination with a titratable acid, in this case PO_4^{3-}. The lower portion (**B**) shows conversion of ammonia (NH_3) to ammonium (NH_4^+). O = active transport pump.

to maintain electroneutrality across the membrane. The secreted hydrogen ions react with the tubular fluid bicarbonate ions to form H_2CO_3 and eventually form CO_2 and H_2O. These substances equilibrate across the cell membrane. Inside the cell, CO_2 and H_2O combine to form H_2CO_3 and H^+ and HCO_3^-. This reaction generates hydrogen ion for secretion into tubular fluid, whereas the bicarbonate ion enters the plasma and completes the reabsorption cycle. Although it is not the original filtered bicarbonate ions that are absorbed, an equivalent amount can be regenerated by this process. The rate at which the kidney returns bicarbonate to the body stores depends on the rate of hydrogen ion secretion in exchange for sodium ion.

To conserve body bicarbonate maximally, the rate of hydrogen ion secretion must match the rate of bicarbonate filtration. When the body is presented with an acid load, the kidney must generate more bicarbonate than is filtered, and the opposite must occur when it is confronted by an alkali load. When $[H^+]$ secretion into the tubular fluid exceeds the amount of filtered HCO_3^- present, some of the excess $[H^+]$ remains dissolved in the fluid and increases urinary hydrogen ion concentration. The maximum decrease in urine pH is to 4.0. Hydrogen ions also combine with filtered base components of other buffers. The major component is phosphate, and such complexes are called titratable acids. Finally, excess hydrogen ions in tubular fluid can react with ammonia (NH_3) to form urinary ammonium (NH_4^+). Ammonia is released from renal tubular cells as a product of glutamine metabolism. Ammonia is freely permeable across membranes, is a strong base, and upon forming ammonium is poorly diffusible back out of urine. The rate of ammonia generation depends upon the rate of urine acidification (Fig. 9-9).

Hydrogen ions are normally introduced into body fluids by endogenous acid production. Metabolism of certain dietary substances and the catabolism of body tissues yield strong acids. States of high catabolism or altered diet with increased acid precursor intake can augment the usual hydrogen ion input. Given normal dietary conditions, endogenous acid production is about 1 mEq/kg per day in adults and two to three times that much in children.

Plasma Carbon Dioxide Tension. Cellular metabolism is a process that generates carbon dioxide. The carbon dioxide tension (or partial pressure of CO_2, $PaCO_2$) of arterial blood depends on the rate of production and on the rate of excretion into the external environment by the lungs. The rate of carbon dioxide production is fairly stable in normal people from day to day if the level of exercise stays fairly constant. The stability of carbon dioxide affects H^+ balance through its influence on H_2CO_3 concentration. The regulation of carbon dioxide excretion by alveolar ventilation is very effective. Sensor neurons in the medulla oblongata respond quickly to augment ventilation when arterial $PaCO_2$ increases or reduce ventilation when it decreases.

Acid–Base Imbalances

Interpretation of Acid–Base Disorders. Alterations in acid–base status can result either from imbalances in carbon dioxide elimination relative to production or from disturbances in the ratio of $[HCO_3^-]$ to $[H^+]$. Because carbon dioxide is eliminated by the lungs, inadequate alveolar ventilation resulting in retention of carbon dioxide is called respiratory acidosis. Conversely, excessive alveolar ventilation that decreases arterial carbon dioxide is called respiratory alkalosis. Because carbon dioxide is formed when carbonic acid dissociates, these respiratory disorders are also referred to as carbonic acidosis and alkalosis, respectively. Changes in the ratio of $[HCO_3^-]$ to $[H^+]$ can result from increased cellular acid production or altered hydrogen or bicarbonate elimination. Terminology for such disorders includes metabolic acidosis and alkalosis or noncarbonic acidosis and alkalosis.

Whether "respiratory" or "metabolic" in origin, acute acid–base disturbances alter the arterial pH. Over time, compensatory mechanisms move the pH back toward normal.

Although acid–base disorders can be predicted on the basis of underlying pathophysiological or clinical manifestations, confirmation is possible only by analysis of arterial pH, $PaCO_2$, and HCO_3^- values.* Blood gases can be inter-

*Although not discussed in this chapter, arterial blood gases also include PaO_2.

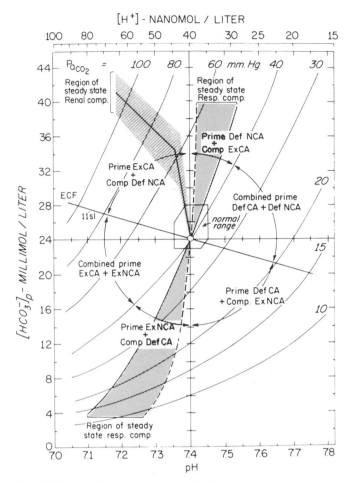

Fig. 9-10. Acid–base nomogram. Acid–base status is determined by plotting any two arterial blood gas values. The pH is plotted on the horizontal axis. The $PaCO_2$ is plotted on the curved isobars. A line drawn from their intersection to the vertical axis indicates the bicarbonate value. Disorders are labeled on the diagram. (Ruch TC, Patton HD: Physiology and Biophysics 2, p 519. Philadelphia, WB Saunders, 1974)

preted by plotting the horizontal and vertical axes on a nomogram (Fig. 9-10). They can also be interpreted by sequential analysis as follows:

1. Look at pH
   For this maneuver, only a pH of 7.4 is considered normal, even though the range of normal is actually 7.35 to 7.45.
   A pH under 7.4 is acidosis.
   A pH over 7.4 is alkalosis.
2. Look at $PaCO_2$ (range of normal: 35–45 mm Hg)
   If $PaCO_2$ is normal, there is no primary respiratory problem and no respiratory compensation for a metabolic problem.
   Abnormal $PaCO_2$ values are interpreted in relation to pH:
   ↑ $PaCO_2$ plus ↓ pH: acidosis of respiratory origin
   ↑ $PaCO_2$ plus ↑ pH: respiratory retention of CO_2 to compensate for metabolic alkalosis
   ↓ $PaCO_2$ plus ↑ pH: alkalosis of respiratory origin
   ↓ $PaCO_2$ plus ↓ pH: respiratory elimination of CO_2 to compensate for metabolic acidosis

3. Look at HCO_3^- (range of normal: 22–26 mEq/liter)
    If HCO_3^- is normal, there is no primary metabolic problem and no metabolic compensation for a respiratory problem.
    Abnormal HCO_3^- values are interpreted in relation to pH:

    ↓ HCO_3^- plus ↓ pH: acidosis of metabolic origin

    ↓ HCO_3^- plus ↑ pH: renal retention of (H^+) or elimination of (HCO_3^-) to compensate for respiratory alkalosis

    ↑ HCO_3^- plus ↑ pH: alkalosis of metabolic origin

    ↑ HCO_3^- plus ↓ pH: renal retention of (HCO_3^-) or elimination of (H^+) to compensate for respiratory acidosis.

4. Use above finding to diagnose acid–base status
    Possible disorders include compensated or uncompensated respiratory acidosis, compensated or uncompensated respiratory alkalosis, compensated or uncompensated metabolic acidosis, compensated or uncompensated metabolic alkalosis. Simultaneous respiratory and metabolic disorders are also possible.
    If $PaCO_2$, HCO_3^-, and pH are *all* within their normal ranges, acid–base status is normal.[1]

Respiratory Acidosis. Alveolar ventilation inadequate to "blow off" all the carbon dioxide produced by cell metabolism results in respiratory acidosis. Specific causes of alveolar hypoventilation may be respiratory or nonrespiratory in orgin. For example, alveolar hypoventilation may result from a respiratory disease such as chronic bronchitis but may also result from a nonrespiratory cause such as impingement of abdominal contents upon the diaphragm. Selected causes of respiratory acidosis include the following:

Lung diseases
  Chronic bronchitis
  Severe pneumonia
  Status asthmaticus
Chest wall disorders
  Cervical spine injury
  Guillain-Barré syndrome
  Multiple rib fractures (flail chest)
  Myasthenia gravis
Central nervous system dysfunction
  Head injury affecting mid or lower pons
  Narcotic or barbiturate overdose
Abdominal problems
  Ascites
  Upper abdominal incision
Immobility

Manifestations of respiratory acidosis result from the response of various tissues to a decreased pH. The most prominent symptoms are those due to effects on the cardiovascular and central nervous systems. Early cardiovascular manifestations include tachycardia and increased blood pressure. These effects are compounded by hypoxemia. If the pH continues to drop, eventually myocardial depression occurs, resulting in decreased cardiac output.[21] The central nervous system manifestations are believed to result from dilation of cerebral vessels leading to an increase in intracranial pressure. Manifestations include headache, personality changes, somnolence, and finally coma.

An additional result of acidosis is the potential development of hyperkalemia due to compensatory cellular buffering. Potassium shifts out of cells and excess hydrogen moves in. Manifestations of hyperkalemia have been described previously. Appropriate management of hyperkalemia demands interpretation of potassium values in relation to pH (Fig. 9-11). For each 0.1 unit decrease in the arterial pH, the plasma potassium value is increased by 0.6 mEq/liter.[13] When the hyperkalemia is known to be a result of cell buffering, treatment is directed toward

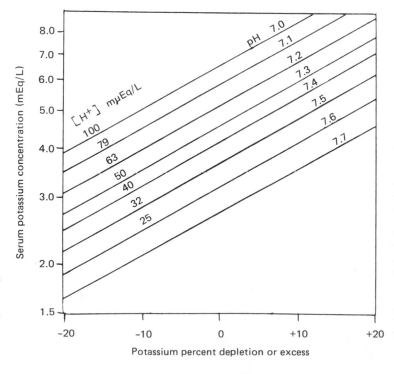

Fig. 9-11. The relationship between serum potassium concentration, blood pH, and percent change in content-capacity. Serum potassium is plotted on the vertical axis and a horizontal line is drawn to intersect with the pH. The percent of total body potassium depletion or excess can then be determined. (Scribner BH: Teaching Syllabus for the Course on Fluid and Electrolyte Balance, p 76. Seattle, University of Washington School of Medicine, 1969)

correction of the causative acidosis. If the potassium elevation is life-threatening, maneuvers to shift potassium back into the cells are also indicated.

Respiratory acidosis also affects tissue oxygenation. Severe respiratory acidosis leads to the development of hypoxemia because of the disturbed relationship between oxygen consumption and carbon dioxide production. Hypoxemia that occurs for this reason can be managed by oxygen administration. Both the decreased pH and elevated carbon dioxide also shift the oxygen–hemoglobin dissociation curve to the right, so oxygen is more easily unloaded at systemic capillary beds. Quantitatively, the effect is greater for the decreased pH.[10] When individuals with respiratory acidosis are also hypoxemic, this compensatory offloading is less, because both loading and unloading occur on the steep portion of the oxygen–hemoglobin dissociation curve.[21]

Within several hours of the onset of respiratory acidosis, the kidneys begin to increase bicarbonate reabsorption and elimination of hydrogen ion. Eventually, the pH moves close to normal. Because the cerebral manifestations, cardiovascular signs, and hyperkalemia resulted from the decreased pH, these effects are no longer apparent. However, hypoxemia, when present, persists.

Treatment for respiratory acidosis includes maneuvers to increase alveolar ventilation and, when necessary, correction of acidosis by the administration of bicarbonate. Although intubation and mechanical ventilation may be required in severe cases, aggressive nursing interventions can in many instances reverse hypoventilation. Such maneuvers include coached deep breathing, ambulation, and incentive spirometry. Concomitant hypoxemia is treated with oxygen, according to its severity. It should be recalled that for persons with chronic respiratory acidosis, the medullary respiratory center may have become insensitive to the elevated carbon dioxide. Persons with chronic respiratory acidosis depend on partial pressures of below 60 mm Hg for the stimulus to breathe. Oxygen therapy for such persons is administered at low liter flows.

Respiratory Alkalosis. In contrast to respiratory acidosis, respiratory alkalosis is a result of alveolar hyperventilation, such that more carbon dioxide is eliminated than is produced. A common and well-recognized cause is anxiety. In addition, alveolar hyperventilation may result from damage to the medullary respiratory center or may be iatrogenic, for example, when mechanical ventilation is excessive.

A major manifestation is neuromuscular irritability caused by a change in calcium binding to albumin. As the pH rises, albumin–calcium binding increases, so the proportion of ionized calcium declines. As a result, manifestations of calcium deficit occur, despite no actual calcium depletion.

Other manifestations include a feeling of lightheadedness or altered consciousness, both of which are related to the increase in pH in the cerebrospinal fluid.[13] As with acidosis, cellular buffering occurs. In this instance, potassium moves into cells and hydrogen moves out, so hypokalemia results. Because these manifestations are related to the elevated pH, they are often absent in chronic states, that is, when the

kidneys have compensated by excreting bicarbonate.[13] Treatment of respiratory alkalosis is most effectively directed toward elimination of the underlying cause.

Metabolic Acidosis. Although similar to respiratory acidosis in most of its effects, metabolic acidosis is produced by a relative gain in noncarbonic acids. Again, potential causes are many. When inadequate oxygen is available to fuel the conversion of pyruvic acid to carbon dioxide and water, it is instead converted to lactic acid.[7] Therefore, such a sequence is possible whenever cellular ischemia exists, as in shock, diabetic acidosis, and following cardiac arrest. Ineffective renal hydrogen ion elimination, as in renal failure, also results in metabolic acidosis. Another common cause is the excessive gastrointestinal loss of pancreatic bicarbonate, such as occurs in diarrhea. In this situation, acidosis is due to a relative rather than an actual gain in hydrogen ion. Metabolic acidosis can also result from expansion of extracellular fluid volume with isotonic fluids, so the bicarbonate buffer system is dilute.[7]

As with respiratory acidosis, manifestations include the aforementioned central nervous and cardiovascular effects and hyperkalemia. Neurologic dysfunction is usually less obvious than with respiratory acidosis, presumably because carbon dioxide diffuses across the blood–brain barrier more readily than does hydrogen.[13] Decreased contractility and potentially lethal arrhythmias are likely when the pH drops below 7.20.[13] Respiratory compensation by increased ventilatory elimination of carbon dioxide begins in minutes. Management, in addition to treatment of the underlying disorder, includes the administration of bicarbonate.

Metabolic Alkalosis. Either loss of hydrogen ion or retention of bicarbonate may result in metabolic alkalosis. Vomiting and nasogastric suction commonly cause hydrogen loss in the form of hydrochloric acid. Chloride loss often underlies the renal retention of bicarbonate. When chloride is depleted, the only available anion to be reabsorbed with sodium is bicarbonate. As a result of continued sodium and bicarbonate reabsorption, metabolic alkalosis ensues. Another cause is depletion of extracellular fluid volume, so the relative proportion of bicarbonate increases. This condition is referred to as contraction alkalosis. In addition, when volume is depleted, the kidneys retain more sodium and with it bicarbonate ion to maintain electroneutrality. This sequence also can cause metabolic alkalosis, particularly when chloride is already depleted.[13] Finally, hyperaldosteronism causes excessive hydrogen ion excretion and also results in metabolic alkalosis.

Manifestations of metabolic alkalosis are often related to volume depletion. Neurologic symptoms are less frequent than in respiratory alkalosis, because carbon dioxide diffuses more readily across the blood–brain barrier than does bicarbonate ion.[13] Paresthesias and occasionally tetany may occur as a result of the change in calcium binding.

Metabolic alkalosis is usually associated with hypokalemia, partly as a result of cell buffering, as described previously. In addition, metabolic alkalosis increases sodium and potassium exchange in the distal tubule.[3]

Compensatory respiratory retention of carbon dioxide begins in minutes. Treatment of metabolic alkalosis involves restoration of extracellular fluid volume and replacement of chloride ion as well as management of any other initiating causes.

REFERENCES

The selections marked with an asterisk (*) are helpful for further reading.

1. Broughton JO: Understanding blood gases. Ohio Medical Products Medical Article Reprint Library, Aug, 1971*
2. Carrol HJ, Man S Oh: Water, Electrolyte and Acid-Base Metabolism. Philadelphia, JB Lippincott, 1978
3. Cohen JJ: Disorders of potassium balance. Hosp Pract 14, No. 1:119–128, 1979
4. Cohen JJ, Kassirer JP: Acid-base metabolism. In Maxwell MH, Kleeman CR (eds): Clinical Disorders of Fluid and Electrolyte Metabolism, 3rd ed, pp 181–232. New York, McGraw-Hill, 1980
5. Davenport HW: The ABC of Acid-Base Chemistry, 5th ed. Chicago, University of Chicago Press, 1969
6. Gault MH, Dixon ME, Doyle M et al: Hypernatremia, azotemia, and dehydration due to high-protein tube feeding. Ann Intern Med 68(4):778–791, 1968
7. Goldberger E: A Primer of Water, Electrolyte and Acid-Base Syndromes, 6th ed. Philadelphia, Lea & Febiger, 1980*
8. Hays RM: Dynamics of body water and electrolytes. In Maxwell MH, Kleeman CR (eds): Clinical Disorders of Fluid and Electrolyte Metabolism, 3rd ed, pp 1–36. New York, McGraw-Hill, 1980
9. Kleeman K, Singh BN: Serum electrolytes and the heart. In Maxwell MH, Kleeman CR (eds): Clinical Disorders of Fluid and Electrolyte Metabolism, 3rd ed, pp. 145–180. New York, McGraw-Hill, 1980
10. Lenfant C: Gas transport and gas exchange. In Ruch TC, Patton HD (eds): Physiology and Biophysics: Circulation, Respiration and Fluid Balance, 20th ed, pp 325–357. Philadelphia, WB Saunders, 1974*
11. Reineck HJ, Stein JH: Regulation of sodium balance. In Maxwell MH, Kleeman CR (eds): Clinical Disorders of Fluid and Electrolyte Metabolism, 3rd ed, pp 189–212. New York, McGraw-Hill, 1980
12. Reynolds TB: Water, electrolyte, and acid-base disorders in liver disease. In Maxwell MH, Kleeman CR (eds): Clinical Disorders of Fluid and Electrolyte Metabolism, 3rd ed, pp 1251–1265. New York, McGraw-Hill, 1980
13. Rose BD: Clinical Physiology of Acid-Base and Electrolyte Disorders. New York, McGraw-Hill, 1977
14. Schultze RG, Nissenson AR: Potassium: Physiology and pathophysiology. In Maxwell MH, Kleeman CR (eds): Clinical Disorders of Fluid and Electrolyte Metabolism, 3rd ed, pp 113–143. New York, McGraw-Hill, 1980
15. Schwartz AB, Lyons H: Acid-Base and Electrolyte Balance. New York, Grune & Stratton, 1977
16. Schwartz WB, Cohen JJ: The nature of the renal response to chronic disorders of acid-base equilibrium. Am J Med 64(3):417–428, 1978
17. Scribner BH: Teaching Syllabus for the Course on Fluid and Electrolyte Balance. Seattle, University of Washington School of Medicine, 1969*
18. Valtin H: Renal Dysfunction: Mechanisms Involved in Fluid and Solute Imbalance, 7th ed. Boston, Little, Brown, 1979
19. Weitman R, Kleeman CR: Water metabolism and the neurohypophyseal hormones. In Maxwell MH, Kleeman CR (eds): Clinical Disorders of Fluid and Electrolyte Metabolism, 3rd ed, pp 531–645. New York, McGraw-Hill, 1980
20. Welliams GH, Dluhy RG: Fluid electrolyte and acid-base abnormalities in hypertensive disease. In Maxwell MH, Kleeman CR (eds): Clinical Disorders of Fluid and Electrolyte Metabolism, 3rd ed, pp 703–744. New York, McGraw-Hill, 1980
21. Zwillich C, Kryger M, Weil J: Hypoventilation: Consequences and management. Adv Intern Med 23:287–306, 1978

ADDITIONAL READING

Keyes, JL: Basic mechanisms involved in acid-base homeostasis, Part I. Heart Lung 5(2):239–246, 1976

Keyes JL: Blood gas analysis and the assessment of acid-base status. Heart Lung 5(2):247–255, 1976

Kubo WM, Grant MM: The syndrome of inappropriate secretion of antidiuretic hormone. Heart Lung 7(3):469–476, 1978

Siegel PD: The physiologic approach to acid-base balance. Med Clin North Am 57(4):863–879, 1973

Stroot V, Lee C, Schaper CA: Fluids and Electrolytes: A Practical Approach, 2nd ed. Philadelphia, FA Davis, 1977

Trunkey DB: Review of current concepts in fluid and electrolyte management. Heart Lung 4(1):115–121, 1975

Zeluff GW, Suki WN, Jackson D: Hypokalemia: Cause and treatment. Heart Lung 8(5):854–860, 1978

CORONARY ARTERY DISEASE

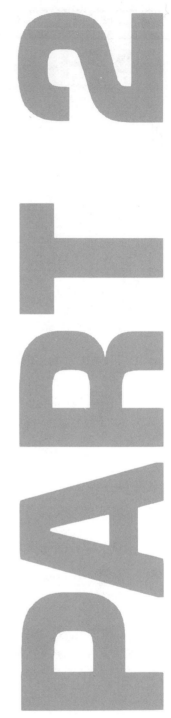

SECTION A
PATHOPHYSIOLOGY

10

Pathogenesis of Atherosclerosis

MARIE J. COWAN, R.N., Ph.D.

Arteriosclerosis means hardening of the arteries and is a general term describing three diseases:

1. atherosclerosis, in which there is proliferation of smooth muscle cells and accumulation of lipids in the intima of the large and middle-size muscular arteries;
2. medial calcific sclerosis, or Mönckeberg's sclerosis, in which there is an accumulation of calcium in the media of medium-sized arteries;
3. arteriolar sclerosis in which there is thickening of the walls and narrowing of the lumen of the small arteries and arterioles and which is often associated with hypertension.

Atherosclerosis is the most frequent cause of death in the United States and Western Europe. It is an arterial disease, most commonly affecting the aorta and the coronary, cerebral, femoral, and other large or middle-sized arteries. Myocardial infarctions (MI) and cerebral infarction (cerebrovascular accidents) are the two major consequences of the disease. The pathogenesis of atherosclerosis is unknown. One of the problems is that the disease progresses for many years before symptoms develop, making it difficult to relate causally the early development with mechanisms of disease. Much of the research in the area of atherosclerosis has been to identify its risk factors. The incidence of atherosclerosis increases with age. The major risk factors are high blood pressure, hyperlipidemia, and cigarette smoking. These factors operate both independently and synergistically. The focus in this chapter is on pathogenesis as the mode of origin of atherosclerosis. Before the different hypotheses can be presented, it is helpful to review the morphology of the normal artery and the atherosclerotic lesion.

MORPHOLOGY OF THE NORMAL ARTERIAL WALL

The walls of the normal musculoelastic arteries contain three layers: the intima, the media, and the adventitia. The *intima* is enclosed by a single layer of endothelial cells on the luminal surface and a continuous boundary of elastic fibers, the internal elastic lamina. Between these confines, the space contains various components of the extracellular connective tissue matrix. The endothelial cell barrier normally is impermeable to proteins in the blood. The *media* consists almost entirely of smooth muscle cells, and the extracellular space consists of collagen, elastin, and proteoglycans. The *adventitia* consists mostly of fibroblasts with a few smooth muscle cells in loose connective tissue. The adventitia is separated from the media by a discontinuous boundary of elastic fibers, the external elastic lamina (Fig. 10-1).

MORPHOLOGY OF THE ATHEROSCLEROTIC LESION

The intima of the arterial wall is principally involved with atherosclerosis, although secondary changes are occasionally found in the media resulting in arterial dilatation and localized aneurysm formation. The lesions associated with atherosclerosis can be divided into three different morphologic types: the fatty streak, the fibrous plaque, and the complicated lesion.

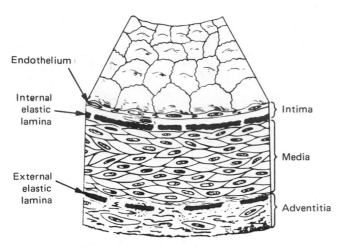

Endothelium

Internal
elastic
lamina

External
elastic
lamina

Intima

Media

Adventitia

Fig. 10-1. Structure of normal muscular artery. (Ross R, Glomset JA: N Engl J Med 295:370, 1976. Reprinted by permission from the New England Journal of Medicine)

Fatty Streak

The fatty streak is a yellowish, smooth lesion protruding slightly into the arterial lumen. It does not obstruct blood flow and is not associated with any clinical symptoms. The lesion is characterized histologically by the presence of lipid desposits within the smooth muscle cells and macrophages in the intima of the artery. These cells "balloon out" because of the lipid in them and are commonly referred to as foam cells. The lipid is mostly cholesterol and cholesterol esters. Fatty streaks have been observed in people of all ages from infancy to senility. In a study of young children, of those from 1 month to 1 year of age, 43% had fatty streaks; and in the children over the age of 1 year, fatty streaks were universal.[19] Whether these lesions are irreversible and, also, whether the fatty streak is the precursor of the fibrous plaque are controversial.

Raised Fibrous Plaque

The characteristic lesion of atherosclerosis is the raised fibrous plaque. The fibrous plaque is a yellowish-gray elevated lump on the surface of the artery (Fig. 10-2). It protrudes in varying degrees into the arterial lumen, sometimes completely obstructing arterial blood flow. There are three major histologic characteristics of the fibrous plaque: proliferation of smooth muscle cells, accumulation of collagen, and accumulation of lipid within the intima. The plaque consists principally of smooth muscle cells. Smooth muscle cells ordinarily are located in the media and give the artery its contractility. The smooth muscle cells in the intima of the plaque probably are derived from those in the media. The smooth muscle cells secrete collagen, elastin, and glycosaminoglycans.

The plaque's dense connective tissue consists mostly of collagen fibers. With progression of the lesion, there is fibroplasia resulting in a fibrous cap over the atheroma. There may be no difference in the concentration of glycosaminoglycans between normal arterial walls and fibrous plaques.[3] Glycosaminoglycans may be associated with the trapping of lipid in the atheroma.[3] Plaques contain small amounts of elastin, but the amount may be less than what is normally present in the arterial wall.[3]

In the fibrous plaque, there is progressive accumulation of lipids, principally cholesterol in the form of lipoproteins, and cholesterol esters; usually more lipid is found extracellularly than in the smooth muscle cells. Debris from dead cells and varying amounts of crystals of cholesterol collect deep in the lesion along the intima–media border. Droplets of lipids may be seen along the elastic fibers and in pinocytotic vesicles within the endothelial cells.

Lastly, various components of the plasma have been found within the fibrous plaque. These include fibrin, fibrinogen, albumin, white blood cells, and lipoproteins. All the lipids in the serum have been found in the fibrous plaques except the large chylomicrons.

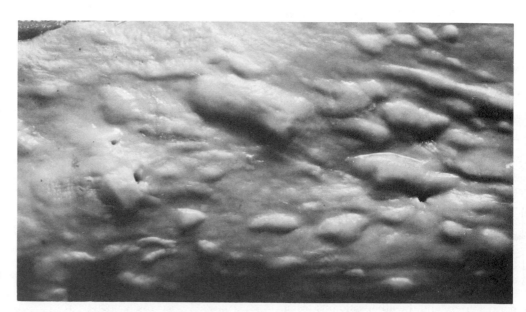

Fig. 10-2. Atherosclerotic inner surface of an artery (magnification × 2.5)(Benditt E: Sci Am 236:75, 1977 Courtesy of E. P. Benditt)

Most pathologists believe that the fibrous plaque is irreversible; that is, no regression is possible. However, it may be possible to alter further progression of the atheroma.

Complicated Lesion

The complicated lesion is a fibrous plaque with calcification, rupture of the plaque, hemorrhage into the plaque, and/or thrombus formation. The complicated lesion most often is associated with the clinical sequelae caused by complete occlusion of arterial blood flow resulting in infarction or by inadequate perfusion of the organ resulting in ischemia.

The fundamental controversy about the pathogenesis of an MI is whether or not an MI is caused by a coronary artery thrombus. There is no question that an MI is associated with atherosclerotic coronary artery disease (CAD). In the majority of postmortem cases an acute MI is related to the presence of a coronary artery thrombus. However it is conceivable that, in the presence of a severely stenosed coronary artery without a thrombus present, any increase of work demand on the heart or any decrease in oxygen supply to the heart could result in coronary occlusion long enough to cause an MI.

PATHOGENESIS OF ATHEROSCLEROSIS

There are six hypotheses of the pathogenesis of atherosclerosis: response-to-injury hypothesis; monoclonal hypothesis; clonal-senescence hypothesis; lipid-insudation hypothesis;

Fig. 10-3. Endothelial desquamation caused by several different forms of injury, possibly resulting in exposure of the underlying intimal connective tissue. (Ross R, Glomset JA: N Engl J Med 295:420, 1976. Reprinted by permission from the New England Journal of Medicine.)

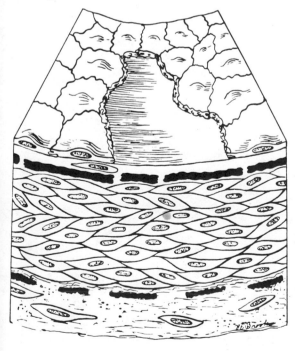

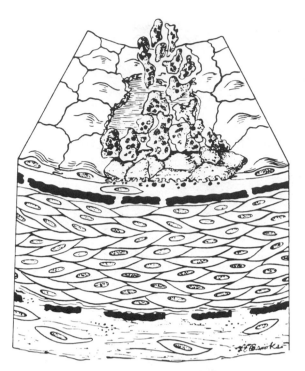

Fig. 10-4. Platelet aggregates, or microthrombi, may form as a result of adherence of the platelets to the exposed subendothelial tissue. Platelets that adhere to the connective tissue release granules whose constituents may gain entry into the artery wall. Platelet factors thus may interact with plasma constituents in the artery wall and stimulate intimal smooth muscle proliferation and formation of new connective tissue. (Ross R, Glomset JA: N Engl J Med 295:421, 1976. Reprinted by permission from the New England Journal of Medicine.)

thrombogenic hypothesis; and hemodynamic hypothesis. The hypotheses are not mutually exclusive; and they have been combined, modified, and extended so that currently the two dominant hypotheses are response-to-injury and monoclonal.

Response-to-Injury Hypothesis

The response-to-injury hypothesis holds that a nonspecific injury (mechanical, chemical, hormonal, immunologic) to the endothelial cells of the luminal arterial surface results in a change of permeability of the intimal membrane (Fig. 10-3). Thus platelets, lipoproteins, and other substances of the blood can diffuse into or come in contact with the intimal layer. Supporters of this hypothesis suggest that humans can suffer endothelial injury, for example, from the increased shear stress in hypertension, from hydrocarbons in cigarette smoking, from carbon monoxide, plasma cholesterol, hemodynamic stress, catecholamines, angiotension, or hormones.

Injury to the arterial endothelium causes an immediate platelet response with platelet adherence to the subendothelial connective tissue, aggregation, and release of the contents of platelet granules (Fig. 10-4). Ross and coworkers have reported that a growth-stimulating factor is released from platelets when they aggregate.[15-17] When smooth muscle cells from primates are grown in tissue culture, this growth-stimulating factor causes the cells to

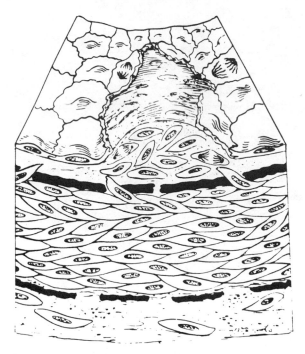

Fig. 10-5. Smooth muscle cells migrating from the media into the intima through fenestrae in the internal elastic lamina and actively multiplying within the intima. Endothelial cells regenerate in an attempt to recover the exposed intima, which thickens rapidly owing to smooth muscle cell proliferation and formation of new connective tissue. (Ross R, Glomset JA: N Engl J Med 295:421, 1976. Reprinted by permission from the New England Journal of Medicine.)

divide and the number of cells doubles. The smooth muscle cells normally would be protected from this platelet factor by the endothelial cell barrier. Thus, with endothelial injury, the platelets may release a factor that causes the smooth muscle cells to proliferate in the intima. The smooth muscle cells secrete collagen and may form large amounts of new

connective tissue (Fig. 10-5). In addition, endothelial injury causes regeneration of endothelial cells, which is an adaptation of the tissue to recover the hole made by the injury.

According to this hypothesis, the injury may be reversible. After the endothelium of an artery has been experimentally removed by a balloon catheter, the endothelial cells slowly grow back from the periphery of the lesion. As the endothelium grows back, the amount of smooth muscle cells in the intima decreases, for unknown reasons.[15,16] However, if the endothelial injury is not limited, but is continuous or repeated, the balance between reendothelialization and smooth muscle cell proliferation may be tipped. This balance, possibly affected by risk factors, may determine whether the lesion progresses or stays the same size. Thus, continuous hyperlipidemia, hypertension, or smoking may cause repeated bouts of injury resulting in continued proliferation of smooth muscle cells and formation of new connective tissue; continued deposition of lipid in the intima from the blood; and prevention of healing by reendothelialization (Fig. 10-6). This hypothesis is supported by the fact that in experimental animals, almost any kind of chronic damage to the artery—chemical, mechanical, or immunologic—will induce lesions that resemble human atherosclerotic lesions.

Monoclonal Hypothesis

The monoclonal hypothesis holds that the atherosclerotic plaque is due to a proliferation of smooth muscle cells that are monoclonal.[1–3] In other words, each atherosclerotic lesion is started by a single smooth muscle cell, and the rest of the proliferative cells are the progeny or descendants or clones of that cell. Benditt proposed that some mutagenic event (*i.e.*, aryl hydrocarbons from cigarette smoking, cholesterol epoxide, virus) provides the single cell with a selective advantage and that the progeny of that altered cell have increased capacity for growth (Fig. 10-7).[1,2]

Benditt used a genetic technique to acquire data for the monoclonal hypothesis.[2] This technique is based on the fact

Fig. 10-6. Two possible cycles of events in the response-to-injury hypothesis. The large cycle may represent what occurs in all persons at varying times. Endothelial injury may lead to desquamation, platelet adherence, aggregation, and release, followed by smooth-muscle proliferation and connective-tissue formation. If the injury is a single event, the lesions may go on to heal and regress, leaving a slightly thickened intima. The smaller, inner cycle demonstrates the possible consequences of repeated or chronic injury to the endothelium; lipid deposition may occur and smooth-muscle proliferation may continue after a sequence of proliferation, regression, proliferation, and regression. This leads to a complicated lesion, containing newly formed connective tissue and lipids, which may eventually calcify. This sequence of events could lead to a complicated lesion that goes on to produce clinical sequelae, such as thrombosis and infarction. (Ross R, Glomset JA: N Engl J Med 295:423, 1976. Reprinted by permission of the New England Journal of Medicine)

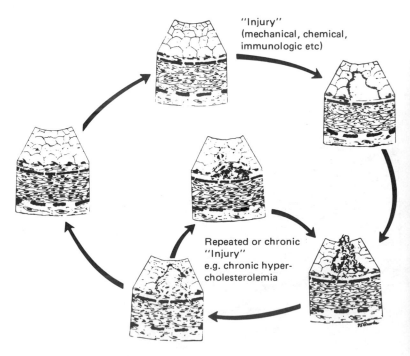

"Injury" (mechanical, chemical, immunologic etc)

Repeated or chronic "Injury" e.g. chronic hypercholesterolemia

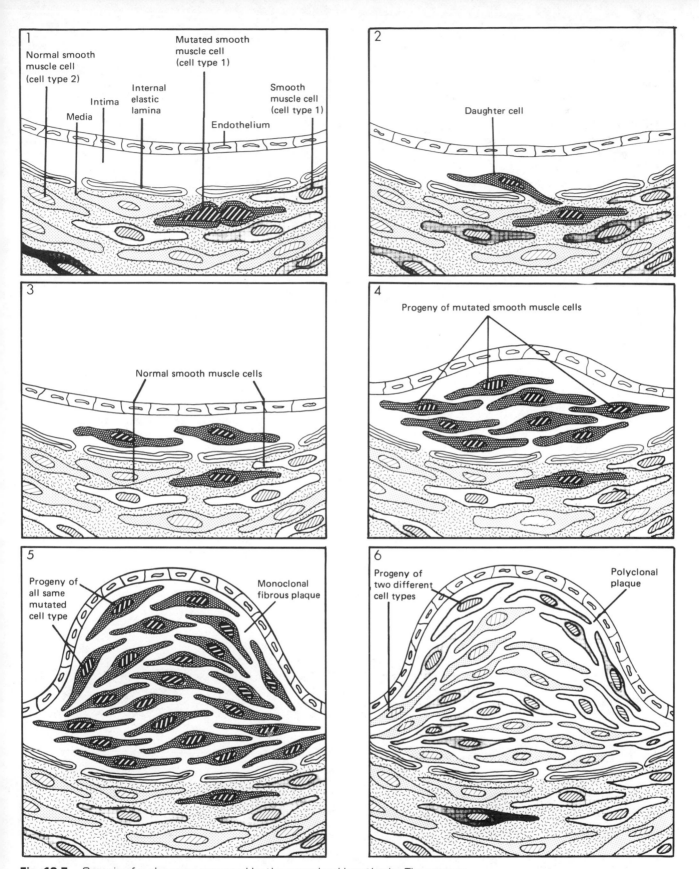

Fig. 10-7. Genesis of a plaque as proposed by the monoclonal hypothesis. The process begins in the inner media. There are two cell types. A single cell (*dark color*) has undergone mutation that gives it a selective advantage, and some stimulus causes the mutated cell to divide (**1**). Its daughter cell migrates into the intima (**2**). The progeny of the mutated cell, having a selective advantage and perhaps somehow freed of some curb on proliferation, continue to multiply, thickening the intima (**3,4**) and eventually forming a lumpy plaque (**5**), all of whose cells are progeny of the original cell that mutated. The last drawing (**6**) shows, by way of contrast, a polyclonal plaque, which is the kind that would arise from the migration and proliferation of many cells of both cell types. (Benditt E: Sci Am 236:80, 1977. Copyright © 1977 by Scientific American, Inc. All rights reserved.)

that human (mammalian) females are "mosaics" because their tissues are made up of small "patches" composed of two cell populations that have either an active maternal or an active paternal X chromosome. In the cells of females, there are two X chromosomes, one derived from the father and the other from the mother. Only one is active in adult life; the other one is inactivated during embryonic development. Therefore, either the maternal or the paternal X chromosome remains in a given cell and the progeny of that cell. The two cell types normally are well mixed in tissues (*i.e.,* polyclonal); it is considered an abnormal growth pattern if a patch of tissue is made up of one cell type (monoclonal).

The two cell types can be differentiated by "marker" genes. The X chromosome codes for the enzyme glucose-6-phosphate dehydrogenase (G-6-PD). G-6-PD has two phenotypes, A and B, which can be distinguished by electrophoresis. Type A moves faster in an electric field than type B. About 40% of black females are heterozygous for G-6-PD, that is, one X chromosome codes for type A, whereas the second X chromosome codes for type B. Progenitor cells of one or the other of the two X chromosomes replicate to form "patches" of cells containing only one of the G-6-PD phenotypes.

Benditt has shown that out of 15 fibrous plaques from one heterozygous female, four plaques produced only type A enzyme; eight plaques produced only type B enzyme; three plaques showed a mixed population.[2] In 27 samples of normal tissue from the same person, there are an even mixture of both A and B types. Thus Benditt has shown that fibrous plaques consist of cells of one type (monoclonal) A or B, but not mixed A and B. The three plaques that showed the mixed population probably were "contaminated" during sampling, that is, probably a normal cell mixture that was close to the plaque. Benditt reported the same results in three other patients, and these results have been confirmed by other investigators.[14,20,21]

In addition, Benditt has reported that inflicting endothelial injury in the aorta of animals produces a proliferative response made up of mixed cell population.[1] Thomas and co-workers have found that fatty streaks are not monoclonal, but polyclonal.[21] Thus these data give rise to questions of whether or not the "plaques" induced in experimental animals by endothelial injury or by high-cholesterol diets are the same as the fibrous atherosclerotic plaques seen in humans. It also gives rise to the question of whether or not fatty streaks represent the early development of the atherosclerotic fibrous plaque. Assuming that the fatty streak is the precursor of the fibrous plaque, it has also been argued that lesions are not monoclonal in origin, thus excluding a mutatation type origin; rather, a tumor progression type of development (like cervical cancer) might be indicated.

The monoclonal hypothesis represents a departure from the traditional viewpoint of atherogenesis. Consideration is given to factors that transform cells. These mutagenic factors may include some or all of the risk factors such as cigarette-derived hydrocarbons, cholesterol and other dietary carcinogens, and viruses.

Clonal-Senescence Hypothesis

The clonal-senescence hypothesis relates atherosclerosis to age, which is one of its risk factors.[11-13] The hypothesis holds that smooth muscle proliferation in the intima is due to an age-dependent decline in replication of stem cells in the media (*i.e.,* clonal-senescence of media cells) and an age-dependent failure of a negative feedback control system regulated by chalones, which are substances secreted by smooth muscle cells that may be able to inhibit mitosis of the stem cells, thus decreasing the yield of new differential progeny of smooth muscle cells.[5,11-13] The stem cell is a cell that gives rise to differentiated, specific cell types, in this case smooth muscle cells.

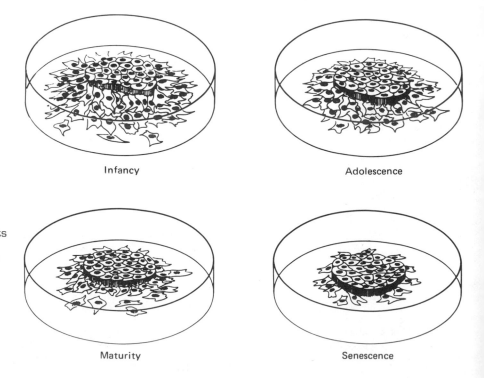

Infancy

Adolescence

Maturity

Senescence

Fig. 10-8. Migration time of fibroblasts growing out from a tiny scrap of living tissue placed in culture varies inversely with age of the source. This has been ascertained for fibroblasts from chickens, rats, and human beings and from several tissues, including heart, lung, and skin. (Hayflick L: Sci Am 242:65, 1980. Copyright © 1979 by Scientific American, Inc. All rights reserved)

The hypothesis is based on studies of the replicative ability of fibroblast cells in culture and upon the fact that atherosclerosis is more prevalent in the abdominal aorta than in the thoracic aorta. There is a greater age-related decline in replication for cells in the abdominal aorta than for cells in the thoracic aorta.[13] When human fibroblasts are grown in laboratory glassware, they divide a multiple finite number of times, then slowly stop replicating and eventually die. Their ability to replicate declines with age (Fig. 10-8).[9]

Martin and Sprague hypothesized that with advancing age, as the number of stem cells diminishes in the media, the concentration of chalones decreases.[11–13] The decreased concentration of chalones that diffuses into the intima from the media releases feedback inhibition and increases the replication of intimal stem cells, resulting in smooth muscle proliferation and atherosclerosis. Hypothetically, these proliferations would be monoclonal and would be consistent with the monoclonal hypothesis.[1–3]

Lipid-Insudation Hypothesis

The lipid-insudation hypothesis holds that lipoproteins that infiltrate into the arterial intima from the blood act as an irritant and induce proliferation of smooth muscle cells. The hypothesis has been supported by many epidemiologic studies, research on plasma lipoprotein metabolism, and pathologic observations. The reader is referred to Chapter 13 for a discussion of elevated serum lipids as a risk factor of atherosclerosis.

The exact mechanism by which cholesterol is transported across the endothelial wall is unknown. Local injury to the endothelium may be induced by serum low-density lipoproteins (LDL) in animals. Feeding primates a high-cholesterol diet increases serum cholesterol and causes endothelial injury.[18] All sizes of plasma lipoproteins, except chylomicrons and large LDL, can be transported across the endothelial cells in vesicles about 750 Å in diameter[20,22] (Fig. 13-2). Serum LDL from primates causes arterial smooth muscle cells to proliferate in tissue culture.[10]

Goldstein and Brown have described a lipoprotein receptor in cultured fibroblast cells.[7] The functions of the LDL receptor are to transfer LDL into the cell, stimulate cholesterol esterification in the cell, suppress 3-hydroxy-3-methylglutaryl coenzyme A (HMG CoA) reductase activity and cholesterol synthesis, and enhance degradation of the protein component of the LDL.

Patients with type II familial hypercholesterolemia may have a genetic functional lack of LDL receptors. In normocholesterolemic people, it is thought that when the endothelial cells are damaged (by any mechanism), lipids pass readily into the intima. Because there is a higher concentration of intimal extracellular lipids, the LDL receptors on the cell surfaces bind more LDL, which stimulates intracellular esterification. Consequently, there is an abnormal accumulation of cholesterol within the smooth muscle cells resulting in formation of foam cells and plaques.

Thrombogenic Hypothesis

The thrombogenic or encrustation theory holds that the fibrous plaque begins as a mural thrombus that is converted to a mass of dense connective tissue, as fibroblasts and possibly smooth muscle cells migrate into the thrombus from the arterial walls. This is one of the oldest hypotheses of atherogenesis, and most of the evidence supporting it is intermixed with the evidence for the response-to-injury hypothesis.

With endothelial injury, there is platelet adherence, aggregation, and release of granules (Fig. 10-4). That is, a thrombus is formed. Platelets release a growth-promoting factor that causes proliferation of smooth muscle cells.[17] In experimental animals, it has been demonstrated that atherosclerotic lesions that follow endothelial injury can be prevented by preventing platelets from releasing their growth-stimulating factor or by increasing platelet survival time.[10,17] Platelet survival times decrease when platelets aggregate and break down at the site of arterial injury.[10] The platelet survival times of patients with homocysteinurea, a genetic disease in which people are predisposed to early, extreme atherosclerosis, were 50% lower than those of normal persons. Their platelet survival times were increased by giving dipyridamole (Persantine) or the vitamin, pyridoxine.[10]

Hemodynamic Hypothesis

Hemodynamic factors such as turbulence, shearing stresses, and pressures tangential to the vessel circumference have been used to explain why plaques are more often situated about arterial branchings, bends, and taperings, and why some arteries or arterial segments are regularly more severely involved by atherosclerosis than others.

In a straight vessel with laminar flow, flow velocity is greatest at the center and least near the wall where contact with the intima results in frictional resistance. Departures from laminar flow tend to occur at abrupt changes in vessel configuration or diameter. For example, turbulence develops where blood leaves a stenosed segment and enters a dilation; or, conceivably, turbulence occurs about normal branch orifices and curves. Turbulence results in more than the usual amount of energy of the flowing blood dissipated in collisions between circulating elements and the intimal wall. As a result, turbulence is thought to aid in the formation of fibrous plaques by favoring the formation of thrombi or by causing endothelial injury.[6] In experimental animals, the lesion exposed to turbulence shows an intimal thickening of smooth muscle cells, connective tissue cells, poorly oriented collagenous fibers, and a predilection for lipid deposition.[4]

Even when flow is laminar, the flowing blood exerts a dragging force on the intimal surface in the direction of flow. The media and adventitia are held by the periarterial tissues and are fixed at such points as branching of the arteries. The intima thus tends to be displaced relative to the media, producing endothelial detachment.

In the experimental animal, a shear stress applied for a long time results in intimal fibrosis characterized by dense, oriented collagenous fibers with few smooth muscle cells, lipids, or connective tissue cells.[4] This type of lesion, mediated by an increase in shearing force, is thought to be one of the cellular mechanisms of hypertension, which is known to be one of the risk factors of atherosclerosis.

Tangential tension is greatest where the vessel radius is

the greatest. Thus the tension is increased at bends and branches of the arteries. Increased mural tension conceivably would favor atherogenesis by rendering the stretched intima more permeable to circulating substances.[6]

Atherosclerosis occurs more in the abdominal aorta than the thoracic aorta.[8] Glagov has defined a basic lamellar structural unit in the medial layer of the aorta.[6] At birth, the thoracic segment and the abdominal segment of the aorta are of the same width; however, the thoracic segment has more lamellar units. With development, the width of both segments doubles. The lamellar units in the thoracic segment increase in number, but the number of the lamellar units in the abdominal segment remains the same. Hypothetically, this limitation renders the abdominal aorta less adaptable to mechanical tension with age. In addition, the medial layer of the thoracic segment is vascular, whereas that of the abdominal segment is avascular. The medial abdominal aorta depends on diffusion of oxygen and nutrients across the intima from the arterial blood flow. Any increase in thickness or change of composition of the intima would render the media ischemic and conceivably promote smooth muscle proliferation. The same hypothesis has been used regarding atherogenesis in the coronary arteries where there is a relative absence of penetrating vasa vasorum.

REFERENCES

1. Benditt E: The origin of atherosclerosis. Sci Am 236:74–85, 1977
2. Benditt E, Benditt JJ: Evidence for a monoclonal origin of human atherosclerotic plaques. Proc Natl Acad Sci 70:1753–1756, 1973
3. Benditt EP, Gown AM: Atheroma: The artery wall and the environment. Int Rev Exp Pathol 21:155–118, 1980
4. Davignon J: The lipid hypothesis. Arch Surg 113:28–34, 1978
5. Florentin RA, Nam SC, Jana Kideui K et al: Population dynamics of arterial smooth muscle cells. II. In vivo inhibition of entry into mitosis of swine arterial smooth muscle cells by aortic tissue extracts. Arch Pathol 95:317–320, 1973
6. Glagov S: Mechanical stresses on vessels and the non-uniform distribution of atherosclerosis. Med Clin North Am 57:63–77, 1973
7. Goldstein J, Brown M: Lipoprotein receptors, cholesterol metabolism and atherosclerosis. Arch Pathol 99:181–184, 1975
8. Haimovici H, Mailer N: Role of arterial tissue susceptibility in experimental canine atherosclerosis. J Atherosclerosis Res 6:62–74, 1966
9. Hayflick L: The cell biology of human aging. Sci Am 242:58–65, 1980
10. Kolata G: Atherosclerotic plaques: Competing theories guide research. Science 194:592–594, 1976
11. Martin GM: Cellular aging—clonal senescence. Am J Pathol 89:484–512, 1977
12. Martin GM: Cellular aging—post replicative cells. Am J Pathol 89:513–530, 1977
13. Martin GM, Sprague CA: Symposium on in vitro studies related to atherogenesis: Life histories of hyperplastoid cell lines from aorta and skin. Exp Mol Pathol 18:125–141, 1973
14. Pearson TA, Wang A, Salezo K et al: Clonal characteristics of fibrous plaques and fatty streaks from human aortas. Am J Pathol 81:379–837, 1975
15. Ross R, Glomset JA: The pathogenesis of atherosclerosis, Part I. N Engl J Med 295(7):369–377, 1976
16. Ross R, Glomset JA: The pathogenesis of atherosclerosis, Part 2. N Engl J Med 295(8):420–425, 1976
17. Ross R, Glomset J, Karuja B et al: A platelet-dependent serum factor that stimulates the proliferation of arterial smooth muscle cells in vitro. Proc Natl Acad Sci USA 71:1207–1210, 1974
18. Ross R, Harker L: Hyperlipidemia and atherosclerosis. Science 193:1094–1100, 1976
19. Schwartz CJ: Gross aortic sudanophilia and hemosideria deposition: A study on infants, children, young adults. Arch Pathol 83:325, 1967
20. Stein V, Stein O: Lipid synthesis and degradation and lipoprotein transport in mammalian aorta. Ciba Found Symp 12:165–184, 1973
21. Thomas WA, Florentin RA, Reiner JM et al: Alterations in population dynamics of arterial smooth muscle cells during atherogenesis. Exp Mol Pathol 24:244–260, 1976
22. Watts H: Basic aspects of the pathogenesis of human atherosclerosis. Hum Pathol 2:31–55, 1971

11

Pathophysiology of Myocardial Ischemia and Infarction

SANDRA D. SOLACK, R.N.,M.S.N.

PHYSIOLOGIC DETERMINANTS IN ISCHEMIA AND INFARCTION

The pathophysiologic events in the myocardium that occur with coronary artery disease (CAD) range from potentially reversible injury of the muscle cells to the irreversible destruction of all cellular components in a tissue area. An energy imbalance underlies these events. It may follow an increased demand for oxygen in a setting of limited coronary reserves or may result from an abrupt decrease in flow due to hypotension, thrombi, and arterial spasm.[79]

The determinants of myocardial oxygen consumption ($M\dot{V}O_2$) and the myocardial response to varying metabolic demands are discussed in Chapter 2. Three points in that chapter are significantly related to the coronary ischemic response.

1. The myocardium matches metabolic demands by altering coronary blood flow (flow = change in pressure/vessel resistance). Flow can be increased by decreasing resistance (vasodilation) or by increasing the driving pressure (pressure gradient between aortic root and right atrium) in the vessel.
2. Coronary flow is a function not only of metabolic requirements but also of wall tension and neurogenic influences from the sympathetic system.
3. The coronary vessels are capable of autoregulation. This inherent characteristic allows them to respond to local environmental conditions, so that blood flow can be constantly maintained.

Ischemia is defined as an imbalance between the need and supply of blood flow. The result is an inadequate provision of O_2 and nutrients and the deficient removal of metabolic end products from the tissue. This situation differs from hypoxia, wherein arterial O_2 content is reduced (as in anemia) but flow is adequate or even increased.[36,86] Myocardial ischemia is accompanied by a shift from aerobic to anaerobic metabolism. It can result from an occlusion followed by recirculation (return of blood flow) or from flow inadequate to meet increased metabolic needs.[36] When the ischemia is severe and prolonged, irreversible injury or infarction of tissue results. This usually accompanies complete interruption of flow. At this stage, biochemical energy processes are unable to preserve cellular boundaries.[8] Infarction is identified pathologically as a central area of coagulation necrosis. This means that all cells (e.g., interstitial, nervous, muscle) in this zone are functionally and electrically silent.[22]

Beyond the infarcted core are numerous gradations of ischemic injury with structural and biochemical features. These areas are identified pathologically as selective myocardial cell necrosis. This term describes death of myocardial cells alone, whereas the supportive neural, interstitial, and other cells remain viable.[64] These "twilight zones" are responsible for many of the metabolic and electrical sequelae of a myocardial infarction (MI).[21] In addition, some may include areas of potentially viable muscle cells. Therapeutic goals are directed toward preserving these cells.

The preservation of cells after an ischemic event requires a determination of components critical to the reversibility of an injury.[8] Biochemical defects in adenosine triphosphate (ATP) synthesis, changes in cell volume regulation, cellular membrane dysfunction, and altered ionic environments are postulated to be important factors in tissue necrosis.[8,36,82]

111

The degree of anaerobic metabolism, the extent of collateralization, and large demands on the heart in early recovery may also influence the size of the necrotic zone.[78]

ALTERATIONS IN CORONARY BLOOD FLOW PATTERNS

Altered coronary blood flow patterns are significant in determining the outcome of an MI. This is reflected in the distribution and degree of injury in the cardiac ventricular wall. Transmural MIs are those with necrosis across the wall of the myocardium. They occur with almost a 40% frequency and are usually associated with occlusion of an epicardial artery. The necrotic area may extend through the entire thickness of the wall or may involve just the subendocardial and midcardiac layers.[22] Nontransmural MIs are usually defined as those occurring in the inner half of the subendocardial myocardium. Intramyocardial and subepicardial MIs without subendocardial involvement are infrequent. In contrast, there is a 60% probability that an MI is subendocardial.[22] MIs are rarely associated with total coronary occlusion, and the lesion involves a mix of infarcted and noninfarcted myocardial fibers.[21]

Subendocardial Blood Flow

The subendocardium is particularly vulnerable to changes in left venticular mechanics. If an abrupt change in coronary blood flow occurs, the subendocardial region is the most severely affected. This happens for mechanical and for metabolic reasons. The intraventricular wall tension is greatest there, and, as a result, external compression of its vessels is maximal.[72] In addition, the most distal branches of the coronary system feed the subendocardium. Blood flow decreases progressively as distance from the source increases, because of the added resistances of the intervening vessels.[25] Oxygen consumption is also higher in the subendocardium than in the other layers of the heart.[37] Therefore, a transmural gradient of O_2 need and supply exists. This is further reflected in greater lactate accumulation, creatine phosphokinase (CK) and phosphate depletion, and a wider distribution of infarcted tissue as it proceeds from epicardium to subendocardium.[34]

Flow in Stenotic Vessels

Normal coronary vessels provide a homogeneous flow of blood throughout the myocardium. However, significant stenosis (more than 75% occlusion) in a vessel compromises flow, and a nonuniform distribution of O_2 supply results.[34] The stenotic coronary artery may adapt by maximally dilating (autoregulation response), even under resting conditions. As a result, further vasodilation may not occur when metabolic demands increase or when the driving pressure falls (as in systemic arterial hypotension). The muscle supplied by the stenotic artery subsequently becomes ischemic.[42] The mechanical resistance created by the lesion also hinders flow. In addition, local ischemia is associated with a greater increase in resistance, so flow may be further compromised.

A positive feedback system may be initiated in which ischemia breeds more ischemia. Although the etiology of the resistance response to ischemia is unclear, it has been implicated as a factor in the evolution of an MI following total vessel occlusion.[34]

Collateral Vessels

The outcome of redistribution patterns of flow in the heart during ischemia and after infarction depends on collateralization as well as on cardiac metabolic demands. Collateral vessels serve as alternative interconnecting channels and may be recruited when a parent vessel is unable to meet flow requirements.[32] Coronary collaterals may result from the transformation of cells into new vessels in response to ischemic stress.[9] Another alternative is that they are dormant in normal hearts and expand and undergo intimal growth when the need arises.[76] Enlargement of collateral vessels is often demonstrated by coronary arteriography in patients with CAD, ventricular hypertrophy, and cor pulmonale.[9]

The extent of protection, if any, afforded by collateral vessels is an unanswered question. It is difficult to interpret autopsy data, since it is often unknown whether collaterals precede or succeed infarction. One study, however, demonstrated collaterals in dogs about one week after complete coronary occlusion.[6] Evidence to support the protective influence of collaterals comes from autopsy demonstrations of completely occluded vessels without infarction. This suggests collateral augmentation.[2] In addition, infarct size may be smaller in an area fed by an occluded vessel because of collaterals.[9]

The significance of augmented collateral flow lies in its presumed ability to reestablish flow to ischemic tissue before irreversible damage occurs. In dogs, infarct size is correlated to reperfusion after abrupt surgical occlusion. This relation is more significant in the marginal zone where reflow patterns can predict extent of viable tissue several days after ischemia. Reflow does not influence viability in the central necrotic zone, however, because this is an area of irreversible damage.[85] Evidence of augmented collateral flow after progressive occlusion of coronary arteries has also been shown to prevent MIs in dogs.[27] Higher ejection fractions, better regional wall motion, and fewer MIs have also been observed in patients with well-developed collaterals.[73] In both dogs and humans with augmented collateral flow, however, a stress-induced increase in myocardial metabolism still produces ischemic changes in the ECG.[26,70] Therefore, collaterals may serve the myocardium well at "rest" but may have limited capacity under stress.[71].

Competitive Redistribution of Coronary Blood Flow

Competitive redistribution is another mechanism by which flow can be altered in the ischemic myocardium. As metabolism accelerates, increased blood flow through normal vessels may alter flow through collaterals. Autoregulation in normal coronaries lowers the resistance in the large vessels from which distal collaterals are fed. This, in turn, reduces the driving pressure of blood through the collaterals so that flow through them decreases. On the other hand, flow is increased in normal vessels as vasodilation occurs. In effect, normal vessels may "steal" flow from collaterals during stress.[60]

Coronary Artery Spasm

Coronary artery spasm is a source of reversible myocardial injury in patients with Prinzmetal's variant angina.[30] It is due to variable smooth-muscle contraction in a coronary artery and results in increased resistance and decreased flow to the distal bed. Several factors may be involved in the mechanism that produces spasm. Increased sympathetic activity associated with rapid-eye-movement sleep has been correlated with coronary spasm. Mechanical irritation of the arterial wall from an atheroma is another possible mediating factor.[45] The relation of spasm to the pathogenesis or sequelae of an MI, however, is unclear. Coronary arterial spasm has been documented in acute recovery after MI in some patients.[54] Its occurrence may be secondary to intimal hemorrhage, catecholamine excess, or the release of vaso-active substances from platelets in response to injury.[54]

ISCHEMIC PAIN: ANGINA PECTORIS

The majority of patients with myocardial ischemia or infarction develop symptoms of angina. About 90% of patients with recurrent angina pectoris have hemodynamically significant stenosis or occlusion of a major coronary artery.[84] Symptomatic MI without chest pain can occur, however, and the reported frequency is as high as 25%.[84]

The precise mechanism responsible for exciting visceral afferent fibers during angina is unknown.[72] Plasma kinins have been implicated as chemical mediators in pain production. A kinin activation sequence is initiated in response to tissue injury. Bradykinin has produced pain when injected into limb vasculature of animals and humans. In addition, release of bradykinin from the myocardium has been measured after ischemia. Serotonin may sensitize pain receptors to bradykinin as well.[84]

The cause of the pain may also be mechanical. Stretch of the myocardium due to ischemic injury, edema formation, and altered local contractility may stimulate pain receptors. Ischemic pain may also be due to altered mechanics of the coronary vessels themselves.[72]

Once the pain receptor is stimulated, impulses are carried by the visceral afferent fibers accompanying the sympathetic nerves. They enter the spinal cord through the eighth cervical to the first four thoracic dorsal root ganglia.[64] The dermatomes (peripheral axonal fields supplied by single dorsal roots) innervating the heart are also shared by other cutaneous and somatic structures. When the brain receives a pain impulse from those dermatomes, the input may be registered as coming from any of those structures. In addition, the brain uses past experience to integrate information. Because neck or arm pain is more commonly experienced than is cardiac visceral pain, the cardiac afferent input may be interpreted as jaw, neck, or arm discomfort. This explains the mechanism of referred pain frequently observed with angina associated with MI.[62]

Exertional and stress-related ischemic episodes heralded by angina may be accompanied by dyspnea and other symptoms related to altered hemodynamics. The initial pain with exercise may be due to the direct vasoconstrictive effect of catecholamines and sympathetic stimulation of the coronary vessels. Spontaneous relief of pain sometimes may follow as exercise continues. This phenomenon of "walk-through" angina may be due to vasodilation resulting from delayed autoregulation of stenotic vessels.[72]

The syndrome of Prinzmetal's angina is the occurrence of severe, often prolonged chest pain in the absence of precipitating factors such as exercise and stress. Coronary artery spasm is the apparent etiologic mechanism. The ischemic nature of spasm is supported by measured increases in coronary vascular resistance, lactate production, and arteriovenous O_2 difference.[30]

LOCAL PHYSIOLOGIC ALTERATIONS

The physiologic determinants of the degree to which ischemic injury evolves are emphasized in the first two sections of this chapter. The description of an MI as an ongoing process and dependent on a number of factors is stressed. The pathophysiologic consequences of an MI are also evolutionary and interrelated. They include local changes in biochemical, mechanical, and electrical processes as well as systemic responses aimed at maintaining circulatory integrity.

Metabolic Events

The heart depends on an adequate supply of O_2 and on dietary substrates to form the energy molecule, ATP. Breakdown of ATP into its constituents, adenosine diphosphate (ADP) and inorganic phosphate (P_i), liberates large amounts of energy used for a number of metabolic and reparative processes. The steps by which glucose and free fatty acids (FFA) generate ATP are explained in Chapter 2. Four factors are emphasized in that chapter. First, the myocardium depends on an aerobic environment to produce adequate amounts of ATP. Second, the predominant metabolic fuel depends on the dietary state of the individual. FFA are primarily metabolized when the person is in the unfed state, whereas glucose is readily degraded under postprandial conditions. Third, the tricarboxylic acid (TCA) cycle is the major link between substrate supply and production of ATP through oxidative phosphorylation in the mitochondria. Fourth, glycolysis is the only metabolic pathway that can produce ATP without a net consumption of O_2 (Fig. 2-15).

Sequence in Ischemic Metabolism. Whereas sufficient ATP supplies can be maintained in skeletal muscle for prolonged periods under anaerobic conditions, the myocardium is severely limited. BEsides deficient supplies of O_2, the ischemic heart faces decreased supply of substrate, loss of glycolytic enzymes, and deficient removal of metabolites.[86] Hypoxia severely limits oxidation of FAA, because the transport of their activated intermediates into the mitochondria requires ATP. The production of acetyl CoA is also

TABLE 11-1 ENERGY BALANCES

Reaction	ATP (moles generated per mole of glucose)
Anaerobic glycolysis	
glucose → lactate	2
TOTAL	2
Oxidative metabolism	
Aerobic glycolysis	2
TCA cycle	2
Oxidative phosphorylation	32
TOTAL	36

limited when O_2 is reduced. Therefore, oxidation of any substrate by the TCA cycle is hindered, and oxidative phosphorylation comes to a halt.[56] Hence, the ischemic myocardium becomes solely dependent on glycolysis for its energy.

Immediately after the onset of ischemia, ATP levels are maintained by accelerated use of ATP and creatine phosphate (CP) stores. Within seconds these resources are expended and glycolysis increases. Glycogen depletion occurs minutes later, but anaerobic glycolysis continues.[78] Because acetyl CoA production requires O_2, pyruvate is metabolized by an alternative route to form lactate. This reaction is catalyzed by lactic dehydrogenase (LDH) and is a consequence of increased levels of pyruvate. A net 2-mole yield of ATP occurs (Table 11-1).[56] Although energy production through anaerobic glycolysis is only 5% of normal, it is critical to the survival of ischemic tissue.[56] Canine studies have demonstrated that glycolysis may be able to maintain viability of myocardial cells for up to 20 minutes after occlusion.[78]

Glycolytic Supports. Several compensatory mechanisms support anaerobic glycolysis in the myocardium. Hypoxia itself augments glucose transport into the cell by increasing glucose metabolism and creating a favorable concentration gradient for diffusion.[57] Local catecholamine release stimulates production of cyclic adenosine monophosphate (c-AMP). This activates protein kinases and phosphorylase, which increase glycolysis.[41] Increased levels of ADP and P_i potentiate phosphofructokinase (PFK) activity. This enzyme is a catalyst in the production of pyruvate.[59]

Consequences of Anaerobic Glycolysis. Although anaerobic glycolysis is vital, it does create environmental consequences for the myocardial cell. Accelerated production of lactate and accumulation of P_i from hydrolysis of ATP lead to an excess of hydrogen ions (H^+). Because flow is deficient, the H^+ concentration increases and acidosis results. This may alter cellular permeability to lactate, so its intracellular accumulation is also encouraged.[36] Acidosis may also depress contractility[52] ands potentiate intravascular coagulation in poorly perfused areas.[55] The sensitivity of myocardial tissue to lyosomal enzymes may also be greater during acidosis.[78]

Glycolysis may be inhibited by an accumulation of its degradation products. This biochemical feedback inhibition may limit some of the intracellular consequences of excess metabolites.[1] Acidosis inhibits glycolysis by depressing the activity of PFK.[78] Excess lactate and pyruvate may indirectly restrain anaerobic glycolysis as well.[55]

Deficient FFA Metabolism. The deficient metabolism of FFA may also have consequences for the energy state of the ischemic myocardium. Because the activated state FFA, acyl CoA, cannot enter the mitochondria when ATP supplies are low, it accumulates in the cytoplasm. This may prevent ADP uptake by the mitochondria and limit ATP synthesis. Increased breakdown of myocardial triglycerides also occurs and is due to catecholamine stimulation in ischemia. However, more FFA are incorporated into stored fat. Pathologic studies have demonstrated accumulation of triglycerides in the border zones of necrotic tissue. The mechanism responsible for this observation may be the increased level of glycolytic intermediates noted to stimulate fat synthesis.[57]

Ion Alterations. An important sequel to deficient energy supplies is the inhibition of intracellular ion pumps. the sodium/potassium (Na^+/K^+) pump uses ATP to maintain high K^+ and low Na^+ intracellular concentrations. Defective pumping leads to equilibration of ions, leading to intracellular Na^+ accumulation and efflux of K^+ from the cell. Consequences of this altered ionic ratio include membrane depolarization and conduction abnormalities, inhibition of enzyme processes, cellular edema, and anomalous excitation–contraction coupling.[76]

The calcium (Ca^{2+}) pump also uses ATP as an energy source. After excitation–contraction coupling has occurred, Ca^{2+} in the sarcoplasm is pumped into the sarcoplasmic reticulum. Relaxation of muscle follows. With inadequate ATP supplies, pumping is defective and Ca^{2+} accumulates in the sarcoplasm. This may lead to changes in contractility and relaxation of the muscle, and prolong the action potential.[72] Ca^{2+} deposits in the mitochondria have also been detected by histologic methods after impairment of oxidative phosphorylation.[60] A possible beneficial effect of intracellular Ca^{2+} accumulation, however, may be its stimulation of phosphorylase, the enzyme responsible for activating glycolysis.[82]

Correlations Between Metabolic and Pathologic Events. The heterogeneity of pathologic changes in MI may be related to the dynamic metabolic alterations in the ischemic process (Fig. 11-1). The core of the infarct is functionally dead, and glycolysis and cellular respiration are absent. Adjacent zones of graded anaerobic and aerobic respiration progress peripherally from the necrotic area. Opie represents the zone surrounding the core as one of total ischemia wherein inhibited anaerobic metabolism is accompanied by lactic acidosis, ionic equilibration, and intracellular Ca^{2+} accumulation. Surrounding this, zones of subtotal and mild ischemia are supplied by waxing and waning collateral flow. Their energy is maintained through combined aerobic and anaerobic metabolism. Still further from the necrotic zone is the area of normal cellular respiration. This is characterized by oxidative phosphorylation and metabolism of FFA and glucose. Notably, the ischemic zone is variable in size and depends on the volume of O_2 delivered relative to O_2 needs for its survival.[57]

Tissue analysis of enzyme activity in central and peripheral zones of infarcted muscle in dogs also demonstrates differential metabolic properties. Glycolytic and oxidative enzymes are markedly depressed in the peripheral zone

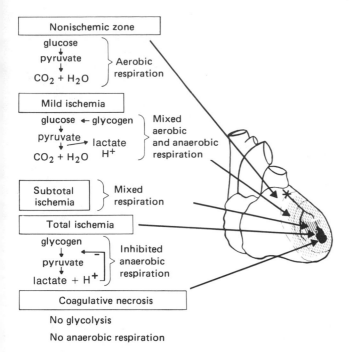

Fig. 11-1. Scheme of regional metabolic changes after an acute coronary occlusion. See text for details. (Adapted from Opie LH: Am J Cardiol 36:945, 1975)

from 24 hours to 6 months after the acute event. Permanent depression of enzyme activity occurs in the necrotic zone where scar tissue forms.[7]

Protein synthesis is initially depressed because of loss of intracellular K[+] and possible defects in ribosomal activity (ribosomes are involved in the transfer of DNA). Within 48 hours after occlusion, the incorporation of protein as well as lipid increases in the infarcted and ischemic areas.[7]

Mechanical Alterations

Contractile Changes. The functional changes that occur with an MI originate in the contractile elements and vary on a continuum from mild to severe alterations in hemodynamics. The size rather than location of left ventricular infarction is the most important factor determining the degree of impairment in contractility and ejection. However, location can be an important factor in that equivalent tissue damage in the apex versus papillary muscle can have quite different consequences. Necrosis of 40% of the left ventricle is usually associated with fatal cardiogenic shock.[43] A transmural MI is more likely to produce changes in stroke volume (SV) and left ventricular end-diastolic volume (LVEDV) than is one that is confined to the subendocardium. Moreover, loss of functional muscle from previous infarctions has additive effects on impairment from subsequent infarctions.[43]

Contractility diminishes within seconds after a coronary occlusion. This occurs prior to ST-segment elevation.[63,68,77] Impeded shortening of muscle fibers reduces the development of contractile tension. In addition, passive lengthening of necrotic fibers replaces shortening during systole.[63] These alterations create a zone of asynergy that acts as a slack element in series with contractile proteins (Fig. 29-1).

Wasted contractile effort results.[43] The most marked contractile changes take place in the subendocardium, because its perfusion is most compromised by compression during systole.[31]

A mixture of normal and necrotic fibers in the marginal zone produces a hypokinetic area.[68] Abnormal contraction of these elements together with holosystolic expansion in the central zone creates asynchronous movement. Aortic flow decreases, energy is dissipated, and further ischemia can result.[43,68]

Increased diastolic length and systolic shortening in normal muscle may compensate for the contractile defects in injured muscle.[68] Augmented activity of glycolytic and oxidative enzymes in normal muscle illustrate the biochemical counterpart of mechanical compensation.[7]

The distribution of contractile changes after MI is associated with alterations in wall thickness. The degree and rate of thickening of the ventricular wall during systole are proportionate to the extent of fiber shortening. A progressive decrease in systolic wall thickness from normal through marginal and necrotic zones occurs. It is assumed that this represents loss of functional myocardium.[68]

The effects of ischemia on myocardial contractile mechanisms may be mediated directly or indirectly by Ca^{2+}. The degree of contractility is probably determined by the extent of interaction between actin and myosin filaments. The development of tension is also related to the duration of the action potential. Ca^{2+} is necessary for both of these processes. It is significant that Ca^{2+} transport within the cell also requires energy. Therefore, the loss of energy resources that occurs in ischemia may affect Ca^{2+} interactions.[86]

A diminished ATP supply due to ischemia may prevent Ca^{2+} interaction with contractile proteins by inhibiting the Na^+/K^+ pump. The intracellular accumulation of Na^+ that results may lead to competition between Na^+ and Ca^{2+} at receptor sites.[72] Contractile losses paralleling reductions in ATP have been demonstrated in dog hearts.[1] Other studies demonstrate better correlations between contractility and CP.[43,63]

The role of acidosis in the myocardial consequences of ischemia is controversial. Several hypotheses have been proposed to describe apparent correlations between pH changes and myocardial mechanics. Acidosis may directly depress contractility by altering the speed of tension development and decreasing the inward Ca^{2+} current with depolarization. Excess H[+] may displace Ca^{2+} from contractile proteins or alter its release from the sarcoplasmic reticulum during cardiac excitation.[82,83]

Relaxation Changes. Postischemic impairment of relaxation is another mechanical alteration documented in dogs after short periods of coronary occlusion.[68] The time course of decline in relaxation velocity parallels contractile dysfunction. However, the reversal of relaxation defects is more prolonged than recovery of contractility after reperfusion takes place. It is possible that this prolonged tension is due to decreased uptake of Ca^{2+} by the sarcoplasmic reticulum.[1]

Compliance Changes. Mechanical alteration of the ischemic myocardium is also reflected in changes in compliance of the left ventricle. As presented in Chapter 1, compliance is

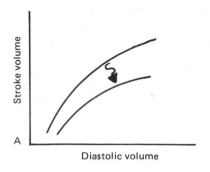

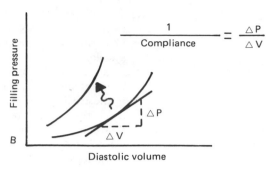

$$\frac{1}{\text{Compliance}} = \frac{\triangle P}{\triangle V}$$

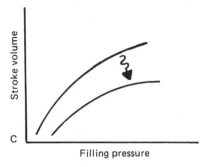

Fig. 11-2. Mechanisms for depressing the left ventricular function curve. A decrease in contractility (**A**) or compliance (**B**) can produce a similar alteration in the ventricular function curve (**C**). Compliance can be found at any one end-diastolic pressure by calculating the slope of the diastolic tension curve. (Adapted from Diamond G, Forrester JS: Circulation 45:18, 1972 by permission of the American Heart Association, Inc.)

a general description of the pressure/volume relation and can be represented by the Starling curve. Compliance changes can follow alterations in ventricular size, geometry, and wall stiffness.[19]

The usual finding after an MI is decreased compliance. The implication is twofold: A smaller volume of blood is ejected per increment of pressure change in the ventricle, or the ventricle must develop greater pressure for each increment in volume (Fig. 11-2b). A decrease in compliance can be a result of increased preload following an increase in end-diastolic volume. The Starling curve shows that an increased end-diastolic volume can lead to greater tension and SV. However, this compensatory mechanism has a maximum beyond which tension falls. It is at this point that compliance decreases.[43] Fibers are overstretched, and interactions between actin and myosin filaments are altered.[3] As fiber length increases, the radius of the ventricle and wall tension also increase (Laplace's law). $M\dot{V}O_2$ rises as a result.

An increase in left ventricular wall stiffness can also contribute to loss of compliance. Wall stiffness describes the passive stress character of the ventricle and is a determinant of diastolic pressure.[19] Thinning of the wall, scar tissue formation, tissue edema, and muscle fiber disarray increase stiffness.[68]

It is important to note that changes in contractility and compliance can alter the ventricular function curve. A contractility change may signal a need for alteration in medical therapy. A change in compliance due to wall stiffness, however, is often transient and is part of the process of scar-tissue formation (Fig. 11-2).[19] The differentiation of these mechanisms partly accounts for the increased use of hemodynamic monitoring of the patient with acute MI.

Change in Left Ventricular Parameters. The changes in left ventricular parameters subsequent to ischemia and infarction generally parallel alterations in contractility and compliance (Fig. 11-3). The rate of pressure development correlates with shortening velocity, and both are depressed after infarction. The amplitude of systolic pressure may decrease (because of decreased contractility), increase (because of catecholamine release), or remain the same. As a consequence of depressed contractility and ejection speed, the fraction of blood expelled with each ventricular contraction diminishes. SV falls, and an increase in end-diastolic volume and fiber length results. Indirect indicators of left ventricular function may also change. Left atrial, pulmonary artery wedge, and pulmonary artery end-diastolic pressures may rise as contractility and compliance decrease.[3,72,76] Hemodynamic monitoring is discussed in Chapter 21.

Systemic Hemodynamic Changes. The diversity of systemic hemodynamic patterns after an MI may be due largely to variations in peripheral vascular resistance (PVR).[72] Transient hypertension with elevated PVR and normal cardiac output (CO) has been noted and may be due to catecholamine excess. The resultant increase in afterload may depress SV while increasing $M\dot{V}O_2$.[43] Hypotension with normal CO and normal or decreased PVR is sometimes observed. This finding may represent active vasodilation of peripheral arterioles or decreased sympathetic tone.[76] Most often, changes in left ventricular contractility and compliance precipitate the onset of sympathetic compensation. Increases in heart rate (HR) help to maintain CO. Elevations in PVR help sustain arterial blood pressure (BP). If contractility is severely depressed, compensatory mechanisms fail. As peripheral resistance and afterload increase, $M\dot{V}O_2$

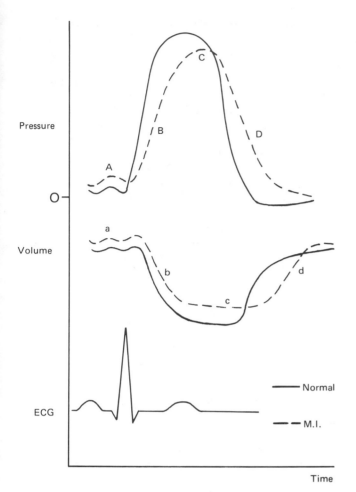

Fig. 11-3. An approximation of changes in left ventricular pressure and volume that may occur after an MI. This figure is only a simulation. Each phase of the curve is subject to numerous influences. An increased LVEDP (**A**) may result from decreased compliance or increased preload, or both.[3,4,18] An increased LVEDV (**a**) may be a compensatory change resulting from decreased contractility.[19,43] A decreased rate of shortening velocity and pressure development (**B**) and emptying (**b**) may result from altered actin–myosin interactions.[68] Lowered contractility may also reduce the amplitude of systolic pressure (**C**) and reduce volume ejected (**c**).[50,63,65,72] A slowed relaxation rate (**D**) and filling rate (**d**) may result as well.[33,65] Changes from an increased EDV (Starling mechanism) and the influence of catecholamines may compensate, so that hemodynamic changes are minimal. (After Scher AM: Mechanical events in the cardiac cycle. In Ruch TC, Patton HD (eds): Physiology and Biophysics: Circulation, Respiration and Fluid Balance pp 102–116. Philadelphia, WB Saunders, 1974)

rises, more ischemia ensues because of inadequate perfusion, and contractility is further depressed. This process is cyclical and leads to pump failure and cardiogenic shock (Chap. 27).

Mechanical Evolution. The pathologic evolution of an MI involves polymorphonuclear leukocyte infiltration, necrotic cell removal, and scar formation. The temporal sequence of these events has been determined by postmortem studies. The clinical manifestation of this time course is variable and depends on many factors. The repair process ends when damaged muscle is replaced by fibrous tissue.[18] Although

the heart is healed, the noncontractile scar creates functional abnormalities. These alterations are discussed in the preceding section.

The injury response begins 24 hours after occlusion and is marked after 5 days. Cells and surrounding interstitium swell, and leakage of intracellular enzymes and K^+ occurs. Leukocytes and macrophages infiltrate the area and engulf necrotic cells.[6,18,44] A fever and leukocytosis commonly accompany this stage of repair. In cases of transmural MI, damage to the epicardium may allow lymphocytes and fibrin to enter the pericardial space as well. Fibrinous pericarditis may then result.[47]

Necrotic tissue is degraded throughout the first week. This progresses from the periphery to the core of the infarct. Fibroblasts appear after 4 days and synthesize a collagen matrix. Small capillaries bud from surviving vessels and grow into the damaged zone.[18,44,47] These vessels remain very small and differ from collaterals.[44]

The infarct is most thin during the second week because progressive removal of necrotic tissue occurs more rapidly than collagen formation. Aneurysmal dilation of a transmural MI may develop. Ventricular rupture, though rare, may also occur in the second week as fibers are rapidly degraded.[47] Contraction of normal muscle against necrotic tissue may separate fibers. Dissecting blood may follow the shear line created in the myocardium and may cause a rupture.[21]

Grossly visible signs of scarring are present from the second through the fourth weeks. The bulk of necrotic cells are removed, and the density of tiny capillaries increases.[47] The endocardium overlying the infarct may show a gradual increase in its thickness.[18,21]

The final product of the repair process is a tough white fibrous scar. The time during which the MI has formed a mature scar is variable.[49] Estimates from autopsy data and healing from experimental MIs range from 2 to 3 months. Very large infarcts may still have some necrotic muscle bundles in the central zone for longer periods. Between 3 and 6 months, the scar contracts.[18,21,44,47]

Progressive increase in the function of normal muscle and stabilization of the infarcted zone usually occur as scar formation evolves.[21] End-diastolic dimensions decrease in the central zone. Dyskinesia (outward movement) of this area may evolve into akinesia (absent movement).[68] Stiffening of this zone may improve left-ventricular performance, because the loss in compliance may prevent systolic bulging, energy loss, and sequestration of blood.[3,43] A gradual increase in dimensions of normal tissue takes place and may be due to compensatory lengthening or hypertrophy of muscle.[68]

Electrical Alterations

Alterations in the cardiac resting and action potentials are a consequence of ischemia. These changes are due to abnormal permeability of cell membranes and diminished ATP supplies leading to defects in the Na^+/K^+ and Ca^{2+} pumps. The location of the infarction is an important determinant of electrical sequelae. Although the necrotic zone is electrically silent, it may produce ECG changes correlating with infarct location.

Variations in depolarization, duration of action potential, and refractoriness contribute to random dispersal of electrical impulses in the cells of the marginal zone. This can produce arrhythmias.[16] These arrhythmias can be significant because they may alter hemodynamics. In addition, they may extend the infarction by increasing the energy imbalance in the heart. Tachycardias may also increase the amount of K+ lost to the extracellular space.[12]

Changes in the Single Cell. The ischemic cell undergoes changes in its resting membrane potential, phase 0 depolarization, action potential duration and amplitude, and phase 4 depolarization. The composite of electrical alterations in all these cells is manifested as arrhythmias, conduction abnormalities, and morphologic changes in the surface ECG (Fig. 11-4).

The resting membrane potential of the ischemic cell decreases from -90 mV to near -60 mV because of a reduction in the gradient between intracellular and extracellular K+.[15] A less negative potential brings the cell closer to threshold. This partly inactivates the fast Na+ channel and unmasks the effects of the slow Ca^{2+} current on the action potential.[58] As a result, the upstroke of phase 0 depolarization slows, and conduction velocity decreases.[20,58] Abnormal intracellular concentrations of Na+ and K+ may also be responsible for decreasing the amplitude of the action potential in the ischemic cell.[15] In the necrotic zone cells are permeable equally to Na+ and K+, and ionic equilibration occurs. These cells are continually depolarized to values near zero, so electrical excitability is absent.[16]

The duration of the action potential shortens; this may be due to several mechanisms.[87] Although the mechanism is not completely understood, high extracellular K+ increases the outward K+ current. Repolarization may, then, occur more quickly, and the width of the action potential decreases.[38] Glycolytic inhibitors such as lactate and FFA

Fig. 11-4. Changes in the action potential of a ventricular myocardial cell immediately after ischemia occurs. Highlighted is a decreased resting membrane potential (**a**) and slope of phase 0 (**b**). Phase 2 (**c**) and the action potential (**d**) shorten. The rate of repolarization (**e**) may increase or decrease. (Adapted from Kleiber AG, Janse MJ, van Capelle FJL, et al: Circ Res, 42:606, 1978 by permission of the American Heart Association, Inc.)

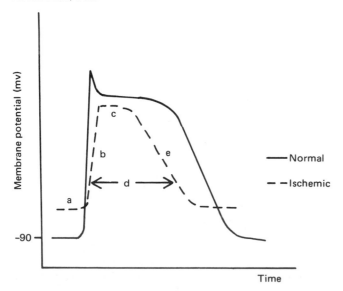

shorten the action potential as well.[58] An abbreviated plateau period may also decrease the span of the action potential. This implies that the slow inward Ca^{2+} current may be impaired.[38]

The slope of phase 4 depolarization determines heart rate. This slope increases in the ischemic pacemaker cell and may be due to the influence of c-AMP and catecholamines. Spontaneous depolarization can also be initiated in nonpacemaker tissue (*e.g.*, Purkinje cells) when the resting potential decreases. This source of automaticity may generate tachyarrhythmias.[58] A decreased slope of phase 4 depolarization sometimes may follow pronounced vagal activity after infarction. Bradycardia and escape rhythms may subsequently occur.

The changes in the ischemic cardiac cell may correlate to specific alterations in the ECG. Reduction of the resting membrane potential may be associated with T-Q depression. ST-segment elevation may relate to a reduced amplitude and duration of the action potential and delayed depolarization. T-wave inversion may result from prolonged repolarization in ischemic cells relative to repolarization in normal tissue.[60]

The described changes in the ischemic cell are additive throughout the myocardium in varying degrees. In general, conducting tissue is resistant to ischemia because of its relatively low O_2 consumption and high supply of glycogen.[58] Purkinje cells also have longer survival than the surrounding muscle because of their proximity to oxygenated ventricular cavity blood.[5,16] The variations in ischemia and survival time set the stage for arrhythmias. Reentry and increased automaticity are the primary mechanisms responsible for electrical disturbances. The influence of each correlates with the time course of the MI and may be related to site as well as extent of injury.[16]

Reentry. Reentry is the most common cause of ectopy and is due to asynchronous recovery of excitable cells. Reentrant mechanisms are noted in the earliest period after MI and may be due to instability of collateral flow to ischemic cells. Recurrence of arrhythmias, caused by reentry, days to weeks after the acute event, may be due to functionally disrupted Purkinje cells that are no longer ischemic.[16,87]

The normal heart acts as a syncytium in which electrically coupled cells pass impulses without decrement. The ischemic heart, however, has adjacent zones of cells that are unequal in refractoriness and excitability.[5,16,58] The abnormal conduction in these cells is the cellular mechanism responsible for reentry. It is a function of decreased membrane potential and a slowed rise of the action potential.[49,58] Additional requirements for reentry include unidirectional block, prolonged impulse propagation distal to the block, and restimulation of cells proximal to the block.[16,48]

The reentrant sequence is illustrated in Figure 26-2. It can occur in two ways. First, an electrical impulse reaches an ischemic zone. It conducts normally around the area and excites the ventricle. At the same time, the impulse is slowly propagated through the ischemic zone, reaches normal tissue, finds it nonrefractory, and reexcites the ventricle.[5,26] Second, unidirectional block in the ischemic area prevents antegrade conduction of an impulse. Then, the impulse passes through normal tissue. However, slow retrograde conduction through the zone occurs. Once it reaches non-refractory normal tissue proximal to the block, it conducts normally and reexcites the ventricle.[5,26]

Reentrant mechanisms produce ectopic foci coupled to preceding complexes and may result in single extrasystoles, sustained tachycardias, or fibrillation.[5,16,49] The significant condition is that an impulse is propagated through a zone slow enough to meet repolarized tissue distal to the zone.[16]

Automaticity. Automaticity is a property of pacemaker cells and is due to a spontaneous loss of diastolic potential.[26] The role of abnormal automaticity after acute MI is unclear. It implies that nonpacemaker cells can spontaneously generate action potentials at a rate sufficient to override the dominant pacemaker (usually the sinoatrial node).[16] This focus can trigger extrasystoles as well as tachycardia.

Abnormal automaticity may account for arrhythmias in the period 12 to 24 hours after acute MI[16] and also in the late recovery period.[87] This time course may be related to delayed ischemia of Purkinje cells.[12] Abnormal automaticity may be due to partial depolarization of ischemic cells. This increases the potential difference between normal and ischemic tissue. A flow of current results and may excite nearby nonrefractory fibers.[5,12] Excitation of Purkinje fibers, due to stretch from ventricular dilation or interstitial edema, is another postulated mechanism.[49]

Increased or decreased automaticity of pacemaker fibers may also be a source of arrhythmias. Catecholamine release and vagal stimulation produce opposite effects on phase 4 depolarization. These responses have been described earlier.

NONSPECIFIC SYSTEMIC STRESS RESPONSE

The systemic stress response influences cellular events in the ischemic myocardium. It is nonspecific and its magnitude reflects the physiologic and psychologic character of the individual. The neurohumoral activation that results is, in part, responsible for many of the clinical changes observed in the early recovery after MI.

The signal for the stress response may have two sources: the psychologic distress associated with pain, fear, and anxiety and the inhibition of the baroreceptor reflex when BP falls as a consequence of reduced myocardial contractility and SV. The hypothalamus stimulates the anterior pituitary to release adrenocorticotrophic hormone (ACTH). In turn, glucocorticoids are liberated from the adrenal cortex. Protein catabolism is enhanced and insulin release is suppressed. As a result, serum glucose levels rise, providing a substrate supply for myocardial glycolysis.[56,58]

The hypothalamus influences cardiovascular centers in the medulla during the stress response. Simultaneous activation of the sympathetic nervous system (SNS) and inhibition of the parasympathetic nervous system (PNS) occur. Postganglionic release of norepinephrine follows. Measurement of circulating catecholamines demonstrates peaks in norepinephrine and epinephrine within the first few hours after MI,[40] and after transfer from cardiac to intermediate care units.[28,74,75] Norepinephrine augments lipolysis and increases cardiac contractility and peripheral resistance.[56]

Maintenance of the stress response is supported by adrenal medullary release of catecholamines—primarily, epinephrine. The duration of the response varies with the severity of the physical or psychologic stress and hormonal stores. Epinephrine inhibits pancreatic beta-cell insulin production, stimulates liver and muscle glycogenolysis, and enhances platelet aggregation. It also increases myocardial contractility. Its effects on peripheral resistance are variable.[56]

The net effect of plasma catecholamine activity on the ischemic myocardium is related to the degree of adrenergic overload. The positive inotropic actions of norepinephrine and epinephrine increase $M\dot{V}O_2$. Alpha adrenergic stimulation elevates PVR and systolic BP. Afterload increases, and cardiac work is further extended. Diastolic BP also increases and may enhance coronary perfusion. However, O_2 supply may be surpassed by the O_2 demand induced in the ischemic myocardium.[56,58]

Arrhythmias may be generated because of catecholamine excess. Sympathetic stimulation can lead to tachycardia and increased automaticity of nonpacemaker cells.[5] Shortening of the refractory period with catecholamines may not be uniform throughout the ischemic myocardium and initiate reentrant arrhythmias.[16] In addition, the increased production of c-AMP from norepinephrine excess is correlated with ventricular fibrillation in dogs.[11]

Catecholamines also induce lipolysis. This increases circulating FFA. Arrhythmic as well as hemodynamic sequelae may be related to this elevation.[52] A reduced level of total serum lipids is also found in the acute recovery period.[48]

The stress response elevates epinephrine, serotonin, and ADP levels. These substances enhance platelet clumping.[53] Significant increases in circulating platelet microthrombi have been documented in patients during the acute period of MI.[50] Disrupted flow due to an occlusion and increased catecholamine activity may induce platelet aggregation and contribute to extension of the infarction.[51] Increased fibrinogen levels are also noted during the first week after MI.[29] Fibrinogen-induced fibrin formation helps solidify a thrombus, once it is generated by platelet clumping.[53]

A subgroup of patients after acute MI have increased vagal activity. This most frequently occurs after inferoposterior MI.[72] These individuals have bradycardia and an inappropriately low PVR with normal or low CO.[76] A similar response has been noted in people who respond to stress with vasovagal syncope.[23] A possible source for this finding may be the left ventricular stretch receptors. These receptors may be activated in the ischemic zone and lead to increased vagal afferent activity.[24]

Increased parasympathetic activity after MI may be a protective mechanism. By decreasing HR and contractility, it lowers $M\dot{V}O_2$ and may protect against arrhythmias.[24] Decreased activity in isolated sympathetic nerves in the first hour after MI has been noted in dogs.[24] In addition, disruption of PNS fibers after coronary occlusion in cats leads to greater frequency of ventricular fibrillation.[13]

A summary of the systemic response after MI is presented in Figure 11-5. It illustrates that psychologic and physiologic stress sequelae may modify the combined metabolic, electrical, and mechanical response of the heart to ischemia.

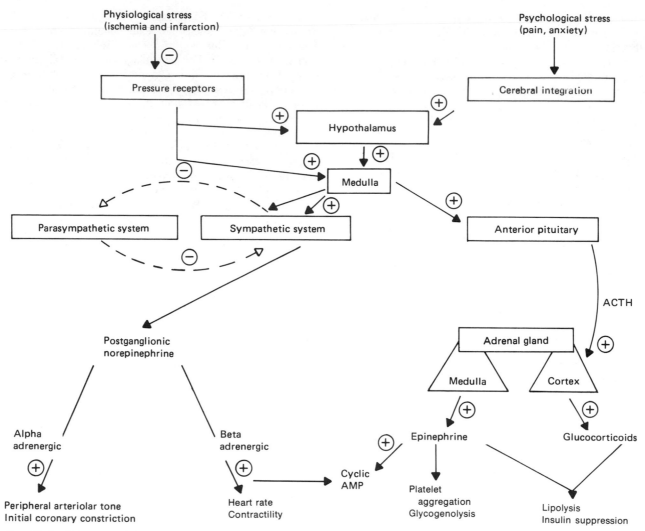

Fig. 11-5. Summary of the systemic stress response that may occur after an MI. The diagram emphasizes net excitatory influences in the sequence. Feedback mechanisms may exist between each step (not shown). (Adapted from Oliver MF: In Dickinson CJ, Marks J, (eds): Developments in Cardiovascular Medicine. Lancaster, England, MTP Press Ltd, 1978)

SITE OF INFARCTION

The site of an MI is usually determined by the occlusion of a coronary artery supplying a specific muscle area. The most frequent and hemodynamically significant infarctions involve the left ventricle. Clinical interest in infarction site relates to correlations between site and arrhythmias, prodromal symptoms, and to a lesser extent, hemodynamic sequelae.

The size of an MI is the most important determinant of power failure. Methods used to quantify size include measurement of serum enzymes, ST-segment mapping, measurement of QS waves, radionuclide imaging, and angiography.[79]

Clinical determination of infarct location is usually done by ECG analysis. Damage to the left ventricle is usually implied when the site of an MI is described. The ECG gives clues to the general location of healed MIs but may be imprecise in determining the exact site of transmural damage. It is usually not a good predictor of subendocardial

infarction.[66,70,80] Previous MIs, extent of collateral supply, and degree of occlusion influence the accuracy of the ECG diagnosis of location.[18,79] On the other hand, the ECG has an approximate 60% sensitivity in denoting the general presence of an MI or ischemic damage.[17]

The description of the infarction site includes a presumed knowledge of the vessel occluded. The reader is referred to Chapter 1 for a review of the details of coronary anatomy and supply. Primary sites based on pathologic descriptions can be categorized as anterior, inferoposterior, and lateral aspects of the left ventricle.

Anterior Location

An anterior MI usually involves occlusion of the left anterior descending (LAD) artery.[79] Minimal involvement includes the apical half of the left ventricle,[66] although extension into the septum is common.[76] Atrial or atrioventricular (AV) block with anterior MI may point to associated right coronary artery (RCA) or left circumflex artery (LCA) disease.[76]

However, because the LAD supplies the anterior two-thirds of the septum, its occlusion can produce ischemia of the left and right bundle branches. Variable degrees of fascicular or AV block may result.[67] Sympathetic hyperactivity presented by transient hypertension and sinus tachycardia has been significantly correlated with anterior MI in cats.[14] It is not known if this relationship holds true for humans.

Inferior/Posterior Location

Inferior and posterior MIs result from occlusion of the RCA in 80% to 90% of the patients. In 10% to 20% of the people, LCA occlusion is the cause.[18,76] The extent of muscle damage ranges from apical-diaphragmatic through posterobasal involvement of the left ventricle.[66]

Associated supply of the AV junction and His bundle by the occluded artery also leads to ischemia of the conduction system. Second- and third-degree AV blocks and escape rhythms may result. In 55% of the population, the RCA also has a branch to the sinoatrial (SA) node and atria. Subsequent to RCA occlusion, SA block and atrial arrhythmias may develop.[35] Associated symptoms with inferoposterior MI include fainting, hiccoughing, and nausea.[35] Parasympathetic overactivity may also occur and manifest itself as sinus bradycardia and hypotension.[14]

Lateral Location

Myocardial infarction confined to the lateral wall of the left ventricle is the least common and is usually due to occlusion of the LCA. More common is the association of lateral wall damage with anterior and inferoposterior MIs.[79] The LCA also supplies the AV junction, His bundle, and anterior and posterior papillary muscles in 10% of the population. Hence, LCA occlusion may herald conduction abnormalities. The LCA supplies the SA node and atria in 45% of the population.[76] The advent of atrial arrhythmias with lateral MIs may signify proximal occlusion of the LCA near the left main coronary artery. Extension of the thrombus may lead to left main occlusion, with serious consequences.[35]

Other Locations

Isolated right ventricular infarctions are rare. More common is the association of right ventricular injury with inferoposterior MI, due to occlusion of the RCA.[66,76] Neck vein distention, hypotension, and elevated right atrial pressure may signal a right ventricular infarction.[10]

Subendocardial infarction damages the inner layer of the myocardium and is infrequently related to coronary occlusion.[3] The susceptibility of the subendocardium to ischemia is described in an earlier section of this chapter. Subendocardial MIs may be related to subsequent transmural events. A prospective study of 50 patients with subendocardial infarction demonstrated a relatively benign inhospital course. However, in a medically treated subgroup, 21% suffered an acute transmural infarction within 1 year of discharge from the hospital.[45,46]

REFERENCES

1. Apstein CS,, Deckelbaum L, Magopian L et al: Acute cardiac ischemia and reperfusion: Contractility, relaxation, and glycolysis. Am J Physiol 235(6):H637–H650, 1978
2. Baroldi G: Cornary thrombosis: Facts and beliefs. Am Heart J 91(6):683–688,1976
3. Bertrand ME, Rousseau MF, LaBlanche JM: Cineangiographic assessment of left ventriculor function in the acute phase of transmural myocardial infarction. Am J Cardiol 43(3): 472–480, 1979
4. Bertrand ME, Rousseau MF, Lefebvre JM et al: Left ventricular compliance in acute transmural myocardial infarction in man. Eur J Cardiol (Suppl)7:179–193, 1978
5. Bigger JT: Antiarrhythmic drugs in ischemic heart disease. In Braunwald E (ed): The Myocardium: Failure and Infarction, pp 295–306 New York, HP Publishing, 1974
6. Bloor CM, Ashraf M: Pathogenesis of acute myocardial infarction. Adv Cardiol 23:1–13, 1978
7. Braasch W, Gudbjarnason S, Bing RJ: Biochemical changes in the myocardium during the reparative processes following coronary artery occlusion. In DeHaas JH, Hemker HC, Snellen HA (eds): Ischaemic Heart Disease, pp 26–35. Leiden, The Netherlands, Leiden University Press, 1970
8. Braunwald E, Maroko PR: Protection of the ischemic myocardium. In Braunwald E (ed): The Myocardium: Failure and Infarction, pp 329–342. New York, HP Publishing, 1974
9. Cohen MV: The functional value of coronary collaterals in myocardial ischemia and therapeutic approach to enhance collateral flow. Am Heart J 95(3):396–404, 1978
10. Cohn JN, Guiha NH, Broder MI: Right ventricular infarction: Clinical and hemodynamic features. Am J Cardiol 32(2):209–214, 1974
11. Corday F, Heng MK, Meerbaum S et al: Derangements of myocardial metabolism preceding onset of ventricular fibrillation after coronary occlusion. Am J Cardiol 39(5):830–889, 1977
12. Corday E, Lang T: Altered physiology associated with cardiac arrhythmias. In Hurst JW, Logue RB, Schlant, RC et al (eds): The Heart, 4th ed, pp 628–633. New York, McGraw-Hill, 1978
13. Corr PB, Gillis RA: Role of the vagus nerves in the cardiovascular changes induced by coronary occlusion. Circulation 49(1): 86–97, 1974
14. Corr PB, Pearle DL, Hinton JR et al: Site of myocardial infarction: A determinant of the cardiovascular changes induced in the cat by coronary occlusion. Circ Res 39(6):840–847, 1976
15. Corr PB, Sobel BE: The importance of metabolites in the genesis of ventricular dysrhythmias induced by ischemia. I. Electrophysiological considerations. Mod. Concepts Cardiovasc Dis 48(8):34–47, 1979
16. Corr PB, Sobel BE: The importance of metabolites in the genesis of ventricular dysrhythmias induced by ischemia. II. Biochemical factors. Mod Concepts Cardiovas Dis 48(9): 48–52, 1979
17. Cowan MJ: Quantification of Myocardial Infarction Size by Spatial Vectorcardiography. Ph.D. dissertation, University of Washington, 1979 available through microfilms, Ann Arbor, Michigan
18. Crawford T: Pathology of Ischaemic Heart Disease, pp 80–100. London, Butterworth, 1977
19. Diamond G, Forrester JS: Effect of coronary artery disease and acute myocardial infarction on left ventricular compliance in man. Circulation 45(1):11–19, 1972
20. Durrer D, Janse MJ, Lie KI et al: Human cardiac electrophysiology. In Dickinson CJ and Marks J (eds): Developments in Cardiovascular Medicine, pp 53–75. Baltimore, University Park Press, 1978
21. Eliot RS, Edwards JE: Pathology of coronary atherosclerosis and its complications. In Hurst JW, Logue RB, Schlant RC et al (eds): The Heart, 4th ed., pp 1121–1130. New York: McGraw-Hill, 1978
22. Eliot RS, Holsinger JW: The pathophysiologic panorama of myocardial ischemia and infarction. Adv Cardiol 9:2–15, 1973
23. Epstein SF, Stampfer M, Beiser GD: Role of the capacitance

and resistance vessels in vasovagal syncope. Circulation, 37(4):524–533, 1968

24. Feola M, Arbel ER, Glick G et al: Attenuation of cardiac sympathetic drive in experimental myocardial ischemia in dogs. Am Heart J 93(1):82–88, 1977
25. Fiegl EO: The coronary circulation. In Ruch TC, Patton HD (eds): Physiology and Biophysics: Circulation, Respiration and Fluid Balance, pp 247–261. Philadelphia, WB Saunders, 1974
26. Fisch C: Electrophysiologic basis of clinical arrhythmias. Heart Lung 3(1):51–56, 1974
27. Flameng W, Schwarz F, Schaper W: Coronary collaterals in the canine heart: Development and functional significance. Am Heart J 97(1):70–77, 1979.
28. Gentry WD, Musante GJ, Haney T: Anxiety and urinary sodium/potassium as stress indicators on admission to a coronary care unit. Heart Lung 2(6):875–877, 1973
29. Gidron E, Margalit R, Oliven A et al: Effect of myocardial infarction on components of fibrinolytic system. Br Heart J 39(1):19–24, 1977
30. Goldberg S, Lam W, Mudge G et al: Coronary hemodynamic and myocardial metabolic alterations accompanying coronary spasm. Am J Cardiol 43(3):481–487, 1979
31. Gorlin R, Herman M: Physiology of the coronary circulation. In Hurst JW, Logue RB, Schlant RC et al (eds): The Heart, 4th ed, pp 101–106. New York, McGraw-Hill, 1978
32. Gregg DE: The natural history of coronary collateral development. Circ. Res 35(9):335–344, 1974
33. Grossman W, Mann J: Evidence for impaired left ventricle relaxation during acute ischemia in man. Eur J Cardiol (Supp)7:239–249, 1978
34. Guyton RA, Daggett WM: The evolution of myocardial infarction: Physiologic basis for clinical intervention. In Guyton AC, Cowley AW (eds): International Review of Physiology: Cardiovascular Physiology II, pp 305–339. Baltimore, University Park Press, 1976
35. James TN: Anatomy of the coronary arteries and veins. In Hurst JW, Logue RB, Schlant RC et al (eds): The Heart, 4th ed, pp 32–47. New York, McGraw-Hill, 1978
36. Jennings RB: Relationship of acute ischemia to functional defects and irreversibility. Circulation (Suppl I)53(3):I26–I29, 1976
37. Jesmok GJ, Gross GJ, Hardman HF: Effect of propranolol and nitroglycerin plus methoxamine on transmural creatine kinase activity after acute coronary occlusion. Am J Cardiol 42(11):769–773, 1978
38. Katz AM: Physiology of the Heart, pp 35–72; pp 229–256; pp 419–433. New York, Raven Press, 1977
39. Kleber, AG, Janse MJ, van Capelle FJL et al: Mechanism and time course of S-T and T-Q segment changes during acute regional myocardial ischemia in the pig heart determined by extracellular and intracellular recordings. Cir Res 42(5):603–613, 1978
40. Klein RF, Troyer WG, Thompson HK: Catecholamine excretion in myocardial infarction. Arch Intern Med 122(6):476–482, 1968
41. Kleitke B, Wollenberger A, Krause EG et al: Effect of acute ischemia on cyclic AMP levels and other parameters in the cytosol and in mitochondria of hypertrophied and nonhypertrophied hearts. Adv Cardiol 18:27–40, 1976
42. Knoebel SB, Rasmussen S: Myocardial blood flow: Newer clinical considerations. Heart Lung 3(1):78–82, 1974
43. Kones RJ: Cardiogenic Shock: Mechanism and Management. Kisco, NY, Futura, 1974
44. Lodge-Patch I: The ageing of cardiac infarcts, and its influence on cardiac rupture. Br Heart J 13(1):37–42, 1951
45. Luchi RJ, Chahine RA Raizner AE: Coronary artery spasm. Ann Intern Med 91(3):441–449, 1979
46. Madigan NP, Rutherford BD, Frye RL: The clinical course, early prognosis and coronary anatomy of subendocardial infarction. Am J Med 60:634–641, 1976
47. Mallory GK, White PD: The speed of healing of myocardial infarction. Am Heart J 18(6):647–671, 1939
48. Markiewicz K, Lutz W, Pelka W et al: Dynamics of serum lipid changes in acute myocardial infarction. Acta Med. Pol 17(3):193–201, 1976

49. Mazzoleni A: Electrophysiologic mechanisms of sudden death in patients with coronary artery disease. Heart Lung 2(6):841–846, 1973.
50. Mehta M, Mehta J: Platelet function studies in coronary artery disease: Evidence for enhanced platelet microthrombus formation activity in acute myocardial infarction. Am J Cardiol 43(4):757–760, 1979
51. Moore S: Platelet aggregation secondary to coronary obstruction. Circulation (Suppl I)53(3):I66–I69, 1976
52. Mueller HS, Ayres SM: Metabolic responses of the heart in acute myocardial infarction in man. Am J Cardiol 42(9):363–371. 1978
53. Mustard, JF: Platelets and thrombosis in acute myocardial infarction. In Braunwald E (ed): The Myocardium: Failure and Infarction, pp 177–190. New York, HP Publishing, 1974
54. Oliva PB, Breckinridge JC: Arteriographic evidence of coronary arterial spasm in acute myocardial infarction. Circulation 56(3):366–374, 1977.
55. Oliver MF: Metabolism of the normal and ischaemic myocardium. In Dickinson CJ, Marks J (eds): Developments in Cardiovascular Medicine, pp 145–164. Lancaster, Eng, MTP Press, 1978
56. Oliver MF: The metabolic response to a heart attack. Heart Lung 4(1):57–60, 1975
57. Opie LH: Metabolism of free fatty acids, glucose and catecholamines in acute myocardial infarction: Relation to myocardial ischemia and infarct size. Am J Cardiol 36(12):938–953, 1975
58. Opie LH, Nathan D, Lubbe WF: Biochemical aspects of arrhythmogenesis and ventricular fibrillation. Am J Cardiol 432(1):131–148, 1979
59. Opie LH, Owen P, Lubbe W: Estimated glycolytic flux in infarcting heart. Recent Adv Stud Cardiac Struct Metab 7:249–255, 1976
60. Page E, Polimeni PI: Ultrastructural changes in the ischemic zone bordering experimental infarcts in rat left ventricles. Am J Pathol 87(1):81–92 1977
61. Patton HD: Somatic sensation and its disturbance. In Patton HD, Sundsten JW, Crill WE (eds): Introduction to basic neurology, pp 169–193. Philadelphia, WB Saunders, 1976
62. Patton HD: Visceral sensation and referred pain. In Patton HD, Sundsten JW, Crill WE (eds): Introduction to Basic Neurology, pp 194–198. Philadelphia, WB Saunders, 1976
63. Puri PS: Correlation between biochemical and contractile changes after myocardial ischemia and revascularization. Recent Adv Stud Cardiac Struc Metab 7:161–169, 1976
64. Reichenbach DD, Benditt ED: Catecholamines and cardiomyopathy: The pathological potential importance of myofibrillar degeneration. Hum Pathol 1(1):125–150, 1970
65. Richards AF, Seabra-Gomes R: Observations on the effect of angina on the left ventricle, with special reference to diastolic behavior. Eur J Cardiol (Suppl)7:213–238, 1978
66. Roberts WC, Gardin JM: Location of myocardial infarcts: A confusion of terms and definitions. Am J Cardiol 42(11):868–871, 1978
67. Roffman JA, Fieldman A: Ventricular conduction defects: Significance and prognosis. Heart Lung 9(1):111–121, 1980
68. Ross J, Franklin D: Analysis of regional myocardial function, dimensions, and wall thickness in the characterization of myocardial ischemia and infarction. Circulation (Suppl I)53(3):I88–I92, 1976.
69. Rowe GG: Inequalities of myocardial perfusion in coronary artery disease ("coronary steal"). Circulation 42(8):193–194, 1970
70. Savage RM, Wagner GS, Ideker RE et al: Correlation of postmortem anatomic findings with electrocardiographic changes in patients with myocardial infarction: Retrospective study of patients with typical anterior and posterior infarcts. Circulation 55(2):279–285, 1977
71. Scher AM: Mechanical events in the cardiac cycle. In Ruch TC, Patton HE (eds): Physiology and Biophysics: Circulation, Respiration and Fluid Balance. pp 102–116. Philadelphia, WB Saunders, 1974
72. Schlant RC: Altered cardiovascular physiology of coronary atherosclerotic heart disease. In Hurst JW, Logue RB, Schlant

RC et al (eds): The Heart, 4th ed, pp 1134–1156. New York, McGraw-Hill, 1978

73. Schwarz F, Flameng W, Ensslen R et al: Effect of coronary collaterals on left ventricular function at rest and during stress. Am Heart J 95(5):570–577, 1978

74. Shannon VJ: The transfer process: An area for concern for the CCU nurse. Heart Lung 2(3):364–367, 1973

75. Siggers DC, Salter C, Fluck DC: Serial plasma adrenaline and noradrenaline levels in myocardial infarction using a new double isotope technique. Br Heart J 33(6):878–883, 1971

76. Silber EN, Katz LN: Heart Disease, pp 780–789. New York, Macmillan, 1975

77. Smith HJ, Kent KM, Epstein SE: Relationship between regional contractile function and S-T segment elevation after experimental coronary artery occlusion in the dog. Cardiovasc Res 12(7):444–448, 1978

78. Sobel BE: Biochemical and morphologic changes in infarcting myocardium. In Braunwald E (ed): The Myocardium: Failure and Infarction, pp 247–260. New York, HP Publishing, 1974

79. Sokolow M, McIlroy MB: Clinical Cardiology, pp 135–142. Los Altos, Calif, 1977

80. Sullivan W, Vlodaver Z, Tuna N et al: Correlation of electro-cardiographic and pathologic findings in healed myocardial infarction. Am J Cardiol 42(11):724–732, 1978

81. Torstila I: The plasma kinin system in acute myocardial infarction. Acta Med Scand (Suppl)620:1–62, 1978

82. Trump BF, Mergner WJ, Kahng MW et al: Studies on the subcellular pathophysiology of ischemia. Circulation (Suppl I)53(3):I17–I25, 1976

83. Tsien RW: Possible effects of hydrogen ions in ischemic myocardium. Circulation (Suppl I) 53(3):I14–I16, 1976

84. Uretsky BF, Farquhar OS, Berezin AF et al: Symptomatic myocardial infarction without chest pain: Prevalence and clinical course. Am J Cardiol 40(4):498–503, 1977

85. White FC, Sanders M, Bloor CM: Regional redistribution of myocardial blood flow after coronary occlusion and reperfusion in the conscious dog. Am J Cardiol 42(2):234–243, 1978

86. Williamson JR, Schaffer SW, Ford C: Contribution of tissue acidosis to ischemic injury in the perfused rat heart. Circulation (Suppl I)53(3):I3–I14, 1976

87. Wit AL, Bigger JT: Possible electrophysiological mechanisms for lethal arrhythmias accompanying myocardial ischemia and infarction. Circulation (Suppl III)51, No. 52:III96–III115, 1975

12

Sudden Cardiac Death

MARIE J. COWAN, R.N., Ph.D.

Atherosclerotic coronary artery disease (CAD) is the main cause of death in the United States. From January to August, 1979, the death rate due to ischemic heart disease was 252.9 per 100,000.[32] Sudden cardiac death (SCD) is the major health problem in the United States because 30% to 66% of the patients who die from CAD die of sudden cardiac death. Depending upon the availability of a mobile life-support unit, 40% or more die before reaching the hospital.[2,6,26,30,35,47] There is no completely reliable long-term treatment to prevent further episodes of ventricular fibrillation for those survivors of SCD; and there are no reliable physiologic predictors available to foretell the first event of ventricular fibrillation.

DEFINITION OF SUDDEN DEATH

Sudden cardiac death is neither a clinical nor a pathologic diagnosis, but a descriptive term to indicate death from cardiac causes that has occurred within seconds to hours after the onset of symptoms. The time period between the onset of symptoms and death ranges from "instantaneous deaths" occurring 30 seconds or less after onset of symptoms[15] to "sudden death" occurring minutes to 24 hours after onset of symptoms.[26,52] Although sudden cardiac death is most commonly defined as occurring within 6 hours after the onset of symptoms,[39] this is probably too long a time to fit the definition and encompasses a heterogeneous group of patients.

Coronary artery disease is related to 75% of all sudden deaths, and other causes contribute to about 25% of the cases. Causes of sudden death are listed in Table 12-1. The main objective of this chapter is to discuss the relationship of SCD to CAD, to selective myocardial cell necrosis, and to primary ventricular fibrillation.

SIGNS AND SYMPTOMS OF SUDDEN CARDIAC DEATH

Electrocardiographic Signs

Data from out-of-hospital mobile coronary care units indicate that primary ventricular fibrillation (VF) is the clincial diagnosis responsible for SCD in approximately 98% of the patients.[9] A smaller subgroup (1%–5%) has asystole, bradycardia, or heartblock. In patients who have been resuscitated from VF, repolarization abnormalities on the resting ECG are more prevalent than in patients with CAD but without VF. In 46% of the SCD cases the ECG showed ST-segment depression; 52% showed T-wave flattening; and 35% showed prolongation of the QTc interval.[21]

More importantly, these survivors of SCD showed a high prevalence of ventricular ectopic activity during months to years of follow-up. In 92% of the cases, the ECG showed unifocal ventricular premature beats (PVCs); 70% had multiform PVCs; 48% had ventricular couplets; 47% had bigeminy or trigeminy; and 9% had ventricular tachycardia.[9]

In persons who are resuscitated from ventricular fibrillation, electrocardiographic confirmation of myocardial necrosis is difficult. It is conceivable that selective myocardial cell necrosis can mimic the ECG criteria for an acute

TABLE 12-1 CAUSES OF SUDDEN DEATH

Cardiac Causes

Atherosclerotic coronary artery disease
    Selective myocardial cell necrosis
    Myocardial infarction

Aortic stenosis

Cardiomyopathies

Acute myocarditis

Aortic or ventricular aneurysm with dissection or rupture

Congenital heart disease

Prolapsed mitral valve syndrome

Iatrogenic causes: Digitalis and other drug causes

Accessory atrioventricular conduction syndromes

Noncardiac Causes

Pulmonary hypertension (primary, particularly during pregnancy)

Pulmonary embolism

Cerebral or subarachnoid hemorrhage

Sudden infant death syndrome (SIDS; should at least in part be included in cardiac causes)

Choking

Jervell and Lange-Nielson syndrome (syndrome of prolonged Q-T interval, congenital deafness, syncope and ventricular fibrillation following emotional or physical stresses)

Romano-Ward syndrome (similar to Jervell and Lange-Nielson syndrome without congenital deafness)

Electrolyte abnormalities (*i.e.*, hypokalemia)

Acid–base abnormalities (*i.e.*, alkalosis)

---

myocardial infarction.[11] A pathologic Q wave indicates necrosis, regardless of the pathogenesis of the lesion. However, only about 17% of the SCD cases exhibit Q wave changes;[5] and it is difficult to distinguish how many are associated with selective myocardial cell necrosis and how many are associated with myocardial infarction.

Physical Signs and Symptoms

The physical signs of SCD are collapse and unconsciousness. Approximately 80% of the patients who have SCD were noted to have had other cardiovascular symptoms and had visited a physician within one month prior to VF. Angina was reported in 43% of the cases prior to the development of VF; signs and symptoms of congestive heart failure were reported in 20% of the cases.[9] There is a definite lack of symptoms such as dyspnea, faintness, weakness, palpitation, nausea, vomiting, or fatigue immediately before collapse.[15]

Types of Activity Preceding Event

Types of activity that have been reported to precede immediately the terminal episode are extreme physical exertion; sitting or reclining; and sleeping. There was no relationship between the incidence of SCD and eating, automobile driving, sexual intercourse, or defecation.[15]

Serum Enzyme Changes

Cobb reported lactate dehydrogenase (LDH) isoenzyme patterns for 172 survivors who had been resuscitated from primary ventricular fibrillation.[8] Selective myocardial cell necrosis was considered present when the percentage distribution of alpha-1 LDH (type I LDH isoenzyme) was both increased and greater than alpha-2 LDH (type II LDH isoenzyme). Reliance on the diagnostic use of serum glutamic oxaloacetic transaminase (SGOT), total creatine phosphokinase (CK), and total LDH enzyme activities is not wise because cardiopulmonary resuscitation (CPR) alone commonly results in elevated total serum enzyme activity. A serum increase of alpha-1 LDH is specific to myocardial cell injury,[49] as is the CK_2 isoenzyme increase (or MB positive). A rise in the CK_2 level would detect an injury 24 to 48 hours old, whereas a rise in the alpha-1 LDH level would detect an injury 72 to 120 hours old (see Chap. 15). However, in approximately 60% of the cases of primary ventricular fibrillation, there is no diagnostic rise in CK_2 or alpha-1 LDH.[9] This probably depends on (1) the size of the pathologic lesions, which tend to be small focal areas of myocardial cell necrosis surrounded by viable capillaries, and (2) the rapid "wash-out" of the enzymes from the injured area to the serum.

PATHOLOGY RELATED TO SUDDEN CARDIAC DEATH

A high proportion of people who die from sudden cardiac death have severe atherosclerotic coronary artery disease. Severe coronary artery disease is defined as one or more coronary vessels with 75% or greater stenosis. Reichenbach reported that in a sample of people who died suddenly, 59% had an old complete occlusion in one or more coronary vessels; 8% had single vessel stenosis of over 90%; 18% had double vessel stenosis of over 90%; 13% had triple vessel stenosis of over 90%. Only 8% did not have significant coronary artery disease.[38]

A survey of several reports show that, although approximately 55% of the people studied post mortem after SCD had old myocardial infarctions, there is evidence that sudden cardiac death is not usually associated with acute myocardial infarction. Acute thrombosis of the coronary arteries is not a common finding after sudden cardiac death.[4,15,38,39,46] The frequency of pathologic evidence of acute myocardial infarction after sudden cardiac death (19%) is relatively low.[13,33] A large percentage of patients who have been resuscitated from primary ventricular fibrillation do not develop clinical evidence of acute myocardial infarction, diagnosed either by enzyme or electrocardiographic criteria.[5,8] Thus sudden cardiac death appears not to be causally related to acute myocardial infarction and/or acute coronary thrombus.

Selective Myocardial Cell Necrosis

Selective myocardial cell necrosis is the pathologic lesion that most frequently has been associated with sudden cardiac death and with the clinical syndrome of primary ventricular fibrillation.[37,38] In 50 patients who died suddenly and had documented ventricular fibrillation, 44 (88%) showed evidence of necrosis selectively involving myocardial cells.[37] Selective myocardial cell necrosis has also been referred to as myofibrillar degeneration, myocytolysis, or catecholamine cardiomyopathy.

Selective myocardial cell necrosis is a lesion in which focal myocardial cells are injured but in which the surrounding interstitial cells, nerves, and capillaries remain viable. It implies that the injury occurred without complete occlusion of coronary blood flow. There may have been decreased coronary blood flow or complete occlusion with recirculation of flow such as could occur with spasm of a severely stenosed coronary artery. It is different from the center core of myocardial infarction, which is coagulative necrosis. Coagulative necrosis refers to an area of complete cell death: necrosis of myocardial cells, interstitial cells, capillaries, and nerves. It is caused by complete occlusion of coronary arterial blood flow. Selective myocardial cell necrosis is similar to peripheral areas of ischemia surrounding the core of myocardial infarction. Myocardial ischemia is defined as a condition in which the oxygen needs of the myocardium are not met and the conversion from aerobic to anaerobic glycolysis takes place. It implies a reduced coronary blood flow resulting in tissue hypoxia but not complete occlusion. There may be complete occlusion with anoxia for a short period followed by resumption of blood flow. Irreversible injury occurs at different rates for different cells and can be caused by degrees of hypoxia and different intervals of anoxia. For instance myocardial cells are irreversibly injured earlier than endothelial cells lining capillaries. Within the population of myocardial cells, there seems to be different susceptibilities to injury. Therefore, in ischemia, there are various zones of cellular injury: In some areas there may be selective myocardial cell necrosis, and in other areas some interstitial cells, capillaries, and/or nerves may also be injured. In summary, the injured myocardial cells seen in selective myocardial cell necrosis and in the ischemic peripheral zone of myocardial infarction appear histologically different from the injured myocardial cells seen in the core of a myocardial infarction.

The histologic features of selective myocardial cell ne-

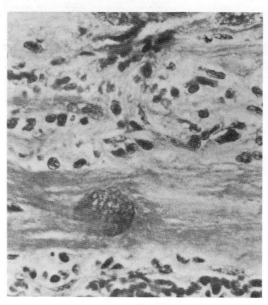

Fig. 12-2. Infiltration of lymphocytes and histiocytes in the interstitial tissue in development of selective myocardial cell necrosis. A myocardial cell displays enlargement of the nucleus. Tissue from *Macaca nemestrina*. (Original magnification × 640) (Cowan M: Heart Lung 8:560, 1979)

crosis have been described by Reichenbach and Benditt.[36] The myocardial cell characteristically shows a transverse "banding" and a loss of the linear arrangement of myofibrils. Conversely, in the core of the myocardial infarction, the myocardial cell does not have "banding," and the striations remain intact (Fig. 12-1). The "banding" is seen histologically in less than 24 hours after the injury and can last for 6 to 8 days until the macrophages infiltrate and phagocytose the necrotic cells. It is hypothesized that the "banding" is due to an influx of calcium into the injured myocardial cell. The calcium could be supplied to the injured area by way of the coronary blood supply. Dense granular basophilic material appears in the injured myocardial cell cytoplasm by the second through the fifth day. This is evidence of calcification of the mitochondria and "shut-down" of oxidative phosphorylation.

In selective myocardial cell necrosis, the lesion as well as the injured myocardial cell differs from that seen in myocardial infarction. The former lesion is made of multiple, small focal areas of necrosis randomly located in the myocardium. Myocardial infarctions are large, confluent areas of necrosis in areas distal to an occluded coronary artery. The interstitial cellular response is much smaller in selective myocardial cell necrosis than in infarction. There are few polymorphonuclear leukocytes and a small mononuclear cell response (Fig. 12-2). By the ninth day, there is interstitial fibrosis with myocytolysis (Fig. 12-3). On cross section, myocytolysis appears as empty sarcolemma sheaths. Some myocardial cells adjacent to the interstitial fibrosis have enlarged nuclei with enlarged nucleoli (Fig. 12-4). These cells are interpreted to represent an increase of protein synthesis suggesting a reparative response. It is conceivable that these myocardial cells represent viable but injured cells capable of generating ectopic ventricular beats.

Fig. 12-1. Dense transverse bands in the early development of selective myocardial cell necrosis in tissue from *Macaca nemestrina*. (Original magnification × 160) (Cowan M: Heart Lung 8:560, 1979)

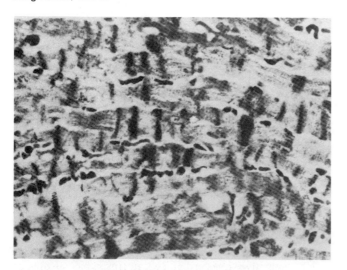

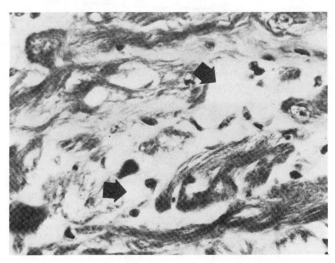

Fig. 12-3. Myocytolysis resulting in empty sarcolemmal sheaths (*arrows*) in tissue from *Macaca nemestrina*. (Original magnification × 640) (Cowan M, Heart Lung 8:561, 1979)

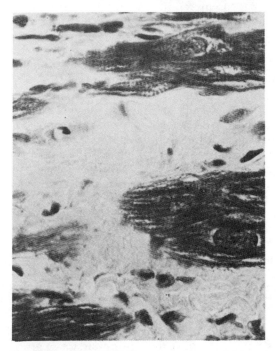

Fig. 12-4. Interstitial fibrosis and myocardial nuclear enlargement associated with the chronic stage of selective myocardial cell necrosis in tissue from *Macaca nemestrina*. (Original magnification × 640) (Cowan M: Heart Lung 8:561, 1979)

Pathogenesis of Selective Myocardial Cell Necrosis

The pathogenesis of selective myocardial cell necrosis is a complicated problem because many conditions can induce the lesion in experimental animals; and the lesion has been associated with other diseases besides sudden cardiac death in humans. There was a 26% incidence of selective myocardial cell necrosis in a randomly selected group of patients with different pathologic diagnoses undergoing autopsy.[36] The lesion has been reported to occur in patients after open-heart surgery;[36] in patients who died from subarachnoid hemorrhage,[17] and in patients who died from pheochromocytoma.[24]

Catecholamines are significant in the pathogenesis of selective myocardial cell necrosis. The lesion is induced in animals with various catecholamines: isoproterenol,[13] epinephrine,[7] norepinephrine,[48] methoxamine,[40] and metaraminal.[3] The lesion can be induced by stimulation of the stellate ganglia[25] and by stimulation of specific areas in the midbrain reticular formation with accompanying sympathetic physiologic responses.[17]

Selective myocardial cell necrosis can also be induced in experimental animals by hypokalemia;[12,16] sodium salts and corticoids in combination with hypokalemia; papain; trypsin; streptokinase; plasmocid; magnesium deficiency; cobalt; freezing; and cardiac defibrillation.[36]

Selective myocardial cell necrosis can be induced by hypoxia, low coronary artery perfusion states, or both. Selective myocardial cell necrosis can be seen in the ischemic peripheral zone around a myocardial infarction. Jennings has demonstrated that within 10 to 15 minutes of ischemia in dogs, changes characterized by early swelling can be observed in the mitochondria of the ischemic myocardial cells.[22] With reinstitution of flow, these changes could be returned to normal, that is, the cell injury was reversible. With occlusion of flow for longer than 20 minutes, the reinstitution of arterial blood flow resulted in irreversible cell injury as indicated by tissue swelling, contraction bands, and granular calcium densities in the mitochondria. The concentration of cellular potassium and glycogen fell rapidly. There was a decrease in both extracellular and intracellular pH.[53] These metabolic events occurring within the first few seconds and minutes of ischemia have pathologic effects on the contractility and electrophysiology of the heart.

Mechanism by Which Catecholamines Induce Selective Myocardial Cell Necrosis

Fleckenstein induced selective myocardial cell necrosis in rats by subcutaneous injection of isoproterenol (Isuprel).[13] He showed that there was an increase in radioactive calcium uptake by the injured myocardial tissue, a decrease in adenosine triphosphate (ATP) and creatinine phosphate (CP), and an increase in serum enzyme levels: LDH, SGOT, and lactate-I-isoenzyme. He proposed the hypothesis that catecholamines caused myocardial cell injury by causing an intracellular calcium overload that initiates low ATP levels by excessive activation of calcium-dependent intracellular ATPases and by upcoupling the oxidative phosphorylating capacity of the mitochondria.

PATHOPHYSIOLOGY OF VENTRICULAR FIBRILLATION RELATED TO SUDDEN CARDIAC DEATH

The cause of SCD is usually attributed to VF. There is direct evidence that VF induced in dogs by ischemia, catecholamines, or both, is associated with a decreased threshold to

VF.[23,33] There is also direct evidence that catecholamines, hypoxia, or both cause selective myocardial cell necrosis[41] and that selective myocardial cell necrosis is seen in people who die suddenly.[39] However, it is still controversial whether automaticity, reentrant mechanisms, or both are the electrophysiologic mechanisms of ventricular fibrillation in SCD. Thus, the pathophysiologic mechanisms of SCD are not yet known.

Mechanism by Which Sympathetic Stimulation and Ischemia Induce Ventricular Fibrillation

Schwartz and co-workers have done a series of studies to show that (1) stimulation of the left stellate ganglion decreased the ventricular fibrillation threshold, thus promoting fibrillation; (2) ablation or cooling of the left stallate ganglion increased the ventricular fibrillation threshold; (3) stimulation of the right stellate ganglion increased the ventricular fibrillation threshold; (4) ablation or cooling of the right stellate ganglion decreased the ventricular fibrillation threshold.[42-45] Other researchers also have described the cardiac adrenergic effects on ventricular vulnerability and the production of arrhythmias.[1,18,20,50,54] From their data it appears that stimulation of the left stellate ganglion will promote ventricular fibrillation; however, the stimulation of the right stellate ganglion offers a protective mechanism. If the adrenergic neurogenic effects on the heart become imbalanced, then the heart becomes vulnerable to ventricular fibrillation. It should be noted that there is not necessarily a direct relationship between ventricular fibrillation threshold (VFT) and the spontaneous occurrence of ventricular fibrillation. The VFT is a model that has been seriously challenged as a test for the propensity to spontaneous arrhythmias.

The two ganglia differ in their distribution and effects on the heart. The left stellate innervates predominantly the posteroinferior surface of the left ventricle, whereas the right stellate ganglia innervates the anterior wall.[54] There was a difference of ventricular recovery times between the two areas. The posteroinferior area had a reduced ventricular recovery time. It is significant that acute ischemia, which also reduces ventricular recovery time, resembles the effect of excess sympathetic activity of the left stellate ganglion. Despite the vastly different origin of the short recovery times of two states (ischemia and excess sympathetic activity), the similar electrophysiologic states can result in similar ventricular arrhythmias. Stimulation of the left and right stellate ganglion exert reciprocal effects on the Q-T interval and T waves of the electrocardiogram. Yanowitz and co-workers had shown that stimulation of the left stellate ganglion or removal of the right stellate ganglion in animals increases the magnitude of the T wave and prolongs the Q-T interval.[54] Schwartz and Wolf have reported that the QTc was prolonged in 57% of patients who had SCD (these patients also had had a recent MI).[42]

There is evidence that experimental coronary occlusion affects sympathetic cardiac innervation. Malliani and co-workers reported that transient coronary occlusion increased the firing rate of left stellate preganglionic nerve fibers.[33,34]

Kliks and colleagues have shown that coronary occlusion for two minutes in dogs decreased ventricular fibrillation threshold by 35% of control values.[23] Stimulation of the left stellate ganglion decreased the threshold by 42%. The combination of the two procedures reduced the threshold an average of 63%. After left stellate ganglionectomy, coronary occlusion reduced ventricular fibrillation threshold by only 11% of control values.

Mechanisms of Ventricular Fibrillation

The mechanisms of ventricular fibrillation have not been established. Automaticity and/or reentrant mechanisms could be involved. It has been demonstrated that manipulation of the sympathetic tone and myocardial ischemia influence the incidence and severity of ventricular fibrillation in animals. It is well established that *nonuniform cardiac recovery properties* reduce the threshold for ventricular fibrillation. A variety of states, including ischemia and sympathetic stimulation, increase the degree of inequality of refractory periods in ventricular muscle. Although the mechanism of ventricular fibrillation is not known, probably the degree of inequality of recovery times is related to the duration of the vulnerable period and to the occurrence of excitation propagating in a nonuniform manner so that reentry may occur at varying cardiac locations.

Ventricular arrhythmias that occur within minutes after coronary occlusion depend on the multiple effects of hypoxia, pH changes, anaerobic metabolites, adenosine, potassium, calcium, and catecholamines on the electrical properties of cardiac fibers. An abnormal "slow response" action potential of myocardial cells induced by calcium, potassium, and catecholamines may be one of the causes of ventricular fibrillation in SCD.[53] An increased interstitial potassium concentration may exist because of the leakage of potassium out of the injured myocardial cell. The increased interstitial potassium concentration causes the resting membrane potential to become less negative, inactivating the sodium channels. Thus, no "normal" action potential can be generated. In the presence of a less negative membrane potential caused by high extracellular potassium concentration in addition to an increased concentration of catecholamines, the voltage threshold of the Ca^{2+} channel (that is, about -40 mV) is activated. Hence, the slow inward Ca^{2+} current produces the "slow response" action potential. The slow response action potential is blocked by verapamil and magnesium, which are specific calcium channel blockers. The slow response action potential is slowly propagated and promotes unidirectional block. These characteristics allow reentry to occur in very short conduction path lengths.

Automaticity describes the behavior of cardiac cells that can spontaneously depolarize during diastole and generate action potentials. Normal automaticity can be enhanced in the His–Purkinje system by an increased catecholamine concentration or in tissues adjacent to an ischemic zone.[53]

Environmental stress of diverse types can affect the heart, lower the threshold of vulnerability to ventricular fibrillation, and in animals with coronary occlusion, provoke ventricular fibrillation. Undue anxiety and bereavement appear to increase vulnerability to sudden cardiac death in man.[28]

THERAPEUTIC CARE OF PEOPLE PRONE TO SUDDEN CARDIAC DEATH

The main concepts of therapeutic intervention of people prone to SCD are prediction, prevention, and clinical care after resuscitation.

Predictors of Sudden Cardiac Death

Those persons who are likely to develop SCD are those who have been previously resuscitated from primary ventricular fibrillation. In 1974, Baum and co-workers reported that patients resuscitated from ventricular fibrillation without associated acute myocardial infarction are prone to sudden death, most likely from ventricular fibrillation.[5] They have a high mortality rate: 47% within 2 years after resuscitation. Those who have been resuscitated from ventricular fibrillation secondary to acute myocardial infarction had a mortality rate of 14% after 2 years. In 1977, the mortality rates were lower after SCD.[9] The mortality rate at 1 year was 26% and at 2 years, 36%. People who have had a myocardial infarction also remain at risk for sudden cardiac death.

Bruce and colleagues reported that three variables have high correlations with the risk of sudden death measured during exercise testing.[6] They are the presence of cardiomegaly; exercise duration of less than 3 minutes or failure to attain level II on the Bruce treadmill protocol (see Chap. 18); and exertional hypotension or failure to increase systolic pressure above 130 mm Hg. Depression of the ST segment in the left precordial leads, indicating ischemia, is not a good predictor of sudden cardiac death.

The Framingham studies described the coronary profile of 109 persons who had suffered sudden death.[10] The coronary profile was made up of serum cholesterol concentration, systolic blood pressure, relative body weight, smoking, and electrocardiographic evidence of left ventricular enlargement. There was no combination of these risk factors that significantly separated the persons who died suddenly.

The presence of frequent ventricular ectopic beats as monitored continuously on a Holter monitor is not considered to be a predictor of SCD. Ventricular arrhythmias are present in 85% of the patients with coronary disease.[29] The presence of complicated ventricular ectopic beats (*i.e.*, multifocal or R-on-T phenomenon) probably will prove to be better predictors of SCD.[51]

Prevention of Sudden Cardiac Death

Measures to prevent sudden cardiac death can be divided into several general areas:

1. Prompt and effective cardiac resuscitation from ventricular fibrillation through community emergency medical aid units and through education of lay persons in cardiopulmonary resuscitation (CPR) techniques (Chaps. 23 and 26)
2. Long-term prophylactic antiarrhythmic drugs and beta-adrenergic blocking drugs (Chaps. 34 and 35)
3. Continuous 24-hour electrocardiographic monitoring for complicated ventricular arrhythmias (Chap. 26)
4. Coronary bypass surgery (Chaps. 24 and 25)
5. Left stellate ganglionectomy
6. Psychologic stress reduction techniques (Chaps. 22 and 43)
7. Aneurysm removal (Chap. 29)
8. Valve surgery (Chap. 48)
9. Electrophysiologic studies to assess the adequacy of antiarrhythmic therapy (Chap. 26)
10. Other studies to identify high-risk patients, including exercise testing (Chap. 18), radionuclide scanning (Chap. 20), cardiac catheterization (Chap. 19), and echocardiography (Chap. 20)

At present, there are no drugs that have proved long-term prophylactic ability for the prevention of sudden death.[28] Some of the drugs being tested with varying degrees of success are aprindine;[14] quinidine; procainamide; methyl lidocaine;[31] bretylium;[31] verapamil;[14] propanolol; alprenolol;[27] dimethyl propranolol;[31] and disopyramide.

Reports on results of coronary bypass surgery appear to indicate that the procedure can reduce the incidence of sudden cardiac death. The medical and surgical sample groups in Hammermeister's study were not randomized;[19] however, the sudden death rates for subgroups of medically treated patients were 1.8 to 10.9 times higher than the rates for subgroups of surgically treated patients with a comparable extent of coronary disease and ejection fraction.

Research for the prevention of sudden cardiac death using sympathectomy or left stellate ganglionectomy has been usually confined to animals, although Schwartz has been applying this technique to patients.[28,42-45] In humans, sympathetic blockade has been achieved by beta-adrenergic blocking agents such as propanolol, alprenolol,[27] and dimethyl propranolol.[31]

Clinical Care

The clinical care for the patient who has been resuscitated from primary ventricular fibrillation is much the same as that for the patient who has had an acute myocardial infarction, except that there is a higher incidence of anoxic encephalopathy in the former group. The reader is referred to Part II, Sections C and D for further discussion of the nursing interventions and evaluation of the clinical course of patients with myocardial infarction and to Section E for pharmacologic treatment of arrhythmias.

The role of prompt CPR, bystander-initiated CPR, and early defibrillation cannot be minimized. For techniques that have been used to improve CPR and to prevent anoxic encephalopathy and for other general supportive measures of the patient who has been resuscitated, refer to Chapters 23 and 26.

REFERENCES

1. Armour JA, Hageman GR, Randall WC: Arrhythmias induced by local cardiac nerve stimulation. Am J Physiol 223:1068–1075, 1972
2. Bainton CR, Peterson DR: Deaths from coronary heart disease

in persons fifty years of age and younger. N Engl J Med 268:569–575, 1963

3. Bajusz E, Jasmin G: Influence of variations in electrolyte intake upon the development of cardiac necrosis produced by vasopressor amines. Lab Invest 13:757–766, 1964

4. Baroldi G: Acute coronary occlusion as a cause of myocardial infarct and sudden coronary heart death. Am J Cardiol 16:859–880, 1965

5. Baum R, Alvarez H, Cobb L: Survival after resuscitation from out-of-hospital ventricular fibrillation. Circulation 50:1213–1235, 1974

6. Bruce R, DeRouen T, Peterson D et al: Non-invasive predictors of sudden cardiac death in men with coronary artery disease. Am J Cardiol 39:833–840, 1977

7. Chappel C, Rona G, Balazs T et al: Comparison of cardiotoxic actions of certain sympathomimetic amines. Can J Biochem 37:35–42, 1959

8. Cobb L, Baum R, Alvarez H et al: Resuscitation from out-of-hospital ventricular fibrillation: 4 years follow-up. Circulation (Suppl III)51 and 52:223–228, 1975

9. Cobb L, Hallstrom AP et al: Clinical predictors and characteristics of the sudden cardiac death syndrome. Proceedings USA–USSR First Joint Symposium on Sudden Death, DHEW Publication No. (NIH) 78-1470, 1977

10. Doyle J, Kannel W, McNamara P et al: Factors related to suddenness of death from coronary disease: Combined Albany–Framingham Studies. Am J Cardiol 37:1073–1078, 1976

11. Düreen DR, Becker AE: Focal myocytolysis mimicking the electrocardiographic pattern of transmural anteroseptal myocardial infarction. Chest 69:506–511, 1976

12. Emberson JW, Nuir AR: Changes in the ultrastructure of rat myocardium induced by hypokalemia. Q J Exp Physiol 54:36–40, 1969

13. Fleckenstein A, Janke J, Doring H et al: Myocardial fiber necrosis due to intracellular calcium overload: A new principle in cardiac pathophysiology. Recent Adv Stud Cardiac Struct Metabol 4:563–680, 1973

14. Foster P, King R, de B Nicholl A et al: Suppression of ouabain induced ventricular rhythms with aprindine HCl: A comparison with other antiarrhythmic agents. Circulation 53:315–321, 1976

15. Freidman M, Manwaring J, Rosenmann R et al: Instantaneous and sudden deaths: Clinical and pathological differentiation in coronary artery disease. JAMA 255:1319–1328, 1973

16. French J: A histological study of the heart lesion in potassium-deficient rats. AMA Arch Pathol 53:485–496, 1952

17. Greenhoot J, Reichenbach D: Cardiac injury and subarachnoid hemorrhage. J Neurosurg 30:521–531, 1969

18. Hageman G, Goldbert J, Armour J et al: Cardiac dysrhythmias induced by autonomic nerve stimulation. Am J Cardiol 32:823–830, 1973

19. Hammermeister K, De Rouen T, Murray J et al: Effect of aortocoronary saphenous vein bypass grafting on death and sudden death. Am J Cardiol 39:925–934, 1977

20. Han J, De Jalon P, Moe G: Adrenergic effects on ventricular vulnerability. Circ Res 14:516–524, 1964

21. Haynes RE, Hallstrom AP, Cobb LA: Repolarization abnormalities in survivors of out-of-hospital ventricular fibrillation. Circulation 57:654–658, 1978

22. Jennings R: Early changes of myocardial ischemic injury and infarction. Am J Cardiol 24:753–765, 1969

23. Kliks B, Burgess M, Abildskov JA: Influence of sympathetic tone of ventricular fibrillation threshold during experimental coronary occlusion. Am J Cardiol 36:45–49, 1975

24. Kline I: Myocardial alterations associated with pheochromocytomas. Am J Pathol 38:539–551, 1961

25. Klouda M, Brynjolfsson G: Cardiotoxic effects of electrical stimulation of the stellate ganglia. Ann NY Acad Sci 156:271–280, 1969

26. Kuller L, Lilienfeld A, Fisher R: Epidemiological study of sudden and unexpected deaths due to atherosclerotic heart disease. Circulation 34:1056–1068, 1966

27. Lowell R: Arrhythmias prophylaxis: Long-term suppressive medication. Circulation (Suppl III)51 and 52:236–240, 1975

28. Lown B, Verrier R, Rabinowitz S: Neural and psychological mechanisms and the problem of sudden cardiac death. Am J Cardiol 39:890–902, 1977

29. Lown B, Calvert A, Armington R et al: Monitoring for serious arrhythmias and high risk of death. Circulation (Suppl III)51 and 52:189–210, 1975

30. Lown R, Wolf M: Approaches to sudden death from coronary heart disease. Circulation 44:130, 1971

31. Lucchesi B, Kniffen F: Pharmacological modification of arrhythmias after experimentally induced acute myocardial infarction. Circulation (Suppl III)51 and 52:247, 1975

32. Monthly Vital Statistics Report. DHEW Publication (PHS) 80-1120, Vol 28, No. 9. Washington DC, U.S. Government Printing Office, 1979

33. Malliani A, Recordati G, Schwartz PJ: Nervous activity of afferent cardiac sympathetic fibers with atrial and ventricular endings. J Physiol 229:457–469, 1973

34. Malliani A, Schwartz P, Zanchetti A: A sympathetic reflex elicited by experimental coronary occlusion. Am J Physiol 217:703–709, 1969

35. McNally RH, Pemberton J: Duration of last attack in 998 fatal cases of coronary artery disease and its relation to possible cardiac resuscitation. Br Med J 3:129–142, 1968

36. Reichenbach D, Benditt EP: Catecholamines and cardiomyopathy: The pathogenesis and potential importance of myofibrillar degeneration. Hum Pathol 1:125–150, 1970

37. Reichenbach D, Moss N: Myocardial cell necrosis and sudden death in humans. Circulation (Suppl III)51 and 52:60–62, 1975

38. Reichenbach D, Moss N, Meyer E: Pathology of the heart in sudden cardiac death. Am J Cardiol 39:865–872, 1977

39. Roberts W, Buja M: The frequency and significance of coronary arterial thrombi and other observations in fatal acute myocardial infarction. Am J Med 52:425–443, 1972

40. Rosenblum I, Wohl A, Stein A: Studies of cardiac necrosis: Production of cardiac lesions with sympathomimetic amines. Toxicol Appl Pharmacol 7:1–8, 1965

41. Schroeder J, Lamb I, Harrison D: Patients admitted to the coronary care unit for chest pain: High risk subgroup for subsequent cardiovascular death. Am J Cardiol 39:829–832, 1977

42. Schwartz P, Wolf S: QT interval prolongation as predictor of sudden death in patients with myocardial infarction. Circulation 57:1074–1077, 1978

43. Schwartz P, Snebold M, Brown A: Effects of unilateral cardiac sympathetic denervation on the ventricular fibrillation threshold. Am J Cardiol 37:1034–1040, 1976

44. Schwartz P, Malliani A: Electrical alternation of the T wave: Clinical and experimental evidence of its relationship with the sympathetic nervous system and with the long Q-T syndrome. Am Heart J 89:45–50, 1975

45. Schwartz P, Periti M, Malliani A: The long Q-T syndrome. Am Heart J 89:378–390, 1975

46. Spain D, Bradess V: The relationship of coronary thrombosis to coronary atherosclerotic and ischemic heart disease (A necropsy study covering a period of 25 years). Am J Med Sci 240:701–710, 1960

47. Spiekerman RE, Brandenberg JT, Achor RWP et al: The spectrum of coronary heart disease in a community of 30,000: A clinicpathologic study. Circulation 25:57–65, 1962

48. Szakacs J, Mehlman B: Pathologic changes induced by L-norepinephrine: Quantitative aspects. Am J Cardiol 5:619–627, 1960

49. Vasudevan G, Mercer D, Varat M: Lactic dehydrogenase isoenzyme determination in the diagnosis of acute myocardial infarction. Circulation 57:1055–1057, 1978

50. Verrier R, Thompson P, Lown B: Ventricular vulnerability during sympathetic stimulation: Role of heart rate and blood pressure. Cardiovasc Res 8:602–610, 1974

51. Vismara L, Zakauddin V, Foerster J et al: Identification of sudden death risk factors in acute and chronic coronary artery disease. Am J Cardiol 39:821–828, 1977

52. WHO Scientific Group: The pathological diagnosis of acute ischemic heart disease. WHO Tech Rep Ser 441:5–27, 1970

53. Wit A, Bigger JT: Possible electrophysiological mechanisms for lethal arrhythmias accompanying myocardial ischemia and infarction. Circulation (Suppl III)51 and 52:96–115, 1975

54. Yanowitz F, Preston J, Abildskov JA: Functional distribution of right and left stellate innervation to the ventricles. Circ Res 18:416–428, 1966

ADDITIONAL READING

Cobb LA, Werner JA, Trobaugh GB: Sudden cardiac death, Parts 1 and 2. Mod Concepts Cardiovasc Dis 49:31–42, 1980

Cowan M: Sudden cardiac death and selective myocardial cell necrosis. Heart Lung 8:559–563, 1979

13

Coronary Artery Disease Risk Factors

SANDRA L. UNDERHILL, R.N., M.N.

The presence of coronary artery disease (CAD) is associated with one or more characteristic findings that are known as risk factors. Risk factors have been determined on the basis of systematic observations of relationships between certain characteristics and the subsequent development of CAD. Current research is finding physiologic explanations for these relationships.

Effective patient teaching requires a knowledge base for recognizing the risk factors, criteria for evaluating their importance, and interpretation of data from studies that identify risk factors. However, there is not complete agreement about the importance of modifying risk factors in patients with known CAD nor whether it is effective.

Risk factors can be classified in a number of ways. For the purposes of both patient and professional education, we use here the categories of unavoidable risk factors, atherogenic personal attributes (for some people these are also unavoidable), life-style habits, signs of preclinical cardiovascular disorders, and questionable risk factors.[14,78]

EPIDEMIOLOGY

Risk factors are determined by interpretation of data from epidemiologic studies, which have shown that an epidemic of CAD exists in the United States and other Western industrialized countries. Over 600,000 deaths occur from CAD each year in the United States, representing one-third of all deaths. Approximately one million persons a year experience myocardial infarction (MI) or sudden cardiac death (SCD),[132] but in recent years the death rates from coronary and cerebral vascular disease, hypertension, rheumatic fever, and rheumatic heart disease have been declining. For unknown reasons, from 1969 to 1977, the death rate from cardiovascular diseases per 100,000 population dropped 19% among white males and 24% among white females.[135] This trend is unique to the United States, occurs in all age groups and in both sexes, and is accompanied by a decline in deaths from all causes.

Scientists are currently speculating about what is happening in the United States to account for these changes, especially in regard to possible contributions made by modifying the risk factors. At the recent Conference on the Decline in Coronary Heart Disease Mortality, it was decided that the decrease in CAD mortality is real, that contributions from primary risk-factor modification and from fundamental and clinical research have contributed to the decline but do not fully explain the decrease, and that further research regarding its decline is needed. Risk-factor reduction could be responsible if the number of all MIs is decreasing or if the severity of the clinical illness is lessening. Fundamental and clinical research resulting in better patient care could be the cause of the decline if the incidence of total CAD is unchanged.[59] It is interesting to note that CAD-related deaths began to decline in 1964, the year that the U.S. Surgeon General first warned of the hazards of cigarette smoking and that the American Heart Association first recommended dietary reductions of saturated fats and cholesterol.[153]

Etiologic Criteria

Before a risk factor can be implicated in causing CAD it must meet several criteria. First, the habit, trait, or finding must be consistently associated with CAD independently of other factors. Second, these factors must be present prior to the occurrence of CAD. Third, they should have disease predictability. Last, epidemiologic data must be consistent with the findings of other research and have plausible pathogenic pathways.[130-131] All of these criteria have been met for the three major risk factors of CAD: elevated serum cholesterol, elevated blood pressure, and cigarette smoking.

Geographic Distribution

Industrialized European countries and the United States have the highest incidence of CAD in the world (Fig. 13-1). Only Finland has a death rate from CAD higher than that of the United States. Because most American families have a European heritage, the explanation is not a difference in ethnic background. It has been noted that in countries with a fast-rising standard of living, the incidence of heart disease rapidly increases.[35] This might be explained by the changes in diet and life-style that are usually associated with more affluent communities.

Framingham Study

One of the most important prospective studies of CAD risk factors was initiated in Framingham, Massachusetts in 1948. It continues to the present with a study group of 5209

men and women. This study has provided a major source of data for assessing CAD risk factors. Its purpose was to study factors associated with development of atherosclerosis and hypertensive cardiovascular disease during long-term surveillance of a sample of Framingham's adult population.[4] Volunteer subjects aged 30 to 59 years living in the Framingham area were selected and given periodic clinical examinations. As a result of this study, seven characteristics that affect development of cardiovascular disease have been determined: age, sex, elevated serum cholesterol, elevated blood pressure (BP), cigarette smoking, left ventricular hypertrophy (LVH) by electrocardiogram (ECG), and the presence of glucose intolerance. In order to base study results on a very large population, data from this study[57,123] were combined with data from seven other longitudinal studies [25, 26, 36, 37, 42, 86, 108, 128, 143] to form the national cooperative Pooling Project.[112]

UNAVOIDABLE RISK FACTORS

Unavoidable risk factors include age, sex, family history of CAD, and ethnic background. Current research indicates, however, that unavoidable risk factors are often influenced by those that can be avoided and thereby become modified to some degree.

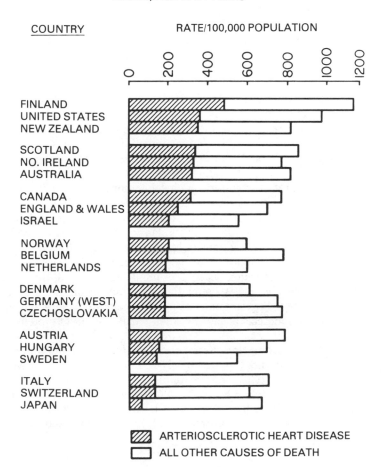

MALES, AGE 45-54 YEARS

ARTERIOSCLEROTIC HEART DISEASE
ALL OTHER CAUSES OF DEATH

Fig. 13-1. Rates of mortality from arteriosclerotic heart disease and all other causes of death in 21 countries, 1967, in males aged 45 to 54 years. (DiGirolama M, Schlant RC: p 1104. In *The Heart*, 4th ed, Hurst JW, Logue RB, Schlant RC et al (eds). New York, McGraw-Hill, 1978). Reproduced, with permission, from the Annual Review of Pharmacology, Volume 12, ©1972 by Annual Reviews Inc.)

TABLE 13-1 INCIDENCE OF CARDIOVASCULAR DISEASE* IN WOMEN†

Age at Examination	Menopausal Status	Incidence per 1000 per Year
Less than 40 years	Premenopausal	0.6
	Postmenopausal	2.2
40 to 44 years	Premenopausal	0.6
	Postmenopausal	3.6
45 to 49 years	Premenopausal	2.0
	Postmenopausal	4.0
50 to 55 years	Premenopausal	3.6
	Postmenopausal	6.5

* CAD, stroke, CHF, or intermittent claudication
† (Adapted from Kannel WB, Hjortland MC, McNamara PM et al: Menopause and risk of cardiovascular disease. The Framingham Study. Ann Intern Med 85:447–452, 1976)

Age and Sex

Increasing age is associated with an increasing incidence of CAD. In men, the occurrence of CAD increases steadily with age, but in women its incidence increases sharply after menopause. For unknown reasons, CAD in postmenopausal women still remains less than for men. Premenopausal women in the Framingham study developed cardiovascular disease at less than one-half the rate of men. Women in that study had a 10% probability of having a cardiovascular event before age 60, as compared with a 27% probability for men.[80] The incidence of cardiovascular disease in women is shown in Table 13-1.

Family History

A positive family history, or a history of CAD among blood-related family members, is important in predicting the occurrence and prognosis of CAD. Individuals have a greater chance of developing CAD at a young age if parents or siblings developed the disease before age 50.[35] Early parental death from CAD is associated with fatal CAD in men aged 40 to 59.[34]

Ethnic Background

Ethnic background may contribute to some risk factor development. For example, hypertension is more prevalent in black men than in white men (see Chap. 47). However, ethnicity, in a broader sense, implies life-style as well as ethnic origin. Japanese men living in Japan have a lower incidence of CAD than Japanese-American men living in Hawaii or California.[113] Although ethnic origin is not modifiable, the life-styles associated with particular cultures can be altered.

ATHEROGENIC PERSONAL ATTRIBUTES

Atherogenic personal attributes include elevated serum lipids and lipoproteins, elevated BP, and glucose intolerance. Lipid disorders are described in greater detail because they are not presented elsewhere in this text.

Elevated Serum Lipids and Lipoproteins

Lipids are naturally occurring organic substances that include triglycerides (neutral fats), phospholipids, and plant and animal sterols. Fatty acids are the building blocks of triglycerides and phospholipids. Triglycerides contain three fatty acids bound to glycerol and are usually composed of at least two different fatty acids. They may be saturated (no double bonds) or unsaturated (various numbers of double bonds). Phospholipids consist of two fatty acids bound to glycerol. These are found almost entirely in cell membranes and are usually bound with protein. This combination is known as a lipoprotein. Cholesterol is a sterol found in animal tissue.[19]

Serum lipids are derived from the breakdown and synthesis of fats and carbohydrates from exogenous and endogenous sources. Although there does not appear to be a chemical relationship between fats and carbohydrates, they are related by a complex series of enzyme-catalyzed reactions that allow glucose to be converted to glycerol and palmitic acid, a fatty acid.[19] To be absorbed, fats must first be broken down into free fatty acids (FFA) and monoglycerides.

Lipids synthesized by the liver that circulate in the blood as part of lipoprotein complexes are triglycerides, cholesterol (both free and esterified with fatty acids), and phospholipids. These are bound to the plasma proteins albumin, alpha (α)-globulin, and beta (β)-globulin. Chylomicrons also circulate in the blood, but, because they are composed of 90% triglyceride with only a small amount of protein, they are generally considered separately from the complexes. Chylomicrons, formed in the small intestine from long-chain fatty acids, are absorbed into the lymphatic system and travel to the peripheral circulation. The milky appearance of plasma after meals (lipemia) is due to the presence of large numbers of chylomicrons.

Classification of Lipoproteins. Classification of the lipoprotein complexes is based on their various densities and mobilities as determined by lipoprotein electrophoresis (Fig. 13-2) (see Chap. 15).[50] Lipoprotein density varies with the proportion of fat to protein. The larger the particle size, the greater is the ratio of fat to protein, and the lower the density. The fat-to-protein ratio of chylomicrons is 99:1, whereas for high-density lipoprotein (HDL) cholesterol, it is 1:1.[13] Serum cholesterol is highest in the low-density lipoprotein (LDL) fraction, and serum triglyceride is greatest in chylomicrons and the very low density lipoprotein (VLDL) fraction. The mobilities demonstrated by lipoproteins during electrophoresis are classified as α, β, or pre-β, with α being the most mobile and pre-β being the least mobile of the moving particles. Chylomicrons do not demonstrate mobility during electrophoresis because of their small amount of protein.

Fat Consumption. Estimates of the fat consumption in the American diet (approximately 2500 calories daily, but with great variability) range from 65 to 160 grams* per day. Approximately 39% of the total calories are thought to be derived from fat. Of the total fat intake, 42% is saturated, 41% is monounsaturated, and 16% is polyunsaturated.[45]

---

*One gram of fat yields nine calories.

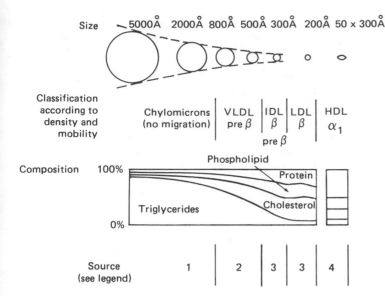

Size 5000Å 2000Å 800Å 500Å 300Å 200Å 50 x 300Å

Classification according to density and mobility

Chylomicrons (no migration) | VLDL pre β | IDL β | LDL β | HDL α₁

pre β

Composition 100%

Phospholipid
Protein
Triglycerides
Cholesterol

0%

Source (see legend) 1 | 2 | 3 | 3 | 4

Fig. 13-2. Classification of plasma lipoproteins by physical and chemical properties. Size is shown in angstrom (Å) Units. The larger the particle size, the greater is the ratio of fat to protein, and the lower the density. Mobility of lipoprotein electrophoresis ranges from α, the most mobile, to pre-β, the least mobile. Chylomicrons do not migrate. *VLDL* = very low density lipoprotein (predominantly triglyceride), *IDL* = intermediate-density lipoprotein, *LDL* = low-density lipoprotein (predominantly cholesterol), and *HDL* = high-density lipoprotein. Sources: *1.* dietary *2.* liver synthesis from carbohydrates and endogenous triglycerides, *3.* by-products of VLDL catabolism, *4.* the protein remaining after VLDL catabolism. (Adapted from Bierman EL: Hyperlipoproteinemia p. 4. Current Concepts, Kalamazoo, Upjohn, 1976)

Contributions to total caloric intake would, therefore, be 16% to 17% each for saturated and monounsaturated fats, and 6% for polyunsaturated fats. Figure 13-3 shows the percentage of fatty acid composition of some commonly used dietary fats.

Saturated Fats. Saturated fatty acids (SFA) have no double bonds because they have been saturated by hydrogen. They can occur naturally or may be produced by hydrogenation of monounsaturated or polyunsaturated fats. Hydrogenation affects the hardness, spreadability, melting point, and shelf-life of fats and oils. Hydrogenation is used commercially to manufacture solid shortenings and produce margarines that imitate many of the characteristics of butter.

Fig. 13-3. Fatty acids in some representative food fats. Most marine oils, like menhaden oil, have a high content of compounds with 3–6 double bonds. Most seed oils sold in the United States have compositions similar to that of corn oil. However, some are highly saturated; coconut oil, shown here, is the most highly saturated. Seed-coat fats, of which olive oil is an example, contain less PUFA than do the common commercial seed oils. Other poultry fats resemble chicken fat in composition, and fats of most red meats resemble beef fat. (Adapted from Dayton S: In Feldman EB (ed): Nutrition and Cardiovascular Disease, p. 61. New York, Appleton-Century Crofts, 1976)

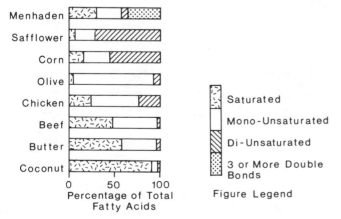

Menhaden
Safflower
Corn
Olive
Chicken
Beef
Butter
Coconut

0 50 100
Percentage of Total Fatty Acids

Saturated
Mono-Unsaturated
Di-Unsaturated
3 or More Double Bonds

Figure Legend

In a study of CAD in seven countries it was shown that SFA intake was strongly correlated to serum cholesterol levels ($r = 0.89$). In this same study, the correlation of development of CAD and percentage of SFA in the diet was also high ($r = 0.84$). The correlation between development of CAD and the percentage of total fat in the diet was not as great ($r = 0.38$).[83]

Polyunsaturated Fats. Polyunsaturated fatty acids (PUFA) contain two or more double bonds. Because of their molecular structure, close molecular packing is prevented so that they remain liquid at room temperature. Large amounts of PUFA are found in vegetable-seed oils, such as corn, sunflower, and safflower, and in fish oils, which are even more unsaturated than the seed oils. (The oils of seed coats, such as olive oil, are monounsaturated or contain only one double bond.) The notable exceptions to predominantly PUFA-containing vegetable-seed oil are coconut oil, palm oil, and palm-kernel oil; these are the primary vegetable oils contained in most nondairy creamers. They are the most highly saturated of the dietary fats, including natural cream. Some PUFA lower serum cholesterol levels and are termed physiologically active PUFA (PAPUFA). The reasons for the serum cholesterol-lowering effects of PAPUFA are unclear and controversial.[67] As documented in Table 13-2, the PAPUFA content of margarine is extremely variable, depending on the oil base used and the degree of hydrogenation. When choosing oils and margarines, select those highest in PAPUFA to receive the greatest serum cholesterol-lowering effect.

All PUFA are prone to oxidation at their double bonds. This causes formation of lipid peroxides that taste rancid and are toxic when ingested. Vitamin E protects PUFA from oxidation and, fortunately, is found in many PUFA-rich oils, such as corn oil and soybean oil. The vitamin E content in safflower oil is adequate but is not as bioavailable as in other oils.[12] A high-PUFA diet leads to development of larger PUFA stores and consequently to a larger vitamin E requirement.[32,63]

TABLE 13-2 OIL AND PAPUFA* CONTENT OF MARGARINES

Margarines	Oil	% PAPUFA
Regular		
Land O Lakes	Soybean	10
Promise	Sunflower	45
Fleishmann's Corn Oil	Corn	35
Imperial	Soybean, palm, sunflower, corn, cotton-seed	33
Parkay	Soybean	19
Saffola	Safflower	42
Mazola	Corn	36
Blue Bonnet	Soybean	32
Nucoa	Soybean	33
Soft		
Soft Parkay	Soybean	38
Soft Fleishmann's	Corn	44
Soft Parkay Corn Oil	Corn	44
Mrs. Filbert's 100% Corn Oil	Corn	44
Soft Imperial	Soybean, palm, sunflower, corn, cotton-seed	36
Soft Chiffon	Soybean	44
Promise	Sunflower, soy-bean, cotton-seed	51
Squeeze Parkay	Soybean, cotton-seed	45

* PAPUFA = physiologically active polyunsaturated fatty acids

(Adapted from Margarine—The Better Butter? Consumer Reports 44(2):66–72, 1979)

Serum Cholesterol. It has been firmly established that an elevated serum cholesterol level greatly increases the risk of CAD development.[75,83] The correlation between serum cholesterol level and the 5-year incidence of CAD development in the Seven Countries Study was high ($r = 0.76$).[83] The level of serum cholesterol is raised by diets high in cholesterol and SFA.[83] However, because cholesterogenesis is generally unaffected by diet (producing 500 to 1000 mg of cholesterol daily in the liver and small intestine), controversy over the contribution of a diet high in cholesterol and SFA to the development of CAD still exists.[151]

In the United States, serum cholesterol levels are low at birth (64 mg/dl), rise to 180 to 200 mg/dl by age 30, increase by approximately 2 mg/dl per year from age 20 to 45, and peak by age 50.[149] These data are also supported by the Lipid Research Clinics Program Prevalence Study.[61] In societies whose members tend not to gain weight with age, the trend of rising serum lipids with age is absent or less pronounced. Serum cholesterol levels are different in men and women.[149] Table 13-3 lists mean plasma* cholesterol levels in the United States by age and sex. Although such values may not be optimal, "norms" have been established for various countries, based on the average level of serum cholesterol for each population. In general, serum cholesterol levels are lowest among vegetarian populations and highest where

* Values for serum cholesterol average about 3% higher than values for plasma cholesterol.[90]

large amounts of animal fats are consumed regularly. Norms in Japan and Greece are among the lowest, whereas norms in Finland, the United States and the Netherlands are among the highest.[83] The Framingham data have shown that a man with a serum cholesterol level of more than 259 mg/dl is three times more likely to develop CAD than one whose serum cholesterol is less than 200 mg/dl.[75] In an attempt to define what the ideal serum cholesterol level should be, a questionnaire was sent to investigators in the United States and other countries. The averages from 35 replies were 146 mg/dl, 174 mg/dl, and 185 mg/dl for males aged 10, 30, and 50, respectively.[161] Blackburn suggests that the ideal mean serum cholesterol level in adults should be even lower: 160 mg/dl.[14]

Serum Triglyceride. Refined carbohydrates, especially sucrose, have the greatest influence over the level of serum triglyceride. Serum triglyceride is elevated by diets high in refined carbohydrates and SFA, lowered by PUFA, and unaffected by monounsaturated fats. Repeated daily alcohol consumption also raises serum triglyceride,[9,24] as does stress.

Serum triglyceride levels also vary by age and sex (Table 13-3).[149] Experts have defined the ideal fasting serum triglyceride levels as 87, 100, and 100 mg/dl for both sexes at ages 10, 30, and 50, respectively.[159] In both men and younger women (under age 50), serum triglyceride alone does not correlate to the risk of CAD development, but appears to be implicated only when serum cholesterol is also elevated.[56] However, in women over age 50, serum triglyceride is superior to serum cholesterol in predicting risk from CAD,[77] perhaps because elevated serum triglyceride is highly correlated to a low serum HDL level.[56,58]

TABLE 13-3 MEAN PLASMA CHOLESTEROL AND TRIGLYCERIDE IN THE UNITED STATES POPULATION IN RELATION TO AGE, SEX, AND SEX HORMONE THERAPY

Sex	Age	Cholesterol (mg/dl)	Triglyceride (mg/dl)
White men	15–19	150	78
	35–39	201	145
	40–44	206	151
	45–49	212	152
	50–54	213	152
	55–59	214	141
	60–64	213	142
	65–69	213	137
White women not taking sex hormones	15–19	157	72
	35–39	184	86
	40–44	193	98
	45–49	202	104
	50–54	218	115
	55–59	230	125
	60–64	231	127
	65–69	233	131
White women taking sex hormones	15–19	169	106
	35–39	194	126
	40–44	199	129
	45–49	209	130
	50–54	218	130
	55–59	218	126
	60–64	224	126
	65–69	222	130

(Adapted from Tyroler HA, Anderson P, Barrett-Connor E et al: Plasma lipid distribution in selected North American populations: The Lipid Research Clinics Program Prevalence Study. Circulation 6(2):302–315, 1980)

TABLE 13-4 HYPERLIPOPROTEINEMIAS

Type	Lipid Abnormality	Causes	CAD Risk	Prevalence	Signs and Symptoms	Treatment
I	↑ Chylomicrons	Chylomicrons not removed by enzymes	Low	Rare	Abdominal pain, eruptive xanthomata, lipemia retinalis, hepatosplenomegaly	Low SFA diet
II	a ↑ Cholesterol b ↑ Cholesterol ↑ Triglyceride	Excess production or inadequate clearance of LDL	Very high	Common	Accelerated atherosclerosis, xanthelasma, tendinous and tuberous xanthomata, corneal arcus	Low SFA diet; for homozygous: drugs and partial ileal bypass surgery; for heterozygous: drugs may be indicated
III	↑ Cholesterol ↑ Triglyceride	Block in metabolism of VLDL and LDL, causing an abnormal "intermediate form" of lipoprotein to circulate	Very high	Infrequent	Palmar and tuberoeruptive xanthomata	Low SFA and calorie diet; drugs
IV	↑ Triglyceride ↑ Cholesterol (slightly)	Excess production or inadequate clearance of VLDL	High	Very common	Obesity, CAD, occasional abdominal pain	Low calorie and carbohydrate diet; restrict alcohol intake; weight reduction
V	↑ Chylomicrons ↑ Triglyceries	VLDL excess combined with poor removal of chylomicrons	Low	Rare	Obesity, abdominal pain, eruptive xanthomata, lipemia retinalis, hepatosplenomegaly	Low SFA diet, weight reduction, followed by drugs

(Adapted from Schlant RC, DiGirolama M: Modification of risk factors in the prevention and management of coronary atherosclerotic heart disease. In Hurst JW, Logue RB, Schlant RC et al (eds): The Heart, 4th ed, pp 1311–1344. Copyright © 1978. Used with the permission of McGraw-Hill Book Company, New York; Schatz IJ: Classification of primary hyperlipidemia—Observations on 214 patients. JAMA 210(4):701–704, 1969)

HDL Cholesterol. High concentrations of HDL in the serum seem to have a protective effect against development of atherosclerosis.[75,101] Women have higher HDL concentrations than men. Of all the lipid risk factors, low serum concentrations of HDL have the highest correlation to high LDL and to CAD risk. Persons with HDL concentrations below 35 mg/dl have eight times the incidence of CAD of those with HDL concentrations of 65 mg/dl. Some studies have shown a positive correlation between alcohol intake and serum HDL levels,[24,160] whereas others have not.[58] Dietary habits do not affect HDL levels.[58] Physical activity increases serum HDL.[92,158] In a recent study of men with three different patterns of physical exercise, serum HDL levels varied with the amount of physical activity (marathon runners, 65 mg/dl; joggers, 58 mg/dl; inactive men, 43 mg/dl).[58] Levels of HDL are also associated with body weight; the higher the weight, the lower is the HDL level.[58,92]

Hyperlipidemia and Hyperlipoproteinemia. Hyperlipidemia (elevated serum cholesteral and triglyceride) and hyperlipoproteinemia (elevated serum lipoproteins, as diagnosed by lipoprotein electrophoresis) may be familial or induced by factors such as diet, alcohol intake, stress, drugs, and certain endocrine abnormalities.[121] Table 13-4 summarizes the hyperlipoproteinemias. For familial hyperlipoproteinemias, the term homozygous implies that the disease was transmitted by both parents, and the term heterozygous implies that the disease was transmitted by only one parent. The development of CAD is associated with types IIa, IIb, III, and IV. Treatment of hyperlipoproteinemia is by diet, weight reduction, drug therapy (see Chap. 39), and partial ileal bypass surgery (see Chap. 22). Any underlying cause, such as diabetes mellitus, must also be treated. Homozygous

hyperlipoproteinemias are very severe and are refractory to most therapies.

Recommendations. Primary prevention of the development of CAD could greatly improve morbidity and mortality rates in the United States. Genetic counseling for those with known familial hyperlipoproteinemias is advised. On the basis of both animal and epidemiologic studies, recommendations to reduce total consumption of fat and cholesterol and to substitute PUFA for SFA in the diet have been made by the American Heart Association,[65] the American Health Foundation, the Food and Nutrition Board of the National Research Council, and the American Medical Association.[3] Table 13-5 lists some specific recommendations for changing dietary habits.

Elevated Blood Pressure

Elevated systolic and diastolic BP is a major contributor to the development of cardiovascular disease, particularly stroke and congestive heart failure (CHF).[17,75,79,83,112] Chapter 47 contains a complete discussion of hypertension and the nurse's role in its control. Drugs used in the management of hypertension are presented in Chapter 37.

Glucose Intolerance

Glucose intolerance* is evidence of diabetes mellitus, which is known to occur in people who also develop atherosclerotic disease.[41,114,139] In the Framingham study, those who devel-

---

* Glucose intolerance is demonstrated by a fasting blood glucose level above 130 mg/dl or by an abnormal response to a glucose tolerance test, with blood glucose levels at one hour, two hours, or three hours, higher than 195, 140, or 130 mg/dl, respectively.[121]

TABLE 13-5 SPECIFIC DIETARY RECOMMENDATIONS FOR PREVENTION OF CORONARY ARTERY DISEASE

Do

Maintain ideal body weight

Eat moderate portions

Use lean meat, poultry, fish

Cook by methods that reduce SFA content (broiling, roasting, braising in liquid)

Skim off fat during cooking

Use salad and cooking oils and margarine high in PUFA (in conjunction with adequate vitamin E in diet)

Use fat-modified (made with reduced SFA and cholesterol) processed meat products, dairy products, baked goods

Use grains, fruits, vegetables, legumes

Season with lemon, wine, vinegar, spices, herbs rather than butter

Prepare salad dressings with vinegar, tomato juice, fruit juice

Restrict commercial baked goods to bread

Restrict intake of refined carbohydrates

Do Not:

Do not add SFA when cooking

Do not use dairy products high in SFA (butter, whole milk, whole milk cheese)

Do not use margarines or shortening high in SFA

Do not use egg yolks, nuts, bacon, lard, suet

Do not use baked goods and candies high in SFA and cholesterol

Do not use nondairy products made with coconut oil

(Data from Feldman EB: Saturated fats. In Feldman EB (ed): Nutrition and Cardiovascular Disease, pp 30–58. New York, Appleton-Century-Crofts, 1976; Inter-Society Commission for Heart Disease Resources: Report of primary prevention of atherosclerotic diseases. Circulation 42:A55–A95, 1970; Symposium: Status of fat in food and nutrition. J Am Oil Chem Soc 51:244–264, 1974)

oped diabetes mellitus had at least a doubled risk of cardiovascular mortality.[75] Arterial wall exposure to abnormally high levels of circulating insulin may be directly related to the development of CAD. High insulin levels are found in persons with obesity, elevated serum triglycerides, and uremia, and in those taking oral contraceptives. High insulin levels may be inappropriate to the blood sugar levels found in cases of mild diabetes or may be induced by the insulin therapy for insulin-dependent diabetics. Proliferation of smooth muscle cells, inhibition of glycolysis, and synthesis of cholesterol, triglyceride, and phospholipid all occur in response to elevated serum insulin.[139] However, glucose intolerance is not easily isolated as a CAD risk factor because most people who have diabetes also are hypertensive, hyperlipidemic, and overweight.

LIFE-STYLE HABITS

Life-style habits include cigarette smoking, physical inactivity, obesity and weight change, emotional stress, and use of oral contraceptives. Each of these risk factors can be eliminated or modified by persons concerned with their health.

Cigarette Smoking

Cigarette smoking is one of the three greatest CAD risk factors in both men and women.[81,112] Cigarette smoking has been proved to cause more deaths from CAD (MI and SCD) than from either lung cancer or chronic obstructive airway disease. Factors related to the cigarette-smoking habit that influence CAD incidence and mortality are the number of cigarettes smoked (Fig. 13-4), duration of smoking, [expressed simply as a pack-year history (packs per day multiplied by number of smoking years), for example, 2 packs per day × 10 smoking years = 20 pack-years] age at initiation of smoking, and pattern of inhaling. A typical high-risk individual has smoked several packs per day for many years, began smoking at a young age, and inhales. Male cigarette smokers, regardless of the number of cigarettes smoked, have a 70% higher mortality rate than male non-smokers.[126] In young women (under age 50) who smoke 35 cigarettes or more per day, the rate of MI is 20 times that of young women who never smoked.[125] Women who smoke and use oral contraceptive agents or estrogens for other reasons are at increased risk (Table 13-6).[6,72,73,155] Pipe and cigar smokers, although at greater risk than nonsmokers, run less risk of developing CAD than cigarette smokers, probably because they inhale less smoke. The risk of death from CAD is reduced when cigarette smoking is stopped. After ten years of not smoking cigarettes, the risk of mortality from CAD approaches that of a nonsmoker.[126]

Pathophysiology of Cigarette Smoking. The exact pathologic mechanism that causes cigarette smoking to result in CAD has not been identified (see Chap. 10). Cigarette smoke contains about 2000 compounds that separate into gas and particulate matter. Although many of these compounds are suspected to be detrimental to health, only three have been judged most likely to contribute to the health hazards of smoking: "tar," nicotine, and carbon monoxide. Tar, the particulate matter left when water and nicotine are removed from cigarette smoke, contains hydrocarbons and other carcinogenic substances. Nicotine, also particulate, causes release of epinephrine and norepinephrine, resulting in arrhythmias and in increased heart rate (HR), BP, cardiac output, stroke volume, contractility, oxygen consumption, and coronary blood flow.[126] However, some experimental evidence suggests that left ventricular ejection fraction is diminished, possibly from a change in the elastic elements in cardiac muscle.[2] There is also an enhanced mobilization and utilization of FFA and hyperglycemic effects. Smokers of low-tar (less than 17.6 mg) and low-nicotine (less than 1.2 mg) cigarettes may experience less risk of CAD than smokers of high-tar and -nicotine cigarettes, although this risk is still considerably greater than the risk to nonsmokers. Carbon monoxide, which reduces the O_2-carrying capacity of the blood, cannot be selectively filtered, and in smokers with CAD, exposure to it can reduce the duration of their exercise capacity prior to the onset of angina.[126]

The Nonsmoker Involuntarily Exposed to Cigarette Smoke. Even when ventilation is adequate, carbon monoxide levels are raised above the Ambient Air Quality Standard of nine parts per million by cigarette smoking in enclosed spaces. The effects of involuntary exposure to smoking on morbidity and mortality from CAD are not known. However maximum exercise capacity of older non-smokers can be altered as a result of exposure to carbon monoxide levels found in involuntary smoking situations. In nonsmokers with CAD, exposure to the carbon monoxide levels of smoke-filled environments may curtail exercise duration before angina is precipitated.[5,126]

The Smoking Habit. The prevalence of smoking for adult males has declined from 53% in 1964 to 38% in 1978. The prevalence among women has remained at 30%. However, among younger women, especially teenagers, cigarette smoking has increased. The smoking habit may result from the need to maintain a serum nicotine level. It has been suggested that nicotine, the strongest pharmacologic agent found in cigarette smoke, is responsible for being the primary

Fig. 13-4. Smoking status and 10-year, age-adjusted rates per 1000 men for any major coronary event (nonfatal MI, fatal MI, SCD), SCD, any coronary death, death from all causes. Data from Pooling Project (Stamler J, Epstein FH: Preventive Med 1(1-2):31, 1972. Adapted from Inter-Society Commission for Heart Disease Resources: *Circulation*, 42:A67, 1970)

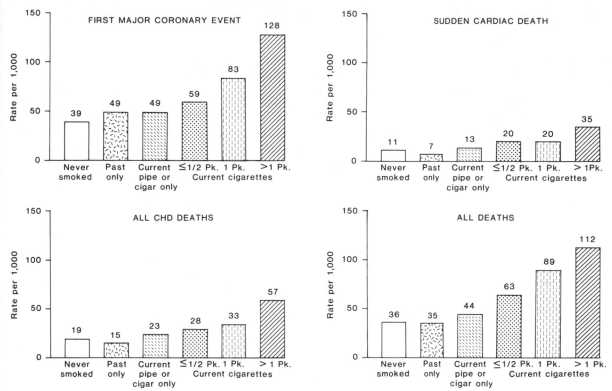

TABLE 13-6 ESTIMATES OF INCIDENCE OF NONFATAL AND FATAL MYOCARDIAL INFARCTION IN YOUNG WOMEN IN RELATION TO USE OF ORAL CONTRACEPTIVE AGENTS* AND SMOKING

INVESTIGATOR	AGE RANGE (YEARS)	RISK FACTOR	INCIDENCE
	Nonfatal Myocardial Infarction		
Mann, Vessey, Thorogood et al., 1975[96]	30–39	(No OCA)	2.1/100,000
	30–39	OCA	5.6/100,000
	40–44	(No OCA)	9.9/100,000
	40–44	OCA	56.9/100,000
Jick, Dinan, Rothman 1978[73]	27–37	Cigarette smoking *or* OCA	1/190,000
	27–37	Cigarette smoking *and* OCA	1/8400
	38–40	Cigarette smoking *or* OCA	1/47,000
	38–40	Cigarette smoking *and* OCA	1/920
	41–43	Cigarette smoking *or* OCA	1/23,000
	41–43	Cigarette smoking *and* OCA	1/540
	44–45	Cigarette smoking *or* OCA	1/16,000
	44–45	Cigarette smoking *and* OCA	1/250
	Fatal Myocardial Infarction		
Mann and Inmann, 1975[95]	30–39	(No OCA)	1.9/100,000
	30–39	OCA	5.4/100,000
	40–44	(No OCA)	11.7/100,000
	40–44	OCA	54.7/100,000

* OCA = oral contraceptive agent

incentive to smoke and for establishing the smoking habit. For heavy smokers, the smoking habit consists of smoking 20 to 30 cigarettes each day, or approximately one every 20 to 40 minutes of the waking day. In humans, the biologic half-life of nicotine is 20 to 30 minutes. Even though many children begin smoking at an early age, the onset of addictive smoking does not appear to begin until the high-school years. During attempts to stop smoking, a tobacco-withdrawal syndrome (craving for tobacco) is commonly experienced, more so by women than by men. Abrupt withdrawal causes this syndrome to subside quickly, whereas in partial abstinence, the state of withdrawal remains chronic.[126]

Recommendations. Assessment of psychologic aspects of smoking behavior is important when designing strategies for prevention and cessation of smoking. Psychologic needs are met by smoking, for the following reasons: Smoking reduces tensions, provides sensory stimulation, enhances self-image (especially in the young), and is a social act. Primary prevention of cigarette smoking-induced CAD must begin with education of children and young adults. Because most youth are oriented to the present, the type of educational programs designed should not dwell on future consequences alone. Strategies to resist peer pressure, the negative role-modeling of parents who smoke, and the various advertising and media campaigns should be included in these programs. Many formal programs that help adults to stop smoking are available, but of the 29 million smokers who have stopped since 1964, 95% have done so on their own.[27,126]

Physical Inactivity

Traits associated with physical deconditioning, such as obesity, a low vital capacity, and a rapid HR, are all associated with increased risk of MI in men.[75] Most practitioners feel that physical exercise has merit in preventing or minimizing coronary atherosclerosis. It has been shown that CAD mortality after MI can be reduced in patients participating in cardiac rehabilitation exercise programs.[74] However, a review of the literature prior to 1972 by Froelicher and Oberman and prior to 1977 by Froelicher suggests contradictory and controversial evidence concerning the contribution of physical inactivity to the development of CAD.[53,54] Many studies, including the Framingham study,[75] support the CAD-protective properties of physical exercise,[18,21,43,49,98,103,105–107,116,144,157,161] whereas other studies

refute a difference in CAD incidence or mortality based on physical activity alone.[1,47,84,102,104,122,127,134] The method used to assess the physical activity of those participating, which was done either retrospectively or by questionnaire, was a limitation in many of these studies. Retrospectively, most recent occupation determined whether physical activity was categorized as sedentary, moderately active, or very active. This classification did not always take into account the fact that persons with angina, CHF, hypertension, obesity, or diabetes might change from an active job to a more sedentary one, or might choose a less demanding job to begin with. In addition, assessing on-the-job work activity does not take into account the level of leisure-time activity. Questionnaires, which also made categorization of physical activity difficult, often could not be replicated and were judged grossly inaccurate.[161]

The Protective Effect of Physical Activity. The exact mechanism by which physical activity may protect against CAD development and mortality is not known. Recently, a larger percentage of HDL cholesterol, known to be protective against development of CAD[56] has been noted in persons who are physically very active.[58,92,158] However, the amount of physical exercise necessary to raise serum HDL levels has not been determined. The suggested mechanisms by which physical activity may protect against the development and severity of CAD are summarized in Table 13-7.

Recommendations. Persons without known heart disease should exercise regularly. Their minimum physical activity should consist of active participation, in a relaxed atmosphere, in one or more forms of exercise, such as walking at a fast pace, jogging, running, swimming, playing tennis, or bicycling. Activity should last for 15 to 60 minutes (continuous) and be performed three to five times weekly. The HR should increase by 60% to 90% of its maximum (usually 30 to 50 beats per minute).[109,121] Persons with known heart disease or who are over 40 years of age should consult with their physician for an exercise prescription before beginning to exercise (see Chap. 42).

Obesity and Weight Change

Obesity. There is an increased risk of CAD development and mortality in overweight or obese individuals. Obesity is defined as a body-mass index (weight/height^2) greater than

TABLE 13-7   MECHANISMS BY WHICH PHYSICAL ACTIVITY MAY REDUCE THE OCCURRENCE OR SEVERITY OF CORONARY ARTERY DISEASE

Increases in	Decreases in
Serum HDL levels[92,158]	Serum lipid levels[91,158]
Coronary collateral vascularization[39]	Triglycerides
Vessel size[136,145]	Cholesterol (total)
Myocardial efficiency[30,33,44,51,91]	Glucose intolerance[40,55]
Efficiency of peripheral blood distribution and return[87,91]	Obesity and adiposity[121]
Electron transport capacity[48]	Platelet stickiness[64,124]
Fibrinolytic capability[44,91]	Arterial blood pressure[33,44,91]
Arterial O$_2$ content[33]	Heart rate[33,44]
Red blood cell mass and blood volume[48]	Vulnerability to dysrhythmias[110]
Thyroid function[152]	Neurohormonal overreaction[110]
Growth hormone production[55]	"Strain" associated with psychic "stress"[48]
Tolerance to stress[60,91]	
Prudent living habits[121]	
Joie de vivre[121]	

(Adapted from Fox SM III, Naughton JP, Gorman PA: Mod Concepts Cardiovasc Dis 41 (4):20, 1972)

20% above the ideal value.[148] A controversy exists regarding the contribution to CAD risk of obesity alone versus other known risk factors that frequently accompany obesity, such as advancing age, elevated BP, and elevated serum cholesterol. The Seven Countries Study followed up men aged 40 to 59 years without apparent CAD for a 5-year period and concluded that obesity did not make a significant contribution to development of CAD when the factors of age, BP, serum cholesterol, and smoking were equal.[85] However, data from the Manitoba study refute these findings.[111] The incidence of CAD in young men was examined over a 26-year period. After 16 years of follow-up, body-mass index alone was identified as a CAD risk factor. A high body-mass index was highly correlated to development of MI, SCD, coronary insufficiency, and suspected MI; the correlation was strongest to SCD. Of all patients with MI, those that were obese ran the greatest risk of having SCD.

Weight Change. The Framingham study examined the effect of weight change on the atherogenic traits of serum cholesterol, systolic BP, glucose intolerance, and serum uric acid. They found that all these traits in all age groups, without age trends, were positively correlated to weight gain. These associations were greater in men than in women. For serum cholesterol, systolic BP, glucose intolerance, and serum uric acid, the Framingham data indicate that changes over time in relation to relative weight are more strongly related to change in weight rather than to the general level of adiposity.[7]

Recommendations. Persons should attain and maintain optimal body weight. Weight tables for men and women according to height and age can be found in the Metropolitan Life Insurance Bulletin.[135] Weight correction should reduce risk from CAD and may improve exercise tolerance in persons with known CAD.[7] Weight gain can be controlled by eating well-balanced meals that do not exceed the daily caloric requirement, which is based on age, height, body build, and activity level. Ideal weight is best achieved by primary prevention of obesity: not overfeeding infants and children, so that excess numbers of fat cells are not formed, and not overeating, especially during middle-age when metabolism slows and the calorie requirement is reduced. Overweight individuals should ask a health care professional, such as a nurse, physician, or dietician, for a diet prescription. Fad diets do not usually result in permanent weight loss. The best way to lose weight is by changing eating habits.

Emotional Stress

The etiology of CAD cannot always be explained by the presence of one or more of the major risk factors alone. Data from the Pooling Project have shown that 42% of the cases of CAD that developed over a 10-year period occurred among men who did not have as many as two of the major risk factors.[132] Therefore, another causative factor appears to be involved in the development of CAD. Many scientists feel that this risk factor is "stress," defined in this context by the American Heart Association's Committee on Stress, Strain and Heart Disease as "any stimulus, physical or emotional, internal or environmental, that evokes a response by the cardiovascular system."[120] (See Chapters 7 and 11 for descriptions of the physiology of physical stress and the cardiovascular effects of the stress response, respectively.)

Emotional stress is considered by many to be a factor in the incidence and mortality of CAD. Even though stress is highly associated with the "American way of life," it must be remembered that stress of one kind or another has been present in almost every civilization, and that what is stressful for one individual may not be stressful for another. Those components of our life-style that appear to affect CAD development and mortality are sociocultural mobility, socioeconomic status, status incongruity, educational level, anxiety and neuroses, life dissatisfaction, life change, and behavior patterns.[22,68-71,141]

Sociocultural Mobility. It appears that major changes in place of residence, occupation, and cultural situations increase the incidence of CAD. Rates of CAD development are at least twice as high in men experiencing several lifetime job changes and geographic moves than in those who experience no changes.[140] In a study of Israeli men, rates of MI were higher in the group who immigrated to Israel than in the group who was born there.[99] In a study of a rural community in which the population remained stable but the community became urban, the incidence of CAD in that population was increased above the predicted rate.[150] It is not known whether risk increases because of mobility, the new situation, or the characteristics that predispose some people to move.[141]

Socioeconomic Status. In the past, a higher socioeconomic status in the United States was associated with increased CAD risk, whereas persons with a lower socioeconomic level had less incidence of CAD. This was also true in other countries.[94] More recently, it has been shown that, although white males remain the single highest group affected, persons of lower socioeconomic status are no longer appreciably less subject to CAD than are persons in the middle and upper socioeconomic levels.[23]

Status Incongruity. Status incongruity, defined by Jenkins as simultaneously possessing characteristics of one or more different social classes, is also associated with increased CAD risk. Status incongruity reflects movement, either upward or downward, in certain aspects of a person's life. This inconsistency is thought to result in more frequent conflicts and tensions.[70]

Education Level. The higher the level of education, the lower is the incidence of CAD mortality. This is especially true among women.[88] A study of males with confirmed MI revealed that those with more education were more likely to report the presence of chest pains before the actual MI occurred than those with less education.[31]

Anxiety and Neuroses. The incidence of CAD appears to be associated with anxiety,[10,100,147] depression,[20] psychophysiologic complaints ("somaticizing"),[154] complaints of sleep disturbances,[52] and emotional drain.[82] However, many of these findings were absent or equivocal in other studies.

Life Dissatisfaction. Life dissatisfactions are associated with development of angina pectoris but not of MI. It appears that the intensity of the problem rather than the content is the critical issue.[99] The reason for this discrepancy is not known. It may be that these different presentations of CAD have different precursors.[70]

Life Change. Life change has been implicated as a causative factor in CAD development. Holmes and Rahe designed a rating scale to measure the importance of life changes to development of illness.[62] Unfortunately, many studies concerning life changes and CAD have been retrospective and without a control group, but a large prospective study has shown no association between an increased number of life changes and incidence of acute MI over a 12- to 15-month period.[146] Increased life changes were, however, associated with development of neuroses and chronic, disabling diseases.[71]

Behavior Pattern. A CAD-prone behavior pattern, the type A personality, has been identified. It is characterized by aggressiveness, ambitiousness, competitive drive, preoccupation with deadlines, impatience, and time urgency. The opposite pattern, the type B, has none of these personality traits.[117] The Western Collaborative study group has shown that type A men have a higher incidence of CAD than type B men.[118]

Recommendations. Awareness of the effects of stress on the body and the heart and of the types of situations that induce stress may provide an incentive to avoid emotional stressors when possible. Unfortunately, many stress-inducing situations cannot be avoided, but responses to these situations may be altered. Stress-reduction techniques are discussed in Chapters 22 and 43. In addition, regular physical activity, such as running, swimming, or bicycling and more leisure-time activity may help to dispel some of the effects of emotional stress on the cardiovascular system.

Use of Oral Estrogens for Contraception and Other Purposes

Myocardial infarction among young, healthy women is rare. Use of oral contraceptive agents (estrogen and progestin) is associated with an increased risk of nonfatal and fatal MI in young women. In women aged 30 to 39, the incidence of nonfatal MI among oral contraceptive users is 2.7 times greater than in nonusers. For women aged 40 to 44, this risk among users is 5.7 times that among nonusers.[96] The incidence of fatal MI is similar: 2.8 times greater risk for women aged 30 to 39 who use oral contraceptives than for those who do not, and 4.7 times greater risk for women aged 40 to 44 who use oral contraceptive agents than for those who do not.[95] The risk from cigarette smoking acts synergistically with the risk from oral contraceptive agents (see Table 13-6).[73] Other major risk factors, such as hyperlipidemia, hypertension, and glucose intolerance, also appear to have additive effects.[96] For oral-contraceptive users, the death rate from all types of circulatory disease increases with age, duration of oral contraception used, and cigarette smoking.[11]

The incidence of acute MI in women under age 46 taking supplementary estrogens is similar to the incidence of MI from oral contraceptive agents.[72] However, no positive correlation between acute MI and estrogen therapy in older women has been found.[115]

Theories of the Pathophysiologic Mechanism. How oral contraceptive agents contribute to MI incidence and mortality is not known.[6] Serum lipids, specifically triglyceride, cholesterol, LDL, and VLDL levels, are elevated by oral contraceptives.[8,138] The level of HDL varies with the type and dose of various combination oral contraceptives, generally increasing with higher estrogen doses and decreasing with higher progestin doses.[16] Increased serum lipids could contribute to atherosclerosis, but this has not been documented angiographically. Smooth, rounded lesions that are proximal to the major coronary arteries but spare the remaining coronary tree are seen, rather than the diffuse, irregular lesions typical of atherosclerosis.[155] Intimal proliferation of the coronary arteries has been noted, with or without thrombosis.[66,93,95] Abnormalities of clotting factors (increases in Factor VII and, to a lesser extent, in Factor X[155]) and platelet functions cannot be discounted as contributing to these vascular changes.[38] Mean BP, systolic more than diastolic, increases among users of oral contraceptives.[46,89] Some users develop hypertension, but BP tends to normalize after discontinuation of these agents. Changes in BP are thought to be due to increased angiotensinogen, plasma renin activity, and aldosterone secretion and excretion rates.[29,156]

Recommendations. Women over 37 years of age who smoke cigarettes and have a positive family history of CAD or who have other known risk factors should seek alternative methods of birth control.[6,73,96] Postmenopausal women 39 to 45 years of age should avoid all estrogen use if they smoke or have other MI risk factors.[72] Women taking estrogens should have their BP monitored at regular intervals.

SIGNS OF PRECLINICAL CARDIOVASCULAR DISEASE

Electrocardiographic Characteristics

Left ventricular hypertrophy (LVH) on ECG has been associated with increased CAD risk.[15,76] According to the Framingham study, those with "possible" LVH-ECG (principally an increase in R-wave potential without prominent S-T and T-wave abnormalities) face twice as much risk of developing CAD as those with normal ECGs. Definite LVH-ECG increases CAD risk threefold. It is thought possible that LVH is an expression of hypertensive hypertrophy, whereas marked voltage increases with S-T and T-wave changes indicate ischemic myocardial involvement.[76] Nonspecific T-wave changes on the resting ECG are also predictive of CAD development. Other electrocardiographic findings suggestive of future CAD development are prominent left axis deviation (beyond −30°), first-degree atrioventricular block (PR .22 seconds or longer), and frequent resting premature beats (10% of recorded beats or more). Sinus tachycardia at rest was not predictive of CAD development in men originally free of CAD.[15]

Blood and Tissue Characteristics

Factors related to blood characteristics appear to affect risk of CAD. In the Framingham study, persons with type O blood had the lowest serum cholesterol levels and less intermittent claudication than did persons with other ABO groups, especially type A.[75] Abnormalities of the blood's components and clotting mechanisms may also influence risk. Current research areas include the effect on the development of CAD of hematocrit level, leukocyte count, platelet stickiness, erythrocyte sedimentation rate, coagulation disorders, and carboxyhemoglobin levels.[35] Recently, the HLA antigen BW38 has been associated with premature CAD. It is not known whether this antigen is directly related to CAD pathogenesis or acts as a marker for immune response genes or other genetic factors.[137]

QUESTIONABLE RISK FACTORS

There may be other factors that contribute in a minor way to the development of CAD, but a direct cause–effect relationship has not been established.[35]

COMBINED RISK FACTORS

The greater the number of risk factors, the greater is the risk of developing CAD. Combinations of risk factors have a synergistic effect (Fig. 13-5). The *Coronary Risk Hand-book* provides the clinician with a simple method of predicting CAD risk, based on the seven characteristics identified in the Framingham study.[28] For example, the following single risk factors for a 40-year-old man indicate a slight probability of CAD development in six years: systolic BP of 150 mm Hg (1.3% probability) or serum cholesterol of 285 mg/dl (2.4% probability). If both risk factors are present, the individual's probability of developing CAD increases to 4.1%, which is greater than the sum of the two risks. Smoking cigarettes increases his risk to 6.3%. His risk is raised to 8.1% with the addition of glucose intolerance, and 15.6% if LVH-ECG is present.[28] At this point, the individual's risk of developing CAD is considerable.

Recommendations. The importance of eliminating combined risk factors cannot be overemphasized. Primary prevention and reduction of further risk in patients with known CAD requires an understanding of atherosclerotic disease. The American Heart Association distributes educational literature that is aimed toward the lay population. In addition, their recently published *Heartbook* is an excellent source for patient education.[14]

Primary prevention of CAD should be the goal. Because many of the risk factors are directly related to acquired habits (over-eating, a "taste" for cholesterol-rich foods, smoking, lack of exercise), children should be taught a different style of living. Family role-modeling may be the most effective method of instilling healthful habits in young children.

For many adults, decreasing the risk of CAD represents a major change in life-style: in eating habits (decreasing calories, cholesterol, saturated fats, carbohydrates), in smoking habits, and in physical activity. Because most people cannot accomplish all these changes at once, a *realistic* and attainable plan of action that is mutually agreeable and provides the greatest reduction in risk should be initiated.

Fig. 13-5. The major risk factors and 10-year, age-adjusted rates per 1000 men for any major coronary event, SCD, any coronary death, and death from all causes. Data from the Pooling Project. (American Health Foundation Position Statement on Diet and Coronary Heart Disease: *Preventive Medicine*, 1(1-2):267, 1972. Adapted from Inter-Society Commission for Heart Disease Resources: *Circulation*, 42:A68, 1970) Reprinted by permission from Academic Press.

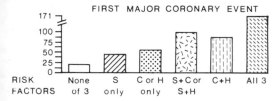
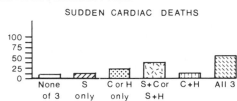
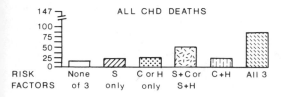
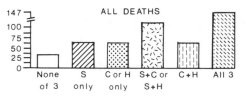

CODE: S = Cigarette smoking, any use at entry
C = Serum cholesterol, ≥ 250 mg/dl
H = Diastolic blood pressure, ≥ 90 mm Hg

These individuals should be closely followed up and given a great deal of encouragement to continue modifying CAD risk.

NURSING INTERVENTION IN MODIFICATION OF CORONARY ARTERY DISEASE RISK FACTORS

Nurses can play an important role in both primary prevention and therapeutic management of CAD. Many nurses are assuming expanded roles in hypertension control programs, in many instances improving patient adherence to the prescribed therapeutic plan (see Chap. 47). School nurses can provide education programs to young people regarding CAD and its prevention. Nurses working in the adult community can offer classes concerning CAD risk factor modification. Cardiac nurses have the opportunity and obligation to teach cardiac patients and families about the implications of CAD and ways to modify life-style in order to maintain optimal cardiac functioning. (Refer to Part II, Section G, for a complete discussion of cardiac rehabilitation.) American Heart Association educational literature is available for use in these programs.

The author wishes to acknowledge Karen E. Krueger for assistance with review of the literature

REFERENCES

1. Adelstein AM: Some aspects of cardiovascular mortality in South Africa. Br J Preventive Social Med 17:29–40, 1963
2. Ahmed SS, Moschos CB, Lyons MM et al: Cardiovascular effects of long-term cigarette smoking and nicotine administration. Am J Cardiol 37(1):33–40, 1976
3. American Health Foundation: Position statement on diet and coronary heart disease. Prev Med 1(4):559–561, 1972
4. An Epidemiological Investigation of Cardiovascular Disease. The Framingham Study. Sections 1 and 2, 1978
5. Aronow WS: Effect of passive smoking on angina pectoris. N Eng J Med 299(1):21–24, 1978
6. Arthes FG, Masi AT: Myocardial infarction in younger women: Associated clinical features and relationship to use of oral contraceptive drugs. Chest 70(5):574–583, 1976
7. Ashley FW, Kannel WB: Relation of weight change to changes in atherogenic traits: The Framingham Study. J Chronic Dis 27:103–144, 1974
8. Aurell M, Cramér K, Rybo G: Serum lipids and lipoproteins during long-term administration of an oral contraceptive. Lancet i:292–293, 1966
9. Barboriak JJ, Hogan WJ: Preprandial drinking and plasma lipids in man. Atherosclerosis 24:323–325, 1976
10. Bengtsson C, Hällström T, Tibblin G: Social factors, stress experience and personality traits in women with ischaemic heart disease, compared to a sample population of women. Acta Med Scand (Suppl) 549:823–92, 1973
11. Beral V, Kay CR: Mortality among oral contraceptive users. Lancet ii:727–731, 1977
12. Bieri JG, Evarts RP: Vitamin E adequacy of vegetable oils. J Am Diet Assoc 66:134–139, 1975
13. Bierman EL: Hyperlipoproteinemia. Current Concepts. Kalamazoo, Mich, Upjohn, 1976
14. Blackburn H: Risk factors and cardiovascular disease. In American Heart Association Heartbook, pp 2–20, New York, EP Dutton, 1980
15. Blackburn H, Taylor HL, Keys A: The electrocardiogram in prediction of five-year coronary heart disease incidence among men aged forty through fifty-nine. In Keys A (ed): Coronary Heart Disease in Seven Countries, Circulation (Supp I) 41:154–161, 1970
16. Bradley DD, Wingerd J, Petitti DB et al: Serum high density lipoprotein cholesterol in women using oral contraceptives, estrogens and progestins. N Engl J Med 299(1):17–20, 1978
17. Brand RJ, Rosenman RH, Sholtz RI et al: Multivariate prediction of coronary heart disease in the Western Collaborative Group Study compared to the findings of the Framingham Study. Circulation 52(2):348–355, 1976
18. Breslow L, Buell P: Mortality from coronary heart disease and physical activity of work in California. J Chronic Dis 11(4):421–444, 1960
19. Brown WH: Introduction to Organic and Biochemistry. Boston, Willard Grant Press, 1972
20. Bruhn JG, Paredes A, Adsett CA et al: "Psychological predictors of sudden death in myocardial infarction. J Psychosom Med 18:187–191, 1974
21. Brunner D: The influence of physical activity on incidence and prognosis of ischemic heart disease. In Raab W (ed): Prevention of Ischemic Heart Disease, pp 236–243. Springfield, Ill, Charles C Thomas, 1966
22. Buell JC, Eliot RS: Stress and cardiovascular disease. Mod Concepts Cardiovasc Dis 48(4):19–24, 1979
23. Cassel J, Heyden S, Bartel AG et al: Incidence of coronary heart disease by ethnic group, social class, and sex. Arch Intern Med 128:901–906, 1971
24. Castelli WP, Gordon T, Hjörtland MC: Alcohol and blood lipids: The Cooperative Lipoprotein Phenotyping Study. Lancet ii:153–155, 1977
25. Chapman JM, Goerke LS, Dixon W et al: The clinical status of the population group in Los Angeles under observation 2–3 years. Am J Public Health Part 2, 47:33–42, 1957
26. Chapman JM, Massey FJ, Jr: The interrelationship of serum cholesterol, hypertension, body weight, and risk of coronary disease: Results of the first ten years follow-up in the Los Angeles Heart Study. J Chronic Dis 17(10):933–949, 1964
27. Colby AO: What does smoking really do to the heart? Mod Med 46:53–58, 1977
28. Coronary Risk Handbook. Dallas, American Heart Association, 1973
29. Crane MG, Harris JJ, Winsor W: Hypertension, Oral Contraceptive agents, and conjugated estrogens. Ann Intern Med 74:13–21, 1971
30. Crews J, Aldinger EE: Effect of chronic exercise on myocardial function. Am Heart J 74:536–542, 1967
31. Croog SH, Levine S: Social status and perceptions of 250 men after myocardial infarction. Public Health Reports 84:989–997, 1969
32. Dayton S: Polyunsaturated fats. In Feldman EB (ed): Nutrition and Cardiovascular Disease, pp 59–84. New York: Appleton-Century-Crofts, 1976
33. Detry J-MR, Rousseau M, Vandebroucke G et al: Increased arteriovenous oxygen difference after physical training in coronary heart disease. Circulation 44:109–118, 1971
34. Deutscher S, Ostrander LD, Epstein FH: Familial factors in premature coronary heart disease—A preliminary report from the Tecumseh Community Health Study. Am J Epidemiol 91(2):233–237, 1970
35. DiGirolama M, Schlant RC: Etiology of coronary atherosclerosis. In Hurst JW, Logue RB, Schlant RC et al (eds): The Heart, 4th ed, pp 1103–1121. New York, McMillan, 1978
36. Doyle JT: Risk factors in coronary heart disease. NY J Med 63:1317–1320, 1963
37. Doyle JT, Haslin AS, Hilleboe HE et al: A prospective study of degenerative cardiovascular disease in Albany—Report of 3 years' experiences. I. Ischemic heart disease. Am J Public Health, Part 2, 47:25–32, 1957
38. Dugdale M, Masi T: Hormonal contraception and thromboembolic disease: Effects of the oral contraceptives on hemostasis mechanisms. J Chronic Dis 23:775–790, 1971
39. Eckstein RW: Effect of exercise and coronary artery narrowing on coronary collateral circulation. Circ Res 5(3):230–235, 1957

40. Epstein FH: Epidemiological investigations of cardiovascular disease and related disorders in a complete, natural community—Tecumseh, Michigan, USA. In Schettler G, Sanwald R (eds): Pathophysiological and Clinical Aspects of Lipid Metabolism, pp 149–160. Stuttgart Georg Thieme Verlag, 1966
41. Epstein FH: Hyperglycemia, a risk factor in coronary heart disease. Circulation 36:609–619, 1967
42. Epstein FH, Ostrander LD Jr, Johnson BC et al: Epidemiologic studies of cardiovascular disease in a total community—Tecumseh, MI Ann Intern Med 62(6):1170–1187, 1965
43. Epstein L, Miller GJ, Stitt FW et al: Vigorous exercise in leisure time, coronary risk factors, and resting electrocardiogram in middle-aged male civil servants. Br Heart J 38:403–409, 1976
44. Epstein SE, Redwood DR, Goldstein RE et al: Angina pectoris: Pathophysiology, evaluation and treatment (NIH Conference). Ann Intern Med 75:263–296, 1971
45. Feldman EB: Saturated fats. In Feldman EB (ed): Nutrition and Cardiovascular Disease, pp 30–58. New York, Appleton-Century-Crofts, 1976
46. Fisch IR, Freeman SH, Myatt AV: Oral contraceptives, pregnancy, and blood pressure. JAMA 222:1507–1510, 1972
47. Forssman O, Lindegard B: The post coronary patient. A multidisciplinary investigation of middle-aged Swedish males. J Psychosom Res 3(2):89–169, 1958
48. Fox SM III, Naughton JP, Gorman PA: Physical activity and cardiovascular health. I. Potential for prevention of coronary heart disease and possible mechanisms. Mod Concepts Cardiovasc Dis 41(4):17–20, 1972
49. Frank CW, Weinblatt E, Shapiro S et al: Physical inactivity as a lethal factor in myocardial infarction among men. Circulation 34(6):1022–1033, 1966
50. Frederickson DS, Lees RS: A system for phenotyping hyperlipoproteinemia. Circulation 31(3):321–327, 1965
51. Frick MH: Coronary implications of hemodynamic changes caused by physical training. Am J Cardiol 22:417–425, 1968
52. Friedman GD, Ury HK, Klatsky, AL et al: A physchological questionnaire predictive of myocardial infarction: Results from the Kaiser–Permanente epidemiological study of myocardial infarction. Psychosom Med 36:327–343, 1974
53. Froelicher VF: Does exercise conditioning delay progression of myocardial ischemia in coronary atherosclerotic heart disease. Cardiovasc Clin 8:11–30, 1977
54. Froelicher VF, Oberman A: Analysis of epidemiologic studies of physical inactivity as risk factor for coronary artery disease. Prog Cardiovasc Dis 15(1):41–65, 1972
55. Ganong WF: Review of Medical Physiology, 8th ed. Los Altos, Lange Medical Publications, 1977
56. Gordon T, Castelli WP, Hjörtland MC et al: High density lipoprotein as a protective factor against coronary heart disease. The Framingham Study. Am J Med 62:707–714, 1977
57. Gordon T, Moore FE, Shurtleff D et al: Some methodologic problems in long-term study of cardiovascular disease—Observations in the Framingham Study. J of Chronic Dis 10(3):186–206, 1959
58. Hartung GH, Foreyt JP, Mitchell RE et al: Relation of diet to high-density-lipoprotein cholesterol in middle-aged marathon runners, joggers, and inactive men. N Engl J Med 302(7):357–361, 1980
59. Havlik RJ, Feinlaub M, Thom T et al: Proceedings on the Conference on the Decline in Coronary Heart Disease Mortality. Washington, DC, U.S. Department of Health, Education, and Welfare, DHEW Publication No. (NIH) 79–1610, 1979
60. Heinzelmann F, Bagley RW: Response to physical activity programs and their effects on health behavior. Public Health Reports 85:905–911, 1970
61. Heiss G, Tamir I, Davis CE et al: Lipoprotein-cholesterol distributions in selected North American populations: The Lipid Research Clinics Program Prevalence Study. Circulation 61(2):302–315, 1980
62. Holmes TH, Rahe RH: The social readjustment rating scale. Journal Psychosom Res 11:213–218, 1967
63. Horwitt MK: Vitamin E. In Goodhart RS, Shils ME (eds):

Modern Nutrition in Health and Disease, 5th ed, pp 175–185. Philadelphia, Lea & Febiger.
64. Ikkala E, Myllylä, G, Sarajas HSS: Platelet adhesiveness and ADP-induced platelet aggregation in exercise. Ann Med Experimentalis et Biologiae Fenniae 44:88–89, 1966
65. Inter-society Commission for Heart Disease Resources: Report on primary prevention of atherosclerotic diseases. Circulation 42:A55–A95, 1970
66. Irey NS, Norris HJ: Intimal vascular lesions associated with female reproductive steroids. Arch Pathol 96:227–234, 1973
67. Jackson RL, Taunton OD, Morrisett JD et al: the role of dietary polyunsaturated fat in lowering blood cholesterol in man. Brief Reviews in Circ Res (Monograph 64), pp 11–17. Dallas, American Heart Association, 1979
68. Jenkins CD: "Psychologic and social precursors of coronary disease. Part I. N Eng J Med 284(5):244–255, 1971
69. Jenkins CD: Psychologic and social precursors of coronary disease. Part II. N Eng J Med 284(6):307–317, 1971
70. Jenkins CD: Recent evidence supporting psycholoic and social risk factors for coronary disease, Part I. N Engl J Med 294(18):987–994, 1976
71. Jenkins CD: Recent evidence supporting psychologic and social risk factors for coronary disease, Part II. N Eng J Med 294(19):1033–1038, 1976
72. Jick H, Dinan B, Rothman KJ: Noncontraceptive estrogens and nonfatal myocardial infarction. JAMA 239 (14):1407–1408, 1978
73. Jick H, Dinan B, Rothman KJ: Oral contraceptives and nonfatal myocardial infarction. JAMA 293(14):1403–1406, 1978
74. Kallio V, Hämäläinen H, Hakkila J et al: Reduction in sudden deaths by a multifactorial intervention programme after acute myocardial infarction Lancet ii:1091–1094, 1979
75. Kannel WB: Recent findings of the Framingham Study. Resident and Staff Physician 24:56–71, 1978
76. Kannel WB, Gordon T, Castelli WP et al: Electrocardiographic left ventricular hypertrophy and risk of coronary heart disease. Ann Intern Med 72(6):813–822, 1970
77. Kannel WB, Castelli WP, Gordon T et al: Serum cholesterol, lipoproteins, and the risk of coronary heart disease. Ann Intern Med 74(1):1–12, 1971
78. Kannel WB, McGee D, Gordon T: A general cardiovascular risk profile: The Framingham Study. Am J Cardiol 38(1):46–51, 1976
79. Kannel WB, Gordon T, Schwartz MJ: Systolic versus diastolic blood pressure and risk of coronary heart disease. The Framingham Study. Am J Cardiol 27(4):335–345, 1971
80. Kannel WB, Hjörtland MC, McNamara PM et al: Menopause and risk of cardiovascular disease. The Framingham Study. Ann Intern Med 85:447–452, 1976
81. Kannel WB, McNamara PM, Schwartz MJ: Blood pressure and risk of coronary heart disease. The Framingham Study. Dis Chest 56(1):43–52, 1969
82. Kavanaugh T, Shepard RJ: The immediate antecedents of myocardial infarction in active men. Can Med Assoc J 109:19–22, 1973
83. Keys A (ed): Coronary Heart Disease in Seven Countries. Circulation (suppl I) 41:1–211, 1970
84. Keys A (ed): Physical activity and the epidemiology of coronary heart disease. In Brunner D (ed): Medicine and Sport, Vol. 4: Physical Activity and Aging, pp 250–266. Baltimore, University Park Press, 1970
85. Keys A, Aravanis C, Blackburn H et al: Coronary heart disease: Overweight and obesity as risk factors. Ann Intern Med 77:15–27, 1972
86. Keys A, Taylor HL, Blackburn H et al: Coronary heart disease among Minnesota business and professional men followed 15 years. Circulation 28(3):381–395, 1963
87. Kilbom À: Physical training in women. Scand J Clin Lab Invest (Suppl 119) 28:1–34, 1971
88. Kitagawa EM, Hauser PM: Differential Mortality in the United States: A Study of Socioeconomic Epidemiology. Cambridge, Harvard University Press, 1973

89. Kunin CM, McCormack RC, Abernathy JR: Oral contraceptives and blood pressure. Arch Intern Med 123:363–365, 1969

90. Laboratory Methods Committee of the Lipid Research Clinics Program: "Cholesterol and triglyceride concentrations in serum/plasma pairs. Clin Chem 23:60–63, 1973

91. Larsen OA, Malmberg RO (eds): Coronary Heart Disease and Physical Fitness. Baltimore, University Park, Press, 1971

92. Lehtonen A, Viikari J: The effects of vigorous physical activity at work on serum lipids with a special reference to high-density lipoprotein cholesterol. Acta Physiol Scand 104(1):117–121, 1978

93. Maleki M, Lange RL: Coronary thrombosis in young women on oral contraceptives: Report of two cases and review of the literature. Am Heart J 85:749–754, 1973

94. Malhotra SL: Epidemiology of ischaemic heart disease in India with special reference to causation. Br Med J 29:895–905, 1967

95. Mann JI, Inman WHW: Oral contraceptives and death from myocardial infarction. Br Med J 2:245–248, 1975

96. Mann JI, Vessey MP, Thorogood M et al: Myocardial infarction in young women with special reference to oral contraceptive practice. Br Med J 2:241–245, 1975

97. Margarine—The Better Butter?: Consumer Reports 44(2):66–72, 1979

98. McDonough JR, Hames CG, Stulb SC et al: Coronary heart disease among negroes and whites in Evans County, Georgia. J Chronic Dis 18(5):443–468, 1965

99. Medalie JH, Kahn HA, Neufeld HN et al: Myocardial infarction over a five-year period. I. Prevalence, incidence and mortality experience. J Chronic Dis 26:63–84, 1973

100. Medalie JH, Snyder M, Groen JJ et al: Angina pectoris among 10,000 men. 5 year incidence and univariate analysis. Am J Med 55:583–594, 1973

101. Miller, NE, Førde OH, Thelle DS et al: The Thromsø Heart Study. High density lipoprotein and coronary heart disease: A prospective case control study. Lancet i:965–967, 1977

102. Mitrani Y, Karplus H, Brunner D: Coronary atherosclerosis in cases of traumatic death. The influence of physical occupational activity on the development of coronary narrowing. Medicine and Sport, Vol. 4: Physical Activity and Aging, pp 241–248. Baltimore, University Park Press, 1970

103. Morris JN: Epidemiology and cardiovascular disease in middle age. Parts I and II. Mod Concepts Cardiovasc Dis 29(12):625–632, 1960

104. Morris JN, Crawford MD: Coronary heart disease and physical activity of work. Br Med J ii:1485–1496, 1958

105. Morris JN, Heady JA, Raffle PA et al: Coronary heart disease and physical activity of work. Lancet 265:1111–1120, 1953.

106. Paffenbarger RS, Laughlin ME, Gima MS et al: Work activity of longshoreman as related to death from coronary heart disease and stroke. N Engl J Med 282(20):1109–1114, 1970

107. Paffenbarger RS Jr, Wing AL, Hyde RT: Physical activity as an index of heart attack risk in college alumni. Am J Epidemiol 108(3):161–175, 1978

108. Paul O, Lepper MJ, Phelen WH et al: A longitudinal study of coronary heart disease. Circulation 28(1):20–31, 1963

109. Pollack M, Gettman L, Milesis C et al: Effects of frequency and duration of training on attrition and incidence of injury. Med Sci Sports 9(1):31–36, 1977

110. Raab W: Preventive Myocardiology. Springfield, Ill, Charles C Thomas, 1970

111. Rabkin SW, Mathewson FAL, Hsu P-W: Relation of body weight to development of ischemic heart disease in a cohort of young North American men after a 26 year observation period: The Manitoba Study. Am J Cardiol 39:452–458, 1977

112. Relationship of blood pressure, serum cholesterol, smoking habit, relative weight and ECG abnormalities to incidence of major coronary events: Final report of the Pooling Project. J Chronic Dis 31(4):201–306, 1978

113. Robertson TL, Kato H, Rhoads GG et al: Epidemiologic studies of coronary heart disease and stroke in Japanese men living in Japan, Hawaii, and California. Am J Cardiol 39(2):239–243, 1977

114. Robertson WB, Strong JP: Atherosclerosis in persons with hypertension and diabetes mellitus. Lab Invest 18(5):538–551, 1968

115. Rosenberg L, Armstrong B, Jick H: Myocardial infarction and estrogen therapy in post-menopausal women. N Engl J Med 294:1256–1259, 1976

116. Rosenman RH: The influence of different exercise patterns on the incidence of coronary heart disease in the Western Collaborative Group Study. Medicine and Sport, Vol. 4: Physical Activity and Aging, pp 267–273. Baltimore, University Park Press, 1970

117. Rosenman RH: The role of behavior patterns and neurogenic factors in the pathogenesis of coronary heart disease. In Eliot RS (ed): Stress and the Heart, pp 123–141. Mt Kisco, Futura Publishing Co, 1974

118. Rosenman RH, Friedman M, Strauss R et al: Coronary Heart Disease in the Western Collaborative Study Group: A follow-up experience of 4½ years. J Chronic Dis 23:173–190, 1970

119. Schatz IJ: Classification of primary hyperlipidemia—Observations on 214 patients. JAMA 210(4):701–704, 1969

120. Scherlis S, Levenson RM, Sagall EL et al: Report of the Committee on Stress, Strain and Heart Disease, American Heart Association. Circulation 55(5):825A–835A, 1977

121. Schlant RC, DiGirolama M: Modification of risk factors in the prevention and management of coronary atherosclerotic heart disease. In Hurst JW, Logue RB, Schlant RC et al (eds): The Heart, 4th ed, pp 1311–1344. New York, McGraw-Hill, 1978

122. Shanoff HM, Little JA: Studies of male survivors of myocardial infarction due to 'essential' atherosclerosis. I. Characteristics of the patients. Can Med Assoc J 84:519–530, 1961

123. Shurtleff D: Some characteristics related to the incidence of cardiovascular disease and death: The Framingham Study. 18 Year follow-up. U.S. Department of Health, Education and Welfare, DHEW Publication No. (NIH) 74-599, 1974

124. Simpson MT, Hames CG, Meier D: An epidemiological study of platelet aggregation and physical activity. Circulation (suppl II) 43–44:1971

125. Slone D, Shapiro S, Rosenberg L et al: Relation of cigarette smoking to myocardial infarction in young women. N Engl J Med 298(23):1273–1276, 1978

126. Smoking and Health, A Report of the Surgeon General: Washington, DC, U.S. Department of Health, Education and Welfare, DHEW Publication NO. (PHS) 79-50066, 1979

127. Spain DM, Bradess VA: Occupational physical activity and degree of coronary atherosclerosis in "normal" men. Circulation 22(2):239–242, 1960

128. Stamler J: Cardiovascular diseases in the USA. Am J Cardiol 10(3):319–340, 1962

129. Stamler J: Epidemiology of coronary heart disease. Med Clin North Am 57(1):5–46, 1973

130. Stamler J: Introduction to risk factors in coronary artery disease. In McIntosh HD (ed): Baylor College of Medicine Cardiology Series. Northfield, Medical Communications, 1978

131. Stamler J: Lifestyles, major risk factors, proof and public policy. Circulation 58(1):3–19, 1978

132. Stamler J, Beard RR, Connor WE et al: Primary prevention of the atherosclerotic diseases. Circulation 42:A55–A94, 1970

133. Stamler J, Epstein FH: Coronary heart disease: Risk factors as guides to preventive action. Prev Med 1(1–2):27–48, 1972

134. Stamler J, Kjelsberg M, Hall Y: Epidemiologic studies on cardiovascular–renal disease. I. Analysis of mortality by age–race–sex–occupation. J Chronic Dis 12(4):440–455, 1960

135. Stat Bull Metropol Life Ins Co 60(2):1–15, 1979

136. Stevenson JA, Feleki V, Rechnitzer P: Effect of exercise on coronary tree size in the rat. Circ Res 15(3):265–269, 1964

137. Stone PH, Sherrid M, Cohn K: Correlation of HLA types in premature coronary artery disease: An attempt to define independent genetic risk factors (abstr). Circulation (Suppl II) 59 and 60:46, 1979

138. Stokes T, Wynn V: Serum lipids in women on oral contraceptives. Lancet ii:677–680, 1971

139. Stout RW: The relationship of abnormal circulating insulin levels to atherosclerosis. Atherosclerosis 27:1–13, 1977

140. Syme SL, Hyman MM, Enterline PE: Some social and cultural

factors associated with the occurrence of coronary heart disease. J Chronic Dis 17:277–289, 1964

141. Syme SL: Social and psychological risk factors in coronary heart disease. Mod Concepts Cardiovasc Dis 44(4):17–21, 1975

142. Symposium: Status of fat in food and nutrition. J Am Oil Chem Soc 51:244–264, 1974

143. Taylor HL, Blackburn H, Keys A et al: Five year followup of employees of selected U.S. railroad companies. In Keys A (ed): Coronary Heart Disease in Seven Countries, Circulation (Suppl I) 41:1–20, 1970

144. Taylor HL, Klepetar E, Keys A et al: Death rates among physically active and sedentary employees of the railroad industry. Am J Public Health 52(10):1697–1707, 1962

145. Tepperman J, Pearlmen D: Effects of exercise and anemia on coronary arteries in small animals as revealed by the corrosion-case technique. Circ Res 9(3):576–584, 1961

146. Theorell T, Lind E, Flodérus B: The relationship of disturbing life changes and emotions to the early development of myocardial infarction and other serious illnesses. J Epidemiol 4:281–293, 1975

147. Thiel HG, Parker D, Bruce TA: Stress factors and the risk of myocardial infarction. J Psychosom Res 17:43–57, 1973

148. Thomas AE, MacKay EA, Cutlip MB: A nomograph method for assessing body weight. Am J Clin Nutr 29:302–304, 1976

149. Tyroler HA, Anderson P, Barrett-Connor E et al: Plasma lipid distribution in selected North American populations: The Lipid Research Clinics Program Prevalence Study. Circulation 61(2):302–315, 1980

150. Tyroler HA, Cassel J: Health consequences of culture change. II. Effect of urbanization on coronary heart mortality in rural residents. J Chronic Dis 17:167–177, 1964

151. Vahouny GV, Treadwell CR: Cholesterol: Some aspects of its metabolism and balance in man. In Feldman EB (ed): Nutrition and Cardiovascular Disease, pp 85–116. New York, Appleton-Century-Crofts, 1976

152. Vander AJ, Sherman JH, Luciano DS: Human Physiology, 2nd ed. New York, McGraw-Hill, 1975

153. Walker WJ: Editorial: Changing United States life-style and declining cardiovascular mortality: Cause or coincidence? N Engl J Med 297(3):163–165, 1977

154. Wardell WI, Bahnson CB: Behavioral variables and myocardial infarction in the Southeastern Connecticut Heart Study. J Chronic Dis 26:447–461, 1973

155. Waxler EB, Kimbiris D, Van Den Brock H et al: Myocardial infarction and oral contraceptive agents. Am J Cardiol 28:96–101, 1971

156. Weinberger MH, Collins RD, Dowdy AJ et al: Hypertension induced by oral contraceptives containing estrogen and gestagen. Ann Intern Med 71:891–902, 1969

157. Werkö L: Can we prevent heart disease? Ann Intern Med 74(2):278–288, 1971

158. Wood PD, Haskell W, Klein H et al: The distribution of plasma lipoproteins in middle-aged male runners. Metabolism 25(11):1249–1257, 1976

159. Wynder EL, Hill P: Blood lipids: How normal is normal? Prev Med 1(1–2):161–166, 1972

160. Yano K, Rhoads GG, Kagan A: Coffee, alcohol and risk of coronary heart disease among Japanese men living in Hawaii. N Engl J Med 297:405–409, 1977

161. Zukel WJ, Lewis RH, Enterline PE et al: A short term community study of the epidemiology of coronary heart disease. Am J Public Health 49(12):1630–1639, 1959.

organ and cellular development. Am J Pathol 58(2):185–199, 1970

Capocaccia AM, Conti S, Farchi S et al: Identifying subsets of major risk factors in multivariate estimation of coronary risk. J Chronic Dis 30:557–565, 1977

Castelli WP: CHD risk factors in the elderly. Hosp Pract 11(10):113–121, 1976

Crawford MD, Clayton DG, Stanley F et al: An epidemiologic study of sudden death in hard and soft water areas. J Chronic Dis 30:69–80, 1977

Davignon J: The lipid hypothesis. Arch Surg 113:28–34, 1978

Dayton S, Pearce ML, Hashimoto S et al: A controlled clinical trial of a diet high in unsaturated fat in preventing complications of atherosclerosis. Circulation (Suppl II) 40:1–63, 1969

Dillon D, Seasholtz J: Oral contraceptives and myocardial infarction. Cardiovasc Nurs 15(2):5–9, 1979

Dolder MA, Oliver MF: Myocardial infarction in young men: Study of risk factors in nine countries. Br Heart J 37:493–503, 1975

Elmfeldt D, Wilhelmsen L, Wedel H et al: Primary risk factors in patients with myocardial infarction. Am Heart J 91(4):412–419, 1976

Epstein FH: Hereditary aspects of coronary heart disease. Am Heart J 67(4):445–456, 1964.

Epstein FH: Predicting, explaining, and preventing coronary heart disease. Mod Concepts Cardiovasc Dis 48(2):7–12, 1979

Final Report of the Heart Disease in the Young Study Group. Seattle, American Heart Association of Washington, 1979

Fisher WR, Truitt DH: The common hyperlipoproteinemias. Ann Intern Med 85:497–508, 1976

Fox SM, III, Naughton JP, Gorman PA: Physical activity and cardiovascular health. II. The exercise prescription: Intensity and duration. Mod Concepts Cardiovasc Dis, 41(6):25–30, 1972

Fox SM, III, Naughton JP, Gorman PA: Physical activity and cardiovascular health. III. The exercise prescription: Frequency and type of activity. Mod Concepts Cardiovasc Dis 41(6):25–30, 1971

Frerichs RR, Webber LS, Voors AW et al: Cardiovascular disease risk factor variables in children at two successive years: The Bogalusa Heart Study. J Chronic Dis 32(3):251–262, 1979

Goldstein JL, Hazzard WR, Schrott H et al: Hyperlipidemia in coronary heart disease. J Clin Invest 52:1533–1577, 1973

Gordon T, Kannel WB, Halperin M: Predictability of coronary heart disease. J Chronic Dis 32:427–440, 1979

Gotto AM, Nichols BL, Jr, Scott LW et al: Obesity: Risk factor No. 1. Heart Lung 7(1):132–136, 1978

Havel RJ: Classification of the hyperlipidemias. Ann Rev Med 28:195–209, 1977

Holme I, Helgeland A, Hjermann I et al: Coronary risk factors and socioeconomic status: The Oslo Study. Lancet ii:1396–1398, 1976

Horenstein S: Oral contraceptives, stroke, and related phenomena, Parts I and II. Curr Concepts Cerebrovasc Dis—Stroke 10:25–33, 1975

Hunter S McD, Frerichs RR, Webber LS et al: Social status and cardiovascular disease risk factor variables in children: The Bogalusa Heart Study. J Chronic Dis 32:441–449, 1979

Irey NS, Manion WC, Taylor HB: Vascular lesions in women taking oral contraceptives. Arch Pathol 89:1–8, 1970

Jenkins CD, Zyzanski SJ, Rosenman RH: Risk of myocardial infarction in middle-aged men with manifest coronary heart disease. Circulation 53(2):342–347, 1976

Katz LN: Physical fitness and coronary heart disease. Circulation 35(2):405–414, 1967

Levy RI: Progress toward prevention of cardiovascular diseases. Mod Concepts Cardiovasc Dis 47(10):103–108, 1978

McIntosh HD, Eknoyan G, Jackson D: Hypertension: A potent risk factor. Heart Lung 7(1):137–140, 1978

McIntosh HD, Entman ML, Evans RI et al: Smoking as a risk factor. Heart Lung 7(1):145–149, 1978

McIntosh HD, Stamler J, Jackson D: Introduction to risk factors in coronary heart disease. Heart Lung 7(1):126–131, 1978

Medalie JH, Levene C, Papier C et al: Blood groups, myocardial infarction and angina pectoris among 10,000 adult males. N Engl J Med 285(24):1348–1353, 1971

ADDITIONAL READING

Alexander JK, Fred HL, Wright KE et al: Exercise and coronary artery disease. Heart Lung 7(1):141–144, 1978.

Blackburn H: Coronary risk factors: How to evaluate and manage them. Eur J Cardiol 2(3):249–266, 1975

Bloor CM, Pasyk S, Leon AS: Interaction of age and exercise on

Menotti A, Capocaccia R, Conti S et al: Identifying subsets of major risk factors in multivariate estimation of coronary risk. J Chronic Dis 30:557–565, 1977

Miettinen OS, Neff RK, Jick H: Cigarette smoking and nonfatal myocardial infarction: Rate ratio in relation to age, sex and predisposing conditions. Am J Epidemiol 103:30–36, 1976

Morris JN, Ball KP, Antonis A et al: Controlled trial of soya-bean oil in myocardial infarction. Lancet ii:693–699, 1968

Paul O: Physical activity and coronary heart disease. II. Am J Cardiol 23(2):303–306, 1969

Primary prevention of atherosclerotic diseases. Circulation 42:A84–A87, 1970

Risk factors and coronary disease: A statement for physicians. Circulation 62(2):449A-455A, 1980

Russek HI, Zohman BL: Relative significance of heredity, diet and occupational stress in coronary heart disease of young adults. Am J Med Sci 235(3):266–275, 1958

Salel AF, Fong A, Zelis R et al: Accuracy of numerical coronary profile: Correlation of risk factors with arteriographically documented severity of atherosclerosis. N Engl J Med 296(25):1447–1450, 1977

Salky N, Dugdale M: Platelet abnormalities in ischemic heart disease. Am J Cardiol 32(5):612–617, 1973

Shekelle RB, Shryock AM, Paul O et al: Diet, serum cholesterol, and death from coronary heart disease. N Engl J Med 304:65–70, 1981

Simborg DW: The status of risk factors and coronary heart disease. J Chronic Dis 22:515–552, 1970

Swyer GIM: The pharmacologic action of oral contraceptives. In Wrong O (ed): Fourth Symposium on the Advancement of Medicine, p 165. London, Pitman, 1968

Tomanek RJ: Effects of age and exercise on the extent of the myocardial capillary bed. Anat Rec 167(1):55–62, 1970

White JR, Froeb HF: Small-airways dysfunction in nonsmokers chronically exposed to tobacco smoke. N Engl J Med 302(13):720–723, 1980

SECTION B
ASSESSMENT

14

History-Taking and Physical Examination of the Patient with Cardiovascular Disease

SANDRA L. UNDERHILL, R.N., M.N.

This chapter is not meant to be a complete guide to history-taking or to physical examination. Although emphasis is placed upon the general techniques that are important for the nurse to acquire, the rationale for in-depth assessment skills is also discussed.

Competence in obtaining a history and in performing a physical examination cannot be achieved simply by reading the material presented. It is vitally important to become actively involved in clinical assessment, ideally with a qualified nurse or physician who can provide guidance through a preceptorship. Many hours of practice are required before the beginning learner becomes skilled in assessment techniques.

NURSING ASSESSMENT

A nursing assessment includes both history-taking and a physical examination. A complete assessment should begin upon the patient's admission to the emergency room or cardiac care unit (CCU). Because of emergency conditions, the history may need to be completed over the next several shifts, but the physical examination should be accomplished as soon as possible after the patient is admitted and repeated at frequent intervals thereafter. The nursing assessment differs from the medical assessment in terms of identifying the patient's problems and establishing goals and a workable plan of care. Rather than concentrating on a pathophysiologic problem (such as congestive heart failure) that is the concern of the physician, the nurse should be concerned mainly with those problems that interfere with the patient's ability to carry out activities of daily living. Such a problem might be shortness of breath. This does not imply that a knowledge of the underlying medical problem is not important. In critical care settings, the nurse should be able to elicit pertinent histories and interpret physiologic findings in order to be of benefit to the patient. It is always important to include the medical regime in the patient's overall plan of care. However, whereas the medical goal is to cure the disease, the nursing goal is to help the patient and family* to cope with the illness.

Nursing Process

The nursing process consists of five components: assessment, diagnosis, prescription, implementation, and evaluation.[20] In order for nursing problems to be correctly diagnosed and treated it is imperative that the assessment be both complete and accurate.

According to Little and Carnevali, there are four criteria for developing a nursing assessment. First, the information obtained must allow the nurse to begin immediately to plan realistic, individualized nursing care. Next, the care plan must be applicable to a particular setting, for example, the nursing care delivered in the CCU. Third, the assessment should be gathered in a reasonable length of time. Last, the data gathered by the nurse should not duplicate information collected by others unless their information is obtained too late to be useful to the nurse planning care, or if the focus of the interviewing is different.[20]

---

* Family also refers to others with whom the patient has a close relationship.

Problem-Oriented Nursing Records

For any assessment to be useful, it must be systematically charted. Weed suggests recording *subjective* information first (what the patient tells you; for example, his symptoms), followed by *objective* data (what you observe about the patient; for example, physical findings and laboratory results).[32] To complete Weed's problem-oriented medical records (POMR) approach, *analysis* and *planning* should also be included.

The acronym SOAP (subjective, objective, analysis, and plan) is often used to indicate the four steps of the POMR. The title of the problem heads the SOAP format but is actually written after the first three components are completed. Initially, the title of the problem is an abnormal physiologic or laboratory finding, or a symptom—for example, chest pain for 24 hours. This is later replaced by the confirmed diagnosis—for example, acute anterior myocardial infarction (MI). This POMR method of charting is designed for use during the initial assessment and in subsequent progress notes. However, it is medically oriented. In order for the nursing process to be implemented, the SOAPE format, which includes *evaluation* of the plan, should be used. This format is appropriate for problem-oriented nursing records, which includes the initial assessment and nursing notes.

TAKING A CARDIOVASCULAR HISTORY

It is important that the nurses working in CCUs understand how to obtain both medical and nursing histories.

Medical history taking is divided into three main areas:

- The patient's chief complaint (CC)
- The history of the present illness (PI)
- The past medical history (PH)

The medical history obtained by the nurse in the CCU does not necessarily need to be complete but must provide enough data to make informed clinical judgments. If physicians are present on admission and take the medical history, the nurse's responsibilities are to be aware of the data collected, validate her own findings and compare episodes of the same symptoms that occur during hospitalization in the CCU with the patient's previous experiences. However, the nursing history cannot be taken from the medical data base and must be gathered by the nurse from the patient or family, or both.

Chief Complaint

The chief complaint is the reason why the patient came to the hospital and represents his priority for treatment. It should be recorded within quotation marks exactly as stated. The chief complaint should also indicate duration, for example, "shortness of breath for one week."

Occasionally a patient may have more than one chief complaint. These should be listed in order of importance to the patient. If the patient has more than three chief complaints, they should be recorded with the history of the present illness.[12,21]

History of the Present Illness

To describe history-taking, a sample symptom, chest pain, will be used throughout. Obtaining the history of the present illness starts with a more detailed discussion of the chief complaint, for example, "Tell me more about your chest pain." There is a wide range in patients' abilities to express thoughts accurately, chronologically, and succinctly. Some patients need guidance more than others. Listen to the patient. It is best to let him tell his story in the most comfortable manner. However, patients who appear to be rambling need to be redirected by clarifying or leading questions.

The information that must be obtained when describing any symptom is: the time and manner of onset, duration, frequency, location, quality, quantity, setting, associated phenomena, and alleviating or aggravating factors. Pertinent negative answers should also be listed.[12,21]

The *time of onset* should be recorded when possible with both the date and time, for example, "9:00 P.M. on December 22nd." The *manner of onset* is the factor, or factors, which usually precipitates the symptom; for instance, "chest pain brought about by an unusually heavy meal." *Frequency and duration* should be stated specifically rather than generally. A response such as "I have the chest pain a lot of the time" has meaning only to the patient. "Once a week," "once a day," or "more than three times a day" provides much more information. Likewise, a response that "the pain lasts just a short time" is subjective and should be restated as, for example, "2 minutes," "15 minutes," or "1 hour."

The patient describes the *exact location* of the symptom by pointing to it with one finger. If the pain radiates, the patient should trace its path with a finger tip. The *quality* of a symptom refers to its unique properties, such as color, appearance, and texture. Pain, the most common symptom of cardiovascular disease, is so subjective that its quality is particularly difficult to describe. Thus, it is important to use the patient's own words in quotation marks whenever possible. Terms such as sharp, dull, stabbing, burning, aching, crushing, or throbbing are frequently used. To better understand the meaning of the quality of the symptoms to the patient, his response to it should be recorded: for example, "It makes me stop what I'm doing and sit down," or "I can continue my activities without stopping."

Quantity refers to the size, extent, or amount of the symptoms. The quantity of chest pain is described in terms of its severity. Again, this is extremely subjective and might best be rated on a five-point scale, ranging from "barely noticeable" (1) to "worst pain ever" (5).

The *setting* is used to describe the patient's whereabouts and whether he was alone, with someone else, or always in the presence of the same person. This information may be useful later in counseling or teaching a patient to develop greater insight into the development of symptoms.

The patient should be asked if any other symptoms are associated with the chief complaint. For example, palpitations and dizziness might always precede the chest pain. If he mentions associated symptoms, these should be described in the same manner as the chief complaint. It is also important to note whether they are always associated with the chief complaint and whether they occur independently, at other times.

Factors that improve the symptom, for instance, resting, changing position, or taking medication, should be noted. Likewise, conditions that make the chief complaint worse, for example, eating, exercise, or a cold climate, must also be recorded. These factors can provide helpful diagnostic information. To complete the present illness history, it is also important to record any negative responses to the interviewer's questions, for example, "The pain is not made worse by strenuous exercise."

Past Medical History

The past medical history is divided into two sections: personal and family. The personal history includes past illnesses, allergies, immunizations, habits, social history, and medications taken regularly. Usual childhood diseases, injuries, operations, or other major illnesses should be recorded under past illnesses. When discussing childhood diseases, the cardiac nurse should specifically question the patient about streptococcal infection and the possibility of rheumatic fever. The major illnesses that should be specifically asked about are previous chest pain or heart attack, high blood pressure, chronic obstructive airway disease, diabetes mellitus, or bleeding disorders.

Any allergic reaction, for example, to drugs, food, environmental agents, or animals, should also be noted. The examiner should always ask if the patient has an allergy to penicillin. The cardiac nurse should also inquire about allergic reactions to emergency drugs commonly used in the CCU, such as lidocaine hydrochloride and morphine sulfate. Both the allergen and the reaction should always be noted, because some patients confuse an allergic reaction with a drug's side effect. Alcohol, drug, and tobacco habits must also be recorded. The smoking history should always be known prior to oxygen administration and recorded as the number of pack-years (packs per day multiplied by the number of years) the patient has smoked.

Social history includes marital status, number of children, occupation, and hobbies. Any other pertinent life-style pattern can also be noted here, for example, particular dietary habits. It is important that all prescription and over-the-counter drugs that the patient takes be known. If the patient has brought his medication with him, these can be sent to the pharmacy for verification and safe-keeping.

A family history is taken to determine the health status of the patient's immediate family (parents, siblings, and children). Notations regarding the age and health status of each family member are made: living and well, deceased, and the possible or confirmed diagnosis, now or at death. This information can be written into the health record or outlined on a family tree.[12,21]

Functional and Therapeutic Classification

After the medical history is completed, it may be possible to categorize the patient according to the New York Heart Association's functional and therapeutic classification (Table 14-1).[23] This classification may be helpful in the management of the patient's activities.

Nursing History

The format for obtaining a nursing history is not standardized as is that for obtaining a medical history. Most hospitals have developed a style that is appropriate to their needs. There may be as many varied history forms as there are number of hospitals.

Whatever the format, the four major content areas that must be included in any nursing history are:[20]

- Identifying information
- The patient's perception of coping challenges
- Resources and support systems
- Functional assessment

Table 14-2 presents a suggested nursing assessment format.

TABLE 14.1 FUNCTIONAL AND THERAPEUTIC CLASSIFICATIONS OF PATIENTS WITH DISEASES OF THE HEART

New York Heart Association

Functional Classification		Therapeutic Classification	
Class I.	Patients with cardiac disease but without resulting limitations of physical activity. Ordinary physical activity does not cause undue fatigue, palpitation, dyspnea, or anginal pain.	Class A.	Patients with cardiac disease whose physical activity need not be restricted in any way.
Class II.	Patients with cardiac disease resulting in slight limitation of physical activity. They are comfortable at rest. Ordinary physical activity results in fatigue, palpitation, dyspnea, or anginal pain.	Class B.	Patients with cardiac disease whose ordinary physical activity need not be restricted, but who should be advised against severe or competitive efforts.
Class III.	Patients with cardiac disease resulting in marked limitation of physical activity. They are comfortable at rest. Less than ordinary physical activity causes fatigue, palpitation, dyspnea, or anginal pain.	Class C.	Patients with cardiac disease whose ordinary physical activity should be moderately restricted, and whose more strenuous efforts should be discontinued.
Class IV.	Patients with cardiac disease resulting in inability to carry on any physical activity without discomfort. Symptoms of cardiac insufficiency or of the anginal syndrome may be present even at rest. If any physical activity is undertaken, discomfort is increased.	Class D.	Patients with cardiac disease whose ordinary physical activity should be markedly restricted.
		Class E.	Patients with cardiac disease who should be at complete rest, confined to bed or chair.

TABLE 14.2   SAMPLE NURSING ASSESSMENT FORM

Name _____ Age _____ Date _____
Prefers to be called _____ Assessment Made by: _____ RN

Areas	Subjective/Objective Data
Patient Perceptions of Current health status Goals Needed/usable services	
Functional Abilities Breathing/circulation Elimination Emotional/cognitive Mobility/safety Nutrition Hygiene/grooming Sensory input Sexuality Sleep/rest	
Resources and Support Systems Environmental Personal/social Other	

Identifying Information. The patient's name, the name he prefers to be called by, his age and birth date, admission date, and date and time of the interview are all recorded under identification of the patient. Some of this information may be obtained from the medical history. The nurse obtaining the history should also be identified on the form.

The Patient's Perception of Coping Challenges. The patient's appreciation of his current health status as either good or bad is helpful in assessing how he views its effect upon his daily living. For example, a 42-year-old man with an old anterior MI is admitted to the CCU. His chief complaint is extreme fatigue that prevents him from working a full 8-hour day at the office. The medical investigation initially focuses upon ruling out any new process affecting the adequacy of cardiac output (CO), such as a left ventricular aneurysm. The nursing approach centers upon non-pathophysiologic causes for fatigue, for example, fear of over-stressing his heart and dying suddenly, changes in the work situation, family difficulties, or any other reason to be depressed.

Being aware of the patient's goals in terms of his health and life-style are important in determining whether his expectations are realistic. "What do you see yourself doing three months from now?" is a good way to ask the patient to define his goal. Another approach is ascertaining what changes he would be willing to make in his life if he was unable to achieve his plan.

One must understand what the expectations of health care are for the patient. For example, is the patient with unstable angina pectoris who has been admitted for "tests" able to explain what the tests are for and how they are done?

Communication between the medical team and the nursing staff is essential prior to planning any teaching.

Resources and Support Systems. It is important to consider the patient's support system when planning nursing care: environmental resources, such as the proximity to the hospital; personal–social support, such as a spouse to provide home care; and economic support, such as an adequate pension, are all examples. Needed resources that are not readily available must also be considered.

Functional Assessment. The functional assessment of the patient's ability to perform activities of daily living (ADLs) within his own life-style provides much of the data necessary to plan nursing care for the acutely ill patient. Table 14-2 provides a complete list of the areas to be assessed. Although all are important, the CCU nurse must first assess those items concerned with the heart and cardiac output. Both subjective and objective assessments are ideally obtained at the same time. However, in acute situations, physical assessment (which is discussed in great detail later in the chapter) takes priority over the nursing history. The extent of the nursing history obtained depends in large part upon the physical and emotional readiness of the patient to answer questions. A few pertinent medically oriented questions may be all that time permits.

To facilitate the gathering of subjective information for a cardiovascular nursing history, examples of questions to ask the patient follow. However, it is important to phrase questions according to the appropriateness of the situation and to pursue logically areas where further clarification is necessary.

1. Breathing.
   - Are you ever short of breath?
   - When do you become short of breath?
   - How do you make your breathing better?
   - What makes it worse?
   - How long has breathing been a problem?
   - What activities are necessary for you to do that you are no longer able to do because of your breathing?
   - Are you on any medication?
   - What time of day do you prefer to take your medication or treatment?
2. Circulation. These symptoms could be examined using the same types of questions listed above:
   - Chest pain
   - Weight gain or loss
   - Swelling in the hands, feet, or legs
   - Dizziness
   - Fatigue
   - Palpitations
   - Manifestations of high blood pressure
   - Coldness in hands or feet in warm weather
3. Urination.
   - Is the amount of your urine output normal for you?
   - Do you ever have to get up at night to use the bathroom?
   - How many times?
   - When did you notice a change?
   - Do you take a water pill?
   - When do you take it?
4. Mentation.
   - Do you think as fast as you used to? As clearly?
   - Do you laugh or cry more easily than before?
   - When did you notice the change?
   - Are you taking any medication that might affect your thinking?

If the patient is able, the foregoing areas should be more completely assessed for problems other than those of a cardiovascular nature. Additionally, other functional abilities must also be assessed. Before finishing the nursing history, or after each interviewing period, it is important to ask "Is there anything that I have not covered that you would like to tell me about?" This allows the patient the opportunity to reveal anything else that comes to mind.

PERFORMING A CARDIOVASCULAR PHYSICAL EXAMINATION

Every qualified CCU nurse should be able to perform a basic cardiovascular physical examination. Nurses spend 24 hours a day with patients and are, therefore, in a good position to identify changes in the patient's condition. It is to the patient's benefit to detect changes early, before serious complications develop. The CCU nurse who telephones a physician to report that the patient "Just does not look good"

lacks the credibility of the nurse who identifies "A new S_3 gallop, bilateral crackles half way up the lung fields posteriorly and jugular vein distention of 14 centimeters (cm)."

A cardiovascular physical assessment should include an evaluation of the following items:
- The heart as a pump
- Filling volumes and pressures
- Cardiac output (CO)
- Compensatory mechanisms

Factors that reflect a *reduced contractility* are reduced pulse pressure, cardiac enlargement, and presence of murmurs and gallop rhythms.

Filling volumes and pressures are estimated by the degree of jugular vein distention (JVD), and the presence or absence of crackles, peripheral edema, and postural changes in blood pressure (BP).

Cardiac output is reflected by heart rate (HR), pulse pressure, peripheral vascular resistance (PVR), urine output, and central nervous system manifestations.

An example of a *compensatory mechanism* is an increased filling volume.

After the initial assessment in the CCU, a physical examination should be done routinely along with vital signs, at least every four hours. The order of examination precedes logically from head to toe:

1. General appearance
2. Blood pressure
3. Pulse
4. Hand
5. Head and neck
6. Precordium
7. Posterior chest
8. Abdomen
9. Feet and legs

With practice, this assessment can be done in approximately 10 minutes.

General Appearance

The patient is observed to be either in acute distress or not in acute distress (NAD). Level of consciousness should be noted and described. Appropriateness of thought content, reflecting the adequacy of cerebral perfusion, is particularly important to evaluate. Family members who are most familiar with the patient can be of help in alerting the examiner to subtle behavioral changes. The nurse should also be aware of the patient's anxiety level, not only to attempt to put him more at ease, but to realize its effects upon the cardiovascular system.

Blood Pressure

Equipment. Systemic arterial BP is measured indirectly, using a stethoscope and a sphygmomanometer. Any stethoscope that is in good condtion can be used. A sphygmomanometer consists of a manometer, an inflatable bag inside a pressure cuff, and a bulb attached to the bag for inflation. The cuff must fit the extremity properly in order for accurate measurements to be obtained. The BP cuff should be approximately 20% wider than the diameter of the limb (usually an arm), and should be long enough to encircle it. Normal-sized adults can use an arm cuff 12 cm to 14 cm in width and 30 cm in length. Pediatric cuffs, which are available in various widths, should be used for patients who have very thin arms. Cuffs that are too narrow will reflect a falsely elevated BP. Conversely, falsely low readings are obtained from cuffs that are too wide. The inflatable bag should be long enough to go half way around the arm.[2,18]

A manometer is attached to the inflatable bag. There are two types of manometers: mercury and aneroid. The mercury type, which is the most reliable, can be mounted either on a portable stand or on the wall above the bed or table. A reservoir of mercury (Hg) is attached to the bottom of the manometer, which is calibrated in millimeters (mm). In response to pressure exerted upon the bulb, mercury rises vertically in the manometer. As pressure is released from the bag, the column of mercury falls and BP can be measured in mm Hg. It is important that the meniscus of the mercury be at eye level when the BP is measured. The BP reading should be taken at the top of the meniscus. If the wall mounting is too high or the portable stand too low, errors in BP determinations will be made.

The aneroid type has a round gauge calibrated in mm Hg, or torr,* and affixed to the BP cuff. Advantages of the aneroid sphygmomanometer are that it is easily seen, conveniently portable, and with the cuff, comprises one unit. Unfortunately, the calibration of the dial frequently becomes inaccurate. It is important before each use to check that the indicator needle is pointing to the zero mark on the dial. If the needle is either below or above this mark, the BP reading will be incorrect by that number of torr. These sphygmomanometers should be recalibrated by qualified personnel yearly and as needed.

Technique for Obtaining BP by Palpation. The deflated cuff is placed snugly around the arm, with the bag covering the inner aspect of the arm and the brachial artery. The lower margin of the cuff should be 2.5 cm above the antecubital space. As long as the patient's arm is at heart level, the BP can be determined with the patient in any position. Errors up to 10 mm Hg, both systolic and diastolic, can be made if the arm is not at the correct level: Falsely elevated pressures are obtained if the arm is lower than the heart; falsely low pressures are measured if the arm is higher than the heart. The arm must be supported during pressure determination. The patient's position should always be recorded; symbols such as those shown in Figure 14-1 are frequently used. On the initial examination, the BP should be recorded in both arms. Subsequently, the arm with the highest BP should be used. One should also indicate whether the BP was taken in the right arm (RA) or left arm (LA).

After the cuff is in place, the brachial artery is palpated continuously. Once the brachial pulse is obtained, the cuff is inflated rapidly. The pressure at which the pulse disappears should be noted, but the cuff inflation should continue for another 30 mm Hg before the actual measurement of the BP begins. For example, if the brachial pulse disappears

* 1 torr = 1 mm Hg

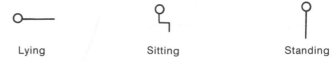

Fig. 14-1. Record of a patient's position during blood pressure determination.

when the cuff pressure is 110 mm Hg, the cuff should be pumped to 140 mm Hg before starting. The cuff should not be inflated further than necessary, because high cuff pressures are extremely uncomfortable, create undue anxiety in the patient, and tend to raise the patient's BP. The pressure in the cuff should be reduced gradually by 2 to 3 mm Hg per second. The point at which the brachial pulse is first detected on expiration is the systolic BP. Diastolic BP cannot be determined accurately by this method.[13] Once measurement is made, the cuff should be deflated rapidly. There should be a minimum of 1 to 2 minutes before the BP is measured again in order to release venous blood.[18]

Systolic BP is measured by palpation in patients whose BPs cannot be heard, for example, patients in shock. It is also useful when checking BPs frequently, for instance, every 1 to 2 minutes. Palpated BPs are charted using P as diastolic pressure, for example, 90/P.

Technique for Obtaining BP by Auscultation. Preparation of the patient and use of the BP apparatus are identical in the auscultatory method. After the brachial pulse has been located, the diaphragm of the stethoscope is applied firmly over the artery, using light pressure. Heavy pressure might partially occlude the artery, creating turbulence in the blood flow, prolonging phase IV (see below), and falsely lowering the diastolic BP. Care must be taken to avoid causing extraneous noise, for example, the stethoscope touching the cuff or any other material.

There are five sounds that are heard when auscultating the BP, called Korotkov sounds (Table 14-3). These sounds are created by constriction of the BP cuff, which causes turbulence of blood flow within the vessel (Fig. 14-2). Korotkov sounds are heard after each heart beat. Systolic pressure is recorded at the highest point at which two consecutive beats are heard on expiration (phase I). In adults, diastolic pressure is equated with the *disappearance* of Korotkov sounds (phase V).[22] Muffling of sound (phase IV), which for many years was considered to represent diastolic BP, can also be recorded between the systolic and diastolic values, but must not be used as the diastolic pressure. Pressures are recorded as either 120/70 or 120/80/70.

A preliminary palpable pressure should be obtained prior to auscultation to avoid the auscultatory gap. In the auscultatory gap, which occurs more commonly in hypertensive patients, sounds indicating the true systolic pressure fade away in phase II and reappear at a lower pressure point (Fig. 14-3). If the cuff has not been inflated 30 mm Hg beyond the palpable pressure, the listener may hear the systolic pressure at a point below the auscultatory gap (the beginning of phase III) and record an erroneously low systolic pressure.

"Normal" BP for adults less than 45 years of age in our society ranges from 110 to 140 mm Hg systolic and 65 to

TABLE 14.3 PHASES OF KOROTKOV SOUNDS

Phase	Sound	Recorded as
I	First appearance of faint, clear tapping sounds that gradually increase in intensity	Systolic BP
II	Sounds assume a swishing or murmurlike quality.	
III	Sounds become crisper and increase in intensity.	
IV	Distinct muffling abruptly occurs, and the sounds become soft and blowing.	
V	Disappearance of sounds	Diastolic BP

(Kirkendall WM, Burton AC, Epstein FH et al: Recommendations for Human Blood Pressure Determination by Sphygmomanometers. New York, American Heart Association, 1967)

95 mm Hg diastolic. However, there is a wide physiologic variation. After a baseline BP is obtained, changes in the BP should be compared with that individual's normal pressure.[24]

Determination of Pulse Pressure. The pulse pressure is the difference between systolic and diastolic pressure (Fig. 14-4). For example, a patient with a BP of 120/70 mm Hg has a pulse pressure of 50 mm Hg. Pulse pressure reflects stroke volume (SV), ejection velocity, and (PVR).

Pulse pressure is increased in many situations. A widened pulse pressure is seen in sinus bradycardia, complete heart block, aortic regurgitation, anxiety, exercise, and catecholamine infusion, which are examples of situations characterized by increased SV. Examples of conditions that increase pulse pressure by reducing PVR are fever, hot environment, and exercise. Conditions such as atherosclerosis, aging, and high blood pressure widen the pulse pressure because of decreased distensibility of the aorta, arteries, and arterioles. A narrowed pulse pressure can also be caused by many factors: reduced ejection velocity in congestive heart failure,

shock, and hypovolemia; mechanical obstruction to systolic outflow in aortic stenosis, mitral stenosis, and mitral insufficiency; peripheral vasoconstriction in shock and with certain drugs; and artifactually from an auscultatory gap.[24]

Determination of Postural BP Changes. Postural (orthostatic) hypotension occurs when the BP drops after an upright position is assumed and is usually accompanied by dizziness, lightheadedness, or syncope. Although there are many causes of postural hypotension, only three will be discussed here: saline depletion, inadequate vasoconstrictor mechanisms and autonomic insufficiency. Saline depletion is thoroughly discussed in Chapter 9.

- However, it must be stressed that a frequently overlooked cause of saline depletion in the CCU patient is diuretic therapy. Any CCU patient receiving diuretics should be assessed for a postural BP drop daily or before each diuretic dose.

- If saline depletion is present but has not been detected, and nitroglycerin, or any other vasodilating agent, is administered, syncope and cardiac arrest could occur.

Inadequate vasoconstrictor mechanisms can occur independently or as part of the syndrome of primary autonomic insufficiency. For years, prolonged bed rest has been thought to contribute to inadequate vasoconstriction although this recently has been questioned (see Chap. 30). Other causes of inadequate vasoconstrictor mechanisms are vasovagal reactions, sympathectomy, diseases of the central and peripheral nervous system, and carotid sinus syncope.[1]

Postural changes in BP can help the clinician differentiate saline depletion or inadequate vasoconstrictor mechanisms from the syndrome of primary autonomic insufficiency.

Blood pressure is always checked first with the patient lying down. He should be supine and as flat as possible for at least 10 minutes. This allows any BP changes that have occurred in the upright posture or during exercise to return to baseline. Both BP and apical HR are recorded. Without removing the cuff, the patient is then asked to sit on the edge of the bed with his feet dangling. Any symptoms, such

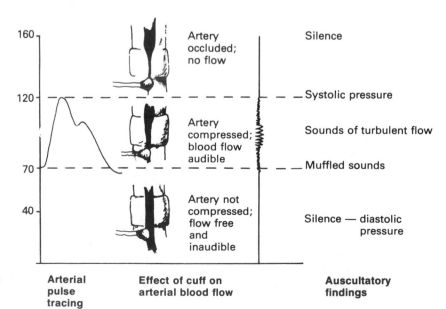

Fig. 14-2. Auscultation of the blood pressure. (Adapted from Bates B: A Guide to Physical Examination, 2nd ed, p 179. Philadelphia, JB Lippincott, 1979)

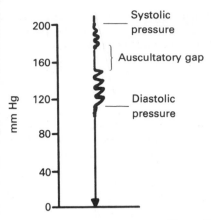

Fig. 14-3. Auscultatory gap. (Bates B: A Guide to Physical Examination, 2nd ed, p 181. Philadelphia, JB Lippincott, 1979)

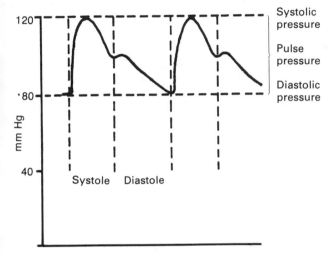

Fig. 14-4. Pulse pressure. (Bates B: A Guide to Physical Examination, 2nd ed, p 173. Philadelphia, JB Lippincott, 1979)

as dizziness or lightheadedness, are noted. If the patient is prevented from remaining upright by his symptoms, he must be allowed to return to bed without completing the test. If he is able to continue, wait 1 to 3 minutes before rechecking *both* BP and HR. The reflex mechanism that maintains BP in the upright position should equilibrate the pressure within that period. One should make certain that the patient's arm is at heart level and that the cuff has not slipped out of position. If necessary, this same procedure is repeated in the standing position.

Normal postural responses are an increased HR[7] usually by 15%;[30] variable systolic BP changes, ranging from slight[28] to a 15-mm Hg drop;[12] and diastolic BP changes ranging from a 5-mm Hg-or-less decrease[12] to a 5-to-10 mm Hg increase.[28] However, mean arterial BP is thought to vary by less than 10 mm Hg.[30] The increase in HR helps to offset the reduced SV and to maintain the CO.

Saline depletion should be suspected (in the presence of an appropriate history) when, in response to sitting or standing, the HR increases and either the diastolic BP drops by 10 mm Hg or the systolic pressure decreases by 15 mm Hg.

The systolic drop is more important if the diastolic pressure is difficult to hear.[28] Some authorities do not state

a specific HR increase,[7,28,30] whereas others feel that an increase of 20 beats per minute is necessary to diagnose saline depletion.[3,26]

It is difficult to differentiate saline depletion from inadequate vasoconstrictor mechanisms. With the latter, the HR again responds appropriately, but because of diminished peripheral vasoconstriction, both the systolic and diastolic BP drop.

Following is an example of a postural BP recording showing either saline depletion or inadequate vasoconstrictor mechanisms:

BP	HR	
120/70	70	o—
100/55	90	⚲
98/52	94	⚲

In autonomic insufficiency, the HR is unable to increase to compensate for the gravitational effects of upright posture.[7] Peripheral vasoconstriction may be diminished or may not occur at all. The presence of autonomic insufficiency does not rule out concurrent saline depletion.

Following is an example of autonomic insufficiency as demonstrated by a postural BP drop:

BP	HR	
150/90	60	o—
100/60	60	⚲

Determination of Paradoxical BP. Paradoxical BP is an exaggerated decrease in the systolic BP upon inspiration. The mechanism is complex and controversial. Normally, during inspiration, blood flow into the right heart is increased, right ventricular output is enhanced, and pulmonary venous capacitance is increased, resulting in less blood reaching the left ventricle. This reduces left ventricular SV by approximately 7% and arterial pressure by approximately 3%.[27]

During cardiac tamponade, effects of respiration on both right and left ventricular filling appear to be greater than normal, causing a reduction of 10 mm Hg or more in systolic pressure during inspiration (Fig. 14-5). It has also been suggested that this finding may be due to an increase in intrapericardial pressure as a result of augmented right

Fig. 14-5. Paradoxical blood pressure in cardiac tamponade. The paradox is greater than 20 mm Hg. (After Fowler NO: Examination of the Heart, Part 2. Inspection and Palpation of Venous and Arterial Pulses, p 33. New York, American Heart Association, 1972, by permission of the American Heart Association, Inc.)

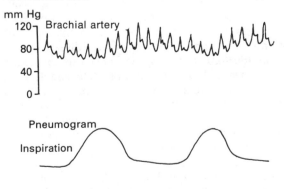

ventricular filling within the taut pericardial sac.[6,29] However, other authorities found that cardiac tamponade does not interfere with the normal inspiratory fall in intrapericardial pressure.[29]

Another theory, supported by echocardiography, is that selective left ventricular impairment during inspiration occurs. There appears to be a shift of the interventricular septum toward the left ventricle in tamponade as a result of overdistention of the right ventricle.[11,17]

Chronic obstructive airway disease, constrictive pericarditis, pulmonary emboli, restrictive cardiomyopathy, and cardiogenic shock have also been associated with an abnormal inspiratory decline of BP. Echocardiographic studies of patients with emphysema demonstrate both an augmented inspiratory filling of the right ventricle as well as an exaggerated inspiratory decline of left ventricular filling.[11]

The patient should breathe normally and must not exaggerate his respiratory effort during an examination for a paradoxical BP. As before, one should inflate and gradually deflate the cuff until the first systolic sound is heard on expiration and continue slowly releasing the cuff pressure until sounds are heard both on inspiration and expiration. The difference between the two is termed the paradox, and normally is less than 10 mm Hg.[2,9]

For example, if the first systolic sound occurs at 140 mm Hg during expiration and Korotkov sounds begin appearing with both inspiration and expiration at 120 mm Hg, the paradox is 20 mm Hg. Paradoxical BPs should be determined as a baseline in all CCU patients and routinely in all patients with pericarditis or with heart catheters, such as a temporary pacing wire.

The Effect of Arrhythmias on BP Determination. Any arrhythmia that alters SV and CO can be detected during BP measurement. Because of decreased diastolic filling time, *premature ectopic beats* usually have a smaller SV than do normal sinus beats. If there is a compensatory pause following the early ectopic impulse, the postextrasystolic beat has an even greater SV because of the extra diastolic filling time.

In *bigeminal rhythms,* as the BP cuff is deflated, Korotkov sounds of the alternate strong beats are heard first and are half as fast as the HR. Further reduction in cuff pressure enables the listener also to hear the alternating weaker sounds produced by the ectopic impulses.

True *pulsus alternans,* indicative of severe organic heart disease and left heart failure, is also manifested by alternating strong and weak pulses, but with a regular cadence. It is detected in the same manner. Pulsus alternans can occur with ectopic bigeminal rhythms that are on time and interpolated rather than premature, and in this instance does not necessarily indicate severe organic disease.[24]

In *atrial fibrillation,* the SV is constantly changing, resulting in a beat-to-beat variation in systolic and diastolic pressure. Blood pressure readings in atrial fibrillation should be noted as only approximate.[18,24]

Ventricular tachycardia can also be detected during BP auscultation. Many patients are, of course, too ill for this maneuver; but, rarely, a patient will have stable ventricular tachycardia. In ventricular tachycardia, an occasional well-timed atrial contraction contributes to diastolic ventricular filling. This atrial kick augments the SV for that beat. As

the cuff is deflated, the systolic pressure is periodically increased. For the same reason, this finding is also present in *complete heart block,* but the rate of the Korotkov sounds is much slower.

Radial Pulse

The radial pulse should be assessed for quality and rate. One must become familiar with the *normal pulse contour* (Fig. 14-6A) before appreciating abnormal pulse waves. Normally, the upstroke of the pulse is rapid and smooth, and the dicrotic notch is not palpable.

Small, weak pulses (Fig. 14-6B) have a diminished pulse pressure, which is indicative of a reduced SV and ejection fraction and of increased PVR.

Large, bounding pulses result in an increase of pulse pressure (Fig. 14-6C). Increased pulse pressure is caused by increased SV and ejection velocity and by diminished peripheral vasoconstriction. (Refer to the description of pulse pressure in the preceding section on BP.)

In *pulsus alternans,* strong pulse waves alternate with weak ones (Fig. 14-6D). Note that the cadence of the rhythm is regular.

Bigeminal pulses (Fig. 14-6E), which should not be confused with pulsus alternans, are caused by a bigeminal, premature ectopic rhythm. Note that every other pulse wave is not only diminished, but is also early. (Refer to the discussion of the effects of arrhythmias upon BP in the preceding section.)

Fig. 14-6. Normal and abnormal pulses. (**A**) Normal; (**B**) small and weak; (**C**) large and bounding; (**D**) pulsus alternans; (**E**) bigeminal; (**F**) pulsus paradoxus. (Bates B: A Guide to Physical Examination, 2nd ed, p 185. Philadelphia, JB Lippincott, 1979)

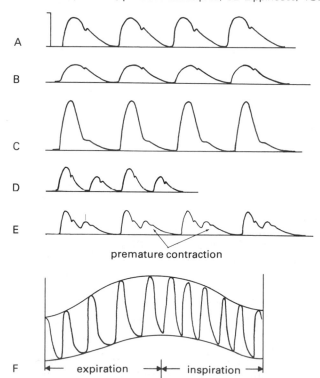

premature contraction

F |← expiration →|← inspiration →|

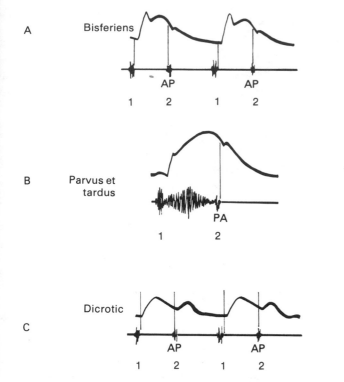

A Bisferiens

AP AP

1 2 1 2

B Parvus et tardus

PA

1 2

Dicrotic

C

AP AP

1 2 1 2

Fig. 14-7. Double pulses. **(A)** Pulsus bisferiens (AP indicates that aortic valve closure precedes pulmonic valve closure). **(B)** Pulsus parvus et tardus (PA indicates that pulmonic valve closure precedes aortic valve closure). **(C)** Dicrotic. (After Hurst JW, Schlant RC: In Hurst JW, Logue RB, Schlant RC et al, (eds): The Heart, 4th ed, pp 188–189. New York, McGraw-Hill, 1978)

Pulsus paradoxus (Fig. 14-6F) is the reduction in strength of the arterial pulse that can be felt during abnormal inspiratory decline of left ventricular filling. However, it is more apparent and can be quantified if sphygmomanometry is used. (Refer to the discussion of the determination of paradoxical BP.)

There are three types of double pulse beats: pulsus bisferiens, pulsus parvus et tardus (anacrotic), and dicrotic. *Pulsus bisferiens* (Fig. 14-7A) is characterized by a rapid upstroke and double systolic peak. This pulse may be present in idiopathic hypertrophic subaortic stenosis, aortic stenosis with regurgitation, and pure aortic insufficiency. *Pulsus parvus et tardus* (Fig. 14-7B) is found in severe aortic stenosis. It resembles the double systolic beat in pulsus bisferiens, but its upstroke is more gradual and the pulse pressure is smaller. Usually it is palpable only in the carotid artery. When the pulse is *dicrotic* (Fig. 14-7C), the pulse waves are palpable during both systole and diastole. It can usually be felt in peripheral arteries as well as in the carotid artery. A dicrotic pulse is associated with reduced PVR and low diastolic pressure, the latter two also being associated with fever.[17]

The HR can be determined by counting the radial pulse. If the rhythm is regular, the HR can be counted for 15 seconds and multiplied by four to determine the rate per minute. If it is irregular, the pulse should be counted both apically and radially for a full minute. By auscultating the

heart and palpating the radial pulse at the same time, the examiner can determine if all cardiac contractions are perfused peripherally. Those that are not perfused are usually premature, without adequate SV. Apical–radial differences, commonly occurring in atrial fibrillation and with premature ventricular contractions, must be recorded. If the difference is very large, it is helpful to have two people count for the same minute.

Hand

The color of the hand is noted first. Cyanosis, a blue tint that occurs when at least 5 g of hemoglobin become desaturated, can be either peripheral or central.

Peripheral cyanosis can be detected easily in the nailbeds of light-skinned individuals, but it may be more difficult to detect in those with darker skin. Peripheral cyanosis implies that because of reduced blood flow in the periphery, more time is available for the tissues to extract oxygen from the hemoglobin molecule, widening the arteriovenous oxygen difference. It may occur normally with the peripheral vasoconstriction associated with a cold environment or anxiety, or pathologically in conditions that reduce blood flow, for example, cardiogenic shock. *Pallor* can denote anemia or an increased PVR.

Capillary refill time provides an estimation of the rate of peripheral blood flow. When the tip of the fingernail is depressed, the nail bed blanches. When it is quickly released, the area is reperfused and becomes pink. With a normal rate of peripheral blood flow, reperfusion occurs almost instantaneously. More sluggish return of color indicates a slower peripheral flow.

Hand temperature and moistness, which are controlled by the autonomic nervous system, should be noted. Normally, the hands should be warm and dry. In peripheral vasoconstriction from a high level of circulating catecholamines (for example, with low CO), the extremities also become cold and clammy. In the individual under stress, the hands typically are cool and the palmar surfaces moist.

Skin mobility and turgor can be assessed by lifting a fold of skin and noting how easily it is moved and how rapidly

Fig. 14-8. Clubbing is not diagnosed from appearance, but from the angle at the base. **(A)** A clubbed finger. **(B)** The normal base angle in degrees. (After Winslow EH: Heart Lung 4(3):421–429, 1975)

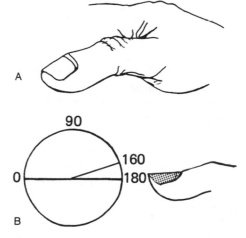

A

90

0

160

180

B

it returns to place. Edema decreases mobility. Dehydration and aging reduce turgor.

The presence or absence of *clubbing*, which is associated with chronic hemoglobin desaturation, should be noted. The ends of the fingers and toes enlarge diffusely, assuming the appearance of clubs (Fig. 14-8A). However, the diagnosis of clubbing is not made by shape, but rather by the angle between the base of the nail and the skin next to the cuticle. When viewed from the side, this base angle normally, is 160 degrees. In clubbing, the angle becomes 180 degrees or greater (Fig. 14-8B).[33] Congenital clubbing is not associated with chronic hemoglobin desaturation and has no known cause.

Examination of the Head and Neck

Head. In examining the head, a CCU nurse needs to be concerned primarily with checking the lips and earlobes for peripheral cyanosis and the buccal mucosa for central cyanosis. In *central cyanosis*, hemoglobin does not become fully saturated with oxygen. It implies serious heart or lung disease and is accompanied by peripheral cyanosis. In severe heart disease, a right-to-left shunt exists in which blood passes through the lungs without being oxygenated, as happens in severe congestive heart failure with interstitial pulmonary edema. In severe lung disease, changes produced by chronic obstructive airway disease or fibrosis prevent oxygenation.

Neck. Jugular vein distention (JVD) is caused by increased filling volume and pressure on the right side of the heart. It is a late finding in left ventricular failure. Jugular veins act like manometers and can be used to measure central venous pressure (CVP), which reflects right atrial or right ventricular end-diastolic pressure. The normal CVP is 4 to 10 cm of water.

- To measure the CVP noninvasively, begin with the patient supine. The backrest position can be elevated for patient comfort.
- Determine the heart level by finding the phlebostatic axis [fourth intercostal space (ICS) at the sternum, intersecting the mid-anterior–posterior line] (Figs. 14-9A, 21-1).
- Locate the neck veins; either the internal or external jugular veins can be used (Fig. 14-9 B and C). Blood assumes the level that corresponds to the CVP when the neck veins are occluded by the examiner's fingertip at the angle of the jaw.
- Do not strip the veins first; backfilling of the blood in the vein may be prevented by a valve in the jugular vein.
- The patient should be positioned at an angle that will allow the meniscus to be seen below the angle of the jaw.
- Measure the vertical distance between the phlebostatic axis and the meniscus with a centimeter ruler.

The distance in centimeters corresponds to the CVP (Fig. 14-9 D). For example, a distance of 10 cm equals a CVP of 10 cm water. If the patient's neck veins collapse on deep inspiration, which creates a negative intrathoracic pressure of −5 cm water, the CVP is less than 5 cm water.

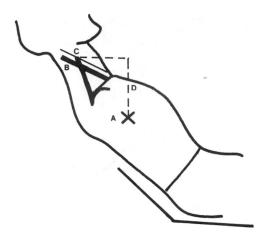

Fig. 14-9. Noninvasive determination of central venous pressure. (**A**) Phlebostatic axis. (**B**) Internal jugular vein. (**C**) External jugular vein. (**D**) Vertical distance in centimeters from the meniscus to the phlebostatic axis equals the CVP in cm H_2O. (Courtesy of Dr. R.E. Wills)

Precordium

The precordium should be assessed in an orderly fashion. Seven precordial areas should be examined (Fig. 14-10). Those named for the heart valves are actually located over the valvular outflow tracts rather than over the valves themselves:

- The aortic area is the second ICS to the right of the sternum.
- The pulmonic area is the second ICS to the left of the sternum.
- The tricuspid area is at the lower left sternal border.
- The mitral area is at the apex of the heart.
- The right ventricular area is over the lower half of the sternum and the left parasternal area.
- The third left ICS, known as Erb's point, is where selected abnormalities of the aortic or pulmonic valves may be detected.
- The epigastric area is where aortic or right ventricular pulsations can be seen and palpated.

Inspection, palpation, percussion, and auscultation should be used in that order when performing a cardiac examination. The patient's room should be quiet and permit privacy. For the cardiac nurse, it is most important to establish a baseline so that change can be documented rather than to diagnose a particular problem.

Inspection.

- For proper inspection of the precordium, the patient should be supine and flat, with chest bared.
- Tangential lighting or light shone from the side, rather than overhead lighting, should be used so that shadows are cast on the anterior chest wall, allowing the examiner to detect any movement.
- It may also be helpful for the examiner to crouch down so that the chest wall is at eye level. Any pulsating movement over each of the seven areas should be noted.

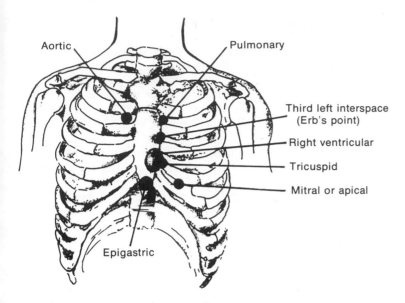

Aortic

Pulmonary

Third left interspace
(Erb's point)

Right ventricular

Tricuspid

Mitral or apical

Epigastric

Fig. 14-10. The areas to assess in the precordial examination. (Adapted from Bates B: A Guide to Physical Examination, 2nd ed, p 150. Philadelphia, JB Lippincott, 1979)

Except at the mitral area, *movement over any of the valvular outflow tracts* is *abnormal*. For example, pulsation over the right second ICS may represent an aortic aneurysm, and pulsation over the second left ICS could represent increased filling pressure or flow in the pulmonary artery. Slight movement of the sternum can be normal in thin individuals and in those with hyperdynamic heart beats as may be found in fever or anemia. A sternal rise which is sustained after cardiac contraction indicates right ventricular enlargement.

Normally, the *point of maximal impulse* (PMI) can be seen at the apex. It should lie within the fifth ICS, inside the midclavicular line (MCL), and should have a rapid upstroke and downstroke. The PMI cannot be seen in every patient. In thin patients, it is easily detected whereas in those who have large breasts or who are obese it may not be visible. A PMI that is below the fifth ICS, lateral to the MCL, or can be seen in more than one ICS represents left ventricular enlargement.

Paradoxical movement of the left anterior chest is suggestive of a left ventricular aneurysm. With paradoxical movement, as the apex contracts, the aneurysmic area bulges out. This ectopic impulse is usually seen above the PMI. Pulsations in the epigastric area normally may be seen in very thin individuals, but may also represent an abnormality.

Palpation. Abnormal movement that was not visible on inspection may be detected by palpation. However, some movement is more easily seen than felt. All seven areas should be palpated by using either the heel of the hand (the palmar surface of the hand at the wrist), the ulnar surface of the hand, or the fingers. The heel or the ulnar surface of the hand is more sensitive to thrills (vibrations), whereas the fingers are more sensitive to pulsations. Thrills indicate turbulence of blood flow and are associated with murmurs.

- Examine the sternal area for a right ventricular lift or heave.
- Palpate the PMI for location, size, amplitude, and duration. The normal PMI is felt as a light tap, extending over 1 cm

to 2 cm or less. It immediately follows the first sound and lasts halfway through systole. An impulse that is diffuse (felt over two ICSs) or sustained (holosystolic) represents left ventricular enlargement.

- Also palpate for paradoxical movement.

If the PMI cannot be felt with the patient lying flat, he should be examined in the left lateral position, which brings the apex against the chest wall. The quality of the apex beat can still be determined even though the location cannot. Aortic or right ventricular pulsations can be felt in the epigastric area. By placing the palmar surface of the hand over the epigastrum and sliding the fingers under the rib cage, the examiner can differentiate these pulsations. Pulsations beating downward against the fingertips indicate right ventricular movement, whereas those pushing forward against the fingers originate in the aorta. An increased aortic pulse could indicate abdominal aortic aneurysm or aortic regurgitation.[2]

Percussion. Percussion is used to evaluate the size of the heart. The technique of mediate percussion involves the examiner placing a passive hand firmly over the area to be percussed and striking the distal interphalangeal joint of the middle finger of that hand (the pleximeter) with the middle finger of the opposite hand (the plexor) (Fig. 14-11). Table 14-4 lists the five sounds that are produced by percussion.

- Percuss the left heart border in the third, fourth, and fifth ICSs.
- Firmly place the pleximeter finger either parallel or perpendicular to the ICS and lightly tap with the plexor finger.
- Move medially at 1-cm intervals from the area of resonance (lung tissue) to the area of dullness (heart tissue).

The heart border should be within the MCL. Left ventricular enlargement displaces the cardiac border to the left. Determination of heart size is not thought to be as accurate with percussion as with palpation.[2] More accurate information can be obtained from a good chest film.

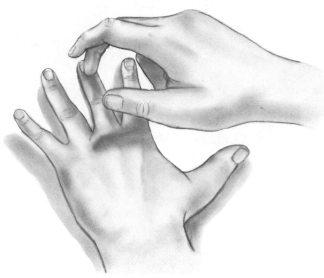

Fig. 14-11. The technique of percussion. (Bates B: A Guide to Physical Examination, 2nd ed, p 125. Philadelphia, JB Lippincott, 1979)

TABLE 14.4 SOUNDS PRODUCED BY PERCUSSION

Finding	Characteristics	Anatomic Locations
Tympany	Musical note that is sustained the longest; higher pitch than resonant	Air in closed structures, which vibrates with the surrounding tissue: stomach, intestines
Hyperresonance	Sustained longer than resonance; moderate-to-high pitch	Air-filled lungs
Resonance	Sustained moderate time; moderate pitch	Lung tissue
Dullness	Short sound; high pitch	Relatively airless solid tissue: heart, liver
Flatness	Short sound; high pitch	Solid tissue with least amount of trapped air; arm or leg muscles

(From Malasanos L, Barkauskas V, Moss M et al: Health Assessment. St. Louis, CV Mosby, 1977)

Auscultation. A good quality stethoscope is required for cardiac auscultation. Although the human ear is able to hear sounds ranging in frequency from 20 cycles per second, or Hertz (Hz), to 20,000 Hz, it is most sensitive to 1000 to 5000 Hz. The frequency of most heart sounds is less than 1000 Hz. The stethoscope must transmit these low-frequency sounds to the ear. The parts of the stethoscope are the earpieces, the tubing, and the chest pieces. The earpieces should fit comfortably into the ear canal and be snug enough so that extraneous sound cannot enter. They must also be kept free of ear wax. Double tubing with a small internal diameter (3 mm) should extend from the earpieces to the chest pieces. Additionally, the tubing should be reasonably

short (25–30 cm), so that the sound is not "diluted," and thick, to minimize room noise.[16]

There are two basic types of chest pieces: the diaphragm and the bell. The *diaphragm,* which brings out higher frequencies and filters out the lower ones, is useful for listening to the first and second heart sounds (S_1 and S_2) and high-frequency murmurs. It should be pressed firmly against the skin. The *bell* filters out high-frequency sounds and accentuates the low-frequency ones. Diastolic filling sounds and low-frequency diastolic murmurs are heard best with the bell. It should rest lightly on the chest; if firm pressure is applied, the skin becomes taut and acts like a diaphragm.

All areas identified in Figure 14-9 should be auscultated except the epigastric area. The listener's goals when auscultating the precordium are to identify S_1 and S_2, the HR and its characteristics, murmurs, extrasystolic sounds, and diastolic sounds.

There are two basic heart sounds, S_1 and S_2. The period between S_1 and S_2 is systole, and the time between S_2 and S_1 is diastole (Fig. 14-12). In normal sinus rhythm, the two sounds are easily identified by the cadence. However, in more rapid rhythms, systole and diastole may be equal in time, or if the rate is very fast, diastole may become shorter than systole. In this instance, in order properly to identify systole from diastole, the examiner can palpate the carotid artery while listening to the heart. Carotid upstroke slightly precedes the second sound.

If the clinician wants to validate the auscultatory findings, a phonocardiogram can be done.[31] In a phonocardiogram, heart sounds, electrocardiogram, and carotid pulse tracings are recorded simultaneously (see Fig. 20-20). Because of the equipment needed and the necessity for a quiet room, phonocardiograms usually are not taken at the bedside.

The *first heart sound* is thought to be due to closure of the mitral and tricuspid valves and is, therefore, heard loudest at the apex of the heart. Phonetically, if the heart sounds are "lub-dup," S_1 is the "lub." Usually, mitral and tricuspid closure is heard as a single sound.[19]

The intensity of the S_1 has little clinical applicability to nursing care but may be of interest. The intensity of the S_1 depends upon leaflet mobility, position of the atrioventricular valves at the onset of systole, and the rate of ventricular upstroke. A loud S_1 is noted clinically in mitral stenosis when the cusps are mobile; with a short PR interval (0.11–0.13 seconds), because the leaflets are wide open when systolic contraction begins; and in tachycardia, hyperthyroidism, or exercise, because of an increased rate of pressure rise. Most commonly, a soft S_1 is due to poor conduction of sound through the chest wall, but other causes include a fixed or immobile valve; a long PR interval (0.20–0.26 seconds), which allows the atrioventricular valves to float back into position without systolic intervention; and low flow at the end of diastole. The intensity of S_1 varies in atrial fibrillation because diastolic filling time is not constant.

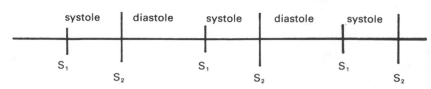

Fig. 14-12. The normal heart sounds.

In a regular rhythm with a variable S_1 intensity, complete heart block should be suspected.[19]

The *second heart sound* results from closure of the aortic and pulmonic valves and is, therefore, heard best at the base of the heart. Phonetically, the "dup" of the "lub-dup" is the S_2 sound. Physiologic (normal) splitting of the S_2 occurs during inspiration. During inspiration an increased amount of blood is returned to the right side of the heart. Pulmonic closure (P_2) is delayed because of the extra time needed for this increased blood volume to pass through the valve. On expiration the split sounds merge (Fig. 14-13A). Because aortic closure (A_2) is loud and easily transmitted, and P_2 is soft, split S_2s are heard best using the diaphragm in the second left ICS. A delay in A_2 results in a paradoxically split S_2, an abnormal finding. Causes are electrical (*e.g.,* left bundle branch block, right ventricular pacing, or right ventricular ectopy) and mechanical (*e.g.,* aortic stenosis, systolic hypertension, left ventricular failure, or left ventricular ischemia) (Fig. 14-13B).

Normally, A_2 is always louder than P_2, even in the pulmonic area. In pulmonary hypertension from mitral valve disease, or in primary, embolic or respiratory pulmonary hypertension, the intensity of P_2 increases so that A_2 is less than P_2 or A_2 is equal to P_2. The intensity can usually be evaluated best at the apex, because both sounds radiate to that area in pulmonary hypertension.[19]

Diastolic filling sounds (S_3 and S_4) occur during the two phases of rapid ventricular filling: protodiastole, the passive rapid filling; and with atrial contraction, the active rapid filling. Sudden changes in volume inflow cause vibration of the valves and supporting structures. These sounds, which are very low in frequency, can arise from either side of the heart.

The S_3 *sound*, ventricular sound or physiologic S_3, can be normal in healthy children or young adults but disappears by 30 years of age. In older people it is called a ventricular or S_3 gallop and usually signifies loss of ventricular compliance. Lack of myocardial distensibility produces the vibrations heard during passive filling. It is one of the first clinical findings associated with cardiac decompensation, such as congestive heart failure from any cause. A ventricular gallop is heard after the S_2 in a "lub-dup-ta" cadence (Fig. 14-14). A left ventricular gallop is heard best using the bell at the apex, with the patient in the left lateral position. Right ventricular gallops are heard at the lower left sternal border.[14]

The S_4 *or atrial gallop* is commonly heard in older people. It occurs after atrial contraction as the blood is ejected into the noncompliant ventricle. Even though this is the fourth heart sound, it is heard immediately before S_1 and sounds like "ta-lub-dup" (Fig. 14-15). Atrial gallops are heard in the majority of patients who have had an MI and in a large number of patients experiencing angina pectoris. It may

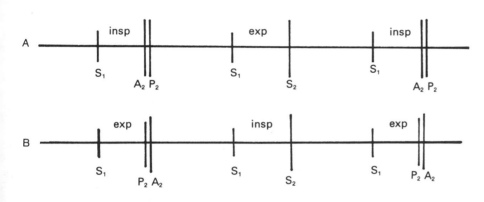

Fig. 14-13. Splitting of the S_2. (**A**) Physiologic splitting; during inspiration the P_2 sound is delayed. (**B**) Paradoxical splitting of the S_2; during expiration A_2 is delayed.

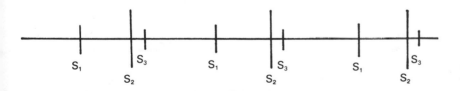

Fig. 14-14. An S_3 gallop immediately follows the S_2.

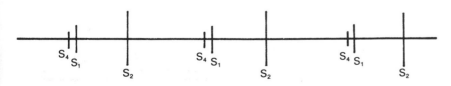

Fig. 14-15. An S_4 gallop immediately precedes the S_1.

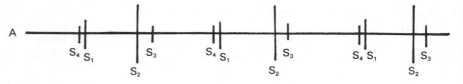

Fig. 14-16. Both an S₃ and S₄ gallop can occur during the same cardiac cycle. (**A**) Quadruple rhythm.

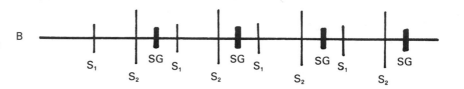

Fig. 14-16. Both an S₃ and S₄ gallop can occur during the same cardiac cycle. (**B**) Summation gallop (SG)—the S₃ and S₄ merge in middiastole.

also be detected in patients with coronary artery disease, hypertensive cardiovascular disease, cardiomyopathy, and aortic stenosis. An S₄ gallop does not necessarily imply cardiac failure.

Left atrial gallops are heard best using the bell at the apex of the heart with the patient in the left lateral position. Gallops originating from the right side, for example, with primary pulmonary hypertension and cor pulmonale, are heard best over the right ventricular area. Because atrial contraction is necessary to produce an S₄ gallop, atrial gallops are not heard in atrial fibrillation.[14]

A *quadruple rhythm* is heard if both gallop sounds occur (Fig. 14-16A). However, if the patient is ill enough to have a quadruple rhythm, he is usually also tachycardic. The S₃ and S₄ sounds fuse in mid-diastole to one loud diastolic sound, a *summation gallop,* which resembles the sound of a galloping horse (Fig. 14-16B).[14]

Heart murmurs are sounds produced in the heart or great vessels by increased or turbulent blood flow. Figure 14-17 illustrates the mechanisms of heart murmurs. Murmurs are classified according to timing (systolic or diastolic), intensity, location, radiation, configuration, and quality. Figure 14-18 demonstrates systolic and diastolic murmurs.

A description of the grading of the intensity of murmurs is found in Table 14-5. Intensity is always expressed as a fraction in Roman numerals, with the denominator being VI, for example, grade II/VI. It is important to note that the intensity of the murmur does not necessarily correlate with the severity of the valvular lesion. The location is the area where the murmur is heard the loudest; areas of radiation should also be noted. Configuration of a murmur is described as crescendo, decrescendo, crescendo–decrescendo (dia-

→

Fig. 14-17. Mechanisms of heart murmurs. (**A**) Flow across a partial obstruction, such as a stenotic valve. (**B**) Flow across a valvular irregularity without obstruction. (**C**) Increased flow through normal structures. (**D**) Flow into a dilated chamber. (**E**) Backward or regurgitant flow across an incompetent valve or defect. (**F**) Shunting of blood out of an area of high pressure into a chamber or artery through an abnormal passage. (Bates B: A Guide to Physical Examination, 2nd ed, p 166. Philadelphia, JB Lippincott, 1979)

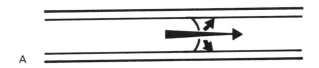

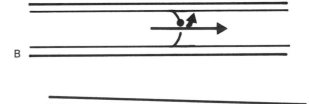

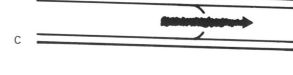

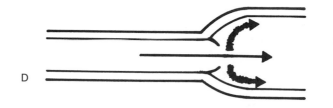

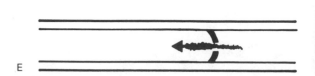

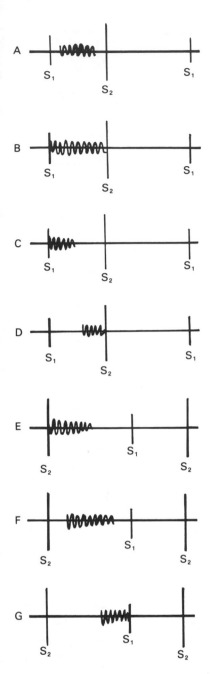

Fig. 14-18. Systolic and diastolic murmurs. (**A–D**) Systolic: (**A**) midsystolic; (**B**) holosystolic; (**C**) early systolic; (**D**) late systolic. (**E–G**) Diastolic: (**E**) early diastolic; (**F**) middiastolic; (**G**) late diastolic. (Adapted from Perloff JK: In Hurst JW, Logue RB, Schlant RC et al: *The Heart,* 4th ed, p 269. New York, McGraw-Hill, 1978)

mond-shaped), or plateau (sustained) (Fig. 14-19). The quality of a murmur is best described by using such terms as harsh, rough, rumbling, blowing, squeaking, or musical.[25]

- The CCU nurse must be particularly concerned with changes in murmurs rather than in the diagnosis of them. The one exception to this is the diagnosis of the murmur of mitral regurgitation, which is indicative of papillary muscle dysfunction (see Chap. 48).

A pericardial friction rub is a characteristic finding in pericarditis, which occurs in more than 15% of patients with

acute MI. Approximately 7% of patients with MI develop a pericardial friction rub, which commonly occurs within the fourth day of hospitalization.[15] The rub occurs with heart movement: atrial systole, ventricular systole, and ventricular diastole. Each of these three components creates its own short, scratchy sound (Fig. 14-20). Rubs are classified as three component, two component (ventricular systole and diastole), or one component (ventricular systole). The last may be difficult to differentiate from a murmur. Rubs are best heard with the patient either sitting upright and leaning

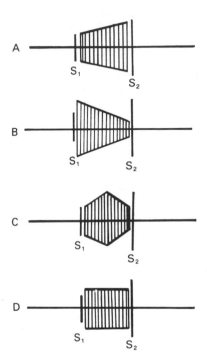

Fig. 14-19. Configurations of murmurs. (**A**) Crescendo; (**B**) descrescendo; (**C**) crescendo–decrescendo; (**D**) plateau.

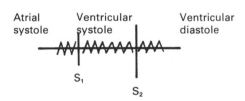

Fig. 14-20. A three-component pericardial friction rub.

TABLE 14.5   GRADING THE INTENSITY OF A MURMUR

Grade	Clinical Findings
I/VI	Very faint; only heard with special effort
II/VI	Faint but readily recognized
III/VI	Prominent but not loud
IV/VI	Loud; accompanied by a thrill
V/VI	Very loud; accompanied by a thrill
VI/VI	Exceptionally loud; can be heard with stethoscope just removed from contact with the chest; accompanied by a thrill

(Perloff JK: Systolic, diastolic, and continuous murmurs. In Hurst JW, Logue RB, Schlant RC et al (eds): The Heart, 4th ed, pp 268–287. New York, McGraw-Hill, 1978)

forward with the breath expelled (most appropriate for the patient with an acute MI) or on his hands and knees in bed. A pericardial friction rub can be heard with or without a pericardial effusion.[10]

Posterior Chest

The lung examination described in this chapter is very elementary. Its function is to help identify the respiratory manifestations of atelectasis and congestive heart failure. In order for the examiner properly to assess the lungs, the room should be quiet and the patient's back should be exposed. Ideally, the patient should be in a sitting position.

Inspection.

- Note rate, depth, rhythmicity, and ease of the patient's respirations. Normally the respiratory rate is less than 16 per minute and the rhythm is regular.

  Tachypnea is associated with pain or anxiety.

  Bradypnea can be noted during sleep or after administration of respiratory depressant drugs, such as morphine sulfate.

  Cheyne-Stokes respirations, characterized by periods of alternating depth and apnea, occur in patients with left ventricular failure (Fig. 14-21).

- Note presence of cough, production of sputum.
- Look for use of accessory muscles, especially the neck or intercostal muscles.
- Note any deformity of the chest.

  With a barrel chest, which is associated with pulmonary emphysema and normal aging, anteroposterior (A-P) to lateral diameter ratio of the chest is 1:1. Normally, the A-P to lateral ratio is 1:2 or 5:7. Kyphoscoliosis, an abnormal spinal curvature, may prevent the patient from fully expanding his lungs (Fig. 14-22).

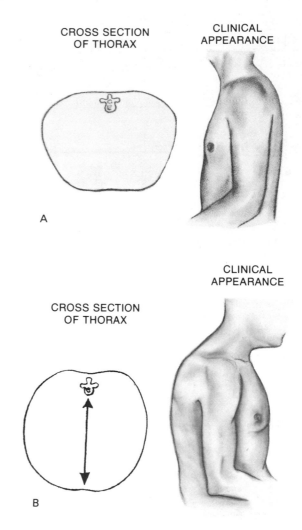

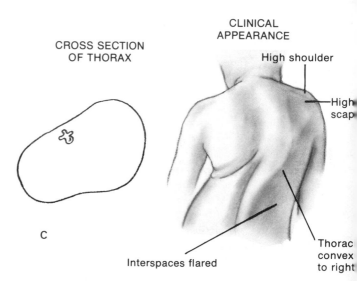

Fig. 14-21. Abnormalities in rate and rhythm of breathing compared to normal. (**A**) Normal; (**B**) tachypnea; (**C**) Cheyne-Stokes. (Bates B: A Guide to Physical Examination, 2nd ed, p 133. Philadelphia, JB Lippincott, 1979)

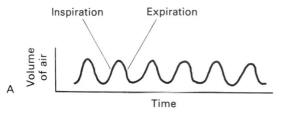

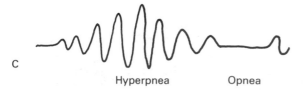

Fig. 14-22. Deformities of the thorax compared to normal. (**A**) Normal adult; (**B**) barrel chest; (**C**) kyphoscoliosis. (Bates B: A Guide to Physical Examination, 2nd ed, p 132. Philadelphia, JB Lippincott, 1979)

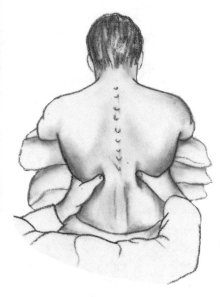

Fig. 14-23. Assessment of respiratory excursion. (Bates B: A Guide to Physical Examination, 2nd ed, p 121. Philadelphia, JB Lippincott, 1979)

Palpation.

- Assess respiratory excursion by placing your thumbs slightly to either side of the spine and parallel to the tenth ribs.
- As the patient inhales deeply, evaluate the depth and symmetry of his breath by the movement of your thumbs (Fig. 14-23).[2]

Percussion. Respiratory excursion can also be identified by percussion. Normally, the tenth rib is the lower lung border posteriorly. On deep inspiration, the lower border shifts to the twelfth rib.

- Percuss downward from areas of resonance or hyperresonance to dullness to determine lung position or excursion (Fig. 14-24).

Auscultation.

- During auscultation the patient is asked to breathe slowly and deeply through his mouth (nose-breathing changes the pitch of the sounds). The examiner listens with the diaphragm of the stethoscope pressed firmly enough against the back to leave a blanched ring on the skin after the stethoscope is removed.
- Auscultation of the posterior chest should be done in an orderly fashion, starting at the apices and moving down to the bases (Fig. 14-25).
- The examiner should listen for one full breath in each location.
- Note the quality and intensity of lung sounds.

Normal breath sounds, which formerly were called vesicular breath sounds, are heard in peripheral lung tissue away from the large airways. They are soft, blowing sounds with a low pitch. The inspiratory–expiratory time ratio is 5:2 (Fig. 14-26A). These sounds normally are somewhat diminished at the lung bases. They may also be decreased in obese patients, with shallow breathing, or with pleural effusion. They are increased with exercise.

Bronchovesicular sounds have moderate pitch and intensity. The inspiratory–expiratory time ratio is 1:1. They are heard in the areas around the mainstem bronchi—below the clavicles and between the scapulae (Fig. 14-26B).

Bronchial sounds, heard over the bronchial areas, are loud and high pitched. Expiratory time is greater than inspiratory time (Fig. 14-26C). Bronchovesicular or bronchial sounds heard in the peripheral lung tissue are abnormal.[2,21]

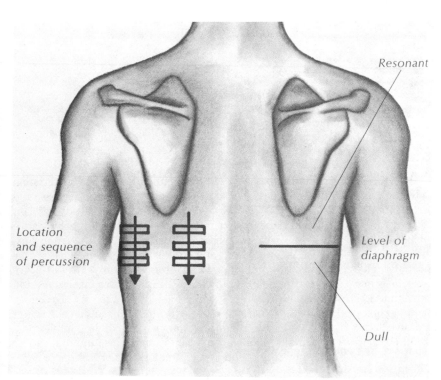

Resonant

Location and sequence of percussion

Level of diaphragm

Dull

Fig. 14-24. Percussion of the posterior chest. (Bates B: A Guide to Physical Examination, 2nd ed, p 127. Philadelphia, JB Lippincott, 1979)

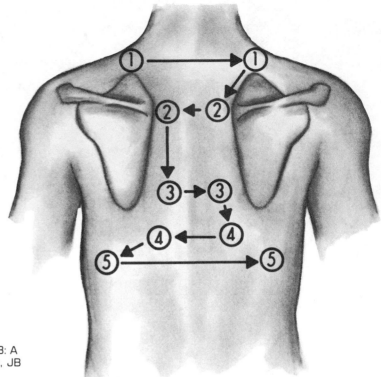

Fig. 14-25. Auscultation of the posterior chest. (Bates B: A Guide to Physical Examination, 2nd ed, p 122. Philadelphia, JB Lippincott, 1979)

Upstroke represents inspiration

Downstroke represents expiration

Length of upstroke or downstroke
   represents duration

Thickness represents amplitude

A   Angle represents pitch

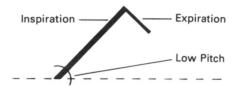

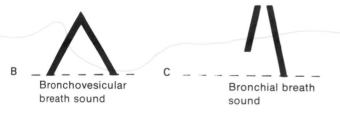

Fig. 14-26. Diagrammatic representation of normal lung sounds. **(A)** Normal breath sound. **(B)** Bronchovesicular breath sound. **(C)** Bronchial breath sound. (Brown MS, Hudak CM, Brenneman J et al: *Student Manual of Physical Examination*, pp 83—85. Philadelphia, JB Lippincott 1977)

Adventitious sounds are sounds superimposed over normal breath sounds. There are two categories of adventitious sounds: discontinuous and continuous. Discontinuous sounds are short and intermittent. Their crackling and bubbling is similar to the sound generated by rubbing hairs between the fingers in front of the ear. These are now termed *"crackles"* (the old term was *"rales"*), and, although they are nonspecific, they can indicate either atelectasis or pulmonary edema. Crackles are generally attributed to fluid in the alveoli. However, studies have shown that crackling can be due to the explosive reopening of closed alveoli.[5,8] Crackling from atelectasis or pulmonary interstitial edema occurs during late inspiration (Fig. 14-27A).

Continuous adventitious sounds have a longer duration than crackles. They are commonly called *"wheezes"* and *"rhonchi."* Wheezes, which have been called "sibilant rhonchi" in the past, are high pitched and are indicative of airway narrowing, as in asthma (Fig. 14-27B). A *rhonchus*, which is low pitched and sounds like a snore, is caused by airway obstruction, usually from sputum (Fig. 14-27C). Both continuous sounds are heard during inspiration and expiration.[5]

A *pleural friction rub* results from inflamed pleura rubbing together and is a characteristic finding in pleuritis. A pleural friction rub is a coarse, grating sound that can be heard on inspiration and expiration (Fig. 14-28).

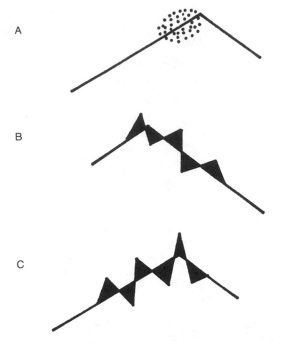

Fig. 14-27. Adventitious breath sounds. (**A**) Crackles. (**B**) Wheeze superimposed over an asthmatic breath sound (inspiration<expiration). (**C**) Rhonchus.

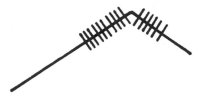

Fig. 14-28. Pleural friction rub.

Abdomen

In cardiac nursing, the abdominal examination has only two purposes: first, to determine if the liver is of normal size or is enlarged from right heart failure; second, to palpate for an overdistended urinary bladder in a patient complaining of urinary retention or with reduced urinary output, possibly resulting from an obstructed urinary catheter, low CO, or administration of atropine sulfate.

Percussion. Percussion of the liver should start in the MCL, at or below the umbilicus, and proceed upward from an area of tympany (intestinal) to one of dullness (liver).
- Identify the lower edge of the liver in the MCL.
- Next, percuss downward at the MCL from resonance (lungs) to dullness.
- Measure the distance from the upper edge to the lower edge in centimeters. The normal liver span is 6 cm to 12 cm. A right pleural effusion or lung consolidation (dullness) may obscure the upper border. Gas in the colon (tympany) may obscure the lower edge.[2]
- To assess for a distended urinary bladder: percuss downward from the umbilicus to the symphysis pubis. Supra-

pubic dullness may indicate a distended urinary bladder. If ascites is present, abdominal percussion may not reveal bladder distention.

Palpation. Deep palpation is necessary to feel the liver. It is imperative that the patient be relaxed.
- Place your left hand under the patient's 11th and 12th ribs for support. It also makes the liver easier to palpate if you push up with this hand.
- Place the right hand on the abdomen below the lower edge of dullness, with the fingers pointing toward the right costal margin.
- As the patient takes a deep abdominal breath and then exhales, gently but firmly push in and up with the fingers (Fig. 14-28).
- With each expiration move your hand further toward the liver. The liver edge should come down to meet the fingers. Normally, it feels firm with a smooth surface. It should not be tender. Venous engorgement of the liver produces a smooth, tender edge (Fig. 14-29).

If right heart failure is suspected, check for hepatojugular reflux:
- Position the patient so that the meniscus of the jugular vein is visible.
- Press gently but firmly over the liver for 30 to 60 seconds.
- If the patient complains about right upper quadrant tenderness, press a different abdominal area.
- If the jugular vein pressure rise is greater than 1 cm, a hepatojugular reflux is present, suggesting congestive heart failure.[2]

If percussion does not confirm suspicions of a distended urinary bladder, it will be necessary to palpate gently above the symphysis pubis. Normally, a bladder cannot be detected during palpation. Again, the presence of ascites fluid may make assessment of bladder distention difficult or impossible.

Feet and Legs

Although it is not necessary for the CCU nurse to perform a complete peripheral vascular examination, she should assess the patient's feet and legs for the presence of edema and adequacy of peripheral circulation. The patient should be lying in bed with legs exposed.

Inspection.
- Assess the size, symmetry, color, appearance, and hair distribution. A shiny appearance or lack of hair on the lower legs, feet, and toes can indicate chronic, diminished arterial circulation.
- Note any other abnormalities, such as pigmentation, ulceration, or edema.

(Assessment of the patient with acute thrombosis is discussed in Chapter 28.)

Palpation.
- Assess for unilateral or bilateral edema by pressing firmly with your thumb over a bony surface, for example, behind the medial malleolus, or over the dorsum of the foot or

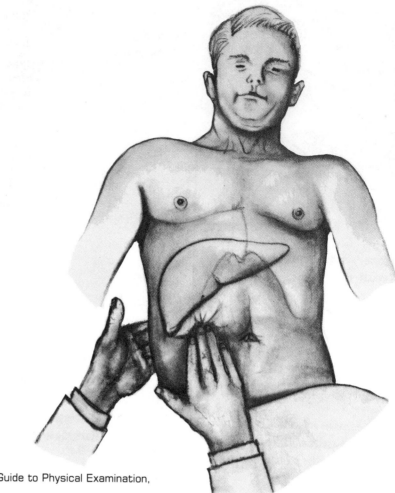

Fig. 14-29. Deep palpation of the liver. (Bates B: A Guide to Physical Examination, 2nd ed, p 208. Philadelphia, JB Lippincott, 1979)

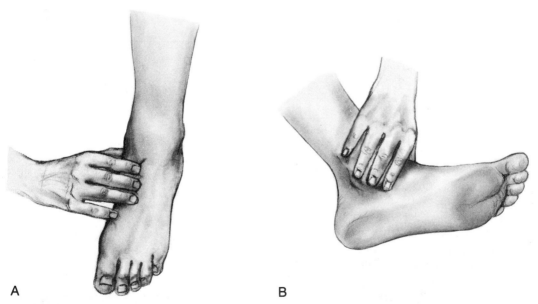

A   B

Fig. 14-30. Palpation of peripheral pulses. (**A**) Dorsalis pedis. (**B**) Posterior tibial. (Bates B: A Guide to Physical Examination, 2nd ed, p 265. Philadelphia, JB Lippincott, 1979)

shin, for at least 5 seconds. Pitting occurs in dependent areas* with the saline excess of congestive heart failure.

To assess the adequacy of peripheral circulation, one should always compare one foot or leg with the other.

- Begin by determining temperature by touching the skin with the back of your hands.
- Palpate for pulses.

  Femoral pulse is palpated deeply below the inguinal ligament, midway between the anterior iliac spine and the pubic tubercle.

  Dorsalis pedis pulse is located on the dorsum of the foot, lateral to the extensor tendon of the great toe.

  Posterior tibial pulse can be found behind and slightly below the medial malleolus (Fig. 14-30).[2]

REFERENCES

1 Adams RD, Braunwald E: Faintness, syncope and episodic weakness. In Thorn GW, Adams RG, Braunwald E et al (eds): Harrison's Principles of Internal Medicine, 8th ed, pp 75–81. New York, McGraw-Hill, 1977
2. Bates B: A Guide to Physical Examination, 2nd ed. Philadelphia, JB Lippincott, 1979
3. Bookman LB, Simoneau JK: The early assessment of hypovolemia: Postural vital signs. J Emergency Nurs 3(5):43–45, 1977
4. Brown, MS, Hudak CM, Brenneman J et al: Student Manual of Physical Examination. Philadelphia, JB Lippincott, 1977
5. Cugell DW: Sounds of the lungs. Chest 73(3):311–312, 1978
6. Dornhorst AC, Howard R, Leathart GL: Pulsus paradoxus. Lancet i:746–748, 1952
7. Dustin HP, Tarazi RC, Hinshaw LB: Mechanisms controlling arterial pressure. In Frohlich ED (ed): Pathophysiology, 2nd ed, pp 49–82. Philadelphia, JB Lippincott, 1976
8. Forgacs P: The funcional basis of pulmonary sounds. Chest 73(3):399–405, 1978
9. Fowler NO: Examination of the Heart, Part 2. Inspection and Palpation of Venous and Arterial Pulses. New York, American Heart Association, 1972
10. Fowler NO: The recognition and management of pericardial disease and its complications. In Hurst JW, Logue RB, Schlant RC et al (eds): The Heart, 4th ed, pp 1640–1659. New York, McGraw-Hill, 1978
11. Fowler NO: Physiology of cardiac tamponade and pulsus paradoxus. I. Mechanisms of pulsus paradoxus in cardiac tamponade. Mod Concepts Cardiovasc Dis 47(11):109–113, 1978
12. Frank MJ, Alvarez-Mena SV: Cardiovascular Physical Diagnosis. Chicago, Year Book, 1973
13. Geddes LA: The Direct and Indirect Measurement of Blood Pressure. Chicago, Year Book, 1970
14. Harvey WP: Gallop sounds, clicks, snaps, whoops, honks, and other sounds. In Hurst JW, Logue RB, Schlant RC et al (eds): The Heart, 4th ed, pp 255–268. New York, McGraw-Hill, 1978
15. Hurst JW, Logue RB, Walter PF: The clinical recognition and medical management of coronary atherosclerotic heart disease. In Hurst JW, Logue RB, Schlant RC et al (eds): The Heart, 4th ed, pp 1156–1290. New York, McGraw-Hill, 1978
16. Hurst JW, Schlant RC: Principles of auscultation. In Hurst JW, Logue RB, Schlant RC et al (eds): The Heart, 4th ed, pp 226–237. New York, McGraw-Hill, 1978
17. Hurst JW, Schlant RC: Examination of the arteries and their pulsation. In Hurst JW, Logue RB, Schlant RC et al (eds): The Heart, 4th ed, pp 183–192. New York, McGraw-Hill, 1978
18. Kirkendall WM, Burton AC, Epstein FH et al: Recommenda-
19. Leatham A: The first and second heart sounds. In Hurst JW, Logue RB, Schlant RC et al (eds): The Heart, 4th ed, pp 237–255. New York, McGraw-Hill, 1978
20. Little DE, Carnevali DL: Nursing Care Planning, 2nd ed, pp 125–146. Philadelphia, JB Lippincott, 1976
21. Malasanos L, Barkauskas L, Ross M et al: Health Assesment. St Louis, CV Mosby, 1977
22. Moser M, Guyther JR, Finnerty F et al: Report of the joint national committee on detection, evaluation and treatment of high blood pressure. JAMA 237(3):255–261, 1977
23. New York Heart Association Criteria Committee: Diseases of the Heart and Blood Vessels: Nomenclature and Criteria for Diagnosis, 6th ed, pp 110–114. Boston, Little, Brown, 1964
24. Nutter DO: Measuring and recording systemic blood pressure. In Hurst JW, Logue RB, Schlant RC et al (eds): The Heart, 4th ed, pp 217–226. New York, McGraw-Hill, 1978
25. Perloff JK: Systolic, diastolic, and continuous murmurs. In Hurst JW, Logue RB, Schlant RC et al (eds): The Heart, 4th ed, pp 268–287. New York, McGraw-Hill, 1978
26. Price SA, Wilson LM: Pathophysiology, p 668. New York, McGraw-Hill, 1978
27. Ruskin J, Bache RJ, Rembert JC et al: Pressure–flow studies in man: Effect of respiration on left ventricular stroke volume. Circulation 48:79–85, 1973
28. Scribner BH: Fluid and Electrolyte Balance, 7th ed. Seattle, University of Washington, 1969
29. Shabetai R, Fowler NO, Fenton JC et al: Pulsus paradoxus. J Clin Invest 44:1882–1898, 1965
30. Tarazi RC, Gifford RW, Jr: Systemic arterial pressure. In Sodeman WA Jr, Sodeman WA (eds): Pathologic Physiology, 5th ed, pp 177–205. Philadelphia, WB Saunders, 1974
31. Tavel ME: Clinical Phonocardiography and External Pulse Recordings, 3rd ed. Chicago, Year Book, 1978
32. Weed LL: Medical Records, Medical Education, and Patient Care. Chicago, Year Book, 1971
33. Winslow EH: Visual inspection of the patient with cardiopulmonary disease. Heart Lung 4(3):421–429, 1975.

ADDITIONAL READING

Bates B, Lynaugh J: Teaching physical assessment. Nurs Outlook 23(5):297–302, 1975
Cochran PT: Bedside aids to auscultation of the heart. JAMA 239(1):54 55, 1978
Delaney MT: Examining the chest, Part I. The lungs. Nurs 75, 5(8):12–14, 1975
Hobson LB: Examination of the Patient. New York, McGraw-Hill, 1975
Hurst JW, Logue RB, Schlant RC et al (eds): The Heart, 4th ed. New York, McGraw-Hill, 1978
Jarvis CM: Vital signs: How to take them more accurately and understand them more fully. Nurs 76, 6(4):31–37, 1976
Jarvis CM: Perfecting physical assessment, Part 2. Nurs 77, 7(6):38–45, 1977
King GE: Measurement of blood pressure. In Frank MJ, Alvarez-Mena SV (eds): Cardiovascular Physical Diagnosis, pp 53–61. Chicago, Year Book, 1973
Kostis, JB: Ventricular fibrillation during rectal examination in a patient with acute myocardial infarction. Chest 72(2):265–266, 1977
Lehman Sr J: Auscultation of heart sounds. Am J Nurs 72(7): 1242–1246, 1972
Littman D: Stethoscopes and auscultation. Am J Nurs 72(7): 1238–1241, 1972
Patient assessment: Examination of the abdomen. Am J Nurs 74(9):1702, 1974
Patient assessment: Examination of the chest and lungs. Am J Nurs 76(9):1453–1475, 1976

---

* If the patient is bedridden, the most dependent area is usually the sacrum.

Patient assessment: Examination of the heart and great vessels, Part I. Am J Nurs 76(11):1807–1830, 1976

Patient assessment: Auscultation of the heart, Part II. Am J Nurs 77(2):275–298, 1977

Patient assessment: Abnormalities of the heart beat. Am J Nurs 77(4):647–672, 1977

Pierce L: Anatomy and physiology of the liver in relation to clinical assessment. Nurs Clin North Am 12(2):259–273, 1977

Powell AH: Physical assessment of the patient with cardiac disease. Nurs Clin North Am 11(2):251–257, 1976

Pulmonary terms and symbols: A report of the American College of Chest Physicians–American Thoracic Society Joint Committee on Pulmonary Nomenclature. Chest 67(5):583–593, 1975

Reports from the American Thoracic Society Ad Hoc Committee on Pulmonary Nomenclature. Am Thoracic Society News 3(4):5–6, 1977

Robard S: The clinical utility of the arterial pulses and sounds. Heart Lung 1(6):776–784, 1972

Sauvé MJ, Pecherer A: Concepts and Skills in Physical Assessment. Philadelphia, WB Saunders, 1977

Taggert E: The physical assessment of the patient with arterial disease. Nurs Clin North Am 12(1):109–117, 1977

Thompson PL: Physical examination in ischemic heart disease. Med J Aust 1(14):492–495, 1976

15

Laboratory Tests Using Blood and Urine

SUSAN L. WOODS, R.N., M.N.

and

DEBRA LAURENT-BOPP, R.N., M.N.

Laboratory tests used in the evaluation of cardiac patients are presented in this chapter. The following serum enzymes will be discussed: (1) serum glutamic oxaloacetic transaminase (SGOT); (2) lactic acid dehydrogenase (LDH) and LDH isoenzymes; (3) creatine kinase (CK) and CK isoenzymes. Hematologic studies include the following: (1) complete blood count (CBC); (2) sedimentation rate and; (3) prothrombin time (PT); (4) recalcification (recal) time; (5) partial thromboplastin time (PTT). Specific blood chemistries include: (1) electrolytes (sodium, potassium, chloride, carbon dioxide, calcium, magnesium); (2) lipoproteins (cholesterol, triglycerides, phospholipids) and lipid electrophoresis; and (3) nonelectrolytes and nonlipids (bilirubin, catecholamines, creatinine, glucose, protein, urea nitrogen, uric acid). Routine urinalysis and blood levels of selected cardiac drugs are also discussed.

Some of these tests are used to diagnose myocardial infarction (MI). Others are used as general screening tests, or are tests done to determine concurrent disease. Still other tests are obtained to establish a patient's baseline and to evaluate the effect of treatment.

SERUM ENZYMES

Enzymes are catalytic proteins that accelerate biochemical reactions in living cells.[7] Each organ contains a variety of enzymes, with biochemical analysis tending to show an enzyme or group of enzymes characteristic of that organ. The organ-specific enzymes are those found in relatively high concentrations in a particular tissue, for example, in heart, kidney, liver, and skeletal muscle.

Enzyme activity is high in cells and low in serum. When cells become hypoxic or injured, the injured cell membrane leaks cytoplasmic enzymes into the serum. The pattern of enzyme elevation in serum can reflect the degree of cell injury, because some enzymes are confined to cell cytoplasm, and others are bound to mitochondria.[5]

The diagnosis of acute MI is made with the following information: the patient's history, his electrocardiogram, and the enzyme studies. Angiography and nuclear studies may also be performed. The rationale in using serum enzyme studies is that the heart muscle is rich in enzymes which catalyze different biochemical reactions. The serum activity of these enzymes is increased markedly after MI because enzymes are released by injured or dead myocardial cells.

The enzyme assays most commonly used to detect MI are (1) serum glutamic oxaloacetic transaminase (SGOT); (2) lactic acid dehyrdrogenase (LDH) and (3) creatine kinase (CK), formerly known as creatine phosphokinase. Because these enzymes are relatively nonspecific a combination of serum enzyme tests as well as serial sampling is used in establishing the presence of acute MI.

Specificity can be improved by measuring isoenzyme activity. Isoenzymes are electrophoretically distinct forms of enzymes; they have the same catalytic function as do enzymes but different physical and chemical properties.[29] With electrophoresis the enzymes migrate in an electric field at different rates and to different electric poles. Isoenzymes can be detected and quantified by methods other than electrophoresis, such as ultracentrifugation, radio-immunoassay, and column chromatography. The tissue distribution of one isoenzyme can be different from the tissue distribution of another isoenzyme. The specificity of an isoenzyme is far greater than the specificity of total enzyme activity.[20] Isoenzyme fractions of both LDH and CK are extremely useful in establishing the diagnosis of acute MI.[17,41]

In a series of 125 patients with MI, Coodley found a direct relationship between the amplitude of rise of CK, SGOT, and LDH enzymes and early mortality in MI. In 56% of hospital deaths from MI (14 of 25), enzyme levels were six times normal. Enzyme activity was also correlated with the incidence of arrhythmias (Table 15-1). In 81.8% of cases with ventricular arrhythmias, enzyme levels were four times

TABLE 15-1 RELATION OF ENZYME ELEVATION TO ARRHYTHMIAS

ARRHYTHMIAS NOTED	Number of Patients (N = 125) with Enzyme Elevation 2× Normal			Number of Patients (N = 125) with Enzyme Elevation 4× Normal		
	CK	SGOT	LDH	CK	SGOT	LDH
79 Patients Experienced						
Multifocal ectopic ventricular contractions (N = 77)	8	11	15	69	66	62
Bigeminy (N = 27)	5	6	8	22	21	19
Ventricular tachycardia (N = 21)	3	2	6	18	19	15
Ventricular fibrillation (N = 7)	1	2	2	6	5	5
29 Patients Experienced						
Atrial tachycardia (N = 22)	10	11	8	12	11	14
Atrial fibrillation (N = 24)	10	11	10	14	13	12

(Coodley EL: JAMA 225(6):597–605, 1973)

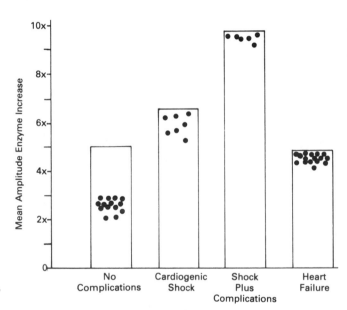

Fig. 15-1. Relationship between enzyme rise and complications of infarction. (Coodley EL: JAMA 225(6):598, 1973)

TABLE 15-2 RELATION BETWEEN AMPLITUDE OF ENZYME RISE AND COMPLICATIONS OF MYOCARDIAL INFARCTION (N = 125)

Enzyme Level IU*	Ventricular Arrhythmias (N = 79)	Heart Failure (N = 17)	Shock (N = 13)	No complications (N = 16)
CK				
120	4†	1	0	1
160	55	9	1	1
200	20	7	12	1
SGOT				
120	5	1	0	2
160	57	11	1	1
200	17	5	12	1
LDH				
750	7	2	0	2
1,000	51	10	2	2
1,250	21	5	11	2

* IU indicates international units; normal ranges of enzymes; CK—5 to 40 IU; SGOT—4 to 40 IU; LDH—150 to 250 IU.
† Number of patients.
(Coodley EL: JAMA 225(6):597–605, 1973)

normal. In most patients who developed congestive heart failure, the initial enzyme levels were 4 to 5 times normal. Cardiogenic shock in 10.4% (13 of 125) of the cases was associated with an enzyme level at least five times the upper limit of normal. In shock associated with multiple complications, a rise seven to ten times the normal enzyme level was seen (Fig. 15-1; Table 15-2).[10]

Serum Glutamic Oxaloacetic Transaminase

Serum glutamic oxaloacetic transaminase (SGOT) was the first enzyme to be used extensively to confirm MI.[28] The highest tissue concentration of this enzyme is in cardiac muscle, followed by skeletal muscle, brain, liver, kidney, testis, lung, spleen, in descending order.[7] After MI, the activity of SGOT rises sharply within the first 12 hours, peaks in 24 to 48 hours, and returns to normal by the fifth or sixth day (Fig. 15-2).

With MI, the level of SGOT can be correlated with prognosis. Levels over 700 units usually indicate a massive MI, levels over 300 units are associated with high mortality, whereas levels under 100 units are associated with a low mortality.[8]

Extremely high levels of this enzyme are also found in fulminating hepatitis, in which there is massive destruction of liver tissue, and in skeletal muscle damage.[51] Other factors affecting SGOT level are shown in Table 15-3. SGOT does not add to specificity or sensitivity of LDH or CK determinations. Current recommendations of the World Health Organization and the American Heart Association are to obtain only LDH and CK levels and those of their isoenzymes.

Normal Values of SGOT

8–33 Units/ml[51]
5–55 Units[2]

Lactic Dehydrogenase (LDH)

This enzyme is distributed widely throughout most tissues of the body but is concentrated primarily in the liver, striated muscles, red blood cells, and kidney (Fig. 15-3). Increased serum LDH activity after MI generally appears within 24 hours, reaches its peak between 48 and 72 hours, and may take as long as 7 to 10 days to return to baseline (Fig. 15-4). A rise in serum LDH usually begins somewhat later than the rise in serum SGOT and remains elevated for a longer period. The highest values of LDH are usually seen in patients with MI, hemolytic disorders, and pernicious anemia. As with SGOT, LDH renders a nonspecific picture,

TABLE 15-3 FACTORS ELEVATING SGOT LEVELS

After cardiac surgery
After thoracic surgery
Rarely after prostatic surgery
Occasionally with use of anabolic steroids, oxacillin, ampicillin, nalidixic acid, methyldopa, cephalothin, and narcotics
After cholecystectomy
In status asthmaticus
Occasionally with anticoagulants
Heart failure and heart necrosis
Shock
Physical stress
Muscle disease or injury
Visceral emboli
Occasionally in pancreatitis
Pericarditis with sanguinous effusion
Liver disease including mononucleosis
After biliary tract surgery

(Coodley EL: Enzymes and isoenzymes in myocardial infarction. In Brest AN (ed): Coronary Heart Disease. Cardiovasc Clin 1(2):139–153, 1969)

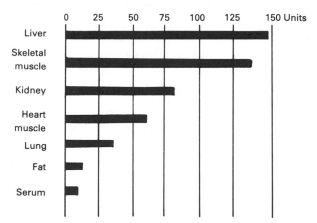

Fig. 15-3. LDH content in the body organs. (Coodley EL: Textbook of Coronary Care, p 84. Philadelphia, Charles Press, 1972)

with elevations occurring in a variety of disease states (Table 15-4). LDH determinations without LDH isoenzymes are less specific than is SGOT for myocardial tissue. One should be aware of the possibility of falsely elevated LDH levels caused by hemolysis of blood specimens.

Normal Values of Serum LDH

80–120 Wacker Units[51]
71–207 IU/L[51]
150–450 Wroblewski Units[51]
63–155 units (male); 62–131 units (female)[2]

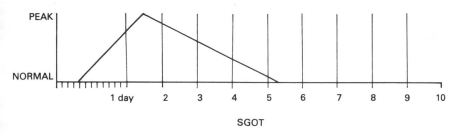

Fig. 15-2. SGOT elevation occurs within 12 hours after MI, peaks, in 24 to 48 hours, and returns to normal by the fifth or sixth day. (Adapted from Jackson VD: Myocardial Infarction, p 35. Fort Lauderdale, Saturn Scientific, 1977)

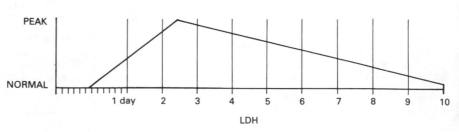

Fig. 15-4. LDH elevation occurs within 24 hours after infarction, reaches a peak between 48 to 72 hours after, and may take from 7 to 10 days to return to baseline. (Adapted from Jackson VD: Myocardial Infarction, p 35. Fort Lauderdale, Saturn Scientific, 1977)

TABLE 15-4 DISEASE STATES THAT MAY ELEVATE LDH

Hemolytic anemia
Pernicious anemia
Liver disease (including patients with congestive heart
   failure and hepatic congestion)
Pulmonary embolism and infarction
Renal diseases (especially infarction)
Hemolosis associated with prothetic heart valves
Neuromuscular disorders (i.e., muscular dystrophy)
Neoplastic and myeloproliferative disorders

(Galen RS: Diag Med 1:40–52, 1978)

Lactic Dehydrogenase (LDH) Isoenzymes

Lactic dehydrogenase has five isoenzymes, numbered 1 to 5, in order of rapidity of movement toward the positive pole of an electrical field (Fig. 15-5).[5] The distribution of LDH isoenzymes is shown in Table 15-5. Lactic dehydrogenase 1, the fastest-moving isoenzyme, is the predominate isoenzyme in heart, renal cortex, and red blood cells; the slowest moving enzyme, LDH_5, is found in the liver and skeletal muscle.[5] LDH_2 is also present in these tissues; its

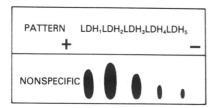

Fig. 15-5. Isoenzyme distribution. Isoenzymes numbered 1 to 5 in order of rapidity of movement toward positive (+) pole of electrical field. (Burke M: Postgrad Med 64(1):169, 1978)

TABLE 15-5 DISTRIBUTION OF LDH ISOENZYMES IN HUMAN TISSUES

	LDH_1	LDH_2	LDH_3	LDH_4	LDH_5
Normal serum	25%	35%	20%	10%	10%
Heart	40	35	20	5	0
Kidney	35	30	25	10	0
Brain	25	35	30	10	0
Lung	5	10	35	35	15
Thyroid	5	10	30	30	25
Bladder	5	10	40	35	10
Uterus	5	20	50	20	5
Bowel	5	30	45	10	10
Spleen	5	15	30	30	20
Liver	0	5	10	15	70
Skeletal muscle	0	0	10	30	60

(Galen RS: Resident and Staff Physician 23:67–75, 1977)

activity in serum is greater than that of LDH_1. The normal ratio of LDH_1 to LDH_2 is less than one in normal serum; that is, the amount of LDH_1 is less than that of LDH_2. After MI, the ratio reverses, because LDH_1 is liberated as a result of myocardial necrosis (Fig. 15-6). This "flipped" pattern occurs in one to three days, usually between 12 and 24 hours, and is present in 80% of MI patients within 48 hours after the acute episode.[17] Vasudevan noted that the "flipped" pattern is not essential for a diagnosis of MI. If the LDH_1 increases to 76% of LDH_2 in the absence of renal infarction or hemolysis, the specificity for MI is 95%.[53]

Other conditions associated with the "flipped" LDH pattern include renal infarction and hemolysis such as is associated with prosthetic heart valves or hemolytic anemia.[17]

Serum LDH isoenzymes are relatively sensitive and specific, but not so accurate as CK isoenzymes for determining or excluding a diagnosis of MI (Table 15-6).[54] Serum for LDH iosenzyme determination must be kept at room temperature.

Normal Values of Serum LDH Isoenzymes[2]

ISOENZYME	ACTIVITY
LDH_1	17–27%
LDH_2	28–38%
LDH_3	19–27%
LDH_4	5–16%
LDH_5	5–16%

Creatine Kinase

Creatine kinase (CK) is generally regarded as the most sensitive and reliable enzyme used in the diagnosis of MI. Heart and skeletal muscle are its richest source (Table 15-7).[9] Appearance of CK occurs as early as three to six hours after the onset of an MI, and peaks at approximately 24 hours. The enzyme has usually returned to the normal range after 72 to 96 hours (Fig. 15-7).

According to Beeler, the sensitivity of CK is 96%. Its specificity, however, is much lower, because CK can also be

Fig. 15-6. Isoenzyme pattern in acute MI with LDH_1 greater than LDH_2. (Burke M: Postgrad Med 64(1):169, 1978)

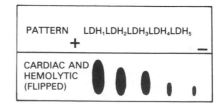

TABLE 15-6 PARAMETER SENSITIVITY AND SPECIFICITY

Diagnostic parameter	False-negative (%)	Sensitivity (%)	False-positive (%)	Specificity (%)
ECG	34	66	0	100
Total CK	2	98	15	85
$LDH_1 : LDH_2$	10	90	5	95
CPK-MB	0	100	1	99

The incidence of both falsely positive and falsely negative parameters is shown. A parameter was considered falsely positive when all others (3) were negative. Likewise, a parameter was considered falsely negative when all others (3) were positive. Lack of false positives is indicative of a specific parameter, whereas lack of false negatives indicates high sensitivity.

(Wagner GS, Roe CR, Limbird, LE et al: The importance of identification of the myocardial specific isoenzyme of creatine phosphokinase (MB form) in the diagnosis of acute myocardial infarction. Circulation 47:263–269, 1973)

TABLE 15-7 RELATIVE CONTENT OF CK IN TISSUES*

Skeletal muscle	3
Heart	1
Cerebral cortex	0.75
Nonpregnant uterus	0.15
Gall bladder	0.1
Pylorus	0.035
Adrenal	0.025
Thyroid	0.015
Lung	0.0001
Liver and red blood cells	0

* Heart muscle content regarded as 1
(Coodley EL: In Brest AN (ed): Coronary Heart Disease. Cardiovasc Clin 1(2):139–153, 1969)

elevated due to strenuous exercise[50] in patients with primary disease of the muscle,[11] with convulsions,[3] with chronic alcoholism,[35] with intramuscular injections,[34] and by major surgery (unrelated to the type of operative procedure).[13] Approximately 50% of patients with acute cerebrovascular diseases have abnormally high serum CK levels.[1] The time course of serum CK in MI and in cerebrovascular diseases reveals two major differences. In MI, there is an early appearance of abnormal levels of CK, whereas it takes approximately two days before the onset of abnormal levels in the cerebrovascular group. Second, the abnormal levels in the cerebrovascular group seem to last longer, and the levels are not so high as those found in MI.

Controversy about elevated CK in relation to cardioversion still persists, with most findings being of infrequent to modest elevation, seemingly dependent upon the number of shocks delivered and watt-seconds used.[14,38] Elevation of CK has been described in association with coronary angiography and cardiac catheterization. Matlof and co-workers[33] have shown the CK rise associated with coronary angiography is primarily the result of parenteral premedication and can be avoided by the use of oral premedication.

Infarction size can be assessed quantitatively in patients

with MI by analysis of serial CK changes, or by determination of CK peak values.[49]

However, large contributions to elevated serum CK from other tissues can spuriously influence calculations of infarction size.

Normal Values of Serum CK

Female—up to 2.5 units[2]; 5–35 mU/ml[51]
Male—up to 4.3 units[2]; 5–55 mU/ml[51]

Creatine Kinase Iosenzymes

Creatine kinase has three isoenzymes: fast-moving CK-1 (BB), intermediate moving CK-2 (MB), and slow moving CK-3 (MM). These isoenzymes can be identified by column chromatography, electrophoresis, or radioimmunoassay.

Normal serum contains only the MM fraction, although an occasional trace of MB activity may be seen.[5,37] The BB fraction is almost never seen in serum, even after a cerebrovascular accident, because the enzyme does not cross the blood-brain barrier (Fig. 15-8)[17]

The CK-MM is found predominantly in skeletal and cardiac muscle. The CK-BB is predominantly present in brain. The myocardium contains predominantly CK-MM, but 15% to 20% of the total CK activity is contributed by the MB portion. Table 15-8 shows the distribution of CK isoenzymes in human tissue. Thus, myocardial necrosis results in the appearance of significant amounts of the CK-MB isoenzyme. Elevation of the CK-MB is found in the 48-hour period following MI in all patients.[18] After an MI, CK-MB appears approximately four to eight hours after chest pain and reaches peak activity at 24 hours. The CK-MB level never exceeds 40% of the total CK activity, the remainder being CK-MM.[17] The CK-MM remains elevated for four to five days after the episode. Three blood samples should be obtained within the 48 hours after MI symptoms: on admission, at 24 hours, at 48 hours.[17] It is suggested by others that in order to predict rate of isoenzyme rise, blood samples should be obtained during the 24 hours following the onset of symptoms from MI at 3 hours, at 6 hours, at 12 hours, and at 24 hours.

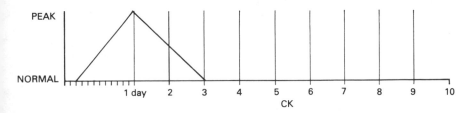

Fig. 15-7. CK elevation occurs 3 to 6 hours after MI, reaches a peak approximately 24 hours later, and returns to normal after about 3 days. (Adapted from Jackson VD: Myocardial Infarction, p 35. Fort Lauderdale, Saturn Scientific, 1977)

Despite the increasing use of CK-MB fraction in the diagnosis of MI, the current medical literature contains conflicting reports. Opinions differ as to whether

1. CK-MB is present only in the myocardium.
2. CK-MB is released only with MI.[21]

Other tissues reported to have CK-MB fraction include aorta, diaphragm, and tongue, all of which contain the CK-MM as the predominant isoenzyme.[24] The bladder, intestine, pancreas, prostate, stomach, and uterus are reported to contain CK-MB but predominantly CK-BB.[24,56] In contrast, Roberts and co-workers[43] and Galen and Gambino[18] surveyed a variety of human tissues obtained at surgery and identified CK-MB only in the myocardium. Differences are probably due to the use of different laboratory methods.

Serum CK-MB release has also been reported to occur in the absence of an MI. Table 15-9 lists some causes of a CK-MB release. Table 15-10 lists some causes that are known not to elevate CK-MB activity.

A rise in serum CK-MB is less useful as an indication of MI after cardiac surgical procedures, such as coronary bypass grafting, valve replacement, or repair of congenital defects. The CK-MB release occurs intra-operatively; therefore, the CK-MB cannot reliably indicate the occurrence of an acute MI in the perioperative period of cardiac surgery.[36]

TABLE 15-9   PROCEDURES AND DISEASES RESULTING IN SERUM CK-MB RELEASE

Atrial fibrillation[14]
Cardiac catherization[18]
Cardiac contusion[32]
Cardiopulmonary resuscitation[52]
Cardioversion[14]
Congestive heart failure[19,20]
Multiple trauma[18]
Muscular dystrophy[18]
Myoglobinuria[18]
Polymyositis[4,18]
Pulmonary emboli[20]
Tachyarrhythmias[14]

TABLE 15-10   DISORDERS AND PROCEDURES NOT RESULTING IN CK-MB RELEASE

Cardiac catherization[42,43]
Cardioversion[27]
Pulmonary embolism[27]
Acute rhabdomyolysis[41]
Thoracic, abdominal, genitourinary surgery[43,44]
Trauma[25]

Estimation of infarction size by means of measuring accumulated CK-MB release can be a valid and reliable clinical measure for assessing the extent of left ventricular necrosis in the setting of acute MI.[40] It is less valid and reliable in certain cases of inferior wall MI because there may be concomitant right and left ventricular necrosis.

A combined analysis of isoenzymes during the initial 48 hours after an acute MI offers a substantial amount of information. The presence of an elevated CK-MB fraction and the "flipped" LDH isoenzyme pattern is helpful in the diagnosis of MI (Table 15-11). The predictive values of combined isoenzyme profiles is shown in Table 15-12.

Serum CK-MB appears to be the most specific and sensitive indicator of an acute MI available at this time. Failure to detect this isoenzyme virtually excludes the diagnosis of MI, provided blood samples are drawn on admission, and at 8-hour intervals for the next 24 hours.[31] Because of the heat lability of the CK-MB isoenzyme, the blood sample should be frozen after it is obtained.

Normal Value of Serum CK-MB

Not detected in serum

Use of enzyme analysis has proved valuable in the diagnosis of MI. Serial blood samples of multiple enzymes lend greater sensitivity and specificity to the test. Creatine kinase appears to be the most helpful enzyme in diagnosing MI, but it must be kept in mind that CK is elevated in other clinical states. Serum LDH isoenzymes are relatively sensitive and specific, but not so accurate as CK-MB isoenzyme for defining or excluding the diagnosis of acute MI. A combined analysis of isoenzymes will increase the amount of information needed to make the clinical diagnosis of acute MI.

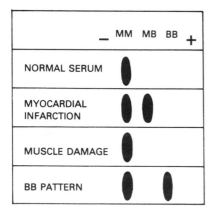

Fig. 15-8. CK isoenzymes normally present in MI, with muscle damage, and BB pattern. BB pattern appears with acute brain injury, gastric carcinoma, and stage D prostatic carcinoma and in patients undergoing long-term hemodialysis or aortocoronary bypass surgery. Symbols indicate positive (+) and negative (−) poles of electrical field. (Burke M: Postgrad Med 64(1):169, 1978)

TABLE 15-8   DISTRIBUTION OF CK ISOENZYMES IN HUMAN TISSUES

	CK-1(BB)	CK-2(MB)	CK-3(MM)
Normal serum	0%	0%	100%
Skeletal muscle	0	0	100
Heart	0	40	60
Brain	90	0	10
Lung	90	0	10
Bladder	95	0	5
Bowel	100	0	0

(Galen RS: Resident and Staff Physician 23:67–75, 1977)

TABLE 15-11 ENZYME PATTERNS AND PROBABILITY OF MYOCARDIAL INFARCTION (DURING THE 48-HOUR PERIOD FOLLOWING THE ACUTE EPISODE)

Enzyme Pattern	CK-MB absent Usual LDH	CK-MB present Usual LDH	CK-MB present Flipped LDH
Probability of MI	100% no MI	Equivocal for MI*	100% MI

* The non-MI cases show clinical and ECG evidence of ischemia.
(Galen RS: Resident and Staff Physician 23:67–75, 1977)

TABLE 15-12 PREDICTIVE VALUE OF COMBINED ISOENZYMES FOR MI AND NON-MI PATIENTS

Isoenzyme	Number of subjects	Combined clinical and ECG classification		Predictive value of the result
		MI	NON-MI	%
CK-MB present, LDH isoenzymes flipped	36	36	None	100
CK-MB present, LDH isoenzymes not flipped	17	10	7	60
CK-MB absent	41	None	41	100

(Galen RS, Reiffel JA, Gambino SR: JAMA 232(2):145–147, 1975)

HEMATOLOGIC STUDIES

In a complete blood count (CBC), the following determinations are included: red blood cell (RBC) count, hemoglobin (Hb), hematocrit (Hct), corpuscular indices, white blood cell count (WBC), and a differential WBC count (Diff.). Other hematologic studies include sedimentation rate, prothrombin time, recalcification time, and partial thromboplastin time.

Complete Blood Cell Count

Red Blood Cell Count. The RBCs (erythrocytes) are formed in the red bone marrow. The production of RBCs is inhibited by a rise in circulating RBC levels, and stimulated by anemia and hypoxemia. The RBC represents the number of RBCs in 1 microliter (μl) of whole blood.

Normal Red Blood Cell Count[51]

4.6 and 6.2 × 10[6] μl(male); 4.2 and 5.4 × 10[6] μl(female)

Hematocrit. The hematocrit (Hct) is the volume of packed RBCs found in 100 ml of blood.

Normal Hematocrit[51]

Men—40–54%
Women—38–47%

Hemoglobin. The RBCs contain a complex protein compound called hemoglobin. Hemoglobin (Hb) is the oxygen-carrying protein of the RBC and is reported in grams per 100 ml. A deficiency in the total Hb is termed anemia. Normochromic normocytic anemia (normal cell size, normal color) is commonly caused by chronic disease and extensive hemorrhage and hemolysis. Hemolysis in the cardiac patient may be due to prosthetic heart valves. Hypochromic microcytic anemia (smaller than normal cells, less than normal color) is most frequently caused by iron deficiency. Macrocytic anemias (larger than normal cells) are often associated with folic acid deficiency and vitamin B_{12} deficiency. Anemia from any cause must be looked for in the cardiac patient, because it may manifest itself as angina, aggravate congestive heart failure, and contribute to a diagnosis of subacute bacterial endocarditis.[51]

Normal Hemoglobin

men 13.5 to 18.0 g/100 ml; in women, 12.0 to 16.0 g/100 ml.[51]

Corpuscular Indices. With the erythrocyte count, the quantity of hemoglobin, and the hematocrit, one can describe the characteristics of individual RBCs in terms of cell size [mean corpuscular volume (MCV)], in terms of amount of hemoglobin present in a single cell [mean corpuscular hemoglobin (MCH)], and in terms of the proportion of each cell occupied by hemoglobin [mean corpuscular hemoglobin concentration (MCHC)]. The indices are calculated by these formulas:[55]

$$MCV = \frac{Hematocrit\ (as\ \%) \times 10}{RBC\ count\ (millions\ per\ cubic\ mm)}$$

$$MCH = \frac{Hemoglobin\ (as\ g/100\ ml) \times 10}{RBC\ count}$$

$$MCHC = \frac{Hemoglobin}{Hematocrit}$$

Normal Values[51]

MCV—82–98 cu microns
MCH—27–31 pg
MCHC—32–36%

White Blood Cell (WBC) Count

The white blood cell count expresses the number of WBCs in 1 microliter of whole blood. For five to seven days after MI the WBCs may be 12,000 to 15,000/cu mm. Elevation of the WBC also occurs in patients with bacterial endocarditis and Dressler's syndrome, or any other disease process which has an inflammatory component.

Normal White Blood Count[51]
4500 and 11,000/cu mm.

Differential Count

An important part of the WBC count is the differential count, so-called because it is a tabulation of the various types of WBCs that constitute the total count.

As mentioned previously, an acute MI, bacterial endocarditis, and Dressler's syndrome can all cause an elevated WBC count. This elevation is due to increased amounts of neutrophils and is termed neutrophilic leukocytosis.

Adult WBC Differential Counts[16]

CELL	AVERAGE* (ABSOLUTE)	RANGE* (ABSOLUTE)	(PERCENT OF TOTAL)
Total leukocytes	7,000	5,000–10,000	100
Total neutrophils	4,300	3,000–7,000	60 to 70
Lymphocytes	2,100	1,500–3,000	20 to 30
Monocytes	375	285–500	2 to 6
Eosinophils	200	50–400	1 to 4
Basophils	25	0–50	0.1

* Figures are in terms of number of cells per cubic millimeter of whole blood.

Sedimentation Rate (Sed Rate)

The sedimentation rate reveals the speed of sedimentation of RBCs; it is elevated in inflammatory processes. The sedimentation rate is elevated in MI, in bacterial endocarditis, and in Dressler's syndrome and is low in congestive heart failure.[51] Because many other factors affect the sed rate, it is considered a nonspecific test, having neither disease nor organ specificity.

Normal Sedimentation Rate (Westergren)

Men under 50 years	15 mm/hour
Men over 50 years	20 mm/hour
Women under 50 years	20 mm/hour
Women over 50 years	30 mm/hour

Prothrombin Time (PT)

Used in initiating and maintaining patients on oral anticoagulants such as warfarin, this test measures the activity of prothrombin, fibrinogen, and Factors V, VII, and X. Warfarin inhibits vitamin K-dependent synthesis activation of clotting Factors II, VII, IX, and X. Therapeutic PTs are considered to be 1.5 to 2 times normal, or a 15 to 50% change in the normal value.

Normal Prothrombin Time[51]
12 to 15 seconds

Recalcification (recal) Time

Anticoagulants found in the blood-collecting tube prevent coagulation by binding calcium ions needed at various stages of clotting. The ionized calcium can be restored under controlled conditions and the time required for clotting of recalcified plasma measured. The therapeutic range for the recal time is 1.5 to 2 times normal.

Normal Recalcification Time[55]
69 to 122 seconds

Partial Thromboplastin Time (PTT)

This test is used in assessing patients receiving heparin. It measures deficiencies in all plasma clotting factors except VII.[16] Heparin sodium acts directly with antithrombin III to prevent the formation of thrombin and fibrin. Low dosages of heparin diminish production of clotting Factor X and thus limit the clotting factor substrates available to form thrombin and fibrin. The therapeutic range for PTT is kept at 1.5 to 2.5 times the normal.

Normal Partial Thromboplastin Time[51]
60 to 70 seconds

BLOOD CHEMISTRIES

Blood specimens for biochemical testing are drawn by venipuncture when the patient is in the postabsorptive state (not having eaten for 10 or more hours). Blood is drawn at a consistent time of day in order to provide a patient's baseline when comparing repeated tests. A single sample of 2.5 ml of serum is required to obtain 12 blood chemistries when the multichanneled analyzer, SMA (sequential multiple analysis), is used. The 12 tests usually include (1) sodium, (2) potassium, (3) chloride, (4) carbon dioxide, (5) total protein, (6) albumin, (7) urea nitrogen, (8) glucose, (9) calcium, (10) bilirubin, (11) alkaline phosphatase, and (12) glutamic oxaloacetic transaminase. Results of the SMA 12 can be recorded on a graph form. In addition to these 12 tests, other chemical tests may be needed to evaluate a patient with cardiac disease. Some of these tests may include measurement of catecholamines, creatinine, lipoprotein and lipid electrophoresis, magnesium, and uric acid.

Normal values may differ from laboratory to laboratory, because individual differences in procedure affect actual ranges. Ranges of normal values of selected blood chemistries can be found in Table 15-13.

TABLE 15-13 NORMAL RANGES OF SELECTED BLOOD CHEMISTRIES

Blood Chemistry	Normal Range	Comments
Bilirubin (total)	Up to 1.5 mg/100 ml	
Calcium: total	4.6–5.5 mEq/l	Serum protein level
ionized	1.9–2.25 mEq/l (pH 7.4 and 37°C)	may affect results.
Carbon dioxide content	24–34 mEq/l	
Chloride	98–109 mEq/l	
Cholesterol	135–315 mg/100 ml (at age 40)	Fasting
Creatine kinase	Up to 4.3 units (male) Up to 2.5 units (female)	
Creatinine	0.9–1.4 mg/100 ml (male) 0.8–1.2 mg/100 ml (female)	
Epinephrine	0.48–0.51 μg/l[16]	
Glucose	70–110 mg/100 ml	Fasting
Lactic dehydrogenase	63–155 units (male) 62–131 units (female)	
Magnesium	1.3–2.1 mEq/l	
Norepinephrine	1.55–3.73 μg/l[16]	
Osmolality	278–305 mOsm/kg serum water	
Phosphate, alkaline	35–148 units	
Potassium	3.6–5.5 mEq/l	
Protein (total)	6.6–8.3 g/100 ml	
Sodium	135–155 mEq/l	
Transaminase glutamic- oxalacetic	13–55 units	
Triglyceride	30–135 mg/100 ml	Fasting
Urea nitrogen	8–26 mg/100 ml	
Uric acid	4.0–8.5 mg/100 ml (males) 2.8–7.5 mg/100 ml (females)	

(A Pocket Guide to Text Requirements: Van Nuys, CA, Bio Sciences Laboratories, May 1978)

Electrolytes

Electrolyte balance and electrolyte imbalances in cardiac patients are discussed in depth in Chapter 9. The electrolytes discussed below are those commonly measured in cardiac patients. Most of them are measured when an SMA-12 is obtained.

Calcium. Calcium is essential for the formation of bones and for blood coagulation. Calcium ions affect neuromuscular excitability and cellular and capillary permeability;[55] they also contribute to anion–cation balance.

Carbon Dioxide. Carbon dioxide is a part of the alkali reserve of the body. The amount of carbon dioxide indicates the amount of bicarbonate available to combine with cations.[46] Carbonic acid and bicarbonate are measured to obtain carbon dioxide content.

Chloride. Chloride influences the osmotic pressure of the blood, tissues, and intersititial fluids. Chloride maintains electrical neutrality.

Sodium. Sodium concentration reflects relative water balance.

Magnesium. Magnesium is essential in many enzymatic activities involving lipid, carbohydrate and protein metabolism. It is predominantly an intracellular ion.

Potassium (K+). Potassium is important in anion-cation balance and is essential to proper muscular function and electrical conductance. Small increases and decreases in serum K+ affect heart function. When drawing blood, care should be taken to avoid hemolysis.

Other Selected Chemistries

Alkaline Phosphatase. Alkaline phosphatase is an enzyme released in liver and bone disease. An increased serum level suggests an abnormality in the liver or in bones.

Bilirubin. Bilirubin is a product of hemoglobin breakdown and is removed from the body by the liver. An elevated bilirubin level may indicate abnormal liver function.

Catecholamines. Epinephrine and norepinephrine are elevated in pheochromocytoma, a tumor of the adrenal medulla. Pheochromocytoma is a cause of hypertension.

Creatinine. Creatinine is a waste product formed from creatine and phosphocreatine. Individuals with large muscle mass have higher serum creatinine levels than do those with less muscle. Creatinine is easily excreted by the kidney. An elevated serum level implies severe long-standing kidney function impairment.

Glucose. Glucose is elevated whenever endogenous epinephrine is mobilized. Mild hyperglycemia would be expected during stress states. Blood specimens for glucose determination should be drawn when the patient is fasting. Hyperglycemia is often precipitated by myocardial infarction.[12] Diabetes mellitus is frequently the cause of marked hyperglycemia. Myocardial infarction may precipitate diabetes in a person with latent diabetes.[46]

Protein. Total protein measurement includes addition of the following serum proteins: albumin (53%); globulin (14% alpha, 12% beta, and 20% gamma); and fibrinogen (1%). Protein components (albumin and globulins) can be quantitated with the use of protein electrophoresis. Albumin (4 to 5.5 g/100 ml) contributes to the balance of osmotic pressure between blood and tissues. Globulins (2 to 3 g/100 ml) influence osmotic pressure and include the immunoglobulins (antibodies). Fibrinogen (0.2 to 0.4 g/100 ml) is the precursor of fibrin which forms the blood clot. Since albumin is produced in the liver, a low serum albumin level is seen in liver disease. The half-life of albumin is 18 days. If albumin is reduced, edema results, because albumin accounts for 90% of the serum colloid-osmotic pressure. Albumin is reduced in congestive heart failure because of hypervolemic dilution. Alpha and beta globulins tend to decrease with abnormal liver function. The gamma globulins, the body's antibodies, increase with chronic disease.[55] Fibrinogen, a large globulin, is manufactured by the liver; it is reduced in disseminated intravascular coagulation and increased in some bacterial infections.[55]

Urea Nitrogen. Urea nitrogen is the nitrogen fraction of urea and is excreted by the kidney. Blood urea nitrogen (BUN) increases when the kidney is diseased, or in diseases that affect kidney function. The BUN increases with gastrointestinal hemorrhage, with saline depletion, and with reduced renal perfusion.

Uric Acid. Uric acid is the end product of purine metabolism. Uric acid is increased in gout. Severe renal disease results in a high level of serum uric acid, because excretion is reduced. Large doses of salicylates may interfere with accurate test results.[55]

Lipid Categories

Plasma normally contains insoluble lipid elements: free fatty acids; exogenous triglycerides; endogenous triglycerides, which are manufactured in the liver; cholesterol; and phospholipids. To be transported, each is attached to a protein.

Free Fatty Acids. Free fatty acids (FFA) are rapidly turned over and provide the body with an energy supply. Measurement of FFA is not part of clinical lipid evaluation.

Triglycerides. Lipids from the diet appear in plasma as the triglyceride portion of chylomicrons. Clearance of chylomicrons from the blood should be complete six hours after a fat-containing meal. Chylomicrons contain 81% triglycerides, 10% cholesterol, 7% phospholipids, and 2% protein. Endogenous triglycerides are triesters of glycerol and fatty acids synthesized from carbohydrates by the liver and are transported primarily in very low density (pre-beta) lipoproteins (Fig. 15-9).[16]

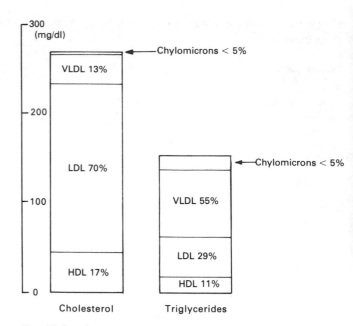

Fig. 15-9. Contribution of each lipoprotein class to total plasma cholesterol and triglycerides in the normal subject. (Lees RS, Wilson DE: N Engl J Med 284(4):187, 1971)

Cholesterol. The cholesterol level is important in the evaluation of the tendency toward atherosclerosis. The liver has a prominent role in the metabolism of cholesterol. Each major lipoprotein fraction carries cholesterol. Cholesterol is transported largely in the low density (beta) lipoprotein. Small amounts are transported in the high density (alpha) lipoproteins and in the low density (pre-beta) lipoproteins (Fig. 15-9).

Phospholipids. Phospholipids are important in membrane metabolism. The principal circulating phospholipids (150 to 375 mg per 100 ml) are lecithin and sphyngomyelin. Phospholipids are transported in the alpha and beta lipoproteins, chiefly as high density alpha molecules. The relationship between the phospholipids and the other serum lipids can be determined by electrophoresis. Lipoprotein electrophoresis is extremely valuable in the identification of individuals who are likely to develop atherosclerosis or coronary artery disease, or both.

Lipoprotein Electrophoresis

Electrophoresis separates the lipoproteins into the stationary chylomicrons (least dense) and the remaining mobile lipoproteins. The alpha (high-density) lipoproteins move the farthest; the beta (low-density) move least; and the pre-beta (very low density) fall between the alpha and the beta lipoproteins. (Fig. 15-10). The bands of lipoprotein produced permit qualitative evaluation. The densitometer has been used for quantitation.[39]

There are five major abnormal patterns of lipoprotein electrophoresis as classified by Frederickson and Lee. Each is produced by a familial hyperlipoproteinemia. The five types are summarized in Table 15-14. The electrophoresis pattern is shown in Figure 15-10. Distinguishing lipoprotein abnormalities is useful, since diet and drug therapy varies with each type.

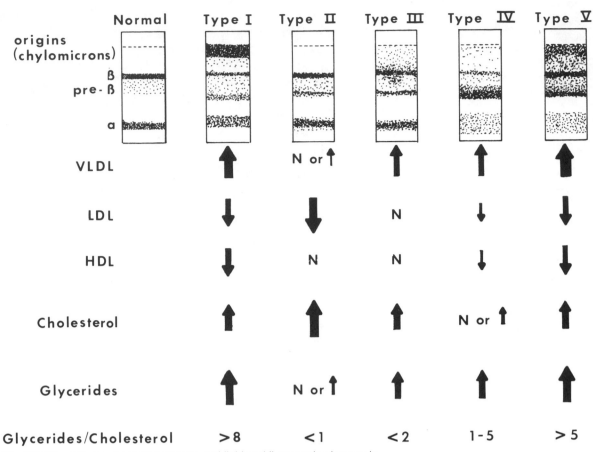

Fig. 15-10. Electrophoresis patterns and lipid and lipoprotein changes in hyperlipoproteinemia. The width of the arrows is proportional to the extent of the deviation from normal, and the direction of the arrows indicates increase or decrease of lipids. The usual glyceride—cholesterol ratio is given as an aid to diagnosis. (Lees RS, Wilson DE: N Engl J Med 284(4):187, 1971)

TABLE 15-14   TYPES OF FAMILIAL HYPERLIPOPROTEINEMIAS

Lipoprotein	Electrophoresis	Comments
I	Prominent chylomicron band; other lipoprotein bands decreased.	Plasma creamy in appearance (it develops a top cream layer with clear plasma below) Uncommon type
II	Prominent beta bands; other bands normal	Plasma appears clear Common type Seen in severe, early coronary artery disease (CAD)
III	Broad beta band; other bands normal	Clear to milky appearing plasma Uncommon type Seen in accelerated atherosclerotic disease, especially peripheral
IV	Pre-beta band increased; other bands decreased	Clear to milky appearing plasma Most common type CAD is pronounced
V	Pre-beta band increased; chylomicron band present	Plasma is creamy Uncommon to fairly common type

(Data from Frederickson DS, Lees RF: Circulation 31:321–327, 1965; French RM: The Nurse's Guide to Diagnostic Procedures. New York, McGraw-Hill, 1971; Roberts R, Sobel BE: Arch Intern Med 138:421–424, 1976; Widmann, FK: Goodale's Clinical Interpretation of Laboratory Tests. Philadelphia, FA Davis, 1973)

A nomogram using serum levels of triglycerides and cholesterol for determining types of hyperlipidemia has been proposed by Harlan (Fig. 15-11). It does not replace electrophoresis.

When blood specimens for lipid studies are obtained, the patient should be fasting, should have eaten only a normal diet for two weeks, have had no alcoholic beverages for the preceding 24 to 48 hours, and have had no recent radiologic examinations that used contrast media. The usual screening test includes cholesterol and triglyceride levels and lipoprotein electrophoresis. Since lipids may be abnormal if drawn when the patient is having an acute MI, it is recommended

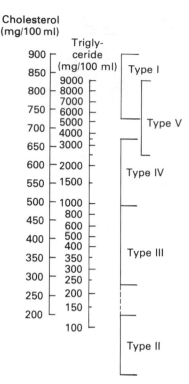

Fig. 15-11. Nomogram for determining types of hyperlipidemia. The type of hyperlipidemia is determined by placing a straightedge over the cholesterol and triglyceride values; the Frederickson classification is then indicated on the right hand scale. (Harlan WR: Arch Intern Med 124:64—65, 1969)

that lipid studies be done at another time. The amount of serum needed for selected chemistries can be found in Table 15-15.

URINALYSIS

A urine specimen for a routine urinalysis is obtained from all patients admitted to the cardiac care unit and refrigerated at once to inhibit bacterial growth. The usual tests done are (1) description of the color; (2) degree of cloudiness; (3)

TABLE 15-16   NORMAL RESULTS OF A ROUTINE URINALYSIS

Color	Pale straw to dark amber
Degree of cloudiness	Clear
pH	4.5 to 7.5
Specific gravity	1.010 to 1.025
Protein	None to a trace
Glucose	None

Microscopic Examination

Epithelial cells	Squamous only
White blood cells	Fewer than 4 cells/high power field
Red blood cells	Occasional cells/high power field
Casts	None

(French RM: The Nurse's Guide to Diagnostic Procedures. New York, McGraw Hill, 1971)

pH: (4) specific gravity; (5) tests for protein and glucose; and (6) a microscopic examination of the sediment. Certain drugs artifactually change the color of the urine. Phenazopyridine (pyridium) causes the urine to turn orange, riboflavin causes it to turn bright orange, phenacetin may turn the urine brownish-grey or black, and diphenylhydantoin and phenothiazines may turn it pink, red, or reddish brown.[51] Normal results of a routine urinalysis can be found in Table 15-16. Abnormal findings may indicate the need for other tests.

SERUM CONCENTRATIONS OF SELECTED DRUGS

Serum levels of cardiac drugs are frequently obtained to determine the effectiveness of drug therapy. Usual ranges of therapeutic and toxic ranges of serum concentrations of selected drugs are given in Table 15-17.

The serum concentrations must always be interpreted in the context of all the clinical data. For example, digitalis intoxication can occur within the usual range of therapeutic serum concentrations, if the patient has hypokalemia, hypercalcemia, hypomagnesemia, acid-base imbalances, in-

TABLE 15-15   AMOUNT OF SERUM NEEDED FOR SELECTED LABORATORY TESTS AS REQUIRED BY BIOSCIENCE LABORATORIES

Albumin	1 ml		Lactic dehydrogenase (LHD)	1 ml—room temperature only
Alkaline phosphatase	1 ml		LDH isoenzymes	1 ml—room temperature only
Bilirubin	1 ml protect from light		Lipoprotein electro-	
Calcium	1 ml		phoresis	1 ml
Carbon dioxide	3 ml		Magnesium	1 ml
Chloride	1 ml		Potassium	1 ml
Cholesterol	1 ml		Procainamide	4 ml
Creatine kinase (CK)	1 ml		Propranolol	5 ml
CK isoenzyme	2 ml		Protein	1 ml
Creatinine	1 ml		Quinidine	2 ml
Dilantin	2 ml		Sodium	1 ml
Enzyme electrophoresis	1 ml		Uric acid	1 ml (phosphotung state method)
Globulin	1 ml			
Glucose	1 ml		Urea nitrogen	1 ml

(A Pocket Guide to Test Requirements. Van Nuys, CA, Bio Science Laboratories, May, 1978)

TABLE 15-17 THERAPEUTIC AND TOXIC SERUM CONCENTRATIONS OF SELECTED DRUGS

	Therapeutic	Toxic
Digitoxin	Up to 20 ng/ml	Over 26 ng/ml
Digoxin	0.5–2.0 ng/ml	Over 2.0 ng/ml
Diphenylhydantoin	10–20 μg/ml	20–50μg/ml
Disopyramide	2–4 ng/ml[51]	
Lidocaine	1.2–5.5 μg/ml	Over 9 μg/ml
Procainamide	4–8 μg/ml	Over 12 μg/ml
Propranolol	40–85 ng/ml	Over 85 ng/ml
Quinidine sulfate	2.3–5.0 μg/ml	Over 6 μg/ml
Theophylline	10–20 μg/ml	Over 20 μg/ml
Tocainide	6–12 ng/ml[51]	
Verapamil	2–4 ng/ml[51]	

(A Pocket Guide to Test Requirements: Van Nuys, CA, Bio Science Laboratories, May, 1978)

creased adrenergic tone, hypothyroidism, hypoxemia, or myocardial ischemia.[26]

Digitoxin, diphenylhydantoin, and quinidine and chiefly bound to serum albumin. Bound fractions have no pharmacologic effect. The determination of a drug in the serum is usually the total amount bound and unbound. Usually the amount of unbound drug is a fairly constant percentage of the total. In situations where there is less albumin, or when the drug-binding ability of the albumin is depressed (such as uremia), or where other drugs that are highly bound to protein are also given, then the amount of drug bound will be less. Thus, serious toxicity can result even within the normal therapeutic range because of an increase in non-protein bound drug.[26]

The blood specimen to determine serum concentration of a drug should be drawn one to two hours after an oral drug is given, since absorption and distribution are usually complete by this time. The serum concentration is lowest shortly after the administration of an oral dose.[26]

REFERENCES

1. Acheson J, James DC, Hutchinson EC et al: Serum-creatine-kinase levels in cerebral vascular disease. Lancet 1:1306–1307, 1965
2. A Pocket Guide To Test Requirements: Van Nuys, CA, Bio Science Laboratories, May, 1978
3. Belton NR, Backus RE, Millichap J: Serum creatine phosphokinase activity in epilepsy. Neurology 17(11):1073–1076, 1967
4. Brownlow K, Elevitch FR: Serum creatine phosphokinase isoenzyme (CPK₂) in myositis. JAMA 230:1141–1144, 1974
5. Burke MD: Clinical enzymology. Postgrad Med 64(1):165–170, 1978
6. Burke MD: Laboratory tests: Basic concepts and realistic expectations. Postgrad Med 63(4):53–60, 1978
7. Cardiac Enzymes in Perspective: Nutley, Roche Diagnostics, Hoffman–LaRoche, 1976
8. Coodley EL: The diagnosis of myocardial infarction by enzyme analysis. In Meltzer LE, Dunning AJ (eds): Textbook of Coronary Care, pp 82–92. Philadelphia, Charles Press, 1972
9. Coodley EL: Enzymes and isoenzymes in myocardial infarction, In Brest AN (ed): Coronary Heart Disease. Cardiovasc Clin 1(2):139–153, 1969
10. Coodley EL: Prognostic value of enzymes in myocardial infarction. JAMA 225(6):597–605, 1973
11. Danowski TS, Sabeth G, Vester JW et al: Serum CPK in muscular dystrophy and myotomia dystrophica. Metabolism 17:808–817, 1968
12. Datey KK, Nanda NC: Hyperglycemia after acute myocardial infarction: its relation to diabetes mellitus. N Eng J Med 276(5):262–265, 1967
13. Dixon SH, Fuchs JC, Ebert PA: Changes in serum creatine phosphokinase activity following thoracic, cardiac and abdominal operations. Arch Surg 103:66–68, 1971
14. Ehsani A, Ewey GA, Sobel BE: Effects of electrical countershock on serum creatine phosphokinase isoenzyme activity. A J Cardiol 37:12–18, 1976
15. Frederickson DS, Lees RS: A system for phenotyping hyperlipoproteinemia. Circulation 31:321–327, 1965
16. French RM: The Nurse's Guide to Diagnostic Procedures. New York, McGraw-Hill, 1971
17. Galen RS: Myocardial infarction: A clinician's guide to the isoenzymes. Resident and Staff Physician 23:67–75, 1977
18. Galen RS, Gambino SR: Isoenzymes of CPK and LDH in myocardial infarction and certain other disease. Pathobiol Annu 5:283–315, 1975
19. Galen RS, Gambino SR: Creatine kinase isoenzyme MB and heart disease. Clin Chem 21:1848–1849, 1975
20. Galen RS, Reiffel JA, Gambino SR: Diagnosis of acute myocardial infarction. JAMA 232(2):145–147, 1975
21. Guzy PM: Creatine phosphokinase–MB (CPK–MB) and the diagnosis of myocardial infarction. West J Med 127:455–460, 1977
22. Harlan WR: A nomogram for determining types of hyperlipidemia. Arch Intern Med 124:64–65, 1969
23. Jackson VD: Myocardial Infarction. An Introduction for Nurses. Fort Lauderdale, Saturn Scientific, 1977
24. Jockers-Wretou E, Pfeiderer G: Quantitation of creatine kinase isoenzymes in human tissues and sera by an immunological method. Clin Chim Acta 58:223–232, 1975
25. Klein MS, Shell WE, Sobel BE: Serum creatine phosphokinase (CPK) isoenzymes after intramuscular injections, surgery and myocardial infarction: Experimental and clinical studies. Cardiovasc Res 7:412–418, 1973
26. Koch-Weser J: Serum drug concentrations as therapeutic guides. N Engl J Med 287(5):227–231, 1972
27. Konttinen A, Somer H: Specificity of serum creatine kinase isoenzymes in diagnosis of acute myocardial infarction. Br Med J 1:386–389, 1973
28. LaDue JS, Wroblewski F, Karmen A: Serum glutamic oxalo-acetic transaminase activity in human acute transmural myocardial infarction. Science 120:497–499, 1954
29. Latner A, Shillen AW: Isoenzymes in Biology and Medicine. New York, Academic Press, 1968.
30. Lees RS, Wilson DE: The treatment of hyperlipidemia. N Engl J Med 284(4):186–195, 1971
31. Lester RM, Wagner GS: Acute myocardial infarction. Cardiovasc Clin North Am 63(1):3–24, 1979
32. Lindsey D, Navin RT: Transient elevation of serum activity of MB isoenzyme of creatine phosphokinase in drivers involved in automobile accidents. Chest 74(1):15–18, 1978
33. Matlof HJ, Buhl J, Wexler L et al: Serum enzymes and electrocardiograms after coronary arteriography. N Engl J Med 288:142–143, 1973
34. Meltzer HY, Mrozak S, Boyer M: Effect of intramuscular injections on serum creatine phosphokinase activity. Am J Med Sci 259:42–48, 1970
35. Nygren A: Serum creatine phosphokinase in chronic alcoholism. Acta Med Scand 182:383–387, 1967
36. Oldham HN, Roe CR, Young WG, et al: Intraoperative detection of myocardial damage during coronary artery surgery by plasma creatine phosphokinase isoenzyme analysis. Surgery 74:917–925, 1973
37. Rapaport E: Serum enzymes and isoenzymes in the diagnosis of acute myocardial infarction. Part I: Serum enzymes. Mod Concepts Cardiovasc Dis 46(9):43–46, 1977
38. Reiffel JA, Gambino SR, McCarthy DM et al: JAMA 239(2):122–124, 1978
39. Remp D, Schatz IJ: Quantitation of Paper Electrophoretic Lipoprotein Patterns (abstr) Circulation (Suppl 2)36:33, 1967
40. Roberts R, Gowda KS, Ludbrook PA et al: Specificity of elevated serum MB creatine phosphokinase activity in the diagnosis of acute myocardial infarction." Am J Cardiol 36:433–437, 1975
41. Roberts R, Ludbrook PA, Weiss ES et al: Serum CPK isoenzymes after cardiac catheterization. Br Heart J 37:1144–1149, 1975

42. Roberts R, Sobel BE: CPK isoenzymes in evaluation of myocardial ischemic injury. Hosp Pract 11(1):55–62, 1976
43. Roberts R, Sobel BE: Elevated plasma MB creatine phosphokinase activity. Arch Intern Med 138:421–424, 1976
44. Roberts R, Sobel BE: Editorial: Isoenzymes of creatine phosphokinase and diagnosis of myocardial infarction. Ann Intern Med 79:741–743, 1973
45. Schatz IJ: Classification of primary hyperlipidemia—Observations on 214 patients. JAMA 210(4):701–704, 1969
46. Sharp L, Rabin B: Nursing in the Coronary Care Unit. Philadelphia, JB Lippincott, 1970
47. Smith AS: Separation of tissue and serum creatine isoenzymes on polyacrylamide gel slabs. Clin Chim Acta 39:351–350, 1972
48. Sobel BE: Enzymatic diagnosis of infarction. West J Med 127(6):505–508, 1977
49. Sobel BE: Estimation of infarct size in man and its relation to prognosis. Circulation 46:640–648, 1972
50. Swaiman KF, Awad EA: Creatine phosphokinase and other serum enzyme activity after controlled exercise. Neurology 14(11):977–980, 1964
51. Tilkian SM, Conover MB, Tilkian A: Clinical Implications of Laboratory Tests, 2nd ed. St. Louis, C.V. Mosby, 1979
52. Tonkin AM, Lester RM, Guthrow CE et al. Persistance of MB isoenzyme of creatine phosphokinase in the serum after minor iatrogenic cardiac trauma-absence of postmortem evidence of myocardial infarction. Circulation 47:627–631, 1973
53. Vasudevan G, Mercer DW, Varat MA: Lactic dehydrogenase isoenzyme determination in the diagnosis of acute myocardial infarction. Circulation 57(6):1055–1057, 1978
54. Wagner GS, Roe CR, Limbird, LE et al: The importance of identification of the myocardial specific isoenzyme of creatine phosphokinase (MB form) in the diagnosis of acute myocardial infarction. Circulation 47:263–269, 1973
55. Widmann FK: Goodale's Clinical Interpretation of Laboratory Tests. Philadelphia, FA Davis, 1973
56. Yasmineh WG, Pyle RB, Hanson NQ et al: Creatine kinase isoenzymes in baboon tissues and organs. Clin Chem 22:63–66, 1976

ADDITIONAL READING

Apps MCP, Tinker J: The measurement and control of myocardial infarct size. Intensive Care Med 4(21):21–27, 1978
Beeler MF: Interpretation in Clinical Chemistry. Chicago, American Society of Clinical Pathology, 1978
Bigger JT Jr, Schmidt DH, Kutt H: Relationship between the plasma level of diphenylhydantoin sodium and its cardiac antiarrhythmic effects. Circulation 38:363–374, 1968
Koch-Weser J, Klein SW: Procainamide dosage schedules, plasma concentrations, and clinical effects. JAMA 215:1454–1460, 1971
Scheer E: Enzymatic changes and myocardial infarction: A nursing update. Cardiovasc Nurs 14(2):5–8, 1978
Vesell ES, Passananti GT: Utility of clinical chemical determinations of drug concentrations in biological fluids. Clin Chem 17:851–866, 1971

16

Radiologic Examination of the Chest

JON S. HUSEBY, M.D.

A cardiac care nurse may be the first health-care professional to see the chest radiograph of a patient in acute distress. Valuable time may be saved if the nurse is able to recognize the presence of an abnormality. Knowledge of chest radiograph interpretation and the disease processes that an abnormal film indicates can help additionally in the nurse's understanding of disease pathophysiology thereby allowing for better patient care. This chapter will be divided into five sections:

1. How x-rays work
2. Interpretation of chest radiographs
3. Chest-film findings in MI or conditions that may mimic an acute MI
4. Chest-film findings in complications of acute MI
5. Miscellaneous uses of the chest radiograph

HOW X-RAYS WORK

X-rays are radiant energy, like light, except that these waves are shorter and can pass through opaque objects. They are produced by bombarding a tungsten target with an electron beam and are channeled so that a narrow but diverging beam is emitted from the tube. When an x-ray exposure is taken, the tube is usually aimed so that the rays pass through the subject to the x-ray film in either a posterior to anterior (PA) or anterior to posterior (AP) direction (Figs. 16-1, 16-2). Because the x-rays are diverging and subject to reflection (scatter), structures more distant from the film will be magnified and less distinctly outlined. Generally, chest radiographs are taken PA because this places the heart, an anterior structure, closer to the film, resulting in less

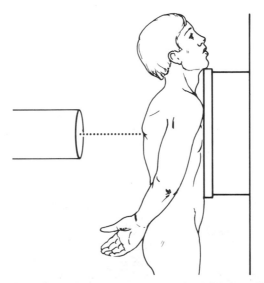

Fig. 16-1. Positioning a patient for a PA frontal chest radiograph. The x-ray tube is behind the patient and the x-ray film is close to his anterior chest.

magnification and allowing the cardiac outline to be seen clearly.

Anteroposterior chest radiographs are often taken in cardiac care units because it is difficult to put the x-ray tube behind the patient. The x-ray film is therefore placed behind the patient. Because the heart is relatively far away from the x-ray film, its outline is somewhat less distinct and the heart size is magnified. Moreover, the distance between the tube and the patient in cardiac care units (CCU) is shorter than usual, in order to cut down x-ray scatter. This also results in greater magnification.

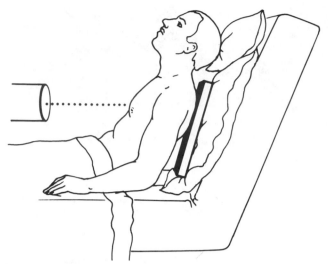

Fig. 16-2. Typical CCU patient positioned for an AP chest radiograph. Note that, as often occurs in the CCU, the patient's chest is not perfectly perpendicular to the x-ray tube. This causes the lung fields to appear large and indistinct. This is called a lordotic position.

The degree of darkness of the x-ray film depends on how much x-ray energy traverses the patient and exposes the film. This depends upon the density of the material through which the x-ray beam passes. The chest has four major types of tissue densities through which rays must pass: bone, water, fat, and air. Because bone is the densest of these, fewer and less energetic x-rays pass through this substance. Thus, the shadow on the x-ray film cast by bone is light. (An x-ray picture is like a photographic negative, with white color indicating lack of exposure and black color indicating intense exposure.) The lung, which is largely air, is least dense; therefore it appears black on a chest radiograph. Soft tissues and blood are largely water, with similar densities, between those of bone and air. Fat is usually visibly less dense than other soft tissues. Thus, a chest radiograph is actually a shadowgram.

The reason a structure can be outlined is that the shadow of one density contrasts with that of an adjacent density. If two structures are of equal density and adjacent to each other, a single combined shadow will result. If two structures of similar density are in different planes, or are separated by a structure of a different density, then the two structures are seen on x-ray film to be separated. This property of the x-ray shadowgram is helpful in determining where a certain density lies. For example, if a density on a PA chest radiograph is inseparable from and therefore adjacent to the descending thoracic aorta, then the observer knows that this abnormal density is in the posterior chest; if the density is inseparable from the right heart border, then the density is in an anterior position, because the heart is an anterior structure.

INTERPRETATION OF CHEST RADIOGRAPHS

A chest radiograph is usually read as though the reader were looking at the patient. The x-ray film is placed on a viewbox so that the patient's right side is to your left and the patient's

Fig. 16-3. (**A**) Normal PA chest radiograph. (**B**) Outline of structure visible on normal PA chest radiograph. The diagrammatic overlay shows the normal anatomic structures. (1) trachea; (2) right main bronchus; (3) left main bronchus; (4) left pulmonary artery; (5) right upper-lobe pulmonary artery; (6) right interlobar artery; (7) right lower and middle lobe vein; (8) aortic knob; (9) superior vena cava. (Fraser RG, Pare JAP: Diagnosis of Disease of the Chest, pp 92—93. Philadelphia, WB Saunders, 1970)

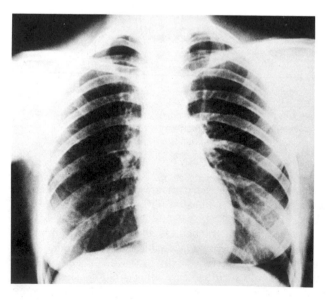

A

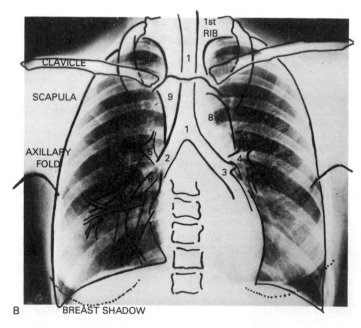

B

left side is to your right. To ensure that all anatomic structures are seen, radiographs are read according to a certain pattern. It is common practice to look at soft tissues, bones, and diaphragms first, then at the lungs, and finally at the outline of the heart and the aorta. Most structures in the chest, except the heart, are bilateral. Thus, if an abnormality is found on one side of the chest, the other side should be observed to ensure that this "abnormality" is not present there also. Figure 16-3A is a normal PA chest radiograph and Figure 16-3B indicates what structures the shadows represent. Figure 16-4A shows the location of various lung lobes on a frontal projection and Figure 16-4B, a lateral film, shows the location of these lobes when the chest is viewed from the side.

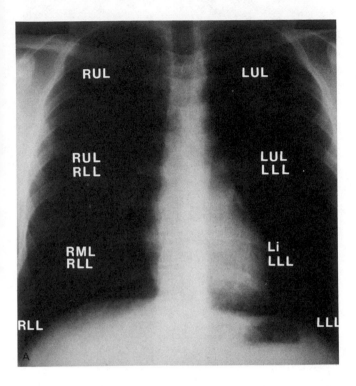
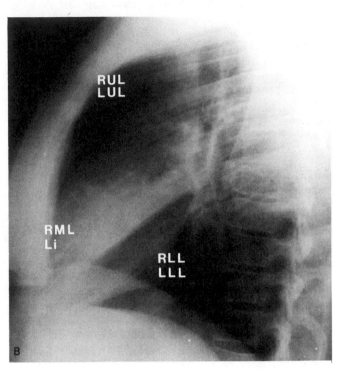

Fig. 16-4. **(A)** Location of the lung lobes on the frontal chest radiograph. Because some lobes are anterior and some posterior, an abnormality in a certain area on a frontal chest radiograph can be in one of two lobes. Obtaining a lateral film or noticing whether an anterior or posterior structure is obliterated by an abnormal density, can help with localization. RUL = right upper lobe; RLL = right lower lobe; LLL = left lower lobe; RML = right middle lobe; LUL = left upper lobe; Li = lingula. **(B)** Location of lung lobes in a lateral radiograph. Abnormalities of the right middle lobe and lingula would go undetected with posterior chest auscultation.

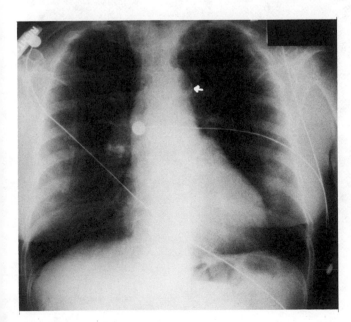

Fig. 16-5. Normal chest radiograph. This is an AP lordotic radiograph of a patient admitted to rule out MI. The lung fields are clear. Because this is an AP film, heart size cannot be assessed (see text). Monitoring leads are noted, and calcium is present in the aortic knob (*arrow*).

CHEST FILM FINDINGS IN MYOCARDIAL INFARCTION AND CONDITIONS THAT MAY MIMIC MYOCARDIAL INFARCTION

A bedside chest film of a patient with an uncomplicated myocardial infarction (MI) is shown in Figure 16-5. Note that this is basically a normal chest film except that, possibly because of pain, the patient has failed to take a deep breath and thus the lung fields are not as large as they would normally appear. This is a lordotic view, which decreases the apparent height of the lung fields as well. Because it is an AP exposure, the patient's heart appears enlarged, although in reality it may not be. Table 16-1 includes conditions that may mimic an acute myocardial infarction (MI). Figures 16-6 through 16-13 are radiographs of some conditions encountered in the differential diagnosis of an acute MI. The treatment for these conditions may differ from that for an MI, and thus it is extremely important to obtain a chest film early in a patient's course to help rule out these conditions.

TABLE 16-1 DIFFERENTIAL DIAGNOSIS OF ACUTE MYOCARDIAL INFARCTION
Pericarditis
Pulmonary embolus
Dissecting thoracic aortic aneurysm
Pleurisy
Pneumonia
Pancoast's tumor
Abdominal problem (ruptured viscus, esophageal spasm, cholelithiasis)
Herpes zoster
Cervical arthritis

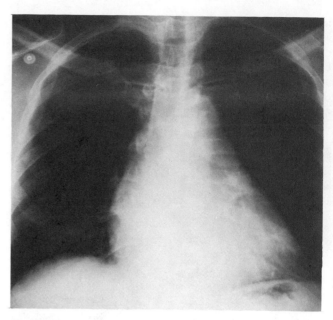

Fig. 16-6. Pericardial effusion. This patient was admitted to rule out myocardial infarction. A pericardial friction rub was present. ST segments were elevated across the precordium, consistent with pericarditis. However, pericarditis was not diagnosed and the patient was heparinized. Subsequently he bled into the pericardium and developed cardiac tamponade. Cardiomegaly may be difficult to distinguish from a pericardial effusion. An echocardiogram (Chap. 20) can differentiate between the two.

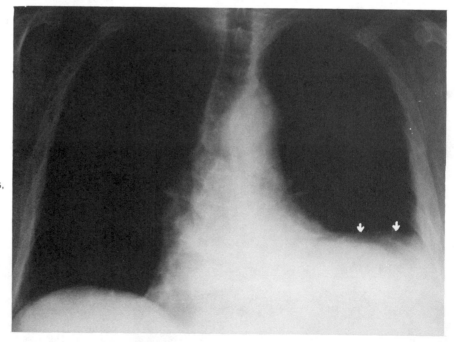

Fig. 16-7. Left pleural effusion. Some common causes of pleural effusion are pulmonary embolus, infection, heart failure, or neoplasm. Pulmonary embolus, an infection in the pleural space, or a neoplasm may cause acute chest pain. Physical findings of pleural effusion include absent breath sounds, dullness on percussion, and possibly (if massive) shift of the trachea to the side away from the pleural effusion. The presence of free pleural fluid can be documented by filming the patient with his left side down and noting that the fluid shifts with gravity. This is known as a left lateral decubitus radiograph.

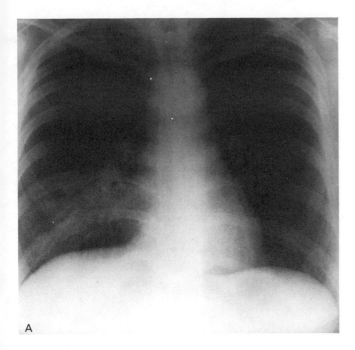

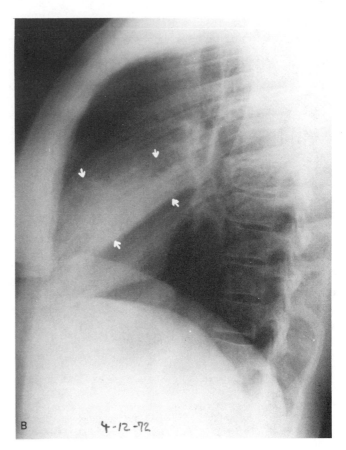

Fig. 16-8. **(A)** Right middle lobe pneumonia. The patient has cough, sputum, fever, chills, and possible chest pain. Physical findings include bronchial breathing, crackles, and dullness over the right anterior chest. The infiltrate obscures the right heart border, indicating that the infiltrate is in an anterior position. **(B)** The middle lobe location is confirmed on the lateral chest radiograph (*arrows*).   →

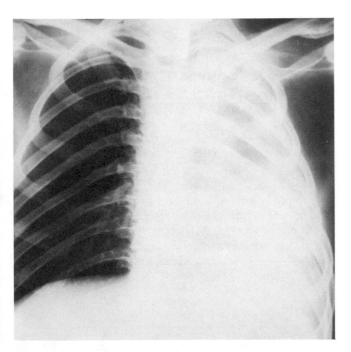

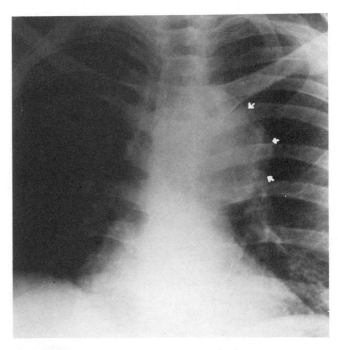

Fig. 16-9. Massive atelectasis of the left lung. The patient may have acute shortness of breath. Volume loss in the left chest is indicated by the shift of the heart to the left (right heart border over spine), tracheal shift (noted by shift of tracheostomy tube), and by elevation of left hemidiaphragm. Physical findings include absent breath sounds, dullness on percussion, and evidence of tracheal shift.

Fig. 16-10. Dissecting aortic aneurysm. The mediastinum is widened (*arrows*). The patient may have chest pain radiating to the neck or through to the back. Blood pressure may be higher in the right arm than in the left. A murmur of aortic insufficiency may be present.

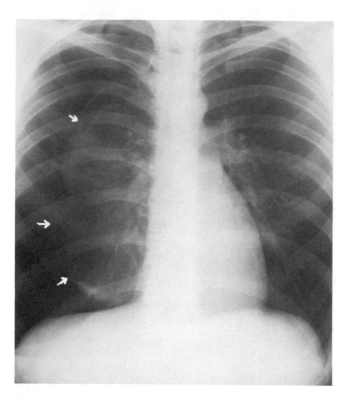

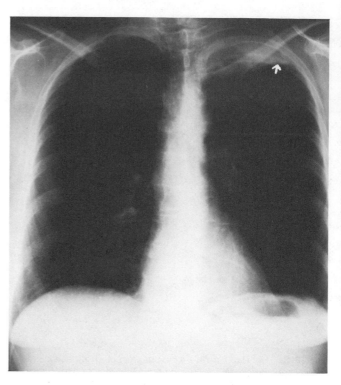

Fig. 16-11. Pneumothorax. The patient may have acute chest pain and shortness of breath. Physical findings include absent or reduced breath sounds on the side of the pneumothorax, tympany or a hollow sound on chest percussion, with possibly a shift of the trachea to the side away from the pneumothorax. The *arrows* indicate the outer border of the right lung. The remainder of the right chest cavity is filled with air in the pleural space.

Fig. 16-12. Pancoast's tumor, a bronchogenic carcinoma situated in the apex of the left lung. In this location it invades the brachial plexus and pleura. Patients may have left-sided chest pain that radiates into the neck and down the left arm, and thus may simulate a myocardial infarction. They frequently have neurologic abnormalities in the involved arm.

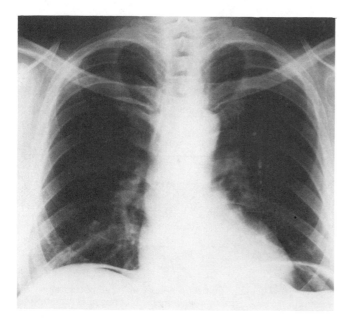

Fig. 16-13. Free air under the diaphragm. This patient had epigastric pain and diaphoresis. The admission radiograph showed free air under the diaphragm consistent with a perforated viscus. At operation a perforated peptic ulcer was found. The patient must be upright for the air to be seen under the diaphragm.

CHEST FILM FINDINGS IN COMPLICATIONS OF ACUTE MYOCARDIAL INFARCTION

Table 16-2 lists some of the complications of MI. *Acute pulmonary edema* (Figs. 16-14 and 16-15) may result from a wide variety of causes, including myocardial dysfunction due to ischemia, fluid overload, arrhythmias, papillary muscle rupture, ruptured interventricular septum, and development of a ventricular aneurysm. *Pericarditis* is usually manifested by a new and pleuritic type of pain different from that of an infarct, although it may seem similar. If pericardial fluid is absent or minimal, a pericardial rub is heard and the cardiac outline may be normal. If a *pericardial effusion*

TABLE 16-2 COMPLICATIONS OF ACUTE MYOCARDIAL INFARCTION

Congestive heart failure
Arrhythmia
Pericarditis, Dressler's syndrome
Pulmonary or systemic emboli
Ventricular aneurysm
Rupture of ventricular septum, papillary muscle, or ventricle

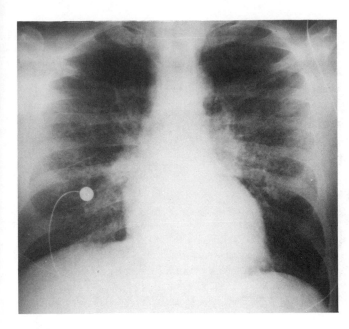

Fig. 16-14. Cardiogenic pulmonary edema. This radiograph shows bilateral fluffy densities. The fact that right and left sides are equally involved somewhat contradicts a diagnosis of pneumonia. Physical findings would include an S₃ gallop, distended neck veins, and bilateral crackles.

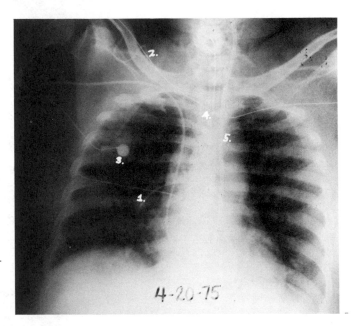

Fig. 16-15. Chest radiograph of a patient with pulmonary edema, showing the position of (*1*) pulmonary artery (Swan-Ganz) catheter; (*2*) central venous pressure catheter; (*3*) cardiac monitoring leads; (*4*) tracheostomy tube; and (*5*) nasogastric tube.

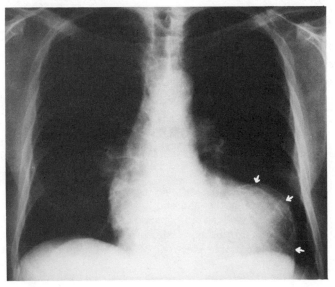

Fig. 16-16. Left ventricular aneurysm. The heart is enlarged. This longstanding aneurysm is outlined by calcium (*arrow*); acutely, the patient may have arrhythmias, intractable angina, left ventricular failure or systemic emboli. Electrocardiogram shows persistent elevation of the ST segment, and physical examination may reveal a rocking or abnormally pulsating precordium.

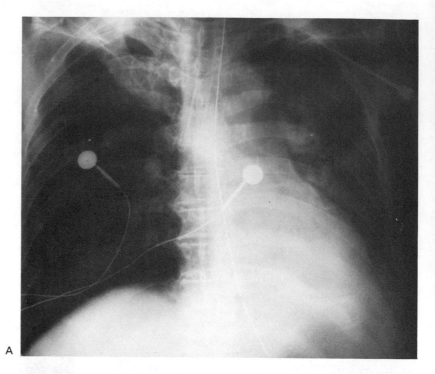

A

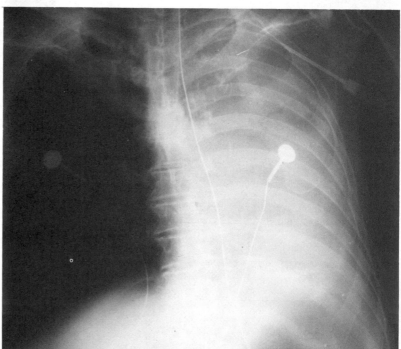

B

Fig. 16-17. **(A)** Endotracheal tube positioned in right mainstem bronchus. **(B)** If left in this position, atelectasis of the left lung would result. The tube should be positioned several centimeters above the carina.

develops, the rub may disappear and the chest film will look like that in Figure 16-6.

Symptoms due to *ventricular aneurysms* (Fig. 16-16) include congestive heart failure, arrhythmias, systemic emboli, and intractable angina. *Pulmonary emboli* may arise from clots within the heart or the deep venous system and may show *pleural effusion* on the radiograph (Fig. 16-7), atelectasis, or consolidation, but commonly the chest roentgenogram is normal.

MISCELLANEOUS USES OF THE CHEST RADIOGRAPH

The chest radiograph can be used to determine proper placement within the bronchus of an endotracheal tube. (Fig. 16-17). A wedged pulmonary artery catheter can result in *pulmonary infarction,* as shown in Figure 16-18. Placement of a pacemaker electrode within the right ventricle

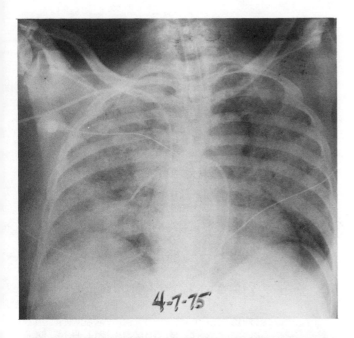

Fig. 16-18.   Pulmonary artery catheter permanently wedged. If the catheter is left in this position, pulmonary infarction can occur.

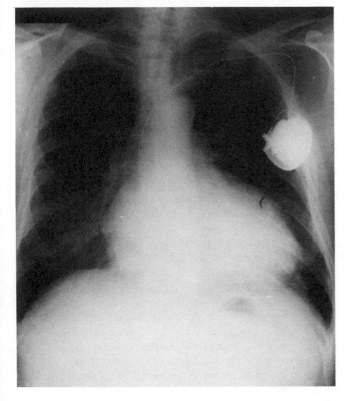

Fig. 16-19.   Proper placement of a right ventricular pacemaker electrode.

can be determined by radiograph (Fig. 16-19). The chest radiograph provides useful data that aid in the total assessment of the patient in the CCU.

REFERENCES

1. Fraser RG, Pare JAP: Diagnosis of Diseases of the Chest, pp 92–93. Philadelphia, WB Saunders, 1970

2. Squire LF: Fundamentals of Roentgenology, pp 16–20. Cambridge, Massachusetts, Harvard University Press, 1966.

ADDITIONAL READING

Felson B: Chest Roentgenology. Philadelphia, WB Saunders, 1973

Tinker J: Understanding chest x-rays. Am J Nurs 76:54–58, 1976

17

Electrocardiography, Vectorcardiography, and Polarcardiography

SUSAN L. WOODS, R.N., M.N.

The section on Polarcardiography was written by
E. S. SIVARAJAN, R.N., M.A.

The purpose of this chapter is to present basic concepts in electrocardiography, vectorcardiography and polarcardiography, and to demonstrate their usefulness.

ELECTROCARDIOGRAM

The electrocardiogram (ECG) is a useful test, in that it assists in the diagnosis of many diseases and provides vital information about a patient's condition and progress.

The ECG is a graphic record of the electrical activity of the heart. Impulse formation and conduction throughout the heart produce weak electrical currents through the entire body.[23] The difference in potential between a positive and a negative area within the body can be measured within the body by a galvanometer, an instrument with a wire between the poles of an electromagnet. As current passes through the wire, the instrument is controlled by the magnetic field. The ECG machine contains a galvanometer that detects changes in surface potential, amplifies the signal, and records these body surface potential changes over time on calibrated moving paper.

By convention, if a positive electrode is placed on the side facing the advancing wave of depolarization, a positive deflection will be produced (Fig. 17-1A). If the poles of the galvanometer are reversed, however, then a negative deflection will be produced. The magnitude of the deflection represents the thickness of the muscle involved. If a positive electrode is placed on the side from which the wave of depolarization is receding, a negative deflection will result (Fig. 17-1B). If an electrode is placed at right angles

(perpendicular) to the wave of depolarization, a biphasic deflection or no deflection (isoelectric) will occur (Fig. 17-1C).[23]

The 12-Lead ECG

Normally, the ECG consists of 12 leads: three bipolar standard leads (I, II, and III); three unipolar leads (aVR, aVL, aVF); and six unipolar chest leads. The three bipolar leads represent a difference of electric potential between two selected sites. Lead I is the difference of potential between the left arm (LA) and the right arm (RA). Lead II is the difference of potential between the left leg (LL) and the RA. Lead III is the difference of potential between the LL and the LA. Einthoven's triangle (1903) is based on the equation, lead II = lead I + III. If leads I, II, and III are bisected by each other, the triaxial reference is produced (Fig. 17-2A, B). Each of these three leads is 60 degrees apart.

The three augmented unipolar extremity leads are aVR (augmented or increased vector of the RA), aVL (augmented vector of the LA) and aVF (augmented vector of the LL). The unipolar leads represent a difference in potential between one site and the average of the potential of two other sites. Lead aVR is the difference of potential between the RA and the average of the potential of the LL and LA. Lead aVL is the difference of potential between the LA and the average of the potential of the LL and RA. Lead aVF is the difference of potential between the LL and the average of the potential of the LA and RA. The three augmented unipolar leads can be superimposed onto the triaxial reference figure, resulting in a hexaxial reference figure (Fig. 17-2C, D).[23] Each of these three leads is 30 degrees apart.

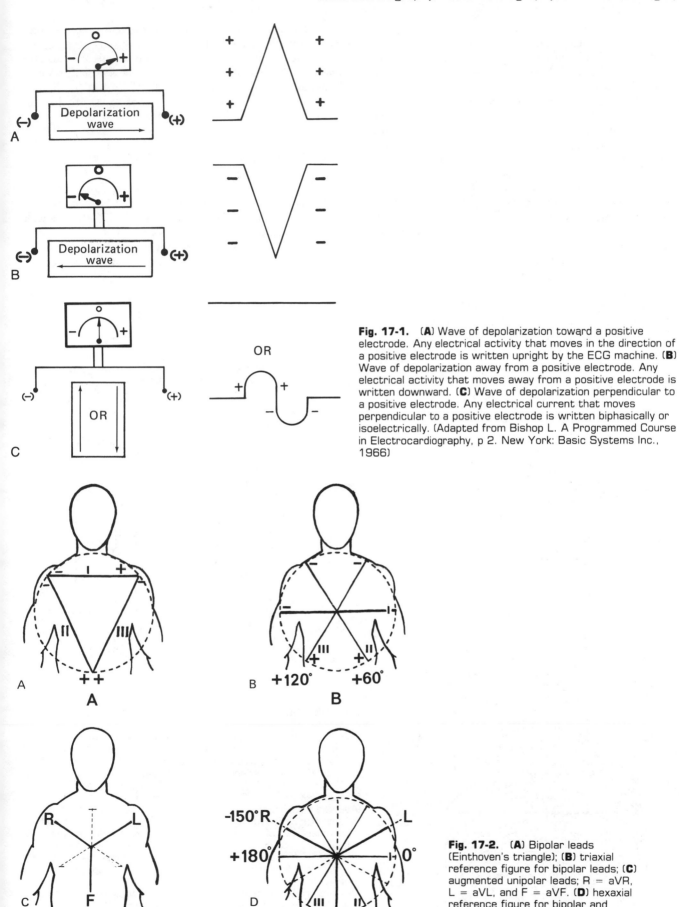

Fig. 17-1. (**A**) Wave of depolarization toward a positive electrode. Any electrical activity that moves in the direction of a positive electrode is written upright by the ECG machine. (**B**) Wave of depolarization away from a positive electrode. Any electrical activity that moves away from a positive electrode is written downward. (**C**) Wave of depolarization perpendicular to a positive electrode. Any electrical current that moves perpendicular to a positive electrode is written biphasically or isoelectrically. (Adapted from Bishop L. A Programmed Course in Electrocardiography, p 2. New York: Basic Systems Inc., 1966)

Fig. 17-2. (**A**) Bipolar leads (Einthoven's triangle); (**B**) triaxial reference figure for bipolar leads; (**C**) augmented unipolar leads; R = aVR, L = aVL, and F = aVF. (**D**) hexaxial reference figure for bipolar and augmented unipolar leads.

The last six leads of the 12-lead ECG are the unipolar precordial (chest) leads and are called "V" leads. The common precordial positions on the chest are shown in Figure 17-3A. Table 17-1 lists the positive and negative electrodes for each of the 12 leads.

Leads other than these 12 leads may be used to interpret more accurately impulse formation and conduction. Other "V" leads may be selected. With an esophageal lead (E lead), the positive electrode is inserted through a nasal catheter into the esophagus so that the tip is positioned behind the left atrium. With a right atrial lead, a transvenous wire is usually inserted percutaneously into the right atrial chamber. With an "atrial" lead (Lewis lead), the positive electrode is placed on the chest to the right of the sternum in the fourth intercostal space, and the negative electrode is placed on the chest to the right of the sternum in the second intercostal space.[23] Other precordial leads in addition to V_1 and V_2 can be used, for example V_{3R} and V_{4R}, so that they correspond with the locations of their opposite numbers on the left side of the chest (Figs. 17-3B, C). Occasionally it is necessary to take chest leads that are further left and toward the back: V_7 (at the posterior axillary line), V_8 (at the angle of the scapula), and V_9 (over the spine). V_{7-9} are the same level as V_{4-6} (Fig. 17-3C).[33]

Generally ECG paper moves at a speed of 25 mm/second. Each small box horizontally is equal to 0.04 second. One large box (5 small boxes) horizontally equals 0.20 second; one large box (5 small boxes) vertically is equal to 5 mm. Ten millimeters is equal to 1 millivolt (mV). The ECG is calibrated to 1 mV vertically, in order to standardize the ECG (Fig. 17-4).

Waves, Complexes, and Intervals

The P wave represents atrial muscle depolarization. It is normally 2.5 mm or less in height and is 0.11 second or less in duration. The atrial repolarization (atrial T wave) is wide and of low amplitude and therefore is not seen or is buried in the QRS complex. The first negative deflection after the P wave is the *Q wave*, which is less than 0.03 seconds in

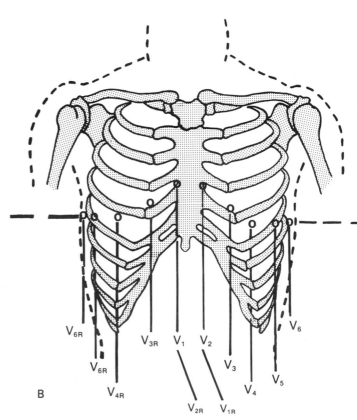

Fig. 17-3. **(A)** Six standard precordial leads—electrode placement:
1. Fourth intercostal space, at *right* side of sternum
2. Fourth intercostal space, at *left* side of sternum
3. Midway between positions 2 and 4
4. Fifth intercostal space, midclavicular line
5. Same level as #4 in the anterior axillary line
6. Same as #4 and #5 in the midaxillary line.
(Adapted from Bernreiter M: Electrocardiography, p 23. Philadelphia, J. B. Lippincott, 1963.) **(B)** Other right precordial leads—electrode placement. V_{3R} to V_{9R} are taken on the right side of the chest in the same location as the left-sided leads V_{3-9}. V_{2R} is the same as V_1. **(C)** Left precordial leads—electrode placement: V_7—posterior axillary line; V_8—posterior scapular line; V_9—left border of spine.
All three are in the same horizontal plane of V_{4-6}. (Adapted from Goldman MJ: Clinical Electrocardiography, p 9. Los Altos, Lange Medical Publication, 1979)

TABLE 17-1   POSITIVE AND NEGATIVE ELECTRODES IN EACH OF THE 12 LEADS

	Positive Electrode	Negative Electrode	Ground Electrode
Lead I	LA	RA	RL
Lead II	LL	RA	RL
Lead III	LL	LA	RL
aVR	RA	Average potential of LA & LL	RL
aVL	LA	RA & LL	RL
aVF	LL	RA & LA	RL
V₁	Fourth intercostal space, at *right* side of sternum	RA & LA & LL	RL
V₂	Fourth intercostal space, at *left* side of sternum	"	RL
V₃	Midway between positions V₂ and V₄	"	RL
V₄	Fifth intercostal space, midclavicular line	"	RL
V₅	Same level as V₄ in the anterior axillary line	"	RL
V₆	Same level as V₄ and V₅ in the midaxillary line	"	RL

Note Code: LA = left arm; RA = right arm; LL = left leg; RL = right leg.
(From Goldman MJ: Principles of Electrocardiography, 10th ed. California, Lange Medical Publications, 1979)

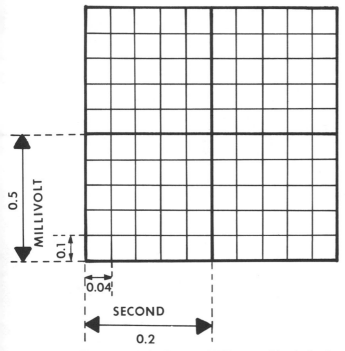

Fig. 17-4. Time and voltage lines on ECG paper. Vertically: 1 mm – 0.1 mV; 5 mm – 0.5 mV; 10 mm = 1.0 mV; Horizontally: 25 little boxes = 1 second; 1500 little boxes = 60 seconds. (Adapted from Bernreiter M: Electrocardiography, p 12, Philadelphia, JB Lippincott, 1963)

duration and less than 25% of the R wave amplitude;[2] the first positive deflection after the P wave is the *R wave;* and the *S* wave is the first negative deflection after the R wave.

The QRS complex (beginning of Q wave to end of S wave) represents ventricular muscle depolarization. Figure 17-5 shows examples of various QRS complex configurations. When a wave is less than 5 mm vertically, small letters (q, r, s) are used; when a wave is greater than 5 mm vertically, capital letters (Q, R, S) are used. When a complex

is all negative, it is called a Q–S complex. Not all QRS complexes have all three waveforms (Fig. 17-6).

The *T wave* represents ventricular muscle repolarization. It follows the QRS complex and is usually of the same deflection as the QRS complex. If a *U wave* is seen, it will follow the T wave. The presence of a U wave may indicate an electrolyte abnormality.

The *ST segment,* which represents early ventricular repolarization of the ventricles, is from the end of the S wave (J point) to the beginning of the T wave (Fig. 17-6).

The *P–R interval* is measured from the beginning of the P wave to the beginning of the Q wave, or to the beginning of the R wave if no Q wave is present, and represents the time required for the impulse to travel through the atria and conduction system to the Purkinje fibers. In adults, the P–R interval normally ranges from 0.12 second to 0.20 second

Fig. 17-5. Examples of various QRS complexes. (Adapted from Bernreiter M: Electrocardiography. p 15, Philadelphia, JB Lippincott, 1963)

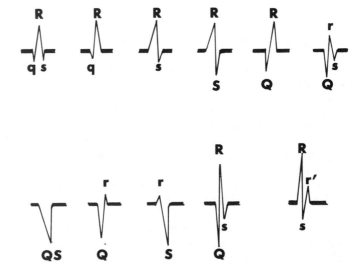

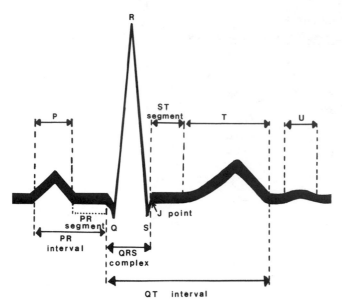

Fig. 17-6. ECG waves, complexes and intervals. (Adapted from Sharp L, Rabin B: Nursing in the Coronary Care Unit, p 101. Philadelphia, JB Lippincott, 1970)

in duration. The *P–R segment* is isoelectric and is measured from the end of the P wave to the beginning of the QRS complex.

The *QRS complex* is measured from the beginning of the Q wave, or the R wave, if no Q wave is present, to the end of the S wave. The QRS complex is normally 0.04 to 0.10 second in duration. The QRS complex in the chest leads can be 0.01 to 0.02 second longer than in the limb leads.[33]

The *Q–T interval,* which represents electrical systole, is measured from the beginning of the Q wave, or R wave, if no Q wave is present, to the end of the T wave. The Q–T interval varies with heart rate and must be corrected to a heart rate of 60 (Q–T$_c$). This is done by use of the nomogram in Figure 17-7. The Q–T interval is usually less than half the R–R interval (measured from the beginning of one R wave to the beginning of the next R wave) and usually is 0.32 to 0.40 second in duration if the heart rate is 65 to 95.[33] The Q–T$_c$ should not exceed 0.42 second in men and 0.43 second in women.[23] The *J point* is the point where the QRS complex ends and the ST segment begins (Fig. 17-6).

Determination of Heart Rate from ECG

Heart rate can be obtained from the ECG strip by several methods. The first, and most accurate if the rhythm is regular, is to count the number of 0.04-second intervals (0.04 second equals one small box) between two R waves, then divide that number into 1500. (There are 1,500 0.04-second interval boxes in a 1-minute strip (Fig. 17-8A). Table 17-2 lists the heart rate according to the number of 0.04-second intervals between R waves. Table 17-3 lists the heart rate depending on the number of 0.20-second boxes (0.20 second equals one large box) between R waves (Fig. 17-8A).

The second method for computing heart rate, especially useful when the rhythm is irregular, is to count the number of R–R intervals in 6 seconds and multiply that number by

10. The ECG paper is usually marked at 3-second intervals (15 large boxes horizontally) by a vertical line at the top of the paper (Fig. 17-8B). The R–R intervals are counted, not QRS complexes. If QRS complexes were counted, the computed heart rate might be inaccurate.

Mean Axis Determination

Impulse formation usually begins in the sinoatrial (SA) node. Conduction of this impulse throughout the heart results in the propagation of thousands of electrical potentials in many directions in space. Over 80% of these potentials are cancelled out by opposing forces and only the net result is recorded. The *mean vector* at a given time in the cardiac cycle represents the sum of electrical potentials as well as the mean magnitude, direction, and polarity.[23] The mean P, QRS, and T vectors can be determined and are usually downward and to the left.

The mean QRS vector (axis) is determined using the frontal plane leads. Each frontal plane lead in the hexaxial reference figure shown in Figure 17-2D is 30 degrees apart. Lead I is 0 degrees at its positive end and 180 degrees at its negative end.

The *QRS axis* can be determined in several ways: First, determine the direction (positive or negative) and magnitude (in millimeters) of the QRS complexes in leads I, II, and III and plot the magnitude and direction on the triaxial reference figure as shown in Figure 17-9; then draw perpendicular

Fig. 17-7. Nomogram for rate correction of QT interval. Measure the observed Q–T interval and the R–R interval. Mark these values in the respective columns of the chart (left and middle). Place a ruler across these two points. The point at which the extension of this line crosses the third column is read as the corrected Q–T interval (Q–T$_c$). (Adapted from Kissin M et al: Am Heart J 35:991, 1948)

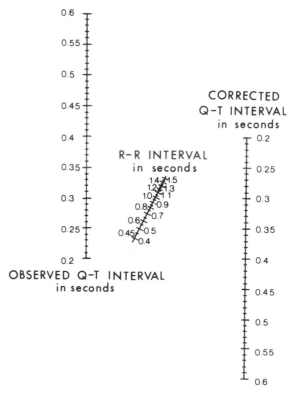

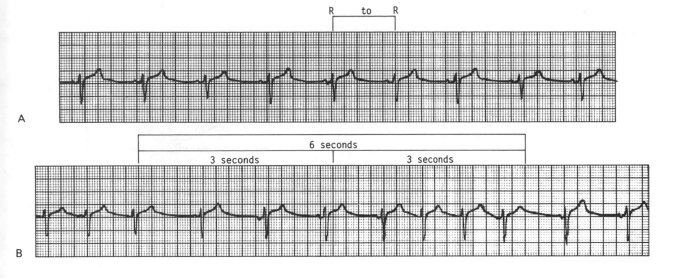

TABLE 17-2 Heart Rate Determination Using the ECG (Small Boxes)

Number of Small Boxes Between R Waves	Heart Rate
1	1500
2	750
3	500
4	375
5	300
6	250
7	214
8	188
9	167
10	150
11	136
12	125
13	115
14	107
15	100
16	94
17	88
18	83
19	79
20	75
21	71
22	68
23	65
24	62
25	60
26	58
27	55
28	54
29	52
30	50
31	48
32	47
33	45
34	44
35	43
36	42
37	40
38	39
39	38
40	38

TABLE 17-2 Heart Rate Determination Using the ECG (Small Boxes) (*Cont.*)

Number of Small Boxes Between R Waves	Heart Rate
41	37
42	36
43	35
44	34
45	33
46	33
47	32
48	31
49	31
50	30

TABLE 17-3 Heart Rate Determination Using the ECG (Large Boxes)

Number of Large Boxes Between R Waves	Heart Rate
1	300
2	150
3	100
4	75
5	60
6	50
7	43
8	38
9	33
10	30

lines from each lead until the lines intersect. The axis is recorded in degrees at this intersection.

Second, the axis can be determined by the following method: (1) From the limb and augmented leads of a 12-lead ECG, select the most isoelectric or biphasic lead. The lead is isoelectric because the current is flowing in a direction perpendicular to that lead (Fig. 17-1C). (2) Determine the lead that is perpendicular to the most isoelectric or biphasic lead. (3) Determine the direction (positive or negative) of

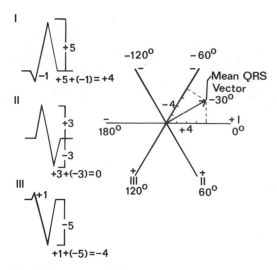

Fig. 17-9.   Mean QRS axis determination.

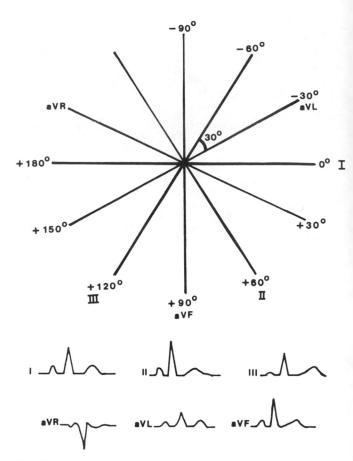

Fig. 17-10.   Mean QRS axis determination. The most isoelectric lead is aVL. The lead perpendicular to aVL is lead II. Lead II is positive; therefore the QRS axis is +60 degrees. (Adapted from Bernreiter M: Electrocardiography, p 22. Philadelphia, JB Lippincott, 1963)

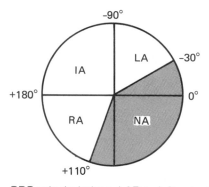

Fig. 17-11.   QRS axis deviations. LAD = left axis deviation; RAD = right axis deviation; NA = normal axis; IA = indeterminate axis. (Adapted from Goldman MJ: Principles of Clinical Electrocardiography, p 33. Los Altos, Lange Medical Publications, 1979)

current flow in this lead. If the QRS complex is positive, then current is flowing toward the positive electrode for that lead; if the QRS complex is negative, then the current is flowing away from the positive electrode. (4) Determine axis in degrees, using the hexaxial reference figure (Fig. 17-10). This method indicates direction, but not magnitude. These same principles and methods can be applied to determine the axis of the P wave and that of the T wave.

The normal QRS axis ranges from +110 degrees to −30 degrees (Fig. 17-11). A left QRS axis deviation (−30 degrees to −90 degrees) can be caused by (1) normal variation; (2) mechanical shifts due to expiration, high diaphragm from pregnancy, ascites, or abdominal tumors; (3) left anterior hemiblock or left bundle branch block; (4) emphysema; and (5) right ventricular ectopic rhythms.[34] A right QRS axis deviation (+110 degrees to +180 degrees) can be caused by (1) normal variation; (2) mechanical shifts due to inspiration or emphysema; (3) right ventricular hypertrophy; (4) left posterior hemiblock; (5) right bundle branch block; (6) left ventricular rhythm; and (7) dextrocardia.[22] An axis of +180 degrees to −90 degrees is indeterminate (Fig. 17-11).

The *P wave axis* is normally between +60 degrees and 0 degrees. The *T wave axis* normally points in the same general direction as the QRS axis. Normally, the QRS axis and T-wave axis are less than 50 degrees apart.[23]

Procedure for Obtaining an Electrocardiogram

To obtain an ECG, the electrodes are placed on the patient as shown in Figure 17-12. With the electrodes in these positions, the first six leads can be obtained. To ensure good contact between the skin and the electrode, the electrodes are placed on a flat surface just above the wrists and ankles; and electrode paste or an alcohol sponge is placed under each electrode. The limb straps are adjusted firmly to hold the electrode in place. These straps should not pinch the patient's skin or be so tight as to decrease circulation distal to the strap. The lead selected on the machine is then turned on to record each of the six leads (Fig. 17-13). Next, the six

"V" leads are obtained by moving the chest leads in the six precordial positions shown in Figure 17-3A. A lead selector switch is turned to "V" to record each of these leads. The arm and leg electrodes must be attached to the patient in order to obtain the "V" leads. There are other ECG machines that record three or six leads simultaneously.

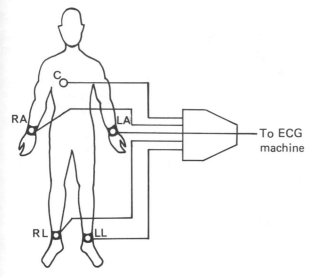

Fig. 17-12. Twelve-lead ECG—electrode placement. (Adapted from Goldman MJ: Principles of Clinical Electrocardiography, p 11. Los Altos, Lange Medical Publications, 1979)

To obtain an esophageal or right atrial chamber lead, the "V" electrode of the ECG machine is attached to the esophageal or right intraatrial electrode with an alligator clamp. The arm and leg electrodes must be attached to the patient. The lead selector is turned to "V".

Each ECG should include the following identifying information:

1. Patient name and identification number
2. Location, date, and time of the recording
3. Patient age, sex, and cardiac medications
4. Race, body build (weight and height measurements), blood pressure, tentative clinical diagnosis, clinical status, and noncardiac medications, such as phenothiazines
5. Any unusual position of the patient during the recording, or the presence of thoracic deformities, amputation, respiratory distress, or muscle tremor[48]

Normal ECG variants are atypical ECG features that exceed a criterion for normality in a person known not to have the disease suggested by the criterion. Some of the normal variants of the adult ECG are as follows:

1. Increased QRS amplitude (depends on body build and chest thickness)
2. Low voltage (depends on body build and chest thickness)
3. Abnormal amplitude of initial QRS deflection, abnormal Q waves (in duration and amplitude) in leads I, II, III, aVL, aVF, V_{4-6}, and abnormal R waves (amplitude) in one or more right (V_{1-2}) and mid precordial "V" leads (V_{3-4})
4. Prolonged Q–T interval (Q–T_c interval plus 15% more, without ST-segment lengthening and without increase in T-wave amplitude)
5. ST-segment elevation (premature repolarization)
6. Horizontal or depressed ST segment (less than or equal to 0.1 mV, usually in women)
7. Inverted T waves (in one or more of leads V_{1-4})
8. Tall T waves
9. Increased U-wave amplitude (corresponding to increase in R–R interval)
10. Notched QRS complex
11. Poor R-wave progression
12. Dextrocardia (heart on right side of body); pattern in limb leads is identical with reversal of right- and left-arm electrodes
13. S wave in leads I, II, III
14. J-point depression (because of atrial repolarization)[48]

The Normal 12-lead ECG

The P wave represents atrial muscle depolarization. The current spreads through the atria in a leftward, slightly forward, head-to-foot direction. The P wave is usually upright in leads I, II, aVF, and V_{3-6}; it is usually inverted in lead aVR and may be inverted in leads V_{1-2}. The P wave in leads III and aVL may be upright, biphasic, flat, or inverted.[24]

The QRS complex represents the three phases of ventricular muscle depolarization: (1) the septum is rapidly depolarized from left to right, in a posterior to anterior and superior direction (the beginning of the QRS complex); (2) the right and left ventricles are depolarized together from endocardium to epicardium, with the dominant direction of depolarization to the left, posterior, and inferior (the midportions of the QRS complex); and (3) the superior portions of the ventricles are depolarized in a left, posterior, and superior direction (the terminal portions of the QRS complex) (Fig. 3-13A–E).

The T wave represents repolarization of the ventricle. It is usually in the opposite direction from ventricular depolarization (see Chap. 3).

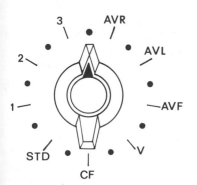

LEAD	SELECTOR				
1	=	LA – RA			
2	=	LL – RA			
3	=	LL – LA			
AVR	=	RA – LL	&	LA	
AVL	=	LA – LL	&	RA	
AVF	=	LL – LA	&	RA	
V	=	C – LL	&	LA	& RA
CF	=	C – LL			

Fig. 17-13. Lead selector switch on an ECG machine.

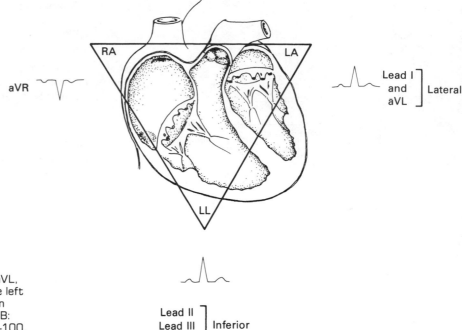

Fig. 17-14. ECG in leads I, II, III, aVR, aVL, aVF. Diagrammed are the surfaces of the left ventricle faced by the positive electrode in each lead. (Adapted from Sharp L, Rabin B: Nursing in the Coronary Care Unit, p 99–100. Philadelphia, JB Lippincott, 1970)

The normal P–QRS–T waveforms in each of the 12 leads are illustrated in Figures 17-14 and 17-15. The surfaces of the left ventricle that the positive electrode of each lead is facing are also diagrammed. Table 17-4 summarizes the normal 12-lead ECG waveform configurations.

Electrocardiographic Apparatus

In addition to the standard 12-lead ECG, the ECG can be used in other ways. One lead of the ECG can be continuously monitored on an oscilloscope (a fluorescent screen). The waveform from this lead can be written out to provide a permanent record. Continuous ECG monitoring is especially useful in the cardiac care unit to detect arrhythmias.

One lead of the ECG can also be monitored by a small tape recorder (Holter Recorder) and recorded on a continuous (1–24 hours) magnetic tape recording. The patient can then be monitored during the day or night to detect arrhythmias or evidence of myocardial ischemia during activities of daily living. The tape recorder weighs approximately 2 pounds and can be carried over the shoulder. The patient keeps a diary of his activity, noting the time of any symptoms, experiences, or any unusual activities performed. The tape recording is then examined, using a specialized instrument called a scanner, analyzed, and interpreted. Evidence obtained in this way is helpful in diagnosing arrhythmias and myocardial ischemia and in evaluating therapy such as antiarrhythmic and antianginal drugs or pacemaker function.[50]

The ECG can also be transmitted by telemetry (telephone lines), thus freeing a patient from a cable connected to the oscilloscope. The ECG signal can then be monitored miles away.

The ECG is useful in diagnosing myocardial infarction (MI), injury, and ischemia; atrial and ventricular enlarge-

ment; electrolyte imbalances; drug effects and toxicity; pacemaker malfunction; conduction abnormalities; effects of systemic disease on the heart; and arrhythmias.

Myocardial Ischemia, Injury, and Infarction

Myocardial Ischemia and Injury. *Myocardial ischemia* causes enlargement and inversion of the T wave due to altered late repolarization. Possibly, the ischemic region remains depolarized, whereas adjacent areas have returned to the resting state.[42] The change is seen in the leads closest to the involved surface of the heart. Ischemia also causes

Fig. 17-15. Normal ECG in the precordial leads. Diagrammed are the surfaces of the left ventricle faced by the positive electrode in each lead. Lateral leads: V_{5-6}; anterior leads: V_{3-4}; septal leads: V_{1-2}. (Adapted from Sharp L, Rabin B: Nursing in the Coronary Care Unit, p 99–100. Philadelphia, JB Lippincott, 1970)

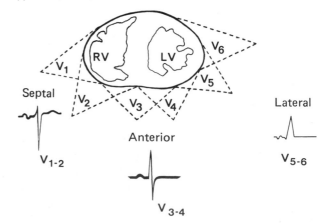

TABLE 17-4 NORMAL ECG WAVEFORM CONFIGURATION IN EACH OF THE 12 LEADS

Lead	P wave	Q wave	R wave	S wave	T wave	U wave	ST segment
I	Upright	Small	Largest wave	Small (less than R wave) or none	Upright		May vary from +1 to −0.5 mm
II	Upright	Small or none	Large (verticle heart)	Small (less than R wave) or none	Upright		May vary from +1 to −0.5 mm
III	Upright, diphasic, or inverted	Usually small or none (for large Q wave to be diagnostic, a Q wave must also be present in aVF).	None to large	None to large (horizontal heart)	Upright, diphasic, or inverted		May vary from +1 to −0.5 mm
aVR	Inverted	Small, none, or large	Small or none	Large (may be QS)	Inverted		May vary from +1 to −0.5 mm
aVL	Upright, diphasic, or inverted	Small, none, or large Q wave (to be diagnostic, a Q wave must also be present in lead I or precordial leads)	Small, none, or large (horizontal heart)	None to large (verticle heart)	Upright, diphasic, or inverted		May vary from +1 to −0.5 mm
aVF	Upright	Small or none	Small, none, or large (verticle heart)	None to large (horizontal heart)	Upright, diphasic, or inverted		May vary from +1 to −0.5 mm
V₁	Upright, diphasic, or inverted	None QS complex	Less than S wave or none	Large (may be QS)	Upright, diphasic, or inverted		May vary from 0 to +3 mm
V₂	Upright	None QS complex (occasionally)	Less than S wave, or none, (progressively larger)	Large (may be QS)	Upright	Upright, lower amplitude than T wave	May vary from 0 to +3 mm
V₃	Upright	Small or none	Less than, greater than, or equal to S wave (progressively larger)	Large (greater than R wave, less than R wave, or equal to R wave)	Upright	Upright, lower amplitude than T wave	May vary from 0 to +3 mm
V₄	Upright	Small or none	Progressively larger wave; R wave greater than S wave	Progressively smaller (less than R wave)	Upright	Upright, lower amplitude than T wave	May vary from +1 to −0.5 mm
V₅	Upright	Small	Progressively larger wave; less than 26 mm	Progressively smaller; less than the S wave in V₄	Upright		May vary from +1 to −0.5 mm
V₆	Upright	Small	Largest wave; less than 26 mm	Smallest; less than the S wave in V₅	Upright		May vary from +1 to −0.5 mm

(From Goldman, MJ: Principles of Electrocardiography, 10th ed. California, Lange Medical Publications, 1979)

ST—segment changes. With *epicardial myocardial injury,* injured cells depolarize normally but repolarize more rapidly than do normal cells. Thus, current flows (during repolarization) from the injured cells to the normal cells, because current flows from positive to negative. This altered current flow results in elevation in the leads facing the area of injury. There is also a decrease (closer to zero) in the resting potential of the injured cells. Current flows from the normal cells into the injured ones during electrical diastole (T–Q segment). This altered current flow produces T–Q-segment depression in the leads facing the area of injury. The ST

segment appears elevated (Fig. 17-16A). Both of these changes are referred to as ST-segment elevation. If the myocardial injury were on the endocardial surface, then the ST segment would appear to be depressed (1 mm or more) in the leads facing the area of injury (Fig. 17-16B). The ST-segment depression is horizontal or slopes downward and is 0.08 second in duration.

Myocardial Infarction. *Myocardial infarction* usually causes Q waves within one to three days because of the absence of depolarization current from necrotic tissue, and

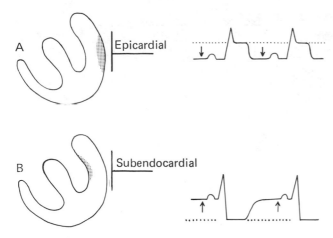

Fig. 17-16. (**A**) ECG effects of epicardial injury. (**B**) ECG effects of subendocardial injury.

opposing currents from other parts of the heart. An abnormal Q wave is 0.04 second or longer in duration and is in depth 25% of the R wave (provided the R wave itself exceeds 5 mm).[2] Old transmural MI can usually be determined by significant Q waves without ST and T wave changes or by reduced voltage of the R wave. In some patients, Q waves disappear. With a transmural MI (involving all three layers of the heart), injury and ischemic changes are also present (Fig. 17-17). The ST-segment elevation lasts a few days to two weeks. The T wave becomes large and symmetric for 24 hours, then inverts within one to three days for one to two weeks. During recovery from an MI, the ST segment often is first to return to normal (1–6 weeks), then the T wave (weeks to months). Q waves are usually permanent.

With an inferior or diaphragmatic transmural MI of the left ventricle, leads II, III, and aVF will have T-wave inversion, ST-segment elevation, and significant Q waves (Fig. 17-18A,B). With a septal MI of the left ventricle, these changes will be seen in leads V_1 and V_2 (Fig. 17-18C); with an anterior transmural MI of the left ventricle, these changes will be seen in leads V_3 and V_4 (Fig. 17-18D); and with a lateral transmural MI of the left ventricle, these changes will be seen in leads I, aVL, V_5, and V_6 (Fig. 17-18E). With a posterior transmural MI of the left ventricle, leads V_1 and V_2 will show changes opposite those of a septal MI: R wave instead of Q wave, ST depression instead of elevation, and upright T wave instead of inversion (Fig. 17-18F).[48] Posterior MI is uncommon. Reciprocal effects are seen in the leads where the positive electrode is located on the opposite side of the infarction.

Infarctions can also occur in more than one area: anteroseptal (V_{1-4}); anterolateral (I, aVL, V_{3-6}) (Fig. 17-19A); posterior–inferior (II, III, aVF, V_{1-2}); and posterolateral (I, aVL, V_{1-2}, V_{5-6}) (Fig. 17–19B). Infarction can occur in one place, with ischemia and injury in another, as shown in Figure 17-19C.

Subendocardial infarction (nontransmural) causes ST-segment depression and T-wave inversion only. No Q waves develop because the epicardial surface is not involved. Epicardial infarction (nontransmural) causes ST-segment elevation and T-wave inversion. No Q waves develop because the endocardial surface is not involved.[33] In atrial infarction the P–R segment is displaced.[35]

Atrial and Ventricular Enlargement (Hypertrophy)

Atrial Enlargement. *Atrial enlargement* (hypertrophy) can also be determined from the ECG. Enlargement can be due to hypertrophy or dilatation. *Left atrial enlargement* (LAE) is caused by conditions that increase the work of the left atrium: mitral stenosis or regurgitation, systemic hypertension, and left heart failure (Fig. 17-20).[38] LAE has the following ECG characteristics:

1. The P wave in leads I, II, aVL is higher than 2.5 mm and longer than 0.12 second in duration (P-mitrale). The Macruz index is greater than 1.6 in lead II (Fig. 17-21).

$$\left(\frac{\text{P-wave duration}}{\text{P–R-segment duration}} = 1.6 \text{ or greater}\right)$$

2. The negative or inverted component of P wave (terminal portion) in leads V_{1-2} is 1 mm or more in depth, greater than 0.04 second in duration, and is directed to the left and posterior.

3. In coarse atrial fibrillation, the fibrillatory waves ("f" waves) in lead V_1 or V_2 are equal to or greater than 1 mm in amplitude.

Right atrial enlargement (RAE) is commonly caused by conditions that increase the work of the right atrium: pulmonary hypertension, pulmonary or tricuspid stenosis or regurgitation (Fig. 17-22).[38] RAE has the following characteristics:

Fig. 17-17. ECG effects of infarction, injury, and ischemia as they correspond to the zones of infarction. 1. Ischemia causes inversion of T wave because of altered repolarization. 2. Muscle injury causes elevation of ST segment. 3. Death (infarction) of muscle causes Q or Q–S waves because of the absence of depolarization current from dead tissue and opposing currents from other parts of heart. During recovery (subacute and chronic stages), ST segment often is first to return to normal, then T wave. This recovery corresponds to the disappearance of zones of injury and ischemia.

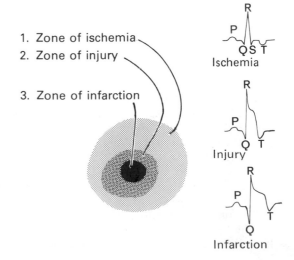

1. Zone of ischemia
2. Zone of injury
3. Zone of infarction

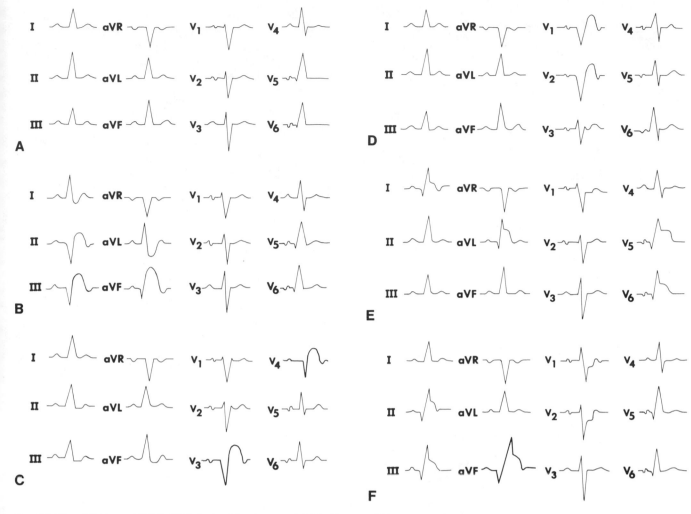

Fig. 17-18. (**A**) Normal ECG. (**B**) Inferior (diaphragmatic) MI. Q wave, ST-segment elevation, T-wave inversion in leads II, III, aVF. Reciprocal changes in leads I and aVL. (**C**) ECG changes with anterior MI. Q waves, ST-segment elevation, T-wave inversion in leads V_{3-4}. Reciprocal changes in leads II, III, aVF. (**D**) ECG changes with septal MI. Q waves, ST-segment elevation, and T-wave inversion in leads V_{1-2}. (**E**) ECG changes with lateral MI. Q waves, ST-segment elevation, and T-wave inversion in leads I, aVL, V_{5-6}. Reciprocal changes in lead V_1. (**F**) ECG changes with posterior MI. R waves, ST-segment depression and upright T wave in leads V_{1-2}. Reciprocal changes in leads II, III, and aVF.

1. The P waves in leads II, III, and aVF are sharp and pointed (3 mm or more) and the P wave in lead aVL maybe inverted. If the P wave meets these criteria, and the P wave axis is greater than +60 degrees, it is called P pulmonale. The Macruz index is less than 1.0 (Fig. 17-21)

2. The P waves in leads V_{1-3} are sharp and pointed. If the P wave meets this criterion and the P wave axis is less than +60 degrees, it is called P congenitale.

3. The positive component of P wave in leads V_{1-2} is greater than 1 mm in height and width.

Biatrial enlargement occurs with mitral valve disease and interatrial septal defect, with multiple valvular defects and biventricular failure. Biatrial enlargement exists if

1. P wave is higher than 2.5 mm in lead II
2. P wave is longer than 0.12 seconds in lead II
3. P wave is notched

Ventricular Enlargement. *Left ventricular enlargement* (LVE), or hypertrophy, is caused by increased volume (diastolic overload or increased preload) and increased pressure (systolic overload or increased afterload) in the left ventricle. The sequence of ventricular activation is shown in Fig. 17-23A.[21,33] Fever, anemia, thyrotoxicosis, and other high-output states can increase voltage, without left ventricular hypertrophy.[23]

If the patient is more than 35 years old, LVE has the following characteristics (Fig. 17-23B):

1. The R wave in lead V_5 or V_6 is equal to or greater than 27 mm.
2. The R wave in lead V_5 or V_6 plus S wave in lead V_1 is equal to or greater than 35 mm.
3. The R wave in lead I is greater than 13 mm.

(text continues on page 209)

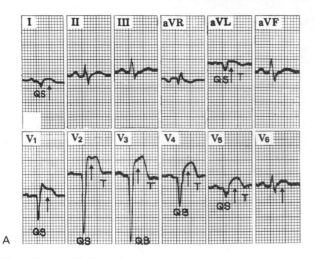

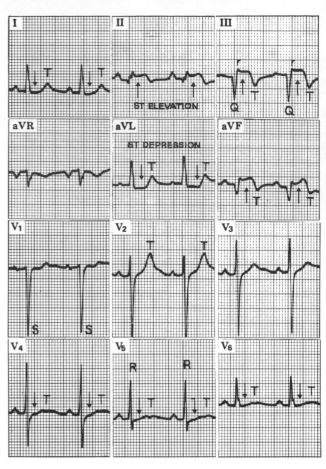

Fig. 17-19. (**A**) ECG changes with anterolateral myocardial infarction. The infarct pattern consisting of Q waves, elevated ST segments and inverted T waves is observed in leads I, aVL and V$_{1-6}$. The ST-segment depressions in leads II, III and aVF are reciprocal. (Mangiola S: Self-Assessment in Electrocardiography, p. 6. Philadelphia, JB Lippincott, 1977). (**B**) ECG changes with Infero-lateral myocardial infarction. The diagnosis of inferior-wall infarction is made on the basis of the findings in leads II, III and aVF. Leads I and V$_{5-6}$ give evidence that this inferior infarct reaches into the lateral wall of the left ventricle. (Bernreiter: Electrocardiography, 131. Philadelphia, JB Lippincott, 1963). (**C**) ECG changes with inferior myocardial infarction with lateral ischemia. (Mangiola S: Self-Assessment in Electrocardiography, p 10. Philadelphia, JB Lippincott, 1979.

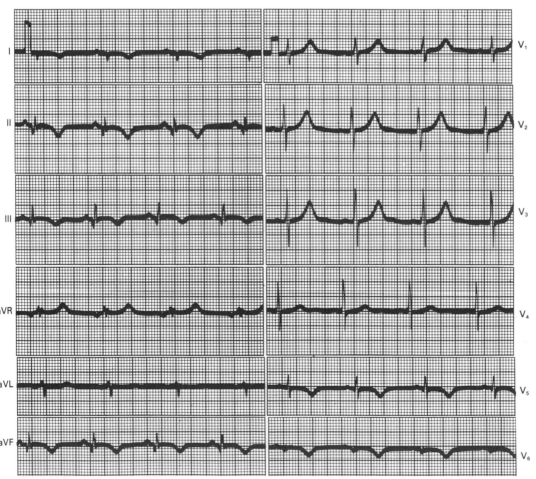

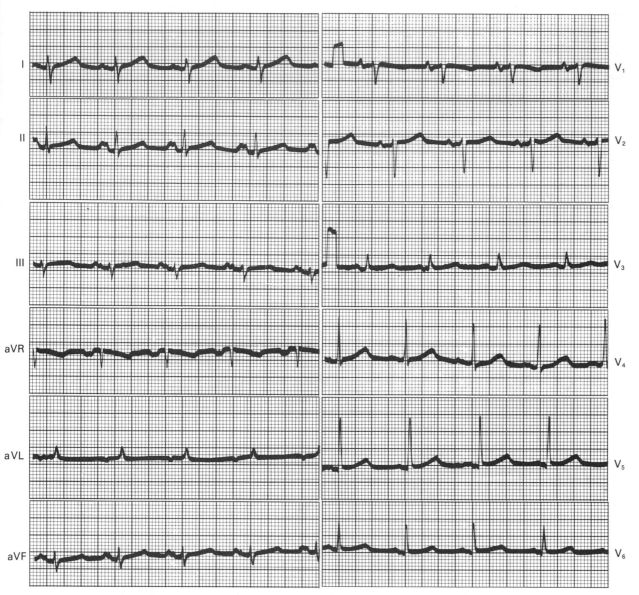

Fig. 17-20. ECG changes with LAE. P mitrale. The notching of the P wave is seen best in leads II and aVF. This patient had clinical evidence of mitral stenosis and mitral regurgitation. (Bernreiter M: Electrocardiography, p 107. Philadelphia, JB Lippincott, 1963)

normal		1.0 − 1.6
RAE		under 1.0
LAE		over 1.6

Fig. 17-21. Macruz index is computed by dividing the P wave duration by the duration of the PR segment.

$$\text{Macruz Index} = \frac{\text{P-Wave Duration}}{\text{PR-Segment Duration}}$$

Normally this index is 1.0 to 1.6. In RAE it is less than 1.0; in LAE, it is over 1.6. (Adapted from Marriott HJL: Practical Electrocardiography, p 87. Baltimore, Williams & Wilkins, 1977)

4. The R wave in lead I plus the S wave in lead III is greater than 26 mm.

5. The R wave in aVL is greater than 11 mm.

6. Secondary ST-segment depression and T-wave inversion appear in leads I, II, V_{4-6}

7. There is a mean QRS axis of 0 to −30 degrees.[23]

8. QRS complex may be prolonged to 0.02 second.

    Another method of determining LVE is by using Estes' Score Card.[21,33]

Criteria	Points

1. R or S wave in limb lead 20 mm or more
   S wave in lead V_1 or V_2 30 mm or more
   R wave in lead V_5 or V_6 30 mm or more
	3

2. Any ST shift (without digitalis) Typical ST strain (with digitalis)	3 1
3. Left-axis deviation −30 degrees or more	2
4. QRS interval 0.09 seconds or more	1
5. Intrinsicoid deflection in V_{5-6} 0.05 second or more (normally 0.035 second)	1
6. P-wave terminal force in V_1 more than 0.04 second	3
	‾13

Total possible score is 13

   5 = LVE
   4 = Probable LVE

Dubin describes another method of determining LVE.[18]

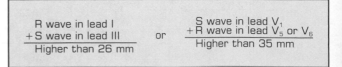

$$\frac{\text{R wave in lead I}}{+\text{ S wave in lead III}} \quad \text{or} \quad \frac{\text{S wave in lead } V_1}{+\text{ R wave in lead } V_5 \text{ or } V_6}$$
$$\text{Higher than 26 mm} \qquad \text{Higher than 35 mm}$$

Right ventricular enlargement (RVE) is caused by any condition that produces a sufficient load on the right ventricle, for example: pulmonary disease or congenital or acquired heart disease. The sequence of ventricular activation is shown in Figure 17-24A.[33] RVE is characterized by the following criteria (Fig. 17-24B):

1. Right-axis deviation of +110 degrees or more
2. Voltage of the R wave in lead V_1 plus voltage of the S wave in lead V_5 or lead V_6 is equal to or greater than 10 mm.

Fig. 17-22. ECG changes with RAE. (Bernreiter M: Electrocardiography, p 105. Philadelphia, JB Lippincott, 1963)

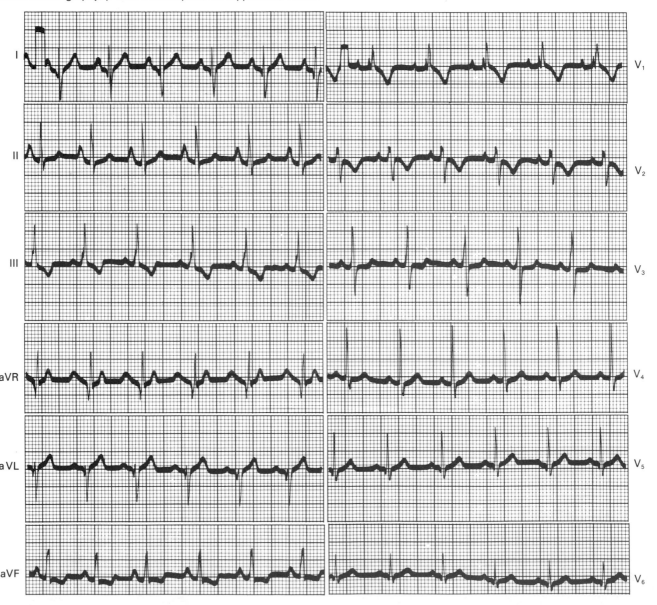

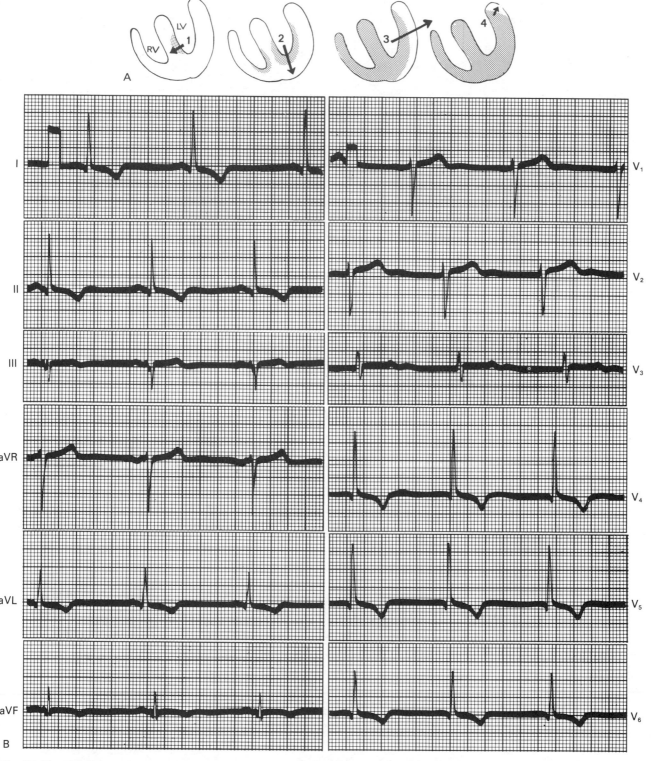

Fig. 17-23. **(A)** Shaded area represents the sequence of ventricular depolarization with LVE.
(B) ECG changes with LVE. Deep S wave (or Q wave) in leads V_{1-2}; tall R wave in leads V_{5-6} and I. (Bernreiter M: Electrocardiography, p 97. Philadelphia, JB Lippincott, 1963)

3. R wave is greater than S wave in lead V_1 or S wave is greater than R wave in lead V_6.

4. S_1, S_2, S_3 (in children). The S wave in leads I, II, and III is greater than the R wave.

5. S wave in leads I, aVL, V_{4-6}; incomplete right bundle branch block; and late intrinsicoid deflection (measured from the beginning of the Q wave to the peak of the R wave) in lead V_1 greater than 0.035 second. Normally this deflection is 0.02 second.

6. Depressed ST segment with upward convexity; inverted

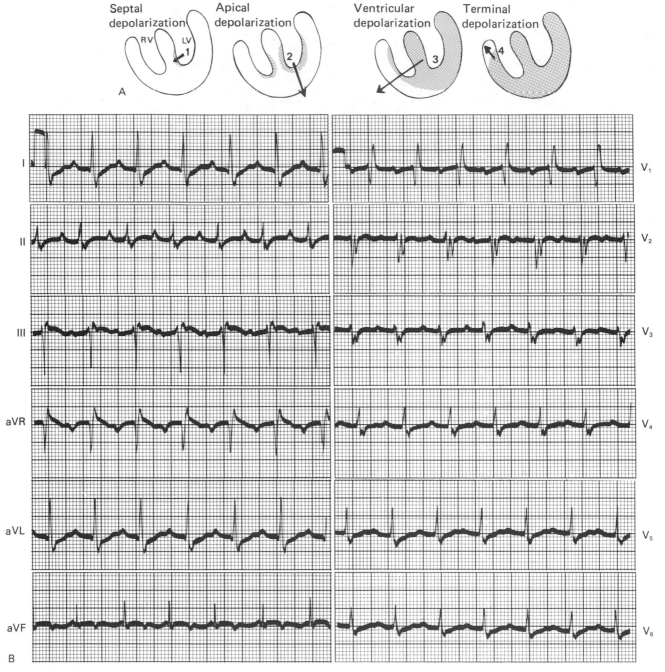

Fig. 17-24. (**A**) The shaded area represents the sequence of ventricular depolarization with RVE. (**B**) ECG changes with RVE; tall R wave in leads V_1; deep S wave in leads V_{5-6} and I. QRS interval is approximately 0.08 seconds. Intrinsicoid deflection (beginning of Q wave to the peak of the R wave) over the right ventricle (V_1) occurs 0.07 seconds after the beginning of the QRS complex. The PR interval is prolonged slightly (first-degree AV block) (Bernreiter M: Electrocardiography, p 102. Philadelphia, JB Lippincott, 1963)

T wave in leads II, III, aVF, and V_{1-3}; due to right ventricular strain.[33,34]

Biventricular enlargement occurs with multiple valvular disease and with biventricular failure. The left ventricular enlargement dominates the electrical picture.[33] Biventricular enlargement has the following characteristics:

1. LVE in precordial leads plus RAD of +90 degrees or greater, or
2. LVE in the left precordial leads plus prominent R waves in the right precordium
3. Shallow S-wave syndrome: lead V_1 has a small S wave; lead V_2 has a large S wave[43]

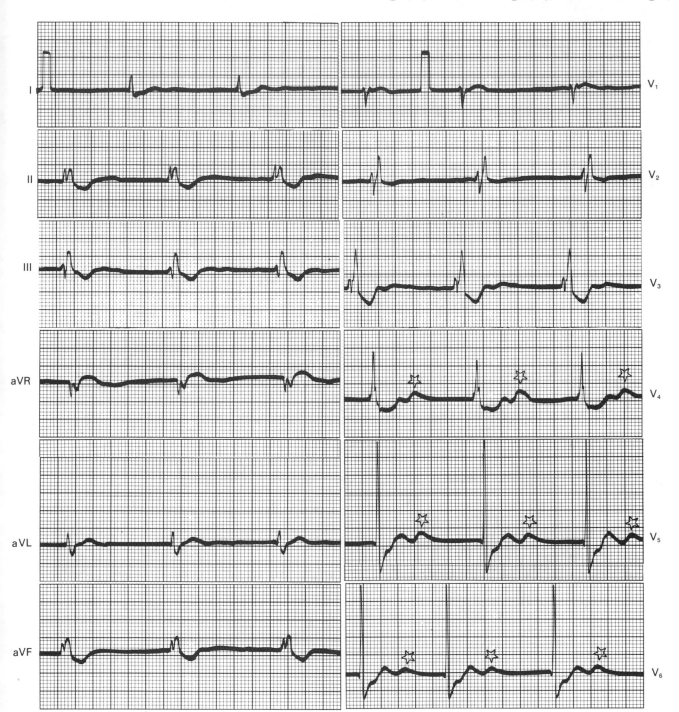

Fig. 17-25. ECG effects of hypokalemia. (Bernreiter M: Electrocardiography, p 158. Philadelphia, JB Lippincott, 1963)

Electrolyte Imbalance

Electrolyte imbalances also affect the ECG. A discussion of electrolyte balance abnormalities can be found in Chapter 9.

Hypokalemia (serum K^+ less than 3.0 mEq/l) may produce the following changes (Fig. 17-25):

1. U wave equal to or higher than T wave (best seen in leads II, III, and V_{1-3})
2. Diminution of T wave (flat or inverted)
3. Peaked P wave in leads II, III, and aVF
4. ST-segment shortening and depression (similar to the effects of digitalis)
5. Ventricular ectopic beats[46,49]
6. QT interval prolonged[28]

The action of digitalis is potentiated by hypokalemia.

Hyperkalemia (serum K^+ greater than 5 mEq/l) will produce the following changes (Fig. 17-26):

1. Tall, tented, symmetric, narrow T waves (seen best in

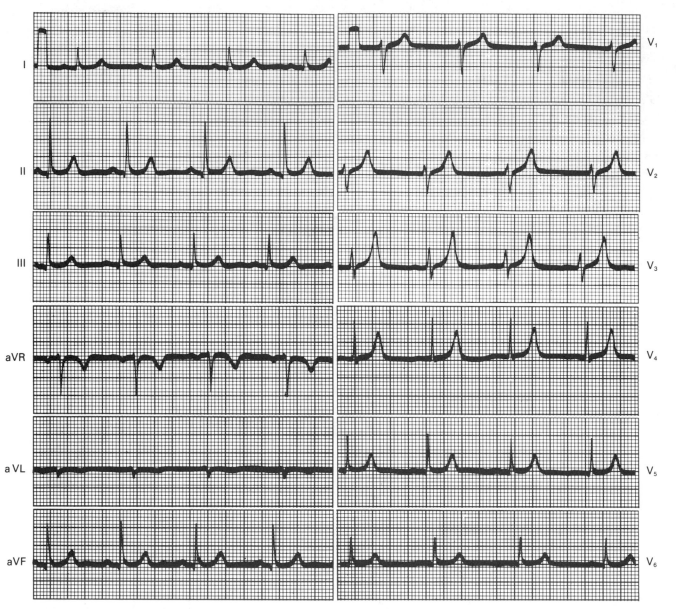

Fig. 17-26. ECG effects of hyperkalemia. (Bernreiter M: Electrocardiography, p 155. Philadelphia, JB Lippincott, 1963)

precordial leads). This requires serum K+ greater than 6 to 7 mEq/l.

2. P waves are flat and broad (serum K+ greater than 7.0 mEq/l) or disappear completely (serum K+ greater than 8.8 mEq/l).

3. Atrioventricular (AV) block (usually first degree)

4. The QRS complex widens (serum K+ greater than 6.5 mEq/l) because of wide S waves in the lateral precordium (V5–6). If the cause goes untreated, the patient may progress from sinus bradycardia to first-degree AV block, through junctional and idioventricular rhythms to ventricular fibrillation or asystole.[46,49]

5. Shortening of the Q–T interval.[28]

Hypocalcemia (serum Ca2+ less than 6.1 mg/100 ml) will produce the following effects (Fig. 17-27):

1. Q–T interval prolonged; increased ST-segment duration[46,49]

2. Flat or inverted T wave

3. Arrhythmias[28]

Hypercalcemia (serum Ca2+ greater than 16 mg/100 ml) may produce these effects, which look like digitalis effect (Fig. 17-28):

1. Q–T interval shortens; ST segments sag and shorten.

2. T waves invert.

3. Ventricular arrhythmias[46,49]

Patients may have both hypocalcemia and hypokalemia. Figure 17-29 demonstrates the ECG findings of these imbalances.

The patient with potassium or calcium imbalances may

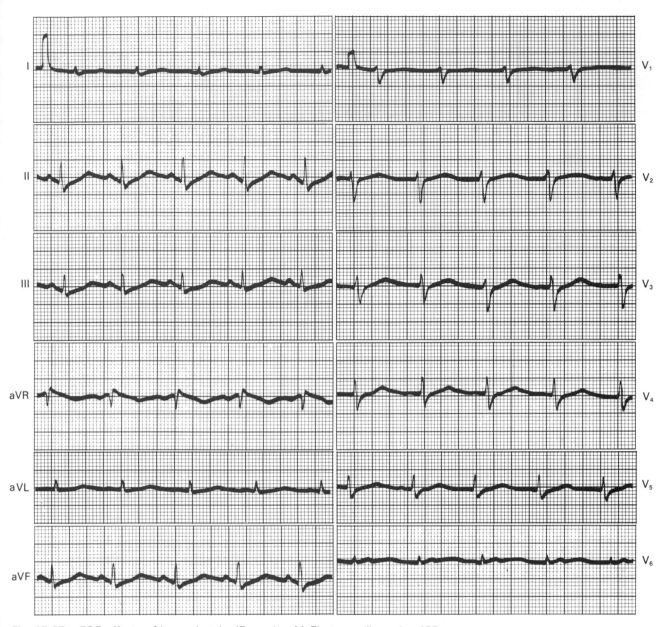

Fig. 17-27. ECG effects of hypocalcemia. (Bernreiter M: Electrocardiography, 162. Philadelphia, JB Lippincott, 1963)

or may not exhibit the ECG changes mentioned. But such changes, if seen, alert the nurse to suspect electrolyte abnormalities. They must be seen in the context of what is already known about the paitent.[52]

Magnesium (Mg^{2+}) concentration in the body does not seem to affect the electrocardiogram. Electrocardiographic changes produced by hypocalcemia are augmented if Mg^{2+} concentration is also low, and they tend to be reversed if Mg^{2+} concentrations are increased above normal.[46]

Effects of Drugs on the ECG

Digitalis slows the heart rate (negative chronotropic effect) and decreases AV conduction (negative dromotropic effect) (Figs. 17-30A, 17-30B). Digitalis also
1. Shortens ventricular activation time

2. Shortens the Q–T interval
3. Depresses the ST segments and makes them sag
4. In large doses, can decrease the T-wave amplitude, cause sinus bradycardia (less than a rate of 50), and prolong the P–R interval greater than 0.24 second
5. In large doses, can cause atrial, junctional, and ventricular extrasystoles (bigeminy) and conduction abnormalities.
6. Increases amplitude of U wave.

Quinidine and procainamide cause the following effects on the ECG (Fig. 17-31):

1. A slightly prolonged PR interval
2. A wide QRS complex thus prolonging the Q–T interval; therapeutic levels can result in a QRS complex of 0.11 second

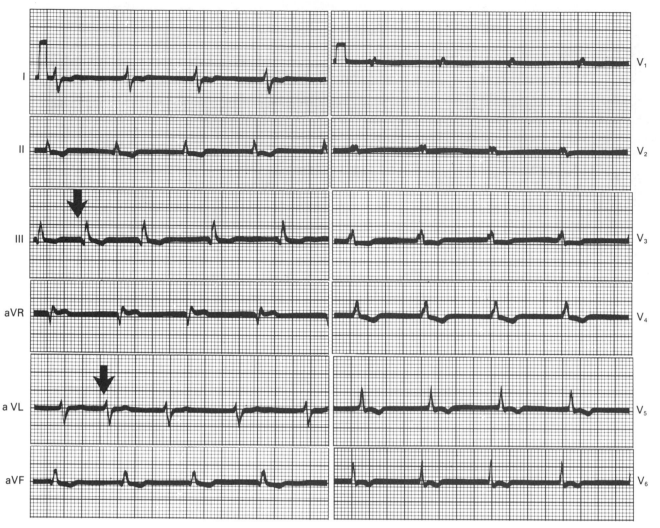

Fig. 17-28. ECG effects of hypercalcemia. (Bernreiter M: Electrocardiography, p 160. Philadelphia, JB Lippincott, 1963)

3. A depressed, widened, and notched T wave
4. Toxicity can cause sinoatrial or AV block, ventricular arrhythmias, and a 50% increase in the QRS complex duration.
5. Inverted T wave

   Phenothiazine can cause the following ECG effects:

1. Minor nonspecific ST-segment and T-wave changes
2. Rarely, prolonged P–R and Q–T intervals
3. Increased U-wave amplitude
4. Decreased T-wave amplitude
5. Intraventricular conduction disturbances
6. Ventricular and supraventricular arrhythmias

   Tricyclic antidepressant drugs have anticholinergic activity and affect the ECG in the following ways:

1. T-wave changes
2. P–R, Q–T, and QRS prolongation
3. Conduction disturbances
4. Supraventricular and ventricular arrhythmias[57]

Conduction Abnormalities.

Abnormalities of Decreased Conduction. Decreased conduction in the (SA) node results in SA block.

Sinoatrial Block (S–A block) or Sinus Exit Block is a conduction disturbance during which an impulse of the SA node is blocked from depolarizing the atria. This block may be caused by excessive vagal stimulation, acute infections, atherosclerosis involving the SA nodal artery, or fibrosis involving the atrium. Digitalis, quinidine, atropine, salicylates, all are reported to cause SA block.[26]

Sinoatrial block has the following characteristics (Fig. 17-32A):

1. Rate: 60 to 100 beats per minute
2. P waves: Normal, but occasionally absent, owing to pause in atrial activity.
3. QRS complex: Usually normal; absent when the P wave is absent, resulting in a pause
4. Ventricular conduction: Usually normal

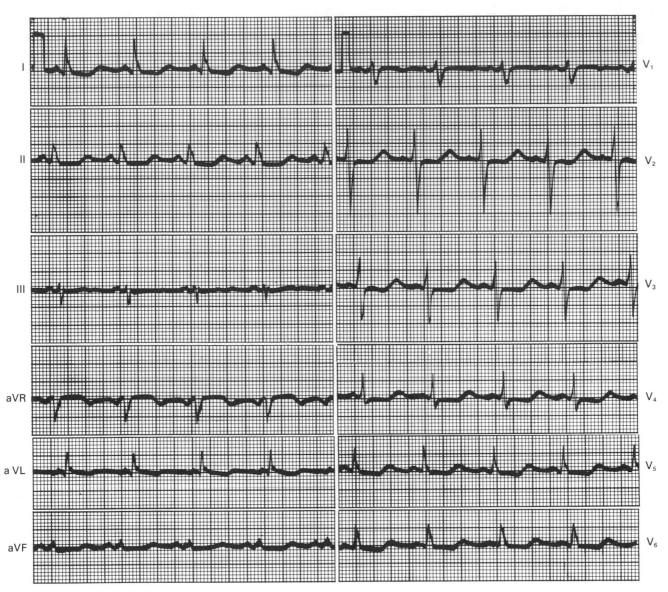

Fig. 17-29. ECG effects of hypocalcemia and hypokalemia. The QT interval was 0.48 seconds (normal for this rate is 0.38 seconds). The prolongation of the QT interval is made up by a prolonged ST segment. (calcium deficiency) as well as a wide T wave (potassium deficiency). (Bernreiter M: Electrocardiography, p 163. Philadelphia, JB Lippincott, 1963)

5. Rhythm: Irregular, because of the occasionally absent P wave and QRS complex. Escape beats from junctional and ventricular areas are common. Type I (Wenckebach) SA exit block may also occur, in which case the P–P interval progressively shortens prior to the pause and the duration of the pause is less than two P–P cycles.

In Type II exit block the length of the pause is a multiple of the basic P–P interval, approximately two, less commonly three or four, times the normal P–P interval.

Treatment depends largely on the cause and the hemodynamic changes produced. If these changes are significant such that syncope or angina occurs, then therapy is directed toward increasing sympathetic tone and decreasing parasympathetic tone.

There are three types of AV block that result from a decreased conduction, usually between the junctional tissue and the Purkinje fibers: first-, second-, and third-degree AV block.

First-Degree AV Block is usually associated with organic heart disease or may be due to the effect of digitalis. It is seen frequently in patients with inferior MI's (if the AV nodal artery is involved.)

First-degree heart block has the following characteristics (Fig. 17-32B):

1. Rate: Variable; usually 60 to 100 beats per minute.
2. P waves: Precede each QRS complex. The PR interval is greater than 0.20 second in duration.
3. QRS complexes: Follow each P wave; are usually normal.
4. Conduction: Delayed conduction, usually anywhere between the junctional tissue and the Purkinje network, produces a prolonged PR interval. Ventricular conduction is usually normal.

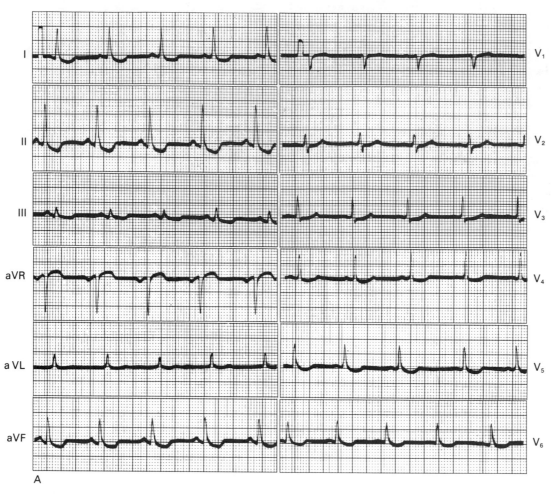

I   II   III   aVR   aVL   aVF   V₁   V₂   V₃   V₄   V₅   V₆

A

Fig. 17-30. **(A)** Digitalis effect. ST segments are depressed slightly, and cupping appears in some of the leads; the T waves are of low voltage. QT interval is 0.32 seconds (average QT interval at this rate 0.36 seconds). (Bernreiter: Electrocardiography p 175. Philadelphia, JB Lippincott, 1963) **(B)** Digitalis intoxication. Every other beat is a ventricular premature contraction—bigeminal rhythm. Bigeminy occurred after complete digitalization. (Bernreiter M: Electrocardiography, p 179. Philadelphia, JB Lippincott, 1963)   →

5. Rhythm: Usually regular

This arrhythmia is important, since it may lead to more serious forms of heart block. It is often a warning signal. His bundle recording may be done to pinpoint the area of block. The patient should be monitored closely for any advancing block.

Second-Degree AV Block or Mobitz Type I (Wenckebach phenomenon) is usually associated with organic heart disease and is frequently due to digitalis intoxication. This block is frequently seen in association with myocardial infarction that involves the AV nodal artery.

Second-degree heart block has the following characteristics (Fig. 17-32C):

1. Rate: Variable. Usually 60 to 100 beats per minute

2. P waves: Precede each QRS complex; the P–R interval becomes increasingly longer until finally a QRS complex is dropped and then the cycle is repeated

3. QRS complex: Follows most P waves, except when QRS complex is dropped

4. Conduction: The P–R interval becomes increasingly longer until an impulse is not conducted through the ventricles because it is blocked somewhere between the junctional tissue and the Purkinje network.

5. Rhythm: Irregular, since the R–R interval becomes progressively shorter until a QRS complex is dropped.

Digitalis intoxication should be ruled out. Depending on the hemodynamic changes produced, efforts to normalize the heart rate may be necessary.

Second-Degree AV Block, Mobitz Type II is also caused by organic heart disease, by myocardial infarctions involving the AV nodal artery, and by digitalis intoxication. This type of block results in a reduced heart rate and usually a reduced cardiac output. Cardiac output is the product of stroke volume and heart rate.

Second-degree heart block has the following characteristics (Fig. 17-32D):

1. Rate: 30 to 55 beats per minute. The artial rate may be two, three, or four times faster than the ventricular rate.

2. P waves: There are two, three, or four P waves for each

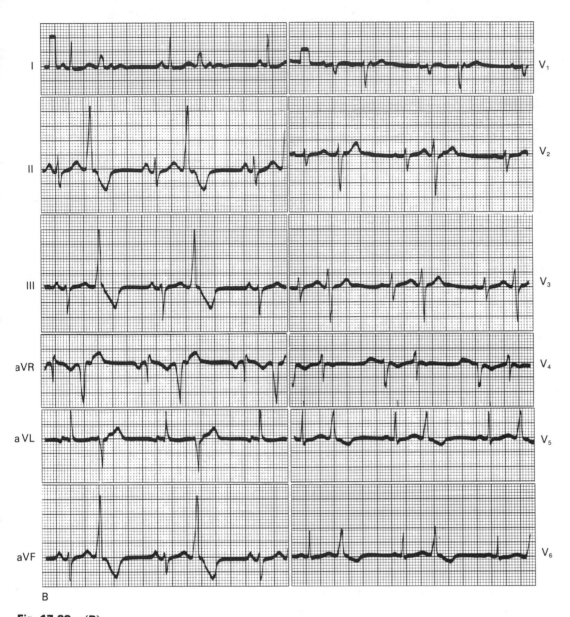

I II III aVR aVL aVF

V₁ V₂ V₃ V₄ V₅ V₆

B

Fig. 17-30. (B)

QRS complex. The PR interval of the conducted beat is usually normal in duration.

3. QRS complex: Usually normal

4. Conduction: One or more of the impulses are not conducted through the ventricles.

5. Rhythm: Usually slow and regular. When an irregularity is seen, it is due to the fact that the block is varying from 2:1 to 3:1 or to some other combination.

Treatment is directed toward increasing heart rate to maintain a normal cardiac output. Digitalis intoxication should be ruled out and myocardial depressant drugs withheld.

Third-Degree AV Block (complete heart block) is also associated with organic heart disease, digitalis intoxication, and MI. The heart rate may be significantly decreased, resulting in a decrease in perfusion to vital organs such as brain, heart, kidneys, lungs, and skin.

Complete block—third-degree AV block—has the following characteristics:

1. Origin: Impulses originate in the SA node but these impulses are not conducted to the Purkinje fibers. They are completely blocked. An escape rhythm from the junctional or ventricular area therefore takes over as the pacemaker.

2. Rate: Atrial rate 60 to 100 beats per minute; ventricular rate 40 to 60 beats per minute if the escape rhythm originated in the junction (Fig. 17-32E), 20 to 40 beats per minute if the escape rhythm originated in the ventricle (Fig. 17-32F)

3. P waves: The P waves originating from the SA node are seen regularly throughout the rhythm, but they have no association with the QRS complexes.

4. QRS complex: If the escape rhythm originated in the junction, the QRS complexes have a normal supraventricular configuration, but have no association with the P waves. QRS complexes occur regularly. If the escape rhythm originated in the ventricle, the QRS complex is longer than 0.10 second in duration, usually broad and

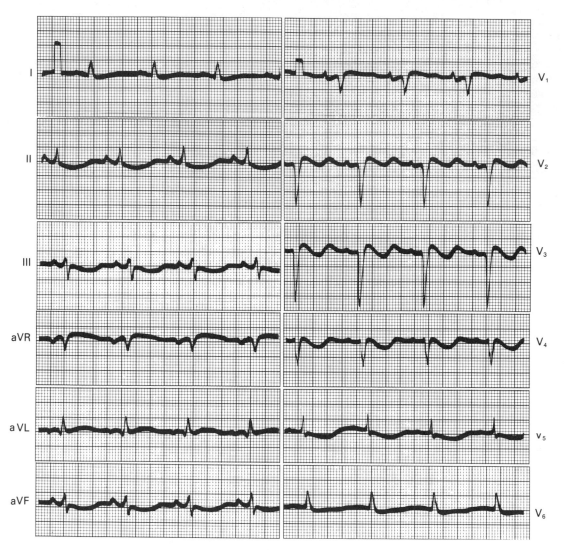

Fig. 17-31. Effects of quinidine on the ECG. The QT interval is prolonged. The "roller coaster" pattern of quinidine effect is typical, particularly in the precordial leads. (Bernreiter M: Electrocardiography, p 183. Philadelphia, JB Lippincott, 1963)

slurred. These QRS complexes have the same configuration as the QRS complex of a premature ventricular contraction.

5. Conduction: The SA node is firing and P waves can be seen. They are all blocked and not conducted to the ventricles. Escape rhythms originating in the junction are usually conducted normally through the ventricles. Escape rhythms from the ventricles are ectopic with aberrant configuration.

6. Rhythm: Usually slow but regular

Treatment is directed toward increasing perfusion to vital organs. This may include increasing rate of escape rhythm; a junctional rhythm can be increased by use of a parasympatholytic (anticholinergic) agent; a ventricular rhythm can be increased by use of a sympathomimetic agent. It may also include insertion of a temporary transvenous pacemaker.

The His Bundle Electrogram (HBE)

The HBE allows the unraveling of complex arrhythmias whose mechanisms were deducted from the 12-lead ECG.

Specific details of the technique can be found in the article by Scherlag and others.[43]

The HBE is obtained from a bipolar or tripolar catheter, which is usually introduced through the femoral vein, advanced into the heart, and positioned across the septal leaflet of the tricuspid valve. The HBE bipolar lead records electrical activity of the specialized tissue of the conduction system. The HBE consists of three deflections:

1. The *A* deflection (initial depolarization of the junction)

2. The *H* deflection (His bundle activity)

3. The *V* deflection (electrical activity from His bundle to the bundle branches; corresponds to the QRS complex on the ECG). From these deflections, two intervals are measured: (a) A–H (atrio–His); (b) H–V His–ventricle (Fig. 17-33).[37]

P–R interval of 0.14 second (140 msec) represents three intervals:

1. P–A time—beginning of P wave to beginning of the A deflection—normal time 25 to 45 msec

2. A–H time—beginning of the A deflection to beginning

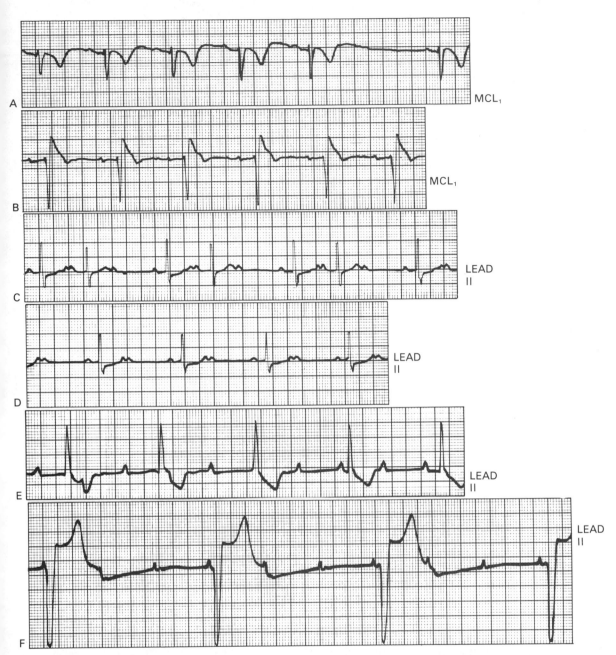

Fig. 17-32. Examples of delayed conduction. (**A**) Sinus exit block. (Type II) (**B**) First-degree AV block. (**C**) Mobitz type I—second-degree AV block. (**D**) Mobitz Type II—second-degree AV block. (**E**) Complete heart block—third-degree AV block—pacemaker in the junction. (Conover M: Cardiac Arrhythmias, p 127. St. Louis, C.V. Mosby, 1978) (**F**) Complete heart block—third-degree AV block—pacemaker in the ventricular.

of the H deflection—normal time 50 to 120 msec; corresponds to conduction time through the AV node (H time is 15 to 20 msec.)

3. H–V time—beginning of the H deflection to onset of the V deflection—normal time 35 to 45 msec; corresponds to conduction time through the Purkinje system[37]

Lesions in different segments of the conducting system can cause varying degrees of AV block (Fig. 17-34):

1. P–A interval   first-degree AV block
      prolongation

2. A–H interval   first-degree AV block
      prolongation   second-degree AV block, Type I

3. H, H–V, and V time   first-degree AV block
      prolongation   second-degree AV block, Type I and II
        third-degree AV block[37]

Intraventricular Conduction Disturbances. These conduction disturbances include right and left bundle branch blocks and left anterior and left posterior hemiblocks. The intraventricular conduction system consists of three fasci-

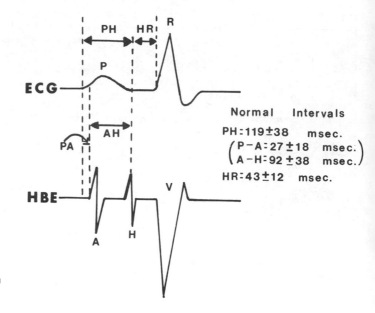

Fig. 17-33. Diagramatic representation of bipolar HBE with simultaneous ECG. (Hecht HH et al: Am J Cardiol 31:232, 1973)

Fig. 17-34. Diagrammatic representation of the A-V conduction system illustrating that the different varieties of the A-V block can occur as a result of lesions in different segments of the conducting system. At the bottom left hand corner are the simultaneous recordings of a standard electrocardiographic lead (L-2) and a typical bipolar electrogram (BE) from the area of the A-V junction. SAN, sinoatrial node: AVN, atrioventricular node; BH, bundle of His; RB and LB, right and left bundle branches; P-A, conduction time through the atrium; A-H, conduction time through the AVN; H-V, conduction time through the His Purkinje system; A, bipolar atrial electrogram; V, the bipolar ventricular electrogram recorded from the area of the A-V junction. (Narula OS: Cardiovasc Clin, 6:135, 1975)

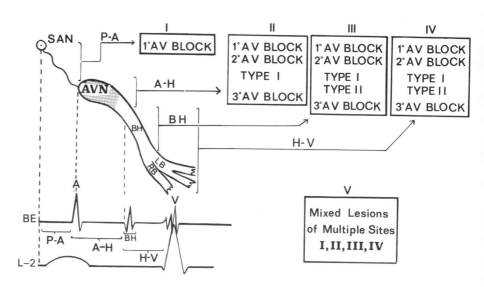

cles: (1) the right bundle branch, (2) the anterior division of the left bundle branch, and (3) the posterior divisions of the left bundle branch. Monofascicular block occurs if one fascicle is blocked, bifascicular block if two fascicles are blocked, and trifascicular block if three fascicles are blocked.

Right Bundle Branch Block (RBBB) is a monofascicular block and may be caused by coronary artery disease or by prolonged right ventricular strain, as in pulmonary stenosis or pulmonary hypertension. The initial and mid-QRS forces are normal, and only the terminal forces are abnormal. This terminal force is directed slowly, anteriorly and to the right (Fig. 17-35).

Right bundle branch block is characterized by (Fig. 17-36):

1. A QRS duration of 0.12 second or longer. Intrinsicoid deflection is greater than 0.07 second in lead V_1 or V_2

2. RSR prime complex (RSR') or R wave in V_{1-2}

3. A late S wave in leads I, II, aVL, and V_5 or V_6

Fig. 17-35. Three steps of ventricular depolarization in RBBB. (Adapted from Marriott HJL: Workshop in Electrocardiography, p 114. Oldsmar, FL, Tampa Tracings, 1972)

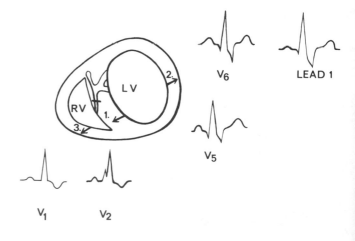

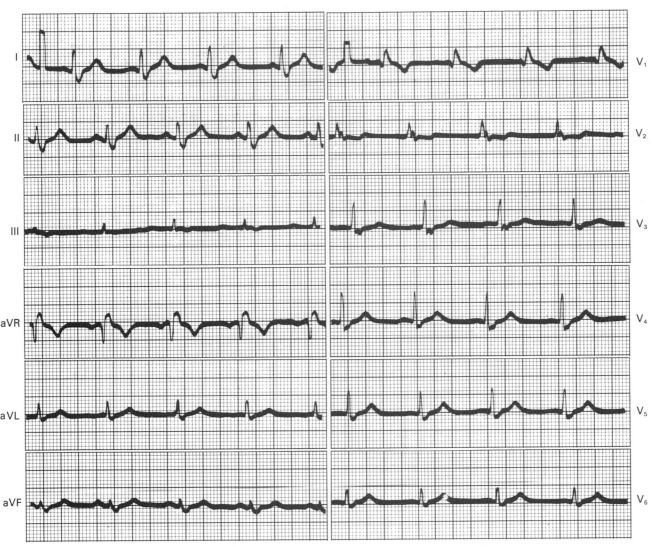

Fig. 17-36. ECG in RBBB. (Bernreiter M: Electrocardiography, p 90. Philadelphia, JB Lippincott, 1963)

4. Secondary ST-segment and T-wave changes V_{1-3}

With incomplete RBBB the QRS complex duration is 0.09 to 0.1 second, and there is an RBBB pattern.[33]

Left Bundle Branch Block (LBBB) is a bifascicular block and may be caused by MI, valvular disease, rheumatic disease, syphilis, trauma, tumors, cardiomyopathy, congestive heart failure, hypertension, coronary artery disease, and fibrosis of the conduction system (Lenegre's disease in the young; Lev's disease in the aged).[34] The early forces are anteriorly directed, but in contrast to the normal pattern, move to the left. The mid- and terminal forces are posterior and more toward the left than normal. Since the initial QRS forces are altered in LBBB, diagnosis of MI from ECG is difficult (Fig. 17-37).

Left bundle branch block is characterized by (Fig. 17-38):

1. A QRS duration of 0.12 second or longer; intrinsicoid deflection greater than 0.07 second in V_5 or V_6

2. rS complex or qS complex in V_{1-2}

3. A broad RSR¹ QRS complex in leads I, aVL, and V_{5-6}

4. Secondary ST-segment and T-wave changes in leads I, aVL, V_{5-6}

With incomplete LBBB, the QRS complex is 0.10 to 0.11 second in duration, and there is a LBBB pattern.[33]

Left Anterior Hemiblock (LAH) is a monofascicular block involving the anterior–superior division of the left bundle branch. Since this portion of the left bundle receives its blood supply from the left anterior descending coronary artery, an anterior MI could result in LAH as well as right bundle branch block. This fascicle is easily damaged, because it receives its blood supply from a single source, is structurally thin, and is located in a highly turbulent area of the left ventricle. Other causes of LAH are left ventricular cardiomyopathies, hypertension, and aortic value disease. Left anterior hemiblock can mimic an anterior MI, lateral MI, or left ventricular hypertrophy. It can mask an anterior MI, inferior MI, left ventricular enlargement, or RBBB.[33]

Left anterior hemiblock is characterized by (Figs. 17-39, 17-40):

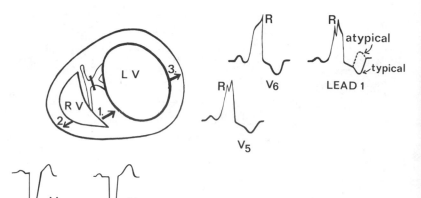

Fig. 17-37. Three steps of ventricular depolarization in LBBB. (Adapted From Marriott HJL: Workshop in Electrocardiography, p 116. Oldsmar, FL, Tampa Tracings, 1972)

1. A mean QRS axis of more than −45 degrees (LAD) because the QRS axis has shifted upward and to the left

2. A Q wave in lead I (because the initial 0.02 second of ventricular depolarization is downward and to the right) and S wave in lead III (because the terminal forces are upward): qI, sIII

3. A QRS duration that is normal or prolonged by 0.02 second

Fig. 17-38. ECG in LLLB. (Mangiola S: Self-Assessment in Electrocardiography, p. 54. Philadelphia, JB Lippincott, 1977)

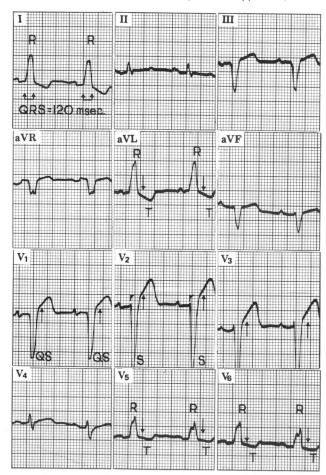

Left Posterior Hemiblock (LPH) is a monofascicular block involving the posterior–inferior portion of the left bundle branch. This fascicle is not easily damaged, because it has a dual blood supply (the left anterior and posterior descending coronary arteries) and is structurally thick, and because of its position in a low-turbulence area of the left ventricle. Left posterior hemiblock is the rarest type of fascicular block. When it does occur, it suggests extensive involvement of the conduction system.[9] Left posterior hemiblock can mimic or mask an anterior MI.[33]

Left posterior hemiblock is characterized by (Figs. 17-41, 17-42):

1. A mean QRS axis of +120 degrees or greater, due to a shift in axis downward and to the right (RAD)

2. An S wave in lead I and a Q wave in lead III, because

Fig. 17-39. Left ventricular depolarization in LAH. (Adapted from Marriott HJL: Practical Electrocardiography 1977, p 82. Baltimore, Williams & Wilkins, 1977)

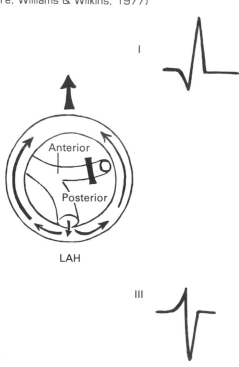

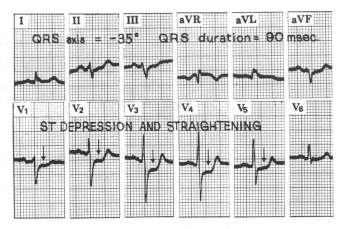

Fig. 17-40. ECG in LAH. The ST-segment depression in V$_{1-5}$ indicates anteroseptal subendocardial injury. (Mangiola S: Self-Assessment in Electrocardiography, p. 88. Philadelphia, JB Lippincott, 1977)

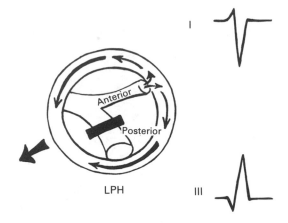

Fig. 17-41. Left ventricular depolarization in LPH. (Adapted from Marriott HJL: Practical Electrocardiography, p 82. Baltimore, Williams & Wilkins, 1967)

the initial 0.02 second of ventricular depolarization is upward and to the left

3. A QRS duration that is normal or prolonged by 0.02 seconds[41]

RBBB with LAH (bifascicular block) is characterized by (Fig. 17-43):

1. An RBBB with mean QRS axis of − 60 degrees to − 120 degrees

2. A Q wave in lead I and an S wave in lead III: qI, sIII

3. A terminal force of around + 180 degrees

4. An intrinsicoid deflection of − 60 degrees[41]

RBBB with LPH (bifascicular block) is characterized by the following, provided that right ventricular enlargement or a vertical heart can be excluded (Fig. 17-44):

1. An RBBB with mean QRS axis of + 120 degrees

2. An rS complex in lead I; a Q wave in lead II and III: rSI, qII, qIII

3. The axis of the first half of the QRS complex is + 120 degrees.

4. Tall R waves in leads II and III

5. AV conduction disturbances

6. The first 0.02 second of the QRS complex is − 45 degrees[41]

Trifascicular block appears as complete heart block. If first-degree AV block develops in a patient with bifascicular block, then one of the following two situations may be occurring: (1) if RBBB with LAH and first-degree AV block occur, this block may be due to impedance to conduction above the bifurcation, or to impedance to conduction through the posterior division of the left bundle branch (Fig. 17-45); or (2) if RBBB with LPH and first-degree AV block occur, this block may be due to impedance to conduction above the bifurcation, or to impedance to conduction through the anterior division of the left bundle branch (Fig. 17-46).

Identification of first-degree AV block in the patient with RBBB with hemiblock (bifascicular block) is an important nursing goal; prompt treatment is necessary if trifascicular block (complete heart block) ensues.

Fig. 17-42. ECG in LPH. (Dubin D: Rapid ECG Interpretation, p 240. Tampa, Clover Publishing Co, 1975)

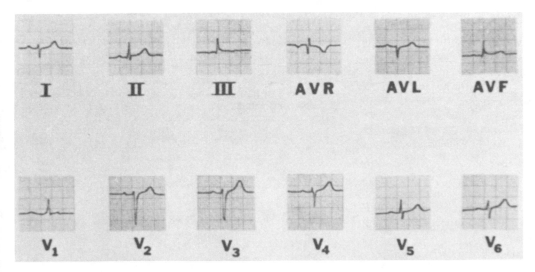

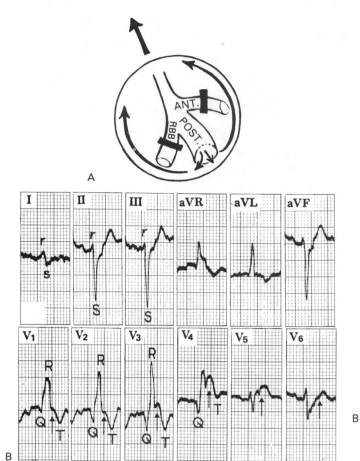

Fig. 17-43. Left ventricular depolarization in RBBB with LAH. (**A**) Schematic drawing; (**B**) ECG. (Adapted from Mangiola S: Self-Assessment in Electrocardiology, p 52. Philadelphia, JB Lippincott, 1977)

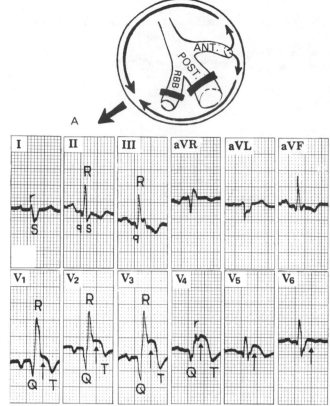

Fig. 17-44. Left ventricular depolarization and ECG in RBBB with LPH. (**A**) Schematic drawing; (**B**) ECG. (Adapted from Mangiola S: Self-Assessment in Electrocardiology, p 52. Philadelphia, JB Lippincott, 1977)

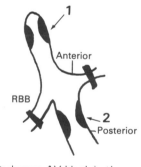

Fig. 17-45. First-degree AV block in the presence of RBBB with LAH may be due to impedance to conduction above the bifurcation (**1**), or to impedance to conduction through the posterior division of the left bundle branch (**2**).

Fig. 17-46. First-degree AV block in the presence of RBBB with LPH may be due to impedance to conduction above the bifurcation (**1**), or to impedance to conduction through the anterior division of the left bundle branch (**2**)

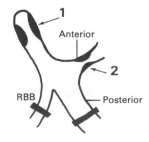

Abnormalities of Increased Conduction

Abnormalities of increased conduction between the atria and ventricles (preexcitation) include the following conditions: accelerated conduction, Wolff–Parkinson–White (WPW) syndrome and Lown–Ganong–Levine syndrome. Accelerated conduction is characterized by a P–R interval of less than 0.12 second in a normal sinus rhythm.

Wolff–Parkinson–White (WPW) Syndrome, premature activation of a portion of the ventricle due to bypass of the AV node by an additional or abnormal anatomical connection, is a congenital disorder that occurs more frequently in males than in females. Of those with WPW syndrome, 60% to 70% have normal hearts. One person in every 666 has WPW syndrome. Because the AV node is bypassed, retrograde conduction to the atria is facilitated and reentry (Chap. 26) more possible. The ECG manifestations may be intermittent

WPW is characterized by (Fig. 17-47):

1. A P–R interval of less than 0.12 second
2. A QRS complex of more than 0.12 second in duration because of initial slurring of QRS (delta wave). The QRS can be the result of a normally conducted beat fusing with the early conducted beat.
3. Paroxysmal atrial tachycardia in 40% to 80% of patients.

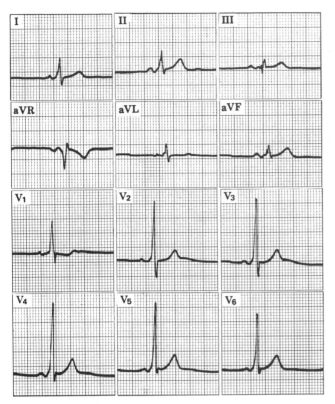

Fig. 17-47. ECG in Wolff-Parkinson-White syndrome, Type A. The PR interval is 0.10 second and there is a delta wave. (Mangiola S: Self-Assessment in Electrocardiography, p 37. Philadelphia, JB Lippincott, 1977)

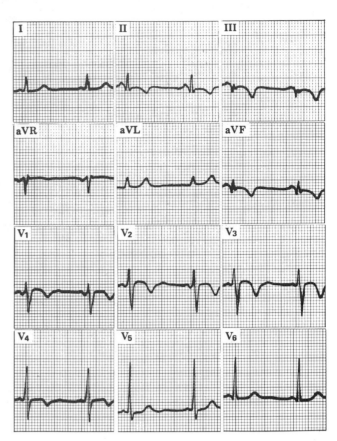

Fig. 17-48. ECG in Lown-Ganong-Levine Syndrome. The PR interval is 0.08 second. (Mangiola S: Self-Assessment in Electrocardiography, p 171. Philadelphia, JB Lippincott, 1977)

4. Secondary ST- and T-wave changes in the opposite direction to the QRS complex and delta-wave axis.

5. A constant P–J interval

6. In Type A (posterior bypass of AV node), a large R wave in V_1; in Type B (anterior bypass of AV node), a large R wave in V_6[19]

Treatment of WPW may include the following: drugs that increase the effective refractory period, such as propranolol; the insertion of a transvenous pacemaker, so that an appropriately timed capture beat can be initiated in order to terminate the tachycardia; and surgical interruption of the accessory pathway.[22,36]

Lown–Ganong–Levine Syndrome is also premature activation of a portion of the ventricle due to bypass of the AV node by a posterior internodal tract entering the lower part of the AV node. This syndrome occurs more frequently in women than in men.

Lown–Ganong–Levine Syndrome (Fig. 17-48) is characterized by

1. A P–R interval of less than 0.12 second

2. A normal QRS complex

3. Supraventricular tachycardia[31]

Effect of Selected Diseases on the Electrocardiogram

Some of the diseases that affect the ECG are myocarditis, pericarditis, pulmonary embolism, pulmonary infarction, central nervous system injury, hypothermia, and myxedema (hypothyroidism).

Myocarditis. Myocarditis, an inflammation of the myocardium, may be associated with many types of infections, nephritis, carbon monoxide poisoning, heat stroke and burns, or may be idiopathic. Myocarditis can affect the ECG in the following ways:

1. Varying AV block

2. Bundle branch blocks

3. LVE

4. Lengthening of Q–T interval

5. ST-segment depression or T-wave inversion

6. Extrasystoles[51]

There are no precise criteria. Usually the T-wave changes are similar to those in pericarditis.[48]

Pericarditis. Pericarditis, an inflammation of the pericardium, may be caused by tuberculosis, mycoses, infection, collagen diseases, uremia, MI, neoplasms, and trauma. Pericarditis (subepicardial inflammation) can affect the ECG in the following ways (Fig. 17-49):

1. Early stage (10 days to two weeks)
   a. ST-segment elevation (concave upward) in many leads
   b. No reciprocal ST-segment depression between leads I and III, or in leads aVL and aVF

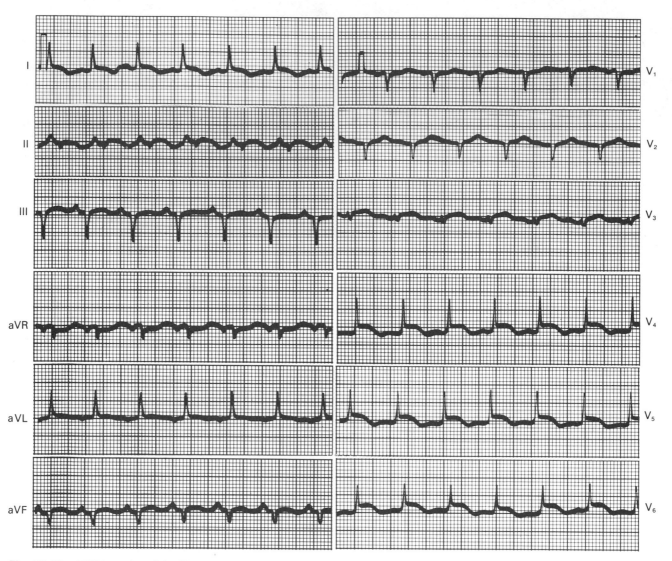

Fig. 17-49. ECG in pericarditis. (Bernreiter M: Electrocardiography, p 120. Philadelphia, JB Lippincott, 1963)

c. Depressed P–R segment in limb leads and leads V_{2-6}

2. Late stage (10 days to weeks after early stage)
   a. Inverted T waves in many leads
   b. Low voltage
   c. No Q waves; evolution takes days or weeks[25,33]

Pulmonary Embolism. Pulmonary embolism, obstruction of a pulmonary blood vessel by a foreign substance, a blood clot, or acute cor pulmonale, affects the ECG in the following ways (Fig. 17-50):

1. P pulmonale (RAE)
2. Right axis deviation
3. Inverted T wave in lead V_1 (suggesting septal ischemia)
4. S wave in lead I; Q wave in lead III (S_1, Q_3); S waves in leads I, II, III (S_1, S_2, S_3); Q wave in leads II, III, aVF (suggesting inferior MI)
5. Transient RBBB
6. Paroxysmal atrial arrhythmias.[21,33]

Central Nervous System Injury. Central nervous system injury may affect the ECG in the following ways (see Chap. 52) (Fig. 17-51 A, B):

1. Elevated ST segments
2. T wave peaked and inverted in all leads
3. Prolonged Q–T intervals
4. U waves
5. Supraventricular arrhythmias. Wandering atrial pacemaker in common.[45]

Hypothermia. Hypothermia affects the ECG by elevating the "J" junction (Fig. 17-52). Temperatures less than 25° Celcius can produce a positive wave, called an Osborn wave, during the terminal QRS complex. Moderate hypothermia can cause bradycardia and Q–T-interval lengthening.[20,48]

Hypothyroidism. Hypothyroidism affects the ECG in the following ways (Fig. 17-53):

1. Flat T waves; no ST-segment shift

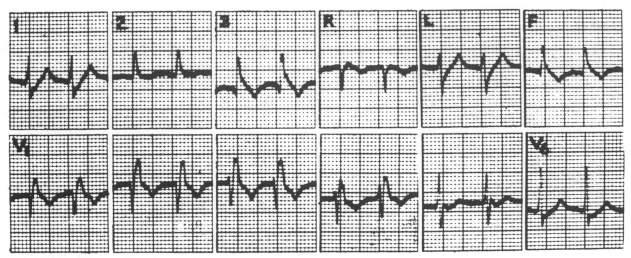

Fig. 17-50. ECG in pulmonary embolism. (Marriott HJL: Practical electrocardiography, p 293. Baltimore, Williams & Wilkins, 1977)

Fig. 17-51. (**A**) Effects of cerebral hemorrhage on the ECG. (**B**) Effects of subdural hematoma on the ECG. (Marriott HJL: Workshop in Electrocardiography, pp 338–339. Oldsmar, FL, Tampa Tracings, 1972)

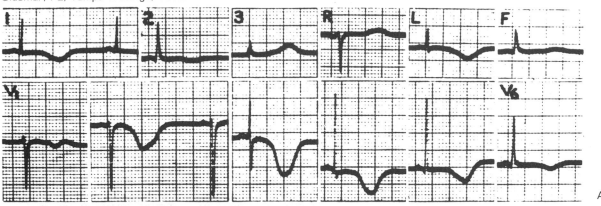

A

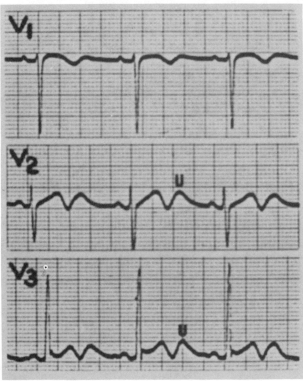

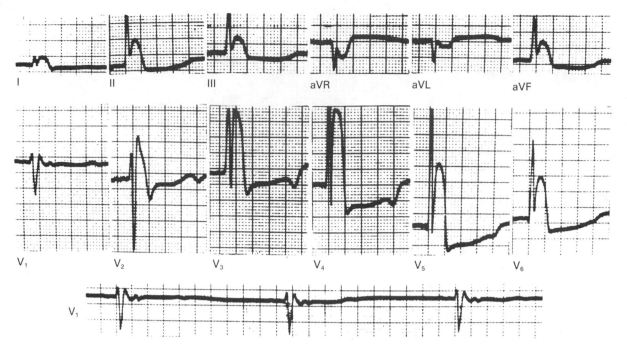

Fig. 17-52. Effects of hypothermia on the ECG. (Marriott HJL: Workshop in Electrocardiography, p 341. Oldsmar, FL, Tampa Tracings, 1972)

Fig. 17-53. Effects of hypothyroidism on the ECG. (Adapted from Bernreiter M: Electrocardiography, p 169. Philadelphia, JB Lippincott, 1963)

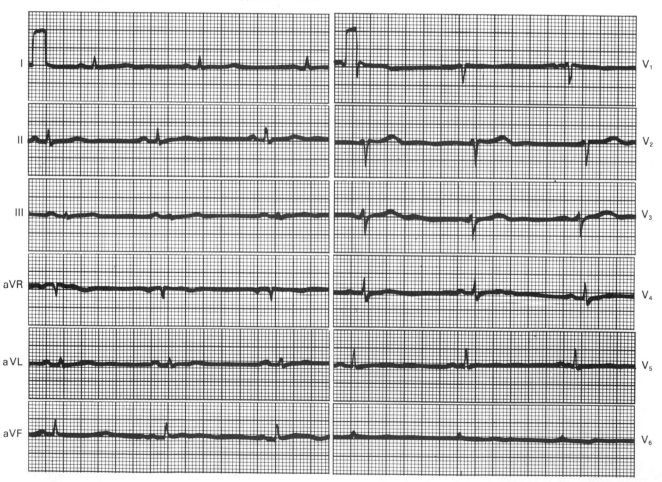

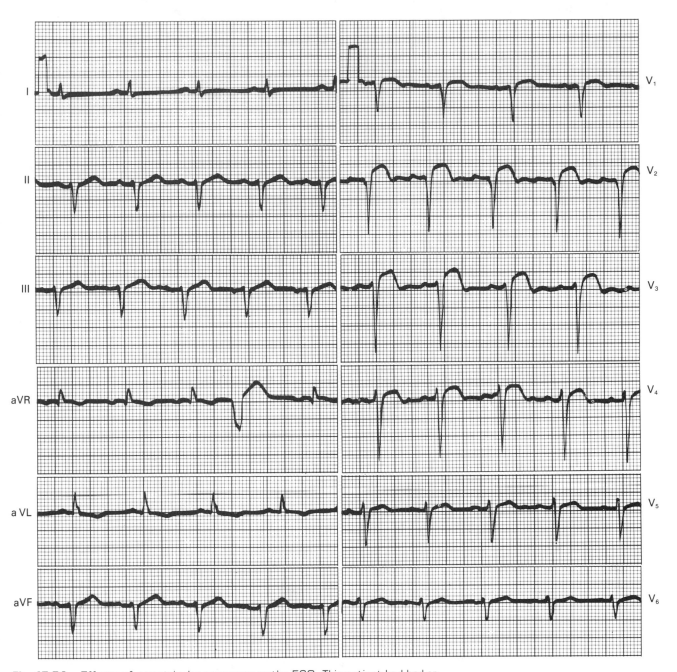

Fig. 17-54. Effects of a ventricular aneurysm on the ECG. This patient had had an anteroseptal MI five years previously. ST-segment elevations, particularly in V_{2-4} had persisted since the acute episode. At the time the tracing was taken the patient had no clinical evidence of infarction. A large ventricular aneurysm involving the anterior wall of the left ventricle was easily demonstrated on fluoroscopic examination. (Adapted from Bernreiter M: Electrocardiography, p 134. Philadelphia, JB Lippincott, 1963)

2. Decreased QRS complex voltage
3. Sinus bradycardia
4. Prolonged P–R interval[34]

Ventricular Aneurysm. Ventricular aneurysm may affect the ECG by elevating the ST segments months or years after MI (Fig. 17-54). This criterion is not precise, and the specificity is limited.

Ventricular Strain. Ventricular strain is determined from ECG by

1. ST-segment depression in lead V_2 (right ventricular strain).
2. ST-segment depression in lead V_5 (left ventricular strain).[18]

Constrictive Disease. Constrictive disease may cause the ECG to have low voltage.

Pleural Effusion. Pleural effusion affects the ECG in the following ways:

1. Low QRS-complex voltage

2. Elevated ST segments
3. Electrical alternans of any of the ECG deflections[33,47]

Arrhythmias

An arrhythmia, any cardiac rhythm that is not normal sinus rhythm at a normal rate, can be determined from the ECG. An arrhythmia may result from altered impulse formation or altered impulse conduction. Discussion of mechanisms of arrhythmias during acute MI can be found in Chapter 26. Before discussing the various types of arrhythmias, I shall outline the characteristics of normal sinus rhythm (Fig. 17-55A):

1. Rate: 60 to 100 beats per minute
2. P waves: precede each QRS complex. The P–R interval is normal (0.12 second to 0.20 second).
3. QRS complex: usually has a normal interval (0.04 second to 0.10 second)
4. Conduction: through the atria, AV node, and ventricles, is usually normal

Arrhythmias Originating in the Sinus Node

Sinus Bradycardia. Sinus bradycardia may be due to vagal stimulation, digitalis intoxication, increased intracranial pressure, or MI involving the SA nodal artery. It is also seen in highly trained athletes, in persons in severe pain, in persons under medication (propranolol, reserpine, methyldopa), in hypoendocrine states (myxedema, Addison's disease, panhypopituitarism), in anorexia nervosa, in hypothermia, and after surgical damage to the SA node.[7]

The following are characteristics of this arrhythmia (Fig. 17-55B):

1. Rate: 40 to 60 beats per minute
2. P waves: Precede each QRS complex. P–R interval usually normal
3. QRS complex: Usually normal
4. Conduction: Usually normal
5. Rhythm: Regular

All aspects of sinus bradycardia should be the same as those of normal sinus rhythm, except for the rate. If slow heart rate is causing significant hemodynamic changes with resultant syncope (insufficient flow of blood to the brain), angina or ectopic arrhythmias, then treatment is directed toward increasing heart rate. If the decrease in heart rate is due to vagal stimulation, attempts should be made to prevent further vagal stimulation. If the patient has digitalis intoxication, then digitalis should be withheld. If atropine does not increase heart rate, then the slow rate is not caused by vagal stimulation.

Sinus Tachycardia. Sinus tachycardia may be caused by fever, acute blood loss, anemia, shock, exercise, congestive heart failure, pain, hypermetabolic states, anxiety, or sympathomimetic or parasympatholytic drugs; it is characterized by the following ECG changes (Fig. 17-55C):

1. Rate: 100 to 180 beats per minute

2. P waves: Precede each QRS complex; may be buried in the preceding T wave; P–R interval usually normal
3. QRS complex: Usually has a normal interval
4. Conduction: Usually normal
5. Rhythm: Regular

All aspects of sinus tachycardia should be the same as those of normal sinus rhythm, except for the rate. Treatment is usually directed at the primary cause. Carotid sinus pressure may be effective in slowing the rate temporarily, and thereby help to rule out other arrhythmias. As heart rate increases, diastolic filling time decreases, resulting in reduced coronary artery filling and in less ventricular diastolic filling (decreased preload).

Sinus Arrhythmia. Sinus arrhythmia is the most frequent heart rhythm and occurs as a normal phenomenon. It commonly occurs in the young or aged, especially with slower heart rates or following enhanced vagal tone from digitalis or morphine. It is absent in the neonate and is commonly found in patients with Cheyne–Stokes respiration. The sinus rate increases with inspiration and decreases with expiration. This arrhythmia is characterized by the following ECG changes (Fig. 17-55D):

1. Rate: 60 to 100 beats per minute
2. P waves: Precede each QRS; PR interval normal
3. QRS complex: Usually normal
4. Conduction: Usually normal
5. Rhythm: May be related to breathing (rate increases with inspiration and decreases with expiration), or, irregularly, may be unrelated to respiration. The irregularity can best be seen by measuring the R–R interval.

Treatment is usually not necessary, but increasing the heart rate with exercise or sympathomimetic drugs will in many cases abolish this arrhythmia.

Sinus Node Arrest. Sinus node arrest can occur from excessive carotid sinus pressure, vagal stimulation, vomiting, straining at stool, involvement of the sinus node or sinus node artery by acute MI, digitalis toxicity, or degenerative forms of fibrosis.

Sinus arrest within normal sinus rhythm has the following characteristics (Fig. 17-55E):

1. Ventricular rate: usually 60 to 100 beats per minute; but frequently in the bradycardia range (fewer than 60 beats per minute)
2. P waves: When P waves are present, the P–R interval is usually normal. If escape beats from the junction or ventricle do occur, the P wave may be absent or inverted before or after the QRS complex
3. QRS complex: Not present during sinus arrest unless escape beat occurs
4. Ventricular conduction: Usually normal when it occurs
5. Rhythm: Irregular. Escape beats from the junctional and ventricular areas are common. The variation will be found by measuring the R–R intervals. The P–P interval will be variable.

Treatment is directed toward normalizing heart rate and eliminating the cause.

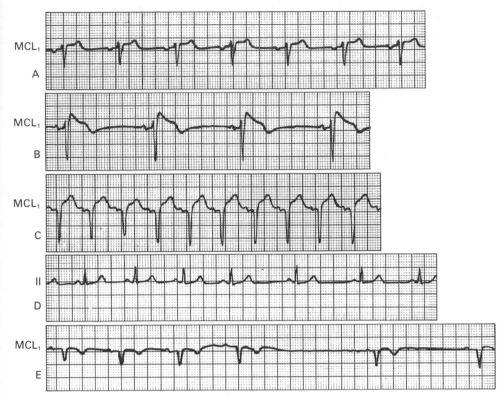

Fig. 17-55. **(A)** Rhythms originating in the sinus node. **(B)** Sinus bradycardia. (Conover M: Cardiac Arrhythmias, p 7. St. Louis, CV Mosby, 1978) **(C)** Sinus tachycardia. **(D)** Sinus arrhythmia. **(E)** Sinus arrest.

Arrhythmias Originating in the Atrial Muscle

Arrhythmias originating in the atrial muscle are these: premature atrial contraction (PAC); wandering atrial pacemaker (WAP); multifocal atrial tachycardia (MAT); paroxysmal atrial tachycardia (PAT); atrial flutter; atrial fibrillation; atrial flutter–fibrillation.

Premature Atrial Contraction (PAC). Premature atrial contractions may be due to atrial muscle irritability caused by caffeine, alcohol, nicotine, stretched atrial myocardium (as in congestive heart failure), stress or anxiety, hypokelemia, atrial ischemia, injury, or infarction, and hypermetabolic states. Premature atrial contractions have these characteristics (Figs. 17-56A, 17-56B, 17-56C):

1. Rate: 60 to 100 beats per minute
2. P waves: Usually have a configuration different from that of the P waves that originate in the SA node. Another site in the atria has become irritable (enhanced automaticity) and fires before the normal firing time of the SA node. P–R interval may vary from the P–R intervals of impulses originating in the SA node.
3. QRS complex: May be normal, aberrant, or absent. If the ventricles have completed their repolarization phase, they can respond to this early stimulus from the atria
4. Conduction: Usually normal
5. Rhythm: Regular, except when the PACs occur. The P wave will be early in the cycle and usually will not have

a complete compensatory pause. (Time between the preceding complex and the following complex is less than the time for two R–R intervals.)

PACs are frequently seen in normal hearts. The patient may say that his heart skipped a beat. A pulse deficit (the difference between apical and radial pulse rate) may exist.

If PACs are infrequent, no treatment is necessary. If they are frequent (more than six per minute) or occur during atrial repolarization, this may herald more serious arrhythmias, such as atrial fibrillation. Again, treatment is directed toward the cause.

Wandering Atrial Pacemaker (WAP). Wandering atrial pacemaker occurs when there is variation in the vagal tone at the SA node or when there are changes in sympathetic stimulation.[38] The patient is usually unaware of the arrhythmia. Wandering atrial pacemaker is characterized by (Fig. 17-56D):

1. Rate: 60 to 100 beats per minute (If the rate is greater than 100, then it is called multifocal atrial tachycardia.)
2. P waves: Will vary from impulse to impulse in size and configuration. Stimulus coming from the SA node or close to it will produce normal-looking P waves. As the pacemaker wanders closer to the AV node, the P waves will become flatter or even inverted. The P–R interval varies, depending on the closeness of the pacemaker to the AV node. At least three different P waves must be seen.
3. QRS complex: Usually normal

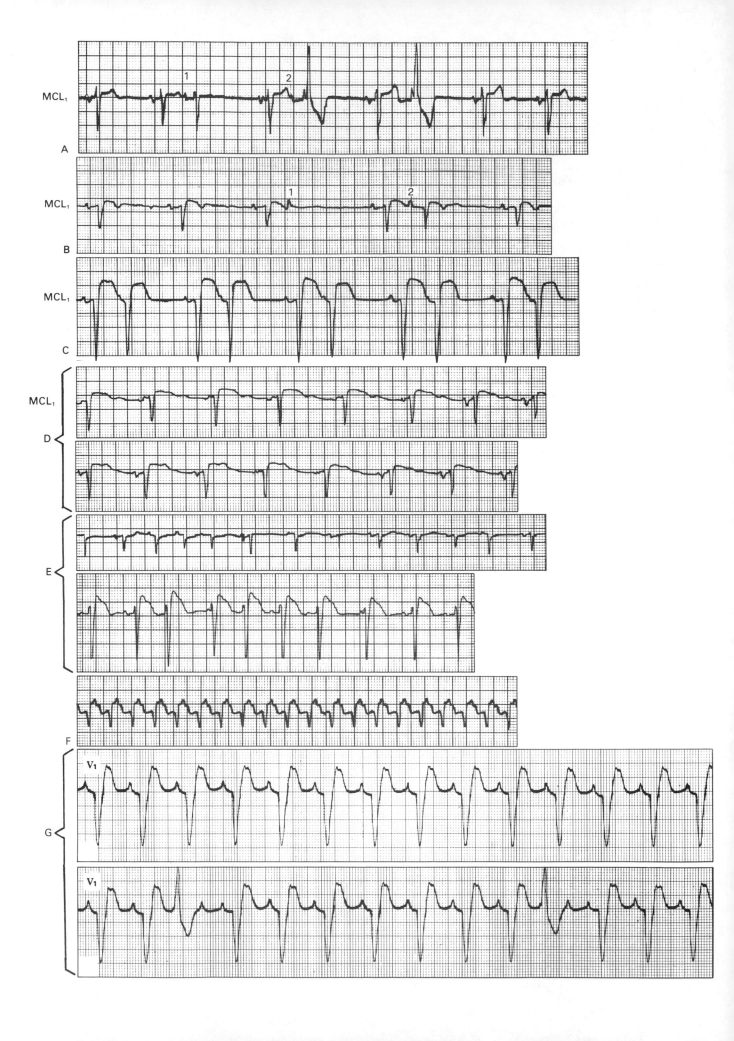

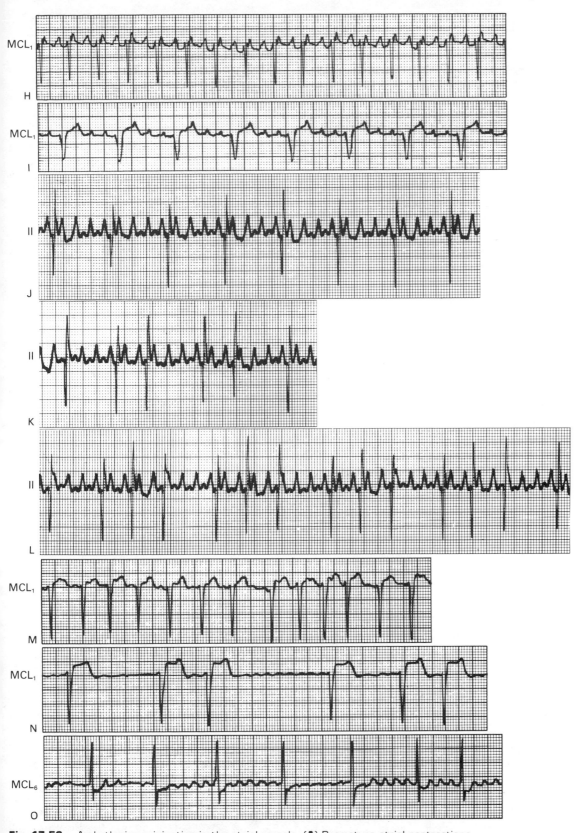

Fig. 17-56. Arrhythmias originating in the atrial muscle. (**A**) Premature atrial contractions. Beat labeled *1* is a PAC with normal ventricular conduction and beat labeled *2* is a PAC with aberrant ventricular conduction. (**B**) Premature atrial contractions. Beat labeled *1* is a PAC without ventricular conduction and beat labeled *2* is a PAC with ventricular conduction. (**C**) Atrial bigeminy. (**D**) Wandering atrial pacemaker (**E**) Multifocal atrial tachycardia (**F**) Paroxysmal atrial tachycardia (**G**) Paroxysmal atrial tachycardia with block. (Mangiola: Self-Assessment in Electrocardiography, p 149. Philadelphia, JB Lippincott 1977) (**H**) Atrial flutter with 2:1 conduction. (**I**) Atrial flutter with 4:1 conduction. (**J**) Atrial flutter with 4:1 conduction. (**K**) Atrial flutter with 3:2 Wenckebach. (**L**) Atrial flutter with 4:3 Wenckebach (**M**) Atrial fibrillation with uncontrolled ventricular response (more than 100 beats/minute). (**N**) Atrial fibrillation with controlled ventricular response (fewer than 100 beats/minute). (**O**) Atrial flutter—fibrillation.

4. Conduction: Conduction from the AV node through the ventricles will usually be normal

5. Rhythm: The R–R intervals may vary because of variations in the P–R intervals

There usually is no need for treatment. Observe for digitalis intoxication. If decreases in heart rate significantly alter cardiac output, then sympathomimetic or parasympatholytic drugs can be used.

Multifocal Atrial Tachycardia (MAT). Multifocal atrial tachycardia is most commonly associated with severe pulmonary disease. Multifocal atrial tachycardia is characterized by (Fig. 17-56E):

1. Rate: More than 100 beats per minute
2. P waves: Impulse may be anywhere from the SA node to the AV node. At least three different P waves are seen. The atrial rate is irregular.
3. QRS complex: Usually normal
4. Conduction: Conduction from the AV node through the ventricles will usually be normal
5. Rhythm: The R–R intervals may vary because of variations in the P–R intervals.

Treatment is directed toward eliminating the cause and decreasing heart rate with a drug such as propranolol.

Paroxysmal Atrial Tachycardia (PAT). Paroxysmal atrial tachycardia is characterized by abrupt onset and abrupt cessation. Rhythm may be triggered by emotions, tobacco, caffeine, fatigue, sympathomimetic drugs or alcohol. Paroxysmal atrial tachycardia is not usually associated with organic heart disease. The rapid rate may produce angina, due to decreased coronary artery filling. Cardiac output is reduced and congestive heart failure may occur. The patient frequently does not tolerate this rhythm for long periods.

Paroxysmal atrial tachycardia is characterized by (Fig. 17-56F):

1. Rate: 150 to 250 beats per minute
2. P waves: Ectopic and slightly to grossly normal. May be found in the preceding T wave. P–R interval shortened (less than 0.12 second)
3. QRS complex: Usually normal, but may be distorted if aberrant conduction is present
4. Conduction: Usually normal
5. Rhythm: Regular

The patient may not be aware of paroxysmal atrial tachycardia. Treatment is directed toward eliminating the cause and decreasing the heart rate. Morphine sedation slows the rate without further treatment. Carotid sinus pressure usually slows the rate or stops the attack, and is usually more effective after digitalis or pressors. The use of vasopressors has a reflex effect on the carotid sinus by elevating the blood pressure and thus slowing the heart rate. Short-acting digitalis preparations may be used. Propranolol may be tried if digitalis is unsuccessful. Quinidine may be effective. Cardioversion may be necessary if the patient does not tolerate the fast heart rate.

Paroxysmal Atrial Tachycardia (PAT) with Block. This arrhythmia can also occur because of the digitalis intoxi-

cation or because the bundle branches cannot repolarize in time to conduct the next impulse through the ventricles.

PAT with block is characterized by

1. Rate: Atrial rate 150 to 250 beats per minute
2. P waves: Usually can be seen preceding each QRS complex; however, when block occurs, there are P waves that are not conducted. The P waves may be buried in the preceding T wave. since the focus point is ectopic, the P waves have a configuration different from those originating in the SA node and are frequently smaller.
3. QRS complex: Normal configuration and interval
4. Conduction: Many of the ectopic impulses from the atria are blocked in the AV node, and those that are conducted through the AV node have normal conduction through the ventricles.
5. Rhythm: Irregular. A QRS complex does not follow each P wave because the atrial rate frequently is too fast. When a block does exist, it is usually varying from 2:1 (Fig. 17-56G) to 3:1, causing the ventricular rate to be irregular.

Treatment is directed toward ruling out digitalis intoxication and reducing the irritability of the atrial myocardium. Stimulation of the vagus nerve by carotid sinus massage may slow or terminate the arrhythmia.

Atrial Flutter. Atrial flutter is usually associated with rheumatic heart disease, atherosclerotic heart disease, thyrotoxicosis, acute cor pulmonale, congestive heart failure, and MI. Any ventricular response of 150 should be suspect for atrial flutter.

Atrial flutter is characterized by

1. Rate: Atrial rate 250 to 350 beats per minute; most commonly 300. The ventricular rate will usually show some degree of block with the ventricle responding in a 2:1 (Fig. 17-56H) or 4:1 (Figs. 17-56I, 17-56J) pattern (rarely 3:1). There may be variations in the block pattern, particularly if treatment has been started.
2. P waves: Characterized by the F waves (flutter waves seen between R waves) occurring in a regular fashion and in a saw-tooth or picket-fence pattern. One F wave usually falls within the QRS–T complex. The inverted F wave is followed by the upright portion of the F wave, which represents the atrial T wave.[38]
3. QRS complex: Usually normal, except where aberrant conduction is present
4. Conduction: Usually normal
5. Rhythm: Usually regular, but irregularities in the block pattern are not uncommon

Wenckebach's periods are common in atrial flutter. With alternating 4:1 and 2:1 conduction, one might expect 3:2 Wenckebach. In 3:2 Wenckebach, every third F wave that is conducted in 2:1 conduction pattern is blocked, and the F–R interval progressively lengthens (Fig. 17-56K, 17-56L).

Treatment is directed toward eliminating the cause, decreasing the rate of ventricular response, and decreasing atrial myocardial irritability. If quinidine is administered, 1:1 conduction could occur unless a negative dromotropic effect is present. Carotid sinus massage may unmask the flutter waves and increase the flutter rate. Cardioversion can usually be achieved with low-DC shock (10–50 joules, or watt-seconds.)

Atrial Fibrillation. Atrial fibrillation is usually associated with atherosclerotic heart disease, rheumatic heart disease, congestive heart failure, thyrotoxicosis, cor pulmonale, and congenital heart disease.

Atrial fibrillation (Figs. 17-56M, 17-56N) is characterized by

1. Rate: An atrial rate of 350 to 600 beats per minute. Ventricular response is usually 120 to 200.
2. P waves: No discernable P waves. Irregular undulation termed fibrillatory or "f" waves are seen; P–R interval cannot be measured.
3. QRS complex: Usually normal
4. Conduction: Usually normal through the ventricles. Characterized by an irregular ventricular response, because the AV node is incapable of responding to the rapid atrial rate. Impulses that are transmitted cause the ventricles to respond irregularly.
5. Rhythm: Irregular and usually rapid, unless controlled. Irregularity of rhythm is due to concealed conduction within the AV node.

A rapid ventricular response reduces the time for ventricular filling and hence the stroke volume. The atrial kick, which is 25% to 30% of the cardiac output, is also lost. Congestive heart failure frequently follows. Coarse atrial fibrillation (slower atrial rate) is more easily converted than fine atrial fibrillation (faster atrial rate). There is usually a pulse deficit.

Treatment is directed toward eliminating the cause, decreasing the atrial irritability and decreasing the rate of the ventricular response. In patients with chronic atrial fibrillation, anticoagulant therapy may be used to prevent thromboemboli from forming in the atria.

Sometimes a mixture of atrial flutter and atrial fibrillation is seen, and some call this atrial flutter–fibrillation (Fig. 17-56O).[33] Some refer to this as coarse atrial fibrillation. Such an arrhythmia is best classified as atrial fibrillation when the criteria for atrial flutter are not satisfied.[48]

Tachycardia–Bradycardia Syndrome

This syndrome is characterized by tachyarrhythmias (paroxysmal atrial fibrillation, flutter, or tachycardia) followed by SA block or sinus arrest, resulting in Stokes–Adams attacks. Clinical correlation with this syndrome has been found with coronary atherosclerosis, amyloidosis, renal insufficiency with azotemia, and trauma following open-heart surgery. Some have used the tachycardia–bradycardia syndrome and sick sinus syndrome interchangeably, but this is not totally accurate, because the sick sinus syndrome includes a variety of sinus and atrial arrhythmias and only indicates a "sick" sinus node. In tachycardia–bradycardia syndrome, not only is the sinus node sick, but the impulse formation at the AV node is depressed as well.[27]

Marked bradycardia (heart rate of fewer than 20 beats per minute or prolonged asystole, exceeding 10 seconds) results in cerebral ischemia. Hence lightheadedness, dizziness, syncope, or convulsions may occur. The tachycardia may cause such symptoms as palpitations, weakness, or chest pain.[27] Treatment is directed toward suppressing the tachycardia with medications (quinidine, procainamide, digitalis, and propranolol) and maintaining an adequate heart rate with a pacemaker.

Arrhythmias Originating in the Junction

Arrhythmias originating in the junction (area between the atria and ventricles around the AV node) are these: junctional rhythm, premature junctional contraction, accelerated junctional tachycardia, and paroxysmal junctional tachycardia.

Junctional Rhythm. A junctional rhythm may occur if there is digitalis intoxication or sinus node disease resulting in a decreased rate of the sinus node. Because the rate is so slow, other irritable sites may compete to be the pacemaker. Junctional rhythm (Fig. 17-57A) has the following characteristics:

1. Rate: 40 to 60 beats per minute
2. P waves: They are usually inverted and may occur before, during, or after the QRS complex, depending on the location of the pacemaker in the junctional tissue. The junctional tissue delays antegrade and retrograde conduction.
3. QRS complex: Normal
4. Conduction: The atria are usually stimulated by the junctional tissue, resulting in an inverted P wave (called retrograde conduction). The conduction from the junctional tissue through the ventricles is usually normal (called antegrade conduction).
5. Rhythm: Usually regular

Retrograde conduction to the atria can be impaired in first-degree retrograde block; the R–P interval (from the beginning of the R wave to the beginning of the P wave) is longer than 0.2 second. In second-degree retrograde block, the R–P interval progressively lengthens, and a ventricular ectopic impulse occurs. The R–P interval progressively shortens until a pause occurs. There is group beating, and beats which initiate each group are equidistant from one another.[7] Or, complete atrioventricular dissociation can occur. The pacemaker within the junctional tissue can wander from subjunctional to junctional. There is usually no need for treatment, unless reduction in heart rate markedly alters cardiac output. If cardiac output decreases so that chest pain syncope or arrhythmias occur, then sympathomimetic or parasympatholytic drugs may be used. Digitalis should be withheld. Quinidine, procainamide, diphenylhydantoin, propranolol, hyperkalemia, and vagal stimulation depress junctional escape centers.

Premature Junctional Contraction (PJC). Premature junctional contractions occur because of increased irritability of the junctional tissue. Irritability can be due to digitalis intoxication or to coronary artery disease, resulting in decreased flow through the AV nodal artery. Premature junctional contractions (Fig. 17-57B) have the following characteristics:

1. Rate: 60 to 100 beats per minute if the basic rhythm is normal sinus rhythm

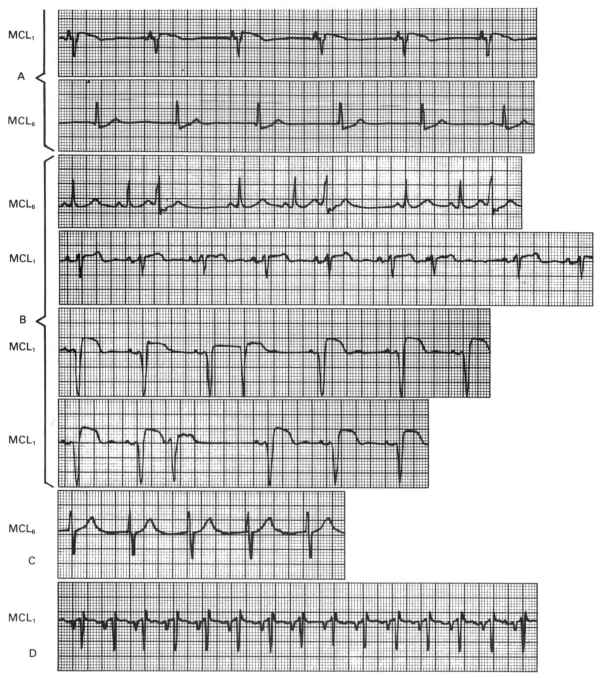

Fig. 17-57. Arrhythmias originating in the junctional area. **(A)** Junctional rhythm. **(B)** Premature junctional contraction. **(C)** Accelerated junctional rhythm. **(D)** Junctional tachycardia.

2. P waves: May occur before, during, or after the QRS complex, depending on the location of the pacemaker in the junctional tissue. The P–R intervals vary and are shorter than normal (less than 0.12 seconds).

3. QRS complex: May be normal or aberrant

4. Conduction: The atria are stimulated in a retrograde fashion. The ventricular conduction is usually normal.

5. Rhythm: Regular, except for the premature contraction. The compensatory pause is usually incomplete.

Usually no treatment is indicated. Digitalis should be withheld. If PJCs occur more frequently than six per minute, an antiarrhythmic drug may be prescribed.

Accelerated Junctional Rhythm and Paroxysmal Junctional Tachycardia. In these rhythms, irritability in the junctional area has increased, resulting in a faster rate. Characteristics of accelerated junctional rhythm (Fig. 17-57C) and paroxysmal junctional tachycardia (Fig. 17-57D) are as follows:

1. Origin: Junctional tissue

2. Rate: Accelerated junctional rhythm, 60 to 100 beats per minute; Paroxysmal junctional tachycardia, 100 to 250 beats per minute

3. P waves: The position of the P wave in relation to the QRS complex will vary according to the location of the pacemaker in the junctional tissue. The configuration of the P wave will also vary accordingly. If the P wave is seen, it is usually inverted.

4. QRS complex: May be normal or aberrant

5. Conduction: Retrograde to the atria. Normal through the ventricles

6. Rhythm: Regular

If the patient is on digitalis, it should be withheld until digitalis intoxication is ruled out, since this is a very common arrhythmia associated with digitalis intoxication. If the patient is not on digitalis, it may be given to increase AV conduction time. If the patient does not tolerate the rate, as demonstrated by signs and symptoms of a decreased cardiac output, then cardioversion may be necessary. This arrhythmia must be documented on the ECG to differentiate from sinus tachycardia or paroxysmal atrial tachycardia. When a rapid junctional rhythm occurs with a bundle branch conduction defect, it is difficult to distinguish this rhythm from ventricular tachycardia (Chap. 26).

Arrhythmias Originating in the Ventricular Muscle

Arrhythmias originating in the ventricular muscle are these: premature ventricular contractions, ventricular bigeminy, accelerated ventricular tachycardia, ventricular tachycardia, ventricular flutter, ventricular fibrillation, ventricular asystole.

Premature Ventricular Contractions (PVCs). Premature ventricular contractions are the result of increased automaticity of the ventricular muscle cells. Premature ventricular contractions can be due to digitalis intoxication, hypoxia, myocardial stretch, hypokalemia, fever, acidosis, exercise, or increased circulating catecholamines (Chap. 26).

Infrequent PVCs are not serious in themselves. Usually the patient feels a palpitating sensation, but has no other complaints. However, the concern lies in that these premature contractions may lead to more serious ventricular arrhythmias.

Premature ventricular contractions are considered serious precursors of ventricular tachycardia and ventricular fibrillation when they

1. Occur in increasing number, more than six per minute

2. Are multifocal (Fig. 17-58A)

3. Occur in pairs of triplets (Fig. 17-58B)

4. Come on the T wave (R-on-T)

Premature ventricular contractions (PVCs) have the following characteristics:

1. Rate: 60 to 100 beats per minute

2. P wave: May be completely obscured, hidden in the QRS complex of the premature beat. The sinus rhythm is usually uninterrupted, resulting in a complete compensatory pause. If a premature P wave is seen before the

wide QRS complex, the impulse is probably a premature supraventricular beat with aberration and not a PVC. If a P wave is seen before the wide QRS complex and is not premature, the impulse is probably a fusion beat (Fig. 17-58C).

3. QRS complex: Usually wide and bizarre. Usually longer than 0.10 second in duration. May have the same focus in the ventricle, or may have a wide variety of configurations if occurring from multiple foci in the ventricles. If unifocal, then these extrasystoles have fixed coupling.

4. Conduction: Occasionally retrograde through the junctional tissue and atria

5. Rhythm: Irregular when the premature beat occurs

In order to decrease the myocardial irritability, the cause must be determined and, if possible, corrected. An antiarrhythmic drug may be useful for immediate and possibly long-term therapy.

Ventricular Bigeminy. Ventricular bigeminy is frequently associated with digitalis excess, coronary artery disease, acute MI, and heart failure. The term bigeminy refers to a condition in which every other beat is premature (Fig. 17-58D).

Ventricular bigeminy has the following characteristics:

1. Rate: May occur at any heart rate; but rate is usually less than 90 beats per minute

2. P waves: The same as described for premature ventricular contractions; they may be hidden within the QRS complex

3. QRS complex: Every other beat is a PVC with a wide, bizarre QRS complex and a complete compensatory pause.

4. Conduction: The sinus beats are conducted from the sinus node in a normal fashion, but alternating PVCs start in the ventricles and may have retrograde conduction through the junctional tissue and atria.

5. Rhythm: Regularly irregular

If the ectopic beats or normal beat occur every third beat, this is termed trigeminy (Fig. 17-58E); every fourth beat, quadrigeminy. A long postectopic interval encourages self-perpetuation of the bigeminy (the rule of bigeminy).[7]

The treatment for ventricular bigeminy is the same as for premature ventricular contractions. Since the underlying cause of ventricular bigeminy is frequently digitalis toxicity, this should be ruled out or treated if present.

Ventricular Parasystole. Ventricular parasystole is an ectopic rhythm with a slower rate than that of the SA node. The parasystolic focus is protected and not inhibited by a faster pacemaker. The sinus rhythm and the parasystolic rhythm occur together. The parasystolic focus may also be found in the atrial or junctional tissue termed atrial parasystole or junctional parasystole.

Ventricular parasystole (Fig. 17-58F) has the following characteristics:

1. Rate: May occur at any heart rate

2. P waves: The normal sinus rhythm P waves are normal; the P waves of the parasystolic impulse are usually hidden within the QRS complex, but may occur in front

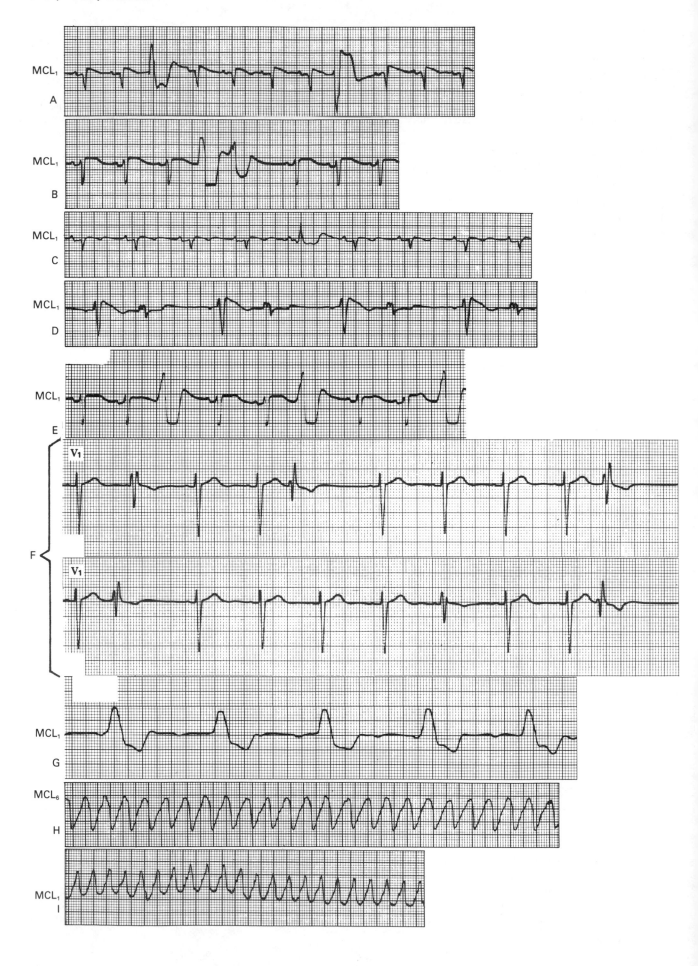

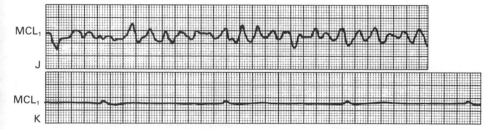

Fig. 17-58. Arrhythmias originating in the ventricle. **(A)** Premature ventricular contractions. Beat labeled *1* shows a left ventricular PVC; beat labeled *2* shows a right ventricular PVC. **(B)** Two left ventricular multifocal PVCs in a row. **(C)** Fusion beats. **(D)** Ventricular bigeminy. **(E)** Ventricular trigeminy. **(F)** Ventricular parasystole (Mangiola S: Self-Assessment in Electrocardiography, p 159. Philadelphia, JB Lippincott, 1977) **(G)** Accelerated ventricular rhythm. **(H)** Ventricular tachycardia. **(I)** Ventricular flutter. **(J)** Ventricular fibrillation. **(K)** Ventricular asystole.

of a fusion beat or after the QRS complex if retrograde conduction occurs

3. QRS complex: The parasystolic QRS complex can be wide and bizarre, or possibly small and narrow if it fuses with a normal sinus QRS complex

4. Conduction: The parasystolic impulse is conducted in a retrograde fashion. It may conduct at the same time as a sinus impulse, resulting in a fusion beat.

5. Rhythm: Regular until the parasystolic impulse interrupts the rhythm, resulting in an irregular rhythm

Parasystole is characterized by varying coupling intervals (the interval between normal beat and ectopic beat), fusion beats, and an ectopic interval that is an exact multiple of the ectopic rate. The parasystolic impulse will not always be seen because the ventricles are receiving stimuli from the sinus node and may be refractory to the ectopic impulse.

Accelerated Ventricular Rhythm and Ventricular Tachycardia. These arrhythmias are caused by increased myocardial irritability, as are premature ventricular contractions. They are usually associated with coronary artery disease, atherosclerotic heart disease, heart disease, and rheumatic heart disease, and may precede ventricular fibrillation. Ventricular tachycardia is extremely dangerous and should be considered an emergency. The patient is generally aware of this rapid rhythm and is quite anxious. Accelerated ventricular rhythm and ventricular tachycardia have the following characteristics:

1. Rate: Accelerated ventricular rhythm 40 to 110 beats per minute (Fig. 17-58G). Ventricular tachycardia 150 to 200 beats per minute (Fig. 17-58H)

2. P waves: Usually buried in the QRS complex; if seen, they do not necessarily fall in the normal pattern with the QRS. The ventricular contractions are disassociated from the atrial contractions. If the atrial beat should capture the ventricle for one beat, a capture beat (Dressler beat) results.

3. QRS complex: Have the same configurations as do those of a premature ventricular contraction: wide and bizarre, with T waves in the opposite direction. A ventricular beat may fuse with a normal QRS, resulting in a fusion beat. Three or more PVCs in a row constitute ventricular tachycardia

4. Conduction: Originates in the ventricle, with possible retrograde conduction to the junctional tissue and atria

5. Rhythm: Usually regular, but irregular ventricular tachycardias are also seen. The ventricular rhythm is rapid. The P waves, if seen, are at a slower rate and are regular. There is no association between the atrial rhythm and the ventricular rhythm (AV dissociation).

The patient's tolerance or lack of tolerance of this rapid rhythm will dictate the therapy to be given. Cardioversion may be indicated if the reduction in cardiac output is marked. Antiarrhythmic drugs may be used. The cause of the myocardial irritability must be determined and corrected, if possible.

Ventricular Flutter. Ventricular flutter has all the characteristics of ventricular tachycardia, but the rate is even faster. The clinical picture is exactly the same as ventricular standstill: the patient may be cyanotic and convulsing; there is no audible heart beat; no palpable pulse; and the patient is not breathing. This arrhythmia is usually fatal without immediate treatment.

Ventricular flutter (Fig. 17-58I) has the following characteristics:

1. Rate: 200 to 400 beats per minute

2. P waves: No visible P waves are seen

3. QRS complex: Rapid, bizarre, picket-fence-like complexes. T waves are not visible.

4. Conduction: originates in ventricles. There may be retrograde conduction through the AV node and atria.

5. Rhythm: Not precisely regular

The treatment for ventricular flutter is similar to that for ventricular tachycardia. However, ventricular flutter is a far more acute emergency, because the patient is without circulation or respiration. This arrhythmia will be fatal unless converted immediately; therefore no initial attempts are made to convert this arrhythmia with drugs. Precordial shock is the first action to be taken and, in the absence of a physician, should be given immediately by the nursing staff. If a defibrillator is not readily available, external cardiac massage, assisted ventilation, and intravenous supportive drugs should be initiated at once. If the nurse present is having trouble discerning if the arrhythmia is ventricular tachycardia or ventricular flutter, her main concern should be the patient's tolerance of the arrhythmia, and she should treat the arrhythmia as the patient's tolerance indicates.

Ventricular Fibrillation. Ventricular fibrillation is a rapid, ineffective quivering of the ventricles. With this arrhythmia, there is no audible heart beat, no palpable pulse, and no respirations. This pattern is so grossly irregular it can hardly be mistaken for another type of arrhythmia. Malfunction of the monitor may produce such a pattern, but in that case, the clinical picture of the patient would rule out the diagnosis of ventricular fibrillation. Ventricular fibrillation is usually fatal without immediate treatment, since only 5% convert spontaneously.

Ventricular fibrillation (Fig. 17-58J) has the following characteristics:

1. Rate: Rapid, uncoordinated, ineffective
2. P waves: Not seen
3. QRS complex: Rapid, irregular undulation without specific pattern (multifocal). The ventricles have only a quivering motion.
4. Conduction: Foci are located in the ventricles, but so many foci are firing at one time that there is no organized conduction: no ventricular contractions occur.
5. Rhythm: Extremely irregular and uncoordinated, without specific pattern

Immediate treatment is defibrillation with 400 watt-seconds. A synchronized machine will not fire on this disorganized rhythm because there are no predominant waves it can recognize. If defibrillation has been unsuccessful, cardiopulmonary resuscitation should be started immediately. Epinephrine and sodium bicarbonate may be used if the fibrillation is fine. Epinephrine may make the fibrillation coarser and thus easier to convert with defibrillation. Blood pressure should be supported, using vasopressors. At no time during the resuscitation should the external cardiac massage and the assisted ventilation be stopped for longer than 5 seconds. Defibrillation and cardiopulmonary resuscitation are discussed in detail in Chapter 26.

Ventricular Asystole. In ventricular asystole there are no QRS complexes. There is no heart beat, no palpable pulse, and no respiration. Ventricular asystole is fatal without immediate treatment. Ventricular asystole (Fig. 17-58K) has the following characteristics:

1. Rate: None
2. P waves: May see them, but they do not conduct through the AV node and ventricles
3. QRS complex: None
4. Conduction: Possibly, through the atria only
5. Rhythm: None

Cardiopulmonary resuscitation is necessary to keep the patient alive. Epinephrine should be administered and repeated at 5-minute intervals. Sodium bicarbonate should be given. These two drugs are not compatible and may not be mixed together. Insertion of a transthoracic or transvenous pacemaker may be necessary.

Analysis of the ECG is complex. A suggested approach to ECG interpretation can be found in Table 17-5.

TABLE 17-5 APPROACH TO ECG INTERPRETATION

1. Determine if the ECG is technically good.
2. Determine the heart rate (atrial and ventricular).
3. Determine the following intervals: PR, QRS, Q-T$_c$.
4. Determine the heart rhythm.
5. Determine the frontal plan axis of the P wave, QRS complex and T wave.
6. Determine from all leads, abnormalities of P wave, PR segment and interval, QRS complex, ST segment, and T wave.
7. Determine the presence of atrial and ventricular hypertrophy, intraventricular conduction defects, myocardial ischemia and infarction, ventricular aneurysm, pericarditis, pericardial effusion, myocarditis, drug effects, and electrolyte abnormalities.

VECTORCARDIOGRAM

The vectorcardiogram (VCG) differs from the ECG in that the net effect of depolarization of the heart is displayed in two-dimensional vector loops with each depolarization of the heart. Loops P, QRS, and T are recorded (Fig. 17-59).

The VCG instrument is an electronic X–Y plotter and it simultaneously plots voltage in two planes at right angles to each other. The electrodes are placed on the body surfaces and the current they pick up leads through amplifiers to a cathode-ray tube (CRT). The CRT discharges an electron beam which passes through a pair of horizontal and vertical plates to a phosphor screen. The loop produced on the CRT screen consists of teardrop dots 2 milliseconds apart. The blunt end of the teardrop is the leading edge.

This loop can be projected on three reference planes: frontal, horizontal, and sagittal (Frank orthogonal X, Y, Z system). The frontal plane is a plot of the X axis (left to right) against the Y axis (head to foot). The horizontal plane consists of a plot of the Z axis (back to front) against the X axis. The sagittal plane consists of a plot of the Y axis against the Z axis (Fig. 17-59).

1. Frontal–X axis against Y axis
2. Horizontal–Z axis against X axis
3. Sagittal–Y axis against Z axis

Seven electrodes are placed in positions on the body surface as described in Table 17-6 (also see Fig. 17-60):

These three loop projections are recorded on photographic film, and from them the three dimensional loop is displayed on a CRT screen. Magnitude as well as direction can be determined with computer aid.

The P loop passes downward, then to the left, and then slightly toward the front. The T loop usually passes slightly toward the front, then downward and to the right of the QRS loop by 0 to 40 degrees.[23]

The QRS loop passes to the left, then downward, and then toward the back. In the frontal plane, the initial deflection is to the right and occasionally upward, then downward and to the left in the 0 to 85 degree range in a clockwise or counterclockwise direction. In the horizontal plane, the initial deflection is toward the front and to the right, then to the left and toward the back in a counterclockwise direction. In the sagittal plane, the initial deflection is

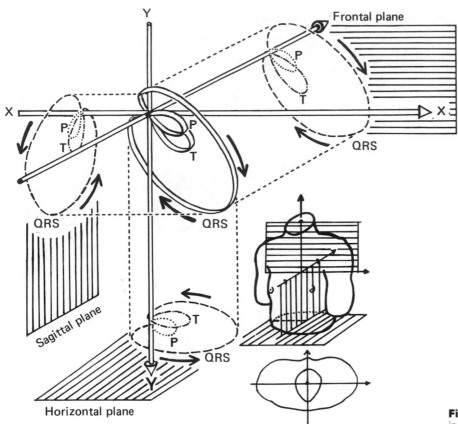

Fig. 17-59. Vectorcardiographic loop in three reference planes.

toward the front and occasionally upward, then downward and toward the back in a clockwise direction.

POLARCARDIOGRAM

A polarcardiogram (PCG) is a continuous recording of spherical polar coordinates of the heart vectors plotted against time.[12] The PCG consists of the spatial magnitude, three planar magnitudes, three longitudinal angles, and three latitude angles.[13] Vectorcardiograms (VCGs) are continuous recordings of the same vector magnitudes and angles, except for the three latitude angles. Furthermore, VCGs differ in that they are not plotted against time. The

Fig. 17-60. Three reference planes of the VCG.

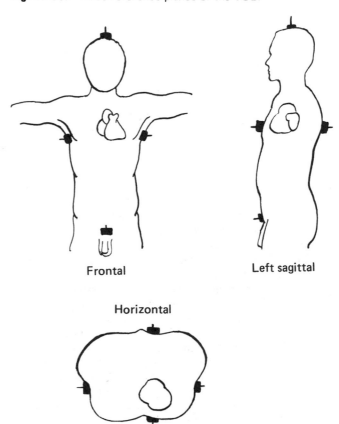

TABLE 17-6 POSITIONS OF ELECTRODES IN VECTORCARDIOGRAM

Direction	Positive Electrode	Negative Electrode
X Axis (left-right)	Left anterior axillary line (A)	Right anterior axillary line (I)
Y Axis (foot-head)	Left ankle (F)	Forehead or neck (H)
Z Axis (front-back)	Posterior chest—immediately behind E (M)	Half-way between center of the sternum, fourth intercostal space if patient is supine; fifth intercostal space if patient is sitting (E)

(From Goldman, MJ: Principles of Electrocardiography, 10th ed. California, Lange Medical Publications, 1979)

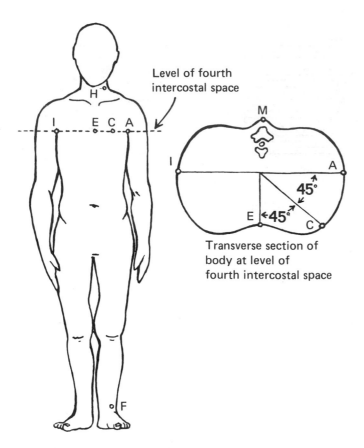

Fig. 17-61. Electrode position for the VCG. (Goldman MT: Principles of Electrocardiography, p 313. Los Altos, Lange Medical Publications, 1979)

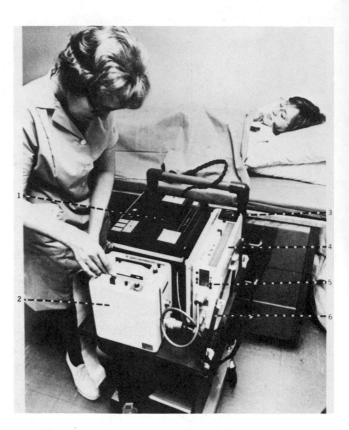

Fig. 17-62. Bedside polarcardiograph equipment. Data acquisition equipment used to record the xyz signals on magnetic tape. The signals are amplified in a patient-interface electronics unit (**4**), monitored on a cathode ray tube (**3**), and pass to a tape recorder (**1**) or to an ECG display unit (**2**) which derives the 12-lead ECG. The ECG display unit may also receive xyz signals recorded on tape. A useful feature of the system is a built-in calibrator with colored pin jacks (**5**) into which the patient cable may be plugged to provide an overall test. Also shown in the picture is a protractor (**6**) for determining electrode position. (Dower GE, Bruce RA: Prog Cardiovasc Dis 19(1):69, 1976)

conventional (scalar) electrocardiograms are representations of vectors in one plane plotted against time.[12,13]

In practice, the Frank lead system or some modification of it is used. For lead placement refer to Figure 17-61.[11] A chest protractor is used to locate the electrode position accurately, so that the adequacy of positioning the "C" electrode near the apex of the heart at 45° to the anterior and left electrodes is obtained. The three simultaneous inputs to the PCG are the x, y, and z signals used in vector cardiography.[12,14] These signals represent the coordinates of the heart vector and can be monitored beat by beat on a cathode ray oscilloscope, just as vector loops in frontal, transverse, and sagittal planes display the interaction of two of these signals at a time. The polarcardiograph transforms them into the corresponding polar coordinates: longitude, latitude, and magnitude.

Instead of a cathode ray oscilloscope, recordings are more recently made on a magnetic tape at the bedside and replayed into a minicomputer. This has several advantages. The bedside equipment is greatly simplified and permanent electrical records of the signals are available for transcription into derived 12-lead ECG and VCG tracings, in addition to the PCG. This system also lends itself well to analysis by a digital computer for various measurement programs (Fig. 17-62). The 12-lead ECGs are derived from x, y, and z signals; they do not exactly match the conventional record-

ing, although the resemblance is close enough for diagnostic purposes.[11,16,17] An advantage of the derived ECG is that ambiguities in rhythm or in ST-segment displacement can sometimes be clarified by deriving the same beats in each of the 12 leads simultaneously and studying them.[10]

Polarcardiography is now established as a clinically applicable and technically feasible method for obtaining ECG information primarily for research purposes. The transformed coordinates do not generate new information, but can bring out relationships not previously suspected, thus making available additional information not previously used.[14] They also provide a unique opportunity for three-dimensional vector orientation with complete time-scale preservation. The latter feature is an advantage over VCG. PCG's are not intended to replace the ECG, but to provide an additional useful display of dynamic changes of the heart vectors.[16,17] It is particularly helpful in the detection and location of an MI[6,8,14,16,30] and the detection of exercise-induced ischemia[5,14,15,39]; it also offers potential for quantification of the size of left ventricular infarction.[8]

REFERENCES

1. Alverez-Mena SC, Martin JF: Phenothiazine induced T wave abnormalities." JAMA 224:1730–1733, 1973
2. Arbelt S: Differential Diagnosis of the Electrocardiogram, 2nd ed. Philadelphia, FA Davis, 1975
3. Bernreiter M: Electrocardiography. Philadelphia, JB Lippincott, 1963
4. Bishop L: The wave of depolarization. A Programmed Course in Electrocardiography, p2. New York, Basic Systems Inc.
5. Bruce RA, Detry JM, Early K et al: Polarcardiographic responses to maximal exercise in healthy young adults. Am Heart J 83:206–218, 1972
6. Bruce RA, Yeon-Bing L, Yun-Lee P et al: Polarcardiographic criteria for myocardial infarction in chinese men. J Electrocardiol 9:309–313, 1976
7. Childers R: Classification of cardiac dysrhythmias. Med Clin North Am 60:3–48, 1976
7a. Conover MH: *Cardiac Arrhythmias*. St. Louis, CV Mosby Co, 1978
8. Cowan MJ: Quantification of myocardial infarction size by vectorcardiogram. Doctoral Dissertation, University of Washington, Seattle, 1979
9. Dhingra, R, Amat-y-Leon, Pouget JM et al: Infranodal block. Med Clin North Am 60:175–192, 1976
10. Dower GE: An arrhythmia clarified by polarcardiography. J Electrocardiol 3(3–4):231–238, 1970
11. Dower GE: A lead synthesizer for the frank system to stimulate the standard 12-lead electrocardiogram. J Electrocardiol 1(1):101–116, 1968
12. Dower GE: Polarcardiography. Springfield, Charles C Thomas, 1971
13. Dower GE: Terminology and standardization in vectorcardiography. J Electrocardiol 7(3):259–264, 1974
14. Dower GE, Bruce RA: Progress in polarcardiography. Prog Cardiovasc Dis 19(1):69–90, 1976
15. Dower GE, Bruce RA, Pool J et al: Ischemic polarcardiographic changes induced by exercise. Circulation 48:725–734, 1973
16. Dower GE, Horn HE, Ziegler WG: The polarcardiographic diagnosis of myocardial infarction. Am Heart J 69:369–381, 1965
17. Dower GE, Horn HE, Ziegler WG: The polarcardiography. Terminology and normal findings. Am Heart J 69:355–368, 1965
18. Dubin Dale: Rapid Interpretation of EKG's. Tampa, Cover Publishing Company, 1975
19. Durrer D, Schuilenburg RM, Wellens HJ: Pre-excitation revisited. Am J Cardiol 25:690–697, 1970
20. Emslie-Smith D, Sladden GE, Stirling GR: The significance of changes in the electrocardiogram in hypothermia. Br Heart J 21:343–351, 1959
21. Estes EH: Electrocardiography and vectorcardiography. In Hurst J (ed): The Heart, 3rd ed. New York, McGraw-Hill, 1974
22. Gallagher JJ, Svenson WC, Sealy WC et al: The Wolff-Parkinson-White syndrome and the Pre-excitation dysrhythmias. Med Clin North Am 60:114–121, 1976
23. Goldman MJ: Principles of Clinical Electrocardiography, 10th ed. California, Lange Medical Publications, 1979
24. Hecht HH, Kossman CE: Atrioventricular and intraventricular conduction: Revised nomenclature and concepts. Am J Cardiol 31:232–244, 1973
25. Hull E: The electrocardiogram in pericarditis. Am J Cardiol 7:21–32, 1961
26. Hurst JW (ed): Cardiac arrhythmias and conduction disturbances. In The Heart, p 482. New York, McGraw-Hill, 1970
27. Kaplan BM, Langendorf R, Lev M et al: The tachycardia–bradycardia syndrome. Med Clin North Am 60:81–99, 1976
28. Katz AM: Physiology of the Heart. New York, Raven Press, 1977
29. Kissin M, Schwarzschild MM, Bakst H: A nomogram for rate correction of the Q–T interval in the electrocardiogram. Am Heart J 35:990–992, 1948
30. Lerman J, Bruce RA, Murray JA: Correlation of polarcardiographic criteria for myocardial infarction with anterio graphic and ventriculographic findings (substantiation of transmural and presentation of nontransmural criteria). J Electrocardiol 9(3):219–226, 1976
31. Lown B, Ganong WF, Levine SA: The syndrome of short PR interval, normal QRS complex and paroxysmal rapid heart action. Circulation 5:693–706, 1952
32. Mangiola S: Self-Assessment in Electrocardiography. Philadelphia, JB Lippincott, 1977
33. Marriott HJL: Practical Electrocardiography, 6th ed. Baltimore, Williams & Wilkins, 1977
34. Marriott HJL: Workshop in Electrocardiography. Florida, Tampa Tracings, 1972
35. Marriott HJL, Myerburg RJ: Recognition and treatment of cardiac arrhythmias and conduction disturbances. In Hurst J (ed): The Heart, 4th Edition, pp 637–694. New York, McGraw-Hill, 1978
36. Massumi RA, Vera Z, Mason D: The Wolff-Parkinson-White syndrome. ModConcepts Cardiovasc Dis 42:41–46, 1973
37. Narula OS: The value of his bundle electrocardiography of cardiac diagnosis. Cardiovasc Clin 6:133–161, 1975
38. Netter F: Ciba-collection heart. In Youkonan F (ed): New Jersey, Ciba Pharmaceutical Company, Vol 5, 1969
39. Niederberger M, Bruce RA, Dower GE et al: Influence of age and ischemic heart disease an spatial ST–T magnitudes at rest and after maximal exercise. J Electrocardiol 6(4):279–284, 1973
40. Pick A: Digitalis and the electrocardiogram. Circulation 15:603–608, 1957
41. Rosenbaum MB: The hemiblocks: Diagnosis and criteria and clinical significance. Mod Concepts Cardiovasc Dis 39:141–146, 1970
42. Ruch TC, Patton HD: Physiology and Biophysics. Philadelphia, WB Saunders, 1974
43. Scherlag B, Lau S, Helfant R et al: Technique for recording his bundle activity in man. Circulation 39:13–18, 1969
44. Sharp L, Rabin B: Nursing in the Coronary Care Unit. Philadelphia, JB Lippincott, 1970
45. Surawicz B: Electrocardiographic pattern of cerebrovascular accidents. JAMA 197:913–914, 1966
46. Surawicz B: Electrolytes and Electrocardiogram. Am J Cardiol 12:656–622, 1963
47. Surawicz B, Lassiter KC: Electrocardiogram in pericarditis. Am J Cardiol 26:471–474, 1970
48. Surawicz B, Uhley H, Borun R et al: Task Force I. Standardization of terminology and interpretation. Am J Cardiol 41:130–145, 1978
49. VanderArk CR, Ballantyne F, Reynolds EW: Electrolytes and the electrocardiogram. Cardiovasc Clin North Am 5:269–294, 1973
50. Weinberg SL: Ambulatory monitoring of arrhythmias. Cardiovasc Clin 6:121–132, 1975
51. Wenger N: Myocarditis. In Hurst J (ed): The Heart, 4th ed. New York, McGraw Hill, 1978, 1529–1556.
52. Wolf PS, Hoffman SJ, Mersch J et al: Assessment skills for the nurse, pp 141–168. In Hudak et al (ed): Critical Care Nursing, Philadelphia, JB Lippincott, 1977

ADDITIONAL READING

ECG In General

Andreoli KG, Fowkes VH, Zipes DP et al: Comprehensive Cardiac Care, 3rd ed. St. Louis, CV Mosby, 1975
Bing, OHL. Clinical EKG Guide, 2nd ed. Newtonville: OHL Bing MD, 1981
Clark, NF: Normal Conduction System and the Electrocardiogram. Philadelphia, FA Davis, 1975
Friedman HH: Diagnostic Electrocardiography and Vectorcardiography, New York, McGraw-Hill, 1977
Grant RT: Clinical Electrocardiography. New York, McGraw-Hill, 1957

Meltzer L: Intensive Coronary Care, 3rd ed. Maryland, The Charles Press Publisher, 1977

Zalis EG, Conover MH: Understanding Electrocardiography, St. Louis, CV Mosby, 1972

Normal Variants

Caird FL, Campbell A, Jackson TFM: Significance of abnormalities of electrocardiogram in old people. Br Heart J 36:1012–1018, 1974

Chou TC: Pseudo-infarction (Non-infarction Q waves). Cardiovasc Clin 5:199–218, 1973

Gottshalk CW, Craige E: A comparison of the precordial ST and T waves in the electrocardiograms of 600 healthy young negro and white adults. South Med J 49:453–457, 1956

Ha D, Draft DL, Stein PD: The anteriorly oriented horizontal vector loop. The problem of distinction between direct posterior myocardial infarction and normal variation. Am Heart J 88:408–416, 1974

Lamonte CS, Freiman AH: The electrocardiogram after mastectomy. Circulation 32:746–754, 1965

Marriott HJL, Slonim R: False patterns of myocardial infarction. Heart Bull 16:71–73, 1967

Parisi AF, Bechman CH, Lancaster MC: The spectrum of ST segment elevation in the electrocardiograms of healthy adult men. J Electrocardio 4:137–144, 1971

Strong WB, Downs TD, Liebman J et al: The normal adolescent electrocardiogram. Am Heart J 83:115–128, 1972

Atrial Enlargement

Abraham AS: P-wave analysis in myocardial infarction, pulmonary edema and embolism. Am Heart J 89:301–304, 1975

Arevalo AG, Spagnuola M, Feinstein AR: A simple electrocardiographic indication of left atrial enlargement: A study of young patients with rheumatic heart disease. JAMA 185:358–362, 1963

Cokkinos DV, Leachman RD, Zamalloa O, et al: Influence of atrial mass on amplitude and duration of the P wave. Chest 61:336–339, 1972

Gross D: Electrocardiographic characteristics of P pulmonale waves of coronary origin. Am Heart J 73:453–459, 1967

Kasser I, Kennedy JW: The relationship of increased left atrial volume and pressure to abnormal P waves on the electrocardiogram. Circulation 39:339–343, 1969

Morris JJ, Estes EH, Whalen BE et al: P-wave analysis in valvular heart disease. Circulation, 29:242–252, 1964

Saunders JL, Calatayud JB, Schulz KJ et al: Evaluation of ECG criteria for P-wave abnormalities. Am Heart J 74:757–765, 1967

Tarazi RC, Miller A, Frohlich E et al: Electrocardiographic changes reflecting left atrial abnormality in hypertension. Circulation 34:818–822, 1966

Ventricular Enlargement

Human GP: Precordial lead patterns in right ventricular hypertension. Circulation 30:562–568, 1964

Manning GW, Smiley JR: QRS-voltage criteria for left ventricular hypertrophy in a normal male population. Circulation 27:224–230, 1964

Murphy ML, Hutcheson F: The electrocardiographic diagnosis of right ventricular hypertrophy in chronic obstructive pulmonary disease. Chest 65:622–627, 1974

Roman GT, Walsh TJ, Massie E: Right ventricular hypertrophy: Correlation of electrocardiographic and anatomic findings. Am J Cardiol 7:481–487, 1961

Romhill DW, Bove KE, Norris RJ et al: A critical appraisal of the electrocardiographic criteria for the diagnosis of left ventricular hypertrophy. Circulation 40:185–194, 1969

Romhill, DP, Estes EH: A point-score for the ECG diagnosis of left ventricular hypertrophy. Am Heart J 75:752–758, 1968

Scott RC: The correlation between the electrocardiographic patterns of ventricular hypertrophy and the anatomic findings. Circulation 21:256–291, 1960

Scott RC: Ventricular hypertrophy. Cardiovasc Clin 5:219–253, 1973

Talbot S: Electrical axis and voltage criteria of left ventricular hypertrophy. Am Heart J 90:420–425, 1975

Drugs

Alexander CS: Cardiotoxic effects of phenothiazine and related drugs. Circulation 38:1014–1015, 1968

Surawicz B, Lasseter KC: Effect of drugs on the electrocardiogram. Progr Cardiovasc Dis 13:26–55, 1970

Electrolyte Imbalances

Bronsky D, Dubin A, Waldstein SS et al: Calcium and the electrocardiogram, I, II, III. Am J Cardiol 7:823–843, 1961

Surawicz B: Electrolytes and the electrocardiogram. Postgrad Med 55:123–129, 1974

Surawicz B: Relationship between electrocardiogram and electrolytes. Am Heart J 73:814–834, 1967

Weaver WF, Burchell HB: Serum K+ and the electrocardiogram in hypokalemia. Circulation 21:505–521, 1960

Effects of Systemic Disease

Abildskov JA, Millar K, Burgess MJ et al: The electrocardiogram and central nervous system. Prog Cardiovasc Dis 13:210–216, 1970

Burch GE, DePasquale NP: The electrocardiographic diagnosis of pulmonary heart disease. Am J Cardiol 11:622–638, 1963

Burch GE, Meyers R, Abildskov JA: A new electrocardiographic pattern observed in cerebrovascular accidents. Circulation 9:719–723, 1954

Fowler NO: The electrocardiogram in pericarditis. Cardiovasc Clin 5:255–267, 1973

Lynch RE, Stein PD, Bruce TA: Leftward shift of frontal plane QRS axis as a frequent manifestation of acute pulmonary embolism. Chest 61:443–446, 1972

Range PJ, Bousuaros G: Giant peaked upright T-waves in cerebrovascular accident. Br Heart J 32:717–719, 1970

Spodick DH: Electrocardiogram in acute pericarditis. Am J Cardiol 33:470–474, 1974

Stein PD, Dafen JE, McIntyre KM et al: The electrocardiogram in acute pulmonary embolism. Prog in Cardiovasc Dis 17:247–257, 1975

Trevino A, Razi B, Beller MB: The characteristic electrocardiogram of accidental hypothermia. Arch Intern Med 127:470–473, 1971

MI, Injury and Ischemia

Cook RW, Edwards JE, Pruitt RD: Electrocardiographic changes in acute subendocardial infarction. Circulation 98:603–613, 1958

Dunn WJ, Edwards JE, Pruitt RD: The electrocardiogram in infarction of the lateral wall of the left ventricle. Circulation 14:540–555, 1956

Horan LG, Flowers NC, Johnson JC: "Significance of the diagnostic Q wave of myocardial infarction. Circulation 43:428–436, 1971

Lewis BS, Schamroth L: The hyperacute phase of true posterior infarction. Heart Lung 6:331–334, 1977

Lui CK: Atrial infarction of the heart. Circulation 23:331–338, 1961

Mills RM, Young E, Gorlin R et al: Natural history of ST segment elevation after acute myocardial infarction. Am J Cardiol 35:609–614, 1975

Savage RM, Wagner GS, Idiker RE et al: Correlation of postmortem anatomic findings with electrocardiographic changes in patients with myocardial infarction: Retrospective study of patients with typical anterior and posterior infarcts. Circulation 55:279–285, 1977

Schamroth L, Perlman MM: The electrocardiographic manifestations of acute true posterior myocardial infarction. Heart Lung 1:658–660, 1972

Shettigar UR, Hultgren HN, Pfeifer JF et al: Diagnostic value of Q-waves in inferior myocardial infarction. Am Heart J 88:170–175, 1974

Accelerated Conduction

Akhtar M, Damato AN, Batsford WP et al: Demonstration of re-entry within the His-purkinje system in man. Circulation 50:1150–1162, 1974

Caracta AR, Damato AN, Gallagher JJ et al: Electrophysiological studies in the syndrome of short PR interval, normal QRS complex. Am J Cardiology, 31:245–253, 1973.

Coumel PH, Waynberger M, Fabiato A, et al: Wolff-Parkinson-White syndrome: Problems in evaluation of multiple accessory pathways and surgical therapy. Circulation 45:1216–1230, 1972

Gallagher JJ, Gilbert M, Svenson RH et al: Wolff-Parkinson-White syndrome: The problem, evaluation and surgical correction. Circulation 51:767–785, 1975

Mandel WJ, Dansig R, Hayakawa H: Lown-Ganong-Levine syndrome. Circulation 44:696–708, 1971

Narula OS: Wolff-Parkinson-White syndrome (a review). Circulation 47:872–887, 1973

Zipes DP, Rothbaum DA, DeJoseph RL: Preexcitation syndrome. Cardiovasc Clin 6:209–243, 1974

Delayed Conduction

Castellanos A, Spence MI, Chapell DE: Hemiblock and bundle branch block. Heart Lung 1:36–44, 1972

Damato AN, Gallagher JJ, Schnitzler RN et al: Use of His bundle recordings in understanding A–V conduction disturbances. J NY Acad Med 47:905–922, 1971

Damato AN, Lau SH, Helfant R et al: A study of heart block in man using His bundle recordings. Circulation 39:297–305, 1969

Dreifus LS, Watanabe Y, Haiat R, et al: Atrioventricular block. Am J Cardiol 28:371–380, 1971

Langendorf R, Pick A: Atrioventricular block, Type II (Mobitz): Its nature and clinical significance. Circulation 38:819–821, 1968

Levites R, Haft J: Significance of first degree heart block in bifascicular block. Am J Cardiol 34:259–264, 1974

Marriott HJ: Electrocardiographic abnormalities, conduction disorders and arrhythmias in primary myocardial disease. Prog Cardiovasc Dis 7:99–114, 1964

Marriott HJ, Hogan P: Hemiblock in acute myocardial infarction. Chest 58:342–344, 1970

Massumi RA, Ali N: Determination of the site of impaired conduction in atrioventricular block. J Electrocardiography 3:193–209, 1970

Narula OS: Wenckebach Type I and Type II atrioventricular block (revisited). Cardiovasc Clin 6:138–167, 1974

Narula OS, Cohen LS, Samet P et al: Localization of A–V conduction defects in man by recording of the His bundle electrogram. Am J Cardiol 25:228–237, 1970

Narula OS, Scherlag BJ, Samet P et al: Atrioventricular block: Localization and classification by His bundle recordings. Am J Med 50:146–177, 1971

Rosen KM, Dhingra RC, Loeb HS et al: Chronic heart block in adults. Arch Intern Med 131:663–672, 1973

Rosenbaum MB, Elizari MV, Kretz A et al: Anatomical basis of AV conduction disturbances. Geriatrics 25(11):132–144, 1970

Rosenbaum MB, Elizari MV, Lazzari JO et al: Intraventricular trifascicular blocks: Review of literature and classification. Am Heart J 78:450–459, 1969

Scholoff LD, Adler L, Donoso E et al: Bilateral bundle branch block. Clinical and electrocardiographic aspects. Circulation 35:790–801, 1967

Uhley HN: The fascicular blocks. Cardiovasc Clin 5:87–97, 1973

His-Bundle Electrograms

Aranda JM, Befeler B, Castellanos A: His bundle recordings: Their contribution of human electrophysiology. Heart Lung 5:907–918, 1976

Damato AN, Lau SH: Clinical value of the electrogram of the conduction system. Prog Cardiovasc Dis 13:119–140, 1970

Dhingra RC, Rosen KM, Rahimtoola SH: Normal conduction intervals and responses in sixty-one patients using His bundle recording and atrial pacing. Chest 64:55–59, 1973

Denes P, Rosen KM: His bundle electrograms: Clinical applications. Cardiovasc Clin 6:69–85, 1974

Haft JI: The His bundle electrogram. Circulation, 47:897–911, 1973

Rosen KM: Catheter recording of His bundle electrograms. Mod Concepts Cardiovasc Dis 42:23–28, 1973

Rosen KM: Evaluation of cardiac conduction in the cardiac catheterization laboratory. Am J Cardiol 30:701–703, 1972

Rosen KM: His bundle electrograms. Circulation 46:831–832, 1972

Scherlag BJ, Samet P, Helfant RH: His bundle electrogram: A critical appraisal of its uses and limitations. Circulation 46:601–613, 1972

Tachycardia—Bradycardia Syndrome

Chung, EK: Sick sinus syndrome: Current view. Mod Concepts Cardiovas Dis 44(11–12):61–70, 1980

Ferrer MI: The sick sinus syndrome. Circulation 47:635–641, 1973

Kaplan B, Langendorf R, Lev M et al: Tachycardia—bradycardia syndrome (so-called "Sick-Sinus Syndrome"). Am J Cardiol 31:497–508, 1973

Arrhythmias

Azevedo IM, Watanabe Y, Dreifus LS: Reassessment of A-V junctional rhythms. Heart Lung 1:626–638, 1972

Baun H and Diettert G: ECG Arrhythmia interpretation. Reston: Reston Publishing Company, 1979.

Childers R: Concealed conduction. Med Clin North Am 60:149–173, 1976

Chung EK: Reappraisal of parasystole. Heart Lung 2:81–89, 1973

Conover MH: Cardiac Arrhythmias, 2nd ed. St. Louis, CV Mosby, 1978

Fisch C, Knoebel SB: Junctional rhythms. Prog Cardiovasc Dis 13:141–158, 1970

Foster W: Principles of Acute Coronary Care. New York, Appleton-Century-Crofts, 1976

Goldreyer B: Sinus node dysfunction—A physiological consideration of arrhythmias involving the sinus node. Cardiovasc Clin 6:179–198, 1974

Krone RJ, Kleiger RE: Prevention and treatment of supraventricular arrhythmias. Heart Lung 6:79–88, 1977

Lipson MJ, Naimi S: Multifocal atrial tachycardia. Circulation 42:397–407, 1970

Marriott JL, Gozensky C: Analysis of arrhythmias in coronary care—A plea for precision. Heart Lung 1:51–55, 1972

Phillips RE and Feeney MK: The Cardiac Rhythms. Philadelphia: WB Saunders Company, 1980

Pick A, Langendorf R: Parasystole and its variants. Med Clin North Am 60:125–147, 1976

Robles de Medina EO, Bernard R, Coumel P et al: Definition of terms related to cardiac rhythm. Am Heart J 95(6):796–806, 1978

Rosen KM: Junctional tachycardia: Mechanisms, diagnosis, differential diagnosis and management. Circulation 47:654–664, 1973

Schamroth L: Some basic principles governing the electrophysiology and diagnosis of heart rhythms. Heart Lung 1:45–50, 1972

Steffens TG, Gettes, LS: Parasystole. Cardiovasc Clin 6:99–110, 1974

Vectorcardiogram

Castellanos A, Lemberg L, Berkovits B: Didactic vectorcardiography: General concepts. Heart Lung 4:697–723, 1975

Chou T, Helm RA: Clinical Vectorcardiography, 2nd ed. New York, Grune and Stratton, 1974

Goldman MJ: Principles of Clinical Electrocardiography, 10th ed. Los Altos, Lange Medical Publications, 1979

Johnston FD: The clinical use of vectorcardiography. Circulation 23:297–303, 1961

Kormbluth AW, Allenstein BJ: The normal direct spatial vectorcardiogram. Am Heart J 54:396–406, 1957

18

Exercise Testing
ERIKA SEIBERLER SIVARAJAN, R.N., M.A.

Exercise testing was first proposed as an adjunct to physical examination 45 years ago, but it was not widely used until the last decade. Its unique advantage as a diagnostic tool is that it provides information about the cardiovascular system in a dynamic state that cannot be obtained by the standard physical examination with a recumbent patient. The increasing use of exercise testing requires that nurses have at least a basic knowledge of this form of evaluation in order to answer questions from the general public and from patients in numerous health-care settings. Low-level treadmill testing has recently been employed to evaluate the readiness of the patient to be discharged from the hospital after acute myocardial infarction (MI). The observations gained from such assessment can be used to determine safe levels of activity during initial days at home.

Exercise testing can be defined as the observation, measurement, and recording of physiological responses to a known amount of physical work. Measuring both the work load and the resultant cardiovascular responses yields important diagnostic and prescriptive information. Exercise tests can be standardized and the results reproduced. Different principles and various types of exercises have been used in exercise testing. There are about as many protocols available as there are exercise laboratories. However, the key points are that the purposes or indications for the test be clearly defined, an appropriate work load selected, and careful assessment of physiological responses be made.

This chapter presents the objectives, the principles and standards, and the various modes of testing. An approach to interpreting the results as well as their nursing implications is also discussed.

OBJECTIVES FOR TESTING

There are two major reasons for exercise testing:

1. *To measure exercise capacity in order to assess fitness for work, sports, and other activities in health and disease.*[3]

Some cardiologists advocate exercise testing as part of a physical examination, particularly for men over 35 years of age with a family history of coronary artery disease (CAD) and who are about to start a physical conditioning program.[8] Similarly, athletes participating in sports undergo exercise tests as part of their training. Results of the test can establish the presence or absence of asymptomatic CAD in apparently healthy men. Exercise testings is also used by the Navy to assess the fitness of divers and Coast Guard rescuers, by the Federal Aviation Administration to test pilots, and by private industry to test persons who hold positions that could potentially jeopardize the public welfare should they suffer a heart attack or sudden death while performing their jobs.

2. *To assess functional impairment and mechanisms of impairment.*

Persons requiring such testing are those with CAD (persons who have angina pectoris, for example, or have had an MI, and those at risk of sudden death) or with valvular heart diseases; the test helps to determine the cause that limits the person's exercise capacity: for example, angina, dyspnea, exertional hypotension, or arrhythmia.

When exercise testing is undertaken in order to evaluate the effects of preventive, therapeutic, and rehabilitation programs, it fulfills one or both of the objectives mentioned. For example, information about work capacity and mechanisms of impairment will document responses to physical conditioning programs, medical therapy, and surgical treatments of CAD. This information will influence future therapy. More specifically, in patients recuperating from MI, exercise testing is used to determine endurance and hemodynamic and electrocardiographic responses during exercise. Decisions about the level of work to which they can return and the amount of exercise that they can safely perform can then be based on these data.

PRINCIPLES OF EXERCISE TESTING

Regardless of the type of test used, the following principles should be observed:[6,7,9,10]

1. In performing the test the level of skill should be uniform and the test familiar to the population being tested.
2. The work done should involve the large muscle groups.
3. A test should begin at a work level considerably below that at which impairment is expected to manifest itself.
4. Multi-level work load tests are preferable to single-level tests.
5. The intensity of the work load should be measurable.
6. The work load should be maintained at each level for sufficient time to ensure that the individual's responses have stabilized. One minute at each level may be sufficient at low intensities, but "steady state" may not be reached before 5 minutes at high exercise intensities. Three minutes represents a reasonable compromise for most people.
7. The increase in work loads to the point of limitation should progress gradually.
8. There should be predetermined criteria for stopping the test.
9. Monitor blood pressure, symptoms, and signs, and continuously monitor ECG (heart rate, arrhythmia and ST segment and T wave changes) during an initial resting period, at each work load, and during recovery.

TYPE OF EXERCISES

There are three types of exercise that can be used. The first is dynamic: a rhythmical contraction of extensor and flexor muscles used for activities such as walking, running, jogging, bicycling, and swimming. The second is isometric: sustained muscle contraction, as in weight lifting and handgripping exercises. The third is a combination of these two.

There is a decided advantage to using dynamic exercise in exercise testing without unduly prolonging exercise time, because the circulatory responses to dynamic exercise are more directly proportional to the relative aerobic requirements.[4,5] Isometric exercise results in a greater increase in systolic blood pressure and heart rate in relation to the aerobic requirement and hence is not often used to assess the cardiovascular system. Use of this form of exercise test would, however, provide more information for a patient whose occupation requires an extensive amount of isometric activity.

MODES OF TESTING

In evaluating exercise tests, the nurse needs to be aware of the major differences in the several test protocols in use (Fig. 18-1).[7] Differences among the types of exercise tests relate to their work loads and the length of time spent at each work load.

Work Load

Tests may have single or multiple stages. A single-stage test is one in which the work load is constant throughout, for example, the step test. This is diagrammatically represented in example 1 of Figure 18-2.[2] In a multi-stage test, the work load is increased at regular intervals until an end point is reached. Examples 2, 3, and 4 of Figure 18-2 are examples of multi-stage tests. The multi-stage test may be continuous or intermittent. In continuous tests the work load may be increased every 3 to 5 minutes (example 3), or every minute

Fig. 18-1. Oxygen requirements increase with work loads from bottom of chart to top in various exercise tests of the step, treadmill, and bicycle ergometer types. (*Nagle FS, Balke B, Naughton JP: Gradational step tests for assessing work capacity. J Appl Physiol 20:745–748, 1965. †Bruce RA: Multi-stage treadmill test of submaximal and maximal exercise. Appendix B, this publication. ‡Kattus AA, Jorgensen CR, Worden RE, Alvaro AF: S–T segment depression with near-maximal exercise in detection of preclinical coronary heart disease. Circulation 41:585–595, 1971. **Fox SM, Naughton JP, Haskell WL: Physical activity and the prevention of coronary heart disease. Ann Clin Res 3:404, 1971. Committee on Exercise, Exercise Testing and Training of Apparently Healthy Individuals: A Handbook for Physicians, p 13. New York, American Heart Association, 1972)

FUNCTIONAL CLASS	CLINICAL STATUS	O₂ REQUIREMENTS ml O₂/kg/min	STEP TEST — NAGLE, BALKE, NAUGHTON* (2 min stages 30 steps/min)	BRUCE† (3-min stages)	KATTUS‡ (3-min stages)	BALKE** (% grade at 3.4 mph)	BALKE** (% grade at 3 mph)	BICYCLE ERGOMETER**
		56.0	(Step height increased 4 cm q 2 min)			26		For 70 kg body weight
		52.5			mph %gr	24		kgm/min
	PHYSICALLY ACTIVE SUBJECTS	49.0		mph %gr	4 22	22		
NORMAL AND I		45.5	Height (cm)	4.2 16		20		1500
		42.0	40		4 18	18	22.5	1350
		38.5	36			16	20.0	1200
		35.0	32		4 14	14	17.5	1050
	SEDENTARY HEALTHY	31.5	28	3.4 14		12	15.0	900
		28.0	24		4 10	10	12.5	
		24.5	20	2.5 12	3 10	8	10.0	750
	DISEASED, RECOVERED	21.0	16			6	7.5	600
II		17.5	12	1.7 10	2 10	4	5.0	450
		14.0	8			2	2.5	300
	SYMPTOMATIC PATIENTS	10.5	4				0.0	
III		7.0						150
IV		3.5						

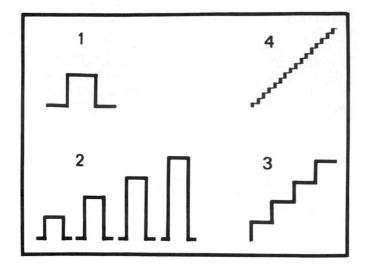

Fig. 18-2. Various principles for exercise test ("abscissa" = time; "ordinate" = rate of work). (Åstrand P: Prog Cardiovasc Dis 19(1):July/August, 1976)

(example 4), whereas intermittent tests incorporate pauses for partial or complete rest between each test stage, thereby prolonging the period of observation.

The work load should be maintained at a given level for sufficient time to permit stabilization of responses or achievement of steady state. The time needed to achieve steady state increases with the intensity of exercise; hence, at low levels one minute may be sufficient, but at higher levels up to 5 minutes may be required. Three-minute stages have been used most frequently; they give maximum yield.

Work loads are best communicated in terms of metabolic equivalents (METs). One MET is the energy expended while sitting quietly and is approximately equivalent to 3.5 to 4.0 ml oxygen per kg/min.[1]

Duration

Both single-stage and multi-stage exercise tests aim at eliciting either maximal performance or some level short of maximal exercise capacity. For example, the test may be terminated at a predetermined work load, or at a certain stage of a protocol which correlates with a known energy expenditure, or on attainment of an age-predicted heart rate. See Figure 18-1 for some commonly used exercise test protocols.

TYPES OF TESTS

Three types of tests are used to provide the work load in exercise testing: (1) the step test; (2) the bicycle or arm-cranking ergometer test; (3) the treadmill test. Regardless of which test is used, the general principles of exercise testing, outlined above, apply to all three. Each test has advantages and disadvantages, as summarized in Table 18-1.[16]

When evaluating reports on exercise testing, it is important to note the following information: the purpose of the test; the specificity of the exercise response; whether the test included weight-bearing or non-weight-bearing activities; and whether there was regional or general muscle involvement during the exercise.

If exercise testing is being used to assess the effects of training, attention needs to be paid to the specific muscles being trained. For example, it would be unwise to use a bicycle ergometer to assess alterations in physiological variables resulting from a running or swimming program. Likewise, if a person is being assessed for readiness to return to work that requires arm strength, then an armcranking ergometer test may give more appropriate information than a treadmill test.

Step Test. This is the simplest, least expensive, and most portable type of exercise testing.[6;13] The two-step apparatus is so designed that each step is 9 inches high, about 10 inches deep, and about 20 to 24 inches wide. The double two-step procedure requires the subject to ascend to the top of the two steps and walk down on the other side. This is counted as one trip. He then retraces his steps to perform his second trip. He is instructed to reverse his direction of turning each time in order to avoid dizziness. Some patients have excessive difficulty with dizziness, so that the test must be terminated. The number of trips is standardized for age, sex, and weight. The patient is instructed to attempt to complete the number of trips in exactly 3 minutes. This can be facilitated by the use of a metronome.

There are certain disadvantages of the step test: Excessive body movement makes measurements difficult; the work load is rate-dependent and requires that the subject maintain a steady pace; the work load is also weight-dependent, because this test overworks the obese and underworks the underweight making it difficult to compare results; it requires strong subject motivation to continue the test.

Although the step test was the pioneer in exercise testing, it has fallen into disuse because more precise methods of exercise testing, such as bicycle ergometry or treadmill testing, are now available.

Bicycle Ergometry. A bicycle ergometer is a device consisting of a wheel operated by a pair of pedals. By altering the resistance or friction on the wheel, a desired work load can be achieved. It can be used for arm cranking, foot pedaling or both, and therefore can be used in the supine as well as the upright position. The cost is relatively low and the device is quite portable. The physiological measurements can be obtained with ease, since the upper body is relatively stable and the test is independent of weight.

The work load is usually started at 150 kilopond meters per minute (KPM/minute) at a constant pedaling frequency of 50 revolutions per minute (RPM), and is increased by 150 to 300 KPM every 3 minutes. In some protocols the work load is increased by 60 KPM each minute. The work load is increased gradually, each level being performed for 3 to 6 minutes until an age-predicted heart rate is reached, or until there are adverse symptoms or electrocardiographic changes.

The major disadvantage with bicycle ergometry is that

TABLE 18-1   ADVANTAGES AND DISADVANTAGES OF STEP TEST, BICYCLE ERGOMETER AND TREADMILL TEST

Test	Advantages	Disadvantages
Step Test	1. Simple 2. Least expensive 3. Most portable	1. Excessive body movement, which complicates measurement 2. Work load is rate-dependent and requires subject to maintain a steady pace 3. Requires strong subject motivation 4. Work load is weight-dependent and results are difficult to compare 5. Difficult to achieve maximum exercise capacity, and reproducibility is questionable. 6 Takes a long time to reach maximum exercise 7. Underworks the obese and overworks the underweight
Bicycle Ergometer	1. Relatively inexpensive 2. Portable 3. Easy to obtain physiological measurements as upper body is quite stable 4. Work load is weight-independent	1. Need for frequent calibration 2. Local muscle fatigue 3. Requires motivation to continue pedaling 4. Rate of pedaling must be constant to maintain constant power 5. Inability to attain maximum oxygen uptake as high as on treadmill 6. Bicycle exercise is a greater stress
Treadmill	1. Walking is familiar to all persons 2. Work rate is constant—the subject either maintains the pace or stops 3. More large muscle groups are involved 4. Relative ease of obtaining clear, accurate measurements 5. Maximum oxygen uptake is the highest attainable 6. Most reproducible and standardized	1. Expensive 2. Bulky and not portable 3. Noisy 4. Potential danger of subject losing balance 5. Habituation—previous treadmill walking may increase duration 6. Work load is weight-dependent. The overweight person must work harder at same speed and gradient

(Sivarajan ES, Halpenny CJ: Am J Nurs 79(12):2164, Copyright © 1979, American Journal of Nursing Company. Reproduced with permission.)

the ergometer requires frequent calibration. The rate of pedaling must be constant to maintain a constant power output. In addition, it may cause quadriceps muscle fatigue, making it difficult to attain maximal oxygen uptake values as high as those that can be attained on a treadmill. Bicycle ergometers are used widely in Europe, whereas the treadmill is more popular in the United States.

Treadmill. The treadmill is a motor-driven device that has variable speeds from 1.0 to 10 miles per hour (1.5 to 16 km per hour) and a slope that can be adjusted from horizontal to a 20% gradient, which permits the subject to walk or run on a level base or on a variety of angles.

There are several advantages of this form of testing over the previous two: the work rate is constant because it is involuntarily regulated—the subject either maintains the pace or discontinues the test; walking is an activity familiar to people of all ages; clear and accurate physiological measurements can be obtained with relative ease; and the maximal oxygen uptake values attainable appear to be higher with the treadmill than with either of the other two devices, making it especially useful for research. These values are also reproducible.

The major disadvantages of the treadmill are that it is expensive and bulky, and lacks portability. It is moderately noisy and there is a potential danger of injury should the subject lose balance and fall. The work load is weight-dependent.

Standards for Exercise Testing

Specifications for exercise testing equipment and standards for exercise testing laboratories have been outlined by the American Heart Association.[6,7,9,10] Personnel responsible for

testing should be familiar with these guidelines. Recommended standards for exercise testing are[6,7,9]

1. The patient should be informed of the purpose, risks, and benefits of the exercise test; a signed consent must be obtained prior to testing.

2. A detailed physical examination, including a resting 12-lead ECG, should be done and interpreted immediately prior to testing.

3. The patient's ECG responses (heart rate, rhythm, and ST segment-T wave changes) should be monitored continuously before, during, and for a specified period after the test. The lead selected should provide high-quality tracings. Single- and multiple-lead systems are in use; the specific choice depends on the purpose of the test. The lead system especially useful in assessing ST segment-T wave responses during exercise is the bipolar CB_5 lead because of its proximity to the left ventricle. The positive electrode is placed in the CB_5 ECG position. The negative electrode is placed below the inferior tip of the right scapula and the ground lead placed anywhere on the patient's back.

4. Reliable equipment for blood pressure measurement should be securely attached to the person's arm and readings obtained at least once during each stage of the test; in persons impaired by heart disease it should be checked at least once every minute.

5. The subject is to be frequently observed and questioned about symptoms, in order to detect unfavorable reactions or signs of impaired circulation.

6. The patient's responses during recovery are monitored for at least 5 to 6 minutes, or until near-resting levels are reached.

7. Appropriate emergency equipment must be kept in the testing room, including a defibrillator and drugs for

dealing with serious arrhythmias, syncope, cardiac arrest, or myocardial infarction.

8. A physician or a qualified person acting as his delegate should continuously monitor the patient's responses to the test.

Criteria for Stopping

The exercise test is usually terminated with the onset of adverse responses such as chest pain, shortness of breath, claudication, or severe arrhythmias, or on attaining the age-predicted heart rate.

Age-predicted heart rates at which the test is stopped are[6,7]

- 170 beats per minute in the 20 to 29 year age group;
- 160 beats per minute in the 30 to 39 year age group;
- 150 beats per minute in the 40 to 49 year age group;
- 140 beats per minute in the 50 to 59 year age group;
- 130 beats per minute in the 60 to 69 year age group.[7,15]

Target heart rate end points are not recommended by all physiologists or cardiologists.

In maximal exercise testing, the development of symptoms (i.e., exhaustion, generalized fatigue, or shortness of breath) is also an end point. However, depending on such factors as the person's health status, the purpose of the test, or the decision of the clinician conducting the test, persons being tested may be stopped at the onset of slight symptoms or be encouraged to continue further.

SPECIFIC PROTOCOLS

Since the treadmill is the most commonly used device for exercise testing in the United States, the remainder of this chapter will be devoted to this form of exercise testing. There are many protocols in use for treadmill testing. Comparison among those most frequently used can be seen in Figure 18-1. In practice, each testing center adopts and becomes familiar and experienced with a given protocol, and uses that to the exclusion of others.

Bruce Protocol Treadmill Test

One familiar treadmill test is the Bruce protocol, described as one example of the many available.[3,5] This is a continuous multi-level maximal exercise test. A physical examination and 12-lead ECG are taken prior to the test. Monitoring follows the standards recommended above. Both speed and gradient are raised every 3 minutes, as follows:

Stage	Speed	Gradient	Duration	METS
I	1.7 mph	10%	3 min	5
II	2.5 mph	12%	3 min	7
III	3.4 mph	14%	3 min	9–12
IV	4.2 mph	16%	3 min	12–14

The test is terminated at the point of marked fatigue or other significant symptoms of exhaustion or if serious untoward effects occur. The instant at which the treadmill is stopped is termed 0-minute recovery, and measurements are re-peated every minute for 6 minutes (6-minute recovery) or until blood pressure and heart rate have returned to near-resting levels.

Low-Level Treadmill Test

In a number of centers, submaximal symptom-limited low-level treadmill testing is used to assess the readiness of the patient for discharge after an MI.[15] By evaluating the cardiovascular responses to low-level treadmill testing, information can be gained for prescribing activity and teaching exercise prior to discharge. One such low-level protocol in use follows:[17,18]

Speed	Gradient	Duration	METS
1.2 mph	0%	3 min	2.14
1.2 mph	3%	3 min	2.35
1.2 mph	6%	3 min	2.74
1.7 mph	6%	3 min	3.30

This test is performed the day before or on the day of discharge from the hospital. By this time, the patient has usually walked in the halls and used stairs for a few days. A 12-lead ECG is taken and interpreted by the cardiologist prior to the test.

The predetermined criteria for stopping this test early are different from those used for regular exercise tests, since this test is performed on patients recovering from a recent MI. They are

- fatigue or chest pain
- a heart rate increase to more than 120 beats per minute (110 beats per minute if on propranolol)
- any other untoward symptoms or signs, such as failure of the systolic blood pressure to rise or a drop in blood pressure below resting levels.[15,18]

APPROACH TO INTERPRETATION OF TEST RESULTS

See Chapter 7 for normal physiological responses to exercise. The exercise test results and differences between the patient's responses and normal responses are evaluated from several parameters, regardless of the test protocol used. The effects of learning and habituation must be considered when evaluating test results.

Exercise Capacity

Exercise capacity is expressed as the duration in minutes or seconds, or the stage of testing attained, and should be noted in relation to the specific test protocol used. The oxygen requirement of a given level of work can be ascertained from Figure 18-1, which lists the oxygen cost for the more frequently used treadmill protocols. This enables the interpreter of the test results to compare the amount of energy expended among a variety of tests. Functional aerobic impairment (FAI) is the term coined by Bruce to denote the degree of limitation expressed as percentage of impairment. This can be determined by nomographic assessment.[5,16] The

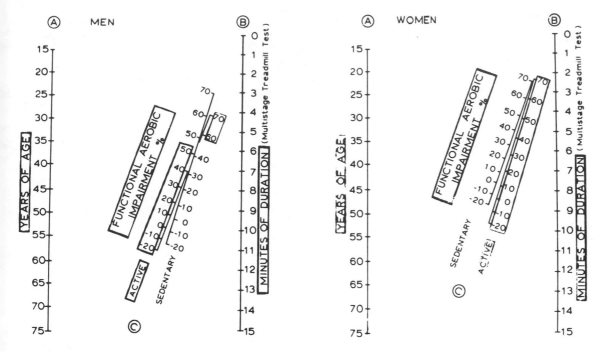

Fig. 18-3. Nomograms for estimating functional aerobic impairment (FAI); nomograms for finding percent deviation of individuals estimated from average predicted values of V_{O_2max}, in healthy middle-aged men (**A**) and women (**B**). (Bruce RA: Ann Clin Res 3:323–332, 1971)

FAI is the difference between the observed duration of the test and the duration expected for a healthy person of the same age, sex, and habitual activity status, expressed as a percentage of the normal.

The nomograms in Figure 18-3 were developed by studying large numbers of normal men and women.[3,5] The column on the right gives minutes and seconds of duration of the Bruce multi-stage treadmill test. Age in years is represented on the left. The two diagonal bars in the center represent percentages of impairment for active and sedentary persons. A person is considered to be active if he exercises vigorously enough to break out in a sweat more than once a week, regularly each week.

To find the FAI of an exercised person, apply a ruler to the duration column on the right, and to the age column on the left. Read the percentage of aerobic impairment at the intersection of the central diagonal line.

- A zero value indicates that the individual's responses are identical to the average maximal oxygen uptake for normal persons of the same age, sex, and habitual physical activity status.
- A variation between the values of +10 and −10 is considered within normal range.
- A value of −10 means that performance was 10% above average for a comparable normal person.
- A value of +10 means that the performance was 10% below average.

The complement of FAI thus serves as an objective index of a person's exercise capacity and can be used to measure changes over time. Another use of the nomogram, when FAI is not zero, is to estimate from the observed duration the physiologically equivalent age. However, the reader needs to be cautioned that nomographic assessment of FAI is applicable only to the Bruce protocol.

Reasons for Stopping

The mechanisms of impairment can be determined from the symptoms or signs manifested. These should be evaluated in relation to the purpose of the test. It is useful to know the level of exercise in terms of METS at which the patient is limited from doing further exercise. The specific manifestations recorded can serve as information on which future therapy can be based. Efficacy of therapy can also be evaluated once objective information on the mechanism of impairment is available. Did the test measure maximal or submaximal performance? It is important to recognize whether a given level of exercise performance represents the patient's maximum performance or some arbitrary level short of it, such as a predetermined heart rate. It is also essential to assess what responses are expected of a given person and whether a limitation in exercise performance represents a pathologic state. Psychologic factors that influence treadmill performance and responses include anxiety, depression, fear and disinterest.

Subjective Symptoms

Reports of symptoms occurring during the test are important as part of the evaluation of the person's capacity for physical exercise.

- Chest pain is an important symptom of myocardial ischemia.
- Shortness of breath in a patient with cardiac impairment is often a symptom of left ventricular failure.
- Claudication is indicative of peripheral vascular disease.

- Leg fatigue is often experienced at maximum exercise.
- Dizziness and lightheadedness may reflect cerebral hypoxia and may coincide with a feeling of exhaustion at maximum exercise.

Dizziness may be accompanied by signs of gray or ashen pallor, diaphoresis, ataxic gait, dyspnea, and strained appearance, as blood is maximally shunted to the heart, brain, and exercising muscle. Trained observers are able to recognize this appearance and expect that the person being tested will very soon say that he can go no further.

Objective Signs

The appearance of an S_3 or *ventricular gallop* during the physical examination that follows the exercise test indicates transient left ventricular dysfunction. *Heart rate* response to exercise decreases with advancing age, and is also affected by such medications as propranolol. Tables on predicted maximum heart rate responses according to age are available (Table 18-2). The increase in heart rate from rest to maximal exercise is considered to define the chronotropic reserve of the heart. In addition to the absolute heart rate achieved, the percentage increase over the resting rate is important as an indication of cardiovascular response to exercise. It is important to note whether heart rate increase is progressive in response to gradually progressive increases in work load or submaximal work loads result in an excessive increase in heart rate.

The increase in *systolic blood pressure* from rest to maximal exercise represents the inotropic reserve of the left ventricle. The inability to raise systolic blood pressure or a fall in systolic blood pressure with increasing exercise indicates an inability of the left ventricle to increase the strength of contraction with increasing exercise. The test should be terminated at the appearance of this sign. Results of large-scale studies show a correlation between inability

to raise systolic blood pressure and ventricular fibrillation or sudden cardiac death.[11] *Diastolic blood pressure* usually does not change greatly with exercise.

The *pressure–rate product* (PRP) is an indirect indicator of myocardial oxygen consumption and is a useful value to calculate.[12] This is obtained by multiplying systolic blood pressure by heart rate and dividing the result by 100 to yield a convenient number. It has been demonstrated that angina pectoris occurs at a constant value of pressure–rate product.[14] Maximal heart rate may be 150 and maximal systolic pressure may be 160 when angina occurs, or the same individual may have a maximal heart rate of 120 and a maximal systolic pressure of 200 when angina occurs; the PRP in each case is 240 units ($150 \times 160/100 = 240$; $120 \times 200/100 = 240$). Because heart rate by itself correlates well with myocardial oxygen consumption,[12] patients can be taught to take their own pulse and regulate their activity to keep their heart rates below the threshold level for angina pectoris or myocardial ischemia.

Electrocardiogram

Until recently, discussions of ECG responses during exercise testing have been overemphasized and have tended to obscure the importance of other clinical responses. The interpretation of ECG responses involves assessing arrhythmias and ischemic changes.

Alterations in the ST segment and T wave of the ECG reflect an imbalance between the demand and supply of oxygen in the myocardium. Figure 18-4 shows the normal and abnormal ST-segment responses.[19] The morphology of the ST-segment depression has been described as taking three forms: upsloping, horizontal, and downsloping. This is normally measured 0.06 to 0.08 mm from the J point (see Fig. 18-4) and is expressed in millimeters of depression. Onset and duration of such depression is also noted.

ST-segment depression occurs during fast heart rates

TABLE 18-2 PREDICTED MAXIMAL HEART RATE BY AGE, AND RECOMMENDED TARGET HEART RATES FOR SUBMAXIMAL EXERCISE TESTING

Note: Different investigators report different maximal heart rates but they are all within similar ranges.

MAXIMAL AND SUBMAXIMAL HEART RATES PREDICTED BY AGE*													
Ages (yrs)	20	25	30	35	40	45	50	55	60	65	70	75	80	85
Maximal heart rate (untrained)	197	195	193	191	189	187	184	182	180	178	176	174	172	170
90% of maximal heart rate	177	175	173	172	170	168	166	164	162	160	158	157	155	153

AVERAGES OF MAXIMAL HEART RATES PUBLISHED BY 10 AMERICAN AND EUROPEAN INVESTIGATORS†					
Ages by Decades	20–29	30–39	40–49	50–59	60–69
Maximal Heart Rate	190	182	179	171	164

RECOMMENDATION FOR TARGET HEART RATES BY DECADES OF AGE, SCANDINAVIAN COMMITTEE ON ECG CLASSIFICATION‡					
Ages by Decades	20–29	30–39	40–49	50–59	60+
Target Heart Rate	170	160	150	140	130

* Data from Sheffield and co-workers.[6]
† This data summarized in Figure 1, Exercise and Stress Testing Workshop Report, in the Myrtle Beach Conference Proceedings.[6]
‡ Data from the Scandinavian Committee on ECG Classification. 1967. The "Minnesota Code" for ECG classification. Adaptation to CR leads and modification of the code for ECG's recorded during and after exercise. *Acta Med Scand* Supp 481:1-26.
(Committee on Exercise. *Exercise Testing and Training of Apparently Healthy Individuals: A Handbook for Physicians*, p. 14) (Dallas, Tx., American Heart Association, 1972).[7]

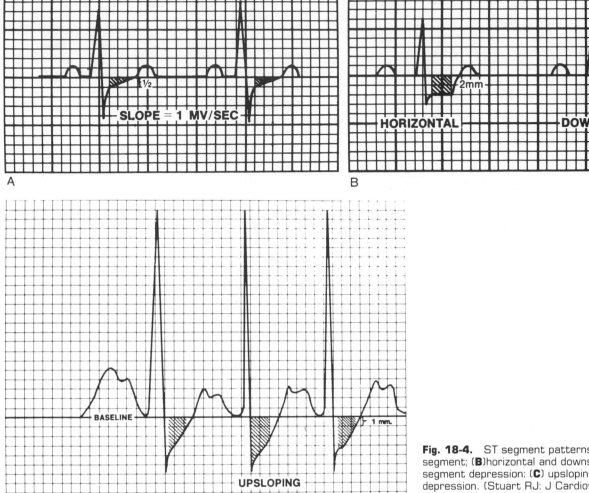

Fig. 18-4. ST segment patterns: (**A**) normal ST segment; (**B**) horizontal and downsloping ST segment depression: (**C**) upsloping ST segment depression. (Stuart RJ: J Cardiovasc Pulmonary Technol April/May:14—17, 1978)

and is commonly seen during normal treadmill testing. There is controversy about what degree of ST-segment depression constitutes an abnormal response. An abnormal response may be defined as one in which ST-segment depression is exaggerated relative to normal during exercise and delayed in returning to the normal ranges during recovery. Widely accepted criteria for an abnormal response consistent with ischemia are 1 mm (0.1 millivolt) or more of ST-segment depression with a horizontal, downsloping or upsloping ST-segment depression measured 0.06 to 0.08 second after the J point.

The significance of upsloping, or horizontal ST-segment depression with T-wave inversion continues to be debated. Infarction, ventricular aneurysm, bundle branch block, hypokalemia, ventricular hypertrophy, and interference with the oxygen-carrying capacity of blood due to anemia, pulmonary disease or hypoxemia, and such drugs as digoxin and quinidine may all influence the ST-segment response.

Exertional arrhythmia may occur during exercise testing or the recovery period. The test may demonstrate the presence of a potentially life-threatening arrhythmia that was undetected on the resting ECG, and may signal the risk of sudden cardiac death. At the moment, there is much concern about management of this finding, because there seems to be no treatment available to prevent this from recurring. Some persons have premature ventricular contractions at rest that are abolished or decreased as heart rate increases with exercise. The significance of this is not fully understood. Various arrhythmias may occur in normal persons as well as in persons with CAD, ventricular hypertrophy, hypertension, and respiratory disease.

The arrhythmias should be assessed in relation to their effects on cardiac output. For example, if a person's heart rate during recovery is 120 beats per minute and every other beat is a *premature ventricular contraction* that does not transmit arterial pulse peripherally, the effective heart rate is 60 beats per minute, and cardiac output may be severely limited.

Adequate baseline information needs to be obtained regarding the type and frequency of arrhythmia at rest in order to enable a comparison to be made between resting and exercise-induced arrhythmias. This is often accomplished by monitoring the patient with a Holter monitor (Chap. 17) prior to treadmill testing.

SENSITIVITY AND SPECIFICITY OF THE TEST

While the exercise test is useful in the diagnostic work-up of a person who may have CAD, ST segment responses do not always correlate with presence of disease.

Sensitivity is the percentage of true positive responses in an exercise tolerance test. Estimations of true positive responses to tests range from 40% to 60%, varying with the cardiac status of the person being tested.

Specificity indicates the percentage of persons with normal responses to exercise tolerance tests who do not have coronary artery disease and who give true negative responses. Specificity is about 90%. The false positive responders are persons with abnormal responses to the exercise tolerance test who have normal coronary arteries. When postexertional ST-segment depression is used as a criterion in the diagnosis of CAD, a problem arises with the responses termed false-negative. These responses are normal, but the person has CAD. Arteriography and subsequent history, when performed, have shown that approximately one-third of the population with CAD have normal but false-negative responses.

NURSING IMPLICATIONS

Nurses in many settings need to be aware of the results of exercise tests and to recognize that information from exercise tests can be used in teaching and counseling patients and the general public. As nurses assume an ever-expanding role in health screening and health maintenance, they take part in preparing patients for exercise tests, interpreting the results, and recommending adjustments in activity and lifestyle. In some settings, nurses may actually do the treadmill testing, with a physician present in the clinic or laboratory.

The nurse needs to be familiar with the setting and the procedures used in order to be able to give the patient a step-by-step description of what he can expect. This is usually helpful in alleviating misconceptions, doubts, and fears the patient may harbor. It is important that the patient come to the treadmill test as calm as possible, since high anxiety may obscure the usual physiological responses to exercise. After the patient has received an explanation from the physician of why a test will be helpful, he may require additional clarification and some extra time to consider the implications. During this time the nurse should be accessible to answer any further questions that may arise.

Instructions to the Patient

1. Get adequate rest and sleep the night before the test.

2. Have breakfast or lunch no earlier than two hours before the test. This meal should be light and without coffee, tea, or alcohol.

3. Wear loose-fitting absorbent clothing (shorts or pants) which are not made of nylon. (Women are further instructed to wear a bra and a short-sleeved, loose-fitting blouse that buttons down the front.) Wear well-fitting comfortable shoes (not slippers) with rubber soles. This is extremely important for stability, comfort, and ease of walking on a moving, inclined surface.

4. Discontinue any medications, as directed by the physi-

cian, before the test. However, some drugs may not need to be discontinued, depending on the purpose of the test. For example, if the physician's objective is to assess the efficacy of a specific drug, such as an antiarrhythmic agent, for preventing exertional arrhythmia, the drug should not be discontinued.

5. Avoid a hot shower for at least two hours after the treadmill test, since this may result in vasodilatation and potentially serious hypotension. The shower should be only tepid.

The specific treadmill results are usually explained by the physician. The nurse may use this information in exercise prescription. This application will be discussed in greater detail in Chapter 42.

REFERENCES

1. Acker J: Early ambulation of post-myocardial infarction patients, early activity after myocardial infarction. In Naughton J, Hellerstein HK (eds): Exercise Testing and Exercise Training in Coronary Heart Disease, pp 311–314. New York, Academic Press, 1973
2. Åstrand P-O: Quantification of exercise capability and evaluation of physical capacity in man. Progr Cardiovasc Dis 19:51–67, 1976
3. Bruce RA: Exercise testing of patients with coronary heart disease. Ann Clin Res 3:323–332, 1971
4. Bruce R, Guy G, Cooper M et al: Seattle heart watch: Initial clinical circulatory and echocardiographic responses to maximal exercise. Am J Cardiol 33:459–469, 1974
5. Bruce R, Kusumi F, Hosmer D: Maximal oxygen uptake and nomographic assessment of functional aerobic impairment in cardiovascular disease. Am Heart J 85:546–562, 1973
6. Committee on Exercise: Exercise Testing and Training of Individuals with Heart Disease or at High Risk for Its Development: A Handbook for Physicians. Dallas, American Heart Association, 1975
7. Committee on Exercise: Exercise Testing and Training of Apparently Healthy Individuals: A Handbook for Physicians, p 11. New York, American Heart Association, 1972
8. DeBusk R: The value of exercise stress testing. JAMA 232:956–958, 1975
9. Ellestad MH, Blomqvist CG, Naughton JP: Standards for adult exercise testing laboratories. Circulation 59:421A–430A, 1979
10. Hellerstein HK: Specifications for exercise testing equipment. Circulation 59:849A–853A, 1979
11. Irving JB, Bruce R: Exertional hypotension and postexertional ventricular fibrillation in stress testing. Am J Cardiol 39:849–851, 1977
12. Kitamura K, Jorgensen CR, Gobel FL et al: Hemodynamic correlates of myocardial oxygen consumption during upright exercise. J Appl Physiol 32:516–522, 1972
13. Master AM: The two-step test of myocardial function. Am Heart J 10:495, 1935
14. Robinson BF: Relationship of heart rate and systolic blood pressure to the onset of pain in angina pectoris. Circulation 35:1073–1083, 1967
15. Sivarajan ES, Bruce RA: Early exercise testing after myocardial infarction. Cardiovasc Nurs January–February 17:1–5, 1981
16. Sivarajan ES, Halpenny CJ: Exercise testing. Am J Nurs 79:2162–2170, 1979.
17. Sivarajan ES, Lerman J, Mansfield LW et al: Progressive ambulation and treadmill testing of patients with acute myocardial infarction during hospitalization: A feasibility study. Arch Phys Med Rehab 58:241–247, 1977
18. Sivarajan ES, Snydsman A, Smith B et al: Low-level treadmill testing of 41 patients with acute myocardial infarction prior to discharge from the hospital. Heart Lung 6:975–980, 1977
19. Stuart RJ: Significance of ST depression patterns in treadmill stress testing. J Cardiovas Pulmonary Tech April–May:14–17, 1978

19

Cardiac Catheterization

KATHERINE M. NEWTON, R.N., M.A.

With the enormous increase in the demand for cardiac surgery in the 1970s, cardiac catheterization has become an increasingly common procedure. The nurse's role in precatheterization teaching and postcatheterization care is well recognized.[9,21,48,51,65] In addition, the Inter-Society Commission for Heart Disease Resources Report for Optimal Resources for Examination of the Chest and Cardiovascular System recommends that a "specially trained nurse should be present to assist with the administration of medications and the preparation and observation of the patient."[46]

Cardiac catheterization has developed to its current state over a period of thirty years of clinical effort. The first documented cardiac catheterization was performed by Werner Forssman in 1929.[25] Guided by fluoroscopy, he passed a catheter into his own right heart through an antecubital vein. He then walked upstairs to the radiology department and confirmed the catheter position by x-ray radiograph. The techniques of right- and left-heart catheterization were developed during the 1940s and 1950s.[16,17,56] In 1953, the percutaneous techniques of arterial catheterization were introduced by Seldinger,[61] and in 1959, selective coronary arteriography was introduced by Sones.[63,64]

The purpose of this chapter is to describe cardiac catheterization procedures and their possible complications together with the nursing care given before and after catheterization, and the interpretation of data as they relate to coronary artery disease (CAD).

As practiced today, cardiac catheterization is a "combined hemodynamic and angiographic procedure undertaken for diagnostic purposes and consisting of the introduction of a catheter or probe into the vascular system and heart in order to perform certain measurements . . . draw blood samples, inject indicators or any combination thereof."[30] Although noninvasive techniques are assuming an important role, cardiac catheterization remains the most definitive procedure for the diagnosis and evaluation of coronary disease.

INDICATIONS

Cardiac catheterization is indicated in a wide variety of circumstances. The most frequent use of cardiac catheterization is to confirm or define the extent of suspected CAD. Anatomic and physiologic severity of the disease is determined and the presence or absence of related conditions is explored.

The indications for cardiac catheterization include:[30,35,69]

1. Known or suspected cardiac disease severe enough to require open-heart surgery
2. Chest pain of unknown etiology for which CAD cannot be ruled out
3. Stable but severe angina pectoris, with or without previous myocardial infarction (MI) and unresponsive to medical management
4. Unstable angina pectoris
5. Uncontrolled congestive heart failure (CHF), ventricular arrhythmias or cardiogenic shock associated with acute MI, septal perforation, ventricular aneurysm, or papillary muscle dysfunction
6. Abnormal electrocardiogram (ECG) in apparently healthy individuals whose occupations involve public

safety, such as airline pilots, air traffic controllers, and truck or bus drivers

7. When "the suspected cardiovascular condition may imply a drastic or at least unquestionable impact on the patient's life expectancy, life style, employment, or insurability or may lead to the institution of a potentially dangerous drug therapy, and there is reasonable doubt as to the accuracy of the clinical diagnosis."[30]

8. History of MI in previously asymptomatic patients 50 years of age or younger [69]

9. Strongly positive indications of CAD from stress-test ECG in individuals with mild or no angina pectoris.[69]

10. Evaluation of aortocoronary bypass graft patency.[69]

CONTRAINDICATIONS

With current levels of safety, there are relatively few contraindications to cardiac catheterization. Any correctable illness or condition, correction of which would improve the safety of the procedure, should be managed prior to catheterization.[35] Acute MI (in situations other than those listed under number 5 above), drug toxicities, and controllable arrhythmias are examples of such conditions. The minimum time that should elapse after MI before performing cardiac catheterization is approximately 3 weeks.[30] Cardiac catheterization is contraindicated in patients whose cardiac diagnosis is certain but in whom cardiac surgery would be deferred because of debilitating illness, including massive obesity or severe cardiomegaly.[30]

Anticoagulation as a contraindication is debated. Some investigators have reported an increase in hemorrhage and other complications in patients receiving anticoagulants,[9,52] whereas others feel that anticoagulants are safe and, at times, beneficial.[50,67] Grossman suggests that patients who are receiving oral anticoagulants should be placed on heparin, which is then withheld for 6 hours prior to catheterization. In patients who must remain on anticoagulants, the use of heparin for catheterization is advisable because its effects may be quickly reversed with protamine sulfate should cardiac perforation or hemorrhage occur.[35]

PATIENT PREPARATION

Patients are usually admitted for cardiac catheterization the day before the procedure. The physician doing the catheterization should explain the procedure and obtain informed consent.

Precatheterization orders usually include

1. Chest x-ray radiograph
2. Hematocrit, hemoglobin, complete blood count, differential
3. Urinalysis
4. Standard 12-lead ECG
5. Nothing by mouth after midnight (or after a liquid breakfast if the catheterization is to take place in the afternoon)

6. Preparation of catheterization site (hexachloraphene scrub of both groin and antecubital areas)
7. Patient to void before going to catheterization laboratory
8. Premedication

A variety of *premedication* is prescribed.[14,35,48] A sedative or sedative hypnotic is frequently ordered.[46] When coronary arteriography is planned, atropine sulphate is often ordered to help prevent the bradycardia and vasovagal reactions which often occur with contrast injections into the coronary arteries. Patients with a history of allergy to iodine-containing substances, such as seafood or contrast agents, may be given an antihistamine such as diphenhydramine hydrochloride before the procedure. The use of prophylactic antibiotics is not recommended.[35,46] If possible, propranolol is discontinued prior to catheterization because of its negative inotropic effect (reduced contractility). This effect could alter the hemodynamic data obtained.[48]

Patients may be sent to the laboratory with[35] or without artificial dentures and glasses. During cardiac output studies using the Fick method, dentures may help the patient obtain a more complete seal around the mouthpiece. The patient is also better able to enunciate when dentures are in place. Glasses allow the patient to view the videotape playback and help keep the patient better oriented to his surroundings.

Nursing Assessment and Patient Teaching

Nursing assessment and teaching are an important part of patient preparation.[29,48,53,65]

- The first step in the nursing assessment must be to evaluate the patient's emotional status and attitude toward catheterization.

- Is this the patient's first cardiac catheterization?

- What are the patient's apprehensions about the procedure?

- What has the patient heard about cardiac catheterization? (With the increase in cardiac catheterization and coronary artery bypass surgery, patients have sometimes heard horror stories from friends or acquaintances about catheterization experiences and may therefore need reassurance about the safety of the procedure.)

- What decisions are being faced? (Patients may be facing good or bad news about the absence or presence and extent of disease. Thus, the period before catheterization will most likely be a time of anxiety and fear for a variety of reasons. Discussion and reassurance may help to relieve some of these feelings.)

The nursing assessment should also include the patient's heart rate and rhythm, blood pressure, evaluation of the peripheral pulses of the arms and legs, and assessment of heart and lung sounds. The site for best palpation of the patient's dorsalis pedis and posterior tibial pulses should be marked on the skin. This information will be used for comparison in evaluating peripheral pulses after catheterization.

The catheterization laboratory confronts the patient with new sights, sounds, and experiences that may be intimidating and frightening. Teaching is aimed at preparing the patient for this experience. In some institutions patients are routinely given a tour of the laboratory the evening before the procedure.[57,65] A printed booklet that the patient can refer to is also helpful. The following points should be covered in patient teaching:

1. The patient will be given nothing by mouth for 8 to 12 hours before the catheterization and will be asked to void before leaving the unit

2. Premedication will be given, if prescribed, but the patient will be awake during the procedure

3. The patient should be instructed in deep breathing without bearing down and in coughing on request. With deep inspiration the diaphragm descends, preventing it from obstructing the view of the coronary arteries in some x-ray projections. Bearing down (the Valsalva maneuver) increases intra-abdominal pressure and may raise the diaphragm, obstructing the view. After the injection of contrast medium, coughing will be requested to help clear the material from the coronary arteries. The rapid movement of the diaphragm also acts as a mechanical stimulant to the heart and helps to prevent the bradycardia that may accompany the injection of contrast medium.

4. The appearance of the laboratory should be explained to the patient, including the general function of the equipment.

5. The patient will wear a gown to the laboratory; both arms will be slipped out of the gown for ECG electrode placement in the laboratory.

6. The patient will lie on a table that tends to be hard and may be turned like a cradle during the procedure.

7. The catheter insertion site(s) will be washed and shaved.

8. The expected length of the procedure should be explained to the patient.

9. The patient will be given a local anesthetic at the catheter entry site but the procedure is rarely totally pain free. The patient should let the staff know if the anesthesic begins to wear off so that more may be given. Pressing the patient's arm or thigh may help him to distinguish pain from pressure.

10. The patient may have "hot flashes" or experience nausea during injection of the coronary arteries with contrast medium.

11. The patient should report angina or other chest pain to the staff.

12. The patient should be told the expected length of bed rest after the catheterization.

In addition to these basic points, the nurse should invite questions about the procedure and discuss the patient's anxieties.

PROCEDURE

The Cardiac Catheterization Laboratory

The cardiac catheterization laboratory is a specially equipped radiologic laboratory for the study of children and adults with known or suspected heart disease. The equipment usually includes

1. A fluoroscope with image intensifier. Fluoroscopy is the continuous presentation of an x-ray image upon a fluorescent screen. This allows the viewing of structures in motion. Traditional fluoroscopy presents a very dim image which cannot be filmed and must be viewed in a darkened room. The image intensifier is a device which receives the fluoroscopic image and increases its brightness, permitting filming of the image as single frames or motion pictures (cinefluoroscopy) and viewing of the image with a television camera,[39] television screen, and videotape recorder.

2. A television camera for filming the fluoroscopic image on videotape for instant replay and for transmitting the image to a television screen so that catheter progression, contrast medium test doses, and so forth, can be monitored.

3. Single or biplane cameras linked to the image intensifier for filming of cineangiograms

4. A large x-ray film changer for recording serial frames on large x-ray film

5. An x-ray table—still or cradle type. With still tables the cameras are mounted on a C-arm which rotates around the patient. With cradle tables the camera is stationary and the patient is turned as necessary by turning the cradle.

6. Pressure transducers and a multichannel recorder

7. Equipment for cardiac output determination

8. Emergency drugs and equipment

9. A defibrillator

10. An ECG with continuous display on television screen or oscilloscope

11. A standby pacemaker including temporary transvenous or intrathoracic electrodes and a pulse generator

Catheterization Approach

Cardiac catheterization can be accomplished by direct exposure of the vein and artery, or by percutaneous methods (the Seldinger technique).[26] Direct exposure is used for the brachial artery and basilic vein, whereas the percutaneous method is used for the femoral artery and vein. All chambers and vessels may be entered using either approach, and both approaches have high degrees of safety.[35]

Although the physician's preference often dictates which approach is used, there are specific factors that may favor the use of one approach over the other. The *direct brachial approach* is indicated in cases of known vascular disease of the abdominal aorta, iliac or femoral arteries, or thrombotic disease of the femoral veins or inferior vena cava.[32,35] Severe hypertension, a wide pulse pressure due to aortic regurgitation, and anticoagulant therapy have been associated with an increased risk of bleeding when the percutaneous approach is used.[52] In cases of severe obesity, the direct approach is used for better visualization and control of bleeding.[35] A disadvantage of the direct approach is that it can be repeated only once or twice.[35] Arterial thrombosis occurs more frequently with this approach,[2] and the patient must return for removal of the sutures.

The *percutaneous femoral approach* is preferred because

of its speed and repeatability and because arteriotomy and arterial repair are not required. Its use is indicated in cases of decreased or absent radial or brachial pulse. When tight aortic stenosis makes retrograde catheterization difficult or impossible, the percutaneous transseptal approach is used for left-heart catheterization.[35]

Direct Brachial Approach. Figure 19-1 illustrates the direct brachial approach. A local anesthesia is used and the brachial pulse is identified. An incision is made over the medial vein for right-heart catheterization, or over both the vein and the brachial artery if right- and left-heart catheterizations are planned. The vein and artery are approached by blunt dissection, and are brought to the surface and tagged with surgical tape. Venotomy and arteriotomy are performed using scissors or a scalpel. The distal segment of the artery is flushed with heparinized saline to prevent clotting from distal arterial stasis. The catheterization is then performed.[34] After catheterization, the distal brachial artery is aspirated until a forceful backflow is achieved and injected with heparinized saline. The arterial incision is then sutured.[29,48] Some laboratories also recommend the routine use of a Fogarty catheter for removal of clots in the distal segment as protection against thrombosis.[28,30] The vein may be tied off, sutured, or used for an intravenous line.

Percutaneous Catheterization. Percutaneous catheterization is accomplished using the technique described by Seldinger (Fig. 19-2).[61] The same technique is used for both arterial and venous entry. The vessels are located and local anesthetic is given. The percutaneous needle has a sharp inner obturator. A small incision is made in the skin over the vein or artery and the needle is passed into the vessel. The obturator is then withdrawn and a guide wire is passed to the right atrium for right-heart catheterization, or to the descending aorta for either left-heart catheterization or coronary arteriography. The needle is then removed, the appropriate catheter is threaded over the guide wire, and the guide wire is removed. The catheter can be changed by reinserting the guide wire through the catheter, removing the catheter and threading the new catheter over the guide wire, which is then removed. This procedure can be repeated several times during the catheterization. Upon completion of the catheterization, the last catheter is removed, and pressure is applied at the site of entry.

Right-Heart Catheterization

Right-heart catheterization (Fig. 19-3) is performed for the purposes of (1) measuring right heart pressures; (2) evaluating the pulmonic and tricuspid valves; (3) sampling of blood oxygen content of right-heart chambers for detection of left-to-right shunt; (4) determining cardiac output by the direct Fick method; and (5) evaluating mitral valve stenosis of mitral valve insufficiency by transseptal approach.[19,21]

The right heart can be approached through the basilic vein and superior vena cava or through the femoral vein and the inferior vena cava. Once the superior or inferior vena cava is reached, the catheter is advanced through the right atrium, right ventricle, and pulmonary artery to a distal pulmonary vessel. Right ventricular irritability is not uncom-

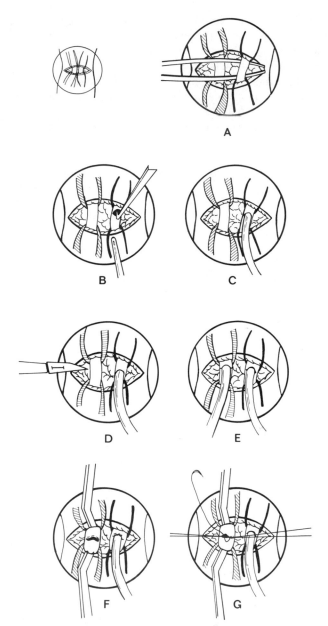

Fig. 19-1. Catheterization by direct exposure of brachial artery and vein. (**A**) Artery and vein are isolated and tagged proximally and distally. The vein rests over a "bridge" formed by straight forceps, giving better control. (**B**) The vein has been incised with scissors, and a catheter is about to be inserted with the aid of a plastic catheter introducer. (**C**) The right heart catheter has been passed through the vein. (**D**) The brachial artery is incised. (**E**) The left heart catheter has been passed. (**F**) The artery is prepared for repair. Concentrated heparinized saline solution is locked in the vessel by clamping the artery as far above and below the arteriotomy as possible. (**G**) The arteriotomy is closed. (After Grossman W: Cardiac Catherization and Angiography, chap. 2, p 16. Philadelphia, Lea & Febiger, 1976)

mon when the catheter tip passes through the right ventricle.[34] The course of the catheter is followed with pressure monitoring through the catheter and with fluoroscopy. When appropriate, blood samples are taken and pressures are recorded as the catheter is advanced. If left-heart catheterization is planned, the catheter may be left in the distal

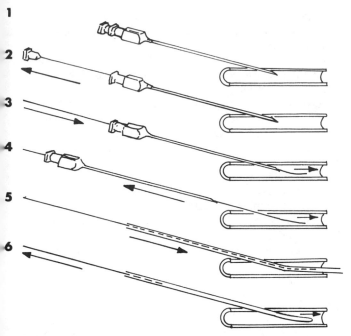

Fig. 19-2. Catheterization by the Seldinger technique. **1.** Arterial puncture; **2.** removal of stylet; **3.** insertion of guide wire through needle; **4.** withdrawal of needle, leaving guide wire in artery; **5.** introduction of catheter into artery over guide wire; **6.** withdrawal of guide wire. (After Schroeder, Daily: Techniques in Bedside Hemodynamic Monitoring, p 96. St. Louis, CV Mosby, 1976)

pulmonary vessel so that simultaneous left ventricular and pulmonary artery wedge pressure waveforms can be recorded.[34] As the catheter is removed, pull-back pressures can be recorded from the pulmonary artery to the right ventricle and from the right ventricle to the right atrium. These pressures are used for evaluating pulmonic and tricuspid valve function. Blood samples can also be taken as

Fig. 19-3. Right heart catheterization through the superior and inferior venae cavae. Catheters are in the wedge position. Chambers and vessels that may be catheterized are numbered: (**1**) Superior vena cava (**2**) Inferior vena cava (**3**) Right atrium (**4**) Right ventricle (**5**) Main pulmonary artery (**6**) Left pulmonary artery (**7**) Right pulmonary artery (**8**) Pulmonary artery wedge. (After Directions in Cardiovascular Medicine 8: Cardiac Catheterization, p. 25. Somerville, NJ, Hoechst Pharmaceuticals, 1973)

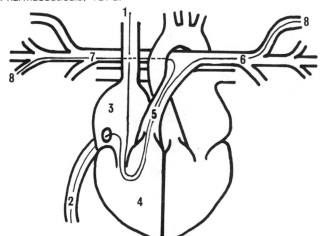

the catheter is withdrawn for detection of left-to-right shunts. If pulmonic or tricuspid valve disease is suspected, contrast can be injected for cineangiograms of the right atrium, right ventricle, or pulmonary artery.

Left-Heart Catheterization

Left-heart catheterization (Fig. 19-4) is performed for the purposes of (1) pressure measurement to evaluate mitral and aortic valve and left ventricular function; (2) angiography to evaluate mitral and aortic valve disease; and (3) left ventriculography.[19,21]

The two main approaches into the left heart are (1) retrograde entry, through the aortic valve by either the direct brachial or percutaneous femoral approach, and (2) transseptal entry, from the right atrium.[15,34] The progress of the catheter in both approaches is followed by fluoroscopy and pressure measurement. In the retrograde approach, the catheter is threaded along the aorta and through the aortic valve to the left ventricle. For mitral valve studies simultaneous pulmonary artery wedge and left ventricular pressures, or simultaneous left atrial and left ventricular pressures are recorded to evaluate pressure differences across the valve. In order to evaluate the aortic valve, pull-back pressure is recorded as the catheter is withdrawn from the left ventricle to the aorta. Cineangiography can be performed during contrast injection of the left atrium, left ventricle, or aortic root to further evaluate valve function.

A third, rarely used, approach to left ventricular catheterization is direct left-ventricular puncture (Fig. 19-4). This

Fig. 19-4. Left heart catheterization, showing the three approaches for catheterizing the left heart: (**A**) Retrograde approach across the aortic valve by way of the femoral or brachial artery; (**B**) transseptal approach through the right femoral vein and inferior vena cava across the atrial septum; (**C**) direct transthoracic puncture. (After Directions in Cardiovascular Medicine 8: Cardiac Catheterization, p 26. Somerville, NJ, Hoechst Pharmaceuticals, 1973)

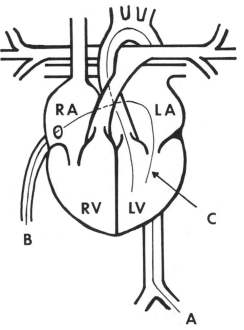

technique is employed only when the other techniques have been unsuccessful, most frequently in cases of severe aortic stenosis.[34,62] Complications occur more frequently with this approach; they include chest pain, cardiac tamponade, pneumothorax, pleural effusion, ventricular arrhythmias, vasovagal responses, and intramyocardial injection of contrast medium.[34,62]

Transseptal Left-Heart Catheterization

The transseptal approach to left-heart catheterization is indicated in the following situations:[15]

1. When left-heart catheterization has not been possible by the retrograde approach or when aortic stenosis suggests that the retrograde approach would be difficult
2. To obtain left-atrial angiograms to study mitral valve motion in mitral stenosis
3. To rule out pulmonary venous obstruction through simultaneous left-atrial and pulmonary artery wedge pressures
4. When pulmonary artery wedge tracings are inaccurate because of pulmonary hypertension or other pulmonary disease

This approach is contraindicated for patients on anticoagulant therapy because of the danger of hemorrhage and tamponade should myocardial puncture occur. When location of the necessary anatomic landmarks is impossible, as in patients who have severe chest deformities or a huge right atrium, or those who cannot lie flat, the transseptal approach is also inadvisable.

Transseptal catheterization is done through the right femoral vein, using percutaneous techniques and the needle described by Brockenbrough (Fig. 19-5).[10] The transseptal catheter is threaded into the right atrium over a guide wire, which is then removed. The transseptal needle, with a blunt stylet extending beyond its tip to prevent the needle from puncturing the catheter, is threaded up the catheter, the stylet is withdrawn, and the needle is connected to a pressure transducer. The catheter and needle are guided together to the fossa ovalis, where the needle is advanced to perforate the atrial septum. After perforation of the septum, left atrial pressure is recorded and a blood sample is drawn to confirm the catheter location. The catheter and needle are advanced well into the left atrium, the needle is withdrawn, and the desired studies are performed.[15]

Ventriculography

Ventriculography (Fig. 19-6) is performed by opacification of the ventricular cavity with contrast medium and, using either serial angiocardiography or cineangiocardiography (see Glossary), filming ventricular motion. Ventriculography can be performed to evaluate valve structure or function, to define ventricular anatomy, and to evaluate ventricular

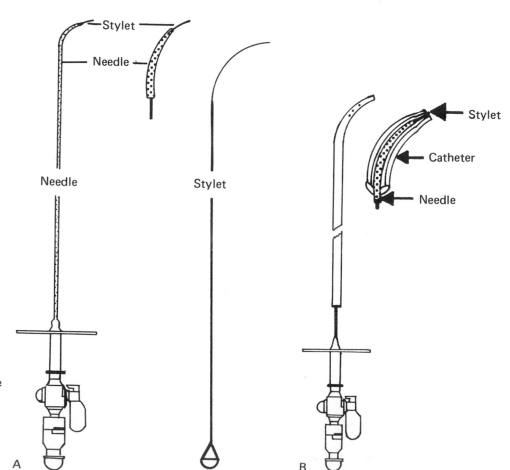

Fig. 19-5. Transseptal needle, stylet, and catheter. **(A)** Brockenbrough transseptal needle and Bing stylet; **(B)** transseptal needle, catheter, and stylet matched before insertion; (After Conti: In Grossman (ed), Cardiac Catheterization and Angiography, pp 35–36. Philadelphia, Lea & Febiger, 1976)

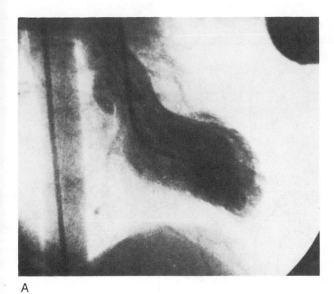
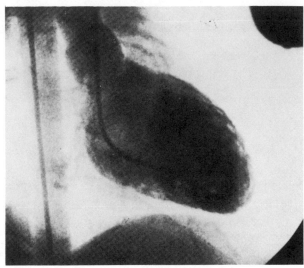

A
B

Fig. 19-6. Left ventriculogram. Two frames, RAO projection, demonstrating left ventricle in systole (**A**) and diastole (**B**). Anterior wall asynergy is visible. (After King, Douglas: In Hurst et al (eds): The Heart, Veins and Arteries, 4th ed, p 411. New York, McGraw–Hill, 1978)

function.[43] The last purpose has become increasingly important in the evaluation of patients for coronary artery bypass surgery.[40,54]

The catheter used for contrast injection during ventriculography must be capable of delivering a large amount of contrast medium in a short period (20 ml/sec for 3 or 4 seconds). Many types of catheters are available for ventricular injections. Catheters with side holes, with or without an end hole, are preferred to end-hole catheters because they have less tendency to recoil. Catheter stability is also important to minimize the risk of ventricular arrhythmias during injection.[43] Arrhythmias change the quality of contraction and thus make it impossible to use the ventriculograms for studies of ventricular function.

Contrast injection is accomplished by power injection. A test dose is first delivered by low-pressure injection to ensure proper catheter placement. The power injection is then made. Patients often feel a "hot flash" and experience nausea with the injection, and occasionally vomit.[43] Ventriculograms can be filmed, using either serial angiocardiography or cineangiocardiography. Single or biplane filming can be used. The principal complications of injection are arrhythmias, intramyocardial or pericardial injection of contrast medium, and embolism from injection of air or thrombi.

Coronary Arteriography

Coronary arteriography can be performed using either the direct brachial approach described by Sones,[63] or the percutaneous femoral approach of Judkins.[45]

With the *direct approach* (Fig. 19-7) a single catheter is manipulated for selective catheterization of both the right and left coronary arteries. During passage of the catheter from the subclavian artery to the aortic arch, the patient may be asked to shrug the shoulders, turn the head to the left, or take a deep breath to assist passage of the catheter.

With the *Judkins technique* (Fig. 19-8) two preformed, polyurethane catheters are used for catheterization of the right and left coronary arteries. The catheters are guided to the distal aortic arch over a Teflon-coated guide wire, the guide is withdrawn, and the catheter is filled with contrast medium and guided to the appropriate coronary artery.

Certain principles apply to both techniques. Premedications may include a sedative, an antihistamine, and atropine. The ventriculogram is usually performed before the coronary arteriogram because of the depressant effects of contrast medium on ventricular function.[14,29] Anticoagulant therapy (heparin) is administered intravenously prior to coronary arteriography to prevent complications from thrombus formation. The ECG and arterial pressure must be closely monitored. Approximately 3 cm to 8 cm of contrast medium is hand-injected. Cineangiograms of both the right and left coronary arteries are done in the left anterior oblique (LAO) and right anterior oblique (RAO) views (Fig. 19-9). Frontal, LAO, and RAO films from axial or lordotic angles may also be taken to view specific lesions more clearly. The patient may be asked to take a deep breath and hold it without bearing down, just prior to the injection, in order to clear the diaphragm from the field. After the injection, the patient is told to cough, which helps clear the contrast medium from the coronary arteries.[48] Cineangiograms of the coronary arteries may also be performed after the administration of nitroglycerin or other vasodilators to evaluate the effects on the coronary circulation, including the collateral vessels.[29,31]

Cardiac Output Studies

The three most commonly used methods of cardiac output (CO) determination are quantitative angiography, the direct Fick method, and the indicator dilution method. Of these, the first is the technique most frequently employed for CO determination when coronary arteriography and ventriculography are performed.

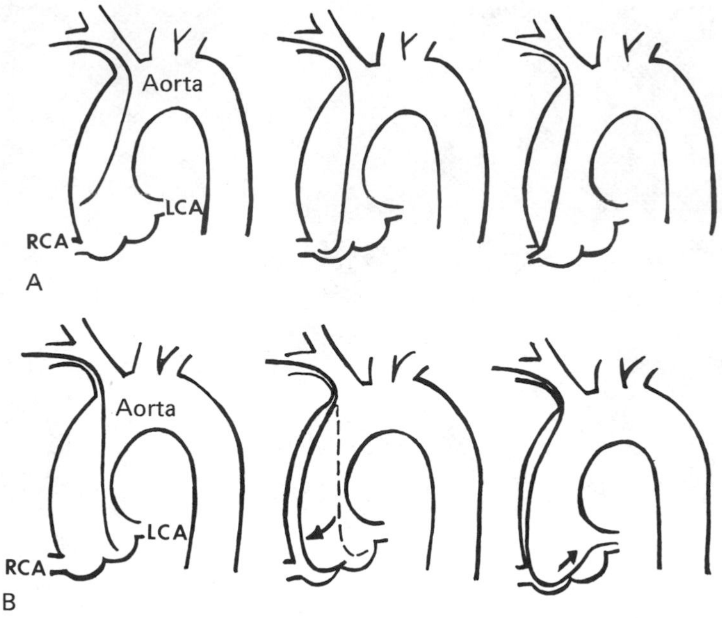

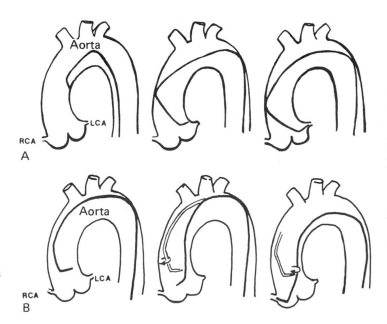

Fig. 19-7. Coronary artery catheterization by the Sones technique, (anterior view). **(A)** Catheter is introduced through the brachial artery to the aortic root and into the right coronary artery (RCA); **(B)** After right coronary catheterization, catheter is rotated and left coronary artery (LCA) is catheterized. (After Conti: In Grossman (ed), Cardiac Catheterization and Angiography, pp 126–127. Philadelphia, Lea & Febiger, 1976)

Fig. 19-8. Coronary artery catheterization by the Judkins technique. **(A)** Catheterization of LCA; **(B)** catheterization of RCA. (After Judkins: Radiol Clin North Am, 6:471, 1968)

Quantitative Angiography. In quantitative angiography, ventricular end-systolic and end-diastolic volumes are determined from the ventriculogram. Single or biplane films can be used. This method assumes the left ventricle to be of a given shape, most commonly elipsoidal.[4,20,59] The ventricular cavity is outlined at end-systole and end-diastole from the ventriculogram (Fig. 19-10). Correction factors are applied to compensate for the magnification and distortion that occur with filming, and then the true dimensions of the ventricle at end-systole and end-diastole are determined.[63] From these dimensions three semidiameters are determined for end-systole and end-diastole, from which the left-ventricular end-systole and end-diastole volumes are calculated.[20,59] Stroke volume is then obtained by subtracting the end-systolic volume from the end-diastolic volume. Computer programs that perform these computations are available.

The advantages and uses of quantitative angiography are multiple. The use of the ventriculogram eliminates the need for right-heart catheterization (which is required in the direct Fick method) and shortens the catheterization time. Because this method reveals the actual ventricular volumes, the ejection fraction can be obtained:

$$\text{ejection fraction} = \frac{\text{stroke volume}}{\text{end-diastolic volume}}$$

This parameter, not obtainable with other methods, is important in evaluating left-ventricular function. The CO obtained by quantitative angiography represents the total CO. In aortic or mitral insufficiency, some of this volume is regurgitant and does not take part in effective circulation. The direct Fick method (preferred over indicator dilution methods in valvular regurgitation) determines the forward cardiac output. These two methods can be used together to

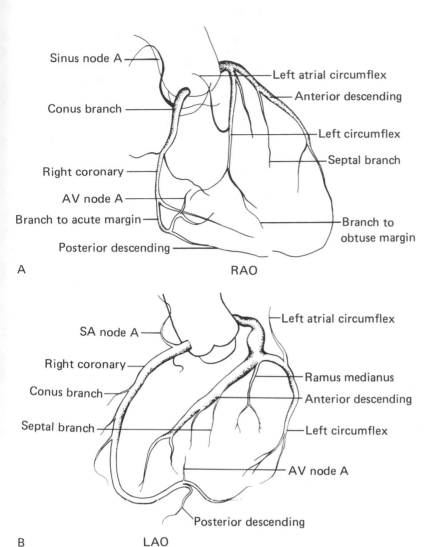

A   RAO

- Sinus node A
- Conus branch
- Right coronary
- AV node A
- Branch to acute margin
- Posterior descending
- Left atrial circumflex
- Anterior descending
- Left circumflex
- Septal branch
- Branch to obtuse margin

B   LAO

- SA node A
- Right coronary
- Conus branch
- Septal branch
- Left atrial circumflex
- Ramus medianus
- Anterior descending
- Left circumflex
- AV node A
- Posterior descending

Fig. 19-9. Spatial appearance of the coronary anatomy in the right anterior oblique (RAO) view (**A**) and in the left anterior oblique (LAO) view (**B**). (After Abrams and Adams: In Abrams (ed), Angiography, 2nd ed, p 402. Boston, Little, Brown & Co, 1971)

determine the regurgitant volume by subtracting the forward CO from the total CO.[58]

Direct Fick Method. The direct Fick method is based on the Fick principle, which states that the amount of substance taken up or released by an organ is equal to the product of the organ's blood flow rate and its arterial–mixed venous oxygen difference.[24] The direct Fick method for CO determination employs the lungs as the organ, oxygen (O_2) as the substance, and CO as the organ's flow. Thus, the formula for CO becomes

$$CO \ (l/min) = \frac{O_2 \ consumption \ (ml/min)}{\left[\begin{array}{c} pulmonary \ venous \ O_2 \\ content \ (ml/l) \end{array} \right] - \left[\begin{array}{c} pulmonary \ arterial \\ O_2 \ content \ (ml/l) \end{array} \right]}$$

Oxygen consumption is measured by having the patient breathe through a mouthpiece that allows inhalation of room air and expiration into a collecting bag (Douglas bag). Expired air is collected during a measured period of at least 3 minutes. The volume of expired air and its oxygen content are measured. Oxygen consumption is computed from the volume and oxygen content of expired air, the oxygen content of the room air, and the time over which the sample was collected.[3]

Pulmonary venous oxygen content can be measured from any systemic artery. Pulmonary arterial oxygen content is measured directly, as the most complete mixing of venous blood occurs in the pulmonary artery. The blood samples are drawn simultaneously during the period of expired air collection. A steady state must exist during the period of air collection because arterial and venous oxygen are sampled at only one point during the collection period.[69]

The mouthpiece must be tightly sealed, the nose clamped, and the collection period carefully timed.[3] The error by this method has been estimated at approximately 10%.[66] Accuracy is higher in patients with a wide arterial–mixed venous oxygen difference and low cardiac output, because there is less relative error in the calculation of the oxygen difference.[3]

Indicator Dilution Method. The indicator dilution method is based on the principle that if a known amount of an indicator is added to an unknown quantity of flowing liquid, and the concentration of the indicator is then measured downstream, the time-course of its concentration gives a quantitative index of the flow.[70] The thermodilution (Chap.

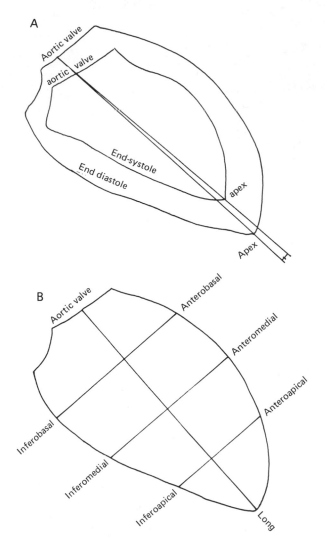

Fig. 19-10. (**A**) End-systolic and end-diastolic endocardiac silhouettes are superimposed with correction for apical rotation; (**B**) This reference system for ventricular wall motion analysis consists of a long axis and six transverse hemiaxes which quadrisect it at right angles. (After Yang: From Cardiac Catheterization Data to Hemodynamic Parameters, 2nd ed, pp 376–377. Philadelphia, FA Davis, 1978)

21) and dye dilution methods represent applications of this principle.[70] Applied to the circulatory system, the amount of indicator, its dilution within the circulation, and the time during which the first circulation of the substance occurs can be used to compute CO. The formula is

$$\frac{\text{cardiac output}}{\text{(l/min)}} = \frac{\text{quantity of indicator in milligrams}}{\bar{c} \times t}$$

where $\bar{c}$ is the mean concentration of indicator and t is the time in minutes between the appearance and disappearance of the dye at the observation site.[3] The indicator used must have the qualities of being easily detectable and must be water-soluble, nontoxic, and stable during the first circulation. Indocyanine green dye is the indicator most frequently used in the catheterization laboratory. Figure 19-11 illustrates the dye dilution method. A known quantity of dye is

rapidly injected into the venous circulation at the inferior or superior vena cava, right atrium, right ventricle, or pulmonary artery. The appearance of dye in the arterial circulation is monitored by withdrawal of arterial blood at a controlled rate through a densitometer, which continuously determines the concentration of the dye. This concentration is plotted as a dye-dilution curve by a recording device to which the densitometer is connected. The dye-dilution curve is recorded through the point of dye recirculation (Fig. 19-11B). The down slope of the initial curve beyond the point of recirculation is extrapolated mathematically.

This method is inaccurate in patients with valvular insufficiency, or with a very low CO, because the down slope of the curve is not exponential and the point of recirculation is not clear.[3]

The benefits of this method are (1) that it is performed over a short period and is therefore more likely to be recorded during a period of steady state and (2) that it is most accurate in patients with normal or high CO.

Hemodynamic Effects of Angiographic Contrast Medium

The hemodynamic effects of contrast agents have been well documented, although they are not fully understood. These effects, both immediate and long-term, vary with the site and quantity of the injection. Immediate effects are seen with both ventriculography and coronary angiography, whereas long-term effects are seen primarily with ventriculography or other injections that require large amounts of contrast medium.

Within three beats after left ventricular injection there are increases in left ventricular end-diastolic pressure and contractile force. These changes are thought to be a direct result of the increase in ventricular volume from the injection itself. Within five to eight beats there is a negative inotropic effect.[47] With coronary arteriography, immediate effects may include sinus bradycardia, a decrease in systemic arterial pressure, and T-wave changes on the ECG.[2,27] Usually these changes quickly revert to normal when the catheter is withdrawn from the coronary ostia and the patient coughs, clearing the contrast medium from the coronary arteries.[14]

The long-term effects of contrast injection reach their peak in 2 to 4 minutes and subside within 15 to 20 minutes. Contrast medium has a direct effect on arteriolar smooth muscle, causing vasodilation in skeletal muscle, decreasing peripheral vascular resistance and systemic arterial pressure.[27,55] The high osmolarity of contrast medium raises serum osmolality. In response, the plasma volume may increase as much as 300 ml when water moves from the extravascular to the intravascular space.[44] Both hematocrit and hemoglobin levels fall, while left-atrial and left-ventricular end-diastolic pressures increase in response to the increased intravascular volume. CO and stroke volume increase as a secondary response to the reduced peripheral vascular resistance (afterload) and increased filling volume and pressures (preload).[11,27,55]

Contrast medium acts as an osmotic diuretic.[11] The profound diuresis that often occurs following catheterization may result in water and saline deficits, which precipitate hypotension.[48] For this reason, patients should be given

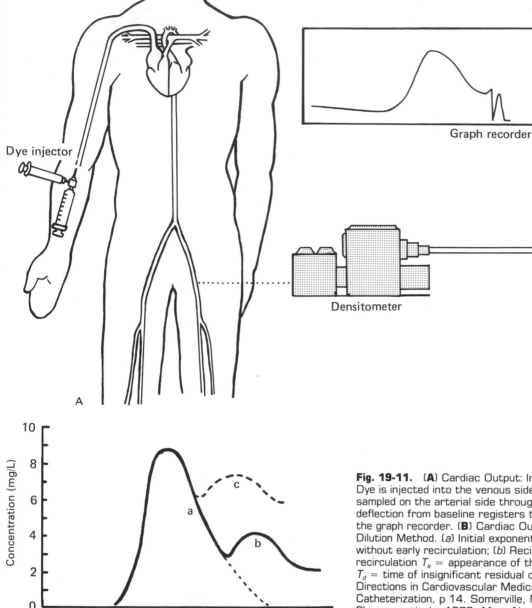

Fig. 19-11. **(A)** Cardiac Output: Indicator Dilution Method. Dye is injected into the venous side of the circulation and sampled on the arterial side through a densitometer. The deflection from baseline registers the cardiac output curve on the graph recorder. **(B)** Cardiac Output Curves: Indicator Dilution Method. (*a*) Initial exponential downslope in curve without early recirculation; (*b*) Recirculation normal; (*c*) Early recirculation T_a = appearance of the dye in the femoral artery T_d = time of insignificant residual dye concentration. (After Directions in Cardiovascular Medicine 8: Cardiac Catheterization, p 14. Somerville, NJ, Hoechst Pharmaceuticals, 1973; After Alpert et al: in Grossman (ed): Cardiac Catheterization and Angiography, p 69. Philadelphia, Lea & Febiger, 1976)

intravenous replacement, or be encouraged to drink liquids on returning from the laboratory.

THE NURSE IN THE CARDIAC CATHETERIZATION LABORATORY

Nurses working in cardiac catheterization laboratories fill many roles. In some laboratories the nurse scrubs and assists in the procedure; in others, she is responsible for monitoring pressure and cardiac rhythm, assisting with hemodynamic studies such as CO determination, and administering medications.[46,65] As indicated earlier, the nurse may visit the patient before the procedure to do teaching and help in preparing the patient.[13,65] In all cases, the nurse plays an important role in providing patient safety and comfort. The nurse ideally has a background in intensive or coronary care and a thorough knowledge of cardiovascular drugs, arrhythmias, sterile technique, cardiac anatomy and physiology, pacemakers, and the concepts of catheter flushing and clot and embolus formation and prevention.[13,46] Changes in the patient's emotional status, alertness, vocal responses, and facial expressions are important indices of his tolerance of the procedure. Alertness on the part of the nurse to these clues and early intervention with reassurance or appropriate medication may help to prevent more serious events, such as vasovagal reactions and coronary artery spasm.[13,48]

COMPLICATIONS AND NURSING CARE AFTER CARDIAC CATHETERIZATION

The nursing care of patients after cardiac catheterization is directed toward the prevention and detection of complications. Although complications are infrequent, they do occur (Table 19-1) and may be life-threatening. Early detection and intervention are essential in preventing permanent disability and death.

Cardiac catheterization is generally performed in patients who are at high risk for intercurrent complications such as MI, stroke, and sudden death. In studying these patients in the 48-hour period before and the 24-hour period after cardiac catheterization, Hilder and his colleagues found the death rate to be twice as high before catheterization (1.2%) as during and afterward (0.6%). Incidence of nonfatal complications was similar in the two periods, including peripheral arterial occlusion, MI, ventricular tachycardia and fibrillation, and cardiac tamponade. These "pseudocomplications" before catheterization underscore the high-risk nature of these patients.[42]

Complications tend to occur more frequently in laboratories that perform fewer cardiac catheterizations. Death, MI, and cerebrovascular thrombosis are more common with the percutaneous femoral approach than with the direct brachial approach. The percutaneous approach requires less experience on the operator's part because of the ease of placement of the preformed catheters, and thus may be used more frequently by operators with less experience. The percutaneous approach also requires the use of more catheters and a guide wire, resulting in increased clot formation as the wire is repeatedly withdrawn and inserted. Arterial thrombosis and reactions to the contrast medium are more frequent with the direct brachial approach than with the percutaneous approach.[2]

The most frequently occurring complication during catheterization is *arrhythmias*. Ventricular arrhythmias often occur in response to catheter manipulation or contrast medium injection and tend not to recur after the predisposing stimulus is removed. Atrial and junctional arrhythmias and varying degrees of blocks also occur in response to these stimuli.[2,48]

Allergic reactions to the contrast medium may occur. Sneezing, itching of the eyes or skin, urticaria, or other beginning signs of allergy are treated with antihistamines and corticosteroids.[7,13,48] Patients with known or suspected allergies to iodine-containing substances such as seafood should receive antihistamines prior to the procedure.[13,48]

Postprocedure Care

When the patient returns from the laboratory, he should be thoroughly assessed. Information about the approach used, the procedures performed and any complications experienced during the catheterization should be obtained from the physician, nurse, or technician. Table 19-2 lists typical postcatheterization protocols. These vary among institutions. The elements of the nursing assessment and intervention and potential findings are listed and explained below.

1. *Psychologic Assessment and Patient Teaching.* Patients are often tired, hungry, and uncomfortable when they return from the laboratory. They are usually relieved that the procedure is over and may already know the preliminary findings of their study. This news may have been good or bad and it is important to find out what the patient has been told and what this means to him. The patient may have questions about surgery or about what is expected of him now. Some are anxious or depressed. Giving the patient the opportunity to express his feelings about the procedure will help to calm and relax him. Reassure him, by describing the sensations he can expect to feel, such as thirst and the frequent need to urinate, even though he has had nothing to eat or drink for several hours. Reemphasize the need for bed rest and the necessity to keep the catheterized limb immobile. Let the patient know that frequent checking of vital signs is routine and not a cause for alarm.

2. *Circulatory Integrity of Entry Site.* The most fre-

TABLE 19-1 COMPLICATIONS OF CARDIAC CATHETERIZATION

	Brachial Approach*	Femoral Approach*	Both Approaches Combined
Major			
1. Thrombosis	0.40–1.67[2,7,12]	0.80–1.19[2,7]	1.20–1.44[2,7,32]
2. Stroke	0.03[2]	0.43[2]	0.20–0.23[2,7]
3. Myocardial infarction	0.22[2]	0.45–1.01[2,32]	0.03–0.60[2,7,48]
4. Death	0.13[2]	0.78[2]	0.15–0.60[2,9,42]
5. Hemorrhage	0.12[2]	0.07[2]	0.16[2]
Minor			
1. Hematoma	—	—	0.50[7]
2. Vomiting	—	—	3.80[7]
3. Headache	—	—	2.00[7]
4. Ventricular fibrillation	1.2[2]	1.15[2]	0.70–1.30[2,7,48]
5. Contrast medium reaction	0.22[2]	0.05[2]	0.14[2]
6. Pseudoaneurysm	0.06[2]	0.06[2]	0.06[2]

TABLE 19-2 POSTCATHETERIZATION PROTOCOLS

1. Check blood pressure, heart rate, temperature, and respiration every 15 minutes for 1 to 2 hours; then every 1 to 2 hours until stable.
2. Check catheterization site for bleeding, hematoma and swelling. Check circulatory status of affected limb(s), including pulses every 15 minutes for 1 to 2 hours, then every 1 to 2 hours until stable.
3. Resume diet and medications.
4. Give pain medication as needed.

Brachial Approach

5. Place patient on bed rest for 2 to 6 hours.
6. Release pressure dressing 30 minutes after return from laboratory and reapply Ace bandage to arm.
7. Instruct patient not to bend, hyperextend, or lie on the affected arm for 3 hours.
8. Instruct patient to remove Ace bandage in 48 hours and to return in 6 days for suture removal.

Femoral Approach

5. Place patient on bed rest for 12 to 24 hours.
6. Apply a sandbag to entry site for 4 to 6 hours.
7. Instruct patient not to flex or hyperextend the affected leg for 12 hours, and to use the bed control to elevate head of bed for use of bedpan.

(Adapted from Cogen R: Am J Nurs 76:401–405, 1976; Kelly AE, Gensini GG: Heart Lung 4:85–98, 1975; Thomas MM, Longo MR Jr: Aviat Space Environ Med 47:192–198, 1976)

quently occurring complication of cardiac catheterization is arterial thrombosis.[2,7,32] Thus, careful assessment of the entry site and of the limb are important elements of postcatheterization nursing care. The site should be checked for visible bleeding, swelling, or tenderness. The arterial pulse at the site and at points distal to it should be compared with pulses on the opposite limb and those recorded before the procedure. Capillary filling and the warmth of the limb should also be evaluated. Blanching, cramping, coolness, pain, numbness, or tingling may indicate reduced perfusion and must be carefully evaluated. A diminished or absent pulse is a sign of serious arterial occlusion.[7,13] The first step, if any of these signs occur, is to check the dressing. A dressing applied too tightly may result in arterial compression if swelling or hematoma occur. If this is not the case, the physician should be notified immediately, and steps should be taken to preserve the limb, as indicated.

Bleeding and hematoma are other complications at the entry site.[2,19] These may occur when a patient moves the limb too vigorously, or when the dressing is not sufficiently tight. Pressure should be applied, the dressing reapplied, if appropriate, and the physician notified. When pressure is applied at an arterial site, the pulse distal to the site should remain palpable.

3. *Blood Pressure Findings.* Evaluation of the blood pressure should include checking for *orthostatic hypotension* and *paradoxical pulse,* as well as comparing the pre- and postcatheterization values. Systolic hypotension of 10% to 15% below baseline is normal after cardiac catheterization.[53] Angiographic contrast medium acts as an osmotic diuretic, and patients frequently return with signs of volume depletion, including orthostatic hypotension. Patients are thus

kept on bed rest until fluid balance is restored with oral liquids or by intravenous replacement.

Hypotension may also be a response to the drugs given during the procedure. Vasodilators are often administered during coronary arteriography or ventriculography.[65] Protamine sulfate, which may be given to reverse the effects of heparin after coronary arteriography, has direct effects on the myocardium and vascular smooth muscle, resulting in vasodilation, bradycardia, and hypotension.[22,23] If the blood pressure is less than 75% to 80% of baseline, other causes such as blood loss or arrhythmias must be considered and assessed, and the physician notified.

TABLE 19-3 NORMAL ADULT VALUES FOR DATA COLLECTED DURING CARDIAC CATHETERIZATION

Pressures (torr)[33]	
Systemic arterial	
peak-systolic	100–140
end-stystolic	60–90
mean	70–105
Left ventricular	
peak-systolic	100–140
end-diastolic	3–12
Left atrial	
left atrial mean (or PAWP)	1–10
"a" wave	3–15
"v" wave	3–15
Pulmonary artery	
peak-systolic	15–30
end-diastolic	4–12
systolic mean	10–20
Right ventricular	
peak-systolic	15–30
end-diastolic	0–8
Right atrial	
mean	0–8
"a" wave	2–10
"v" wave	2–10
Left ventricular volumes[60]	**(biplane angiography)**
end-systolic volume (ml/m^2)	24–36
end-systolic volume (ml/m^2)	70–104
ejection fraction (%)	58–70
Resistance (dynes-sec-cm^{-5})[33]	
total systemic resistance	770–1500
total pulmonary resistance	100–300
pulmonary arteriolar (vascular) resistance	20–120
Flow[60]	
cardiac output (l/min)	4.0–8.0
cardiac index (l/min/m^2)	2.8–4.0
stroke index (ml/beat/m^2)	35–70
stroke volume (ml/min/m^2)	60–130
oxygen consumption (ml/min/m^2)	125
Oxygen saturation (%)[60]	
right atrium	60–75
right ventricle	60–75
pulmonary artery	60–75
left atrium	95–100
left ventricle	95–100
aorta	95–100

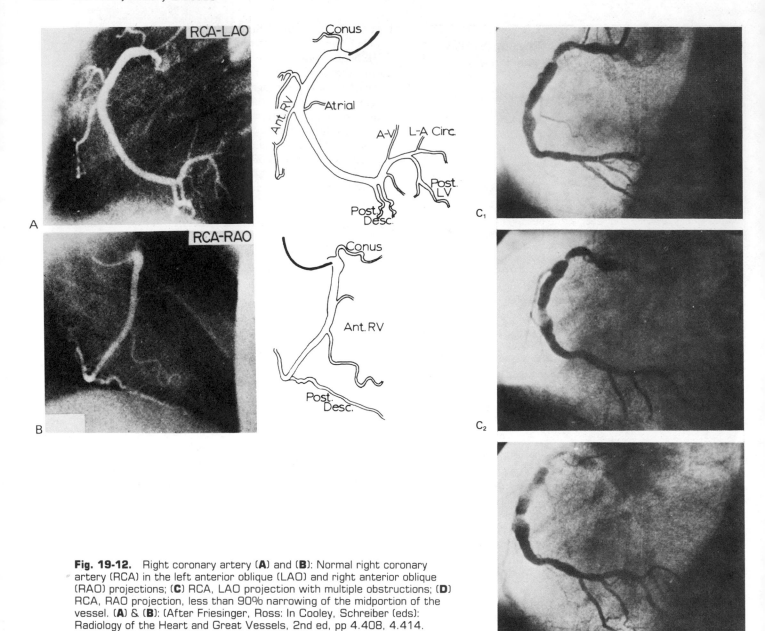

Fig. 19-12. Right coronary artery (**A**) and (**B**): Normal right coronary artery (RCA) in the left anterior oblique (LAO) and right anterior oblique (RAO) projections; (**C**) RCA, LAO projection with multiple obstructions; (**D**) RCA, RAO projection, less than 90% narrowing of the midportion of the vessel. (**A**) & (**B**): (After Friesinger, Ross: In Cooley, Schreiber (eds): Radiology of the Heart and Great Vessels, 2nd ed, pp 4.408, 4.414. Baltimore, Williams & Wilkins, 1967) (**C**) & (**D**): (Gensini: Coronary Arteriography, p 245. Futura, 1975)

Paradoxical pulse suggests pericardial tamponade, which may occur as a result of perforation of the myocardium. In patients with known perforation, this sign should be specifically assessed with each blood pressure measurement, and if it occurs, the physician should be notified.

4. *Heart Rate and Rhythm.* A mild sinus tachycardia (100 to 120 beats per minute) is not unusual following catheterization and may be a sign of anxiety, saline and water loss due to diuresis, or reaction to medication such as atropine. Fluids, time, and reassurance often bring the heart rate down to more normal levels.[65] Heart rates above 120 should be evaluated for other causes, such as hemorrhage, more severe fluid imbalance, fever, or arrhythmias. Bradycardia may indicate vasovagal responses, arrhythmias, or infarction and should be assessed by ECG and correlated with other clinical signs such as pain and blood pressure.[65]

5. *Temperature.* Early increases in temperature may occur because of the fluid loss that occurs with catheterization. More persistent elevations may indicate infection or pyrogenic reactions.

6. *Urinary Output.* Because angiographic contrast medium acts as an osmotic diuretic, patients have an increase in urine output for a short time after catheterization.

Other Possible Problems

Myocardial infarction, pulmonary embolism, stroke, and CHF are all potential complications after cardiac catheterization. The nurse caring for patients after cardiac catheterization should be aware of the signs and symptoms of these complications. Refer to Chapters 11, 27, and 28 for more complete discussion of these specific problems.

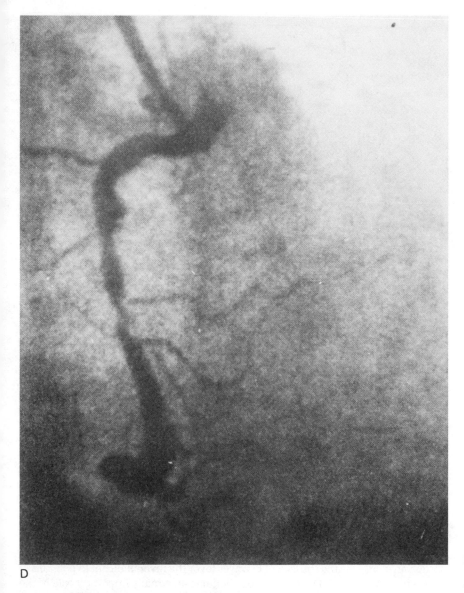

Fig. 19-12. Continued

D

INTERPRETATION OF DATA

Table 19-3 lists normal ranges for some of the data gathered during cardiac catheterization. The assessment of coronary artery disease involves evaluation of the coronary vasculature and left ventricular function.

The first step in evaluating the coronary cinearteriogram is determining whether the coronaries are unobstructed and free of lesions.[29] Each major artery is traced along its entire length, and branches and collaterals are noted and evaluated for irregularities or narrowing.[69] When occlusion is present, the degree of disease and the suitability of the artery for revascularization are of primary concern. The American Heart Association Ad Hoc Committee for Grading of Coronary Artery Disease[5] has recommended the following system for grading of occlusion:

1. Normal: no decrease in lumen diameter
2. 25%:Decrease in lumen diameter up to 25%
3. 50%: Decrease in lumen diameter of 26% to 50%
4. 75%: Decrease in lumen diameter of 51% to 75%
5. 90%: Decrease in lumen diameter of 76% to 90%

6. 99%: Hair-width lumen with greater than 90% narrowing
7. 100%: Total occlusion

In addition to grading the occlusion, the condition of the distal artery must be evaluated. The distal artery may be identified by antegrade or collateral flow, and its caliber and suitability as a recipient for bypass grafting evaluated. Arteries with high degrees of peripheral involvement are less suitable for bypass grafting. The proximity of the occlusion determines the amount of myocardium in jeopardy. A subjective evaluation of the degree of arterial flow is made by observing the time required for perfused arteries to fill and clear. Contrast medium clears faster with higher flow rates. Intermittent luminal obstruction due to systolic constriction from encircling muscle bands or to coronary artery spasm is also observed, and its degree, distribution, and pattern evaluated. If bypass grafts have been injected, they are evaluated in the same manner for patency, flow indices, and the condition of the perfused artery.[69] Figures 19-12 and 19-13 demonstrate normal and abnormal cineangiograms of the right and left coronary arteries.

Evaluation of myocardial function is an important part

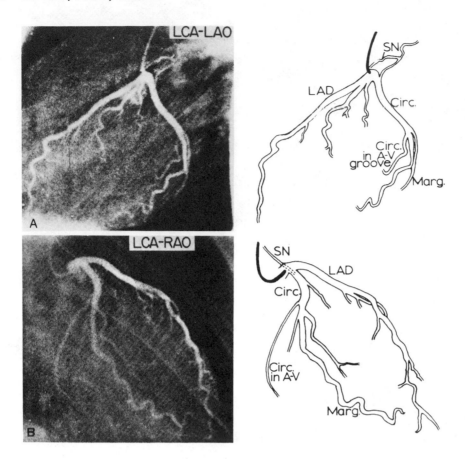

Fig. 19-13. Left coronary artery. (**A**) and (**B**) Normal left coronary artery (LCA) in LAO and RAO projections; (**C**) severe left main lesion shown in LAO projection; (**D**) left coronary artery, RAO projection showing 80% narrowing of the left anterior descending artery. (**A**) & (**B**): (After Friesinger, Ross: In Cooley, Schreiber (eds): Radiology of the Heart and Great Vessels, 2nd ed, p 4.409. Baltimore, Williams & Wilkins, 1967) (**C**) & (**D**) (After King, Douglas: In Hurst (ed): The Heart, Arteries, and Veins, 4th ed, pp 405, 411. McGraw–Hill, 1978)

of the evaluation of coronary artery disease. Patterns of ventricular contraction and the ejection fraction are determined from the ventriculogram. Patterns of ventricular contraction are evaluated by superimposing the systolic and diastolic outlines of the left ventricular chamber in the RAO projection along a long axis. This is drawn from the apex to the aortic valve commissure aligned at the aortic valve or the midpoint of the long axis (Fig. 19-10A). The anterior, inferior, and apical regions of the left ventricle can be examined in the RAO projection. Other methods are used for further subdividing the areas of the ventricular wall by region or by transverse hemiaxis (Fig. 19-10B). The degree of contraction is then evaluated in each region or at each hemiaxis.[69] The ventricular contractile state may be defined as normal, or classified by one or more of five types of asynergy (Fig. 19-14).[41]

1. Hypokinesis—a generalized reduction in myocardial contraction
2. Asyneresis (localized hypokinesis)—a localized or discrete area of reduced wall motion
3. Akinesis—the total absence of wall motion in a discrete area
4. Dyskinesis—paradoxical systolic expansion of a portion of the left ventricular wall
5. Asynchrony—a disturbance in the temporal sequence of left ventricular wall contraction

The reversibility of these contraction abnormalities is an important consideration in the decision for surgery. This can be evaluated with ventriculography after administration of nitroglycerin[38] or catecholamines, or by observing postextrasystolic potentiation following premature contractions.[36] If these maneuvers or events result in improved contractility, revascularization may also improve contractility.[69] Improved function is more common with hypokinesis than with akinesis or dyskinesis.[6,8,57] The presence of collateral vessels and the lack of Q waves favor the reversibility of hypokinesis.[6]

The ejection fraction has an equally important role in the evaluation of coronary artery disease. Since the ejection fraction represents the ratio of the stroke volume to the end-diastolic volume, a decreasing ejection fraction may represent either a decrease in stroke volume or an increase in end-diastolic volume. The latter situation represents the compensatory mechanism for maintaining cardiac output as myocardial function decreases. Thus, the ejection fraction is a reflection of the degree to which contraction abnormalities have compromised myocardial performance. Contraction abnormalities involving 10% to 20 % of the left ventricular outline do not usually change ejection fraction or end-diastolic volume. At 25% to 30% involvement, the end-diastolic volume usually rises with a resultant decrease in ejection fraction.[49] It has been shown that little change in ventricular function occurs with bypass surgery in patients with normal ventricular function or with a markedly reduced ejection fraction and severe akinesis or dyskinesis.[6,69] Surgery may result in improved ventricular function in patients with a slight-to-moderate decrease in ejection fraction and akinesis or hypokinesis.[36,68,69] Similarly, patients studied after bypass surgery show decreases in ejection fraction when grafts are occluded.[8,68]

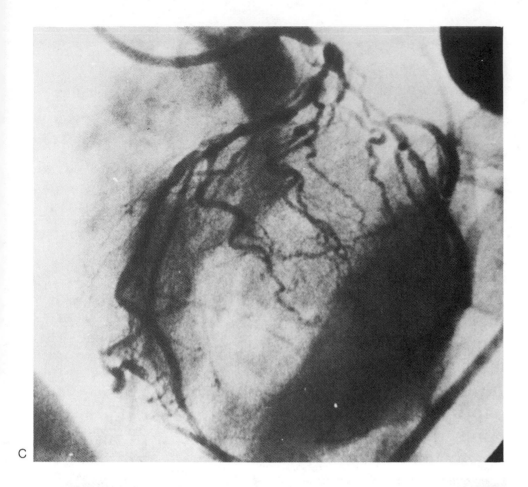

C

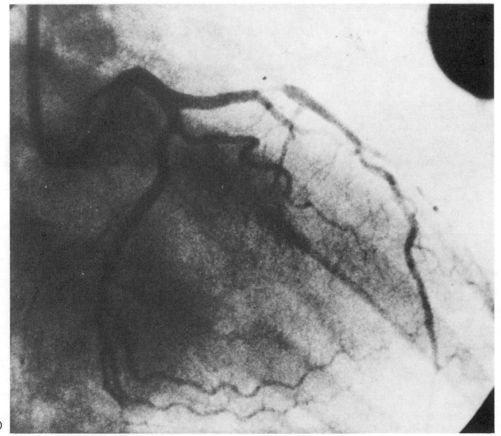

D

Fig. 19-13. Continued

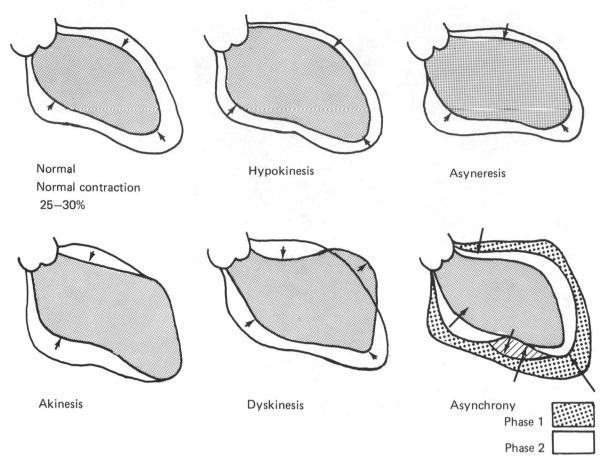

Fig. 19-14. Normal contraction and contraction abnormalities viewed in the RAO projection. *Arrows* illustrate motion from end diastole to end systole. (After Herman: New Engl J Med, 277:225, 1967)

REFERENCES

1. Abrams HL, Adams DF: Coronary arteriography: I. Principles, procedures, interpretation, and applications. In Abrams H (ed): Angiography, 2nd ed, pp 401–428. Boston, Little Brown & Co, 1971
2. Adams DF, Fraser DB, Abrams HL: The complications of coronary arteriography. Circulation 48:609–618, 1973
3. Alpert JS, Dexter L: Blood flow measurement: The cardiac output. In Grossman W (ed): Cardiac Catheterization and Angiography, pp 61–72. Philadelphia, Lea & Febiger, 1976
4. Arvidsson H: Angiocardiographic determination of left ventricular volume. Acta Radiol 56:321–339, 1961
5. Austen WB, Edwards RL, Frye RL et al: A reporting system on patients evaluated for coronary artery disease: Report of the ad hoc committee for grading of coronary artery disease, council on cardiovascular surgery, American Heart Association. Circulation 51:7–40, 1975
6. Banka VS, Bodenheimer MM, Helfant RH: Determinants of reversible asynergy, the native coronary circulation. Circulation 52:810–816, 1975
7. Beckmann CH, Dooley B: Complications of left heart angiography. Circulation 41:825–832, 1970
8. Bourassa MB, Lisperance J, Campeau L et al: Fate of left ventricular contraction following aortocoronary venous grafts, early and late postoperative modifications. Circulation 46:724–730, 1972
9. Braunwald E, Swan HJC: Co-operative Study on Cardiac Catheterization. New York, American Heart Association, 1968
10. Brockenbrough EC, Braunwald E: A new technique for left ventricular angiography and transseptal left heart catheterization. Am J Cardiol 6:1062–1064, 1960
11. Brown R, Rahimtoola SH, Davis GD et al: The effect of angiocardiographic contrast medium on circulatory dynamics in man. Circulation 31:234–240, 1965
12. Campion BC, Frye RL, Pluth JR et al: Arterial complications of retrograde brachial arterial catheterization. Mayo Clinic Proc 46:589–592, 1971
13. Cogen R: Preventing complications during cardiac catheterization. Am J Nurs 76:401–405, 1976
14. Conti CR: Coronary arteriography. In Grossman W (ed): Cardiac Catheterization and Angiography, pp 122–130. Philadelphia, Lea & Febiger, 1976
15. Conti CR: Percutaneous approach and transseptal catheterization. In Grossman, W (ed): Cardiac Catheterization and Angiography, pp 25–40. Philadelphia, Lea & Febiger, 1976
16. Cournand AF, Ranges CS: Catheterization of the right auricle in man. Proc Soc Exp Biol Med 46:462, 1941
17. Cournand AF, Riley RL, Breed ES et al: Measurement of cardiac output in man using the technique of catheterization of the right auricle or ventricle. J Clin Invest 24:106–116, 1945
18. Dalen JE: Shunt detection and management. In Grossman W (ed): Cardiac Catheterization and Angiography, pp. 96–107. Philadelphia, Lea & Febiger, 1976
19. Directions in Cardiovascular Medicine, #8, Cardiac Catheterization. Somerville, Hoeschst Pharmaceuticals Inc., 1973
20. Dodge HT, Hay RE, Sandler H: An angiographic method for directly determining left ventricular stroke volume in man. Circ Res 11:739–745, 1962
21. Edwards M, Payton V: Cardiac catheterization, teaching and technique. Nurs Clin North Am 11:271–281, 1976

22. Egerton WS: The anti-heparin, anticoagulant and hypotensive properties of hexadimethrine and protamine. Lancet 2:632–635, 1961
23. Fadali MA, Ledbetter M, Papacostas CA et al: Mechanisms responsible for the cardiovascular depression effect of protamine. Ann Surg 180:232–235, 1974
24. Fick A: Uber die Messung des Blutquantums in den Herzventrikeln. S.B. Physmed, Wurzburg, p 16, 1870
25. Forssman W: Die sondierung des rechter herzens. Klin Wsch 8:2085, 1929
26. Friesinger GC, Ross RS: Coronary angiography: Review of technique and a report of experience with selective angiography. In Cooley R, Schreiber M (eds): Coronary Angiography, Radiology of the Heart and Great Vessels, 2nd ed, pp 4.403–4.423. Baltimore, Williams & Wilkins, 1967
27. Friesinger GC, Schaffer J, Criley M et al: Hemodynamic consequences of the injection of radiopaque material. Circulation 31:730–740, 1965
28. Gensini G: Coronary Arteriography. Mount Kisco, Futura Publishing Company, 1975
29. Gensini G: Coronary arteriography, role in myocardial revascularization. Postgrad Med 63:121–138, 1978
30. Gensini G: Indications for cardiac catheterization, angiography and coronary arteriography. Geriatrics 30:63–68, 1975.
31. Gensini G, Kelly AE, Da Costa BCB et al: Quantitative angiography: The measurement of coronary vasomobility in the intact animal and man. Chest 60:522–530, 1971
32. Green GS, McKinnon M, Rosch J et al: Complications of selective percutaneous transfemoral coronary arteriography and their prevention. Circulation 45:552–557, 1972
33. Grossman W (ed): Cardiac Catheterization and Angiography. Philadelphia, Lea and Febiger, 1976
34. Grossman W: Cardiac catheterization by direct exposure of artery and vein. In Grossman W (ed): Cardiac Catheterization and Angiography, pp 13–24. Philadelphia, Lea & Febiger, 1976
35. Grossman W: Introduction. In Grossman W (ed): Cardiac Catheterization and Angiography, pp 3–10. Philadelphia, Lea & Febiger, 1976
36. Hamby R, Aintablian A, Wisoff G et al: Response of left ventricle in coronary artery disease to postextrasystolic potentiation. Circulation 51:428–435, 1975
37. Hamby RI, Jabiah F, Aintablion A et al: Left ventricular hemodynamics and contractile pattern after aortocoronary bypass surgery. Am Heart J 88:149–159, 1974
38. Helfant RH, Pine R, Meister SG et al: Nitroglycerin to unmask reversible asynergy, correlation with post coronary bypass ventriculography. Circulation 50:108–113, 1974
39. Hendee WR, Edward CL, Rossi RP: Radiologic Physics, Equipment and Quality Control. Chicago: Year Book Medical Publishers, 1977
40. Herman MV, Gorlen R: Implications of left ventricular asynergy, Am J Cardiol 23:538–547, 1969
41. Herman MV, Heinle RA, Klein MD et al: Localized disorders in myocardial contraction, asynergy and its role in congestive heart failure. N Engl J Med 277:222–232, 1967
42. Hildner JJ, Javier RP, Ramaswamy K et al: Pseudo complications of cardiac catheterization. Chest 63:15–17, 1973
43. Hood WP, Rackley CE: Ventriculography. In Grossman, W (ed): Cardiac Catheterization and Angiography, pp 111–121. Philadelphia, Lea & Febiger, 1976
44. Iseri LI, Kaplan MA, Evans MJ et al: Effect of concentrated contrast media during angiography on plasma volume and plasma osmolality. Am Heart J, 69:154–158, 1965
45. Judkins MP: Percutaneous transfemoral selective coronary arteriography. Radiol Clin North Am 6:467–492, 1968
46. Judkins MP, Abrams HL, Bristow JD et al: Report of the intersociety commission for heart resources, optimal resources for examination of the chest and cardiovascular system. Circulation 52:A1–A37, 1976
47. Karliner MS, Bouchard RJ, Gault JH: Hemodynamic effects of angiographic contrast material in man, a beat by beat analysis. Br Heart J 34:347–355, 1972
48. Kelly AE, Gensini GG: Coronary arteriography and left heart studies. Heart Lung 4:85–98, 1975
49. Kennedy JW: Myocardial function in coronary artery disease. Cardiovasc Nurs 12:23–27, 1976
50. Kloster RE, Bristow JD, Seaman AJ: Cardiac catheterization during anticoagulant therapy. Am J Cardiol 28:675–678, 1971
51. Lamberton MM: Cardiac catheterization: Anticipatory nursing care. Am J of Nurs 71:1718–1721, 1971
52. Mortensen JD: Clinical sequalae from arterial needle puncture, cannulation and incision. Circulation 35:1118–1123, 1967
53. Piazzo D, Jackson BS: Nursing decisions, experiences in clinical problem solving: Sara N., An anxious patient undergoing cardiac catheterization. RN, 39:41–47, 1976
54. Rackley CE, Dear HD, Baxley WA et al: Left ventricular chamber mass, volume and function in severe coronary artery disease. Circulation 41:605–613, 1970
55. Rahimtoola SH, Duffy JP, Swan HJC: Hemodynamic changes associated with injection of angiographic contrast medium in assessment of valvular lesions. Circulation 33:52–57, 1966
56. Richards DW: Cardiac output by catheterization technique in various clinical conditions. Fed Proc: Fed Am Soc Exp Biol, 4:215–220, 1945
57. Saltiel J, Lesperanel J, Bourassa MG et al: Reversibility of left ventricular dysfunction following aorto-coronary bypass grafts. Am J of Roentgenology 110:739–746, 1974
58. Sandler H, Dodge HT: Quantitation of valvular insufficiency by angiocardiography in man. Clin Res 8:191, 1960
59. Sandler H, Dodge HT: The use of single plane angiocardiograms for the calculation of left ventricular volume in man. Am Heart J 75:325–334, 1968
60. Schroeder JS, Daily EK: Techniques in Bedside Hemodynamic Monitoring. St. Louis, The CV Mosby Company, 1976
61. Seldinger SI: Catheter replacement of the needle in percutaneous arteriography. Acta Radiol 29:368–376, 1953
62. Semple T, McGuinness JB, Gardner H: Left heart catheterization by left ventricular puncture. Br Heart J 30:402–406, 1968
63. Sones FM, Shirey EK: Cine coronary arteriography. Mod Concepts Cardiovasc Dis 31:735–738, 1962
64. Sones FM, Shirey EK, Prondflt WL et al: Cine-coronary arteriography. Circulation 20:773, 1959
65. Thomas MM, Longo MR Jr: Care of patients after cardiac catheterization. Aviat Space Environ Med 47:192–198, 1976
66. Visscher MB, Johnson JA: The Fick principle: Analysis of potential errors in its conventional application. J Appl Physiol 5:635–638, 1953
67. Walker WJ, Mundell SL, Broderick HG et al: Systemic heparinization for femoral percutaneous angiography. N Engl J Med 288:826–828, 1973
68. Wolf NW, Kreulen TH, Bove AA et al: Left ventricular function following coronary bypass surgery. Circulation 58:65–70, 1978
69. Yang SS, Bentivoglio LG, Maranhao V, Goldberg H: From Cardiac Catheterization Data to Hemodynamic Parameters, 2nd ed. Philadelphia. FA Davis, 1978
70. Yipintsoi T, Wood EH: The history of circulatory indicator dilution. In Bloomfield DA (ed): Dye Curves: The Theory and Practice of Indicator Dilution. Baltimore, University Park Press, 1974

20

Echocardiography, Radioisotope Studies, and Phonocardiography

MARGARET HALL, R.N., M.D.

Over the years, there has been a great interest in developing reliable and simple tests of the heart and blood vessels, which, in contrast to cardiac catheterization (Chap. 19), do not in themselves present risk of morbidity or mortality to the patient. This is even more important for critically ill patients who tolerate the hemodynamic manipulations or potential complications of invasive studies much less well than those who are not ill. Other important qualities sought in such tests include reduced cost and time and ease of serial repetitions.

Several indirect measurements of cardiovascular status are already in common use. Examples of universally employed and highly analyzed noninvasive tests include the electrocardiogram (ECG) (Chap. 17) and the indirect auscultatory method of blood pressure measurement (Chap 14). Some techniques used more extensively in past years now enjoy a limited popularity. One such technique is ballistocardiography, a test developed to measure cardiac output. This test measures the body's recoil from the ejection of blood with systole. This recoil is similar to a rifle's recoil from the ejection of the bullet. Another test used only on a limited basis in the clinical setting is apexcardiography. It is an attempt to display objectively the impression of left ventricular performance that the experienced clinician can gain from the palpation of the size and contour (in time) of the point of maximum impulse (Chap. 14). Some tests, such as the calculation of systolic time intervals and phonocardiography, continue to serve research or educational purposes. Yet other tests, such as Doppler peripheral vascular imaging, remain in their infancy with respect to widespread application in the identification and quantification of vascular disease.

Two relatively new methods of noninvasive heart examination are the echocardiogram and cardiac radioisotope studies. The major portion of this chapter will be devoted to echocardiography, because it has gained the most widespread clinical acceptance in the evaluation of heart disease. Phonocardiography will also be discussed briefly.

The professional nurse contributes most when she can answer the patient's questions: How is the test done? Why is the test being done? What can it show? Is it painful or uncomfortable? The answers to these questions, rest on an understanding of both the patient's condition and the principles of the examination.

It is useful for the nurse to recognize the important contribution of the trained technician in obtaining diagnostic examinations. These technicians must possess a sophisticated knowledge of cardiac anatomy, physiology, and pathophysiology, and must understand the physics and mechanics that have contributed to the development of the techniques and the machinery. It is also helpful to observe the examination in progress with an opportunity to discuss structure identification with the technician or the physician; this can contribute much to one's understanding of anatomy, physiology, and pathophysiology (Fig. 20-1).

ECHOCARDIOGRAPHY

The study of ultrasound, the designation given to sound waves of higher frequencies than the human ear can detect, began nearly a century ago. The development of SONAR (from sound navigation ranging) probably represents the

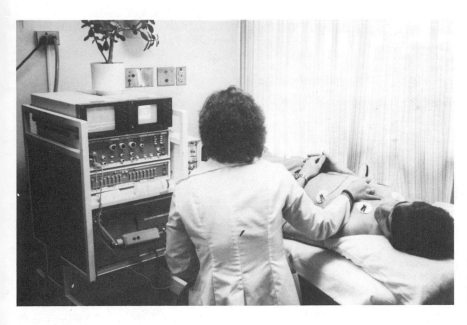

Fig. 20-1. Position of patient and examiner for echocardiogram. Portable machinery permits the examination at bedside with no loss in quality.

first widespread use of pulsed ultrasound for remote object detection.

Technical Aspects

Echocardiography operates very much like SONAR; this analogy is often useful in explaining the test to patients. The ultrasound transducer serves both as a sender of sound waves and a detector of reflected sound waves. These high-frequency (2.5 mHz) waves are generated by the application of changing voltage to a substance called a piezoelectric crystal. This crystal deforms just slightly under the influence of the voltage, and a wave is generated. The waves are generated in very short bursts (for example, 1 microsecond) after which the transducer operates as a receiver for the remainder of 1 millisecond (msec). This is followed by another short burst of sound (Fig. 20-2). These sound waves cannot be heard or felt by the patient, and produce no known damaging effects on the tissues.

The speed of sound through any medium is determined by the density of the medium; denser media transmit sound faster than less dense media. Whenever the ultrasound wave strikes a change in tissue density (such as that between blood and muscle or between soft tissue and bone) a portion of the wave is reflected back to the transducer. The density differences within the body are relatively minor. This means that the speed of the sound wave can be assumed to be nearly constant, and therefore the time between sound emission and sound detection can be used to calculate the distance between the transducer and the reflected tissue interface.

When the ultrasound signal returns to the crystal, it once again deforms it and thereby generates voltage. This voltage

is detected by the echocardiograph and displayed on an oscilloscope or on recording paper.

The transducer has a relatively small diameter (about 1 cm). Its sound "beam" is like a flashlight beam that one might shine into a darkened room. As with the flashlight, changes in the angulation of the transducer will demonstrate different structures or parts of structures. If the objects in the "room" are stationary, then moving the "flashlight" through several degrees of an arc will make visible all the objects in the room.

For moving structures like the heart, such a system would result in an unclear sound signal because, over a period of time, the distance from transducer to tissue density interface would keep changing. This problem led to the development of what is called M-mode (M for motion) echocardiography. A schematic representation of an M-mode scan is shown in Figure 20-3. In the M-mode system, the vertical axis represents the distance from the transducer (which is at the top) to each tissue density interface, and the horizontal axis represents time. Figure 20-4 shows the path of the sound beam for each of the panels of Figure 20-3.

With this brief introduction to the physical and technical aspects of ultrasound, the potential applications of echocardiography to the analysis of both anatomy and physiology (as reflected in the motion of structures) can be appreciated. Much of the research that has already been accomplished in this field accrued as a result of comparing echocardiographic findings with those obtained at cardiac catheterization, surgery, or postmortem examination. Much new information continues to appear in the literature. As with any rapidly growing field, debates arise from time to time among experts over test interpretation. Here will be presented the commonly accepted applications of the test to diagnosis.

Echocardiographic Measurements

It is useful to understand what can be measured by the echocardiogram. As with all tests, there are some drawbacks

Fig. 20-2. Transducer emits short bursts of sound.

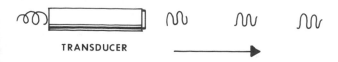

TRANSDUCER

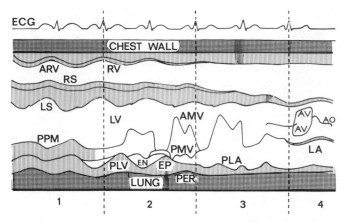

Fig. 20-3. Schematic representation of an echocardiogram from the four transducer positions, illustrated in Figure 19-4. ARV = Anterior right ventricular wall; RS = right side of interventricular septum; LS = left side of ventricular septum; PPM = posterior papillary muscle; RV = right ventricle; LV = left ventricle; PLV = posterior left ventricular wall; EN = endocardium; EP = epicardium; PER = pericardium; AMV = anterior mitral valve leaflet; PMV = posterior mitral valve leaflet; PLA = posterior left atrial wall; AV = aortic valve cusps; AO = aorta; LA = left atrium. (After Feigenbaum H: Cinical application of echocardiography. Prog Cardiovasc Dis 14:531, 1972)

and limitations to echocardiography. Transmission of sound depends greatly on the characteristics of the structure through which the sound must pass. It is difficult or impossible to examine subjects who are obese or in whom there is a large volume of air between the transducer and the heart. Since sound is almost totally reflected by bone, structures cannot be examined through the sternum or the ribs.

Left Ventricular Posterior Wall. In high quality echocardiograms, the endocardial and epicardial surfaces of the posterior wall of the left ventricle can be visualized, and the distance between the two echoes can be measured (Fig. 20-3). The measurement correlates well with the directly measured thickness of the left ventricular wall. When this measurement is increased, it reflects thickening (hypertrophy) of the left ventricular posterior wall, and when it is reduced, particularly in association with reduced wall motion, it may represent thinning of the myocardium, which may occur after myocardial infarction (MI). The anterior and lateral left ventricular free walls cannot be visualized by this technique.

Interventricular Septum. The interventricular septum can be measured from its right ventricular to its left ventricular interface with blood (Fig. 20-3). Just as with the left ventricular posterior wall, thickening indicates hypertrophy. When this occurs in the absence of left ventricular posterior wall thickening, it is called *asymmetric septal hypertrophy.* A thin septum which moves poorly can sometimes be seen when septal infarction has occurred. Functionally, the septum is part of the left ventricle. Therefore it ought to move posteriorly in systole and anteriorly in diastole. When the septal movement is reversed (paradoxical motion) it means that the septum functionally belongs to the right ventricle.

This may occur in right ventricular volume overload. In addition, this same pattern may be seen when there is septal dyskinesis due to MI.

The amplitude of motion of both the left ventricular posterior wall and the interventricular septum from diastole to systole can be measured. The measurement is a reflection of the vigor of local ventricular wall contraction. When the amplitude is increased, it reflects increased vigor of contraction, as may occur in left ventricular volume overload; conversely, when the amplitude is reduced, it means reduced wall motion. This can occur with poor myocardial function from any cause. Occasionally, some parts of the left ventricular wall or septum can be seen to move normally while others move poorly or not at all. Such segmental poor myocardial function is characteristic of coronary artery disease.

The internal left ventricular chamber dimensions are measured from the left septal endocardial echo to that of the left ventricular posterior wall (Fig. 20-3). These dimensions can be correlated with left ventricular volume both at end diastole and at end systole. The change between the two dimensions can be used to calculate an estimate of ejection fraction, much as it is calculated using dye-contrast left ventriculography.

These several characteristics of the left ventricular chamber and its walls can be used to obtain an impression of overall left ventricular function. For instance, an increase

Fig. 20-4. Schematic representation of the course of the ultrasonic beam to achieve the echo represented in Figure 19-3. CW = Chest wall; T = transducer; S = sternum. Other abbreviations are defined in the legend to Figure 20-3. (After Feigenbaum H: Clinical application of echocardiography. Prog Cardiovasc Dis 14:531, 1972)

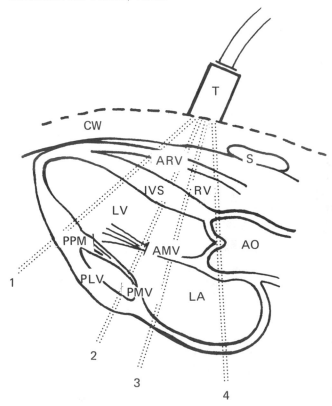

in intracavitary dimensions coupled with increased amplitude of left ventricular wall motion is indicative of left ventricular volume overload.

Right Ventricle. Increased right ventricular internal dimensions reflect increased right ventricular volume. As mentioned, paradoxical septal motion is further evidence of right ventricular volume overload.

Left Atrium. The left atrium is located behind the aorta when the transducer is held in the position equivalent to position 4 of Figure 20-4. The internal dimension of the left atrium from its posterior wall to the posterior wall of the aortic root can be measured. Increased left atrial dimension reflects increased left atrial size. On rare occasions, echo-producing structures can be seen within the left atrium correlating with the presence of tumor or blood clot.

Mitral Valve. The mitral valve is the most vigorously moving structure that can be recorded in most subjects. The motion of the mitral valve is determined by the difference in pressure between the left atrium and the left ventricle at each point in the cardiac cycle. Components of this waveform have been named to facilitate accurate description of excursion of the anterior mitral valve leaflet (Fig. 20-5). Point A corresponds to the peak of atrial systole. With atrial diastole and the onset of ventricular systole, the leaflet passes through point B. At point C, the mitral valve is closed and in its most posterior position. The anterior and posterior leaflets can sometimes be seen in apposition at this point. The distance from C to D represents the period of ventricular systole during which the mitral valve in its annulus is being carried anteriorly toward the transducer. With the onset of ventricular relaxation and the beginning of rapid early diastolic filling, the anterior leaflet once again assumes an extremely anterior position. After early diastolic atrial emp-

Fig. 20-5. Course of the anterior mitral valve leaflet. A = Peak of atrial systole; B = onset of ventricular systole; C = closing point of the mitral leaflets; D = onset of ventricular diastole; E = peak of rapid early diastolic left atrial emptying; F = mid-diastole.

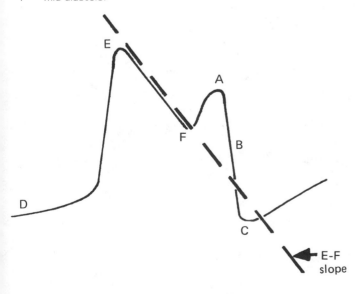

tying, the anterior leaflet once again floats to a near-closed position at point F.

The steepness of the E-F slope is a good measure of the ease of atrial emptying. This slope will be abnormally shallow if atrial emptying is impeded, as might occur with mitral valve stenosis or increased left ventricular diastolic pressure. In addition to changes in motion, the mitral valve can also produce multiple dense echoes, which correlate with the presence of valve thickening and calcification, as occurs in rheumatic mitral stenosis.

Aortic Root. Measurements of the diameter of the aortic root can be made. Increases in this dimension suggest aortic root dilatation. In addition, the amplitude of aortic root excursion from its most posterior position in diastole to its most anterior position at peak systole is another reflection of the force of ventricular systolic ejection. Occasionally, the diagnosis of aortic root dissection can be suspected from the presence of two parallel anterior or posterior aortic "walls" (in conjuction with other supportive clinical and echocardiographic findings).[4]

Aortic Valve. Two of the three aortic valve leaflets can often be recorded, and sometimes the third appears as well. The aortic valve can be evaluated for the presence of multiple dense echoes, suggesting calcification; however, the absence of this finding does not rule out the presence of aortic stenosis. The maximum leaflet separation during systole can be measured. When this is reduced, it may mean that aortic stenosis is present. During diastole, the aortic leaflet echo is a single line between the two walls of the aorta. Ordinarily, this line appears centered between the aortic root walls. It may become eccentrically placed when there is a congenitally bicuspid aortic valve.

Tricuspid and Pulmonic Valves. Occasionally the tricuspid and pulmonic valves may be recorded. It is unusual for the tricuspid valve to be recorded throughout both systole and diastole in adults, and, in fact, its presence on the recording suggests the possibility of right ventricular volume overload. Pulmonic valve motion occurs in response to pressure changes on the right side of the heart. Since this is a low-pressure system, low-pressure events will result in valve motion. The increase in right ventricular pressure which occurs with right atrial systole will, under normal circumstances, be reflected in slight posterior motion in the pulmonic valve. When pulmonary artery pressure is increased, the force of atrial contraction is insufficient to move the pulmonic valve.

Pericardium. The parietal pericardial echoes can be seen as a thin line behind the epicardial left ventricular posterior wall (Fig. 20-3). Multiple dense echoes arising from this structure may be seen when pericardial thickening is present, and an echolucent space between the epicardium and parietal pericardium means that pericardial effusion is present.

Figure 20-6 illustrates a typical M-mode echocardiographic report form. In addition to providing objective measurements of the various structures together with their normal adult values, it gives the echocardiographer–

	ECHO	ADULT NORMAL		ECHO	ADULT NORMAL
NAME		HOSP. NO.		DATE	
SEX	HEIGHT (CM)	WEIGHT(KG)		BSA(M²)	
REFERRED BY		TRANSDUCER			
CLINICAL HISTORY					
REASON FOR ECHO					

DIMENSIONS(MM)	ECHO	ADULT NORMAL	VALVES	ECHO	ADULT NORMAL
LEFT ATRIUM		16-40	AORTIC CUSP SEP.(MM)		>15
AORTIC ROOT		20-37	COMMENT		
RIGHT VENTRICLE		7-26	MITRAL DE AMPLITUDE(MM)		18-26
IV SEPTUM-DIASTOLE		7-11	EF SLOPE(MM/SEC)		> 60
-SYSTOLE			COMMENT		
-MOTION			TRICUSPID		
POST.WALL-DIASTOLE		7-11	PULMONIC "A"WAVE(MM)		2-7
-SYSTOLE			COMMENT		
-MOTION					
LV DIAMETER-DIASTOLE		38-56	DOPPLER QUALITATIVE		
SYST.SHORTENING(%)			FLOWS		
(LVDd-LVDs/LVDd)		25-45%	PROX. AORTA		
PERICARDIAL SPACE			RIGHT PULM. ART.		
			AORTIC VALVE		
*LV EJ.FRACTION EST.(%)			MITRAL VALVE		
- (LVDd³-LVDs³/LVDd³)		50-75%	TRICUSPID VALVE		
			PULMONIC VALVE		

*(ACCURATE ONLY IF NL LV SHAPE & CONTRACTION)

TECHNICAL NOTE		TECH:	EXC	GOOD	FAIR
		QUAL:	POOR	NO INFORMATION	

INTERPRETATION

Fig. 20-6. Echocardiogram report form.

cardiologist the opportunity to interpret the echoes in the light of the clinical history.

Clinical Applications

Cardiomyopathy. Cardiomyopathy (Chap. 49) simply means pathologic changes involving the heart muscle. This condition can be divided functionally into hypertrophic and congestive types.

In *hypertrophic cardiomyopathy,* the echocardiogram demonstrates increased left ventricular wall thickness, usually with normal or reduced intracavitary dimensions. Hypertrophic cardiomyopathy can occur whenever there is increased afterload, such as might occur with aortic stenosis

or systemic hypertension. A special form of cardiomyopathy is idiopathic hypertrophic subaortic stenosis. In this disorder, the ventricular septum grows disproportionately thick, and may even form obstruction to left ventricular outflow. The echocardiographic characteristics of this condition include the thickened septum, narrowing of the outflow tract, abnormal motion of the anterior leaflet of the mitral valve, and occasionally abnormal motion of the aortic valve (Fig. 20-7).

Congestive cardiomyopathy can occur in diffuse coronary disease, in response to alcohol or other toxins, or in a variety of degenerative, metabolic, nutritional, and genetic diseases involving the myocardial cells. The diagnosis of congestive cardiomyopathy is supported by an echocardiogram which shows increased left ventricular intracavitary dimensions associated with a decrease in ventricular wall motion (Fig. 20-8).

Atrial Septal Defect. The defect in the interatrial septum is not demonstrable by ultrasound. However, the primary physiologic consequence of the defect is a left-to-right shunt. This results in right ventricular volume overload, producing increased right ventricular intracavitary dimensions. Easy visualization of the tricuspid valve throughout systole and diastole, and paradoxical septal motion support the diagnosis of right ventricular volume overload (Fig. 20-9).

Mitral Stenosis. In mitral stenosis (Chap. 48), the E-F slope (see Fig. 20-5) is reduced. Calcification of the leaflets may appear as multiple dense echoes. Associated findings include increased left atrial dimension, increased right ventricular dimensions, and sometimes decreased dimensions of the left ventricle. In the presence of mitral stenosis, decreased amplitude in the excursion of the anterior valve leaflet during diastole suggests decreased valve mobility (Fig. 20-10).

Mitral Regurgitation. While mitral regurgitation (Chap. 48) cannot be diagnosed from the pattern of the mitral valve on the echocardiogram, the effects of the valve incompetence

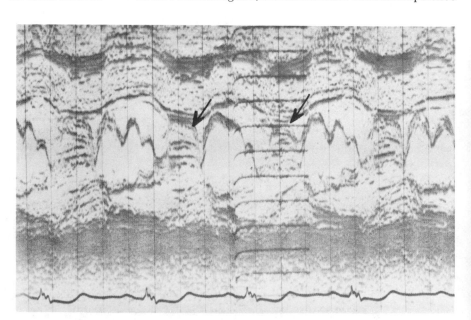

Fig. 20-7. Echocardiogram showing narrowing of the left ventricular outflow tract and systolic anterior motion of the mitral valve (*arrow*) in IHSS. (Clark RD: Case Studies in Echocardiography. Philadelphia, WB Saunders, 1977)

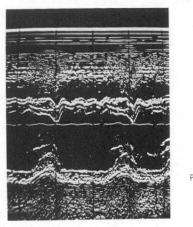
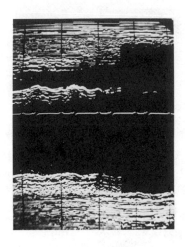

RV
SEPTUM

LV

POSTERIOR LV
WALL

NORMAL

CARDIOMYOPATHY

Fig. 20-8. Echocardiogram showing increased intracavitary dimension and reduced ventricular wall motion in congestive cardiomyopathy.

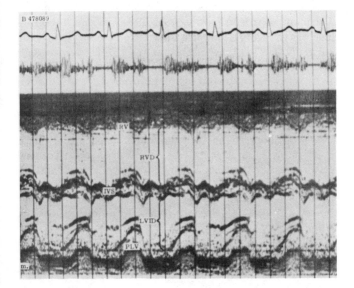

Fig. 20-9. Echocardiogram demonstrating right ventricular dilation and paradoxical septal motion in a patient with atrial septal defect. RV = Right ventricle; RVD = right ventricular dimension; IVS = interventricular septum; LVID = left ventricular internal dimension; PLV = posterior left ventricular wall. (Feigenbaum H: Clinical applications of echocardiography. Prog Cardiovasc Dis 14:531, 1972)

will be evident in increased left ventricular end-diastolic dimension, increased amplitude of left ventricular wall excursion (assuming a healthy myocardium), and increased left atrial dimension.

Mitral Valve Prolapse. Mitral valve prolapse (Chap. 48; click murmur syndrome, floppy valve syndrome, billowing mitral leaflet) is a condition involving prolapse of the mitral valve leaflets into the left atrium abnormally at some point during ventricular systole, thereby giving rise to unusual auscultatory findings. The etiology of this abnormality is variable and it may be seen with myxomatous degeneration of the mitral leaflet tissue, in acute or chronic rheumatic heart disease, in coronary artery disease (where the abnormality may be a result of pathologic changes in the papillary muscles subtending the valve) and in otherwise apparently healthy individuals. Mitral valve prolapse will appear on the echocardiogram as abnormal posterior motion of either anterior or posterior leaflet during ventricular systole (Fig. 20-11).

Aortic Stenosis. In aortic stenosis (Chap. 48), the aortic valve leaflets may demonstrate multiple dense echoes and reduced systolic separation, although lack of these findings does not exclude the presence of aortic stenosis. If aortic

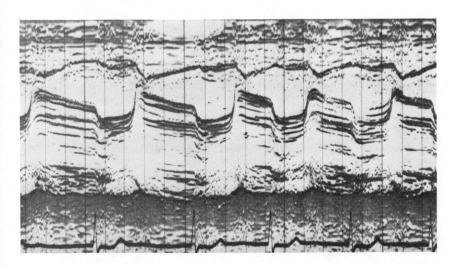

Fig. 20-10. Mitral stenosis. Note flat E—F slope, multiple dense echoes of calcification, and decreased amplitude of anterior mitral leaflet excursion. (Clark RD: Case Studies in Echocardiography. Philadelphia, WB Saunders, 1977)

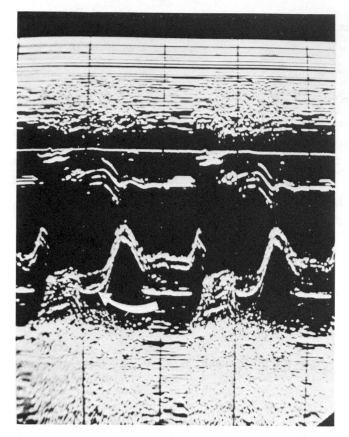

Fig. 20-11. Prolapse of the posterior leaflet of the mitral valve (*arrow*).

stenosis is present to any important degree, it will result in the appearance of a left ventricular hypertrophy pattern (Fig. 20-12).

Aortic Insufficiency. Aortic insufficiency (Chap. 48) represents a volume overload for the left ventricle, and will produce increased internal chamber dimensions and increased amplitude of ventricular wall excursion, unless there is concomitant left ventricular myocardial failure. In addition, the anterior mitral leaflet in diastole is directly in the path of the regurgitant jet of blood. It will "flutter" as further evidence of the regurgitation (Fig. 20-13).

Pericardial Effusion. As mentioned above, the echocardiogram can identify pericardial effusion as an echolucent space between the epicardium and the pericardium. Methods to estimate the volume of pericardial effusion have been suggested. When the clinical diagnosis is pericarditis, the finding of even a small amount of pericardial effusion supports the diagnosis (Fig. 20-14).

Left Atrial Myxoma. A left atrial myxoma can be demonstrated by ultrasound as the prolapse of an echo-producing structure within the left atrium through the mitral orifice and into the left ventricular cavity during diastole. This tumor may result in partial obstruction to the left atrial outflow as in mitral stenosis, and, when severe, can produce all the other intracavitary characteristics of mitral stenosis (Fig. 20-10).

Bacterial Endocarditis. Bacterial endocarditis results in valve destruction, and can produce regurgitation of the affected valve. This will result in the affected ventricle or atrium appearing volume-overloaded. Sometimes the presence of vegetation on the infected valve leaflets can be demonstrated as movable shaggy echoes contiguous with the leaflet.

TWO DIMENSIONAL ECHOCARDIOGRAPHY

Two-dimensional or cross-sectional echocardiography is a relatively new technique which utilizes either many small ultrasound transducers oriented through several degrees of an arc, or a single transducer which moves back and forth through an arc rapidly. The advantage of two dimensional echocardiography is that one can see not only the relationship of structures with respect to their distance from the transducer, as in B-mode, but also the relationships of structures to one another in a plane perpendicular to the transducers. Two-dimensional echocardiography can be displayed as single "stop-frame" pictures, but it provides the most unique information (compared to M-mode), when compiled with a cine display. This combination yields real-time "movies" not unlike contrast cineangiography and is especially useful for segmental abnormalities and congenital defects. The reader is referred to standard echocardiography texts (see Additional Reading) for further discussion. Two-dimensional echocardiography can also be displayed with Doppler sound detection. This combination allows correlation of abnormal heart sounds with the structures from which they arise.

RADIOISOTOPE EVALUATION OF THE HEART

Radionuclides, substances which emit radioactivity, have been used as tracers in the body for more than 50 years. Over the past 15 years, since the development of the gamma-ray camera by Anger, the use of radionuclides to study the heart has been the subject of much research. The great interest in these techniques has been stimulated by scientific advances in the fields of nuclear engineering, as well as the addition of computer technology to evaluation of the acquired data. In addition, development of radiopharmaceuticals has made it possible to locate the tracers selectively in the blood pool or in specific tissues.

Technical Aspects

Radionuclides are atoms in an unstable form. They have a finite probability of spontaneously converting to a more stable configuration, and when they do so, small amounts of energy in the form of gamma rays are emitted. The rate at which the atoms in any given sample will undergo conversion is denoted by the half-life, the time required for one-half of the sample to undergo the conversion. Half-lives of radioactive substances may vary from fractions of a second

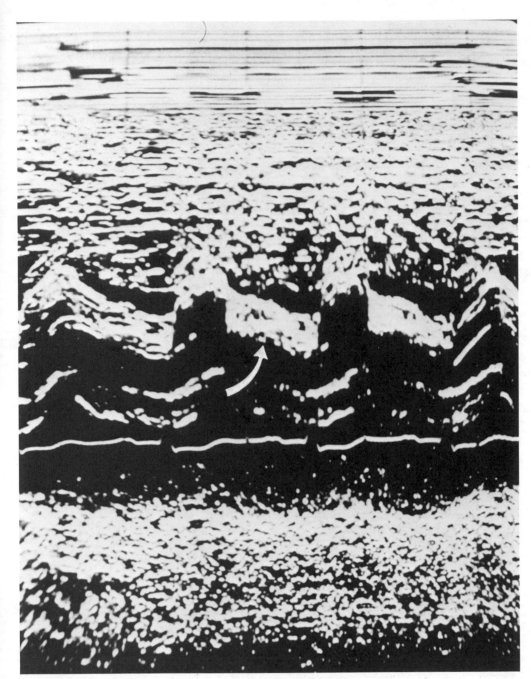

Fig. 20-12. Aortic stenosis. *Arrow* shows thickened apposed leaflets.

to millenia; however, the half-life for any given radionuclide is always the same. In nuclear studies of the heart, certain radionuclides have gained popularity, primarily because their half-lives are appropriate for the study, because of the ability to be complexed with biologic substances and because of the ease with which they can be acquired and stored. Two common radionuclides used in examining the heart and great vessels are thallium and technitium; however, more than a dozen other radionuclides have been employed from time to time. The isotopes can be injected directly as ionic substances, or complexed to such things as albumin microaggregates, red blood cells, or plastic microspheres.

The radioactive decay is detected outside the body as a scintillation (flash of light) and the detector is a gamma-scintillation camera. This camera can function as a scanning device to detect the distribution of radioactivity in relatively stationary structures (as in the lung scan) or, when used with a computer system, can be adjusted to examine the changing intracardiac blood pool throughout the length of the cardiac cycle (Fig. 20-15). In this latter application the computer uses the ECG signal for timing, and divides the cardiac cycle into many small segments. Each of these segments is surveyed individually for radioactivity, and then "summed" to the counts from many more corresponding segments. In this way, the manner in which the radioactivity (and hence the blood pool) changes over the cardiac cycle

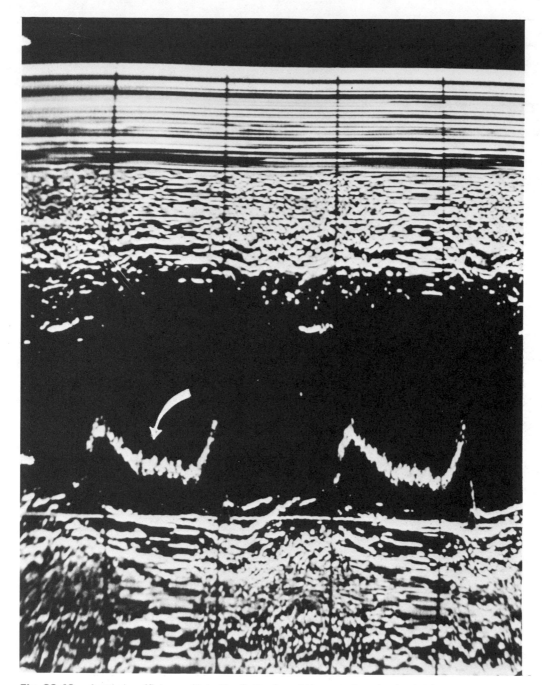

Fig. 20-13. Aortic insufficiency. Note the fluttering of the anterior mitral valve leaflet during diastole due to the regurgitant jet of blood (*arrow*).

can be demonstrated.[7] This "summed" cardiac cycle can be played back as a movie display of a normally recurring heart cycle. The examiner can appreciate the quality of ventricular wall motion, much as is demonstrated with dye-contrast left ventriculography (Fig. 20-16).

Clinical Applications

Myocardial Infarction Imaging (hot spot identification). Technitium pyrophosphate (Tc[99M]) is a radiopharmaceutical used for bone scanning. In acute MI, technitium pyrophosphate is taken up in areas of MI and can be demonstrated

as increased radioactivity as early as 12 hours or as late as six days after the onset of MI. The uptake may be ". . . due to the formation of calcium salt precipitates within the mitochondria of irreversibly-injured myocardial cells, with binding of the phosphate component of the radionuclide to the precipitated calcium deposit."[9] These techniques are most likely to yield positive results when the MI is large and transmural. Sensitivity decreases with small infarctions and nontransmural damage. The overall sensitivity, specificity, and time course of a positive test may not add much to the routine evaluation of possible MI by serial enzymes and ECG's. This technique can prove useful in evaluating

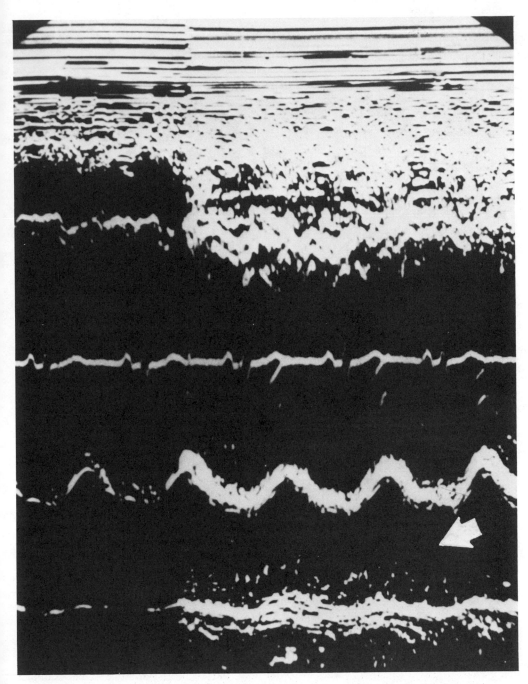

Fig. 20-14. Pericardial effusion showing echolucent space (*arrow*) between epicardium and pericardium.

patients who have had coronary bypass surgery, in the presence of equivocal ECG and enzyme changes, and in patients with left bundle branch block.[9] Unfortunately, the scans of patients with left ventricular dyssynergy (left ventricular aneurysm) may sometimes chronically indicate MI by this technique, thus introducing the potential for making a false-positive diagnosis of MI.[1]

Myocardial Bloodflow Evaluation (cold spot imaging). Intravenously injected potassium analogs such as thallium can be used to evaluate bloodflow through vessels which are distal to and smaller than those visualized with coronary

arteriography. In this technique, "cold spots" correlating to lack of blood flow correspond to areas of infarction. Paired rest-exercise studies can also be performed to evaluate transient ischemia. By this method, patients are exercised to a maximum level, thus inducing a relative (although physiologic) hyperemia through normal, patent coronary arteries. At this point, the radioisotope is injected and initial scanning shows a discrepancy between these hyperemic areas served by the normal vessels and areas with relatively less radioactivity fed by partly obstructed vessels. After recovery from exercise, the patients are rescanned. In the absence of the exercise-induced hyperemia, the heart will

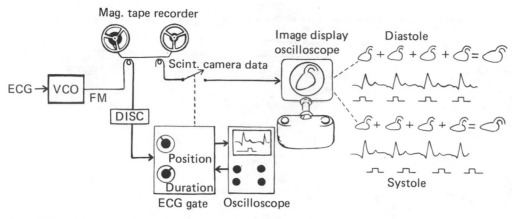

Fig. 20-15. Diagrammatic representation of computer-assisted radioisotope ventriculography. (After Kostuk WJ et al: Circulation 47:242, 1973)

once again show a relatively homogeneous uptake of radioactivity. This test is useful in showing transient segmental reduction in myocardial bloodflow in patients whose clinical evaluation, from the history and the standard exercise test, is equivocal. It may also be useful in making a rough estimate of the volume of cardiac muscle jeopardized by coronary stenosis, and is helpful in evaluating patients before and after coronary bypass surgery.

Fig. 20-16. Systolic and diastolic "frames" from a radioisotope angiogram. (After Kostuk WJ et al: Circulation 47:244, 1973)

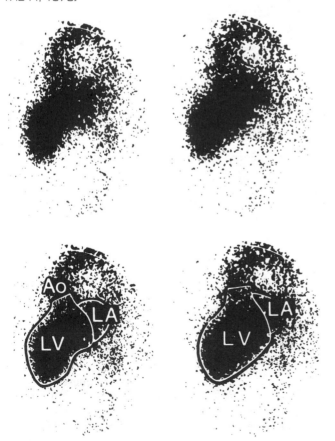

Blood Pool Scanning. As mentioned, gated cardiac blood pool scanning done with computer assistance can be used to evaluate left ventricular function. Calculations similar to those employed with dye-contrast left ventriculography can be used to calculate ejection fraction.[2] These methods can be useful in evaluating ventricular function at rest or during exercise, and in a variety of different types of heart disease.[2] It can also eliminate the need for serial cardiac catheterizations. Blood pool scanning can also be used for identifying the presence of pericardial effusion, although the echocardiogram is more sensitive and less "invasive" for this.

PHONOCARDIOGRAPHY

In phonocardiography, one or more sound-sensitive transducers are placed on the chest so that they can detect the externally audible heart sounds. The impulses thus obtained are recorded on graph paper along with the electrocardiogram. Since heart sounds come in a variety of frequencies from 20 to 400 cycles per second, microphones of different sensitivities can be used so that all audible events may be recorded.

Phonocardiography has been used in conjunction with various other external recording methods, for example, apexcardiography, echocardiography, and carotid pulse recordings. This is done to obtain objective documentation and graphic display of the various physical findings that the experienced examiner might observe (Fig. 20-17).

Phonocardiography has been used as a research tool in conjunction with intracardiac pressure monitoring and other simultaneously recorded data in deducing the exact origins of normal and abnormal heart sounds. It is also occasionally used to document auscultatory findings.

Phonocardiography is also used as an education tool. The phonocardiogram offers a graphic display of the relative timing and duration of cardiac sounds, and assists the student in developing the ability to discriminate not only the presence or absence of sounds, but also the relative intensities, duration, and timing within the cardiac cycle. Because the very exact nature of the heart sounds as

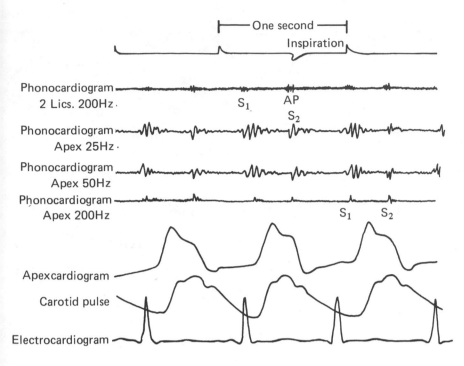

Fig. 20-17. Simultaneous recordings of four phonocardiograms with apex and carotid impulses and ECG simultaneously recorded. (After Seigel W: In Hurst, Logue, Schlant et al (eds): The Heart. New York, McGraw–Hill, 1978)

recorded by the phonocardiogram rarely has clinical importance over the observations that can be made by the experienced clinician, and because the instrumentation requires a certain degree of technical expertise, phonocardiography remains a technique primarily of research and education.

REFERENCES

1. Ahmad M, Dubiel JP, Verdon TA et al: Technitium 99m stannous pyrophosphate myocardial imaging in patients with and without left ventricular aneurysm. Circulation 53:833–838, 1976
2. Ashburn WL, Schelbert HR, Verba JW: Left ventricular ejection fraction—A review of several radionuclide angiographic approaches using the scintillation camera. Prog Cardiovasc Dis 20:267–284, 1978
3. Chang S: M-Mode Echocardiographic Techniques and Pattern Recognition, Philadelphia, Lea & Febiger, 1976
4. Clark RD: Case Studies in Echocardiography. Philadelphia, WB Saunders, 1977
5. Feigenbaum H: Echocardiography. Philadelphia, Lea & Febiger, 1972
6. Goldberg SJ, Allen HD, Sahn DJ: Pediatric and Adolescent Echocardiography. Chicago, Year Book Medical Publishers, 1975
7. Kostuk WJ, Ehsani AA, Karliner JS et al: Left ventricular performance after myocardial infarction assessed by radioisotope angiocardiography. Circulation 47:242–248, 1973
8. Seigel W: Examination by external pulse recording and phonocardiography. In Hurst JW, Logue RB, Schlant RC et al (eds): The Heart, 4th ed. New York, McGraw-Hill, 1978
9. Wynne JB, Holman BL, Lesch M: Myocardial scintigraphy by infarct-avid radiotracers. Prog Cardiovas Dis 20:243–266, 1978

ADDITIONAL READING

Adelstein JS, Maseri A: Radioindicators for the study of the heart: Principles and applications. Prog Cardiovasc Dis 20:3–18, 1977

Bassingthwaite JB: Physiology and theory of tracer washout techniques for the estimation of myocardial blood flow: Flow estimation from tracer washout. Prog Cardiovasc Dis 20:165–190, 1977
Castillo HT: Artifacts in first and second sounds of the phonocardiogram. Circulation 50:360–365, 1974
Coats, K. "Non-invasive cardiac diagnostic procedures," American Journal of Nursing, 75(11):1980–1985, 1975
Curtiss EI, Matthews RG, Shaver JA: Mechanism of normal splitting of the second heart sound. Circulation 51:157–163, 1975
Gramiak R, Waag RC (eds): Cardiac Ultrasound. St. Louis, CV Mosby, 1975
Heymann MA, Payne BD, Hoffman JIE et al: Blood flow measurements with radionuclide-labelled particles. Prog Cardiovasc Dis 20:55–79, 1977
Kriss JP, Enright LP, Hayden WG et al: Radio-isotopic angiocardiography—Wide scope of applicability in diagnosis and evaluation of therapy in diseases of the heart and great vessels. Circulation 43:792–807, 1971
Parker JA, Treves S: Radionuclide detection, localization, and quantification of intracardiac shunts and shunts between the great arteries. Prog Cardiovasc Dis 20:120–150, 1977
Ritchie JL, Hamilton GW, Gould KL et al: Myocardial imaging with indium-113m-and technitium-99m-macroaggregated albumin. Am J Cardiol 35:380–388, 1975
Shaver JA, Nadolny RA, O'Toole JD et al: Sound pressure correlates of the second heart sound. Circulation 49:316–324, 1974
Spodick DH, Quarry VM: Prevalence of the fourth heart sound by phonocardiography in the absence of cardiac disease. Am Heart J 87:11–14, 1974
Strauss HW, Pitt B: Gated cardiac blood-pool scan: Use in patients with coronary heart disease. Prog Cardiovasc Dis 20:207–216, 1977
Tavel ME: The fourth heart sound—A premature requiem? Circulation 49:4–6, 1974
Willerson JT, Parkey RW, Buja LM et al: Are 99m TC-stannous pyrophosphate myocardial scintigrams clinically useful? Clin Nucl Med 2:137–145, 1977

21

Hemodynamic Monitoring in Patients with Acute Myocardial Infarction

SUSAN L. WOODS, R.N., M.N.

and

B. LYNN GROSE, R.N., M.N., CCRN

Hemodynamic monitoring is useful in patients with acute myocardial infarction (MI) because it provides information about vascular capacity, blood volume, pump effectiveness, and tissue perfusion. With this information, therapy can be implemented. Monitoring of central venous pressure, pulmonary artery (PA) pressure, systemic arterial pressure, and cardiac output in the patient with acute MI will be described. Indications, limitations, complications, insertion procedure, measurement of pressures, interpretations, and frequently encountered problems are considered here.

CENTRAL VENOUS PRESSURE MONITORING

Normally, the central venous pressure (CVP) measured in the superior vena cava or the right atrium, is approximately 5 mm Hg.[100] One mm Hg is equal to 1.36 cm H_2O (see Table 21-1).[91] The CVP reflects right-ventricular end-diastolic pressure (RVEDP) or right ventricular (RV) filling pressure (preload).

The CVP is determined by blood volume, vascular tone, and the heart's pumping action. A disturbance in any one of these can alter the CVP. The CVP can be increased by increased circulatory blood volume, by vasoconstriction, or by decreased myocardial contractility. Usually CVP is elevated in RV failure, tricuspid regurgitation, and pericardial tamponade. In patients with acute MI, an increase in CVP is usually caused by RV failure secondary to left ventricular (LV) failure.[30] The CVP may be lowered by hypovolemia, vasodilation, or increased myocardial contractility.[41]

Indications of CVP Monitoring

Monitoring of CVP is indicated when information about RV performance and venous return are needed. The right atrial pressure (RAP) reflects pulmonary artery wedge (PAW) pressure if right and left ventricular function is comparable. The RAP plus 7 is approximately equal to the PAW pressure.[30]

Right atrial pressure (RAP) is needed to calculate systemic vascular resistance (SVR); an estimate of afterload. SVR is equal to mean arterial pressure (MAP) minus RAP, divided by the cardiac output (CO), times 80.

Normal SVR is 800 to 1200 dynes per second per cm^{-5}.

$$SVR = \frac{MAP - RAP}{CO} \times 80$$

Limitations

Central venous pressure (CVP) does not always accurately reflect LV function and, in fact, may actually be misleading.[31,73,76,91] The right ventricle may remain competent despite evidence of LV failure.[77]

In acute MI, LV failure usually occurs before RV failure. An increase in RAP is a late sign of LV failure. Early detection and treatment of this complication of acute MI is essential if myocardial damage is to be minimized.

Complications

Complications associated with CVP monitoring are as follows: infection, arrhythmias, perforation of the right ventri-

TABLE 21-1 WATER AND MERCURY PRESSURE EQUIVALENTS

cm H_2O	=	mm Hg
2.7	=	2
4.1	=	3
5.4	=	4
6.8	=	5
8.2	=	6
9.5	=	7
10.9	=	8
12.2	=	9
13.6	=	10
15.0	=	11
16.3	=	12
17.7	=	13
19.0	=	14
20.4	=	15

cle, vessel laceration, thrombophlebitis, thrombosis, and catheter tip or air emboli. Percutaneous insertion into the subclavian or deep jugular vein can result in pneumothorax.[40,46]

Insertion

The CVP catheter is inserted percutaneously or by way of a vein cutdown. The possible insertion sites include the medial basilic, lateral cephalic, internal or external jugular, and subclavian veins. The physician's skill and the patient's body build, clinical circumstances, age, and thoracic deformities all influence selection of the site.[49]

The selected site is shaved and cleansed with an antiseptic solution such as povidone-iodine (Betadine solution). Lidocaine may be used for local anesthesia. The catheter is inserted into the vein. Aspiration of blood through the catheter during insertion ensures placement within a vein. The distal end of the catheter is usually placed in the right atrium. Placement should be confirmed by chest radiograph. The catheter is secured with a skin suture and attached to an intravenous (IV) setup with a manometer or a transducer and a pressure module. Antiseptic ointment and a dry sterile dressing are applied. This dressing is changed every 24 hours and the site inspected for signs of infection: redness, heat, drainage, and swelling. Any complaints of pain at the site of insertion should also be noted. The IV solution and tubing should be changed every 24 hours.[66]

Pressure Measurement

The CVP can be measured as often as necessary. The patient who is hemodynamically stable can be at backrest elevations of 45 degrees or less when the CVP is measured.[25,87] The zero reference point must remain constant. At least nine different reference points have been recommended for the measurement of venous pressure. Some of these reference points are related to anatomic parts and some to the horizon or the examination table. Winsor and Burch conducted studies to determine the reference level that could be applicable to subjects of any build and in various positions. These investigators described the phlebostatic axis and the

phlebostatic level. Their recommendations have been accepted and widely used for measurement of venous pressure.

The *phlebostatic axis* is the crossing of two reference lines: first, an imaginary line from the fourth intercostal space at the point where it joins the sternum is drawn out to the side of the body beneath the axilla; second, another line halfway between the anterior and posterior surfaces of the chest is drawn (Fig. 21-1A).

The *phlebostatic level* is a horizontal line through the phlebostatic axis. The transducer or the zero mark on the manometer must be level with this line for accurate, comparable measurement. As the patient moves from the flat to erect positions, the chest, and therefore the reference level moves; the phlebostatic level stays horizontal through the same reference point (Fig. 21-1B).[95] A standard reference permits reproducible measurements of venous pressure while the patient moves from flat to erect positions. These reference points should be marked on the patient's chest to ensure consistency of subsequent readings.

With the use of a manometer, the zero mark is positioned on the phlebostatic axis at the correct level, and the CVP line is flushed with IV solution. The stopcock is closed to the patient in order to fill the manometer to approximately 25 cm of water. The stopcock is then closed to the IV source. Normally the fluid in the manometer falls freely. The fluid ceases to fall when the column of water has met an equal pressure. The CVP is measured (in cm of water) from the base of the meniscus of water.[43] The fluid level in the manometer fluctuates with breathing. During inspiration, the fluid falls. The CVP measurement is taken at the end of expiration[49] or averaged over a full respiratory cycle. If the patient is on intermittent positive pressure ventilation (IPPV), the ventilator should be disconnected for CVP measurement, since IPPV can alter CVP as fluid in the manometer increases with inspiration.[41,43] The CVP line is flushed with IV solution and the IV rate adjusted.

With the transducer, the CVP is measured in mm Hg. The transducer dome should be level with the phlebostatic axis. The system is opened to air and adjusted to zero. The system is then closed to air and the mean CVP recorded. The form of the CVP wave gives a clue to the diagnosis of tricuspid regurgitation because giant "V" waves are usually seen.[30] The normal CVP waveform is shown in Figure 21-2A. The giant "V" wave would appear like the giant V wave in the PAW pressure waveform shown in Figure 21-6.

The most common source of error in CVP measurement is failure to place the manometer or transducer at the zero level. The phlebostatic axis must be consistently used. Another source of error is the presence of air or clots in the CVP catheter, resulting in a damped waveform (Fig. 21-2 B–C). The air or clot must be aspirated with a syringe. The catheter should then be flushed and all connections checked for leaks. The catheter can also migrate into the right ventricle, in which case the waveform changes, as shown in Figure 21-2D. If this occurs, the catheter must be repositioned and secured. Because pressure transducers are temperature-sensitive, the zero line may drift. The system amplifier must be rezeroed prior to measurement or once every shift.[40] If the CVP is obtained using a transducer, another source of error could be not converting from mm Hg to cm H_2O.

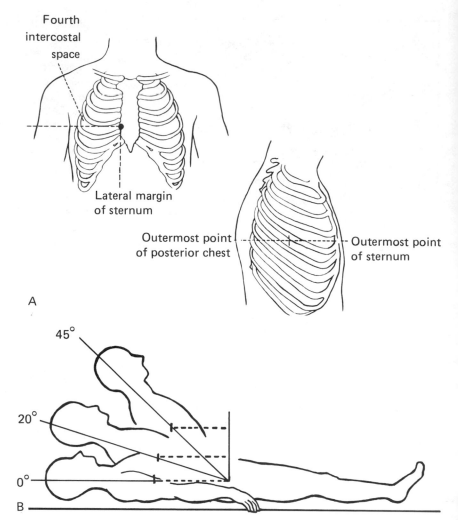

Fig. 21-1. The phlebostatic axis and the phlebostatic level. (**A**) The phlebostatic axis is the crossing of two reference lines: (**1**) a line from the fourth intercostal space at the point where it joins the sternum, drawn out to the side of the body beneath the axilla; (**2**) a line midpoint between the anterior and posterior surfaces of the chest. (**B**) The phlebostatic level is a horizontal line through the phlebostatic axis. The transducer or the zero mark on the manometer must be level with this axis for accurate measurements. As the patient moves from the flat to erect positions, he moves his chest and therefore the reference level; the phlebostatic level stays horizontal through the same reference point. (After Shinn J et al: Heart Lung, 8(2):324, 1979)

PULMONARY ARTERY AND PULMONARY ARTERY WEDGE PRESSURES

Monitoring pulmonary artery and PAW pressures in patients with acute MI is useful because it provides data to guide and evaluate therapy.[29,37] In the absence of pulmonary stenosis, PA pressure is equal to RV pressure during systole. Pulmonary artery pressure increases with increased pulmonary vascular resistance or increased pulmonary flow. Pulmonary artery end-diastolic pressure (PAEDP) is approximately the same as PAW pressure when the pulmonary vascular resistance is normal[30] and when the patient is not mechanically ventilated.[79] The PAW pressure approximates left atrial and left ventricular end-diastolic pressure (LVEDP) in the absence of mitral valve disease. During diastole, the mitral valve is open, and an open column of blood from the pulmonary artery to the left atrium and to the left ventricle exists; the pressure just before contraction (end-diastole) should therefore be approximately equal in the pulmonary arteries, the left atrium, and the left ventricle. (Fig. 21-3).

Knowledge of left-ventricular end-diastolic pressure (LVEDP), the filling pressure prior to contraction, is particularly informative as a guide to therapy.[70,71] In patients with normal compliance (distensibility) of the left ventricle, an increase in the LVEDP indicates an increase in LV volume; a decrease in pressure indicates a decrease in volume. LV failure or hypovolemia can be easily diagnosed and therapy started.[75]

Figure 21-4 demonstrates that PAW pressure and PAEDP are approximately equal to LVEDP. Because an increase in PAW pressure may be an early indication of LV failure, the PAW (or PAEDP) can be used as a guide to therapy. This pressure indicates left heart failure before other signs and symptoms of failure are apparent. Early detection of LV failure is critically important in achieving maximum effectiveness of therapy.

Pressure in the PA is normally 25/9 mm Hg with a mean of 15 mm Hg. The PAW pressure is a mean pressure and is normally between 4.5 to 13 mm Hg.[100]

In 1970 Swan and associates reported their results of catheterizing the right heart with a soft, flexible, radiopaque, flow-directed, balloon-tipped, polyvinyl-chloride catheter of their own design.[90] By means of this catheter, the PA can be rapidly and safely catheterized in the intensive care unit without the aid of fluoroscopy.[90] The PA pressure (systolic, diastolic, and mean) and the pulmonary artery wedge pressure (mean) can be measured. It is important to know the manufacturer's specifications and directions for the catheter used.

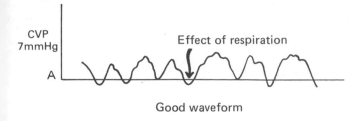

CVP
7mmHg

A

Effect of respiration

Good waveform

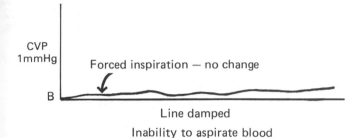

CVP
1mmHg

B

Forced inspiration — no change

Line damped

Inability to aspirate blood

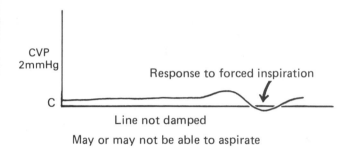

CVP
2mmHg

C

Response to forced inspiration

Line not damped

May or may not be able to aspirate

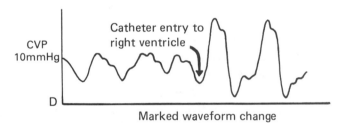

CVP
10mmHg

D

Catheter entry to
right ventricle

Marked waveform change

Fig. 21-2. Troubleshooting central venous pressure waveform. (**A**) Demonstrates good waveform; (**B**) damped pressure; (**C**) pressure appears damped, but is not; (**D**) marked waveform change. (After Guide to Physiological Pressure Monitoring, p 26. Waltham, MA, Hewlett—Packard, 1977)

to the catheter tip, depending on the model. These two specific lumen terminations facilitate placement of the right atrial lumen under varying conditions of cardiac anatomy.[89]

The thermodilution catheter, is 7 French in diameter and 110 cm long, and is marked in 10-cm increments. It serves as a diagnostic tool for rapidly obtaining multiple hemodynamic pressures and for determining cardiac output (Fig. 21-5). This catheter has four lumina:

Lumen 1—The distal catheter lumen terminates at the tip of the catheter. Measurements that can be obtained through this lumen are chamber pressures (as the catheter is inserted), PA and PAW pressures, and blood samples.

Lumen 2—The proximal lumen terminates 30 cm from the catheter tip, which places it in the right atrium when the distal lumen opening is in the PA. Lumen 2 carries the injectate necessary for cardiac output computation. By connecting the proper pressure transducer to the lumen, RAP can be monitored.

Lumen 3—This lumen contains the electrical leads for the thermistor, which is positioned at the catheter surface 4 cm proximal to its tip. This position minimizes the possibility of thermistor contact with the vessel wall, which could cause erroneously high cardiac output readings.

Lumen 4—This lumen is used to inflate and deflate the 1.5 ml capacity balloon. The inflated balloon serves two purposes in the insertion procedure. First, it assists in pulling the catheter through the chambers of the heart because there is a fluid dynamic drag on the balloon. Second, the fully inflated balloon covers the catheter tip; this distributes tip forces over a larger area and minimizes the occurrence of premature ventricular contractions during passage of the catheter.[89]

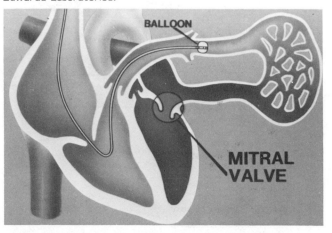

Fig. 21-3. The PA catheter in PAW position measures left heart pressure. During diastole, the mitral valve is open, creating an open column of blood from the pulmonary arteries to the left atrium and left ventricle. When the balloon is inflated, blood flow from behind the catheter (right heart) is obstructed and the catheter tip reflects the pressure in front of the catheter (left heart pressure). (Courtesy of American Edwards Laboratories)

The most commonly used PA catheter, the Swan—Ganz catheter, is available in three designs: double-lumen, triple-lumen, and thermodilution (4-lumen). The double-lumen catheters are designed to monitor PA and PAW pressures, to allow sampling of venous blood, and to allow injection or infusion of solutions. The large lumen terminates at the tip of the catheter. It is through this lumen that pressure tracings are monitored, mixed venous blood samples are taken, or solutions are infused. The small lumen serves to inflate and deflate the balloon.[89]

The triple-lumen catheters are designed to monitor the same parameters as the double-lumen catheters, plus RAP. One large distal lumen terminates at the catheter tip. A small lumen permits inflation and deflation of the balloon. The proximal lumen terminates either 20 or 30 cm proximal

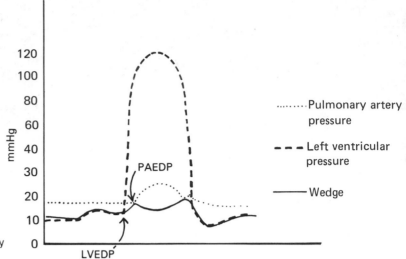

Fig. 21-4. The PA and PAW pressure waves superimposed upon the LV pressure curve. Left ventricular, PAW, and PA pressures are approximately equal at the end of diastole.

Indications for Hemodynamic Monitoring

Pulmonary artery monitoring is indicated for the patient with acute MI in the following situations: to determine the magnitude of pulmonary congestion and peripheral hypo-

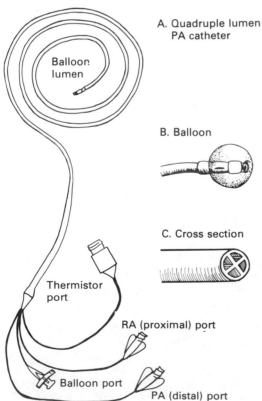

Fig. 21-5. Three views of the Swan-Ganz Catheter. **(A)** The PA catheter with its four ports; **(B)** a close-up of the inflated balloon; **(C)** a cross section of the lumens and the thermistor wires inside the catheter. In the cross section, the wires at the right run the length of the thermistor lumen from the thermistor port to the lumen opening 4 cm from the tip of the catheter. Clockwise from the thermistor lumen are the proximal lumen, distal lumen, and balloon lumen. (After Lalli SM: RN 9:65–77, 1978)

A. Quadruple lumen
PA catheter

Balloon lumen

B. Balloon

C. Cross section

Thermistor port

RA (proximal) port

Balloon port

PA (distal) port

perfusion; to assess LV pump performance; or to determine vascular resistance.

Goals of therapy in acute MI are

1) To relieve pulmonary congestion (PAW pressure greater than 18 mm Hg) by reducing PAW pressure;
2) To relieve peripheral hypoperfusion, (cardiac index [cardiac output divided by body surface area] less than 2.2 liters per minute per meter squared [l/min/m²]) by increasing the cardiac index;
3) To achieve goals 1 and 2 without disturbing the balance between myocardial oxygen supply and demand.[30]

Radiologic manifestations of acute pulmonary congestion correspond to the following PAW pressures:

1) 18 to 20 mm Hg—onset of pulmonary congestion
2) 20 to 25 mm Hg—moderate congestion
3) 25 to 30 mm Hg—severe congestion
4) Greater than 30 mm Hg—onset of pulmonary edema[60]

Cardiac output reduction corresponds to signs and symptoms of peripheral hypoperfusion to the brain, kidney, and skin in the following manner:

1) Cardiac index of 2.7 to 4.3 l/min/m²–normal perfusion
2) Cardiac index of 2.2 to 2.7–subclinical depression
3) Cardiac index of 1.8 to 2.2–onset of clinical hypoperfusion
4) Cardiac index of less than 1.8–cardiogenic shock.[30]

Pulmonary artery monitoring enables one to classify patients with acute MI into four subsets. These subsets enable prediction of short-term prognosis and selection of appropriate therapy to optimize cardiac function. These categories are summarized in Table 21-2.

The morphology of the PA and PAW pressure waves also provides useful information. With acute mitral regurgitation, a giant "V" wave is seen in the PAW pressure waveform (Fig. 21-6).[44,55]

Pulmonary artery monitoring is also useful in the differential diagnosis of cardiogenic shock and pulmonary embolism. In pulmonary embolism, PAEDP is increased and the PAW pressure is normal; in cardiogenic shock both PAEDP and PAW pressure are elevated.[30]

TABLE 21-2   CLASSIFICATION OF PATIENTS WITH ACUTE MI ON THE BASIS OF CARDIAC INDEX AND PAW PRESSURE. THERAPY AND MORTALITY FOR EACH SUBSET ARE PROVIDED

Subset	Cardiac Index	PAW Pressure	Therapy	Mortality
I NO FAILURE	>2.2 L/MIN/M²	<18 MM HG	Sedate, place under observation, order bed rest	3%
II PULMONARY CONGESTION	>2.2 L/MIN/M²	>18 MM HG	Relieve symptoms of pulmonary congestion by decreasing PAW pressure to less than 18 mm Hg. For normal blood pressure: give diuretics For elevated blood pressure: give vasodilators	9%
III PERIPHERAL HYPOPERFUSION	<2.2 L/MIN/M²	<18 MM HG	Relieve hypoperfusion by increasing cardiac index above 2.2 For elevated heart rate: add volume For depressed heart rate: start pacing	23%
IV CONGESTION & HYPOPERFUSION	<2.2 L/MIN/M²	>18 MM HG	Relieve symptoms of pulmonary congestion and hypoperfusion For depressed blood pressure: give inotropes For normal blood pressure: give vasodilators	51%

(Forrester JS et al: N Eng J M 295:1356–1362, 1976)

Limitations

The PAW pressure is an amplitude-damped version of the left atrial pressure (LAP). During diastole, when the mitral valve is open, pressure in the left atrium and left ventricle are the same. Thus the PAW pressure, LAP, and LVEDP are equal. This relationship is changed when mitral stenosis is present as the PAW pressure may no longer equal LVEDP. Also because the mitral valve begins to close before the onset of ventricular systole, PAW pressure may not equal LVEDP. This inequality is marked in patients in whom atrial contribution to ventricular filling is substantial, or in patients with reduced ventricular compliance. Thus, the LVEDP may be higher than the PAW pressure.[30]

Complications

Complications associated with PA monitoring are uncommon but some of these can be identified as follows.

Infection. As with any vascular cannulation, infection can occur. Infection may be caused by lack of aseptic technique during catheter insertion and throughout the time the catheter is in place. If the catheter is not secured to the skin, the nonsterile portion can migrate, resulting in infection.[5] When signs of infection are present, the catheter should be discontinued and the tip sent for culturing.[40]

Dressing, IV solution, tubing, and stopcocks should be changed daily.[51,59]

Pulmonary Artery Rupture. Rupture of the PA can occur.[16,38,53,54] This complication may be caused by an unprotected tip of a migrating catheter passing through the artery wall, or by over-distension of the balloon. This can be prevented by inflating the balloon in small increments until the wedge waveform is observed. If the inflation volume is substantially less than that recommended, the catheter may have migrated. Catheter migration can usually be prevented by securing the catheter to the skin with a suture; it can be detected by chest radiography.[40,89]

Pulmonary Thromboembolism. Pulmonary thromboembolism can occur if a thrombus forms and migrates from the catheter. If clotting of the catheter is suspected, the clotted blood should be aspirated from the catheter and the catheter flushed after removal of the clot. Catheter patency is assured by using a heparinized flush solution. In patients predisposed to thrombus formation, anticoagulation therapy may be advisable.[89]

Pulmonary Infarction. Pulmonary infarction can occur if the catheter migrates to a wedged position, if the balloon is left inflated, or if a thrombus forms in or around the catheter.[72,101] Continuous monitoring of the PA waveform

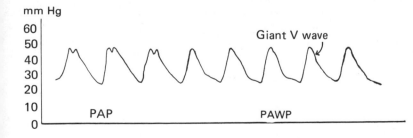

Fig. 21-6. Giant "V" wave in PAW waveform. Giant "V" waves are seen in mitral regurgitation. (Consultant Hemodynamic Training Manual. Santa Ana, American Edwards Laboratories, 1979)

will indicate a change in wave form and pressure if the catheter wedges, or if the balloon is left inflated.[28,60,89]

Catheter Kinking and Intracardiac Knotting. Kinking and knotting of the catheter can be caused by insertion of an excessive length of the catheter.[21] During insertion, the right atrium (RA) should be reached within 60 cm from the right antecubital fossa, 70 cm from the left antecubital fossa, 35 cm from the internal jugular or subclavian veins, or 50 cm from the femoral vein. The catheter should reach the PA after it has been advanced no more than 15 cm from the RA.[89]

Arrhythmias. Arrhythmias can occur if the unprotected tip of the catheter contacts the endocardium or the valves.[2] During insertion and removal, the inflated balloon guards the tip of the catheter. During PA monitoring the catheter can slip back into the right ventricle (RV) and cause RV irritability. Temporary reinflation of the balloon should cause the catheter to return to the PA.[89]

Air Embolization. Air embolization can result if the balloon ruptures. Latex balloons absorb lipoproteins from the blood and gradually lose elasticity, resulting in balloon disintegration and rupture. Air embolization is also a concern when percutaneous placement technique is used to insert the catheter into the internal jugular or subclavian veins. Air can enter the system between the removal of the wire and dilator from the lumen of the introducer, and the insertion of the catheter through the introducer.[18] Air embolization can be reduced by tilting the patient's head down approximately 20 degrees and having him hold his breath at inspiration and perform a Valsalva maneuver during the critical moments.[18] The balloon should never be inflated beyond the recommended inflation volume. If possible, the catheter should not be in place longer than 48 hours.[89] Most balloons can withstand up to 72 inflations without rupturing.[51] Carbon dioxide should be used for balloon inflation instead of air in patients with intracardiac shunt.[51]

Other complications include PA bronchial fistula, intracardiac trauma,[78,81] and systemic venous thrombosis.[26]

Catheter Insertion

The pulmonary artery catheter can be inserted percutaneously or by way of a vein cutdown. The usual sites of insertion include the internal jugular vein, subclavian vein, femoral vein, or the brachial vein. The site of insertion will vary according to the individual practices and skills of the physician. The area selected should be shaved and then scrubbed with hexachlorophene. The skin at the site of insertion is then antiseptically cleaned with povidone-iodine (Betadine) and alcohol. Lidocaine is used for local anesthesia. Before the procedure is started, the integrity of the balloon is checked by submerging the tip in sterile water and inflating it. Then the catheter is flushed with the heparinized solution, and the vein is entered. The external end of the distal lumen is attached to the transducer, which is attached to a pressure module and to heparinized solution (1 to 4 units heparin per ml of 5% dextrose and water or saline) by way of a continuous flush device. The IV bag is placed in

a pressure bag at 300 mm Hg pressure. At this pressure, the device will deliver 3 ml of flush solution per hour, keeping the catheter patent without interfering with continuous pressure measurement. The IV tubing selected should either have in an inline filter or have large drips because minidrops can result in air bubbles entering the system when the continuous flush device is used to irrigate the line. Figures 21-7 and 21-8 illustrate these setups.

The catheter is gently passed to the right atrium with pressure monitoring. The balloon is then inflated, and the catheter carried rapidly and safely by the flow of blood through the tricuspid valve into the right ventricle and then into the PA. When the catheter reaches the PA, it moves into either the right or the left division of the PA and then finally wedges itself in one of the branches of the right or the left PA. The catheter is stopped in a pulmonary vessel of the same size as the inflated balloon. The balloon surrounds the tip, preventing its contact with the vessel wall and leaving the distal lumen open to pressure measurement. The PAW pressure can be measured. With the balloon deflated, the catheter returns to the main PA, and PA pressure can be measured.

In order to prevent necrosis of the pulmonary tissue, the balloon is left deflated except when obtaining a PAW pressure. The catheter is secured in position by closure of the skin incision around the catheter, and a knot can be made in a skin suture a few centimeters distal to the incision, to which the catheter can be tied. A portable anteroposterior chest radiograph will confirm the optimal position of the catheter tip in the main PA.[62]

The *role of the nurse* during catheter insertion is to interpret the procedure to the patient and his family, to assist the physician with the catheter insertion, and to watch the monitor for premature ventricular contractions during catheter insertion.[36,97] Premature ventricular contractions can occur as the catheter comes in contact with the endocardium of the right ventricle and may lead to ventricular tachycardia and fibrillation. A defibrillator and lidocaine bolus should be nearby. The occurrence of significant ventricular arrhythmias is low with the Swan-Ganz catheter.[89]

As the catheter passes through the heart, waveforms can be seen on the oscilloscope (Figs. 21-9, 21-10). Knowledge of these pressure curves is important in determining the position of the catheter. The catheter may become displaced

Fig. 21-7. Transducer, stopcocks, continuous flush device, and IV tubing setup. (After Lalli SM: RN: 9:65–77, 1978)

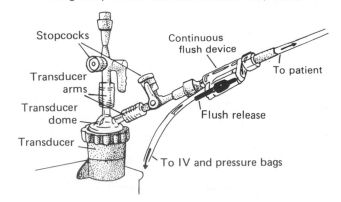

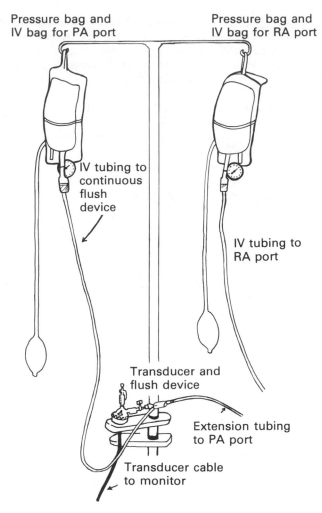

Fig. 21-8. IV solution and pressure bag setup. Transducer is connected to the distal port of catheter for PA and PAW pressure measurements. Proximal port can be attached to a manometer setup (for CVP readings) or to a transducer. A second pressure bag, IV solution, and a continuous flush device can be used to flush the proximal lumen and keep it patent. (After Lalli SM: RN 9:65–77, 1978)

inadvertently, and an observed change in pressure and curve can indicate the position of the catheter.

Pressure Measurements

When obtaining measurements sterility must be maintained and all connections must be secure. Since pressure readings will not be accurate if air bubbles are present, any air in the system must be removed.

Because pressure transducers are temperature-sensitive, it is necessary to check the zero balance, or baseline, frequently. This is performed before and after insertion of the catheter. By "zero the transducer," one means to allow it to equilibrate to air, or to register zero pressure. This maneuver can be done by opening the transducer to air, then bringing it to the level of the patient's heart (the phlebostatic level). Because pressure is monitored through a fluid-filled column, any marked difference between the level of the cardiac chamber where the catheter tip lies and the position of the transducer will result in incorrect pres-

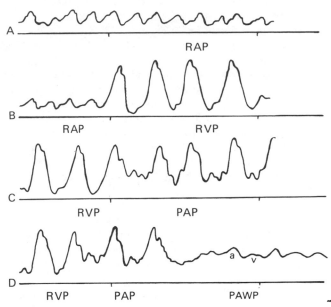

Fig. 21-9. Pressure wave forms as the PA catheter moves through the heart. (**A**) Right atrium (RAP); (**B**) Right ventricle (RVP); (**C**) Pulmonary artery (PAP); (**D**) Pulmonary artery wedge (PAWP). When an RA pressure wave pattern is seen on the oscilloscope, the balloon is fully inflated and blood flow rapidly carries the catheter through tricuspid valve into the right ventricle, and then to the main PA. Catheter finally stops when it wedges into a pulmonary vessel. During this time, the pressure wave patterns on the oscilloscope quickly change from RA to RV to PA to PAW patterns. (Adapted from Woods SL: Am J Nurs, 76:1978, 1976)

sures. The stopcock near the patient is turned off in order to close the catheter's lumen and stop the transmission of pressure impulses to the transducer. At this time, the monitor's meter and wave tracing should read zero. If the monitor does not read zero, the necessary adjustments must be made.[88]

To calibrate the pressure module one must apply a known quantity of pressure to the transducer. Exertion of pressure may be done through built-in mechanisms of the monitor or by a mercury manometer. A mercury manometer with a stopcock and a syringe is attached to the transducer. A zero reading on the manometer should produce a zero reading

Fig. 21-10. PAW waveform: "a" wave = atrial contraction; "c" wave = bulging of the valve into the atrium, secondary to ventricular contraction; "x" descent = a drop in pressure in response to further atrial volume changes during ventricular contraction; "v" wave = during the remainder of systole, continuous venous inflow produces a rise in pressure; "y" descent = a pressure drop in the atrium accompanies the transfer of blood from the atria into the ventricles.

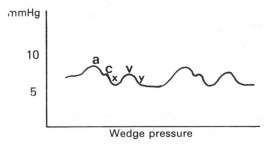

on the instrument. If it does not, then an error has been made in the previous zeroing procedure, and adjustments can now be made to correct this. The level of the mercury is raised to 50 mm Hg and the transducer opened. The monitor meter or wave tracing is adjusted to display 50 mm Hg. The mercury is lowered to zero again and the zero reading is verified. The manometer apparatus may now be removed. The stopcock of the transducer is closed to air. The stopcock nearest to the patient is opened so that pressure impulses may now pass to the transducer. The system is briefly flushed. Zero balancing and calibration should be done frequently—at least once each shift—to ensure accurate monitoring.[88]

Patient Position. It has been assumed that the patient must be flat and supine in order to obtain accurate reproducible measurements. This positioning often requires disturbing patients in order to position them for the reading. However, a study of 10 cardiac patients with normal PA and PAW pressures showed that backrests could be positioned from flat to 45 degrees without markedly affecting the PA and PAW measurements.[98] A further study of 126 critically ill patients determined that backrest position, 20 degrees versus flat, did not markedly affect PA and PAW pressures. On the basis of these findings, it would seem that in patients at backrests of 20 degrees or less, measurements can be obtained without positioning the patient flat.[98a]

IPPV. Patients on ventilators have routinely been taken off for pressure measurements to eliminate the effects of IPPV. It was assumed IPPV would increase the PA and PAW pressures.[12] It has recently been shown that intermittent positive pressure breathing does not markedly affect PA and PAW pressures.[22,79] A recent study of 60 critically ill patients on IPPV showed that in a few individuals PA and PAW pressures did vary according to whether the ventilator was on or off. Most individual differences were small. Thus most patients with IPPV need not be disconnected from the ventilator for these measurements.[38a] The PA diastolic and PAW pressure measurements may be falsely high if the patient is artifically ventilated with positive end-expiratory pressure of 5 cm water pressure or more.[3]

Catheter Position. The question has been raised whether PA and PAW pressures would differ according to catheter position in anterior versus posterior branches of the PA. If the pressures are measured with the transducer properly positioned and with the system calibrated and zeroed at atmospheric pressure, then the measurements are the same regardless of the position of the catheter tip within the PA circulation.[86] West found pressures to vary depending on the position of the catheter within the lungs.[94a]

Recording the PA Pressure. The PA pressures (systolic, diastolic, and mean) are recorded from the digital display on the monitor or from an analog recording. The average pressure over a full respiratory cycle is usually recorded. Others recommend recording PA pressure at the end of expiration.[22] The balloon is inflated slowly until the contour of the PA pressure changes to that of the PAW pressure or until the correct amount of air is used to flow-guide the

catheter distally. The oscilloscope will show the appropriate waveform. The mean PAW pressure is recorded from the monitor. Again the average pressure over a full respiratory cycle or the pressure at end of expiration is recorded. Figure 21-11 shows the method for obtaining PA and PAW pressures from the analog recording.

The balloon is not inflated for more than 15 seconds because this may cause overwedging (falsely high pressure readings) and damage to the PA. To deflate the balloon, the syringe is detached. A PA tracing should then appear on the monitor. The syringe should not be aspirated to deflate the balloon, because this may cause the balloon to rupture. Once the balloon has been deflated, the syringe should not be reattached to the port. Keeping the syringe detached from the balloon port prevents accidental inflation.[51] Measurements are usually obtained and recorded hourly or more often, depending on the need for information regarding the condition of the patient.

Water or saline should never be used to inflate the balloon because adequate deflation may be impossible. Also, the weight of the liquid will impede the passage of the balloon into a distal artery. If there is any possibility of air traveling to the left side of the heart, as in patients with a ventricular septal defect, carbon dioxide should be used to inflate the balloon. Carbon dioxide is absorbed by the blood and will not cause an air embolism.[97]

Fig. 21-11. Method for analog to digital conversion of pulmonary artery and pulmonary artery wedge pressures. (**A**) Selection of pressures within a full respiratory cycle. (**B**) Pulmonary artery systolic and end-diastolic waveforms were read individually throughout the selected respiratory cycle and averaged. The mean pulmonary artery and pulmonary artery wedge pressures are provided by some equipment. These mean lines, for a full respiratory cycle, are bisected so that the areas above and below the line are equal.

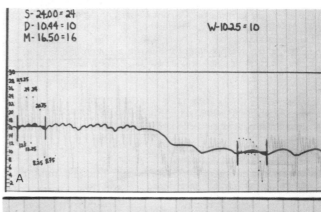

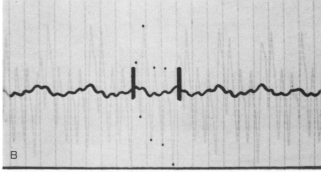

Nursing Care

In addition to the routine care of the patient, the nurse is responsible for calibrating the equipment and for measuring and recording pressures. She is also responsible for using pressure measurements as vital data in assessing the patient's condition and response to therapy.

The dressing at the catheter insertion site should be changed daily and the site inspected for redness, swelling, and drainage. Any signs and symptoms of inflammation or infection should be charted and reported to the physician. Cultures should be made from the site of insertion within 48 hours after insertion, and every 24 hours thereafter.[51] The area should be cleansed with an antiseptic solution of povidone-iodine or alcohol, then antibiotic ointment and a dry sterile dressing should be applied to the incision. The arm can be placed on an armboard wrapped with a guaze dressing, to decrease its mobility. If the catheter was inserted into an antecubital vein, the lower arm should also be assessed for adequacy of circulation. If any impairment in circulation is detached (decreased radial pulse, pallor, or coolness), a tight dressing or armboard compression may be the cause.

If right premature ventricular contractions occur, the catheter tip may have moved from the PA to the RV. The oscilloscope should show an RV waveform. Because the balloon is deflated, the rigid catheter tip is exposed and can irritate the right ventricle. Inflating the balloon will prevent the tip from irritating the ventricle, because the inflated balloon protects the catheter tip. The catheter may even float back into the PA. If this does not occur, then the catheter may need to be repositioned by the physician. When necessary, a chest radiograph can be taken to confirm catheter position.

The fluid-filled pressure catheter provides a direct, low-resistance path to the heart for stray or leaky electrical current and increases the potential for electrically induced ventricular fibrillation.[7] Adherence to the principles of electrical safety is essential to maintain a safe environment for the patient (see Chap. 41).

If the patient requires defibrillation, the transducer may first have to be removed from the catheter to prevent electrical damage to the transducer and monitor. This procedure is especially true of older transducers. Many newer models have built-in safeguards against electrical damage. Manufacturer's specifications should be checked for the transducers being used.

The catheter is usually removed by a physician[51] or a nurse when the patient's condition has improved. Caution must be taken to remove it slowly to prevent ventricular tachycardia. Cultures should be made at the site of the incision and the incision cleansed with Betadine. Antibiotic ointment and a dry sterile dressing should then be applied. Sutures are usually removed in 72 hours.

Attention to the catheter and the monitoring equipment is important at this time. Equally important is the patient's psychologic welfare. The nurse must assess the patient's response to this invasive procedure and to his hospitalization in general.

This assessment is important if one is to individualize the patient's plan of care. An open, caring, supportive approach to the patient is needed if he is to feel that he himself is being cared for, not just his monitoring system.

Data Interpretation

Pressure in the PA is increased under the following conditions: hypervolemia, pulmonary embolism, pulmonary hypertension, increased pulmonary blood flow, and LV failure. Pressure in the PA is decreased in hypovolemia and in pulmonary stenosis. The PAW pressure is increased in LV and LA failure and decreased in hypovolemia. The "a" wave (atrial contraction) is increased with mitral stenosis. The "v" wave (ventricular contraction) is increased with mitral insufficiency and with aortic stenosis (Fig. 21-10).

Monitoring Problems

Some problems that may occur when using PA catheter equipment are discussed here.

Catheter Whip Artifact. Catheter whip artifact can create a measurement 10 mm Hg above or below the real PA pressure. Contraction in the right ventricle causes the catheter to move, which accelerates the fluid in the catheter system, superimposing waves of artifact on the pressure wave.[40] The PA systolic and PA diastolic pressures are not reliable when whip is present. The PA mean is more reliable.[40]

Lack of PAW Pressure Tracings. PAW pressure tracing may be unobtainable. Causes include balloon rupture, overinflation or underinflation, and a catheter that is no longer in proper position within the PA. A chest radiograph will confirm position of the catheter. The balloon should be allowed to deflate spontaneously, then the correct amount of air is injected slowly. If no resistance is met, no more air should be injected.[51,88,97]

A Change in the Configuration of the Pressure Tracing. The configuration of the pressure tracing may change as a result of incorrect position of the catheter, inaccurate transducer calibration, the transducer not being at RA level, or the transducer not being tightly attached to the catheter. A chest radiograph will confirm the position of the catheter; it may need to be repositioned. The transducer should be rezeroed and recalibrated at the RA level. All connections should be checked and secured.[51,88,97]

Pressures May be Damped (decreased amplitude of waveform, lowered systolic pressure, and elevated diastolic pressure). Damped pressures are caused by a clot in the system, blood in the transducer, air in the system, or occlusion of the catheter tip by the balloon or the wall of the PA. Air and blood should be aspirated from the system and all connections secured. If blood is in the transducer, the transducer should be flushed until the blood is off the transducer head. To dislodge the catheter tip from the wall of the PA, instruct the patient to cough and extend his arm perpendicular to his body, or to turn onto his side. A chest radiograph will confirm the catheter position. If the catheter has migrated permanently to a wedge position, the physician should be notified immediately. The catheter may need to be repositioned or replaced.[51,88,97]

Inappropriate Pressures with Proper Waveform. Improper transducer level or inaccurate calibration may produce an incorrect waveform.

No Waveform. A lack of any waveform is the result of one of the following: the monitor not being plugged in or turned on or not being calibrated properly; the transducer not being plugged in or being in the wrong transducer outlet; the dome being loose, or the stopcock being turned in the wrong direction.

CARDIAC OUTPUT MEASUREMENTS

Cardiac output (CO) is a valuable parameter in assessing cardiac function of the acutely ill patient in the cardiac care unit. The measurement provides useful data to quantitate variation in disease states, to evaluate heart function, and to serve as a guide to fluid and drug therapy. In the hands of a well-trained nursing staff, a thermodilution PA catheter can provide frequent measurements of CO.

Measurement of CO by the thermodilution principle was introduced by Fegler[27] in 1954. The method is based on an injection of a quantified cold solution and registration of its dilution by subsequent change in the PA temperature at a point 26 cm farther on in the direction of the bloodstream.[83] A physiologic indicator, unlike dye, mixes well irrespective of the laminar flow in the blood vessels. With the thermodilution method, sterile ice water (saline cooled to 0°C), or solutions at room temperature, can be injected by way of the proximal port (lumen 2) of a thermodilution PA catheter into the right atrium. The temperature is sensed by the thermistor in the PA, and a temperature curve is produced (Fig. 21-12, 13A and B). The blood is temporarily cooled by mixing with the cold injectate. As the cold mixture passes and warm blood follows, heat transfer is reversed. The result of this process is a bidirectional heat exchange. The peak of deflection is reduced, and the downslope of the curve is prolonged.[11] A computer (Model 9520, Edwards Laboratories) which has been connected to the PA catheter, (lumen 3), calculates the area under this curve and the cardiac output is printed on a digital display.

Fig. 21-12. Injection into right atrium.

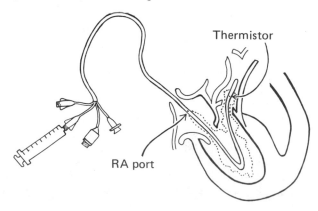

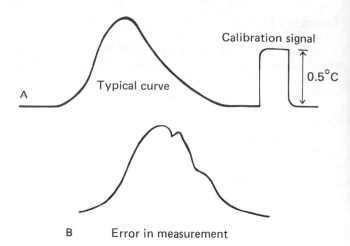

Fig. 21-13. (**A**) Typical thermodilution curve; (**B**) inaccurate thermodilution curve.

Obtaining CO by the thermodilution method has several advantages over the Fick and indicator dye dilution methods. (see Chap. 19). The method depends on a physiologic indicator and does not require any withdrawal of blood.[92] Internal electrical calibration is simple and accurate, and there is minimal recirculation of the indicator.[11] Measurements are repeatable and can be performed as often as one per minute.[93] The reproducibility of CO determination has been demonstrated to be better with the thermodilution than with the dye dilution method.[33] Finally, the nurse is able to perform the thermodilution measurements of CO at the patient's bedside.[93] In addition to its accuracy and the physiologic advantage, the information is immediately available for use in assessing the patient's status and therapy.

Preparation of the Equipment

The most common method for determining CO by thermodilution is by use of an iced injectate. Room temperature injectates (19°C to 25°C) are sometimes used but result in a signal two to three times smaller.[11] One set-up commonly used requires the equipment listed in Table 21-3. A sterile graduate pitcher is nested into an ice bath (a large basin of crushed ice). Wearing a mask and using sterile gloves and sterile syringes, the nurse fills the syringes with 10 ml of 5% dextrose and water, or saline intravenous solution. The syringes are capped with leurtip black caps and are placed in the sterile graduate. An injectate probe is then connected to the bedside computer and the tip is placed into a solution-

TABLE 21-3 LIST OF EQUIPMENT FOR SYRINGE PREPARATION

1. Sterile plastic syringes
2. Rubber caps
3. Large basin
4. Crushed ice to fill large basin
5. Sterile 1000 ml graduate
6. 5% dextrose and water intravenous solution and sterile distilled water for irrigation—refrigerated or room temperature
7. 25-gauge ½-inch needle with cap
8. Mask
9. Sterile gloves
10. Two sterile drapes

filled plungerless syringe placed inside the sterile graduate. To keep the syringe from touching the bottom of the sterile graduate, a 25-gauge needle with cap is placed on the tip of the plungerless syringe. Sterile refrigerated distilled water is then poured into the graduate, leaving the head of the plunger above the solution level. Even though the bath setup is covered with a sterile towel, sterility within the bath is difficult to maintain.[58] A preferable method is one that keeps the syringes cold, but dry (Fig. 21-14). The syringes are kept in the ice bath for about one half hour, to reach a temperature of 0°C to 5°C. These preloaded syringes should be kept for no more than 24 hours. If not used in 24 hours they should be discarded.[14]

Before the CO measurements are obtained, care must be taken to check the equipment.

1. The PA catheter must be in the correct position in the PA, not in the wedged position.

2. The appropriate computation constant must be entered on the side of the computer, by use of the thumb-wheeled switches. The table containing the computation constants accompanies the computer. The constant must be selected on the basis of temperature and volume to be injected. A 10 ml injectate at 0°C to 5°C requires a computation constant of 0.532.

3. The injectate probe cable must be connected to the back of the computer outlet marked "injectate."

4. The PA catheter must be connected to the computer with a cable extension marked "catheter."

5. The computer must be attached to lumen 3, the thermistor coupling of the catheter.

6. Lumen 2, the proximal port must be checked for patency and the presence of vasopressor medications that may be infusing into this line. The line can be checked for patency by drawing blood back through the line and then flushing it with the IV solution. To avoid bolus effects of infusing medications, these medications should be changed from the proximal port to other intravenous lines when the proximal lumen is being used for thermodilution CO measurements.

After the equipment is checked, the patient is placed in the supine position, with the backrest angled from 0 to 20 degrees of elevation.[39] The computer is turned on and the CO mode selected. There is a short wait before the "ready" signal appears on the digital display. When the "ready" signal appears, a syringe preloaded with exactly 10 ml of ice-cold (0°C) saline or 5% dextrose and water is taken from the prepared ice bath. The syringe is attached to a three-way stopcock at the proximal port (lumen 2). At the time of injection the remote "start" foot switch is pushed, which initiates computer calculations and the solution is injected within 4 seconds.

This procedure is performed as quickly as possible in order to avoid alterations in the temperature of the injectate. Also, the syringes are handled by touching only the wing section. With each determination, the start button, or foot switch, should be pushed and injection should begin during the same phase of the respiratory cycle, preferably end expiration.[96]

The computed CO appears on the display in approximately 15 seconds (Fig. 21-15). Forty-five seconds after

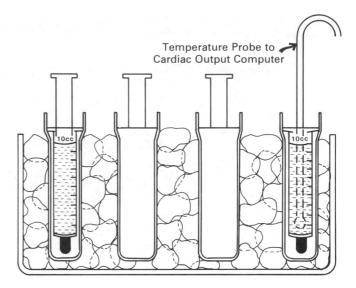

Fig. 21-14. Iced injectate preparation. Preloaded syringes are placed in plastic or metal tubes that are suspended in an ice bath.

display of the first CO, a second CO is measured by repeating the above steps. It is recommended that three CO measurements be taken and an average computed. The measurements should be no greater than 10% apart. To help check the validity of these CO measurements, a strip recorder can be added into the circuitry of the CO computer. Accuracy of the measurement is judged by the shape of the curve. The curve should show a sharp increase to the peak of the curve, and a gradual decrease back to baseline (Fig. 21-13A).

Clinical Application

To evaluate particular therapies, ventricular function curves can be constructed to illustrate the relationship of LVED volume or pressure to stroke volume or CO (Fig. 21-16). The PAW pressure measurements are plotted on the x-axis (horizontal) in mm Hg, and CO measurements are plotted on the y-axis (vertical) in liters per minute. The curve produced describes the Frank–Starling principle. The larger the amount of blood in the ventricles during diastole, the greater is the strength of contraction. Up to a certain limit, the farther the heart is stretched, the greater is the CO. However, there is a point beyond which any further stretching of the fibers results in no improvement of stroke volume and, in fact, stroke volume begins to decrease. An abnormal elevation of PAW pressure without an increase in CO may mean that the shape of the ventricular function curve has changed because of a decrease in contractility or because its position has shifted downward on the y-axis, or both. The slope of the curve reflects the response of the ventricle to an increase in PAW pressure. A flattened curve describes the limit of ventricular function in response to intervention.[74]

Problems with Cardiac Output Measurement

Despite the important diagnostic advantages of using the balloon-tipped, flow-directed PA catheter for thermodilution

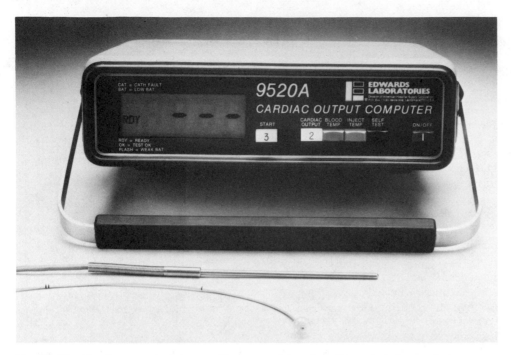

Fig. 21-15. Cardiac output computer. (Courtesy of American Edwards Laboratories)

CO measurements, it is not without problems. Transient arrhythmias have been reported following injection of the cold injectate.[94] Another practical problem reported is that any delay due to handling of the syringe after its removal from the ice bath may cause warming of the injectate temperature, thereby resulting in inaccurate measurements.[83] A third problem which occasionally occurs is the thermistor becoming wedged against the wall of the PA, so

Fig. 21-16. Construction of a left ventricular curve. The following data are plotted on *Curve 1* to determine an individual patient's Starling curve: (**1**) PAW pressure 18 mmHg, cardiac output 3.5 liters/min.; (**2**) PAW pressure 22 mmHg, cardiac output 3.3 liters/min.; (**3**) PAW pressure 13 mmHg, cardiac output 3.0 liters/min.; (**4**) PAW pressure 9 mmHg, cardiac output 2.7 liters/min. A higher cardiac output for the same PAW pressure indicates a change in contractility. See *Curve 2.* PAW pressure 13 mmHg, cardiac ouitput 4.6 liters/min.

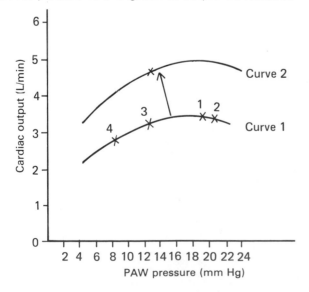

that the area of the curve becomes distorted, the buildup time on the curve is prolonged, the peak deflection is reduced, and the time constant of the downslope is increased.[93] Most reports agree, however, that the value of using the PA catheter for serial thermodilution CO measurements outweighs the drawbacks.[33,82,93,94] Again, to overcome these practical drawbacks it is recommended that three CO measurements be obtained with less than 10% variation.

Several physiologic conditions may also alter the validity and reliability of the thermodilution method. Many critically ill patients may undergo rapid changes in cardiac status, causing wide variation in measurements. An automatic injector can be used; this device provides a constant reproducible rate of injection, and its use is thought to increase reliability of thermodilution CO determinations. Speed of injection is consistent and operator error and fatigue are lessened.[69]

In the mechanically ventilated patient, CO may be altered by measurement at different times during the respiratory cycle. Variations in values are thought to be minimized by injecting the indicator during the same phase in the respiratory cycle,[96] and by using iced indicator rather than room-temperature indicators.[93]

Another source that may alter the validity and reliability of thermodilution CO is mechanical ventilation. Mechanical ventilation elevates intrathoracic pressure, thereby decreasing venous return to the heart.[80] The subatmospheric intrathoracic pressure that occurs in the spontaneously breathing patient on inspiration, due to the pressure gradient between the veins and the right heart, no longer exists.[64] Mechanical ventilation also causes a decrease in CO because the increased inspiratory pressure of mechanical ventilation resists the distending pressure and diastolic filling of the heart. If positive end-expiratory pressure (PEEP) is added to mechanical ventilation, CO may be further reduced. If PEEP

TABLE 21-4 TROUBLESHOOTING TIPS IN THERMODILUTION CO MEASUREMENT

Potential Problems	Causes	Nursing Actions
1. Catheter tracing appears wedged.	Catheter may be wedged in small vessel in the PA	Do not perform CO measurement until catheter is in correct position in PA. Notify physician.
2. Letters "BAT" appear on the digital display.	Battery depleted	Replace battery—unplug old battery from back of computer.
3. Flashing numbers appear on the digital display.	Battery depleted	Replace battery.
4. Letters "CAT" appear on the digital display.	Catheter not connected to computer	Connect computer to catheter.
	Fault in thermistor circuitry	Disconnect thermistor coupling and connect the computer cable to the "test" receptacle on the back of the computer. Push "blood temperature" button. If display shows 37°C ± 0.5°, the computer and cable are functioning properly. Catheter fault caused by catheter rather than by computer circuitry. If numbers on display are outside this range problem is with computer or cable itself.
5. Injectate temperature greater than 5°C.		Add ice to nonsterile basin.
6. Erroneous temperature displayed while computer is in selected "injectate" mode	Fault in injectate probe	Disconnect injectate probe. Computer automatically assumes 0°C, when using ice injectate. If using room temperature injectate, switch to ice solution injectate.
7. Variations in serial CO measurements of greater than 10%	Poor injection technique	Repeat CO measurement. Use strip recorder to check shape of curve.
	Presence of premature ventricular contractions	Observe ECG.
	Patient movement	Keep patient in one position for several minutes.
	Change in cardiovascular hemodynamics	Obtain other parameter, *i.e.*, CVP, PAW or arterial pressure, for comparison.
	Injectate not injected at same time in respiratory cycle	Repeat CO measurements, injecting solution at same point of respiratory cycle—preferably end-expiration.

is added to the respiratory management of the critically ill patient, thermodilution CO measurements must be made with each level of PEEP increase to evaluate the effects of PEEP on the cardiovascular system. Tips for trouble shooting can be found in Table 21-4.

Summary

The measurement of CO by thermodilution permits monitoring of an important parameter of the patient's hemodynamic status. Trends in the patient's cardiovascular status can be observed by using serial thermodilution CO measurements and PAW pressure measurements. In spite of occasional complications and practical problems with its use, the thermodilution method of measuring CO has been shown to be readily available, easily performed, safe, and reliable.

SYSTEMIC INTRA-ARTERIAL MONITORING

Systemic intra-arterial monitoring has become a common method of obtaining direct and continuous blood pressure. It also simplifies obtaining arterial blood gases and serial blood samples. The therapeutic benefits of intra-arterial

monitoring are early recognition of disease complications and assessment of the effects of therapy. In the unstable patient, accurate measurements of cuff blood pressure may be impossible to obtain or reliable arterial blood samples may be impossible to obtain if the patient suddenly becomes hypotensive.

Advantages. The advantages of intra-arterial monitoring are several. This method gives beat-by-beat information which allows more rapid evaluation of changes in the patient's status, quicker visualization of responses to therapy, and more accurate blood pressure measurements, especially in low flow states.[52] The traditional method of blood pressure determination, auscultation and cuff technique, depends on the quality of Korotkoff sounds and normal blood volume to produce audible sounds. In the low-flow or shock states, diminished pulsatile flow may not produce a sound wave and some Korotkoff sounds are lost, making the cuff method unreliable. In patients with severe hypotension or shock, the average systolic pressure is about 33.1 mm Hg less when the cuff pressure is used than when the intra-arterial pressure is used.[17] Thus, low cuff pressure may not indicate arterial hypotension. Coronary blood flow primarily depends on diastolic pressure. An arterial line provides a means of accurately recording the systolic, diastolic, and mean pressures. Prolonged cannulation of an artery is less traumatic to the vessel than are repeated punctures, when serial blood samples are necessary. Prolonged cannulation of the artery is less disturbing to the patient, when multiple samples are required.[20]

Indications. Intra-arterial monitoring is indicated for critically ill patients with hypertension, hypotension, fluctuations in blood pressure, shock (hypovolemic, cardiogenic, or septic), arteriolar vasoconstriction or vasodilation, or for frequent drawing of blood samples. Evaluation of pressures and changes is rapid and accurate.

Sites. Sites for intra-arterial catheterization include the radial, brachial, femoral, and dorsalis pedis arteries. The most common site is the radial artery because the collateral circulation of the hand is distal to the site of cannulation, which minimizes the risk of vascular complications.[15,10,99] Cannulation of this artery will be explained later in depth. The other site used with increasing frequency is the dorsalis pedis artery.[6,84] This artery is used when both radial arteries are inaccessible because of extensive trauma or burns, or because of damage to both radial arteries from numerous catheterizations.[48] Although there is no clinically significant difference in mean arterial pressure between the dorsalis pedis artery and the radial artery, the systolic and pulse pressures are higher in the dorsalis pedis artery.[84] The other two sites, the brachial artery and the femoral artery, are cannulated less often because occlusion of these arteries jeopardizes the circulation of an entire extremity.

Before radial artery cannulation is attempted, collateral circulation to the hand must be determined. If the radial artery is injured during cannulation, continued viability of the hand depends on collateral circulation to that hand. Radial artery cannulation has a low morbidity because the superficial palmar artery is usually formed by continuation of the ulnar artery into the hand (Fig. 21-17).[65]

Two tests have been used to determine collateral circulation to the hand. They are the Allen test and the Ultrasonic Doppler test.[4,65] *The Allen test*[4] begins with the examiner instructing the patient to hold out his hands. The examiner, standing in front or to the side of the patient, checks for obstruction to the ulnar artery, by placing one thumb lightly over the radial artery, and one thumb over the ulnar artery. The patient is then directed to clasp his fist tightly for one minute, and the examiner increases the pressure over these arteries. After one minute the patient is directed to extend his fingers quickly, and the examiner releases his thumb from the ulnar artery, but retains pressure over the radial artery (Fig. 21-18). The examiner notes the return of color to the hand. An intact arterial tree will return the hand to normal color, but if ulnar arteries are obstructed, pallor remains for varying amounts of time. If palmar blush does not appear within five seconds of the patient's extending his fingers, cannulation of the radial artery should not be performed.[9]

The *Ultrasonic Doppler test* is a convenient, simple, and rapid method of evaluating palmar circulation and does not require patient cooperation as does the Allen test. The Ultrasonic Doppler test can be used for critically ill patients in the cardiac care unit who may be unable to cooperate with the examiner. The superficial palmar arch is usually formed by a continuation of the ulnar artery into the hand

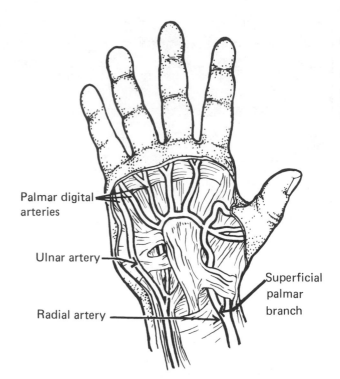

Fig. 21-17. Anatomy of circulation of the palmar surface of the hand. (After Mozersky DJ, Buckley CJ, Hagood CO et al: Am J Surg 126:810–812, 1973)

and is predominantly supplied by the ulnar artery in 88% of the population. The superficial palmar arch is found by positioning the probe of the Doppler ultrasonic velocity detector between the heads of the third and fourth metacarpals. The probe is gradually advanced proximally until a frequency signal (the pulse) is heard. The signal is usually located proximal to a line drawn along the medial edge of the outstretched thumb. When the superficial palmar arch is located, the radial artery is compressed and the effect on the palmar circulation is noted by the examiner. If the signal remains the same or is augmented by radial compression, the radial artery can be used for cannulation without fear of occlusive vascular complication.[65]

Cannulation. Once adequate ulnar circulation is evaluated and equipment is ready, radial cannulation is undertaken. Indwelling arterial cannulation is performed percutaneously or by direct exposure of the artery by surgical cutdown. The hand, wrist, and forearm are placed on an armboard with the wrist hyperextended. The purpose of the armboard is to stablize the extremity. Also, hyperextension fixes the radial artery in a more superficial position, facilitating the insertion of the catheter. The area to be cannulated should be shaved and cleaned with a povidone-iodine. The area closely surrounding the insertion site should be anesthetized with 1% lidocaine (without epinephrine).

Arterial Pressure Monitoring System

The following five components make up the direct pressure-monitoring system: (1) arterial catheter; (2) T-connector; (3) IV solution; (4) transducer; (5) monitor. The setup is similar to that shown in Figure 21-7.

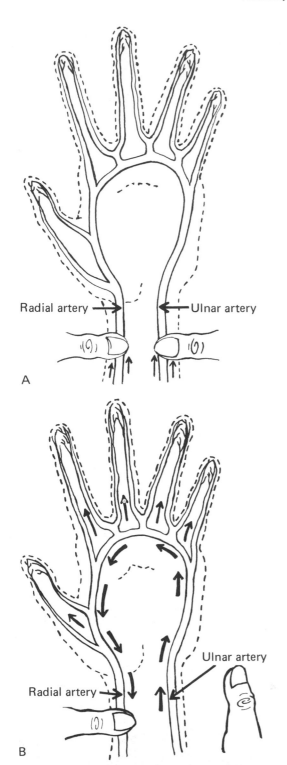

and create a periarterial hematoma.[6] Once the catheter is inserted and flow ascertained, the catheter is secured in place with a suture or adhesive tape, or both.

T-connector. The T-connector[1] provides a method for obtaining blood samples that minimizes suction, aspiration, and syringe vacuum that may cause vasospasm and intimal damage.[52] It is connected between the catheter and the fluid source. The T-connector replaces the use of a three-way stopcock next to the catheter. Replacement by the T-connector prevents such problems as inadvertent air injection, repeated opening of a closed system, and intimal damage from twisting motions of the stopcock for obtaining blood samples.

Intravenous Solution. The IV solution, connected to the T-connector, is used to flush the catheter. The flush system is maintained by use of a pressurized (pressure bag) flush solution (1 to 4 units heparin per ml of 5% dextrose and water or saline by way of a continuous flush device) which delivers 3 ml per hour. This slow, continuous flow minimizes chances of vasospasm, intimal damage, or fluid overload. A stopcock may be placed at either end of the flush device for irrigating the system if air or blood accidentally backs up into the device or transducer.

Transducer. The transducer is connected to the flush device and to the monitor. The transducer changes the mechanical pressure of pulses to an electrical signal. As the pulse bombards the face of the transducer, it pushes and pulls fine wires attached to the back of the transducer; this distortion is converted to electrical impulses which are transmitted to the bedside monitor. The pulse appears as a waveform, rising and falling as it goes across an oscilloscope.

Monitor. The monitor continuously displays, on an oscilloscope, the pressure waveforms (Fig. 21-19). The monitor amplifies the signal coming from the transducer, so that the patient's blood pressure can be observed on the oscilloscope.

There are several major changes in the patient's arterial pressure contour as the wave is transmitted down the arterial system. The changes are due to decreased compliance of the peripheral arteries and to reflection of previous waves.

1. The high-frequency components of pulse are damped out and disappear.
2. Systolic portions of the pressure contour become more narrow and peaked.
3. Systolic pressure becomes higher.
4. The hump becomes more prominent on the descending portion of the pressure wave.
5. The diastolic pressure decreases.[10]

To ensure accurate reading, the monitor must be calibrated to atmospheric pressure. The procedure is outlined in Table 21-5.

Nursing Responsibilities

Besides obtaining accurate pressure information, there is the added nursing responsibility, when caring for a patient with an arterial line, of reducing the incidence of compli-

Fig. 21-18. Allen's test. (**A** and **B**) Compression of radial and ulnar arteries with subsequent release of ulnar artery demonstrates adequate circulation of ulnar artery. (After Lantiegne, KC, Civetta JM: Heart Lung 7:610–621, 1978)

Catheter. A nonreactive Teflon catheter should be used.[8,23] A 20-gauge catheter is the preferred diameter since this size causes less arterial occlusion and less thrombogenicity than larger catheters.[9] Needles such as a butterfly hub should not be used for prolonged cannulation, because any motion of a patient's wrist can cut or damage the radial arterial wall

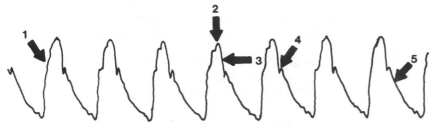

Fig. 21-19. Typical arterial pulse wave on oscilloscope. The initial rapid pressure rise in the artery (**1**) is usually accompanied by some turbulence and is the result of the contraction of the left ventricle forcing its bolus of blood through the open aortic valve into the aorta. As the ventricle empties and relaxes, a peak pressure in the artery is reached (**2**). A notch, called the anacrotic notch, often appears on the upstroke near the peak. Its origin is not well understood. The pressure drops sharply (**3**) as the bolus of blood moves downstream. Meanwhile, the pressure in the ventricle has dropped lower than that in the aorta, allowing aortic intravascular pressure to force the aortic valve closed. The tense aortic walls snap back to their resting mode. This phenomenon is seen on the pressure wave as the dicrotic notch (**4**). It appears whether pressure is measured in the aortic arch itself or far downstream, and is absent only when competent valve action is absent. Closure of the aortic valve is commonly considered the demarcation between the systolic and diastolic phases of the cardiac cycle. There is usually a change in slope (**5**) after the dicrotic notch, as the pressure continues to fall until the next systole. (After Nielsen M: Am J Nurs 74(1):48–53, 1974)

cations. Major and minor complications are listed in Table 21-6. Overall incidence of major complications is less than 1%.[24]

Blood Loss. One of the most common complications of intra-arterial catheterization is blood loss due to faulty connections. Accidental blood loss with a disconnected 20-gauge catheter can be as much as 200 ml in 4 or 5 minutes.[52]

To avoid this complication

1. It must first be assured that all connections of the system are tight.
2. The monitor alarms should be kept with high and low limits set so that alarms will sound when critical values are reached (pressure becomes lower if the system becomes disconnected).
3. It must be certain that the extremity is exposed at all times so that loose connections can be identified quickly.
4. Finally, the patient may need to be restrained if he becomes restless, in order to prevent him from dislodging the catheter or disconnecting the tubing.

Local Obstruction. Another complication to be avoided is local obstruction causing distal ischemia. Incidence of thrombosis is higher if the patient is critically ill, if his blood is hypercoagulable, or if he has impaired tissue perfusion, as in shock.[6]

- The cannulated extremity should be checked every hour for color, temperature, capillary filling, sensation, and blanching.
- If the extremity becomes blanched or cool, or if the patient complains of tingling, the arterial line may be occluded.
- The extremity should be placed below the level of the heart.[67]
- The findings must be reported to the physician and the catheter flow discontinued.

To help prevent vasospasm, medications should never be injected into the line. The extremity should also be checked for cutaneous ischemia. This procedure is performed by observing the response to a bolus of flushing fluid injected by way of the flush device.[47] If the skin blanches as the catheter is flushed, the line should be repositioned or discontinued. Again, the waveform should be checked for a damped tracing. If the waveform becomes damped or the fluctuations are smoothed out, the usual causes are air in the line or transducer, or clotting in the arterial line.

TABLE 21-5 CALIBRATION PROCEDURE FOR INTRA-ARTERIAL MONITORING USING SELF-CALIBRATING EQUIPMENT

Steps

1. Turn monitor alarm off.
2. Turn the stopcock nearest to the transducer away from the transducer (opens transducer to atmosphere).
3. Push in zero calibration button on monitor and turn dial to zero.
4. Push in 100 button on monitor and turn dial to 100.
5. Open stopcock back to original position.
6. Turn monitor alarm on.

TABLE 21-6 LIST OF MAJOR AND MINOR COMPLICATIONS OF INTRA-ARTERIAL CANNULATION

Major	Minor
1. Local obstruction with distal ischemia	1. Pain
2. External hemorrhage	2. Ecchymosis (common)
3. False aneurysm	3. Temporary loss of pulse
4. Massive ecchymosis	4. Arteriospasm
5. Dissection	5. Infection (rare)
6. Air embolism	
7. Blood loss	

(Carrico CJ, Horovitz JH: Monitoring the critically ill surgical patient. Advances in Surgery. Chicago, Year Book Medical Publishers, 1977)

Air Embolism. Air embolism is another complication of intra-arterial catheterization.

● To prevent this complication, the nurse must keep the tubing free of air. The source of the air bubbles may be the drip chamber. When the flush device is released, a high velocity jet of fluid flows through the air-filled drip chamber. Air is thus pulled into the flowing stream and injected into the fluid below. Introduction of a filter into the system and care when filling the flush system have been recommended to eliminate the bubbles.[35] Complete removal of air from the flush bags has also been suggested.[42]

● If an air bubble forms in the tubing, it can be removed by pinch-clamping the T-connector at the catheter site, disconnecting the transmission tubing, and then flushing the entire system until all air bubbles are expelled.[52]

Sepsis. To help prevent sepsis as a complication of intra-arterial monitoring, the nurse has several responsibilities.

● The dressing of the site of entry should be changed every day.[68]

● Povidone iodine, alcohol, and antibiotic ointment in the order mentioned should also be applied to the site daily.

● The dressing should be of waterproof material and be kept dry.

● The tubing and the solution should be changed every 24 hours.[68]

● Sterile caps should be kept over the openings of the stopcocks.

Inaccuracies. There are several sources of inaccuracy in measuring the intra-arterial blood pressure. If there are inaccuracies, the nurse needs to troubleshoot the system (Table 21-7).

Drawing Blood Samples. Sometimes blood samples need to be drawn. The procedure for this is summarized in Table 21-8.

Removal of Catheter. When the need for continuous intra-arterial monitoring has ended, the catheter should be removed by the physician or the nurse.

● First, the procedure is explained to the patient.

● To remove the catheter, the tape or the suture, or both, are removed and the clamp on the T-connector is closed.

● The catheter is quickly removed and the site is immediately compressed for 5 to 10 minutes, or longer if the patient has been anticoagulated or has a coagulopathy.

● At the end of the five to ten minutes, the site is checked for bleeding, possible hematoma, and circulation problems.

● If the patient is thought to be septic, the tip of the catheter should be sent to the laboratory for culturing.

Care of Equipment. Care and cleaning procedures of the intra-arterial monitoring equipment are important.

● The nondisposable transducers should be cultured daily.[6] Anaerobic and aerobic cultures of the infusion fluid should be taken frequently.

● The nondisposable transducers should be cleaned with strong soap, rinsed, and gas-sterilized between patients.

If transducers and pressure gauges are not adequately cleaned between uses, bacteremia, fungemia, and serum hepatitis can result. These conditions occur because the instruments communicate directly with the patient's intravascular space by way of the catheter and tubing.[6]

The invention of sterile disposable transducer domes has reduced the time needed for cleaning, transporting, and sterilizing. With these disposable domes, the blood is contained within the sterile enclosed position of the transducer and does not come into direct contact with the diaphragm of the transducer.[52]

Summary

Intra-arterial catheterization has become a common and important method of assessing the critically ill patient. This method has been shown more accurate in assessing the patient who is in a state of low blood flow or shock. The most common site used is the radial artery, its safety being

TABLE 21-7 INACCURACIES IN BLOOD PRESSURE MEASUREMENT AND NURSING RESPONSIBILITIES

Problem	Causes	Nursing Responsibilities
1. Damped waveform	Prevention of pulses from traveling through fluid-filled catheter, so that pressure waves not sensed	Straighten extremity. Check for kinks in system. Check circulation of extremity. Check for air at transducer. Make sure metal clamp on T-connector is not partly occluding line. Check system for leaks. Draw blood from line. Flush system (after other checks).
2. Large discrepency between cuff pressure and intra-arterial blood pressure	Transducer may not be calibrated. Patient may be going into shock. Air or blood at transducer	Calibrate transducer. Check other vital signs to ensure that patient is not going into shock.
3. Leak in catheter transducer system	Loose connection in system Crack at catheter hub site or in transducer	Check connections. Check for crack in catheter hub and transducer.

TABLE 21-8 BLOOD-DRAWING PROCEDURE FROM AN ARTERIAL LINE

Steps
1. Turn off monitor alarm.
2. Turn stopcock nearest to transducer away from transducer.
3. Close metal clamp on T-connector.
4. Wipe off T-connector membrane with povidone iodine.
5. Draw approximately 2 to 5 ml blood from catheter. Discard this blood.[50]
6. Draw blood sample.
7. Open metal clamp on T-connector.
8. Flush system with flush device.
9. Turn stopcock to original position.
10. Turn on monitor alarm.

---

based on the Allen or Ultrasonic Doppler test. A nonreactive plastic catheter such as Teflon should be used. The intra-arterial monitoring system consists of five parts: catheter, T-connector, fluid source, transducer, and monitor. Once the catheter has been placed, care of the intra-arterial line is primarily the nurse's responsibility.

Major complications of intra-arterial catheterization are accidental blood loss, local obstruction with distal ischemia, air embolism, and sepsis. The nurse has several responsibilities in caring for the patient with an arterial line. Between patients, special care must be taken to ensure sterility of the transducer equipment. Meticulous care of the patient with an arterial line helps avoid complications, thereby making intra-arterial monitoring of the critically ill patient a valuable assessment tool.

REFERENCES

1. Abbott Laboratories, North Chicago, Illinois.
2. Abernathy WS: Complete heart block caused by the Swan–Ganz catheter. Chest 65:349, 1974
3. Adams NR: Reducing the perils of intracardiac monitoring. Nursing 76 6(4):66–74, 1976
4. Allen EV: Thromboangiitis obliterans: Methods of diagnosis of chronic occlusive arterial lesions distal to the wrist with illustrative cases. Am J Med Sci 178:237–244, 1929
5. Applefeld JJ, Caruthers TE, Reno DJ et al: Assessment of the sterility of long-term cardiac catheterization using the thermodilution Swan–Ganz catheter. Chest 74(4):377–380, 1978
6. Baker RJ: Monitoring in critically ill patients. Surg Clin North Am 57:1139–1158, 1977
7. Beall CE, Braun HA, Cheney FW: Physiologic Bases for Respiratory Care. Missoula, Mountain Press Publishing Company, 1974
8. Bedford RF: Percutaneous radial-artery cannulations—increased safety using Teflon catheters. Anesthesiology 42:219–221, 1975
9. Bedford RF: Radial artery function following percutaneous cannulation with 18- and 20-gauge catheters. Anesthesiology 47:37–39, 1977
10. Berne RM, Levy MN: Cardiovascular Physiology. St. Louis, The C.V. Mosby Company, 1977
11. Bloomfield DA: Dye Curves: The Theory and Practice of Indicator Dilution. Baltimore, University Park Press, 1974
12. Bolognini V: The Swan–Ganz pulmonary artery catheter: Implications for nursing. Heart Lung 3(6):979–981, 1974
13. Buchbinder N, Ganz W: Hemodynamic monitoring: Invasive techniques. Anesthesiology 45:146–155, 1976
14. Caldera D, Long MC, Cullen, DJ: Thermodilution technic for cardiac output. N Engl J Med 293:1210, 1975
15. Carrico CJ, Horovitz JH: Monitoring the critically ill surgical patient. In Rob C (ed): Advances in Surgery, pp 101–127. Chicago, Year Book Medical Publishers, 1977
16. Chun GM, Ellestad MH: Perforation of the pulmonary artery by a Swan–Ganz catheter. N Engl J Med 284:1041–1042, 1971
17. Cohn JN: Blood pressure measurement in shock. JAMA 199(13):972–976, 1967
18. Conahan TJ: Air embolization during percutaneous Swan–Ganz catheter placement. Anesthesiology 50(4):360–361, 1979
19. Consultants Hemodynamic Training Manual. Santa Ana, American Edwards Laboratories Division American Hospital Supply Corporation, 1979
20. Dalton B, Laver MB: Vasospasm with an indwelling radial artery cannula. Anesthesiology 34:194–197, 1973
21. Daum S, Schapira M: Intracardiac knot formation in a Swan–Ganz catheter. Anesth and Analg 52(5):862–863, 1973
22. Davidson R, Parker M, Harrison RA: The validity of determinations of pulmonary wedge pressure during mechanical ventilation. Chest 73(3):352–355, 1978
23. Downs JB, Chapman RL, Hawkins IF et al: Prolonged Radial-Artery Catheterization. Arch Surg 108:671–673, 1974
24. Downs JB, Rachstein AD, Klein EF: Hazards of radial artery catheterization. Anesthesiology 38:283–286, 1973
25. Driver CE: The effect of elevating the head of the patient's bed while obtaining the central venous pressure measurement. Circulation, Supplement II (45 and 46): II-241, 1972
26. Dye LE, Segall PH, Russell RO et al: Deep venous thrombosis of the upper extremity associated with use of the Swan–Ganz catheter. Chest 73:673–675, 1978
27. Fegler G: Measurements of cardiac output in anesthetized animals by thermodilution method. Q J Exp Physiol 39:153–164, 1954
28. Foot G, Schabel SI, Hodges M: Pulmonary complications of flow-directed balloon-tipped catheters. N Engl J Med 290(17):927–931, 1974
29. Forrester JS, Chatterjee K, Swan JC: Hemodynamic Monitoring in Patients with Acute Myocardial Infarction. JAMA 226(1):60–61, 1973
30. Forrester JS, Diamond G, Chatterjee K et al: Medical therapy of acute myocardial infarction by application of hemodynamic subsets. N Engl J Med 295:1356–1362, 1976
31. Forrester JS, Diamond G, Freedman S et al: Silent mitral insufficiency in acute myocardial infarction. Circulation 44:877–883, 1971
32. Forrester JS, Diamond G, McHugh TJ et al: Filling pressures in the right and left sides of the heart in acute myocardial infarction. N Engl J Med 285:190–193, 1971
33. Ganz W, Donoso R, Marcus H et al: A new technique for measurement of cardiac output by thermodilution in man. Am J Cardiol 27:392–396, 1971
34. Ganz W, Swan WJC: Measurement of blood flow by thermodilution. Am J Cardiol 29:241–245, 1972
35. Gardner RM, Bond EL, Clark JS: Safety and efficacy of continuous flush systems for arterial and pulmonary artery catheters. Ann Thorac Surg 23:534–538, 1977
36. Gernert CF, Schwartz S: Pulmonary artery catheterization. Am J Nurs 73:1182–1185, 1973
37. Gold HK, Leinbach RC, Dunkman WB: Wedge pressure monitoring in myocardial infarction. N Engl J Med 285:230–231, 1971
38. Golden MS, Pinder T, Anderson WT et al: Fatal pulmonary hemorrhage complicating use of a flow-directed balloon-tipped catheter in a patient receiving anticoagulant therapy. Am J Cardiol 32:865–867, 1973
38a. Grose BL, Woods SL: Effects of mechanical ventilation and backrest position upon pulmonary artery and pulmonary capillary wedge pressure measurements. Am Rev Resp Dis 123:120, 1981
39. Grose BL, Woods SL, Laurent DJ et al: Effects of Backrest position on thermodilution cardiac output measurement in 30 acutely ill patients. Circulation 59 and 60(4):248, 1979

40. Guide to Physiological Pressure Monitoring. Waltham, Hewlett-Packard, 1977
41. Hamilton AJ: Selected Subjects for Critical Care Nurses. Missoula, Mountain Press Publishing Company, 1975
42. Harbort RA, Dalgetty RG: Bubble formation in flush systems. Ann Thorac Surg 25:179–180, 1978
43. Haughey B: CVP lines monitoring and maintaining. Am J Nurs 78(4):635–638, 1978
44. Heikkilä J: Mitral incompetence complicating acute myocardial infarction. Brit Heart J 29:162–169, 1967
45. Hobelman C, Smith DE, Virgilio RW et al: Mechanics of ventilation with positive end-expiratory pressure. Ann Thorac Surg 24:68–76, 1977
46. James PM: Central venous cannulation. Hosp Med 13(5):106–120, 1977
47. Johnson RW: A complication of radial-artery cannulation. Anesthesiology 40:598–600, 1974
48. Johnstone RE, Greenhow DE: Catheterization of the dorsalis pedis artery. Anesthesiology 39:654–655, 1973
49. Knopp R, Dailey RH: Central venous cannulation and pressure monitoring. J Am Coll Emergency Physicians 6(8):358–366, 1977
50. Krueger KE, Underhill SL, Mansfield LW: Obtaining stable hematocrit and plasma sodium values on blood specimens withdrawn from a pulmonary artery catheter. Circulation 59 and 60(Suppl II):246, 1979
51. Lalli SM: The complete Swan–Ganz. RN 9:65–77, 1978
52. Lantiegne KC, Civetta JM: A system for maintaining invasive pressure monitoring. Heart Lung 7:610–621, 1978
53. Lapin ES, Murray JA: Hemoptysis with flow-directed cardiac catheterization. JAMA 220(9):1246, 1972
54. Lemen R, Jones JG, Cowan G: A mechanism of pulmonary-artery perforation by Swan–Ganz catheters. N Engl J Med 242(4):211–212, 1975
55. Lipp H, Gambetta M, Schwartz J et al: Intermittent pansystolic murmur and presumed mitral regurgitation after acute myocardial infarction. Am J Cardiol 30:690–694, 1972
56. Lipp H, O'Donoghue K, Resnekov L: Intracardiac knotting of a flow-directed balloon catheter. N Engl J Med 288:220, 1971
57. Manjuran RS, Agarwal JB, Roy SB: Relationship of pulmonary artery wedge pressures in mitral stenosis. Am Heart J 89:(2)207–211, 1975
58. Mattea EJ, Paruta AN, Worthen LR: Sterility of Prefilled syringes for thermodilution cardiac output measurement. Am J Hosp Phar 36:1156–1157, 1979
59. McArthur BJ, Hargiss C, Schoenknecht F: Stopcock contamination in an ICU: Am J Nurs 75(1):96–97, 1975
60. McCloud TC, Putman CE: Radiology of the Swan–Ganz catheter and associated pulmonary complications. Radiology 116:19–22, 1975
61. McHugh T, Forrester JS, Adler L et al: Pulmonary vascular congestion in acute myocardial infarction: Hemodynamic and radiologic correlations. Ann Intern Med 76:29–33, 1972
62. McNally J: Invasive monitoring with the Swan–Ganz catheter. Ariz Med 31:(6)421–424, 1974
63. Mond H, Hunt D, Sloman G: Haemodynamic monitoring in the CCU using the Swan–Ganz right heart catheter. Brit Heart J 35:635–642, 1973
64. Morgan BC: The hemodynamic effects of change in blood volume during intermittent positive-pressure ventilation. Anesthesiology 30:297–305, 1969
65. Mozersky DJ, Buckley CJ, Hagood CO et al: Ultrasonic evaluation of the palmar circulation. Am J Surg 126:810–812, 1973
66. Murray J, Smallwood J: CVP monitoring: Sidestepping potential perils. Nursing 77 7:42–47, 1977
67. Nielson M: Intra-arterial monitoring of blood pressure. Am J Nurs 74(1):48–53, 1974
68. Nikas D, Konkoly R: Nursing responsibilities in arterial and intracranial pressure monitoring. J Neurosurg Nurs 7:116–122, 1975
69. Normann NA: Thermodilution technic for cardiac output. N Engl J Med 295:48–49, 1976
70. Rackley CE, Russell RO: Left ventricular function in acute myocardial infarction and its clinical significance. Circulation 45:231–244, 1972
71. Rahimtoola SH: Left ventricular end-diastolic and filling pressures in assessment of ventricular function. Chest 63:858–860, 1973
72. Renke RT, Higgins CB, Atkin JW: Pulmonary infarction complicating the use of Swan–Ganz catheters. Br J Radiol 48:885–888, 1975
73. Rice CL, Hobelman CF, John DA et al: Central venous pressure or pulmonary capillary wedge pressure as the determinant of fluid placement in aortic surgery. Surgery 84(3):437–440, 1978
74. Russell RO, Rackely CE: Hemodynamic Monitoring in a Coronary Intensive Care Unit. Mount Kisco, Futura Publishing Company, 1974
75. Rutherford BD, McCann WP, O'Donovan TP: The value of monitoring pulmonary artery pressure for early detection of left ventricular failure following myocardial infarction. Circulation 43:655–665, 1971
76. Samii K, Conseiller C, Viars P: Cental venous pressure and pulmonary wedge pressure. Arch Surg 111:1122–1125, 1976
77. Scheinman M, Abbott JA, Rapaport E: Clinical uses of a flow directed right heart catheter. Arch Intern Med 124:19–24, 1969
78. Schwartz KV, Garcia FG: Entanglement of Swan–Ganz catheter around an intracardiac structure. JAMA 237:1198–1199, 1977
79. Shinn JA, Woods SL, Huseby JS: Effect of intermittent positive pressure ventilation upon pulmonary artery and pulmonary capillary wedge pressures in acutely ill patients. Heart Lung 8(20):322–327, 1979
80. Smith AC: Effect of mechanical ventilation on the circulation. Ann NY Acad Sci 121:733–745, 1965
81. Smith WR, Glauser FL, Jamison P: Ruptured chordae of the tricuspid valve: The consequence of flow-directed Swan–Ganz catheterization. Chest 70:790–792, 1976
82. Solomon HA, San Marco MA, Willis RJ et al: Cardiac output determination: Superiority of thermal dilution. Surg Forum 20:28–30, 1969
83. Sorensen MB, Bille–Brahe NE, and Engell HC: Cardiac output measurement by thermal dilution. Ann Surg 183:67–72, 1976
84. Spoerel WE, Deimling P, Aitken R: Direct arterial pressure monitoring from the dorsalis pedis artery. Can Anaesth Soc J 22:91–99, 1975
85. Stein J, Urdang L: The Random House Dictionary of the English Language. New York, Random House, 1973
86. Stein L, Aberman A, Bernaud JJ: Relationship between pulmonary artery pressure and catheter position. Circulation 48(2):452–453, 1973
87. Strong AB: Effects of patient positioning on central venous pressure measurements: An experimental study. Circulation 51 and 52(Suppl II):II–265, 1975
88. Swan–Ganz Monitoring Systems. Santa Ana, American Edwards Laboratories, 1977
89. Swan HJC, Ganz W: Use of balloon flotation catheter in critically ill patients. Surg Clin North Am 55(3):501–520, 1975
90. Swan HJC, Ganz W, Forrester J et al: Catheterization of the heart in man with use of a flow-directed balloon-tipped catheter. N Engl J Med 283:447–451, 1970
91. Tinker J: Two methods of assessing the critically ill patient. Nursing Times 297:318–320, 1978
92. Warren DJ, Ledingham JGG: Cardiac output in the conscious rabbit: An analysis of the thermodilution technique. J Appl Physiol 34:246–251, 1974
93. Weisel RD, Berger RL, Hechtman HB: Measurement of cardiac output by thermodilution. N Engl J Med 292:682–684, 1975
94. Weisel RD, Vito L, Dennis RC et al: Clinical applications of thermodilution cardiac output determinations. Am J Surg 129:449–454, 1975
94a. West JB: Respiratory Physiology—the Essentials. Baltimore, Williams & Wilkins, 1979
95. Winsor T, Burch GE: Phlebostatic axis and phlebostatic level, reference levels for venous pressure measurements in man. Proc Soc Exp Biol Med 58:165–169, 1945

96. Woods M, Scott RN, Harken AH: Practical considerations for the use of a pulmonary artery thermistor catheter. Surgery 79:469–475, 1976
97. Woods SL: Monitoring pulmonary artery pressures. Am J Nurs 76(11):1765–1771, 1976
98. Woods SL, Mansfield L: Effects of body position upon pulmonary artery and pulmonary capillary wedge pressures in noncritically ill patients. Heart Lung 5(1):83–90, 1976
98a. Woods, SL, Laurent DJ, Grose BL, Mansfield LW: Effect of backrest position on pulmonary artery pressures in acutely-ill patients. Circulation, 62:III–184, October, 1980
99. Wyatt R, Graves I, Cooper DJ: Proximal skin necrosis after radial-artery cannulation. Lancet 1:1135–1138, 1974
100. Yang SS, Bentivoglio GG, Maranhao V et al: Cardiac Catheterization Data to Hemodynamic Parameters. Philadelphia, F.A. Davis, 1978
101. Yorra FH, Oblath R, Jaffe H et al: Massive thrombosis associated with the use of the Swan–Ganz catheter. Chest 65:682–684, 1974
102. Zarins C, Virgilio RW, Smith DE et al: The effect of vascular volume on positive end expiratory pressure: Indirect cardiac output depression and wedge left atrial pressure discrepancy. J Surg Res 23:348–360, 1977

ADDITIONAL READING

Berryhill RE, Benumof JL, Rauscher LA: Pulmonary vascular pressure reading at the end of exhalation. Anesthesiology 49:365–368, 1978
Cayetano TD, Gerzari WA, Barash PG et al: Hand held thermodilution cardiac output injector. Crit Care Med 5:210–212, 1977
Cerra F, Milch R, Lajos TZ: Pulmonary artery catheterization in critically ill surgical patients. Ann Surg 177:37–39, 1973
Civetta JM: Pulmonary-artery-pressure determination: Electronic superior to manometric. N Engl J Med 235:1145–1146, 1971
Civetta JM, Gabel JC: Flow-directed pulmonary artery catherization in surgical patients: Indications and modifications of technic. Ann Surg 176:(6)753–756, 1972
Civetta JM, Gabel JC, Laver MB: Disparate ventricular function in surgical patients. Surg Forum 22:136–139, 1971
Crexells C, Chatterjee K, Forrester JS et al: Optimal level of filling pressure in the left side of the heart in acute myocardial infarction. N Engl J Med 289:1263–1266, 1973
Daily EK, Schroeder JS: Techniques in Bedside Monitoring, St Louis, C.V. Mosby, 1981
Daly JM: Central venous catheterization. Am J Nurs 75:823–824, 1975
DeLaurentis DA, Hayes M, Matsumoto T et al: Does central venous pressure accurately reflect hemodynamic and fluid volume patterns in the critical surgical patient? Am J Surg 126:415–418, 1973
Falor WH, Hansel JR, Williams GB: Gangrene of the hand: A complication of radial artery cannulation. J Trauma 16:713–716, 1976
Feeley TW: Re-establishment of radial artery patency for arterial monitoring. Anesthesiology 46:73–75, 1977
Fisher ML, DeFelice CE, Parisi AF: Assessing left ventricular filling pressure with flow-directed (Swan–Ganz) catheters. Chest 68(4):542–547, 1975
Fitzpatrick GF, Hampson LG, Burgess JH: Bedside determination of left atrial pressure. Can Med Assoc J 106:1293–1298, 1972
Forrester JS, Diamond GA, Swan HJC: Bedside diagnosis of latent cardiac complication in acutely ill patients. JAMA 222:59–63, 1972
Freed MD, Keane JF: Cardiac output measured by thermodilution in infants and children. J Pediatr 92:39–42, 1978
Giordano J, Harken A: Effect of continuous positive pressure ventilation on cardiac output. Am Surg 41:221–224, 1975
Gorlin R: Practical cardiac hemodynamics. N Engl J Med 296:203–205, 1977
Gowen GF: Interpretation of central venous pressure. Surg Clin North Am 53(3):649–653, 1973
Guyton AC, Jones CE: Central venous pressure: Physiological significance and clinical implications. Am Heart J 86(4):431–437, 1973
Hamer JD, Mathews ET, Hardman J: Cannulation of the Radial Artery. Lancet 1:1282, 1974
Hamilton WF, Dow P: An experimental study of the standing waves in the pulse propagated through the aorta. Am J Physiol 125:48–59, 1939
Hodges M, Downs JB, Mitchell LA: Thermodilution and Fick cardiac index determination following cardiac surgery. Crit Care Med 5:182–184, 1975
Homer LD, Moss GS, Herman CM: Errors in measurement of cardiac output with dye-dilution curves in shock. J Appl Physiol 27:101–103, 1969
Kaplan J, Meller E: Insertion of the Swan–Ganz catheter. Anesthesiology Review 11:22, 1976
Katz JD, Cronau LH, Barash PG et al: JAMA 237(26):2832–2834, 1977
King EG, Jones RL, Patakas DA: Evaluation of positive end-expiratory pressure therapy in the adult respiratory distress syndrome. Can Anaesth Soc J 20:546–558, 1973
Malin C, Swartz S: Starling curves as a guide to fluid management. Heart Lung 4:588–592, 1975
Marchiondo K: CVP. The whys and hows of central venous pressure monitoring. Nursing '74 4(1):21–24, 1974
McMichael J, Johnston EA: Postural changes in cardiac output and respiration in man. Q J Exp Physiol 27:55–72, 1937
McMichael J, Sharpey-Schafer EP: Cardiac output in man by a direct Fick method. Brit Heart J 6:33–40, 1944
Mosely P, Roger V, Doty DB: Long-term arterial catheterization for repeated blood sampling. Surgery 67:455–456, 1970
Olsson B, Pool J, Vandermoten P et al: Validity and reproducibility of determination of cardiac output by thermodilution in man. Cardiology 55:136–148, 1970
Pace NL, Horton W: Indwelling pulmonary-artery catheters. JAMA 223:893–894, 1975
Paul DR, Hoyt JL, Boutros AR: Cardiovascular and respiratory changes in response to change of posture in the very obese. Anesthesiology 45:73–78, 1976
Pavek K, Lindquist O, Arfors KE: Validity of thermodilution method for measurement of cardiac output in pulmonary edema. Cardiovasc Res 7:419–422, 1973
Piegas LS, Chissoni de Carvalho H, Marmo do Souza E et al: Use of the Swan–Ganz catheter in the diagnosis of ventricular septal defect after myocardial infarction. Heart Lung 2:539–541, 1973
Powner DJ: Thermodilution technic for cardiac output. N Engl J Med 293:1210–1211, 1975
Prakash R, Parmley WW, Dikshit K et al: Hemodynamic effects of postural changes in patients with acute myocardial infarction. Chest 64(1):7–9, 1973
Rackley CE, Russell RO: Invasive Techniques for Hemodynamic Measurements. New York, American Heart Association, 1973
Reininger E, Troy BL: Error in thermodilution cardiac output measurement caused by variation in syringe volume. Cathet Cardiovasc Diag 2:415–417, 1976
Remington JW: Contour changes of the aortic pulse during propagation. Am J Physiol 199:331–334, 1960
Rodman GH, Civetta JM: Bedside pulmonary artery catheterization: Simplification of technique. Arch Surg 109(6).840–841, 1974
Rotman M, Chen JT, Seningen RP et al: Pulmonary arterial diastolic pressure in acute myocardial infarction. Am J Cardiol 33(3):357–362, 1974
Rushmer RF: Cardiovascular Dynamics. Philadelphia, WB Saunders, 1976
Russell RO, Hunt P, Potanin C et al: Hemodynamic monitoring in the coronary intensive care unit. Arch Intern Med 130:370–376, 1972
Russell R, Rackley CE: Hemodynamic Monitoring in a Coronary Intensive Care Unit. Mt. Kisco, Futura Publishing Company, 1974
Saka E, Lin YT, Oka Y: An unusual cause of false radial artery blood pressure readings during cardiopulmonary bypass. Anesthesiology 43:487–489, 1975
Schroeder JS, Daily EK: Techniques in Bedside Hemodynamic Monitoring. St Louis, C.V. Mosby, 1976

Sokolow M, McIlroy MB: Clinical Cardiology. Los Altos, Lange Medical Publications, 1977

Steele P, Davies H: The Swan–Ganz catheter in the cardiac laboratory. Brit Heart J 35:647–650, 1973

Stenson R, Crouse L, Harrison DC: Computer measurements of cardiac output by dye dilution: Comparison of computer, Fick and Dow techniques. Cardiovasc Res 6:449–456, 1962

Stevens P: Positive end expiratory pressure breathing. American Lung Association 5:1–6, 1977

Swan HJC: Central venous pressure monitoring is an outmoded procedure of limited practical value. In Ingelfinger F et al (eds): Controversy in Internal Medicine, Vol. 2, pp 185–193. Philadelphia, WB Saunders, 1974

Tanner G: Heart failure in the MI patient. Am J Nurs 77:230–234, 1977

Vinsant M, Spence MI, Hagen DC: A Common Sense Approach to Coronary Care. St Louis, C.V. Mosby, 1975

Walinsky P: Acute hemodynamic monitoring. Heart Lung 6:838–844, 1977

Weinstein RA: The design of pressure monitoring devices: Infection control considerations. Med Instrum 10:287–290, 1976

SECTION C
DIAGNOSIS AND TREATMENT

22

Diagnosis and Treatment of the Patient with Coronary Artery Disease and Myocardial Ischemia

SANDRA L. UNDERHILL, R.N., M.N.

Angina pectoris, literally "strangling of the chest," is a symptom of myocardial ischemia as a result of an imbalance in oxygen supply and demand.[27] The focus of this chapter is myocardial ischemia secondary to coronary atherosclerosis. Other causes are coronary artery spasm, a fall in blood pressure, a reduction in extracellular fluid volume, anemia, and drug effect.[10] Myocardial oxygen demands are increased by effort, emotional stress, exposure to cold weather, smoking tobacco, and eating. As long as coronary vasodilation increases blood supply (normally four- to five-fold),[27] this extra demand can be met. However, coronary atherosclerosis prevents adequate vasodilation from occurring.

ASSESSMENT OF THE PATIENT

Angina must be promptly recognized, because complications from myocardial ischemia can be fatal. Accurate history-taking and physical examination by the nurse (Chap. 14) can assist the physician in making an early diagnosis and will also provide important baseline data, useful in evaluating subsequent episodes of chest discomfort. Chest discomfort is associated with many other conditions (Table 22-1). However, it is the role of the physician to make the differential diagnosis.

Angina can be classified as classic or variant (Prinzmetal's). Classic angina is associated with a very characteristic onset, duration, location, radiation, and quality. Prinzmetal's angina is not typically associated with these characteristic findings. Angina can be categorized as stable,

unstable, or prolonged but without recent evidence of infarction. Stable angina is defined as angina that has not changed in frequency, intensity, duration, or character for 60 days, whereas unstable angina has changed within that period and may signify impending infarction. Angina that is considered prolonged lasts 30 minutes or longer.

Clinical Findings

Angina is a subjective symptom which usually lasts 2 to 5 minutes if the precipitating factor is relieved, occasionally 5 to 15 minutes, and rarely 15 to 30 minutes.[18] Patients do not always admit to having chest "pain" and, therefore, pain-equivalents should be used when eliciting the quality of discomfort. Common descriptions used by the patient include: strangling, constriction, tightness, aching, squeezing, pressing, heaviness, expanding sensation, choking in throat, indigestion, and burning.[18] Some patients clench their fist over their sternum when describing the discomfort (Levine's sign). It is rare for patients to experience no chest discomfort as a result of myocardial ischemia.

Location of the discomfort is usually in the retrosternal region, although it may occur anywhere on the chest. It may radiate down both arms, but usually the left; sometimes up to the mandible, maxilla, teeth, to the tongue or hard palate, or to the front or back of the neck (Fig. 22-1). The patient may complain of aching in the left interscapular region or of an aching shoulder, wrist, elbow, or forearm, which is more significant when it is not related to effort involving the shoulder or the arm. Sometimes patients experience discomfort only in an area of radiated pain

TABLE 22-1 CONDITIONS ASSOCIATED WITH CHEST DISCOMFORT[17,18]

Coronary:
Coronary atherosclerotic heart disease
Coronary artery spasm
Coronary arteritis
Fibromuscular hyperplasia of the coronary arteries

Cardiovascular, noncoronary:
Acute pericarditis
Aortic insufficiency
Aortic stenosis
Cardiomyopathy, especially idiopathic hypertrophic subaortic stenosis
Dissecting aortic aneurysm
Extrasystolic beats or premature contractions
Mitral stenosis
Mitral valve prolapse
Superficial thrombophlebitis of pericardial veins

Gastrointestinal:
Acute pancreatitis
"Cafe coronary"
Cholecystitis and cholelithiasis
Diffuse esophageal spasm
Distension of splenic flexure of colon
Esophageal rupture
Peptic ulcer
Reflux esophagitis and hiatal hernia

Pulmonary:
Mediastinal emphysema
Postmyocardial infarction syndrome
Pulmonary embolism
Pulmonary hypertensive pain
Spontaneous pneumothorax

Neuromuscular:
Chest wall pain and tenderness
Herpes zoster
Thoracic outlet syndrome
Tietze's syndrome

Emotional:
Anxiety
Depression
Self-gain

(Hurst JW, King SB III; Hurst JW, Logue RB, Walter PF: In Hurst JW, Logue RB, Schlant RC et al (eds): The Heart, 4th ed, pp 1094–1102 and 1156–1290. New York, McGraw-Hill, 1978)

without any discomfort in the chest itself. The location of the discomfort can change with the natural history of the disease, probably as a result of a new ischemic area.[18] If the patient is able to circumscribe the area of discomfort, an area less than the size of a fingertip does not usually indicate myocardial ischemia.

Classic Angina. There are many factors that characteristically precipitate angina. It occurs frequently during physical exertion. Chest discomfort produced by exertion and relieved by rest is diagnosed accurately as angina by history alone 90% of the time.[18] Occasionally, a patient may experience a "second wind" phenomenon, characterized by discomfort that develops during exertion but disappears while the activity is continued. Early morning activity after a night's sleep sometimes precipitates angina that the same level of activity later in the day does not. The reason for this is not

known. Assuming the recumbent position can cause angina, possibly because of the increased work of the heart in that position (Chap. 30). Chest discomfort can be associated with eating a heavy meal. There is an increase in gastrointestinal oxygen consumption during and after a large meal. Digestion requires increased cardiac output which increases myocardial oxygen demands, often resulting in angina. This is more likely to occur if the meal is followed by exercise. Emotional tension is also a frequent precursor of angina. Chest discomfort from emotional stress tends to last longer than that produced by physical stress, because emotions are not so easily controlled as is activity.[18] For the patient with coronary atherosclerosis who cannot increase coronary blood flow, smoking tobacco, particularly cigarettes, increases myocardial workload, resulting in angina. This effect may be further enhanced by the presence of carboxyhemoglobin in the blood from smoking.[11]

Describing what relieves the discomfort may help the physician to confirm the diagnosis. Chest discomfort that is relieved by nitroglycerin within one to two minutes is probably angina. However, esophageal spasm is also relieved by nitroglycerin. If the pain is worsened by nitroglycerin, the diagnosis may be idiopathic hypertrophic subaortic stenosis. Carotid sinus massage and the Valsalva maneuver, although not recommended, have also been shown to reduce the discomfort of angina.

Prinzmetal's Angina. The chest discomfort of Prinzmetal's angina is similar to but of longer duration than that of classic angina. It is usually not brought on by exertion but may be relieved by rest and nitroglycerin. Interestingly, it appears to be cyclic, frequently occurring at the same time every day, most often on arising or in the early morning. The patient may also complain of palpitations, syncope, or bradycardia during the peak of discomfort. Prinzmetal's angina is caused by spasm of the coronary arteries.

Physical Findings

The physical examination of the patient with ischemic heart disease usually shows normal results. On inspection there may be no alteration in appearance, or the patient may exhibit pallor and cold, clammy skin. Signs are transient. Heart rate and blood pressure may increase at the onset of the ischemic episode. Pulsus alternans may be present. On auscultation an S_3 or S_4 gallop may be noted, and the murmur of mitral regurgitation secondary to ischemia of the papillary muscle may be present. A paradoxically split S_2 may be heard.[18]

Diagnostic Tests

Resting and exercise electrocardiography, radionuclide imaging, and cardiac catheterization with coronary angiography may aid in the diagnosis of ischemic heart disease. Routine chest radiography, echocardiography and serum enzyme determination are not useful in assessing the presence of coronary artery disease and myocardial ischemia.

Electrocardiogram (ECG). The resting ECG is not helpful in diagnosing ischemic heart disease unless taken during

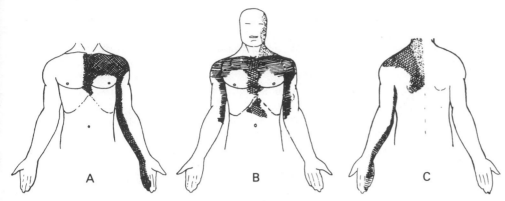

Fig. 22-1. Positions and common points of reference of cardiac pain. (**A**) Area of substernal discomfort projected to left shoulder and arm over distribution of ulnar nerve. Reference of pain may be confined to left shoulder only, or to the shoulder and along the arm only to the elbow. Pain may be referred less frequently to right shoulder and arm (**B**), or to both shoulders, arms, and hands simultaneously. Occasional radiation to the epigastrium and right upper abdominal quadrant may occur. Projection of anginal pain to the back is also encountered less frequently (**C**); reference is usually to the area of the left scapula or the interscapular region. (Smith JR, Paine R: In MacBryde CM, Blacklow RS (eds): Signs and Symptoms, 5th ed, Philadelphia, JB Lippincott, 1970)

an ischemic episode when characteristic ST-segment depression (classic angina) or elevation (Prinzmetal's angina) can be recorded (Chap. 17).

Exercise Tolerance Test (ETT). Depression or normality of the ST-segment during an ETT has been considered a reliable indicator of the presence or absence of ischemic heart disease. Recently, Weiner and associates correlated the description of chest discomfort, ST-segment variation during an ETT, and results of coronary angiography. In men, an ETT added little clinical information for patients with a diagnosis of definite angina by history. A positive response confirmed the presence of coronary artery disease, but false negatives were frequently noted. In women with a definite history of angina, a positive response was highly correlated with the presence of ischemic heart disease. However, a large number of false positive responses were noted, giving this test a low specificity for women, especially those with definite symptoms of angina. In patients with a history of atypical chest discomfort, a large number had false positive responses to the ETT. In women with negative ETT results and nonischemia-like chest discomfort the presence of coronary artery disease can be excluded. Therefore, a thorough clinical history can eliminate the need for the ETT as a diagnostic tool in many instances (Chap. 18).[37]

Cardiac Radionuclide Imaging. Areas of reduced myocardial perfusion can be detected by injecting [201]thallium and comparing rest and postexercise scans. Although of limited availability, radionuclide imaging is useful in the detection of ischemic heart disease (Chap. 20).

Cardiac Catheterization and Coronary Angiography. These tests provide definitive diagnosis of the cause of chest discomfort. However, their use should be limited to clarification of atypical chest discomfort or evaluation of coronary artery anatomy and left ventricular function in order to determine suitability for coronary artery bypass surgery (Chap. 19).

THE NATURE OF ANGINA PECTORIS

To evaluate clinical effectiveness of any intervention for patients experiencing angina, one must first be aware of certain characteristics of this disease process and the influence of the placebo effect. It has been well documented that the severity of angina spontaneously changes without any change in the therapeutic regimen or any recognized interference from extracardiac factors, such as development of anemia, duodenal ulceration, biliary tract disease, or cervical spondylosis, or any changes in body weight or in the weather. Some patients have crescendo angina, which worsens without obvious evidence of progressive coronary disease. Others have complete spontaneous cessation of angina, at least for several months.[31] Because the course of angina is difficult to predict in any given individual, the effectiveness of specific therapies is not easily determined.

Placebo Effect

The placebo effect, also, interferes with demonstration of the efficacy of therapeutic interventions in the treatment of angina. A placebo is a simulated treatment given to improve symptoms but without the ability to act upon the underlying pathophysiologic process, as the real treatment would do. The reaction of the patient to the placebo is termed the placebo effect. A placebo is generally thought of as an inert substance given as a pill in order to provide symptomatic relief, such as relief of pain. However, many other types of placebos exist, for example injections of normal saline, use of complex equipment, and performance of intricate procedures; all seem to have a greater placebo effect than a pill.[29]

Subjective improvement in a patient by means of a placebo has long been recognized. However, the placebo effect may extend to changes in objective responses. In a recent study of patients with angina pectoris, the effects of placebo versus a beta blocking agent on subjective symptoms and ST segment depression during exercise were compared.

After receiving the placebo, 65% of the 37 patients tested said that they felt better, and 27% of these same patients improved upon their exercise tolerance, as demonstrated by an increase in cardiac work before they developed ST-segment depression.[12]

Patients with angina are particularly susceptible to the effects of placebos.[1] A placebo effect is achieved in large part because of the situation in which the placebo is given. First, placebos are administered by authority figures, such as doctors or nurses. These therapists lend credibility to the treatment offered. Second, the establishment of a good therapist–patient rapport, with the therapist expressing warm interest and concern, helps to promote a positive effect. Third, the therapist who communicates belief in the effectiveness of the placebo can readily convince many patients of its worth. Fourth, patients want to believe in the value of the prescribed treatment. For these reasons, any real treatment can also be subject to a placebo effect.[25] Further discussion of the placebo effect is included in Chapter 25.

Evaluating the Relief of Angina Pectoris

The natural course of angina and the interference from the placebo effect make critical evaluation by researchers of any therapy difficult. Similarly, clinicians must also consider these factors when evaluating patient responses. However, for clinicians, the prime concern is to provide symptomatic relief to the patient. Whatever therapy is prescribed, the placebo effect can be a useful adjunct. It should be emphasized that pain that is reduced or relieved by placebo is no less real than pain that is not. Negative reactions on the part of therapists to a patient's placebo effect may not only negate the positive effect achieved by the placebo treatment but also negate the benefits which might have been attained by real therapy.

TREATMENT OF THE PATIENT

In addition to providing symptomatic relief of angina, treatment of myocardial ischemia should improve left ventricular function and prevent myocardial infarction, resulting in improvement in the quality of life and in life expectancy if all goes well. Myocardial ischemia can be reduced or eliminated by increasing blood supply and oxygen delivered to the myocardium or by reducing myocardial oxygen consumption ($M\dot{V}O_2$), or both. Long-term risk-factor modification may help to retard or reverse the basic pathologic process, coronary atherosclerosis (Chaps. 13, 43). Therapy for coronary artery disease is traditionally divided into two modes, surgical and medical, both of which are physician-directed. The disagreement over which is the better mode of treatment is not likely to be resolved for some time (Chap. 25). New interventions have created an expanded role for the nurse and have emphasized some degree of patient control in specific therapeutic modalities.

Medical Intervention

Medical management of the patient with coronary artery disease focuses on activity modification, drugs, and changes in life-style. Any underlying diseases that may promote myocardial ischemia, such as anemia, must also be treated.

Activity. Exercise and physical activity, although very beneficial to the normal heart, can increase ischemia or cause infarction in the patient with angina by producing a further imbalance in oxygen supply and demand. For the patient with angina, activity must be specifically prescribed to gain the most benefit, while preventing complications which might arise.

Patients with stable angina are encouraged to be as active as possible. Walking is a highly recommended form of exercise. Participation in formal cardiac rehabilitation programs is encouraged (Chap. 42). Prolonged, intensive physical training in patients with angina results in markedly reduced pressure-rate product (systolic blood pressure times heart rate) at rest and at work, improvement in frequency and intensity of angina, and improved exercise tolerance.[2] Depending on their job, patients experiencing mild angina can continue to work. However, some patients with disabling, though stable, angina may have to restrict activity severely in order to control chest discomfort.

Activity must be curtailed in patients with unstable angina in order to prevent the progression of myocardial ischemia to infarction. Some selected patients are able to decrease activity at home, but usually the patients are admitted to the hospital, and frequently to a cardiac care unit. Advantages of hospitalization are escape from a potentially stressful home situation; observation of objective data, such as electrocardiographic changes and the effects of medication on the discomfort; identification of complications, such as arrhythmias; and performance of coronary angiography.[18] Unstable angina is a transient phase because it either becomes stable or progresses; activity levels should be appropriately adjusted with any change.

Patients with prolonged ischemia without recent evidence of infarction are admitted to the cardiac care unit and treated as having had a myocardial infarction until proven otherwise (Chap. 23). They are usually comfortable in about 3 days. They may experience further chest discomfort after transfer to the ward, requiring readmission to the unit. If coronary angiography and bypass surgery are not performed, these patients are usually discharged home in about 2 weeks.

Drug Therapy. Drugs specifically given to improve the discomfort of angina act to enhance blood and oxygen supply to the myocardium, either by coronary vasodilation or relief of coronary artery spasm, or by decreasing myocardial oxygen demands, or both. Digitalis can be given to improve congestive heart failure associated with beta blockade therapy (Chap. 34). Antilipid agents are used to manage the long-term hyperlipidemias which may be associated with coronary artery disease (Chap. 39). Opiates and oxygen are not used in the treatment of angina except for patients with prolonged ischemia. Anticoagulants are not indicated. Specific drugs used to alter myocardial oxygen supply and demand in the management of angina are listed in Table 22-2. Actions, indications, contraindications, dosage and administration, side and toxic effects, and nursing implications are presented in Section E of this text.

Changes in Life Style. Information on life-style modification for the patient with myocardial infarction is presented in Chapter 43. For the patient with angina, these same changes may provide symptomatic relief or retard or reverse the atherosclerotic process, helping to prevent the occurrence or recurrence of infarction. Specifically, eating, drinking, and smoking habits may require alteration. Avoidance of stressful situations and improved methods of reacting to them should be encouraged. Stress-reducing techniques are discussed in the section on nursing intervention.

Patients should be encouraged to achieve and maintain optimum body weight. Obesity must be eliminated by a well-balanced, calorie-restricted diet. Angina should improve with weight loss, because the work load of the heart will be less. Diets low in cholesterol, saturated fats, and refined carbohydrates can also be recommended. Specific diet prescriptions should be given (Chaps. 13, 43).

Some patients experience angina during or after large meals. They should be encouraged to eat smaller and more frequent meals. Taking nitroglycerin before eating can eliminate chest discomfort. All patients should be cautioned against exercising immediately after large meals.

Alcohol reduces exercise tolerance in patients with angina. In addition, it may precipitate arrhythmias.[18] The consumption of alcohol is not recommended; for patients who drink in moderation, small amounts may be permitted. Patients with a history of alcohol abuse should be strongly advised not to drink. Treatment for the alcoholic patient should be sought from special agencies, for example, Alcoholics Anonymous.

Smoking tobacco can precipitate angina in patients with coronary atherosclerotic disease. As stated on all cigarette packs, smoking is known to be dangerous to health. Unless the patient relies heavily on tobacco smoking to cope with stressful situations, and has more ischemic episodes without it, tobacco smoking should be prohibited.

Surgical Intervention

There are two surgical interventions which provide treatment for the patient with coronary artery disease. Coronary artery bypass surgery may rapidly reverse the ischemic process, relieving the symptoms of angina; for some patients, partial ileal bypass surgery can impart the long-term beneficial effects of reduced lipid absorption.

Coronary Artery Bypass Surgery. Coronary artery bypass surgery is performed to relieve the symptoms of angina by revascularizing the myocardium. Of patients who have undergone coronary artery bypass surgery, 80% have been relieved of angina and are happier after surgery.[18] This procedure is not indicated for relief of myocardial ischemia that is not manifested by angina, unless a left main coronary lesion has been documented by angiography. In this instance, coronary artery bypass surgery is recommended and has been shown to prolong life.[16] Indications, contraindications, criteria for patient selection, the operative procedure, and pre- and postoperative nursing care are presented in Chapter 24.

Partial Ileal Bypass Surgery. The purpose of partial ileal bypass surgery is to lower blood lipids in patients with high

TABLE 22-2   DRUGS USED TO ALTER OXYGEN SUPPLY AND DEMAND IN THE TREATMENT OF ANGINA PECTORIS

	Increase Blood and Oxygen Supply		Decrease Oxygen Demand
	CORONARY VASODILATATION	RELIEF OF CORONARY ARTERY SPASM	
Classic angina:			
Nitroglycerin and long-acting nitrites	XX[23]		X[23]
Beta adrenergic blockers			
Propranolol			X[23]
Metoprolol			X[23]
Nadolol*			X[13]
Prinzmetal's angina:			
Nitroglycerin and long-acting nitrites		X[17]	
Alpha adrenergic blockers			
Phenoxybenzamine		X[17]	
Phenotolamine		X[17]	
Calcium blockers*			
Verapamil		X[17]	
Nifedipine		X[17]	
Epinephrine-depleting agents			
Guanethidine		X[17]	
Resperine		X[17]	
Parasympatholytic agents			
Atropine		X[17]	
Prostaglandin-synthesis blockers*			
Indomethacin		X[23]	

Key: X = primary action; XX = secondary action; * = experimental.

serum cholesterol in order to retard or reverse the atherosclerotic process, thus maintaining or improving blood supply and oxygen delivery to the myocardium. However, the basic premise of decreasing blood lipids, and in consequence the risk of myocardial infarction, has not been proven (Chap. 13). The terminal third of the ileum is removed and an end-to-end anastomosis is made to the proximal portion of the cecum. This increases fecal bile acid excretion by lowering the reabsorption of bile acids.

After partial ileal bypass surgery, serum cholesterol is decreased 33%[21] to 41%[9] in patients with heterozygous type II hyperlipoproteinemia, but to a lesser degree in those with homozygous type II hyperlipoproteinemia. Reductions in serum cholesterol of 48% in type III and 41% in type IV hyperlipoproteinemias have been documented.[9] The decrease in serum cholesterol following partial ileal bypass surgery has been shown to surpass the reductions attained by diet (6% net)[9] and the antilipid drugs cholestyramine (17%[21] to 22%[9]), clofibrate (15% to 20%), and nicotinic acid (23%)[9] (Chap. 39).

In one study of 55 patients who experienced angina preoperatively, 69% reported some degree of improvement in angina (as noted by the amount of nitroglycerin used) after partial ileal bypass surgery; total remission was reported by 26%. In the same study, 22 patients underwent pre- and postoperative angiography. Nonprogression of atherosclerotic plaques was demonstrated in 12 patients, while regression of plaques occurred in three.[9]

Diarrhea can be an annoying side effect of partial ileal bypass surgery, although the majority of patients have fewer than five bowel movements daily. Firmness and consistency of stools appears to improve with time. There are conflicting opinions regarding the effects upon weight loss.[9,27]

Vitamin B_{12} deficiency develops after partial ileal bypass surgery because the terminal ileum is bypassed. Intramuscular injections of 1000 μg of vitamin B_{12} should be given every two months for life. Interestingly, some patients appear to regain vitamin B_{12} absorption ability between 3 and 12 months after surgery.[9]

Before deciding upon a partial ileal bypass, the risks and benefits must be weighed. At this time most clinicians recommend the surgery only for patients with type II hyperlipoproteinemia who are unable to adhere to prescribed dietary and drug regimens.[18,21,27]

Nursing Implications. Routine pre- and postoperative nursing care is similar to that for any patient undergoing abdominal surgery. Specific preoperative information given should include the expected changes in the frequency, consistency, and amount of stools, and the use of diet and medications that can help control these changes. Lists of foods that may cause diarrhea and gas should be given to the patient. Postoperatively, potential fluid and electrolyte imbalances, particularly saline and water depletion and hypokalemia, should be expected. Patients should be aware of the signs of fluid depletion and of hypokalemia (Chap. 9). If potassium supplements are necessary, instructions regarding their use should be given. The importance of returning to clinic every other month for a vitamin B_{12} injection should be stressed.

NURSING INTERVENTION

Management of the patient with angina is time-consuming. A good therapist-patient rapport, which is essential if the patient is to be expected to adhere to the therapy and if the patient is to believe in the treatment, must be established. Patience, empathy, skill and a great deal of time, spent not only in individual instruction but in development of a program, are needed to make teaching effective. Professional nurses are actively seeking positions that allow them to function more independently in the care of the patient with stable angina. Many physicians are delegating these responsibilities to nurses not only because nurses are educated in these areas and are proving themselves capable in this role, but because nurse time is more cost-effective than is physician time.

Nursing care in the acute situation should be aimed toward minimizing or eliminating myocardial ischemia and preventing progression to infarction. In the chronic situation, nurses must help the patient change his life style in such a way that angina is reduced and risk factors are modifed. A sample nursing care plan for the patient with stable angina pectoris who is hospitalized on a general medical unit is presented in Table 22-3. This care plan should be used only as a guideline for providing nursing care and is not meant to be all-inclusive. In addition, it is not to be used as a standardized care plan, which would defeat the purpose of planning individualized nursing care.

Relief of Anxiety

Patients with angina are understandably very frightened and concerned. They frequently associate the occurrence of chest discomfort with impending death. Most patients have had relatives or friends who have died suddenly from heart problems. In addition, many will need to make radical lifestyle changes in order to help prevent the occurrence of angina.

Anxiety perpetuates the ischemic process of increasing sympathetic nervous system responses, resulting in elevated serum catecholamines, which raise $M\dot{V}O_2$; the increased $M\dot{V}O_2$ can precipitate an anginal attack and further increase anxiety. Anxiety also causes these patients to focus much of their attention on their hearts, resulting in escalation of the severity of the symptoms. The nursing role includes intervention aimed at reducing anxiety in the patient and his family. This can be accomplished by prompt treatment of the chest discomfort, demonstration of clinical expertise, and a caring, reassuring attitude, and also by teaching the patient about angina and how to live with it.

Teaching Plan

Development of a teaching plan enables the nurse to provide standardized content to each patient. (Principles of learning are discussed in Chap. 45). Teaching and learning effectiveness are influenced by the patient's reaction to his diagnosis and its implications, for example, grieving over the loss of good health. Chapter 44 presents psychologic aspects of recovery.

TABLE 22-3   SAMPLE NURSING CARE PLAN FOR THE PATIENT WITH STABLE ANGINA PECTORIS HOSPITALIZED ON A GENERAL MEDICINE UNIT

Problem 1: Myocardial ischemia secondary to reduced coronary blood flow resulting in potential myocardial infarction.
   Goal: To prevent occurrence of myocardial infarction.

Nursing Intervention	Scientific Rationale	Evaluation Criteria
A. Immediately reduce patient's physical activity to the level of activity before occurrence of chest discomfort.	A. Physical activity increases $M\dot{V}O_2$. When myocardial ischemia is severe and prolonged, irreversible injury or infarction of tissue results (Chap. 11).	A. 1. Activity reduced to prechest discomfort level. 2. Patient reports chest discomfort is reduced or relieved.
B. Initially assess, document, and report to the physician the following:	B. These data assist in determining the cause and effect of chest discomfort and provide a baseline so that post-therapy symptoms can be compared.	
1. The patient's description of the chest discomfort including location, radiation, duration, and the factors which affect it.	1. Although there are many conditions associated with chest discomfort (Table 22-1), there are characteristic clinical findings of both classic and variant angina pectoris (see text). (The pathophysiology of ischemic pain is presented in Chapter 11.)	B. 1. Effect on cardiovascular hemodynamics assessed, documented, and reported, as appropriate.
2. The effect of the myocardial ischemia on cardiovascular hemodynamics: perfusion to the heart, to the brain, to the kidneys, and to the periphery.	2. Myocardial ischemia may reduce myocardial contractility and ventricular compliance (Chap. 11) and may produce arrhythmias by promoting reentry and increased automaticity (Chap. 26). Cardiac output is reduced, resulting in reduced blood pressure and oxygen perfusion. The heart rate may increase as a compensatory mechanism to maintain cardiac output.	2. a. Chest discomfort, heart rate, rhythm, conduction, and blood pressure. b. Mentation. c. Urine output and BUN to creatinine ratio. d. Skin color, temperature, and moisture.
C. Obtain a 12-lead ECG during chest discomfort and report marked changes to the physician.	C. ECG changes during myocardial ischemia differ from those during myocardial infarction (Chap. 17).	C. ST-segment and T-wave forms revert to pattern seen prior to onset of chest discomfort within 5 minutes after taking sublingual nitroglycerin.
D. If myocardial infarction is suspected (chest discomfort lasting 30 minutes or longer), draw CK isoenzymes 6 to 12 hours after beginning of chest discomfort. (Chap. 15).	D. Elevated CK-MB is specific to myocardial damage.	D. CK-MB not present.
E. Administer nitroglycerin or other antianginal medications (Table 22-2) as ordered and continuously evaluate the patient's response to therapy.	E. Antianginal agents may increase myocardial blood and oxygen supply, decrease myocardial oxygen demand, or both (Table 22-2 and Chaps. 35 and 36).	E. Within 5 minutes after receiving nitroglycerin: 1. Patient reports relief of chest discomfort. 2. Heart rate and systolic blood pressure return to prechest discomfort levels. 3. Patient appears comfortable: restful, skin warm and dry, respiratory rate at or below prechest discomfort rate.
F. Provide restful environment and allay fear and anxiety by being supportive, calm, and competent.	F. Fear and anxiety precipitate the stress response, which results in increased levels of endogenous catecholamines (Chap. 11). Increased levels of epinephrine reduce pain threshold[39] and elevate $M\dot{V}O_2$.	F. Patient expresses less fear and anxiety.
G. Promote the patient's physical comfort by providing individualized, basic nursing care.	G. Physical comfort promotes the patient's sense of well-being and reduces anxiety.	G. Patient expresses that he is physically comfortable.

TABLE 22-3   SAMPLE NURSING CARE PLAN FOR THE PATIENT WITH STABLE ANGINA PECTORIS HOSPITALIZED ON A GENERAL MEDICINE UNIT (cont.)

Nursing Intervention	Scientific Rationale	Evaluation Criteria
H. Teach the patient to do the following when angina pectoris occurs: 1. Rest and relax. 2. Take nitroglycerin as prescribed (Chap. 36), and if no relief of chest discomfort has occurred within 30 minutes, immediately seek medical attention. 3. Call the physician if a change in the pattern of angina pectoris has occurred.	H. 1. Reduces $M\dot{V}O_2$. 2. Chest discomfort which is not relieved by nitroglycerin may indicate myocardial infarction. 3. Unstable angina pectoris may progress to myocardial infarction (see text).	H. Before discharge, patient describes in own words how he plans to do the following when angina pectoris occurs: 1. Rest and relax. 2. Take nitroglycerin. 3. Call the physician if change in pattern of angina pectoris occurs.

I. Teach the patient to do the following to prevent myocardial ischemia with potential myocardial infarction from occurring:
1. Be aware of precipitating factors:
  a. physiologic, such as activity during cold weather or after a heavy meal, or sexual intercourse
  b. psychologic, such as anger, grief, or sexual intercourse
2. Reduce precipitating factors by, for example:
  a. Regular, active participation in a physical cardiac rehabilitation program (Chap. 42)
  b. Reducing physical activity and psychological stress that usually results in chest discomfort, or by taking prophylactic nitroglycerin in anticipation of these stressors.
  c. Practice a stress-reduction technique of choice.
3. Adhere to the therapeutic plan (such as diet, medications, and activity level) prescribed for control of myocardial ischemia, coronary artery disease risk factors, or any other disease processes.
	I. 1 & 2. Refer to discussion of precipitating factors in text.
	
	3. The therapeutic plan prescribed to control myocardial ischemia promotes reduction of $M\dot{V}O_2$ and improvement in exercise tolerance; the plan designed to control coronary artery disease risk factors (Chap. 13) may prevent the occurrence of myocardial infarction or sudden cardiac death; control of other disease processes, such as congestive heart failure, diabetes mellitus, high blood pressure, peptic ulcer disease, reduces physiologic stress, which can increase $M\dot{V}O_2$.
		I. Before discharge, patient discusses in own words:
		
		1. Precipitating factors.
		
		2. How he could reduce precipitating factors
		
		3. Before discharge, patient describes how he will adhere to the therapeutic plan that has been prescribed for him.

Problem 2: Myocardial ischemia secondary to decreased coronary blood flow resulting in potential chest discomfort, with or without radiation to arms, neck, or jaw.
    Goal: To relieve chest discomfort by restoring balance between myocardial oxygen supply and demand.

Nursing Intervention	Scientific Rationale	Evaluation Criteria
See Problem 1.A-I.	See Problem 1.A-I	See Problem 1.A-I

Problem 3: Myocardial ischemia secondary to decreased coronary blood flow resulting in potential arrhythmias and conduction disturbances.
    Goal A: To prevent occurrence of arrhythmias and conduction disturbances by restoring balance between myocardial oxygen supply and demand.
    Goal B: To detect early and treat aggressively malignant ventricular arrhythmias, conduction abnormalities, supraventricular tachycardia, or bradycardia.

TABLE 22-3   SAMPLE NURSING CARE PLAN FOR THE PATIENT WITH STABLE ANGINA PECTORIS HOSPITALIZED ON A GENERAL MEDICINE UNIT   (cont.)

Nursing Intervention	Scientific Rationale	Evaluation Criteria
A. See Problem 1.A, F, G.	A. Myocardial ischemia may result in arrhythmias by promoting reentry and increased automaticity and in conduction disturbances by impeding or preventing electrical conduction through specialized tissues (Chap. 26).	A. Ideally, normal sinus rhythm without arrhythmia is maintained or restored, or the patient's baseline heart rate, rhythm, and conduction is maintained or restored.
B. 1. Assess and document apical-radial heart rate and rhythm every 8 hours or PRN, or before and after each dose of antiarrhythmic or cardiotonic agent (or any other drug with cardiovascular effects) and report marked changes to the physician (Chap. 34).	B. 1. Changes in apical-radial heart rate and rhythm may be a therapeutic effect of cardiac drug therapy or may be a result of drug toxicity (Chap. 34). Early detection of arrhythmias allows initiation of therapy and may prevent the occurrence of lethal arrhythmias.	B. 1, 2, & 3. Previous heart rate, rhythm, and conduction is restored. All arrhythmias and conduction disturbances are detected as they occur and do not progress to ventricular fibrillation or asystole (Chap. 17).
2. Assess blood pressure and obtain 12-lead ECG if patient complains of palpitations, if changes in the apical-radial heart rate and rhythm are noted, or if other symptoms of decreased organ perfusion occur (Problem 1.B.2.).	2. As above. In addition, palpitations and symptoms of reduced organ perfusion may result from cardiac arrhythmias and conduction disturbances. A 12-lead ECG assists in the diagnosis of arrhythmias and of myocardial damage.	
3. Give antiarrhythmic agents or other drugs as specifically ordered or in accordance with hospital policies and evaluate the response (Chaps. 34 and 35).	3. Refer to Chapters 26, 34, 35.	
4. Assess status of patient to determine other possible causes of arrhythmias and conduction disturbances:		
a. Perform cardiovascular physical examination (Chap. 14).	4. a. Concurrent disease processes, such as left ventricular failure and pulmonary emboli, can result in arrhythmias because of hypoxemia and mechanical stretch.	4. a. Normal heart and breath sounds without adventitious sounds.
b. Obtain venous blood for electrolytes, hemoglobin and, if appropriate, drug levels, as ordered.	b. Electrolyte disturbances may cause arrhythmias or conduction disturbances (Chaps. 9 and 17); lowered hemoglobin levels result in reduced oxygen-carrying capacity of the blood; arrhythmias being treated by antiarrhythmic agents may not be suppressed if serum drug levels are less than therapeutic; arrhythmias and conduction disturbances may result from drug toxicity (Chaps. 15, 34).	b. Serum K^+ level remains between 3.6 and 5.5 mEq/l. Serum Ca^{2+} remains between 4.6 and 5.5 mEq/l. Hemoglobin remains between 12 and 18 g/100 ml. Serum drug levels remain within the therapeutic range (Chaps. 15, 34).
c. Obtain arterial blood for arterial blood gases, as ordered.	c. Hypoxemia and acid-base disturbances can cause arrhythmias and conduction disturbances (Chaps. 9, 17).	c. Arterial blood gases on room air remain between: pH 7.35 — 7.45 PCO_2 35 — 45 mm Hg HCO_3^- 22 — 28 mm Hg PO_2 90 — 100 mm Hg
d. Obtain chest x-ray film, as ordered (Chap. 16).	d. Chest x-ray films may demonstrate concurrent disease processes, such as pulmonary edema or pulmonary emboli, which can cause arrhythmias.	d. Chest x-ray film remains within normal limits (Chap. 16).

TABLE 22-3   SAMPLE NURSING CARE PLAN FOR THE PATIENT WITH STABLE ANGINA PECTORIS HOSPITALIZED ON A GENERAL MEDICINE UNIT   (cont.)

Problem 4: Potential left ventricular dysfunction secondary to reduced myocardial function from myocardial ischemia, or potential myocardial ischemia secondary to left ventricular failure, resulting in transient shortness of breath, dyspnea on exertion, orthopnea, or paroxysmal nocturnal dyspnea.

Goal: To prevent occurrence of respiratory symptoms by reducing $M\dot{V}O_2$, which restores the balance between myocardial oxygen supply and demand.

Nursing Intervention	Scientific Rationale	Evaluation Criteria
A. Initially, every eight hours and during chest discomfort, assess, document, and report to the physician the following:	A. These data are useful in diagnosing left ventricular dysfunction secondary to myocardial ischemia:	A. Patient does not complain of shortness of breath, dyspnea on exertion, orthopnea, or paroxysmal nocturnal dyspnea.
1. Abnormal heart sounds (particularly S_3 and S_4 gallops, and the holosystolic murmur of papillary muscle dysfunction).	1. Diastolic filling sounds (S_3 and S_4 gallops) result from reduced left ventricular compliance associated with myocardial ischemia. Papillary muscle dysfunction (from ischemia of the papillary muscle) indicates mitral regurgitation, which can be a symptom of left ventricular dysfunction, cause left heart failure (diminished stroke volume), or both.	1. Normal heart sounds without gallops or murmurs.
2. Abnormal breath sounds (particularly crackles).	2. The presence of crackles (usually at the lung bases) may indicate pulmonary congestion from elevated left heart pressures.	2. Normal lung sounds without crackles.
3. Patient's intolerance of specific activities.	3. The association of cardiac and respiratory signs and symptoms with activities can be used as a guide for activity prescription and as a basis for teaching the patient.	3. a. Respiratory rate remains less than 16 breaths per minute at rest, and less than 20 breaths per minute with prescribed activity. b. Skin color remains normal. c. PO_2 remains 90–100 mm Hg PCO_2 remains 35– 45 mm Hg d. Heart rate remains less than 60% of maximum (if previously determined by exercise tolerance table). e. Blood pressure remains within this individual's normal limits.
B. See Problem 1.A, F, G.	B. See Problem 1.A, F, G.	B. See Problem 1.A, F, G.
C. Teach patient to do the following to prevent respiratory symptoms secondary to left ventricular failure: 1. Adhere to diet (such as low Na^+, low calorie, low total fat and saturated fat), as prescribed.	C. 1. Low Na^+ diet may reduce the extracellular fluid volume, thus reducing preload, afterload, and $M\dot{V}O_2$. In the obese patient, weight reduction may decrease cardiac work and improve tidal volume. Reduction of saturated fat and cholesterol intake may retard the atherosclerotic process (Chap. 13).	C. Before discharge, patient describes in own words how he will: 1. Adhere to diet.
2. Adhere to activity prescription, but space activities to avoid fatigue.	2. The activity prescription is determined individually to maintain the heart rate and blood pressure within safe limits (Chap. 42). Excessive fatigue is a physiologic stressor, which requires increased $M\dot{V}O_2$, or is a symptom of reduced cardiac reserve.	2. Adhere to activity prescription.
3. Individually modify physical activities which have precipitated respiratory symptoms in the past, such as climbing stairs or lying flat.	3. Physical activity can induce respiratory symptoms by increasing $M\dot{V}O_2$ or altering hemodynamics (increased blood return to the heart).	3. Modify physical activities that have precipitated respiratory symptoms in the past.

TABLE 22-3 SAMPLE NURSING CARE PLAN FOR THE PATIENT WITH STABLE ANGINA PECTORIS HOSPITALIZED ON A GENERAL MEDICINE UNIT (cont.)

Problem 5: Potential reduced cardiac output secondary to left ventricular dysfunction resulting in transient reduced perfusion to vital organs.

Goal: To prevent symptoms of reduced cardiac output by restoring the balance between myocardial oxygen supply and demand.

Nursing Intervention	Scientific Rationale	Evaluation Criteria

A. See Problem 1.A, F, G
B. Initially, every eight hours, and during chest discomfort, assess, document, and report to the physician the following:
  1. Hypotension.
 	
  2. Tachycardia and other arrhythmias.
 	
  3. Fatigue.
 	
  4. Mentation changes (using input from family).
 	
  5. Reduced urine output (less than 250 ml per eight-hour shift).
 	
  6. Cool, moist, cyanotic extremities.
	A. See Problem 1.A, F, G
	B. These data are useful in determining the presence of a low cardiac output state.
		A. See Problem 1.A, F, G.
		
		B. 1. Blood pressure remains within the individual's normal range.
		  2. Ideally, normal sinus rhythm without arrhythmia is maintained, or patient's baseline rhythm is maintained at a heart rate between 60 and 100 beats per minute without further arrhythmia.
		  3. Patient does not complain of excessive fatigue and is able to carry out necessary activities of daily living within prescribed activity limits.
		  4. Patient remains fully alert and oriented, and without personality change.
		  5. Urine output remains greater than 250 ml per eight-hour shift.
		  6. Extremities remain warm, dry and of normal color.

Problem 6: Diagnosis of coronary artery disease manifested by angina pectoris resulting in potential anxiety and fear of death.

Goal: To reduce the patient's fear and anxiety in order to restore balance between oxygen supply and demand.

Nursing Intervention	Scientific Rationale	Evaluation Criteria

A. Assess, document, and report to the physician the patient's and family's level of anxiety and coping mechanisms.	A. These data provide information about the patient's psychologic well-being and a baseline so that post-therapy symptoms can be compared. Causes of individual anxiety are variable and may include: acute illness, hospitalization, pain, daily responsibilities at home and at work, altered role and self-image due to chronic illness. Knowledge of financial resources, if appropriate, and support of successful coping mechanisms are useful (Chap. 44). Because anxious family members can transmit anxiety to the patient, the nurse must also reduce the family's fear and anxiety.	A. 1. Patient (family) reports less anxiety.
		  2. Patient (family) discusses anxieties and fears about death.
		  3. Patient (family) appears less anxious:
		    a. Restful.
		    b. Respiratory rate less than 16 breaths per minute.
		    c. Heart rate less than 100 beats per minute without ectopics.
		    d. Blood pressure within individual's normal limits.
		    e. Skin warm and dry.

B. See Problem 1.F, G.	B. See Problem 1.F, G.	B. See Problem 1.F, G.
C. Assess the need for spiritual counseling, and refer as appropriate.	C. If the patient finds support in a religion, religious counseling may assist in reducing anxiety and fear.	C. Patient expresses less anxiety and fear secondary to religious support.

D. Allow patient (family) to express anxiety and fear by the nurse
  1. Showing genuine interest and concern.
  2. Providing a conducive atmosphere.
  3. Facilitating communication (listening, reflecting, guiding).
  4. Answering questions.
	D. Unresolved anxiety (stress response) increases $M\dot{V}O_2$.	D. Patient (family) expresses less fear and anxiety.

TABLE 22-3   SAMPLE NURSING CARE PLAN FOR THE PATIENT WITH STABLE ANGINA PECTORIS HOSPITALIZED ON A GENERAL MEDICINE UNIT   (cont.)

Nursing Intervention	Scientific Rationale	Evaluation Criteria
E. Teach patient (family) the content necessary for him to modify life style in order to maintain optimal daily functioning (Text and Chap. 43).	E. Improving patient (family) understanding of a disease process or its treatment may assist in reduction of fear and anxiety and in adherance to the individualized therapeutic plan.	E. Patient modifies life style appropriately.
F. Encourage active participation in a cardiac rehabilitation program (Sec. G).	F. Supervised prescribed cardiac rehabilitation may help to eliminate fear of death and may enhance feelings of well-being (Sec. G).	F. Patient participates actively in cardiac rehabilitation program.
G. Teach stress reduction techniques (see text).	G. Stress reduction techniques may help to reduce $M\dot{V}O_2$ and may enhance feelings of well-being (see text).	G. Patient practices stress-reduction technique.

Because the underlying pathologic process is similar, the same basic content can be taught to patients with angina and to those with myocardial infarction. Differences can be pointed out at the time. Specific information that should be taught about medications is discussed in Section II E and in Chapter 45.

Activity. The benefits of participation in physical cardiac rehabilitation programs should be reemphasized. Patients must understand the need to modify activities in cold weather, and to dress warmly on cold days. Those with unstable angina need to understand and cooperate with curtailment of physical activities. Some may need to be placed on complete bedrest and treated as a patient with an acute myocardial infarction (Chap. 23). For those with unstable angina who remain at home, it is imperative that both the patient and the family understand the activity restrictions and the reasons for them.

Sexual activity should be discussed with both patient and spouse. For those with stable angina, resumption of previous sexual activity should be encouraged. Patients with unstable angina should refrain from sexual activity until the angina stabilizes (Chap. 46). Instructions should be given regarding the prophylactic use of nitroglycerin prior to any activity that may precipitate angina (Chap. 36).

Many patients with stable angina are able to keep their jobs, although some will need to switch to part-time employment. Others will seek lighter, less stressful job situations, and some will retire. Chapter 43 discusses how this decision is made and some problems associated with returning to the same job. For those who must seek different employment, vocational rehabilitation counseling may be helpful. A description of community services including financial resources may be particularly helpful to the patient who must retire or limit his work time. Putting the patient in touch with a social worker facilitates use of the community services available.

Awareness of the Precipitating Factors. Patients should be encouraged to identify specific situations that precipitate anginal attacks so that they can learn to avoid them or react differently to them. Daily log sheets with spaces to record time of onset, duration, and associated events may reveal specific patterns of anginal occurrences that are not apparent from interviews.

Precipitating factors can be either physiologic or psychologic, the latter being much more difficult to control. Most patients readily understand the cause-effect relationship between physical stress and angina. In addition to taking prophylactic nitroglycerin, they quickly learn to prevent the occurrence of angina by avoiding, limiting, pacing, and timing physical activities. However, the relationship between emotional stress and angina is usually a more difficult concept for the patient to understand. Emotional stressors can be recognized and acknowledged, but reaction to them is difficult to change. Emotional responses to any given situation are an accumulation of a lifetime of learned reactions, beliefs, and feelings. One way of dealing with emotional stress is by avoiding the situation that caused it, often an impractical solution. The best way to deal with emotional stress is to learn to react to it in a different way. Stress management techniques can help the patient to cope better with psychologic stresses.

Stress Management

Medical or surgical management of angina is not always satisfactory to the patient. He may dislike the headache associated with nitroglycerin or the fatigue that may accompany propranolol. He may prefer not to depend on any drug for well-being. Even if the medical regime is followed, chest discomfort may still occur. Surgery may not be an option, and even if the operation is performed, the grafts may close and the angina may return. Unsatisfactory traditional treatment may leave the patient feeling frightened, depressed, angry, or frustrated, adding to an already stressful situation.

Emotional stress has been implicated as a causative factor in the development of coronary atherosclerotic disease (Chap. 13). In addition, emotional stress is known to precipitate anginal attacks in the patient with coronary atherosclerotic disease. Practicing stress-reduction techniques may help the patient to prevent or minimize episodes of angina and may help to retard the disease process. In most instances these techniques should not be used exclusively but as an adjunct to traditional therapy. General relaxation as a method of reducing stress in the patient after myocardial infarction is discussed in Chapter 43. Table 43-5 lists commonly used relaxation techniques for the post-myocardial infarction patient.

All available methods of learning stress management should be explained to the patient in order that he can select the one best suited to his beliefs and life style. For example, Zen Buddhism or Yoga may be totally unacceptable to the 70-year-old retired banker but very appealing to a 35-year-old artist, and an electrical engineer may be very interested in learning stress management with the help of complex electrical biofeedback equipment. Once the patient agrees to practice a stress-reducing technique and the method is chosen, training should begin. Some forms of stress management, for example a general relaxation technique, can be taught by the nurse while the patient is hospitalized or in a clinic setting after discharge. Classes in transcendental meditation (TM) are offered in most major cities. Hospitals and clinics are beginning to establish biofeedback laboratories. The nurse should facilitate patient entry into the chosen program.

Use of stress-reducing techniques is usually taught in a classroom or laboratory rather than in the learner's living environment. Some require teaching aids, such as tape recordings or biofeedback equipment, for instruction. In order to succeed in utilizing stress reduction techniques, the learner must be able to transfer the ability to perform them into his real life situation.

Relaxation Response. The relaxation response is the opposite of the stress response, which is also known as the defense reaction or flight or fight response (Chap. 11). The relaxation response can be elicited by various mental techniques, including TM, autogenic training, hypnosis, Zen Buddhism, Yoga, and progressive relaxation. It appears to be coordinated by the hypothalamus and results in reduced sympathetic and perhaps increased parasympathetic activity. Physiologic changes induced by the relaxation response are different from those occurring during simple relaxation (sitting quietly with eyes closed) or sleep.[3]

In normal subjects physiologic findings attributed to the relaxation response during meditation are: oxygen consumption and carbon dioxide production during rest and exercise reduced; respiratory rate and minute ventilation reduced, with respiratory quotient unchanged; arterial pH and base excess slightly reduced; heart rate slightly reduced; systolic, diastolic, and mean arterial blood pressures unchanged; arterial blood lactate slightly reduced; arterial PO_2 and PCO_2 unchanged; rectal temperature unchanged; and skeletal muscles relaxed.[3,5,15,36]

Some specific differences in physiologic responses of TM and simple relaxation are important to note. Cardiac output increases by 15% with TM, but declines in simple relaxation. Redistribution of blood flow occurs, as evidenced by reduced liver blood flow (unchanged with simple relaxation) and unchanged renal blood flow (reduced with simple relaxation). It is thought that a marked increase in cerebral perfusion is responsible for the electroencephalographic changes associated with TM.[19]

The effects of TM on $M\dot{V}O_2$ have not been studied. However, pressure-rate product is unchanged or only slightly reduced. The increase in cardiac output with the relaxation response may result from redistribution of blood flow with a subsequent increase in blood return to the heart, or from a decrease in afterload. The net effect can be either a reduced or an unchanged $M\dot{V}O_2$. The Valsalva maneuver, which is done with isometric muscle contraction during progressive relaxation, produces transient changes in heart rate and blood pressure and can result in increased $M\dot{V}O_2$.[14]

For the patient with angina, the physiologic benefit to be derived from stress management is a reduction in $M\dot{V}O_2$ and a lessening of myocardial ischemia. However, little research has been reported using relaxation techniques with angina patients. Normal subjects and hypertensive patients have provided most research data. Opinions differ regarding the effectiveness of using TM for blood pressure reduction in the hypertensive patient. Some studies demonstrate significant blood pressure reductions, systolic more than diastolic, in hypertensives,[4,6] while others showed no significant blood pressure reduction over periods of six months[24] and one year.[33] Because changes in systolic blood pressure affect pressure-rate product, some of this information can be used empirically. Well-controlled scientific studies with anginal patients are necessary before the effectiveness of the relaxation response in the management of myocardial ischemia can be determined.

Use of Biofeedback. Biofeedback is a relatively new method of stress management. The term "biofeedback" implies that during monitoring of a specific body function, the biologic information is returned, or "fed back," to the subject in order to facilitate the modification of that same function by that subject. The biologic information can include brain and muscle potentials, skin temperature, heart rate, or blood pressure. Biofeedback can be displayed as analogue data (specific information, such as the heart rate, is given) or as binary signals (cues, such as lights or sounds, indicate success). Professional interest in biofeedback increased after Miller's reports in 1969 of learned control of autonomic functions (blood pressure, heart rate, salivation, kidney function, peripheral blood flow, and brain potentials) in laboratory animals.[22] Biofeedback of the electromyogram (EMG) can be used as an objective indicator of skeletal muscle relaxation, which occurs during the relaxation response. Use of EMG biofeedback with angina patients has not been reported, but long-term (one year) blood pressure control in hypertensive patients using EMG biofeedback has not been successful.[33]

Biofeedback of heart rate, or systolic blood pressure, or both, for purposes of learned reduction in pressure-rate product may be helpful in lowering $M\dot{V}O_2$. This type of biofeedback may be useful in forestalling or minimizing anginal attacks if learned responses can be used at the first sign of development of chest discomfort. The same basic principle applies to the prompt relief of angina which can be obtained by using carotid sinus massage: reduction of heart rate, cardiac output and $M\dot{V}O_2$.[20]

Learned control of blood pressure has been demonstrated using blood pressure biofeedback. Normal college students learned to increase and decrease blood pressure. Systolic blood pressure changes appeared to be independent of heart rate, and the students could increase or decrease heart rate without changing systolic blood pressure.[30] Using blood pressure biofeedback, hypertensive patients demonstrated reduction of systolic blood pressure by 16 to 34 mm Hg.[28] Systolic blood pressure reductions of this magnitude should lessen MV̇O₂ significantly. However, the baroreceptor reflex might come into play with a systolic blood pressure reduction of this amount; heart rate would increase, and MV̇O₂ might remain unchanged.

Laboratory studies of heart rate biofeedback have demonstrated heart rate control in nine subjects in normal sinus rhythm,[38] and six patients in atrial fibrillation.[7] Increases in heart rate achieved are greater in magnitude than the decreases, which averaged only 1.5-to-2 beats per minute in both studies. In a heart rate biofeedback study of four patients with angina pectoris, decreases averaged 2.6 beats per minute.[34,35] The clinical importance of these small decreases in altering MV̇O₂ is questionable.

Psychologic Benefits of Stress Management. Many persons experience a general feeling of well-being and absence of tension during and after participation in stress-reducing techniques.[3,8,24] This pleasant feeling may certainly contribute to a brighter outlook and help the patient to cope more efficiently with everyday stressful situations.

Selecting a relaxation technique and actively participating in a program of stress management shifts the control away from the therapist, returning at least some control to the patient. For the individual who regards control over self as important, lack of control may contribute to increased stress.

In the study of heart rate control using four patients with angina, two of the four patients met the study criteria for successful heart-rate reduction (decreases of two beats per minute or more). Two patients reported subjective improvement in angina. It is interesting to note that only one of the patients who was subjectively improved had learned to decrease his heart rate. The other was not successful with heart rate reduction using biofeedback, yet improved enough after the training sessions to seek reemployment.[34] Clearly, psychologic benefits are derived from stress management, even though due in part to placebo effects, and can improve the quality of life for the patient with angina.

REFERENCES

1. Amsterdam EA, Wolfson S, Gorlin R: New aspects of the placebo response in angina pectoris. Am J Cardiol 24:305–306, 1969
2. Ari EB, Kellerman JJ, Lapitod C et al: Effect of prolonged intensive training on cardiorespiratory response in patients with angina pectoris. Br Heart J 40(10):1143–1148, 1978
3. Benson H, Beary JF, Carol MP: The relaxation response. Psychiatry 37:37–46, 1974
4. Benson H, Dryer T, Hartley LH: Decreased V̇O₂ consumption during exercise with elicitation of the relaxation response. J Human Stress 4:38–42, 1978
5. Benson H, Marzetta BR, Rosner BA et al: Decreased blood pressure in pharmacologically treated hypertensive patients who regularly elicited the relaxation response. Lancet i:289–291, 1974
6. Blackwell B, Broomfield S, Gartside P et al: Transcendental meditation in hypertension. Lancet i:223–226, 1976
7. Bleeker ER, Engel BT: Learned control of ventricular rate in patients with atrial fibrillation. Semin Psychiatry, 5(4):461–474, 1973
8. Borkovec TD, Grayson JB, Cooper KM: Treatment of general tension: Subjective and physiological effects of progressive relaxation. J Consult Clin Psychol 46(3):518–528, 1978
9. Buchwald H, Moore RB, Varco RL: Ten years clinical experience with partial ileal bypass in management of hyperlipidemias. Ann Surg 180(4):384–392, 1974
10. Clark MC: Chest pain. Heart Lung 4(6):956–962, 1975
11. Doyle JT: Tobacco and the cardiovascular system. In Hurst JW, Logue RB, Schlant RC et al (eds): The Heart, 4th ed, pp 1820–1823. New York, McGraw-Hill, 1978
12. Folli G, Radice M, Beltrami A et al: Placebo effect in the treatment of angina pectoris. Acta Cardiol 33(4):231–240, 1978
13. Furburg B, Dahlqvist A, Raak A et al: Comparison of the new adrenoceptor nadolol, and propranolol in the treatment of angina pectoris. Clin Med Res Opinion 5(5):388–393, 1978
14. Ganong WF: Review of Medical Physiology, 8th ed. Los Altos, Lange Publishing Company, 1977
15. Gash A, Karliner JS: No effect of transcendental meditation on left ventricular function. Ann Intern Med 88(2):215–216, 1978
16. Hultgren HN, Takaro T, Detre K: Veteran's Administration Cooperative Study of surgical treatment of stable angina: Preliminary results. Cardiovasc Clin 8(2):119–130, 1977
17. Hurst JW, King SB III: Definitions and classification of coronary atherosclerotic heart disease. In Hurst JW, Logue RB, Schlant RC et al (eds): The Heart. 4th ed, pp 1094–1102. New York, McGraw-Hill Book Company, 1978
18. Hurst JW, Logue RB, Walter PF: The clinical recognition and medical management of coronary atherosclerotic heart disease. In Hurst JW, Logue RB, Schlant RC et al (eds): The Heart. 4th ed, pp 1156–1290. New York, McGraw-Hill, 1978
19. Jevning R, Smith R, Wilson AF: Alterations in blood flow during transcendental meditation (abstr). Clin Res 24(2):139A, 1976
20. Levine SA: Carotid sinus massage: A new diagnostic test for angina pectoris. JAMA 182(13):1332–1334, 1962
21. Miettinen TA, Lempinen M: Cholestyramine and ileal by-pass in the treatment of familial hypercholesterolemia. Eur J Clin Invest 7(6):509–514, 1977
22. Miller NE: Learning of visceral and glandular responses. Science 163:434–445, 1969
23. Pitt B: Pathophysiology and pharmacology of angina pectoris. Adv Cardiol 26:55–64, 1979
24. Pollack AA, Case DB, Weber MA et al: Limitations of transcendental meditation in the treatment of essential hypertension. Lancet i:71–73, 1977
25. Preston TA: Placebo effect. Coronary Artery Surgery: A Critical Review, pp 81–99. New York, Raven Press, 1977
26. Schlant RC: Altered cardiovascular physiology of coronary atherosclerotic heart disease. In Hurst JW, Logue RB, Schlant RC et al (eds): The Heart, 4th ed, pp 1134–1156. New York: McGraw-Hill Book Company, 1978
27. Schlant RC, Digirolama M: Modification of risk factors in the prevention and management of coronary atherosclerotic heart disease. In Hurst JW, Logue RB, Schlant RC et al (eds): The Heart, 4th ed, pp 1311–1344. New York, McGraw-Hill, 1978
28. Schwartz GE., Shapiro D: Biofeedback and essential hypertension: Current findings and theoretical concerns. Semin Psychiatry 5(4):492–502, 1973
29. Shapiro AK: Factors contributing to the placebo effect. Am J Psychother (Suppl 1) 18:73–88, 1964
30. Shapiro D, Turskey B, Gershon E et al: Effects of feedback and reinforcement on the control of human systolic blood pressure. Science 163:588–589, 1969
31. Short D, Stowers M: Spontaneous changes in the severity of angina pectoris. Am Heart J 96(3):415, 1978
32. Smith JR, Paine R: Thoracic pain. In MacBryde CM, Blacklow RS (eds): Signs and Symptoms, 5th ed, pp 154–180. Philadelphia, JB Lippincott, 1970
33. Surwit RS, Shapiro D, Good MI: Comparison of cardiovascular biofeedback, neuromuscular biofeedback, and meditation in the treatment of borderline essential hypertension. J Consult Clin Psychol 46(2):252–263, 1978
34. Underhill SL: Biofeedback Control to Decrease Heart Rate for Relief of Angina Pectoris. Unpublished Master's Thesis, University of Washington, 1976

35. Underhill SL, Wills RE, Mansfield LW: Biofeedback control of heart rate for relief of angina (abstr). Circulation 56(4):III–102, 1977

36. Wallace RK, Benson H, Wilson AF: A wakeful hypometabolic state. Am J Physiol 221(3):795–799, 1971

37. Weiner DA, Ryan TJ, McCabe CH et al: Exercise stress testing: Correlations among history of angina, ST-segment response and prevalence of coronary–artery disease in the coronary artery surgery study. N Engl J Med 301(5):230–235, 1979

38. Wells D: Large voluntary heart rate changes. Psychophysiology, 10(3):260–269, 1973

39. Wolff HG, Hardy JD, Goodell H: Studies on pain. Measurement of the effect of morphine, codeine, and other opiates on the pain threshold and on analysis of their relation to the pain experience. J Clin Invest 19:659–680, 1940

ADDITIONAL READING

Awan NA, Miller RR, Maxwell KS et al: Cardiocirculatory and antianginal actions of nitroglycerin ointment. Chest 73(1):14–18, 1978

Beecher HK: Evidence for increased effectiveness of placebos with increased stress. Am J Physiol 187:163–169, 1956

Benson H, Epstein M: The placebo effect. JAMA 232(12): 1225–1227, 1975

Brodgen RN, Hill RC, Speight TM et al: Metoprolol: A review of its pharmacological properties and therapeutic efficacy in hypertension and angina. Drugs 14(5):321–348, 1977

Buchwald H, Moore RB, Varco RL: Surgical treatment of hyperlipidemia. Circulation 49 (Suppl I):1–37, 1974

Conti CR, Hodges M, Hutter A et al: Unstable angina—A national cooperative study comparing medical and surgical therapy. Cardiovasc Clin 8(2):167–178, 1977

Duncan B, Fulton M, Morrison SF et al: Prognosis of new and worsening angina pectoris. Br Med J 1:981–985, 1976

Eliot RS (ed): Stress and the Heart. Mt. Kisco, Futura Publishing Company, 1974

Frederickson DS: Disorders of lipid metabolism and xanthomatoses. In Thorn GW, Adams RD, Braunwald E et al (eds): Harrison's Principles of Internal Medicine, 8th ed, pp 670–680. New York, McGraw-Hill, 1977

Greenspan K: Biologic feedback and cardiovascular disease. Psychosomatics 19(11):725–737, 1978

Hurst JW, Logue RB, Schlant RC et al (eds): The Heart, 4th ed. New York, McGraw-Hill, 1978

Jacobsen E: You Must Relax: A Practical Method of Reducing the Strains of Modern Living, 3rd ed. New York, McGraw-Hill, 1948

Johnston D: Clinical applications of biofeedback. Br J Hosp Med 20(5):561–566, 1978

Lesch M, Gorlin R: Pharmacologic therapy of angina pectoris. Mod Concepts Cardiovasc Dis 42(2):5–10, 1973

Paul O: The medical management of angina pectoris. JAMA 238(17):1847–1848, 1977

Peters RK, Benson H, Porter D: Daily relaxation response breaks in a working population: 1. Effects on self-reported measures of health, performance and well-being. Am J Public Health 67(10):946–952, 1977

Putt AM: A biofeedback service by nurses. Am J Nurs 79(1):88–89, 1979

Rahimtoola SH (ed): Coronary artery bypass surgery. Cardiovasc Clin 8(2), 1977

Russell RO Jr, Moraski RE, Kouchoukos N et al: Unstable angina pectoris: National Cooperative Study Group to compare surgical and medical therapy. Am J Cardiol 42:839–848, 1977

Sheldon WC, Loop FD, Proudfit WL: A critique of the VA Cooperative Study. Cleve Clin Q 45(2):225–230, 1978

23

Diagnosis and Treatment of the Patient with an Uncomplicated Myocardial Infarction

SUSAN L. WOODS, R.N., M.N.

Prehospital care of the uncomplicated myocardial infarction (MI) patient includes a community-wide system for optimal cardiac care: 1) continuing public and professional education in basic life support and professional education in advanced cardiac life support, and 2) life-support stations outside of the cardiac care unit (CCU), such as mobile CCU and stationary support stations. Hospital care of the patient with acute MI is commonly provided in a CCU and then in a post-CCU. Hospital care includes diagnosis of MI and medical and nursing management of the patient with MI.

PREHOSPITAL PHASE

In 1977, 4,240,000 Americans had coronary heart disease, of whom 1,000,000 sustained an MI, and 638,427 died. Of those who perished, 350,000, more than half, died before they reached the hospital.[16] The average victim waited 3 hours before deciding to seek help[16] and most of the deaths occurred within the first two hours after the onset of symptoms.[1,2,7,11] A large percentage of the deaths was due to cardiac arrhythmias.[14,34] The greatest advancement in reducing mortality associated with MI was the introduction of the CCU. Here, arrhythmias could be detected early and treated aggressively.

In 1967, nearly 70% of the deaths from MI occurred outside the hospital.[20] In 1977, 55% of the deaths from MI occurred outside the hospital. This reduction in deaths from MI outside the hospital is the result of increased emphasis on prehospital care of the patient with MI.[17] Prehospital care involves bringing medical care to the MI patient as soon as possible after the onset of symptoms, and expediting hospitalization.[27] The most important and frequent cause for delay is the patient's own indecision when he develops oppressive chest discomfort.[15,31,32]

According to Yu and co-workers, this indecision may be related to[41]

1. Lack of information about the significance of the symptoms and the urgency for seeking immediate medical care

2. Denial of the importance of chest discomfort because of the fear of MI and its consequences

3. Misinterpretation of symptoms as reflecting disorders of other organ systems

4. Failure to have an established relationship with a personal physician who can be contacted at the time of an emergency

5. Failure of relatives or co-workers to encourage the patient to seek medical help

6. Ignorance of how to gain access to health care facilities quickly and other psychologic, socioeconomic, and physical barriers hindering rapid entry into the system.

Other causes of delay include inadequate communication systems, transportation problems, traffic problems (such as distance and traffic density), and inadequately equipped emergency rooms. Continuing public and professional education and the out-of-CCU life support stations are two ways of reducing the delay between onset of symptoms and the beginning of treatment. Basic to this community-wide system is an informed public, an efficient communication center, trained medical and paramedical teams, and appropriate vehicles and equipment.[13]

Continuing Public and Professional Education

The American Heart Association has developed a basic life-support program for teaching professionals and the public[16]

1. To recognize early warning signals of MI and provide assistance to persons experiencing them
2. To act quickly to summon emergency care, by having a knowledge of emergency telephone numbers and the emergency service available
3. To perform the basic life-support techniques of cardio-pulmonary resuscitation when necessary.[16]

In addition to the basic life-support program, the Association has developed an advanced cardiac life-support program that teaches professionals

1. Adjuncts for airway and breathing
2. Adjuncts for circulation
3. Arrhythmia interpretation
4. Defibrillation and cardioversion
5. Intravenous techniques
6. Essential cardiac drugs
7. Useful cardiac drugs
8. Acid–base balance and imbalance
9. Stabilization and transportation.

Out-of-Hospital CCU Life Support Stations

Out-of-hospital CCU life support stations include mobile vehicles and stationary areas.

Mobile CCU. Two types of mobile CCU are recommended by the American Heart Association: (1) A basic unit staffed and equipped to handle all emergencies and (2) an advanced unit staffed and equipped to provide definitive measures to stabilize the cardiac patient until he arrives in the CCU. The necessary equipment includes drugs, a battery-powered ECG monitor and defibrillator, and a respirator. Both units should be staffed with specially trained medical or para-medical personnel.[16]

These mobile CCUs can be in a hospital or elsewhere. Hospital-based units may be staffed by physicians[14,34] or by nurses and paramedics, with or without physician contact. Units not based in a hospital may be staffed by paramedics with or without physician contact.[5,21]

The primary purposes of the mobile CCU are to provide basic and advanced cardiac life support at the site of the event and to transport the patient to a hospital CCU under monitoring conditions. In many cities the system is activated by dialing 911 to reach the police or fire department dispatching officer. The dispatcher then calls the mobile CCU and the appropriate hospital. All equipment in the mobile CCU is portable and can be carried anywhere. Upon reaching the site, the mobile unit personnel assess the patient's status and begin oxygen therapy, an IV, and ECG monitoring. If arrhythmias are present the patient is either given antiarrhythmic drugs, or defibrillated before being transported. These units are effective in the management of life-threatening cardiac arrhythmias.[19,24,33]

If the patient is having chest pain, an analgesic is administered. If both basic and advanced life-support measures can be effectively administered at the scene of the incident, they should be continued until the patient is stabilized. If this is not possible, either because of the inability of the rescuer to deliver advanced life support or because of a lack of response by the patient despite competent emergency treatment, then the patient should be transported to continuing professional care without delay.[21]

Stationary Life Support Areas. A stationary emergency life-support unit is one that is located where patients with symptoms suggestive of MI can be given immediate care. Stationary life-support areas may include emergency rooms in hospitals, factories, offices, airports, railroad stations, and athletic stadiums.[4,12,41] The staff may include physicians, nurses, or allied health personnel, but a physician knowledgeable and skilled in the management of cardiovascular emergencies should assume administrative and supervisory responsibility.

Out-of-hospital based life-support stations not based in a hospital are essentially CCUs located in areas where the population density is high (25,000 or more). The purpose of these units is to detect and control arrhythmias and to provide basic and advanced support as needed for cardiac emergencies, and to stabilize the patient with suspected MI before transfer to a CCU for continuing therapy. The staff should be capable of providing continuous ECG monitoring, performing cardiopulmonary resuscitation and initiating appropriate antiarrhythmic therapy, including defibrillation.

The emergency room must be capable of adequately treating a patient with MI. The equipment (ECG monitor, drugs, defibrillator, and oxygen) must be available and the personnel must be skilled in advanced cardiac life support, especially arrhythmia detection and treatment, and cardiopulmonary resuscitation. The middle-aged man with chest pain must be treated as a first-class emergency.[13] He should be placed on continuous ECG monitoring *before* the history is taken.

Since early deaths are most often due to arrhythmias,[41] the patient suspected of having an MI should be transferred as soon as possible to the CCU under continuous ECG monitoring.[28] A portable defibrillator should accompany the patient during transfer. If the stationary unit is outside the hospital, the mobile CCU can then be contacted. Once the patient has been stabilized he can be transported to the CCU.

The specifications for equipment necessary in the delivery of both basic and advanced life support are provided in the Standards and Guidelines for Cardiopulmonary Resuscitation (CPR) and Emergency Cardiac Care (ECC).[38]

HOSPITAL PHASE

Since the early 1960s, CCUs have reduced the in-hospital mortality from acute MI by 30% to 50%.[16,26] Most of the hospitals in this country have a CCU or an intensive care area to care for patients with MI. Early mortality is due most often to ventricular fibrillation, sometimes, but not always, preceded by a bradyarrhythmia or ventricular premature beats.[22,34] The reduced mortality has been associated with prompt detection, effective prevention, and treatment of life-threatening cardiac arrhythmias by means of specific drug therapy, defibrillation, and pacemaker insertion.[41]

Diagnosis of Acute Myocardial Infarction

Subjective data are collected from the patient and his family about his chief complaint, health history, and family and social history (Chap. 14). Objective data are collected from the physical examination (Chap. 14), laboratory studies (Part II, Sec. B) and patient observation. The diagnosis of acute MI is confirmed by a history of chest discomfort, ECG changes, and serum enzyme elevation.

Chest Discomfort Associated with MI. According to Lown, 75% to 85% of patients with acute MI have chest discomfort.[28] The history is typical if severe, prolonged chest discomfort is present. Sometimes the history is atypical and the chest discomfort is mild or even absent. The onset of chest discomfort is abrupt and lasts longer than 15 to 30 minutes. The discomfort is usually midsternal, "crushing" or squeezing and may radiate to the arms, shoulders, back, neck, or jaw. This chest discomfort may be associated with indigestion, nausea and vomiting, diaphoresis, syncope, or palpitations.[36] A detailed description of the chest discomfort associated with ischemia can be found in Chapter 22 (Fig. 22-1) (Table 22-1).

Electrocardiographic Changes with MI. Typical ECG changes are seen in 88% of patients with acute MI. Unequivocal changes in ECG are the development of abnormal, persistent Q waves, and evolving injury lasting longer than 1 day. With unequivocal changes, the diagnosis may be made on the ECG alone.

The ECG may show equivocal changes, consisting of ST-segment elevation, a symmetrical inversion of the T wave, a pathologic Q wave in a single ECG lead, or conduction disturbances. If a small, subendocardial MI exists in the lateral or posterior wall in the presence of an old MI or left bundle branch block, the ECG provides little or no information. Also, when there is a balanced loss of myocardial forces, there are minimal ECG changes.[28] With MI, 62% of patients have classic ECG changes. The area of infarction and subsequent mortality of these patients is as follows:

Area of Infarction	Incidence	Mortality
Anterior (anteroseptal, anterolateral)	26.0%	25.6%
Inferior	16.7%	10.0%
Posteroinferior	8.3%	8.0%
Anteroinferior	6.0%	39.0%
Posterior	2.3%	
Lateral (changes in only leads I and aVL)	2.7%	

Of the remaining 38% of patients with MI, 26% have ST segment–T wave changes that last 24 hours. Of these patients 16.7% have intramural infarction with no mortality and 9.7% have subendocardial infarction with 27.6% mortality. Of patients with MI, 8% have ECG evidence of old MI with no other changes, and have a 25% mortality. The remaining 3.7% have no ECG changes and have an 18.2% mortality.[28]

Enzyme Elevation Associated with MI. Enzyme elevation is seen in 90% of patients with MI (Chap. 15). The enzyme change may not be seen with a small infarction, or because the patient did not live long enough for the rise to occur.

Unequivocal change consists of serial change, or initial rise and subsequent fall of the serum enzymes (SGOT, CK, LDH, and the isoenzymes of CK and LDH). The change must be properly related to the particular enzyme and to the delay time between onset of symptoms and blood sampling.

Equivocal change consists of an enzyme pattern where an initially elevated level is not accompanied by a subsequent fall. Thus the curve of enzyme activity is not obtained. A detailed description of the enzyme pattern with MI is found in Chapter 15.

Summary. A definite diagnosis of MI is usually made in the presence of unequivocal ECG changes or unequivocal enzyme changes, or both; and the history may be typical or atypical. Myocardial infarction is sometimes designated as transmural when unequivocal ECG changes are present, and nontransmural or subendocardial when evolving ST-T changes, in the absence of Q or QS waves, occur together with unequivocal enzyme changes. Possible acute MI is diagnosed when serial, equivocal ECG changes persist more than 24 hours, with or without equivocal enzyme changes; and the history may be typical or atypical.

Medical and Nursing Management: Acute Phase

As the patient enters the hospital, medical and nursing personnel work closely to stabilize the patient with acute MI (cardiac rhythm, blood pressure, pain) and to transfer him to the CCU. Thus, cardiac rhythm, blood pressure, and pain may be treated before the patient is moved.

Goals of Therapy. The goals of treatment in the acute phase are:
(1) rapid management of existing problems (relief of chest discomfort, nausea or vomiting, dyspnea),
(2) prevention or early detection of arrhythmias (Chaps. 17, 26) and other complications of MI (Part II, Sec. C)
(3) beginning rehabilitation (see Part III).[3]
These goals are achieved while attempting to maintain the balance between myocardial oxygen supply and demand.

Cardiac Monitoring in the CCU. The patient is admitted to the CCU and is attached to a cardiac monitor. The electrodes are placed on the chest according to the lead selected for monitoring. Lead MCL_1 (modified left arm lead in the V_1 position), MCL_6 (modified left arm lead in the V_6 position), or M3 (modified Lead III), is commonly used with patients with MI, since it is diagnostically superior to any one other lead. Lead II is also used. Table 23-1 lists the advantages of MCL_1, MCL_6, M3, or Lead II for routine continuous ECG monitoring in the CCU (Fig. 23-1). The electrode site on the skin should be clean (use alcohol), dry

TABLE 23-1   ADVANTAGES OF VARIOUS ECG MONITORING LEADS

Lead	Advantages
MCL$_1$ (modified V$_1$) or MCL$_6$ (modified V$_6$)	1. Allows distinction between (a) left ventricular and right ventricular ectopy, and (b) left ventricular and right ventricular artificial pacing (Chaps. 26, 40).
	2. Allows distinction between right and left bundle branch block (Chap. 17).
	3. Allows distinction between aberration and ectopy (Chap. 26).
	4. Assists in diagnoses that require well-formed P waves (Chap. 17).
	5. Apex of the heart is not covered by an electrode and is clear for auscultation and defibrillation without electrode interference (Fig. 23-1).
M3	1. Allows identification of retrograde P waves.[29]
Lead II	1. Assists in the diagnosis of hemiblock (Chap. 17).

(Marriott JL, Fogg E: Mod Concepts Cardiovasc Dis 39(6):103–108, 1970)

(use gauze) and relatively flat. Hair should be shaved and the skin mildly abraded to reduce the resistance. The electrode with electrode paste is then applied to the chest, the alarm limits for heart rate are set (30% above and below the patient's heart rate),[8] the "beeper" in the patient's room turned off, and the alarm system activated. Sources of artifacts in ECG monitoring are shown in Figure 23-2A–E. Electrodes should be changed often enough (usually about one to three days) to prevent skin breakdown and to provide artifact-free tracings. The patient should be given a brief explanation of the purpose of ECG monitoring while he is in the CCU and his questions should be answered. The patient's heart rate, rhythm, and conduction must be continuously assessed, since most arrhythmias occur within the first two to three days after acute MI, and 90% of these patients will have arrhythmias. Intervention must be directed toward prevention by recognizing and controlling conditions that predispose the patient to arrhythmias. Some of these conditions are: hypokalemia, acidosis, hypoxemia, pain, anxiety, fever, and myocardial stretch (caused by congestive heart failure). Early identification of arrhythmias and prompt, aggressive treatment are necessary if mortality from MI is to be reduced. Arrhythmias can result in reduced

cardiac output and coronary blood flow, increased myocardial oxygen need, and predisposition to a lethal arrhythmia. The cardiac monitor must be under constant surveillance if arrhythmias are to be detected early, and therefore treated early to prevent further problems for the patient (Chap. 26).

Vital Signs and Intravenous Line. Blood pressure, pulse, respiration, and temperature (oral or rectal[30]) should be obtained. An intravenous line (angiocatheter or intracatheter) is established if the patient does not already have one. A scalp-vein needle should be used only temporarily until a more stable intravenous line can be established, since it is easily dislodged. This intravenous line is used to give pain medication and emergency cardiac medications. The intravenous line can be capped and 10 to 100 units heparin in 1 ml of saline injected every 8 hours, and following injection of medications, to maintain patency. Or an intravenous solution of 5% dextrose and water can be attached and infused at a rate to keep the vein open. A simple explanation of procedures is useful to most patients.

Chest Discomfort and Dyspnea. If the patient complains of chest discomfort, he should be given analgesic medication. The anxiety associated with pain increases myocardial oxygen demand. In order to decrease myocardial oxygen need, morphine sulfate is given intravenously in small increments of 1 to 5 mg. Morphine should not be given to patients who have atrioventricular block or sinus bradycardia, since it has a vagotonic effect. Morphine decreases blood pressure, heart rate, and respiratory rate.[35] If the heart rate is less than 70, meperidine may be the drug of choice[28] (Chap. 33). Oxygen

Fig. 23-1. Hookup for constant monitoring with MCL$_1$ (*unbroken lines*). The positive electrode is placed in the V$_1$ position; the negative electrode is placed on the outer one-fourth of the left clavicle; and the ground is placed on the right shoulder. *Dashed lines* show alternative temporary placement of the opposite shoulder to obtain MCL$_6$: The positive electrode is placed in the V$_6$ position. To obtain M3, the positive electrode is placed on the left upper abdomen. (After Marriott JL, Fogg, E: Mod Concepts Cardiovasc Dis 39(6):103–108, 1970)

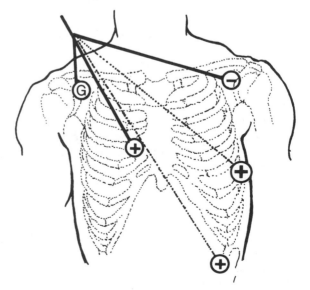

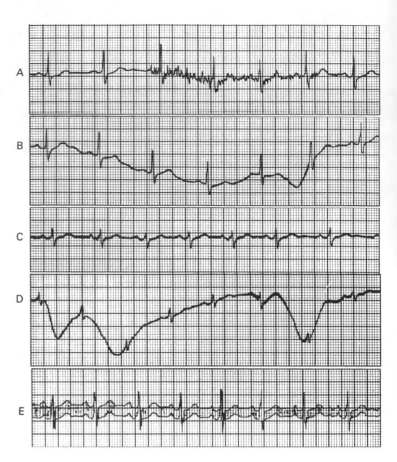

Fig. 23-2. Sources of artifacts in ECG monitored traces. (**A**) Involuntary movement: Usually a result of patient discomfort caused by chill or muscle tremors, coughing, or other nervous reactions to apprehension or discomfort. (**B**) Voluntary movement: Severe baseline deviation caused by gross body movement. (**C**) Poor skin preparation: Failure to "prep" a patient with oily skin causes low amplitude, wandering baseline, and 60-cycle interference. Poor skin "prep" may not show up right away, but affects the signal as the electrodes remain in place. (**D**) Dried-out electrode: The signal usually degenerates with time. Characteristics such as low amplitude, diphasic QRS complexes, 60-cycle interferences, and baseline wandering are usually noted. The trace is consistently rather than intermittently poor. (**E**) Bad grounding: This situation may cause 60-cycle interference, which is distinguishable in the wide baseline. Bad grounding may also create a shock hazard. If in doubt about the grounding connection, do not use it. TV sets, electric cords near the bed, and fluorescent bed lamps may also cause 60-cycle interference. (Medical Products Group, Graphic Controls Corporation, Buffalo, NY 1979)

at 2 to 4 liters per minute by nasal prongs may decrease chest discomfort by increasing oxygen supply to the myocardium.[10,18] Dyspnea can also cause anxiety and can be relieved by the administration of oxygen. Also, the administration of oxygen may diminish the conversion of ischemic myocardium to necrotic tissue. The magnitude of this benefit is not clear, and the primary physiologic mechanisms remain obscure.[6] Arterial blood gases should be used to evaluate effectiveness of oxygen therapy and to assess acid-base balance (Chap. 9).

Physical rest in bed with the backrest elevated, or in a cardiac chair, will assist in decreasing chest discomfort and dyspnea. The head-up position is beneficial for the following reasons: (1) tidal volume is improved, since there is reduced pressure for abdominal contents on the diaphragm, and thus oxygen exchange is improved; (2) drainage of the upper lobes of the lungs is improved;[18] and (3) venous return to the heart (preload) and cardiac output are reduced; thus the work of the heart is reduced.

Throughout this admission procedure, the nurse assesses and documents the patient's cardiovascular, renal, respiratory, neurologic (level of consciousness) and psychologic status. These data provide a baseline. If the patient is anxious, myocardial oxygen demand is increased. Explanations of all the activities and equipment will assist in relieving the patient's anxiety. Patient visiting with family or friends may reduce anxiety, or may cause anxiety. Assessment of the effect of visitors and appropriate intervention is a nursing responsibility. Unit policies should be flexible to provide individual care.

Physician's Orders on Admission. An example of the admitting physician's orders for an uncomplicated MI can be found in Table 23-2. Generally, medical management includes relief of pain, prevention of ventricular fibrillation and other lethal arrhythmias, prescription for rest and exercise, diet limitations, and the prevention and management of anxiety.

Maintenance of the Balance Between Myocardial Oxygen Supply and Demand. The myocardium requires time to recover from the injury of MI. Reduction in myocardial oxygen need will assist the recovery of the myocardium. The size of the infarction is determined by the demand and supply of oxygen to the ischemic and injured zones. Some ways to decrease the patient's myocardial oxygen need are these: (1) promote bed rest with progressive mobilization; (2) assist the patient with activities of daily living; and (3) control the environment to minimize stress.

Bed rest is important to the healing heart but is not without complications. Immobility has many adverse effects (Chap. 30). For the patient with an uncomplicated myocardial infarction activity usually progresses as follows:

CCU Day 1—Bed rest with use of bedside commode.

CCU Day 2—Legs dangling with assistance at bedside, three times a day (at times other than meal time) for five minutes.

CCU Day 3—In chair three times a day (at times other than meal time), as tolerated, for 5 to 15 minutes.

CCU Day 4—Length of time in chair increased as tolerated by patient.

CCU Day 5—Walking in room for five minutes, or as tolerated.

Activities of daily living can pose a problem to the independent person, because he is now dependent on the nurse for assistance. Most CCU staff allow the patients to feed themselves. The diet selected should

1. Minimize myocardial work, to favor adequate myocardial oxygen balance,
2. Maintain normal extracellular volume
3. Minimize patient pain and discomfort

TABLE 23-2   AN EXAMPLE OF AN ADMITTING PHYSICIAN'S ORDERS FOR A PATIENT WITH UNCOMPLICATED MI

1. Bed rest with bedside commode for 24 hours. Activity according to stated protocol.

2. Vital signs—if normal and stable; temperature, pulse, respiration and blood pressure every four hours (while awake).

3. Constant ECG monitoring.

4. Intake and output every shift. Guaiac-test all stools.

5. Weight on admission and daily.

6. Intravenous intracatheter or angiocatheter with injection cap. Heparin 0.15 ml (1000 U/ml) or 100 U heparin IV every 8 hours and PRN to maintain patency of IV catheter.

7. Oxygen 2 to 5 liters/minute per nasal prongs.

8. Diet: Full liquid diet 1-gram sodium for three meals; no coffee or tea; decaffeinated coffee and salt substitute permitted; no extremely hot or cold foods. Advance diet to 3-gram sodium diet, low cholesterol as tolerated. _____ calorie restriction.

9. Chest pain medication:
   Severe—(appropriate analgesia order).
   Minor—(appropriate analgesia order).

10. Minor pain medication: (appropriate analgesia order).

11. Colace 100mg orally twice a day; milk of magnesia 30 ml orally as needed.

12. Sleeping medication: (appropriate order).

13. 12-lead ECG on admission and daily times three and with chest pain or with a new arrhythmia. Place copy on the patient's chart.

14. SGOT, CK, LDH, and LDH isoenzymes on admission and daily times three and with sudden onset of chest pain. CK isoenzymes on admission and every 12 hours (after the onset of symptoms) times three. M-12, complete blood count, sedimentation rate, protime, recalcification time, VDRL, urinalysis, and portable chest film on admission.

15. The qualified CCU nurse is authorized according to stated policy to give complete resuscitation to this patient, including external cardiac massage, defibrillation and administration of intravenous medications as required.

16. No smoking while in CCU.

The following dietary principles during the acute phase are recommended by the American Heart Association:[9]

1. Avoid large meals, which potentially increase demand for splanchnic blood flow and thereby increase postprandial cardiac work

2. Minimize volume of gastric contents in order to decrease the chance of vomiting and aspiration in the event of cardiac emergencies

3. Avoid ingestion of myocardial stimulants, such as caffeine or theobromine

4. Avoid swallowing exceptionally cold or hot food and drink, to help decrease the possibility of cardiac arrhythmias

5. Avoid as much as possible foods that contribute to constipation and resultant straining with bowel movements, which may predispose a patient to vagal cardiac rhythm changes

6. Limit foods known to commonly produce excessive gas in the digestive process, such as dried beans, legumes, and apple juice

7. Offer a diet ample in potassium for all patients except those in renal failure. Most patients on potassium-wasting diuretic therapy will also require supplemental potassium treatment.

The patient's arms should be supported on the overbed table during the meal to prevent him from doing an unconscious Valsalva maneuver. In a Valsalva maneuver, air is forced over a closed glottis, resulting in increased intrathoracic pressure. This increased intrathoracic pressure may be as high as 80 mm Hg[37] and causes a decreased venous return to the heart (decreased preload) and vagal stimulation, resulting in decreased cardiac output. When the forced air is released, the intrathoracic pressure is decreased, and preload is increased, resulting in increased workload for the heart. The patient should be instructed to avoid holding his breath, since this can result in a Valsalva maneuver, and to breathe in and out with the mouth open while engaging in any activity that is normally accompanied by a Valsalva maneuver, such as turning or moving up in bed, reaching, vomiting, pulling, defecating, or coughing.[17]

The use of a bedside commode with assistance is less work than the use of a bedpan. The position one assumes using a commode is more natural and allows for appropriate and optimum utilization of the muscles of defecation (abdominal and rectal). Sufficient fluid intake is necessary to prevent constipation. Stool softeners will decrease the need for straining and possibly prevent a Valsalva maneuver. Initially, the patient will need to be bathed (day 1) and then assisted with the bath (day 2 to 5). The patient with an uncomplicated MI usually can take a warm shower after he is discharged from the CCU. A warm shower is preferred over a hot shower, since a hot shower could result in vasodilation and markedly reduced preload and cardiac output. The patient may need to use a chair in the shower or may need assistance with washing. Discussion of these activities with the patient and physician is necessary to determine their preferences and to develop a workable care plan.

With the daily bath, the intravenous site should be inspected for signs of inflammation (redness, swelling, heat).

Findings should be documented in the patient's chart. The site should be cleaned with an antiseptic, and an antibiotic ointment and a dry sterile dressing should be applied. If the site is inflamed, a new intravenous line should be placed in a different site prior to discontinuing the old line. The intravenous site should be changed at least every three days. Also, electrode sites on the chest should be assessed daily for skin irritation, and washed with soap and water. Different areas of the chest should be selected for application of new electrodes.

An in-depth discussion of activity and exercise can be found in Chapter 42. Table 42-2 gives suggestions for activity progression. It is important to allow the patient as much independence as possible to promote his self-confidence, which in turn facilitates psychologic and physiologic recovery.[35] Behavioral responses of patient and family are discussed in Chapter 44.

To maintain an environment that reduces stress, one must ensure a calm, quiet, optimistic atmosphere. The staff must demonstrate efficiency and competence in their care. In addition, what is stressful to one individual may not be stressful to another. Thus, each must be assessed to determine a suitable environment that reduces stress. Antianxiety drugs such as diazepam may also be useful (Chap. 33).[18] Sensory overload and deficit (Chap. 32) and sleep deprivation (Chap. 31) can occur. (These chapters recommend measures that can be taken to prevent these complications.)

Nursing Care Plan. Table 23-3 contains a sample nursing care plan for the patient in the CCU with an uncomplicated myocardial infarction. Major problems are delineated. This suggested plan of care must be individualized for each patient and is not meant as a standard care plan to be used on all patients. It is meant to demonstrate the use of the nursing process with a patient with this disease, and to provide a guideline for developing an individual plan of care.

Cardiac Care Unit Policies. The CCU must have written policies with the following delineated: (1) purpose of the CCU; (2) admission policies; (3) staffing and duties of each (CCU Director, physician coverage, head nurse, staff nurses); (4) nursing policies and routine care (routine orders); (5) nursing role in an emergency (arrhythmia treatment, pacemaker setting alteration, defibrillation); and (6) record-keeping (charting, log book).

Discharge from the CCU. The patient without complications is usually discharged from the CCU after 3 to 5 days. The nasal oxygen and intravenous line may be discontinued and the patient is transferred by means of a wheelchair to an intermediate care unit or to a medical floor. This transfer should be anticipated and the rationale explained to the patient and family. The anticipation of transfer may reassure the patient. To provide continuity of care, the unit to which the patient is being transferred should be notified of the

TABLE 23-3 SAMPLE NURSING CARE PLAN FOR THE PATIENT IN THE CCU WITH AN UNCOMPLICATED MYOCARDIAL INFARCTION

Problem 1: Myocardial injury, ischemia, and infarction secondary to absent or reduced coronary blood flow resulting in potential chest discomfort with or without radiation to the arms, neck, jaw, shoulders, and back.
  Goal: Relief of chest discomfort by restoring the balance between myocardial oxygen supply and demand.

Nursing Intervention	Scientific Rationale	Evaluation Criteria
1. Initially assess, document, and report to the physician the following:	1. These data assist in determining the cause and effect of the chest discomfort and provide a baseline so that post-therapy symptoms can be compared.	(For 1 through 6) Patient reports relief of chest discomfort within 15 to 30 minutes. Patient appears comfortable: a. seems restful, b. respiratory rate, cardiac rate and blood pressure return to prediscomfort level, c. skin warm and dry.
A. The patient's description of chest discomfort including: location, radiation, duration of pain, and factors that affect it;	A. There are many conditions associated with chest discomfort (Table 22-1). There are characteristic clinical findings of ischemic pain. The pathophysiology of ischemic pain is discussed in Chapter 12.	
B. The effect of chest discomfort on cardiovascular hemodynamic perfusion: to the heart, to the brain, to the kidneys, and to the skin.	B. Myocardial infarction decreases myocardial contractility and ventricular compliance (Chap. 12) and may produce arrhythmias by promoting reentry and increased automaticity (Chap. 26). Cardiac output is reduced, resulting in reduced blood pressure and decreased organ perfusion. The heart rate may increase as a compensatory mechanism to maintain cardiac output.	Effects of chest discomfort on cardiovascular hemodynamics detected to maintain within normal limits: a. heart rate, rhythm, and conduction, b. blood pressure, c. mentation, d. urine output, e. serum BUN and creatinine, f. skin color, temperature, and moisture.
2. Obtain a 12-lead ECG recording during pain, as ordered, to determine extension of infarction or variant angina.	2. An ECG during pain may be useful in the diagnosis of an extension of myocardial ischemia, injury and infarction, and of variant angina.	
3. Administer oxygen as ordered.	3. Oxygen may increase the oxygen supply to the myocardium if actual oxygen saturation is less than normal.	

TABLE 23-3   SAMPLE NURSING CARE PLAN FOR THE PATIENT IN THE CCU WITH AN UNCOMPLICATED MYOCARDIAL INFARCTION (cont.)

Nursing Intervention	Scientific Rationale	Evaluation Criteria
4. Administer narcotic and/or analgesic medications as ordered and continuously evaluate the patient's response.	4. Narcotics are useful in alleviating chest discomfort, decreasing anxiety, and increasing sense of well-being. The side effects of these medications can be dangerous and the patient's status must be assessed (Chap. 33).	
5. Insure physical rest: use of the bedside commode with assistance; backrest elevated to comfort; full liquid diet as tolerated; arms supported during upper-extremity activity; use of stool softener to prevent straining at stool; teach patient to exhale with physical movement to avoid a Valsalva maneuver, and to practice the relaxation response (Chap. 22); individualized visitor privileges, based on patient response; provide a restful environment; and allay fears and anxiety by being supportive, calm, and competent.	5. Physical rest reduces myocardial oxygen consumption. Fear and anxiety precipitate the stress response; this results in increased levels of endogenous catecholamines which increase myocardial oxygen consumption. Also, with increased epinephrine the pain threshold is decreased and pain increases the myocardial oxygen consumption.[40]	
6. Promote the patient's physical comfort by providing individualized basic nursing care.	6. Physical comfort promotes the patient's sense of well-being and reduces anxiety.	

Problem 2: Myocardial ischemia, injury, and infarction secondary to absent or reduced coronary blood flow resulting in potential arrhythmias and conduction disturbances.
Goal 1: Prevent the occurrence of arrhythmias and conduction disturbances by restoring the balance between myocardial oxygen supply and demand.

Nursing Intervention	Scientific Rationale	Evaluation Criteria
1. Same as 3, 5, 6 for Problem 1.	1. Same as 3, 5, 6 for Problem 1.	1,2. Ideally, normal sinus rhythm without arrhythmia is maintained or restored, or the patient's baseline heart rate, rhythm, and conduction are maintained or restored.
2. Administer prophylactic antiarrhythmic medications as ordered.	2. See Chapters 26 and 34.	

Goal 2: Early detection and aggressive treatment of malignant ventricular arrhythmias, conduction abnormalities and supraventricular tachycardia and bradycardia.

Nursing Intervention	Scientific Rationale	Evaluation Criteria
1. Using a cardiac monitor, continuously assess heart rate, rhythm and conduction, and document every four hours, and prior to administration of medications that have a cardiovascular effect. Determine the effect of the arrhythmia on the patient's blood pressure and perfusion to the heart, brain, and kidneys, and report marked changes to the physician.	1. Early detection of arrhythmia allows initiation of therapy and may prevent a lethal arrhythmia. Arrhythmias can result in reduced cardiac output, hypotension, and reduced perfusion to vital organs.	1,2,3. Previous heart rate, rhythm, and conduction restored (Chap. 17). All arrhythmias and conduction disturbances are detected as they occur and do not progress to ventricular fibrillation or asystole.
2. Administer antiarrhythmic and other medications as ordered or according to hospital policy, and evaluate continuously the patient's response to therapy (Chaps. 26, 33, 34, 35).	2. See Chapters 26, 33, 34, 35.	
3. Obtain a 12-lead ECG with any marked change in heart rhythm.	3. A 12-lead ECG assists in the diagnosis of arrhythmias and conduction disturbances and of further myocardial damage.	
4. Assess patient's status to determine other causes of the arrhythmias or conduction disturbances: A. Perform a cardiovascular assessment (Chap. 14).	4. A,B. Data obtained from the history and physical and from laboratory studies can assist in the diagnosis of the disease processes (such as left ventricular failure or pulmonary	4. A,B,C. Normal heart and breath sounds without adventitious sounds (Chap. 14). Serum potassium remains between: 3.6 to 5.5 mEq/L

TABLE 23-3 SAMPLE NURSING CARE PLAN FOR THE PATIENT IN THE CCU WITH AN UNCOMPLICATED MYOCARDIAL INFARCTION (cont.)

Nursing Intervention	Scientific Rationale	Evaluation Criteria
B. Obtain a chest x-ray film (Chap. 16).	embolism) that can cause arrhythmias by the mechanisms of hypoxemia or myocardial stretch. Also, a chest x-ray film provides information regarding the placement of catheters within the heart. Abnormal placement of a catheter within the heart can cause mechanical irritation of the myocardium and result in arrhythmias.	Calcium remains between: 4.6 and 5.5 mEq/L Hb remains between: 12 and 18 g/100 ml Serum drug levels are within the therapeutic range (Chaps. 15, 34). Arterial blood gases on room air remain within the normal limits (Chap. 9). Chest x-ray film remains within normal limits. Incorrect position of heart catheters is detected early.
C. Obtain venous blood (for electrolytes, hemoglobin, appropriate drug levels) and arterial blood (for blood gases) as orderd.	C. Electrolyte imbalance (especially potassium or calcium) can cause arrhythmias and conduction disturbances (Chaps. 9, 17). Reduced hemoglobin decreases the oxygen-carrying capacity of the blood. Hypoxemia, acidosis, alkalosis, and concurrent drug toxicity or subtherapeutic drug levels can cause arrhythmias and conduction disturbances.	

Problem 3: Potential left ventricular failure secondary to reduced myocardial function from myocardial ischemia, injury, and infarction, resulting in: shortness of breath, dyspnea on exertion, orthopnea, and paroxysmal nocturnal dyspnea.

Goal: Prevent pulmonary symptoms by reducing myocardial oxygen consumption, restoring the balance between myocardial oxygen supply and demand.

Nursing Intervention	Scientific Rationale	Evaluation Criteria
1. Initially and every four hours and with chest discomfort, assess, document, and report to the physician abnormal heart sounds (particularly S_3 and S_4 gallops and the holosystolic murmur of left ventricular papillary muscle dysfunction), abnormal breath sounds (particularly crackles), and patient intolerance to specific activities.	1. These data are useful in diagnosing left ventricular failure. Diastolic filling sounds (S_3—S_4 gallop) result from decreased left ventricular compliance associated with myocardial infarction. Papillary muscle dysfunction (from infarction of the papillary muscle) can result in mitral regurgitation and a reduction in stroke volume, leading to left ventricular failure. The presence of crackles (usually at the lung bases) may indicate pulmonary congestion from increased left heart pressures. The association of symptoms and activity can be used as a guide for activity prescription and a basis for patient teaching.	For 1 through 4: Patient does not complain of shortness of breath, dyspnea or exertion, orthopnea, or paroxysmal nocturnal dyspnea. Respiratory rate remains less than 20 breaths per minute with physical activity and 16 breaths per minute with rest. Skin color normal. PaO_2 and $PaCO_2$ within normal range (Chap. 9). Heart rate less than 100 beats per minute with blood pressure within normal limits for this patient. Normal chest film.
2. Same as 5 and 6 for Problem 1.	2. Same as 5 and 6 for Problem 1.	
3. Full liquid diet for 24 hours as ordered.	3. Digestion requires increased cardiac output, which increases the myocardial oxygen consumption. Full liquid diet facilitates digestion because the need to chew has been eliminated, thus requiring less cardiac demand than eating a regular diet.	
4. Teach patient: A. to adhere to the diet prescribed (for example, explain low sodium, low calories); B. to adhere to activity prescription.	4. A. Low sodium diet may reduce extracellular volume, thus reducing preload and afterload, and thus myocardial oxygen consumption. In the obese patient, weight reduction may decrease cardiac work and improve tidal volume. B. The activity prescription is determined individually to maintain the heart rate and blood pressure within safe limits (Chap. 42).	

TABLE 23-3   SAMPLE NURSING CARE PLAN FOR THE PATIENT IN THE CCU WITH AN UNCOMPLICATED MYOCARDIAL INFARCTION (cont.)

Nursing Intervention	Scientific Rationale	Evaluation Criteria

Problem 4: Potential decrease in cardiac output secondary to left ventricular dysfunction resulting in reduced perfusion to vital organs.
   Goal: Prevent symptoms of reduced cardiac output by restoring the balance between oxygen supply and demand.

Nursing Intervention	Scientific Rationale	Evaluation Criteria
1. Initially, and every four hours, and with chest discomfort assess, document and report to the physician the following: A. hypotension B. tachycardia and other arrhythmia C. fatigability D. mentation changes (use family input) E. reduced urine output (less than 250 ml per eight hours) F. cool, moist, cyanotic extremities 2. Same as 5 and 6 from Problem 1.	1. These data are useful in determining a low cardiac output state. An ECG with pain may be useful in the diagnosis of an extension of myocardial ischemia, injury, and infarction, and of variant angina. 2. Same as 5 and 6 from Problem 1.	For 1 and 2: Blood pressure remains within the individual's normal range. Ideally, normal sinus rhythm without arrhythmia is maintained or patient's baseline rhythm is maintained between 60 and 100 beats per minute without further arrhythmia. No complaints of fatigue with prescribed activity. Remains fully alert and oriented and without personality change. Urine output is greater than 250 ml per eight-hour shift. Extremities remain warm and dry with normal color.

Problem 1: Diagnosis of coronary artery disease manifested by myocardial infarction resulting in potential anxiety and fear of death.
   Goal: Reduce the patient's anxiety and fears in order to restore the balance between myocardial oxygen supply and demand.

Nursing Intervention	Scientific Rationale	Evaluation Criteria
1. Assess, document and report to the physician the patient's and family's level of anxiety and coping mechanisms.	1. These data provide information about the psychologic well-being and a baseline so that post-therapy symptoms can be compared. Causes of anxiety are variable and individual, and may include acute illness, hospitalization, pain, disruption of activities of daily living at home and at work, changes in role and self-image due to chronic illness, and lack of financial support. Because anxious family members can transmit anxiety to the patient, the nurse must also reduce the family's fear and anxiety.	For 1 through 7: Patient reports less anxiety. Patient and family discuss their anxieties and fears about death. Patient and family appear less anxious. Patient is restful, respiratory rate less than 16 per minute, heart rate less than 100 per minute without ectopic beats, blood pressure within his normal limits, skin warm and dry. Patient participates actively in a progressive rehabilitation program. Patient practices stress-reduction techniques.
2. Same as 5 and 6 from Problem 1. 3. Assess the need for spiritual counseling and refer as appropriate. 4. Allow patient (and family) to express anxiety and fear: A. by showing genuine interest and concern B. by providing a conducive atmosphere C. by facilitating communication (listening, reflecting, guiding) D. by answering questions. 5. Use of flexible visiting hours allows the presence of a supportive family to assist in reducing the patient's level of anxiety. 6. Encouragement of active participation in a hospital cardiac rehabilitation program (Chap. 42). 7. Teaching of stress reduction techniques.	2. Same as 5 and 6 from Problem 1. 3. If a patient finds support in a religion, religious counseling may assist in reducing anxiety and fear. 4. Unresolved anxiety (the stress response) increases myocardial oxygen consumption. 5. The presence of supportive family members may reduce both patient and family's anxiety. 6. Prescribed cardiac rehabilitation may help to eliminate fear of death, may reduce anxiety and may enhance feelings of well-being (Chap. 42). 7. Stress reduction techniques may help to reduce myocardial oxygen consumption and may enhance feelings of well-being (Chap. 22).	

patient's transfer and the written plan of care, physician orders, and patient's progress should be shared.

Medical and Nursing Treatment: Post-CCU Phase

During the post-CCU phase the risk of complications from MI is markedly reduced. The difference between the intermediate care unit and the medical unit is the intensity and constancy of assessment of cardiac function and assessment of potential complications. For example, in the intermediate care area the patient's heart rhythm should be continuously monitored by telemetry; on the medical floor the patient may be monitored, but less frequently. The area designed for intermediate care should be adjacent to or in continuity with the CCU, thus permitting efficient utilization of manpower and physical resources, and facilitating the transfer of patients to this type of care. The number of beds provided for the area should at least equal or exceed by 50% the number in the CCU. Monitoring and resuscitation capability for intermediate care should be identical with that of the CCU. In some institutions the intermediate care unit is not restricted to patients discharged from CCU but is a place for any patient with cardiovascular disease who may benefit from the monitoring or resuscitative capability of this unit.

The administration of intermediate care should be fully integrated with that of the CCU in order to ensure continuity of optimum management. The training and capabilities of nurses in this unit should be equivalent to that of the CCU nurses.[40]

During this phase the patient is allowed to be more independent in activities of daily living. See Chapter 42 for a detailed discussion of activity and exercise in the post-CCU phase and posthospital phase. Guidelines for patient and family education and sexual counseling can be found in Chapter 45 and 46, respectively.

REFERENCES

1. Adgey AA, Allen JD, Geddes JS et al: Acute phase of myocardial infaction. Lancet 2:501–504, 1971
2. Aldrich RF, Stillerman R, McCormack RC et al: Sudden coronary artery disease (CAD) death in a community and the prospective role of mobile coronary care (MCCU). Circulation (Suppl III) 42:83, 1970
3. Andreoli KG, Fowkes VH, Zipes DP et al: Comprehensive Cardiac Care, 4th ed. St. Louis, CV Mosby 1979
4. Carveth SW: Eight-year experience with a stadium-based mobile coronary-care unit. Heart Lung 3(5):770–774, 1974
5. Cobb LA, Conn RD, Samson WE et al: Early experiences in the management of sudden death with a mobile intensive/coronary care unit. Circulation (Suppl) 42 III:144, 1970
6. Coglman MM: Effects of oxygen on ischemic myocardium. Heart Lung 7(4):635–740, 1978
7. Crampton R, Michaelson SP, Wynbeek A et al: Reduction of pre-hospital, ambulance and coronary death by the pre-hospital emergency cardiac care system: A rationale for training emergency medical technicians, nurses, and physicians. Heart Lung 3(5):742–747, 1974
8. Delano A, Carrel B, Shubin H et al: Monitoring the acutely ill cardiac patient. Cardiovasc Nurs 7(11):61–64, 1971
9. Diet and Coronary Heart Disease. Dallas, American Heart Association, 1978
10. Foster WT: Principles of Acute Coronary Care. New York, Appleton-Century-Crofts, 1976
11. Fulton M, Julian DG, Oliver MF: Sudden death and myocardial infarction. Circulation (Suppl IV) 40:182–193, 1969
12. Goldstein S, Greene W, Moss AJ: Sudden death and hospitalization delay in acute myocardial infarction. A J Cardiol 29:266, 1972
13. Grace WJ: The mobile coronary care unit and the intermediate coronary care unit in the total systems approach to coronary care. Chest 58:363–368, 1970
14. Grace WJ: Pre-Hospital Care of Acute Myocardial Infarction. Dallas, American Heart Association, 1973
15. Hackett TP, Cassem NH: Factors contributing to delay in responding to the signs and symptoms of acute myocardial infarction. Am J Cardiol 24:651–658, 1969
16. Heart Facts 1980. Dallas, American Heart Association, 1980
17. Holland JM: Cardiovascular Nursing: Prevention, Intervention, and Rehabilitation. Boston, Little, Brown & Co, 1977
18. Holloway NM: Nursing the Critically Ill Adult. Mento Park, Addison-Wesley Publishing Co, 1979
19. Kernohan RJ, McGucken RB: Mobile intensive care in myocardial infarction. Br Med J 3:178–180, 1968
20. Kuller L, Lillienfield A, Fisher R: An epidemiological study of sudden death and unexpected deaths in adults. Medicine 46:341–361, 1967
21. Lambrew CT, Schuchman WL, Cannon TH: Emergency medical transport system: Use of ECG telemetry. Chest 63:477–482, 1973
22. Lawrie DM, Higgins MR, Godman MJ et al: Ventricular fibrillation complicating acute myocardial infarction. Lancet 2(7567):523–537, 1968
23. Let's Plug in the Heart. Buffalo, Graphic Controls Corporation, 1979
24. Lewis RP, Frazier JT, Warren JV: Mobile coronary care: An approach to the early mortality of myocardial infarction. Am J Cardiol 26:644, 1970
25. Logue RB, Hurst, JW, Walter PF (eds): The clinical recognition and medical management of coronary atherosclerotic heart disease. The Heart, pp 1252–1260. New York, McGraw-Hill, 1978
26. Lown B, Klein MD, Hershberg PI: Coronary and pre-coronary care. Am J Med 46(5):705–724, 1969
27. Lown B, Ruberman W: The concept of precoronary care. Mod Concepts Cardiovasc Dis 39(5):97–102, 1970
28. Lown B, Vassaux C, Hood WB et al: Unresolved problems in coronary care. Am J of Cardiol 20:494–508, 1967
29. Marriott JL, Fogg E: Constant monitoring for cardiac dysrhythmias and block. Mod Concepts Cardiovasc Dis 39(6):103–108, 1970
30. McNeal GJ: Rectal temperatures in the patient with an acute myocardial infarction. Image 10(1):18–23, 1978
31. Moss AJ, Wynar B, Goldstein S: Delay in hospitalization during the acute coronary period. Am J Cardiol 24:659–665, 1969
32. Olin HS, Hackett TP: Denial of pain in acute myocardial infarction. JAMA 190(11):977–981, 1964
33. Pantridge JF, Adgey AA: Pre-hospital coronary care. The mobile coronary unit. Am J Cardiol 24:666–673, 1969
34. Pantridge JF, Geddes JS: A mobile intensive-care unit in the management of myocardial infarction. Lancet (2):271–273, 1967
35. Rogers DJ, Branyon ME, Kinney MR: Care of the cardiac patient. In Andreoli et al (eds): Comprehensive Cardiac Care, pp 280–334, St. Louis, CV Mosby, 1979
36. Rossi LP, Haines VM: Nursing diagnosis related to acute myocardial infarction. Cardiovasc Nurs 15(3):11–15, 1979
37. Secor J: Coronary Care, A Nursing Specialty. New York, Appleton-Century-Crofts, 1971
38. Standards and guidelines for cardiopulmonary resuscitation (CPR) and emergency cardiac care (ECC). JAMA 244(5):453–509, 1980
39. Wolff HG, Hardy JD, Goodell H: Studies on pain measurement of the effect of morphine, codeine, and other opiates on the pain threshold and on analysis of their relation to the pain experience. J Clin Invest 19:659–680, 1940
40. Yu PN, Bielski MT, Edwards A et al: Report of inter-society

commissions for heart disease resources: Resources for the optimal care of patients with acute myocardial infarction. Circulation 43:A-171–A-183, 1971

ADDITIONAL READING

Baum RS, Alvarez H, Cobb LA: Survival after resuscitation from out-of-hospital ventricular fibrillation. Circulation 50:1231–1235, 1975

Bernard R, Corday E, Eliasch H et al: Nomenclature and criteria of diagnosis of ischemic heart disease. Circulation 59(3):607–608, 1979

Christakis G, Winston M: Nutritional therapy in acute myocardial infarction. J Am Diet Assoc 63(3):233–238, 1973

Cobb LA, Werner JA, Trobaugh GB: Sudden cardiac death. Mod Concepts Cardiovasc Dis 49(6):31–36, 1980

Cromwell RL, Butterfield EC, Brayfield FM et al: Acute Myocardial Infarction: Reaction and Recovery, St. Louis, CV Mosby, 1977

Forrester JS, Chatterjee K, Jobin G: A new conceptual approach to the therapy of acute myocardial infarction. Adv Cardiol 15:111–123, 1975

Forrester JS, Swan HJC: Acute myocardial infarction: A physiological basis of therapy. Crit Care Med 2(6):283–293, 1974

Grace WJ: Out-of-hospital care for cardiac emergencies. Heart Lung 3(5):733–735, 1974

Grace WJ, Chadbourn JA: The first hour in acute myocardial infarction. Heart Lung 3(5):736–741, 1974

Granger J: Full recovery from myocardial infarction: Psychosocial factors. Heart Lung 3(4):600–610, 1974

Gross L, Malaya R: Entrinsically induced arrhythmia in acute myocardial infarction. JAMA 228(8):1021–1024, 1974

Jick H, Miettinen O, Neff R: Coffee and myocardial infarction. N Engl J Med 289:63–67, 1973

Lambrew CT: The experience in telemetry of the electrocardiogram to a base hospital. Heart Lung 3(5):756–764, 1974

Lambrew CT: Stabilization and transportation. In Advanced Cardiac Life Support. Dallas, American Heart Association, 1978

Lester RM, Wagner GS: Acute myocardial infarction. Med Clin North Am 63(1):3–24, 1979

Lewis AJ, Ailshie E, Criley JM: Pre-hospital cardiac care in a paramedical mobile intensive care unit. Cal Med 117:1–8, 1972

Liberthson RR, Nagel EL, Hirschman JC, et al: Prehospital ventricular defibrillation. N Engl J Med 291(7):317–321, 1974

Lie KI, Wellens, HJ, Van Capelle FJ et al: Lidocaine in the prevention of primary ventricular fibrillation: A Double-blind randomized study of 212 consecutive patients. N Engl J Med 291(25):1324–1326, 1974

McNeer JF, Wagner GS, Ginsburg PB et al: Hospital discharge one week after acute myocardial infarction. N Engl J Med 298(5):229–232, 1978

Nolte CT, Grace WJ: Life-support units. Heart Lung 3(5):779–784, 1974

Pace NA: Emergency cardiac care in a metropolitan office building. Heart Lung 3(5):775–778, 1974

Rosati MC, Granatelli A, Lustig GJ et al: Community hospital mobile coronary care unit. NY State J Med 70:2462–2465, 1970

Rose LB: The oregon coronary ambulance project: An experiment. Heart Lung 3(5):753–755, 1974

Rose LB, Press E: Cardiac defibrillation by ambulance attendants. JAMA 219:63–68, 1972

Saltzman HA: Efficacy of oxygen enriched gas mixtures in the treatment of acute myocardial infarction. Circulation 52(3):357–359, 1975

Schroeder JS, Lamb IH, Hu M: The prehospital course of patients with chest pain: Analysis of the prodromal, symptomatic, decision making, transportation and emergency room periods. Am J Med 64(5):742–748, 1978

Swan HJC, Blackburn HW, De Sanctis et al: Duration of hospitalization in uncomplicated acute myocardial infarction, An Ad Hoc Committee Review. Am J Cardiol 37(3):413–419, 1976

Sweetwood HM: Oxygen administration in the coronary care unit. Heart Lung 3(1):102–107, 1974

Trombold JC, Monsen ER, Karkeck JM: Dietary guidelines for hospital cardiac care units. American Heart Association of Washington, Seattle, April, 1976

Uhley HN: Experience with a private ambulance service. Heart Lung 3(5):765–769, 1974

Warren JV, Lewis RP: Beneficial effects of atropine in the prehospital phase of coronary care. Am J Cardiol 37(1):68–72, 1976

Webb SW, Adgey AA, Pantridge JF: Autonomic disturbances at onset of acute myocardial infarction. Br Med J 3(5818):89–93, 1972

Whipple GH, Peterson MA, Haines VM et al: Acute Coronary Care. Boston, Little, Brown & Co, 1972

24

Surgical Intervention for Coronary Artery Disease

KAREN S. WULFF, R.N., M.N., CCRN.

and

PATRICIA A. HONG, R.N., M.A.

Coronary artery disease (CAD) is treated surgically by myocardial revascularization (aortocoronary and internal mammary artery bypass grafting), by cardiac transplantation, and recently, by coronary transluminal angioplasty (dilatation of diseased coronary arteries with a balloon-tipped catheter). Aortocoronary bypass grafting is the most frequent surgical intervention. In 1978, 95,000 myocardial revascularization operations were done nationwide, an incidence of 44.2 procedures per 100,000 people.[20a] This incidence varies regionally depending on the availability of catheterization and surgical facilities and on the therapeutic philosophy. Cardiac transplantation is reserved for certain patients with end-stage CAD.[26] This procedure is currently performed in only a few centers because of the complex surgical and management techniques and because of the infrequency of transplantation. Coronary transluminal angioplasty has had limited clinical trial since 1977, and its clinical value and therapeutic application are yet to be defined.

The intent of this chapter is to provide cardiovascular nurses with information about the surgical procedures, usual therapy, and nursing care requirements of patients undergoing surgical intervention for CAD. The information is important in providing comprehensive care to these patients in the preoperative, intraoperative, and postoperative phases of treatment. Because the exact type of nursing unit where these patients are cared for varies from institution to institution, the term critical care unit will be used to denote these varying units (cardiac care units, surgical intensive care units, cardiac units).

MYOCARDIAL REVASCULARIZATION

Aortocoronary bypass graft surgery connects a segment of a vein or artery between the aortic root and the coronary artery at a point distal to the obstruction or stenosis caused by atherosclerosis (Chap. 10). Most often a portion of the patient's saphenous vein is used for the graft(s). Saphenous veins have greater tensile strength than do upper-extremity veins because they are exposed to greater hydrostatic pressures.[17] Thus, they are better substitutes for arteries than are upper extremity veins. Saphenous vein homografts provide patency similar to that of saphenous autografts and are used when the patient's saphenous veins are not suitable. Segments of cephalic or basilar veins also have been used successfully for aortocoronary bypass.

Although it would seem that segments of arteries would make better arterial grafts than veins, aortocoronary radial artery bypass grafts have been shown to have a high rate of occlusion. These thick-walled arteries develop intimal hyperplasia.[8] In contrast, the thin-walled mammary artery has been used successfully as a segmental graft without hyperplasia and resulting occlusion. Direct bypass of the occluded coronary arteries by attachment of a mammary artery distal to the obstruction has also been effective. Some surgeons have had lower incidence of occlusion with mammary-artery-to-coronary bypass than with aortocoronary saphenous vein bypass.[12] The mammary artery is limited in length and can revascularize only the anterior surface of the heart. This limitation, plus the fact of a more difficult surgical technique, has discouraged surgeons from doing mammary-artery-to-coronary-artery grafts.[18]

CRITERIA FOR PATIENT SELECTION

The question of criteria used in selecting patients for myocardial revascularization has been the subject of much debate (Chap. 25). A general criterion used as rationale for myocardial revascularization is disabling angina pectoris unrelieved by medical therapy. This criterion is subjective. Its interpretation varies with the individual's definition of "disabling" and the physician's protocol for medical treatment of angina. It can serve, however, as a guide for those deciding about surgical intervention.

The location and amount of stenosis in the coronary artery system, the amount of ventricle served by the narrowed coronary artery, and previous infarction related to an obstructed coronary artery are all considered when determining the need for surgical intervention. These are determined by cardiac assessment, with the aid of clinical history, physical (Chap. 14), exercise testing (Chap. 18), ventriculography and coronary cineangiography (Chap. 19), electrocardiogram (Chap. 17), and at times, serum enzyme levels (Chap. 15).

Patients with stenosis of the left main coronary artery exceeding 50% have better prognoses with surgical intervention than with medical therapy.[28] Stenosis of other coronary arteries exceeding 70% is considered significant disease. The area of ventricle supplied by the narrowed vessel generally must also be of significant size before revascularization is considered.

Some of the anatomic indications for myocardial revascularization, particularly in symptomatic patients, are

1. Left main coronary artery disease, more than 50% stenosis

2. Two- and three-vessel disease, more than 70% stenosis and patent distal arteries

3. Single-vessel left anterior descending stenosis, more than 70% stenosis proximal to the first septal branch

4. Single-vessel disease at the site of a previous subendocardial infarction[17]

Generally, unstable angina and postinfarction angina are treated surgically. Myocardial infarction complicated by left ventricular power failure or intractable ventricular arrhythmias are treated by some with revascularization. These conditions are associated with high mortality, whether treated with surgical or medical therapy.

Myocardial revascularization of patients with uncomplicated acute myocardial infarction is done at some centers.[3,4,23] Some of the potential benefits are thought to be interruption of progressive myocardial necrosis, salvage of ischemic myocardium, and bypass of the area of stenosis in the involved coronary artery and in other coronary arteries.[23] This application of revascularization remains controversial. The risks and benefits are difficult to determine. Data from studies where the procedure has been done indicate that surgical mortality is lowest when the revascularization is either performed within the first few hours after onset of symptoms of MI or is delayed until 30 or more days after the occurrence of MI.[3,4,23]

The criteria used to determine when myocardial revascularization is appropriate remain controversial. The process by which the decision is made is critical in ensuring the appropriateness of the decision. Ideally, the assessment and interpretation of all the clinical data are done independently by several physicians and then discussed jointly to determine the therapy that will be recommended to the patient and family. The patient and family must then be informed of the benefits and risks of the proposed therapy and of alternative therapies so that they can be involved in the decision. The patient and family ultimately must define what risks and limitations are tolerable and what therapeutic interventions are acceptable.

PREOPERATIVE PREPARATION OF THE PATIENT

The preoperative phase of patient preparation usually begins prior to hospitalization. This phase focuses on stabilizing any other disease conditions and optimizing cardiac function. The patient with diabetes, hypertension, chronic obstructive pulmonary disease or other respiratory disease, or renal or liver disease should be assessed and medical therapy adjusted to stabilize them. Any sources of possible infection, for example periodontal disease, skin lesions, and stasis ulcer, should be investigated and treated. Therapy should also be adjusted to control any heart failure, arrhythmias, and fluid or electrolyte imbalances to optimize cardiac function. Special consideration should be given to the anxiety associated with waiting for hospitalization and surgery, and a mild tranquilizer should be prescribed as needed to help control increased heart rate, which exacerbates the ischemia.

Nursing Implications

Nursing's role with the patient and family should begin in the prehospitalization phase of preparation with emotional support and teaching. Establishing rapport, answering questions, listening to fears and concerns, clarifying misconceptions, and informing the patient about what to expect, are all interventions the nurse uses to prepare the patient and family emotionally for hospitalization and surgery.

Patient teaching should be based on assessed learning needs. Teaching usually includes information about hospitalization, about the surgery (the preoperative routines, the length of the surgery, what the patient will feel like, the visiting routines in the critical care unit), and about the recovery phase (length of hospitalization, when normal routines such as housework, shopping, and work can be resumed). Any changes made in medical therapy and preoperative preparations will need to be explained and reinforced.

Patients should be instructed to avoid aspirin and any drugs containing aspirin for at least 9 days prior to surgery. Aspirin decreases platelet adhesion and may predispose the patient to surgical hemorrhage. Anticoagulant therapy is usually stopped 5 to 7 days before surgery. The patient is also encouraged to stop or reduce smoking a few weeks prior to surgery. If the patient is on digitalis, a short-acting preparation will be prescribed, but sometimes even this is discontinued 36 to 48 hours prior to surgery. Most antiarrhythmics, nitrates, and propranolol will be continued until the night before surgery.

The patient with nonacute CAD is routinely hospitalized only 1 or 2 days prior to surgery. Most of the preoperative medical evaluation is usually completed before the patient enters the hospital. A new history and physical examination, chest roentgenogram, ECG, serum electrolytes, coagulation screen, and typing and cross-matching of blood may be done at this time. These data provide information about other disease conditions and cardiac problems. Nursing intervention focuses primarily on obtaining a baseline assessment of the patient (Chap. 14), patient teaching, and continued emotional and physical preparation for surgery.

The preoperative assessment (Chap. 14) should be thorough and well documented, since it provides baseline data for postoperative comparison. The history should include a social assessment of family roles and support systems, and a description of the patient's usual functional level and typical activities. This information will assist with emotional care and rehabilitation planning.

Joint teaching of the patient and family may be more effective if the preoperative hospitalization period is very short. The patient's anxiety increases with the admission process and the immediacy of surgery. Unless the nurse has met the patient before the day of hospitalization, the time may be too short to establish a relationship that contributes to patient learning. Joint teaching capitalizes on the established support relationship of the patient and family to increase learning. Teaching in this phase should be directed primarily by the patient's (and family's) questions. Too much detail may only increase anxiety.

The patient may be offered a tour of the critical care unit, the postanesthesia recovery room, or both. (In some hospitals, the patient will initially go to the postanesthesia unit.) The patient recovering from anesthesia is reassured by having already seen and heard the environment and having met someone from the unit. The patient and family should be informed about some of the tubes that the patient will be attached to postoperatively, and their purposes. Most patients will remain intubated and on mechanical ventilation for 6 to 24 hours postoperatively. They need to be aware that this prevents them from talking, but reassure them that the staff are skilled in other means of communication. They should know to expect several intravenous lines, tubes in the chest, and a urinary catheter. Explaining the purpose and approximate time that these will be in place helps to reassure the patient.

The patient's other questions about postoperative routines should be answered. Deep breathing and coughing, using the incentive spirometer or intermittent positive pressure breathing (IPPB), and foot exercises should be explained and practiced by the patient preoperatively. The family's questions at this time will focus primarily on the length of the surgery, on who will discuss the results of the procedure with them and when this may occur, on where to wait during the surgery, on the visiting routines in the critical care unit, and on how they can support the patient preoperatively and in the critical care unit.

Emotional preparation of the patient and family for surgery involves the nurse's skillful communication and teaching techniques. The fears of patients about to undergo cardiac surgery are the same as those facing other surgery. Their fears frequently are intensified because of the special meaning attached to the heart, the realization of a risk of death associated with cardiac surgery, the infrequency with which the public encounters individuals who have undergone this surgery, and the extent to which they are involved in the decision to have surgical or medical therapy for their cardiac disease.

Studies have shown that for patients to be optimally prepared emotionally for surgery, they should be in a moderate state of anxiety.[11] This anxiety enables them to cope with the stresses and discomforts postoperatively. The patient in a moderate state of anxiety presents signs of being anxious, but retains the ability to listen and learn. Preoperative intervention with patients facing cardiac surgery begins with assessment of their level of anxiety. If it is low, the patient may be in denial. Allow the patient more controls (Chap. 44). If the patient exhibits high anxiety, then it is necessary to intervene to lower his anxiety level. This can be done by assessing the fears upon which he is focusing and intervening to lessen them. The fears that most patients express are

1. *Fear of the unknown.* This fear is difficult for the patient to express. Not having past experience with cardiac surgery, the patient does not know enough detail to attach fears to any specific aspect. Instead of specific fears that the patient can identify and begin to cope with, the patient is left with just a generalized dread and anxiety.

   Intervention begins with determining other experiences that the patient has had, with which details of the impending surgery can be compared. Describe what the patient will feel. If the patient has already had a cardiac catheterization, compare the similarities and differences between that and the surgery. Encourage the patient also to talk about any concerns from previous bad experiences.

2. *Fear of pain.* The patient may openly express a fear of pain and the inability to tolerate it or may indirectly express this fear by asking many questions about pain, pain medications, and the state of recovering from anesthesia. Encourage the patient to talk about this fear. Make a comparison between the pain experienced with cardiac surgery and other pain experiences. Inform him about the preoperative sedation, the anesthetic, and the postoperative pain medication. Reassure him that the fear of pain is normal. Admit that he will experience some pain but he will be closely observed and the use of medication, positioning, and relaxation will make the pain tolerable.

3. *Fear of body-image change.* Many patients have a fear of the scarring from surgery. This fear frequently is exaggerated by misconceptions from the communications media or imagined distortions due to lack of knowledge. Patients may talk openly about this fear or indirectly express it through concern about continued love from others or excessive focus on postoperative pain. Discuss this fear with him and correct any misconceptions. Assure

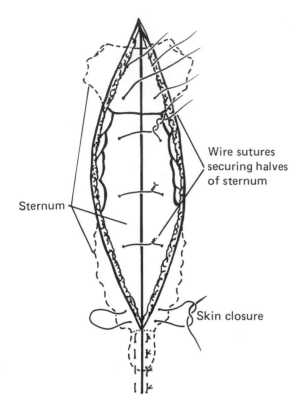

Fig. 24-1. Median sternotomy. (King O: Care of the Cardiac Surgical Patient, p 56. St. Louis, CV Mosby, 1975)

him that the health team members give consistent descriptions of the incisions and the healing process.

4. *Fear of dying.* Some patients directly share their fear of dying. More simply drop clues about their concern, for example, questioning their need for teaching about the surgery and postoperative course, asking for reassurance that someone will care for their family the day of surgery, becoming tearful around their family members, or telling them just to wait at home on the day of surgery. Those who share this fear openly, should be reassured that the fear is normal. Emphasize the postoperative care and routines in teaching, because this indirectly reassures them that they will survive the surgery. Those who only drop clues, despite efforts to encourage them to talk about their fear, should be coached to express this fear, for example, "Are you worrying about not making it through surgery? Most people who have heart surgery at least think about the possibility of dying." Once the fear is expressed, the patient can be helped. By alleviating undue anxiety, emotional preparation of the patient for surgery lessens the chance of preoperative angina or infarction[17] and enhances the patient's involvement in postoperative care and recovery.

Physical preparation of the patient usually involves several showers or scrubs with an antiseptic solution. The patient is medicated for sleep the night before surgery and sedated before going to surgery. With few exceptions, almost all cardiac surgical teams use prophylactic antibiotic therapy for myocardial revascularization, and the antibiotics are started preoperatively.

Patients requiring emergency myocardial revasculariza-

tion may have both coronary cineangiography and surgery within hours. These patients and their families have little opportunity for teaching and emotional preparation. As a result, specific intervention is usually required postoperatively to help them adjust.

Myocardial Revascularization Surgery

Aortocoronary bypass grafting with segments of autogenous saphenous veins accounts for the majority of myocardial revascularization procedures done.[18] The surgical techniques used for this procedure are standardized nationwide.[18] Except for the removal of the vessel segment, the procedure is unchanged when segments of vessels other than the patient's saphenous vein are grafted.

Aortocoronary bypass graft surgery is done through a median sternotomy (Fig. 24-1).[14] While this chest incision is made and the extracorporeal circulation cannulas are being positioned (Fig. 24-2), another member of the surgical team excises the saphenous vein from either the thigh or the lower leg (Fig. 24-3A). The vein is later carefully measured and cut. Veins that are too short occlude early; those that are too long kink.[17]

Almost all surgeons support the patient on extracorporeal circulation (cardiopulmonary bypass) so that the heart can be arrested and a quiet field provided for anastomosis of the saphenous veins to the coronary arteries. Cannulation techniques for the extracorporeal circulation include (Fig. 24-2):

1. One or two cannulas in the right atrium or superior and inferior venae cavae for venous drainage

Fig. 24-2. Cardiopulmonary bypass. Cannulation of the ascending and descending venae cavae, the ascending aorta, the right superior pulmonary vein, and the left ventricle. (Miller DW Jr: Bypass Surgery for Coronary Heart Disease, p 12. Seattle, Univ. Washington School of Medicine, 1978)

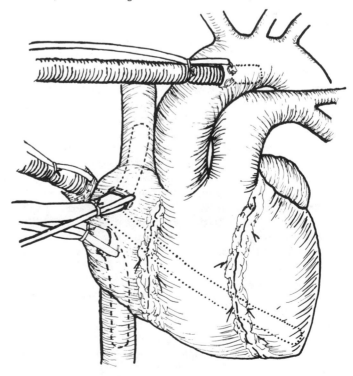

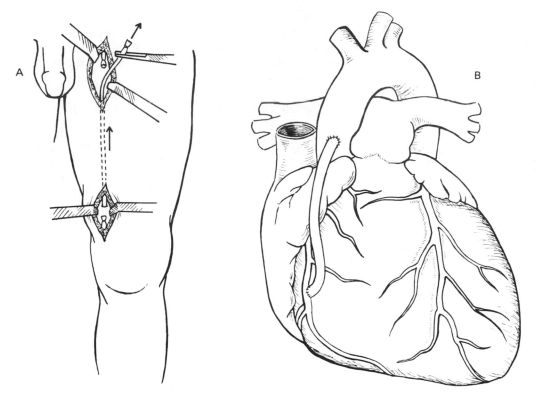

Fig. 24-3.   Direct myocardial revascularization using a coronary artery bypass graft. (**A**) A segment of the saphenous vein is removed and (**B**) anastamosed side-to-end to the aorta and to the coronary artery, distal to the obstruction. (Brunner LS, Suddarth DS: Textbook of Medical—Surgical Nursing, p 435. Philadelphia, JB Lippincott, 1975)

2. A cannula in the ascending aorta to return oxygenated blood from the machine for perfusion

3. A cannula is sometimes placed in the left ventricle by way of the pulmonary vein and the left atrium. This drains blood that returns from the bronchial bed to the left side of the heart, thereby preventing ventricular distention.[17]

In addition to oxygenating the blood, the extracorporeal circulation is used to produce systemic hypothermia.[18] Hypothermia reduces the cellular oxygen consumption and further protects the body while on extracorporeal circulation.

The patient is heparinized to prevent the blood from clotting in the tubing of the extracorporeal (heart–lung) machine. The cardiopulmonary bypass is initiated just prior to the anastamosis of the veins to the coronary arteries. With the patient on cardiopulmonary bypass, the aorta is cross-clamped, and a cold potassium-enriched saline solution is injected into the aortic root. This solution produces prompt electro-mechanical arrest and profound myocardial hypothermia. Instillation of this solution improves myocardial protection during the operative period.[20,24]

The segments of saphenous vein (or of the vessel used for the graft) are implanted in the aortic root with an end-to-side anastomosis. The veins are placed in a reverse position so that their valves do not interfere with blood flow through the vein from the aorta to the coronary arteries. One or several grafts are placed according to the need assessed from the preoperative angiogram. The most widely performed grafts are the single aortocoronary bypass grafts

(simple graft), in which a single vein segment is anastomosed to the aorta, end-to-side, and then attached end-to-side to a coronary artery beyond its stenotic area (Fig. 24-3B).[18] Many surgeons also do sequential grafting, where a single vein segment is anastomosed to the aorta end-to-side and then anastomosed side-to-side to one or more coronary artery branches before terminating in an end-to-side coronary anastomosis (Fig. 24-4).[17] This makes it easier to do multiple bypass grafts, if required, for improved long-term results from aortocoronary surgery.[15] Constructing these anastomoses frequently requires optical magnification in order to connect the saphenous vein (2.5 mm to 4 mm in diameter) to a coronary artery (1.5 mm in diameter) with 10 to 15 fine stitches.

Preoperatively a radial or femoral arterial catheter, a right atrial line (central venous pressure catheter or a pulmonary artery catheter) and a urinary catheter are placed, and cardiac monitoring is initiated. These enable monitoring of the patient during the procedure and postoperatively. Before closing the chest, chest tubes are positioned to evacuate air and drainage from the mediastinum and the thorax.

While the chest is open, epicardial pacemaker wires (atrial and sometimes ventricular) are usually implanted. Commercially available pacer wires are sewn onto the right atrium near the superior vena cava. If atrial pacing is anticipated, two wires are placed about 2 cm apart. If a need for ventricular pacing is anticipated, a wire is implanted on the right ventricle as well. Each pacer wire is sewn through the muscle in several places along the axis in which the wire will be withdrawn. The wires are not fixed to the atrium or ventricle with sutures. These wires are passed through the chest wall and fixed to the skin with a suture.[19] While in place, the wires can be used to pace the heart at an increased rate or to eliminate ectopy by increasing the heart rate. The atrial wires can also be connected to the chest lead of the electrocardiogram (ECG) machine and a recording can be made of the electrical activity in the atria. This tracing is beneficial in differentiating supraventricular arrhythmias and determining effective therapy; for example, atrial flutter can frequently be converted with rapid atrial pacing but atrial fibrillation does not convert with rapid pacing. When the need for pacing is no longer anticipated, the wires are removed by cutting the skin suture and tugging on the wires. The patient should be monitored for hemorrhage and cardiac tamponade for a few hours after the wires are removed. Hemorrhage is rare, however. The patient is transferred to a postanesthesia recovery unit or directly to the critical care unit when the surgery is completed.

Intraoperative risks have been reduced by improved surgical techniques and anesthetic management, identification of preoperative factors that increase operative risk, and use of intraaortic balloon assistance perioperatively. Factors associated with increased operative risk are

Left main coronary artery stenosis

Impaired resting ventricular function

Impending myocardial infarction

Acute and recent myocardial infarction

Postinfarction angina

Cardiogenic shock

Refractory ventricular arrhythmias

Advanced age[17]

Use of intraaortic balloon assistance during cardiac catheterization, during anesthesia induction, and postoperatively has reduced operative mortality with left main coronary artery stenosis, impaired ventricular function, and impending or recent MI.[17] The intraaortic balloon pump increases coronary perfusion and reduces afterload and myocardial oxygen consumption. The system includes a balloon-tipped catheter, which is placed in the thoracic aorta and alternatively inflated and deflated by a pump. The balloon is inflated with either helium or carbon dioxide. The low viscosity of these gases facilitates rapid inflation and deflation of the balloon. The pump is timed to deflate the balloon when the left ventricle begins systole. Deflation of the balloon reduces aortic pressure (afterload) and reduces the pressure work of the ventricle. The pump inflates the balloon as the aortic valve closes and the left ventricle begins diastole. Inflation of the balloon increases diastolic aortic pressure and displaces blood in the aorta, thus increasing flow into the coronary arteries.

To insert the balloon-tipped catheter, a cutdown is made in the groin, using local anesthesia. The femoral artery is isolated and a synthetic vessel graft is anastomosed end-to-side on the artery. The catheter is inserted through the graft and passed up the artery into the aorta (using fluoroscopy) until positioned just distal to the left subclavian artery. Once in place, the catheter is held in position by a tie placed around the synthetic graft. Securing the catheter to the graft rather than to the femoral artery helps to protect the blood

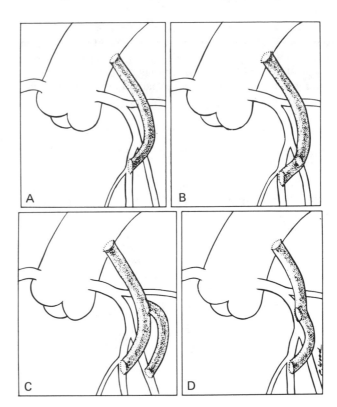

Fig. 24-4. Coronary artery bypass graft. (**A**) Simple graft; (**B**) sequential graft; (**C**) Y graft; (**D**) skip graft; (Miller DW Jr: Practice of Coronary Artery Bypass Surgery, p 207. New York, Plenum, 1977)

flow through the distal femoral artery.[6] The catheter is then connected to the mechanical assist device (pump). Timing for inflation and deflation of the balloon is synchronized with the electrocardiogram. The balloon is inflated during the latter half of the T-wave and is deflated just prior to the QRS complex. Timing is further adjusted by the use of the arterial pressure tracing, that is, inflation-timed with the dicrotic notch; deflation just prior to the aortic valve opening or just prior to systole.

Increased blood flow to the coronary arteries improves perfusion for patients with left main coronary artery stenosis and protects them from ischemia and infarction during catheterization and anesthesia. The increased coronary perfusion may also prevent further myocardial damage perioperatively for patients suffering recent myocardial infarction. Both increased coronary perfusion and reduced afterload can reduce angina and ischemia. Moreover, allowing the failing ventricle a period of working against a decreased afterload pressure may allow it to compensate.

The patient on the intraaortic balloon pump requires careful monitoring and intervention much the same as that outlined for the immediate postoperative period described for the period following cardiac surgery. He may require vasoactive drug therapy and respiratory support. He will need specific positioning and vascular assessment and will be on anticoagulant therapy to reduce thrombus formation on the catheter. In addition, the nurse will be involved in monitoring (and possibly adjusting) the intraaortic balloon pump.

Aortocoronary bypass graft surgery for cardiogenic shock

and refractory ventricular arrhythmias is not universally advocated. These conditions are associated with high mortality, whether treated medically or surgically. Improved surgical and postoperative management techniques have reduced the mortality rates for patients more than 70 years old.[15]

IMMEDIATE POSTOPERATIVE CARE

The primary focus of nursing care initially is acute assessment and prompt intervention to stabilize the patient. Emotional support of the patient (and family) and comfort are equally important. A systems approach is one way purposefully to organize the assessment. Patients facing myocardial revascularization commonly have variations from normal and a potential for greater complications. Table 24-1 presents the parameters monitored for each system, common variations, and potential complications. The possible causes, usual therapy, rationale, and additional nursing interventions are given for each variation and complication. The information presented is typical and must be adapted for the individual patient.

CONTINUED POSTOPERATIVE CARE

The primary focus of nursing care in the postacute phase is gradual rehabilitation toward discharge. The patient without postoperative complications moves from the critical care unit to an intermediate or general care unit one to four days after surgery. This move is a highly anxious time for the patient and family.[27] Ideally, information is shared and consistent care is provided through joint care planning even though the transfer prohibits care by the same nursing personnel.

Before the patient is transferred from the unit, his endotracheal tube, arterial catheters, and probably the chest tubes and urinary catheter are removed. Cardiac monitoring may be continued (usually 72 hours postoperatively or 24 hours after the last arrhythmia).

The care given emphasizes increased independence with activities of daily living, increased ambulation and sitting, and vigorous respiratory care to reduce atelectasis. The patient may be more aware of pain with the increased activity. Pain medications are offered frequently, although the strength of the medication is lessened.

Some of the common problems for which the patient is monitored include supraventricular arrhythmias, hypertension, congestive heart failure, and emotional distress.

About 10% to 30% of patients develop supraventricular tachyarrhythmias after myocardial revascularization.[30] The most common arrhythmias are premature atrial ectopic beats, atrial fibrillation, and atrial flutter. Ordinarily these occur only during the first 8 postoperative days. The patient is monitored for tolerance of the arrhythmia and the presence of congestive heart failure or hypoxia. An atrial rhythm strip is obtained by the use of the atrial pacemaker wire. This lead more clearly differentiates atrial fibrillation and atrial flutter. Atrial fibrillation is treated with inotropic and antiarrhythmic drugs. Atrial flutter is treated with rapid atrial pacing override or cardioversion.

Assessment of fluid and electrolyte balance continues in this phase. Sodium is restricted in the diet and diuretics are given if the patient has congestive heart failure.

Brief periods of confusion are common for the first day or two. Increased intervals of undisturbed rest and sleep eliminate confusion and enhance relaxation. Many patients experience 1 to 2 days of depression in this phase, but are unable to identify a precipitating cause.[13] Perhaps the termination of the high anxiety associated with the preoperative and acute postoperative periods precipitates this letdown or depression. The patient and family need reassurance that the depression is normal and temporary.

Discharge teaching begins for the patient shortly after transfer from the critical care unit because discharge will occur in 3 to 7 days. Joint teaching of patient and family is most effective because of the short interval available for teaching, and the varying emotional state of the patient. Instruction should include pulse taking, wound care, and information about medications, any diet restrictions, and activity adjustments. Some hospitals offer patients a specific cardiac rehabilitation program. The program is similar to the myocardial infarction rehabilitation program (Chap. 42). Since the myocardial revascularization surgery does not treat the underlying atherosclerosis, the patient needs the same cardiac conditioning and reduction of risk factors.

Patients who suffer from some other chronic disease, who are over the age of 70, or who are to have multiple surgical procedures done, for example, myocardial revascularization and valve replacement or revascularization and carotid endarterectomy, have an increased chance of perioperative complications and prolonged phases of recovery.

CARDIAC TRANSPLANTATION

Cardiac transplantation is performed either for advanced idiopathic cardiomyopathy or for inoperable end-stage CAD.[25] Criteria used in selecting patients that favor the success of the transplantation include

Patient under 50 years of age

Cardiac disease duration of fewer than 5 years

Minimal liver and renal dysfunction

Lack of elevated pulmonary vascular resistance

Lack of any infection.[25]

The patient's emotional acceptance of the transplantation and family support systems are important in the long recovery period.

Cardiac Transplantation Surgery

The surgical procedure has changed minimally since 1968.[25] The heart is removed by transecting the great vessels and the atria at a point dorsal to the atrial appendages.[1,7] Some surgeons retain the posterior wall of both atria to provide better anastomosis and to provide some afferent innerva-

(*Text continues on page 351*)

TABLE 24-1   MYOCARDIAL REVASCULARIZATION—IMMEDIATE POSTOPERATIVE PROBLEMS

Cardiovascular

Parameters monitored: Cardiac rate and rhythm, systemic blood pressures, filling pressures (central venous pressure or pulmonary artery and pulmonary artery wedge pressures), heart sounds, peripheral pulses, and sometimes cardiac output. (See Chap. 21 for details on hemodynamic parameters.)

Common postoperative problems:

PROBLEM	POSSIBLE CAUSES	USUAL THERAPY	RATIONALE	ADDITIONAL NURSING INTERVENTIONS
Ventricular ectopic rhythms develop in the initial 24-hour period.	Trauma from handling the heart, or cardioplegia. Serum potassium imbalances. Ventricular distention due to failure.	1. Some physicians initiate a continuous lidocaine infusion for 24 to 48 hours postoperatively to prevent ventricular ectopy. 2. Others treat only if ectopic beats occur. Treatment focuses on determining the cause of the ectopy, *i.e.* hypoxia or hypokalemia, and therapy is directed toward eliminating the cause. If the ectopic beats decrease cardiac output or become malignant (Chap. 26), drug therapy (lidocaine, procainamide) or temporary pacing to overdrive the heart rate is initiated.[31] Note: The critical care nurse should have standing postoperative or unit orders for treating ventricular arrhythmias, including cardioversion and defibrillation for ventricular tachycardia and fibrillation.	1. Prevents ventricular arrhythmias during susceptible period. 2. Cardiac surgery patients are less susceptible to sustained ventricular arrhythmias than are patients with myocardial infarction. Treatment should be more conservative. Focus on finding the cause and treating it.	Quickly assess patient for probable cause. Continued assessment for: a. Effectiveness of therapy b. Recurrence or worsening of problem
Sinus bradycardia or junctional rhythm. Reversal spontaneous in one or two days.	Metabolic problems secondary to extracorporeal circulation.[9]	If the rhythm results in low systemic pressures: a. Pace the patient at an increased heart rate, or b. Medicate to increase heart rate, *i.e.*, with atropine or isoproterenol	Increases heart rate to improve cardiac output and prevent other complications.	
Hypertension	Peripheral vasoconstriction. Increased catecholamines and/or renin-angiotension II[21] Hypothermia	Medicate to control mean arterial pressure less than 110 mm Hg, *i.e.*, nitroprusside drip infusion.	Controls hypertension and thus lessens risk of postoperative hemorrhage and rupture of bypass graft suture line.	Neurologically assess patient for adverse reaction to hypertension *i.e.*, cerebral vascular accident.
Hypotension	Hemorrhage or saline depletion Decreased heart rate Irregular heart rhythm Initial response to vasodilatation (after being vasoconstricted) when fluid balance is marginal Decreased contractility or failure of ventricle	If heart rate and rhythm are normal and filling pressures are low, infuse volume, *i.e.*, blood, plasma, lactated Ringer's solution, saline. If heart rate slow, pace or medicate to increase. If heart rhythm irregular, treat arrhythmia, *i.e.*, digoxin, antiarrhythmics. If saline replacement adequate (filling pressures high), give positive inotropic or vasoactive drugs.	Mean arterial pressure of more than 60 to 70 mm Hg helps prevent bypass graft occlusion. Controls hypotension and maintains adequate tissue perfusion. Digoxin has inotropic effect on myocardium. Adjusts preload and afterload and increases cardiac output. Increases myocardial contractility.	Frequent checks to see that nitroprusside and lidocaine drips are controlled. While administering positive inotropic or vasoactive drugs, monitor for side effects (see Chap. 35).

TABLE 24-1 MYOCARDIAL REVASCULARIZATION—IMMEDIATE POSTOPERATIVE PROBLEMS (cont.)

Potential Complications:

COMPLICATION	POSSIBLE CAUSES	USUAL THERAPY	RATIONALE	ADDITIONAL NURSING INTERVENTIONS
Perioperative MI, usually associated with perioperative ventricular failure or ventricular fibrillation. Diagnosed by new pathologic Q-waves and creatinine phosphokinase isoenzyme (CK-MB or CK-2) more than 40 units/liter.[17] This is the most common complication of myocardial revascularization. Incidence is 5% to 10%.[22]	Occlusion of new graft. Occlusion of stenosed artery that was not bypassed. Embolization of distal coronary artery from plaque loosened during surgery.	For usual therapy for MI, see Chapter 23. A balance must be achieved between rest and decreased activity to reduce myocardial oxygen needs and the mobilization required to prevent atelectasis and pneumonia postoperatively.	Decreases ischemia and promotes myocardial healing. Reduces postoperative atelectasis and prevents pneumonia.	Determine appropriate activity level to: a. Reduce myocardial ischemia b. Prevent postoperative pulmonary complications. The patient and family will have increased emotional distress and will require increased support and understanding. See Nursing Care Plan for MI patient (Chap. 23).
Low cardiac output syndrome[29]	Decreased contractility or failure of ventricle.	If fluid replacement is adequate, i.e., filling pressures are high, give positive inotropic or vasoactive drugs. If pharmacologic intervention is not effective use intra-aortic balloon pump assistance (IABP).	Altering preload and afterload increases cardiac output. Increases contractility of the ventricles. Using intra-aortic balloon pump assistance increases cardiac output and increases myocardial perfusion and decreases afterload.	Clearly monitor affects of therapy and make adjustments in drug infusions as parameters indicate need. Monitor diastolic augmentation, presystolic pressures, and inflation-deflation timing of IABP. IABP assistance requires frequent monitoring of all the usual postoperative parameters. In addition: a. Observe insertion site for edema, hemorrhage, or catheter kinking. b. Monitor color, temperature, and pulses in leg of insertion. c. Keep leg in which IABP catheter is inserted straight immobilized.
Cardiac tamponade. Symptoms which are frequently seen with tamponade include: Decreasing arterial pressure and increasing filling pressures Pulsus paradoxus, greater than 10 mm Hg Narrow or decreased pulse pressure Sudden decrease or cessation of chest tube drainage Cyanosis of head and neck Enlarged cardiac and mediastinal silhouette on x-ray film Persistent unexplained apprehension and restlessness	Occluded chest tube that drains mediastinum Hemorrhage	Vigorous milking or irrigation to open mediastinal drainage Pericardiocentesis Surgical drainage of pericardial sac and ligation of bleeders	Reduces the external pressure on the heart. Stops the hemorrhage.	Immediate notification of surgeons. The time between occurrence of symptoms and the patient's progressing to cardiac arrest is very short (Chap. 29).

TABLE 24-1 MYOCARDIAL REVASCULARIZATION—IMMEDIATE POSTOPERATIVE PROBLEMS (cont.)

Respiratory

Parameters monitored: Respiratory rate, chest excursions, breath sounds, arterial blood gases, amount and quality of sputum, and vital capacity and inspiratory effort (while intubated)

Common postoperative problems:

PROBLEM	POSSIBLE CAUSES	USUAL THERAPY	RATIONALE	ADDITIONAL NURSING INTERVENTIONS
Decreased respiration	Common side effect of anesthesia and surgery in the thorax	Intubation with mechanical ventilation for 6 to 48 hours after surgery	Reexpands lungs. Reverses atelectasis. Compensates for reduced respiratory muscle effort.	
		Adjustment of F_iO_2, rate, and tidal volume according to assessed need for individual		
		Frequent monitoring of arterial blood gases		
		Intermittent hyperinflation and endotracheal suctioning	Compensates for decreased mechanisms of secretion evacuation.	
		Chest tube drainage, usually with 15 to 25 cm of water suction	Evacuates air and drainage from thorax. Reexpands lungs and normalizes negative intraplural pressure.	Intermittently milk or strip chest tubes to keep them patent.
		Patient weaned from mechanical ventilation when: a. Alert enough to cooperate with coughing b. Demonstrates good respiratory parameters, *i.e.,* arterial blood gases, vital capacity, inspiratory effort		
		Weaning may be done by: a. A trial of independent breathing on T-piece prior to extubation b. A trial of intermittent mechanical ventilation (IMV) c. Immediate extubation		Explain patient's role in weaning.
		Respiratory care after termination of mechanical ventilation and extubation includes:		Define extubation as "progress" to patient and family.
		a. Humidified oxygen per mask	Loosens secretions and stimulates cough.	
		b. Frequent deep breathing and coughing		
		c. Use of incentive spirometer or intermittent positive pressure breathing (IPPB) every 1 to 3 hours	Lessens atelectasis, stimulates cough.	Carefully titrate pain medication and sedation so that patient does not restrict coughing and deep breathing as a result of splinting.
		d. Increased mobility, *i.e.,* frequent turning, sitting on the side of bed or up in chair	Enhances deep breathing and mobilization of secretions.	See that his respiratory efforts are not depressed by over-medication.

TABLE 24-1   MYOCARDIAL REVASCULARIZATION—IMMEDIATE POSTOPERATIVE PROBLEMS (cont.)

Potential Complications:

COMPLICATION	POSSIBLE CAUSES	USUAL THERAPY	RATIONALE	ADDITIONAL NURSING INTERVENTIONS
Pulmonary emboli. Sudden onset of dyspnea or unexplained chest pain.	Peripheral thrombophlebitis. Segment of cardiac mural thrombus.	Prevent peripheral thrombus formation by: a. Passive or active foot and ankle exercises during bed rest b. Antiembolic stockings c. Early ambulation Depending on the severity of respiratory compromise, the patient may need increased respiratory support, i.e., increased F_iO_2, mechanical ventilation. Heparinization	Review thromboembolic complications—Chapter 28.	Assess patient for: Cyanosis Hemoptysis Pleural friction rub Cardiac arrhythmias Significant decrease in P_aO_2 Bronchospasm Hypotension Apprehension Calf tenderness or swelling[29] Monitor heparinized patient closely for signs of hemorrhage, i.e., increased chest tube drainage, wound drainage, or vital sign changes.
Respiratory failure	Underlying respiratory disorder, i.e., chronic obstructive disease, asthma, chronic bronchitis Multiple pulmonary emboli Viral or bacterial respiratory infection	Mechanical ventilation with positive end expiratory pressure (PEEP) Frequent hyperinflation and suctioning Medical therapy as needed for bronchospasm or underlying infections Respirator volumes, pressures, and F_iO_2 adjusted by monitoring arterial blood gases frequently	Improvement of oxygenation without prolonging the use of high F_iO_2 Correct treatment for underlying precipitating cause	Sedate patient as needed for tolerance of prolonged intubation and mechanical ventilation. Emotionally support patient and family: a. Provide consistent nursing care. b. Keep progress reports from team members consistent.

Renal

Parameters monitored: Urine output (hourly at first); urine specific gravity, presence of glucose, ketones, protein, and blood (occasionally tested) in urine; serum potassium, creatinine, and blood urea nitrogen (BUN) are checked daily.

Common postoperative problems:

PROBLEM	POSSIBLE CAUSES	USUAL THERAPY	RATIONALE	ADDITIONAL NURSING INTERVENTIONS
Low urine output	Volume depletion Low cardiac output	Patient is hydrated, i.e., with lactated Ringer's solution, dextrose and water, saline solution, plasma, or blood (if hematocrit low) If patient hydrated, but has low cardiac output, inotropic or vasoactive drugs are given. Diuretic therapy	Corrects fluid balance. Urinary output should be maintained at a minimum of 25 ml per hour to prevent tubular damage.[29] Inotropes and vasoactive drugs can improve cardiac output. Urine output decreases with decreased cardiac output or failure.	Observe aseptic care of urinary catheter to prevent infection. Remove catheter when careful urine measurements are no longer needed and patient is able to void.
Increased urine output	Improved cardiac perfusion and output	Fluid balance monitored via systemic and filling pressures Specific gravity checked to verify that patient is not in high output renal failure		

TABLE 24-1 MYOCARDIAL REVASCULARIZATION—IMMEDIATE POSTOPERATIVE PROBLEMS (cont.)

Potential Complications:

COMPLICATION	POSSIBLE CAUSES	USUAL THERAPY	RATIONALE	ADDITIONAL NURSING INTERVENTIONS
Renal failure	Underlying renal disease Perioperative hypotensive crisis	Diuretic therapy Low dose dopamine infusion Peritoneal dialysis or hemodialysis	Review diuretics (Chap. 37) Increase of renal perfusion Prescribed treatment for acute renal failure and possible prevention of chronic failure	Monitor serum potassium and fluid balance closely. Restrict fluid intake. Provide comfort measures, *i.e.,* frequent mouth care. Emotionally support patient and family.

Nervous

Parameters monitored: Level of consciousness, orientation, movement of extremities.

Possible postoperative problems:

PROBLEM	POSSIBLE CAUSES	USUAL THERAPY	RATIONALE	ADDITIONAL NURSING INTERVENTIONS
Decreased level of consciousness (The patient should respond to his name within 1 to 2 hours postoperatively.)	Anesthesia	Frequent assessment of vital signs and neurologic parameters	Allows for early detection of adverse reaction to anesthesia	Protect patient from harm until awake and alert.

Potential Complications:

COMPLICATION	POSSIBLE CAUSE	USUAL THERAPY	RATIONALE	NURSING INTERVENTIONS
Confusion	Perioperative hypotensive crises in a patient with cerebral atherosclerosis Unresolved high preoperative anxiety Alcohol or drug withdrawal Anoxia Prolonged acute care due to postoperative complications can result in confusion, because of a combination of sleep deprivation, abnormal sensory overload, and deprivation of normal sensory input (Chap. 31).	Provision for patient safety. Control of environment: a. Provide undisturbed rest periods. b. Limit people and noise. c. Increase the number of familiar persons and things in environment, *i.e.,* family visiting, pictures, other personal items. d. Provide radio or television for diversion. e. Provide a schedule. f. Have consistency in personnel caring for patient. Frequent reorientation of the patient Sedation as needed to provide sleep Medication for drug withdrawal.	Normalizing the environment lessens fears and increases orientation.	Explain possible causes and outcome of the confusion to family. They in turn can support the patient.
Cerebrovascular accident (CVA)	Thrombus at site of aortosaphenous anastomosis Mural thrombus dislodged by manipulation of the heart Cholesterol emboli dislodged by manipulation of the ascending aorta Microemboli of air, fat, or platelet aggregates shifted from extracorporeal circulation.[17] An unusual accident associated with extracorporeal circulation can cause macroscopic air emboli.	More specific neurologic assessment, *i.e.,* monitor pupillary response, extremity movement and strength, ability to swallow, communicate, and follow commands. Protection of patient from injury to affected extremities, *i.e.,* change position, maintain proper alignment, help patient to do range of motion exercise.	Identifies progression of incident Protects patient from complications of loss of function	Help patient and family cope with the mixed emotions of the perceived loss.

TABLE 24-1 MYOCARDIAL REVASCULARIZATION—IMMEDIATE POSTOPERATIVE PROBLEMS (cont.)

Other Problems

PROBLEM	POSSIBLE CAUSES	USUAL THERAPY	RATIONALE	NURSING INTERVENTIONS
Pain The patient frequently is more aware of pain with increased ambulation than he was in the immediate postoperative period.	Surgical incisions Prolonged immobilization on the operating room table Initial postoperative bed rest Drainage tubes, intravascular catheters, and endotracheal tube	Positioning Analgesics Quiet in the patient's environment	Position changes enhance muscle relaxation.	Assist patient in differentiating between incisional pain and anginal pain. Cautiously medicate patient if he is hypotensive, has neurologic impairment, or is being weaned from the ventilator. Medicate patient prior to periods of deep breathing and coughing or increased mobilization. Encourage patient to express feelings.
Heightened fear and anxiety	Intensive environment of critical care unit Unfamiliar treatments and procedures Physical discomfort and weakness Intubation and inability to talk	Suppression of noise and activity in the environment Reassurance, i.e., surgery is over, progress has begun Anticipation of patient needs Explanation and reexplanation of procedures Identification of examples of progress, i.e., extubation, discontinuation of lines and tubes, increased mobilization Encouragement of short visits from family Sedation of patient for rest and increased tolerance of endotracheal tube Increase mobilization of patient (as tolerated) Preparation of patient (and family) for his transfer to intermediate or general care unit	Reduces stimulation which may increase anxiety. Reassures patient his needs will be met while he is immobilized. Keeping patient informed of progress and what to anticipate increases his trust in the staff and reduces the anxiety caused by fear of the unknown. Family reassurance encourages patient relaxation. Reinforces to patient that he is improving. Transfer from the critical care unit is accompanied by increased anxiety for patient and family.[27]	Support patient's family: a. Explain appearance of patient prior to first visit. b. Provide opportunities away from the bedside for family to express concerns and ask questions. c. Encourage family to get adequate rest. d. Help them understand patient's emotional reactions.[13] Encourage them to visit and support patient. Help patient to anticipate changes in care on the intermediate or general care unit and explain the rationale for the changes.
Hypokalemia.	Postoperative metabolic acidosis with increased urine potassium loss [5] Diuresis Ionic shifts and diuresis due to extracorporeal circulation	Serum potassium monitored and supplemented as needed Potassium added in intravenous fluids		Anticipate need for taking more frequent serum potassium levels and for giving potassium supplements with diuresis.

Other Potential Complications:

COMPLICATION	POSSIBLE CAUSES	USUAL THERAPY	RATIONALE	NURSING INTERVENTIONS
Hemorrhage	Unligated vessel in surgical site. Inadequate reversal of heparinization from extracorporeal circulation	If operative site bleeding, patient is returned to surgery for ligation. Close monitoring of chest tube drainage and replacement of blood loss with blood products initially Blood pressure maintained with volume replacement Control of hypertension	 Maintains adequate cardiac output. Hypertension may increase intrathoracic bleeding.	Answer questions and further explain complications to family (and patient, if alert).

TABLE 24-1   MYOCARDIAL REVASCULARIZATION—IMMEDIATE POSTOPERATIVE PROBLEMS (cont.)
Potential Complications:

COMPLICATION	POSSIBLE CAUSES	USUAL THERAPY	RATIONALE	ADDITIONAL NURSING INTERVENTIONS
	Other coagulopathy	Coagulation screen checked, *i.e.*, platelet count, fibrinogen, fibrin degradation products, prothrombin time, partial thromboplastin time, thrombotest	Determines need for clotting factor replacement.	
		If coagulopathy, appropriate clotting factors replaced, *i.e.*, platelets, fresh frozen plasma, cryoprecipitate, vitamin K, protamine, fresh whole blood	Replacement of deficient clotting factor should control hemorrhage.	
Infection	Atelectasis Pulmonary infection Urinary tract infection Wound infection	Vigorous pulmonary therapy, *i.e.*, suctioning, coughing, deep breathing, and mobilization	Fever in the first one to four days postoperatively frequently is the result of atelectasis.	Assess patient's temperature every 2 to 4 hours. Aseptically care for urinary catheter. Care for wound to prevent wound infection:
		Prophylactic antibiotic therapy	Organism treated with effective antibiotic	a. Clean and aseptically re-dress wounds, daily and when dressing is soiled, until the wound is closed.
		Documented infections cultured and treated with antibiotics Mediastinal wound infection should be surgically drained to prevent sternal infection.[17]		b. After closure, clean wounds daily and leave open to air.

tion.[16] The donor heart is then sutured into place, the vessels are connected to the host vessels, and air is removed from all the cardiac chambers (Fig. 24-5). Two pacer wires are implanted in the donor right atrium prior to closure.[26]

Postoperative Care of Cardiac Transplantation Patients

Postoperative care of the cardiac transplant patient is similar to that of the revascularization patient, except that the patient receives immunosuppressive therapy and must be isolated to protect against infection. Infection and transplant rejection are the two major causes of death of the cardiac recipient.[25] Major emphasis in nursing care is placed on assessment and on reporting of signs of transplant rejection, infection, and complications of treatment or medications.[26]

Critical times that rejection is likely to occur are at 18 to 21 days and at 4 to 6 weeks postoperatively.[26] Signs that have been associated with early transplant rejection are

Demonstration of 20% decrease in QRS voltage on the electrocardiogram and the atrial lead

Presence of third or fourth heart sound

Occurrence of atrial arrhythmias

Evidence of rejection on histologic examination of cardiac biopsy[26]

Development of a technique for doing cardiac biopsies provides a means of detecting rejection at an early stage, evaluating the therapy given against rejection, and adjusting the amount of immunosuppressants given.[25]

The immunosuppressants used to prevent rejection are

Rabbit antihuman thrombocyte globulin (ATG) daily for 3 days and then every other day for 3 doses,

Prednisone (50 mg to 100 mg) in decreasing doses twice a day, and

Azathioprine (100 mg to 200 mg) daily according to peripheral platelet and white blood cell counts, or

Cyclosphosphamide (100 mg to 200 mg) daily if liver disease is present.[26]

The patient is carefully monitored for signs of infection. Amphotericin B solution is used as a gargle to prevent fungal infections in the mouth. Systemic amphotericin B is used to treat fungus infections.[26] Other complications of cardiac transplantation are reactions to ATG, gastrointestinal hemorrhage (due to steroids, thrombocytopenia, or heparinization), and personality changes (due to high doses of steroids).[25]

The cardiac recipient is in protective isolation in the critical care unit for 3 to 4 weeks.[26] The patient wears a sterile gown, mask, gloves, hat, and boots when out of the isolation room. He may walk in the hall a few days after surgery.[26] The isolation routines, the frequent interruptions and stimulation in the critical care unit and the steroid therapy all have an emotional impact on the patient. He may become depressed, withdrawn, compulsive, paranoid, or combative.[26] The nurse can anticipate and prevent these behaviors by controlling the environment, encouraging him to express feelings, keeping him informed, and giving the family support so that they can support the patient.

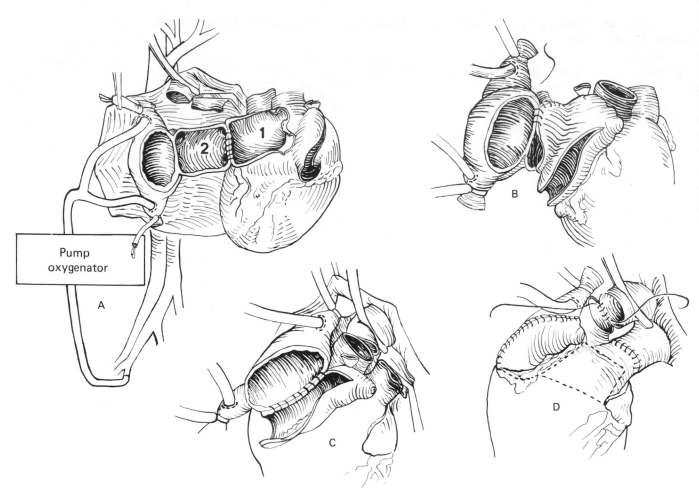

Fig. 24-5. **(A-1)** Cardiac transplantation begins by suturing the donor left atrium **(A-2)** to the posterior wall of the recipient left atrium. **(B)** The first step is completed with the suturing of the intra-atrial septum. **(C)** The right atrial walls are then sutured in place. **(D)** Transplantation is completed by anastamosis of the great vessels. (After Cooley DA, Norman JC: Techniques in Cardiac Surgery, p 220. Houston, Texas Medical Press, 1975)

Cardiac recipients require long-term prednisone therapy and frequent medical follow-up. The goals of patient and family teaching are to promote compliance with this long-term therapy and to promote independence with the care and assessment regimes. Prior to discharge, the cardiac recipient independently manages his medications and dietary and fluid restrictions, assumes responsibility for daily weight and temperature measurements, and learns the signs and symptoms of rejection, infection, and medication side effects. The patient is also encouraged to participate in daily exercise to promote reconditioning.[26]

PERCUTANEOUS TRANSLUMINAL CORONARY ANGIOPLASTY

Percutaneous transluminal coronary angioplasty is an invasive procedure which reduces coronary artery stenosis by applying pressure on the atheromatous plaque with a balloon-tipped catheter.[2] This procedure has had controlled clinical trial since first done by Dr. Andreas Gruntzig at the University of Zurich in 1977.[10]

The criteria used in selecting patients for this therapeutic approach for coronary artery disease include

Patient under 60 years of age

History of angina for less than 1 year

Proximal stenosis of an uncalcified major coronary artery in excess of 70%

Artery of good quality distal to the obstruction

Good ventricular function

Result of exercise thallium scan positive.[2]

The angioplasty procedure is done in the cardiac catheterization facility with surgery backup should emergency myocardial revascularization be required. The angioplasty takes less than 2 hours.

A special balloon-tipped catheter is advanced from the femoral artery into the aortic root and is then threaded through the affected coronary artery to the stenotic area. The balloon is filled by pump with contrast medium to a pressure of 3.5 to 5.0 atmospheres. The pump deflates the balloon after 5 to 15 seconds. The perpendicular force of the inflated balloon compresses the low-density content of a recent atheroma and redistributes it within the wall to reduce the obstruction.[2]

Most patients are hospitalized for only 48 hours and many return to work within a week after the procedure. The long-term effects of percutaneous transluminal coronary angioplasty are yet to be determined. Unanswered questions include

What are the long-term effects on plaque accumulation, resorption, or fibrosis?

What is the type and extent of endothelial damage to the coronary artery?

What is the consequent interaction between the endothelium and blood components?

Clinical trials are being done at centers in order to identify the risks, the indications and contraindications, and the long-term effects of the procedure.

CONCLUSION

Myocardial revascularization and cardiac transplantation are recognized modes of therapy for CAD. Surgical intervention neither reverses nor halts atherosclerotic disease. It has, however, contributed to a decrease in deaths from CAD. Coupled with dietary and exercise modifications, it may serve to reduce pain and return the patient to activity levels previously unattainable, and may aid the patient to achieve a better quality of life.

REFERENCES

1. Barnard CN: Heterotopic versus orthotopic heart transplantation. Transplant Proc 8:15–19, 1976
2. Bentivoglio LG: Bypassing the bypass with percutaneous transluminal coronary angioplasty. Am J Cardiol 43(4):866–867, 1979
3. Berg R Jr, Kendell RW, Duroisin GE et al: Acute myocardial infarction: A surgical emergency. J Thorac Cardiovasc Surg 70:432–439, 1975
4. Bolooki H, Vargas A: Myocardial revascularization after acute myocardial infarction. Arch Surg 111:1216–1224, 1976
4a. Brunner LS, Suddarth DS: Textbook of Medical–Surgical Nursing. Philadelphia, JB Lippincott, 1975
5. Calhoun PL, Bozorgi S: Postoperative care following coronary surgery. Heart Lung 3(6):912–915, 1974
5a. Cooley DA, Norman JC: Techniques in Cardiac Surgery. Houston, Texas Medical Press, 1975
6. Directions in Cardiovascular Medicine 10. Mechanical Circulatory Assistance. Somerville, Hoechst-Roussel Pharmaceuticals, 1974
7. Dong E, Griepp RB, Stinson EB, et al: Clinical transplantation of the heart. Ann Surg 176:503–508, 1972
8. Fisk RL, Brooks CH, Callaghan JC et al: Experience with the radial artery graft for coronary artery bypass. Ann Thorac Surg 21(6):513–518, 1976
9. Futral JE: Postoperative management and complications of coronary artery bypass surgery. Heart Lung 6(3):477–485, 1977
10. Gruntzig A, Myler R, Stertzer S: Percutaneous transluminal coronary angioplasty (PTCA)—Present state of the art. Circulation (abstr) II:264, 1979
11. Jahnke EJ, Love JW: Bypass of the right and circumflex arteries with the internal mammary artery. J Thorac Cardiovasc Surg 71:58–61, 1976
12. Janis IL: Psychological Stress. New York, John Wiley & Sons, 1958
13. Jillings CR: Phases of recovery from open-heart surgery. Heart Lung 7(5):987–994, 1978
14. King OM: Acquired heart disease and trauma of the heart and great vessels. In King OM (ed): Care of the Cardiac Surgical Patient, pp 127–152. St. Louis, CV Mosby, 1975
15. Kirkland JW, Kouchoukos NT, Blackstone EH et al: Research related to surgical treatment of coronary artery disease. Circulation 60(7):1613–1618, 1979
16. Lower RR, Szentpetery S, Thomas FT et al: Clinical observations on cardiac transplantation. Transplant Proc 8:9–13, 1976
17. Miller DW Jr: The Practice of Coronary Artery Bypass Surgery. New York, Plenum Medical Book Co, 1977
17a. Miller DW Jr: Bypass Surgery for Coronary Heart Disease. Seattle, Univ. Washington School of Medicine, 1978
18. Miller DW Jr, Hessel EA II, Winterscheid LC et al: Current practice of coronary artery bypass surgery—Results of a national survey. J Thorac Cardiovasc Surg 73:75–82, 1977
19. Mills NL, Oschner JL: Experience with atrial pacemaker wires implanted during cardiac operations. J Thorac Cardiovasc Surg 66(6):878–886, 1973
20. Mulder DG: Techniques of cardioplegia. J Thorac Cardiovasc Surg 77(2):325–326, 1979
20a. National Hospital Discharge Survey. Washington DC, Division of Health Resources Utilization, National Center for Health Statistics, August, 1980 (unpublished data)
21. Niarchos AP, Roberts AJ, Case DB et al: Hemodynamic characteristics of hypertension after CABG surgery and effects of the converting enzyme inhibitor. Am J Cardiol 43(3): 586–593, 1979
22. Oberman A, Kouchoukos NT, Makar YN et al: Perioperative myocardial infarction after coronary bypass surgery: Four years experience 1971–1974. Am J Cardiol (abstr) 37:160, 1976
23. Phillips SJ, Kongtahworn C, Zeff RH et al: Emergency coronary artery revascularization: A possible therapy for acute myocardial infarction. Circulation 60(2):241–249, 1979
24. Roe BB, Hutchinson JC, Fishman NH et al: Myocardial protection with cold, ischemic, potassium-induced cardioplegia. J Thorac Cardiovasc Surg 73(5):366–374, 1977
25. Russell PS, Cosimi AB: Transplantation. N Engl J Med 301(9):470–479, 1979
26. Sandiford DM: Cardiac transplantation: Eight years's experience. Heart Lung 5(4):566–570, 1976
27. Scalzi C: Nursing management of the behavioral responses following acute myocardial infarction. Heart Lung 2(1):64–69, 1973
28. Tarkaro T, Hultgren HH, Detre KM: VA cooperative study of coronary arterial surgery: Left main disease. Circulation 52(II):563, 1975
29. Thorpe CJ: A nursing care plan—The adult cardiac surgery patient. Heart Lung 8(4):690–698, 1979
30. Tyras DH, Stothert JC, Kaiser GC et al: Supraventricular tachyarrhythmias after myocardial revascularization: A randomized trial of prophylactic digitalization. J Thorac Cardiovasc Surg 77(2):310–314, 1979
31. University Hospital Protocol: Treatment of ventricular electrical instability in adult cardiac surgery patients. University of Washington, Seattle, Spring, 1980

ADDITIONAL READING

Adlkofer Sister RM, Powaser MM: The effect of endotracheal suctioning on arterial blood gases in patients after cardiac surgery. Heart Lung 7(6):1011–1014, 1978
Aspinall MJ: Nursing the Open Heart Surgery Patient. New York, McGraw-Hill, 1973
Barbarowicz P: A comparison of in-hospital education approaches for coronary bypass patients. Heart Lung 9(1):127–133, 1980

Braunwald E: Coronary–artery surgery at the crossroads. N Engl J Med 297:661–663, 1977

Brener ER: Surgery for coronary artery disease. Am J Nurs 72:469–473, 1972

DeBakey ME, Lawrie GM: Aortocoronary–artery bypass: Assessment after 13 years. JAMA 239:837–839, 1978

Effler DB: Myocardial revascularization: A 14-year overview of the Cleveland clinic experience. JAMA 235:828–851, 1976

Gensini GG: Coronary arteriography: Role in myocardial revascularization. Postgrad Med 63:121–138, 1978

Hastillo A, Hess ML, Lower RR: Cardiac transplantation: expectations and limitations. Mod Concepts Cardiovasc Dis. 50(3):13–18, 1981

Johnston BL, Cantwell JD, Watt EW et al: Sexual activity in exercising patients after myocardial infarction and revascularization. Heart Lung 7(6):1026–1031, 1978

Kouchoukos NT, Kirklin JW: Surgical procedures used in the treatment of coronary atherosclerotic heart disease. In Hurst JW (ed): The Heart, pp 1241–1266. New York, McGraw-Hill, 1978

Kurlo-Rose AT: Circulatory Assist: Intra-Aortic Balloon Pumping-Unit 6, in Series 2, Surgical Aspects of Cardiovascular Disease— Nursing Intervention. Continuing Education in Cardiovascular Nursing. New York, Appleton-Century-Croft, 1981

Livelli FD, Johnson RA, McEnany MT et al: Unexplained in-hospital fever following cardiac surgery. Circulation 57(5):968–975, 1978

McIntosh HD, Garcia JA: The first decade of aortocoronary bypass grafting, 1967–1977. Circulation 57:405–431, 1978

Miller P, Shada EA: Preoperative information and recovery of open-heart surgery patients. Heart Lung 7:486–893, 1978

Shinn, JA: Cardiac Transplantation and the Artificial Heart-Unit 7, in Series 2, Surgical Aspects of Cardiovascular Disease—Nursing Intervention. Continuing Education in Cardiovascular Nursing. New York, Appleton-Century-Croft, 1981.

Stack, MC: Coronary Artery Bypass Surgery-Unit 5, in Series 2, Surgical Aspects of Cardiovascular Disease—Nursing Intervention. Continuing Education in Cardiovascular Nursing. New York, Appleton-Century-Croft, 1980.

Tirrell BE, Hart LK: The relationship of health beliefs and knowledge to exercise compliance in patients after coronary bypass. Heart Lung 9(3):487–493, 1980

Whitman G: Intra-aortic balloon pumping and cardiac mechanics: A programmed lesson. Heart Lung 7(6):1034–1050, 1978

25

Treatment of the Patient with Coronary Artery Disease—Medical Versus Surgical

KATHLEEN A. KOMINSKI, R.N., M.N.

and

THOMAS A. PRESTON, M.D.

The coronary atherosclerotic obstructive lesion, with its throttling effect on coronary pressure and flow, is the single most important cause of a myocardial perfusion deficit, which results in myocardial ischemia, injury, or necrosis. By American Heart Association estimates, approximately four million people in this country, or about 20 per 1,000, have had a history of myocardial infarction (MI), angina pectoris, or both, resulting from coronary artery disease (CAD). This is an alarming situation, despite the fact that since the advent of cardiac care units in the early 1960s, the mortality rates from MI were cut by 30%.[22] However, the statistics still show that some 350,000 people, or four persons out of seven (50% to 60%), die suddenly outside of the hospital, usually of cardiac arrhythmias.[12,22] The development of angina pectoris not only represents a precursor of acute MI, but also, because of the metabolic and electrophysiologic pathology involved, portends the possibility of sudden death.[16]

The clinical manifestations of angina pectoris have been known since the late 18th century; it has been only in the last 3 decades, however, that major strides have been made in understanding the pathophysiology of CAD and its management. The current medical regimen (see Chap. 22) used in the treatment of angina pectoris includes modification of life style, behavior modification, treatment of associated diseases, administration of various nitrite compounds and a beta adrenergic blocking agent, and physical conditioning programs.[50,51,59,60]

Previous surgical attempts to improve coronary flow in ischemic states have resulted in many original ideas and numerous disappointments. Although little was gained directly in the treatment of atherosclerosis by sympathectomy, epicardectomy, epicardial abrasion, and internal mammary ligation, the involvement of the surgeon stimulated interest and provided an additional approach in management. With the emergence of aortocoronary bypass graft surgery (CBGS) more than a decade ago, a new era of revascularization surgery was launched. It is no surprise that this surgery has grown to such acclaim and widespread usage. Unlike other revascularization procedures of the past it was the first to make sense physiologically; that is, it reestablished myocardial blood flow by bypassing the atherosclerotic arteries. Also, it provided dramatic symptomatic and objective relief from angina. However, although popular, coronary bypass has not been universally accepted. Reasons for controversy include repeated disappointment with many once highly praised myocardial revascularization procedures, the small number of controlled studies, uncertainty about the natural history of clinical CAD, and lack of evidence that MI is prevented or that life is prolonged. Furthermore, health care planners and third party payers who are picking up increasingly larger tabs for individual patient care foresee a major threat to other health care programs if the number of revascularization operations increases at the present rate. With these facts in mind, it would seem expedient that more critical evaluation be conducted on the results of CBGS. The appropriateness of this procedure has yet to be clearly defined, despite the widespread use and tremendous cost.

GOALS OF THERAPY IN ISCHEMIC HEART DISEASE

The objectives of therapy in ischemic heart disease include relief of symptoms, improved quality of life, improved ventricular function, prevention of MI, and increased life expectancy.

Symptomatic Improvement

There is general agreement about the symptomatic relief of angina and improved quality of life following CBGS, with at least 90% of patients achieving initial freedom from symptoms and 70% to 80% obtaining alleviation of symptoms.[13,25,37,40] This compares with improvement in 30% to 50% of similar patients treated medically.[13,34] Relief of symptoms has been accompanied by a drastic reduction in the use of antianginal medications (nitrites, beta blockers) and improved performance on exercise testing. However, the interpretation of lessened angina and duration of its effect after surgery is beset with many difficulties. The mechanism whereby symptoms are relieved is not always that of improving blood flow to an ischemic segment. Other possibilities include the nonspecific effect of surgery which may include a placebo effect, perioperative infarction of a previously ischemic portion of the myocardium, interruption of perivascular nerves, and natural remission of symptoms.[36,40]

Increased Myocardial Bloodflow. Unlike medical therapy which aims at alleviating the incidence of anginal attacks by reducing myocardial oxygen demands, the theory behind coronary bypass is to revascularize, that is, to reestablish or improve blood flow to an ischemic myocardium. From vein graft blood flow measurements at the time of operation, angiographic documentation of graft patency, the higher pressure-rate product (PRP), and results of the postsurgery exercise tolerance test (ETT), objective evidence has reasonably been secured to support this theory of improved blood flow. The majority of reports of relief of angina seems to substantiate these objective findings. However, what remains uncertain is the duration of the direct results of the surgery. It is becoming increasingly clear that the initial gratifying results do not persist in all patients and that there is a tendency for the level of clinical improvement following coronary bypass to be related to the length of time after surgery.

For example, in a study by Harrison of 350 patients, 85% initially obtained total or marked relief of symptoms. However, after a mean of 30 months after surgery (range 6 to 72 months), though 13% of patients showed further clinical improvement, 47% were unchanged and 40% deteriorated further with respect to chest pain. The investigators concluded that the initial symptomatic benefits may not be maintained in late follow-up studies because of progression of underlying vascular disease.[21] Kloster reported a highly significant difference ($p < 0.01$) in the functional classification between medical and surgical treatment groups 6 months after surgery, but by 2 years there was no longer a significant difference between the two groups.[28] It is noteworthy in this connection to point out that the control

medical groups in various randomized studies[3,28,34] all improved symptomatically and functionally during the course of the study. Thus it appears that with optimal medical therapy, improved quality of life can be attained without subjecting patients to surgical treatment. Sampson and Hyatt report that of 150 successive patients only 4.7% could be considered refractory to medical management.[52]

Improved objective results obtained postoperatively on ETT have been attributed to the extent of graft patency and to the completeness of revascularization: that is, the number of diseased vessels bypassed. Estimates of 60% to 70% improvement in ETT results have been reported, with disappearance of chest pain or ST-segment depression, or both.[31] It is not exactly clear what limits treadmill exercise time in patients with CAD. Chest pain, fatigue, or dyspnea associated with failure to increase heart rate and cardiac output, and acute left ventricular pump dysfunction all play a role.[8] The improvement in exercise tolerance, then, is not clearly dissociated from the relief of symptoms, because it may often be the chest pain that limits exercise tolerance.

The reported correlation between multistage ETT and cinecoronary arteriograms is not perfect, but it is considered relatively good, even though the techniques are examining different facets of the problem of myocardial ischemia; the exercise test measures physiologic function and the coronary arteriogram delineates coronary artery anatomy. Discrepancies have been found between ETT results and angiographic data. For instance, to assess the status of patients with all grafts occluded after CBGS, Block and several associates examined the clinical, angiographic, and exercise-testing data of 23 patients who had no functional grafts at follow-up angiography.[6] Postoperatively, 12 of 23 patients (52%) had related improvement of at least one functional class, and 5 were asymptomatic. Analysis of individual data revealed significant ($p < 0.05$) postoperative improvement in exercise capacity in 13 patients (57%), 5 of whom had had an ischemic ST-segment response preoperatively and no longer had this response postoperatively. Neither preoperative ejection fraction, number of vessels diseased, number of grafts attempted, interval to follow-up study, deterioration in the native coronary circulation, appearance of collateral circulation, control of risk factors, nor medical therapy appeared to separate the patients who did and did not show improvement. However, 11 of these 23 patients (48%) demonstrated angiographic or clinical evidence, or both, of interim myocardial infarction. Postoperatively, this group manifested a mean increase in exercise duration, maximal PRP and heart rate (HR).[6]

Thus it appears that improvement after unsuccessful CBGS is not unknown, and that in some, but not all cases, the improvement may be related to myocardial infarction. Even complete graft patency does not ensure total symptomatic relief. A number of authors have found a discrepancy between the patient's assessment of clinical improvement and the results of exercise testing. Lapin and associates[31] studied 46 patients 3 to 22 months after surgery and reported that 39 of them improved as determined by history, but only 27 patients (59%) showed improved exercise capacity as measured by functional aerobic impairment (the percentage of deviation from expected maximum oxygen consumption[89] (Chap.18). Guiney and co-workers studied 40 patients for

3 to 8 months after a CBGS; 37 improved as determined by history, but only 32 showed improvement in exercise capacity (maximal oxygen consumption).[17] It has been suggested by Helton and others[24] who also found discrepancies between ETT and angiographic data that

1. Demonstration of a patent graft by angiographic techniques is a qualitative assessment of graft patency and as such may bear no relation to quantitative flow in vivo.

2. Neovascularization of the coronary macrocirculation may not uniformly be reflected in ischemic areas owing to obstructions in the microcirculation of the affected areas that are not apparent on preoperative angiograms.

3. Frank infarction of the preoperatively borderline ischemic myocardium may frequently occur during surgery, resulting in an unidentifiable postoperative scar that does not generate ischemic pain and electrocardiogram changes, and as such may be responsible for the abolition of preoperative ischemic changes and pain.[24]

The ultimate fate of venous grafts used in the aortocoronary bypass remains to be determined. Initial optimism notwithstanding, it is well documented that pathologic changes occur in these aortocoronary vein grafts. Grafts obtained at autopsy 7 to 9½ months after operation have been found to develop two distinctive lesions: thrombosis and associated severe distal coronary artery obstruction; and intimal fibrous proliferation with varying degrees of luminal narrowing.[10,15] It has also been noted that atherosclerotic plaques, which are almost never found in the vein when it is in its natural position in the leg, eventually begin to develop when the vein is transplanted into the arterial circulation.[19] This may be because of damage to the endothelial lining caused by the higher arterial blood pressure, or by handling of the vessel during excision and grafting.[19] Comparison figures from one medical center to another differ, but in general it appears that when the veins are examined angiographically in the first month after operation, approximately 70% to 80% are patent, indicating that 20% to 30% become occluded soon after surgery. With longer intervals after operation, as, for example, 6 to 12 months, patency rates of between 70% to 80% still seem to be common. This appears to indicate that the fibrous proliferative process is not apparent during the first year and only produces a total occlusion some time later.

Postoperative evaluation must not be limited to determination of the patency of the bypass. The intrinsic or native circulation of the heart must also be reexamined at the time of postoperative study. The operative procedure does nothing to change the basic atherosclerotic process that afflicts the patient's intrinsic coronary circulation. Several groups that have studied patients after the construction of the vein bypass have been able to demonstrate new obstructive lesions in previously patent segments of the native coronary circulation.[4,15,26,55] In addition several investigators have observed acceleration of the occlusive atherosclerotic process in the native circulation either proximal or distal to the graft.[1,2,4] Intracoronary collaterals have also been observed more frequently to disappear when associated with arteries receiving flow from patent grafts and to persist when the graft is occluded.[38] These observations become important now that it has become common practice to replace arteries

not yet 50% occluded. There are various opinions on the significance or insignificance of progression of the disease in the native circulation. Maurer and associates[35] found that new total occlusions, new obstructive lesions, and progression of preexisting lesions were five times more frequent in grafted than in nongrafted arteries with comparable initial disease.[35] New and progressive lesions were encountered with the same frequency in arteries with patent as with occluded grafts. Progression of proximal occlusion of the native vessel (with either patent or occluded grafts) can have a deleterious effect on myocardial function, including the occurrence of MI with consequent deterioration of left ventricular function.[2,9]

Other Possibilities for Symptomatic Improvement. The incidence of perioperative MI (the period between the operation and 1 month after) with the diagnosis supported by the development of Q waves is 5% to 10%.[13,40] The incidence is even greater when enzymes and radionuclide imaging are used to substantiate the diagnosis.[37] Implications of perioperative MI will be discussed under the section concerning the effect of CBGS in the prevention of MI.

Other mechanisms of symptomatic relief of angina and improved exercise capacity have been attributed to cardiac denervation and the indirect placebo effect of the surgery.[36,40,41,56] Nerve pathways from the heart to the nerve roots are not clearly defined. They traverse a wide pathway and may be transsected during surgery thus abolishing the pain, but without changing the coronary blood flow. The idea of a placebo effect accompanying CBGS cannot be dismissed as a possible cause or as an additive component in the symptomatic relief after bypass surgery. All the necessary attributes are inherent and promoted for such an effect to occur; for example, a distressed patient offered by the physician a promise of relief from angina and possibly an extension of life. Belief is sincere on the part of the patient and the physician that the specific effect of the surgery, relief of symptoms, will occur. "Emotional reaction to the angina sensation is decreased or modified in a therapeutically positive manner, resulting in subjective improvement of symptoms."[47] One of the authors has made this allegation in a study evaluating relief of symptoms in 40 patients following CBGS.[29] When questioned as to the presence of chest pain after surgery, 9 of 31 patients (29%) reported the appearance of a different type of chest pain. However, when further questioned, they often described characteristics of the pain (location, type, precipitating factors) that were identical or similar to chest pain that occured before the surgery. A more frequently reported factor limiting activity after surgery was shortness of breath in 16 of 30 patients (53%), suggesting that a substitution of symptomology should be watched for when evaluating relief of symptoms and improved functional capacity.

Prevention of Myocardial Infarction

There is no evidence that CBGS prevents MI. The incidence of perioperative infarction diagnosed by electrocardiogram (ECG) in 5% to 10% of patients has been reported.[13,40] The magnitude of injury to the myocardium remains the most illusive aspect of CBGS. For instance, disappearance of a Q wave present before surgery may result from the development of a new infarction, electrically opposite to the previous one, with a resulting cancellation of the opposing electrical forces, rather than from an improved coronary blood flow.[36] The ECG remains the best tool for detecting gross infarction, but clearly it does not record lesser degrees of injury. Chemical measurements have shown not only that a patient may survive the operation despite extensive myocardial injury, but also that the injury may not even be clinically recognizable. Therefore injury may not be detected unless selective enzyme measurements are done or a cardiac catheterization is performed some months later.

There is some question concerning the significance of perioperative infarction on the long-term prognosis of the patient. Some investigators imply that surgically induced infarctions are reasonably well tolerated.[14,32] This may not be so, since mortality figures of 12% to 25% for those who have sustained perioperative infarction have been reported to occur within the first year after surgery, a mortality rate comparable to that of patients with spontaneous MI who reach the CCU.[13,26,43,46] In a follow-up study of vein grafts, patients with evidence of perioperative MI had the highest incidence of early and late death. Additionally, they had clinical evidence of myocardial damage and reinfarction at the time of evaluation 1 year after bypass surgery. Thus it appears that although some patients may benefit, in terms of relief of angina, by postoperative infarction, the occurrence of an infarction has a "definitely adverse effect on the long-term functional results and longevity."[44]

The data on the occurrence and prognosis of late infarction (more than 1 year after CBGS) have not been widely reported and remain inconclusive at the present time. The incidence of late MI in a mean follow-up time of 18 months to 3 years has been reported as 6% to 14% (average, 5% per year).[5,11,28,54,57] This closely resembles the incidence of spontaneous MI (approximately 5% to 7% per year) in patients with angina.[27]

Improved Ventricular Function

If myocardial function is limited by ischemia and if CBGS reduces ischemia, then improved left-ventricular perfusion should be one of the benefits of the procedure. However, improvement in symptoms and exercise tolerance after CBGS is far easier to demonstrate than is improvement in ventricular function. There have been reports of patients who have shown dramatic improvement of ventricular function as evidenced by improved hemodynamics, an increase in ejection fraction, decrease in left-ventricular diastolic pressure, and improved contractility as seen cineangiographically.[7,61] However, this is by no means universal, and certainly does not approach the 80% frequency of symptomatic improvement reported by patients.

Measurements of ventricular function promise information about left-ventricular pumping function or systolic fiber shortening. In patients with CAD, an enlarged end-diastolic volume is as serious a prognostic sign as is a low ejection fraction. Left ventricular end-diastolic pressure related to diastolic volume provides information about left-ventricular compliance, which is often reduced in patients with CAD. Segments of the left ventricular wall may contract weakly (hypokinesis) or not at all (akinesis), or may even expand during systole (dyskinesis) (Chap. 19). It is of interest that even though one or more segments of the left ventricular wall contract abnormally, the overall ejection fraction may be normal because other normal segments are compensating for poorly contracting segments. The left ventricle can continue to function at rest with the loss of 30% to 40% of its muscle mass. It is not surprising, then, that resting ventricular function is usually not affected by bypass surgery. In a composite of 40 patients, Hammermeister and others found no marked changes after CBGS in resting measurements of mean ejection fraction or end-diastolic volume. Segmental left-ventricular contraction had improved in 6 (15%), was unchanged in 25 (63%), and was worse in 9 (22%).[20] Ross concluded that bypass surgery improves resting ventricular function in 20%, makes it worse in 20%, and results in no change in 60%.[51]

Since many patients with chronic angina have normal resting ventricular function before surgery, bypass grafts cannot be expected to improve on it. An equally large number of patients have segments of previously infarcted myocardium replaced by scar tissue, which will never regain contractility by increased blood flow through bypass grafts. Poor ventricular function is a contraindication to surgery because it is associated with a consistently high surgical mortality, and the overall results of surgery are questionable. There are patients who have improved resting ventricular function after surgery. These patients have myocardial ischemia that has not progressed to infarction and subsequent hypokinetic wall motion.[7,61] Others suggest that if ventricular function improves with nitroglycerin, the dysfunction is probably due to ischemia and can be improved by surgery.[23] Most authors have concluded that while a small number of patients may experience improved ventricular function after bypass surgery, the frequency with which improvement occurs does not at this time justify recommending the operation for the purpose of improving ventricular function.

Increased Life Expectancy

Does surgical treatment by means of coronary bypass grafting improve the survival of patients with angina pectoris? An answer to this vital and intriguing question must be based on knowledge of the natural history of such patients, which is, unfortunately, rarely available. The two major determinants of a patient's prognosis are the severity of CAD and the quality of his ventricular function. Available information on severity of CAD and chances of survival without surgical treatment can be summarized as follows: the mortality rate for two- or three-vessel disease is 10% in 1 year, or about 50% in 5 years; for single-vessel disease it is probably no more than 2% a year, or less than 10% in 5 years.[27,42]

To determine the role of CBGS in the treatment of CAD, surgical therapy has been compared with medical therapy.[18] Until recently, retrospective or matched comparisons of medically and surgically treated patients have been used. These comparisons are not entirely valid. Although between 250,000 and 300,000 patients in the United States received a bypass graft operation by the summer of 1977, only 1,248 patients were included in controlled studies in which random selection placed them in a "surgery" or "no surgery" group.[36] This random selection used for a large number of reports resulted in the comparison of patients who underwent surgery with patients who were treated medically because they were rejected as surgical candidates, or declined surgery. Many reports also compared surgical results with natural history studies initiated in the mid-1960s, when improved therapy and risk factor reduction programs had recently been added to the medical therapeutic profile. Indeed, since the initiation of improved medical therapeutics, there has been evidence that a gratifying change is occurring in the natural history of coronary heart disease in this country. Data supporting this observation can be found in such reports as that given by the Metropolitan Life Insurance Company, which reported a 19% reduction between 1969 and 1974 in the incidence of death from heart disease in males.[49] In 1975 the Bureau of Census in the Center for National Statistics reported that the death rate from coronary heart disease declined to 2.9% per thousand population for that year alone.[58]

An accurate comparison of survival following medical or surgical treatment obviously requires that treatment be applied to comparable patients in whom favorable and unfavorable prognostic factors (severity of arterial disease, state of ventricular function) are equally distributed or, at least, are readily apparent. The prospective, randomized clinical trial is the technique most likely to produce parity in treatment groups and to yield a convincing comparison of results. Until a recent Veterans Administration (VA) study,[48] the data accumulated from studies using other than a prospective randomized methodology showed a tendency toward increased survival in all subsets of patients with surgical treatment. This frequently approached the 4-year survival rate of 91% (mortality rate of 2% to 4% per year) for the normal population at large.[25,33] However, with the recent VA Cooperative Study these facts have been somewhat altered. In a prospective, randomized study, 596 patients with chronic angina were randomly assigned to a group receiving surgical or medical treatment. They were carefully matched for age, risk factors, and extent of disease. This study is the only one done in the 1970s in which the medical group of patients received treatment. Coronary bypass surgery was found to prolong life in patients with left main CAD and in those with triple-vessel disease and reversible left ventricular dysfunction.

With these exceptions, survival after 3 years was 87% for the medically treated group (a mortality rate of approximately 4% a year) compared with 88% for the surgically treated group. The reported survival data are essentially representative of data collected from similar controlled studies of patients with stable[28,34,35] and unstable[11,39,53] angina. There have been criticisms[25,32,33] of the outcome of the VA study, for example exclusion of patients with poor ventricular function, unstable angina, a higher than usual surgical mortality of 5.8% (average from other studies, 1% to 3%); and a crossover of patients from medical to surgical treatment during the course of the study. However, in spite of the study's shortcomings, it did show, through a randomized controlled protocol, that patients with stable angina, who are suitable for CBGS but not operated upon, live signifi-

cantly longer than was reported in previous studies. Perhaps more important, the VA Cooperative Study has established a precedent to continue more controlled randomized studies to delineate further the indications for CBGS in various subsets of patients not already evaluated.

SUMMARY

Coronary bypass graft surgery has one or more of the following objectives: relief of pain and improvement of quality of life, prevention of myocardial infarction, improved ventricular function, and prolongation of life. Many observers have reported that as many as 70% to 90% of patients are pain free or greatly improved after surgery. In additon, many patients have reported a great improvement in quality of life, for example, improved mental outlook, increased exercise tolerance, and ability to return to work. However, available data do not indicate that initial symptomatic improvement necessarily persists or that relief of symptoms is related to prolongation of life. Furthermore, there is no definite proof that prevention of MI or improved ventricular function results after CBGS. There is valid documentation that CBGS is more effective than medical treatment in prolonging life in certain subsets of patients: those with disease of the left main coronary artery and, to a lesser degree, those with triple-vessel disease and reversible impaired ventricular function.

Finally, it must be realized that CBGS is palliative, not curative. Modern treatment of patients with CAD requires the intensive application of both medical and surgical approaches. Used in a complementary, noncompetitive manner, the likelihood of a continued decline in mortality from ischemic heart disease is already beginning to become a realistic hope for the future.

RELEVANCE OF THE CONTROVERSY TO NURSING

The nurse has many roles with regard to the care of the patient. In caring for physical, emotional, and psychologic needs, the underlying basis for the performance of these functions is often forgotten. It is crucial to know and understand the therapeutic process which occurs with patient therapy. Only in this way is there meaningful communication with a patient who looks to nurses as members of a health profession helping him to recover. Unless critical evaluation is expressed, not only in the nursing profession but in all areas of the health profession, experimental procedures can be detrimental to those who rely on expert opinion and guidance. The nurse therefore has an obligation, acting as teacher, advisor, and adjunct-healer, to participate by critically evaluating methods of treatment as they ultimately affect the patient's care; only then can a state of optimum well-being and satisfaction be achieved.

REFERENCES

1. Aldridge HE, Trimble AS: Progression of proximal coronary artery lesions to total occlusion after aorto-coronary saphenous vein bypass grafting. J Thorac Cardiovasc Surg 62:7–11, 1971
2. Apstein CS, Line SA, Leun DC et al: Left ventricular performance and graft patency after coronary–saphenous vein bypass: Early and late follow-up. Am Heart J 93:547–555, 1977
3. Aronow WS, Stemmer EA: Two year follow-up of angina: Medical or surgical therapy. Ann Intern Med 82:208–212, 1975
4. Barboriak JJ, Batayias GE, Pintar K et al: Late lesions in aorto–coronary artery vein grafts. J Thorac Cardiovasc Surg 73:596–601, 1977
5. Bertolasi CA, Pronge JE, Riccitelli MA et al: Natural history of unstable angina with medical or surgical therapy. Chest 70(5):596–605, 1976
6. Block TA, Murray JA, English MT: Improvement in exercise performance after unsuccessful myocardial revascularization. Am J Cardiol 40:673–680, 1977
7. Bolooki H, Thurer RJ, Ghahrarmani A et al: Objective assessment of late results of aorto–coronary bypass operation. Surgery 76:925–934, 1974
8. Bruce RA: Cardiovascular mechanisms of functional aerobic impairment in patients with coronary heart disease. Circulation 49:696–702, 1974
9. Brundage BH, Anderson WT, Davia JE et al: Determinants of left ventricular function following aorto–coronary bypass surgery. Am Heart J 93:687–698, 1977
10. Bulkley B, Hutchins GM: Accelerated atherosclerosis. A morphological study of 97 saphenous vein coronary artery bypass grafts. Circulation 55(1):163–169, 1977
11. Conti CR, Gilbert JB, Hodges M et al: Unstable angina pectoris: Randomized study of surgical versus medical therapy (National Cooperative Unstable Angina Pectoris Study Group). Am J Cardiol 35:129, 1975
12. The Cooper Colloquium on Sudden Death: Part I. The Nature of the Problem, Wayne, Cooper Laboratories, 1973
13. Dunkman WB, Perloff JH, Kostor JA et al: Medical perspectives in coronary artery surgery. A caveat. Ann Intern Med 81:817–837, 1974
14. Espinoza J, Lipski J, Litwuk R et al: New Q waves after coronary artery bypass surgery for angina pectoris. Am J Cardiol 33:221–224, 1974
15. Glassman E, Spencer FC, Krauss KR et al: Changes in the underlying coronary circulation secondary to bypass grafting. Circulation (Suppl II) 59 and 60:80–83, 1974
16. Goldstein S: Sudden Death and Coronary Heart Disease. Mt. Kisco, NY, Futura Publishing Co, 1974
17. Guiney TE, Rubenstein JJ, Saunders CA et al: Functional evaluation of coronary bypass surgery by exercise testing and oxygen consumption. Circulation (Suppl III) 47–48:141–145, 1973
18. Guinn GA, Mathur VS: Surgery versus medical treatment for stable angina pectoris: Prospective randomized study with 1- to 4-year follow-up. Ann of Thorac Surg 22:524–527, 1976
19. Gunby P: More on coronary bypass surgery. Changes in saphenous veins. JAMA 240(12):1217–1223, 1971
20. Hammermeister KE, Kennedy JW, Hamilton JW et al: The effect of vein bypass grafting on resting left ventricular function. N Engl J Med 290:186–192, 1974
21. Harrison DC: Changes in survival and symptom relief in a longitudinal study of patients after bypass surgery. Circulation (Suppl I) 51 and 52:I–98; I–104, 1975
22. Heart Facts 1980. Dallas, American Heart Association, 1980
23. Helfant RH, Banka US, Bodenheimer MM et al: Left ventricular dysfunction in coronary heart disease: A dynamic problem. Cardiovasc Med 2:557–571, 1977
24. Helton WC, Johnson FW, Hornung J: Treadmill exercise test following coronary artery surgery. In Norman J (ed): Coronary Artery Medicine & Surgery. Concepts and Controversies, pp 868–873. New York, Appleton-Century-Crofts, 1975
25. Hurst JW, King SB, Logue RB et al: Value of coronary bypass surgery, controversies in cardiology: Part I. Am J Cardiol 42:308–329, 1978
26. Itscoitz SB, Redwood DR, Stimson EB et al: Saphenous vein bypass grafts: Long-term patency and effect on the native coronary circulation. Am J Cardiol 36:739–743, 1975
27. Kannel WB, Feinlab M: Natural history of angina pectoris in the Framingham study. Am J Cardiol 21:154–163, 1972
28. Kloster FE, Kremkau EL, Rahimotoola SH et al: Prospective randomized study of coronary bypass surgery for chronic stable angina. Cardiovasc Clin 8:145–156, 1977
29. Kominski KA: Comparison of Physician's Interview and Mail Questionnaire for Evaluating Relief of Angina and State of Well-Being Following Coronary Bypass Surgery. Unpublished Master's Thesis, University of Washington, Seattle, 1977
30. Kuller L, Lillienfield A, Fisher R: An epidemiological study of sudden death and unexpected death in adults. Medicine 46:341–361, 1967
31. Lapin ES, Murray JA, Bruce RA, et al: Changes in maximal exercise performance in the evaluation of saphenous vein bypass surgery. Circulation 47:1164–1173, 1973
32. Lawrie GM, Morris GC, Howell JF et al: Results of coronary bypass more than 5 years after operation in 434 patients. Clinical, treadmill exercise and angiographic correlations. Am J Cardiol 40:665–672, 1977
33. Loop FD, Proudfit WL, Sheldon WC: Coronary bypass surgery weighed in the balance. Am J Cardiol 42:154–156, 1977
34. Mathur VS, Guinn GA, Anastassiades LC et al: Surgical treatment for stable angina pectoris: Prospective randomized study. N Engl J Med 292:709–713, 1975
35. Maurer BJ, Oberman A, Hold JH et al: Changes in grafted and nongrafted coronary arteries following saphenous vein bypass grafting. Circulation 50:293–300, 1974
36. McIntosh HD: Benefits from aorto-coronary bypass graft. JAMA 239:1197–1199, 1978
37. McIntosh HD, Garcia JA: The first decade of aorto-coronary bypass grafting, 1967–1977: A review. Circulation 57:405–431, 1978
38. McLaughlin PR, Berman ND, Morton BC, et al: Saphenous vein grafting changes in native circulation and collaterals. Circulation (Supp 1) 51 and 52:1–66, 1975
39. McNeer JF, Starmer CF, Bartel AG et al: The nature of treatment selection in coronary artery disease. Experience with medical and surgical treatment of a chronic disease. Circulation 49:606–614, 1974
40. Miller D, Dodge HT: Benefits of coronary artery bypass surgery. Arch Intern Med 137:1439–1446, 1977
41. Mnayer M, Crahine RA, Raizner AE et al: Myocardial ischemia without pain in patients with post coronary artery bypass. Circulation (Suppl II) 52:46, 1975
42. Moberg CH, Webster JS, Sones FM. Natural history of severe proximal coronary disease as defined by cineangiography (200 patients, seven year follow-up). Am J Cardiol 29:282, 1972
43. Morton BC, McLaughlin PR, Trimble AS et al: Myocardial infarction in coronary artery surgery. Circulation (Suppl I) 51 and 52:198–201, 1975
44. Mundth ED, Austen WC: Surgical measures for coronary heart disease. N Engl J Med 293:13, 75, 124, 1975
45. Murphy, ML, Hultgren HN, Detae K et al: Treatment of chronic stable angina. A preliminary report of survival data of the randomized veterans administration cooperative study. N Engl J Med 29:621–627, 1977
46. Phillips DF, Proudfit W, Lim J et al: Perioperative myocardial infarction. Angiographic correlation. Am J Cardiol 39:269, 1977
47. Preston Thomas A: Coronary Artery Surgery: A Critical Review. New York, Raven Press, 1977
48. Read RC, Murphy ML, Hultgren HN et al: Survival of men treated for chronic stable angina pectoris. A cooperative randomized study. J Thorac Cardiovasc Surg 75:1–16, 1978
49. Recent Trends in Mortality from Heart Disease: Stat Bull Metropol Life Ins Co 56:3–20, 1975
50. Richtsmeier T, Preston TA: Drug management of stable angina pectoris. Postgrad Med 62(5):91–100, 1977
51. Ross RS: Ischemic heart disease. Am J Cardiol 36:496–505, 1975
52. Sampson JJ, Hyatt KH: Management of the patient with severe angina pectoris. An internist's point of view. Circulation 46:1185–1196, 1972

53. Scheidt SS: Unstable angina: Medical management—or surgery? Cardiovasc Med 2:541–543, 1977
54. Selden R, Neill WA, Ritmann LW: Medical versus Surgical therapy for acute coronary insufficiency, A randomized study. N Engl J Med 293(2):1229–1333, 1975
55. Sheperd RL, Itscoitz SB, Glancy DL et al: Deterioration of myocardial function following aorto-coronary bypass operation. Circulation 49:467–475, 1974
56. Soloff LA: Effects of coronary bypass procedure. N Engl J Med 288:1302–1303, 1973
57. Ullyot DJ, Wisneski J, Sullivan RW et al: The impact of coronary artery bypass on late myocardial infarction. J Thorac Cardiovasc Surg 73:165–175, 1977
58. United States Department of Health, Education and Welfare: Health, United States, 1975, pp 297–301. Public Health Services, Health Resources Administration, National Center for Health Statistics Department of Health, Education and Welfare Publication # (HRA), 76-1232, Rockville, Maryland, 1976
59. Warren SC, Brewer DL, Orgain ES: Long-term propranolol therapy for angina pectoris. Am J Cardiol 32:420–426, 1976
60. Zelis R, Liedtke JA, Leaman DM et al: Angina pectoris, diagnosis and treatment. Postgrad Med 95(5):179–188, 1976
61. Zubiate P, Kay JH, Mendez AM: Myocardial revascularization for the patient with drastic impairment of function of the left ventricle. J Thorac Cardiovasc Surg 73:84–86, 1977

SECTION D
COMPLICATIONS OF MYOCARDIAL INFARCTION

26

Arrhythmias Complicating Myocardial Infarction

SUSAN L. WOODS, R.N., M.N.

Cardiac arrhythmias are disturbances in rate, rhythm, or conduction of the heart's electrical impulses and are the most common complication of acute myocardial infarction (MI). Approximately 90% of all patients with acute MI exhibit an arrhythmia of one type or another.[8] Table 26-1 summarizes some of the reports of incidence and mortality from arrhythmias in patients with MI. An electrocardiographic description of each type of arrhythmia can be found in Chapter 17.

CLASSIFICATION OF ARRHYTHMIAS

Arrhythmias can be classified by heart rate, anatomic origin, blocks, or their presumed mechanisms. Classically, arrhythmias have been classified by anatomic origin and by heart rate. Various conduction disturbances are described according to the anatomy involved and the degree of block manifested.

According to Lown and co-workers, an arrhythmia can be classified as (1) an arrhythmia of electrical instability; (2) a bradyarrhythmia; or (3) an arrhythmia of pump failure.[17] Arrhythmias caused by electrical instability are premature ventricular contractions (PVCs) and ventricular tachycardia. Bradyarrhythmias include sinus bradycardia, junctional rhythm and heart blocks. Arrhythmias due to pump failure are sinus tachycardia, atrial extrasystoles, atrial and junctional tachycardia, atrial flutter, and atrial fibrillation.

Kastor and co-workers have classified arrhythmias according to their presumed mechanisms (Table 26-2).[13] Arrhythmias may also be classified according to three basic electrophysiologic mechanisms (Table 26-3).

MECHANISMS OF ARRHYTHMIAS IN ACUTE MYOCARDIAL INFARCTION

Myocardial ischemia and injury cause the following electrophysiologic changes: (1) reduced threshold of the vulnerable period; (2) presence of electrical gradients at the boundaries of unevenly perfused tissue; (3) enhanced Purkinje fiber automatically; (4) dispersion of refractoriness.[28] Thus, automatically and conduction are both altered. This discussion will follow the classification of arrhythmias shown in Table 26-3.

There seems to be agreement that two basic mechanisms may be involved in the genesis of arrhythmias during acute MI: enhanced automaticity and reentrant activity. Automaticity (spontaneous diastolic depolarization) is enhanced during MI by an increase in circulating catecholamines, myocardial hypoxia, and myocardial stretch. With ischemia, cell membranes become more permeable to sodium, resulting in a decreased intracellular potassium and increased extracellular potassium. These changes lead to a decline (a shift toward zero) in resting membrane potential. The slope of phase 4 of the action potential is increased, and membrane potential is brought to threshold more rapidly,

TABLE 26-1   INCIDENCE (I) OF AND MORTALITY (M) FROM ARRHYTHMIAS
The "I" columns show the percentage of patients with myocardial infarction experiencing an arrhythmia. The "M" columns indicate the percentage of mortality in those so affected.

Type of Arrhythmia		Col 1972	Day 1968		Hindman 1979		Julian 1964		Kleiger 1975		Lown 1967		Mullins 1976	
		I	I	M	I	M	I	M	I	M	I	M	I	M
Sinus tachycardia							43	44	36	53	35	34		
Sinus bradycardia							14	21	22	31	25	4		
Sinus arrest							1							
Supraventricular ectopic PACs							25	24	37	34	52	26		
contractions PJCs									12	11	16	7		
Paroxysmal atrial Tachycardia			7				4	50	4	19	11			
Atrial flutter			3							20	5	44		
Atrial fibrillation			8	3			<2		10	30	13	33		
Junctional rhythm			4				8	25	10	20	5	19		
Premature ventricular contractions			86				67	31	84	32	80	21		
Ventricular tachycardia			23				6	67	31	46	28	20		
Ventricular fibrillation			8	32			10	90	9	57	1			
First-degree heart block			4	0			13	46	10	26				
Second-degree heart block			6	1			10	30	7	32				
Third-degree heart block			6	3			8	37	6	68	7	38		
Bundle branch block	RBBB	7	6	4	11	22	13	62	8	47			2	46
	LBBB	4	8	6	38	24			3	33			5	44
	LAH	9							10	35			5	27
	LPH								2	14			1	42
	RBBB with LAH	8			34	29							5	45
	RBBB with LPH	8			10	38							1	57
Asystole											1			

Abbreviations. PAC = premature atrial contraction; PJC = premature junctional contraction; BBB = bundle branch block; LAH = left anterior hemiblock; LPH = left posterior hemiblock.

TABLE 26-2   KASTOR'S CLASSIFICATION OF ARRHYTHMIAS

Automatic	Fibrillatory	Block	Reentrant	Unknown (Unsettled)
Sinus rhythms	Atrial fibrillation	Sinoatrial (SA)	Supraventricular tachycardia	Flutter
Escape rhythms	Ventricular fibrillation	Intra-atrial	Reciprocal beats	Multifocal atrial tachycardia
Wandering atrial pacemaker		Atrioventricular (AV)	Pre-excitation tachycardia	Multifocal ventricular premature beats
Ectopic atrial tachycardia		Infra-His	Coupled premature beats	Premature beat and tachycardia
Accelerated idioventricular rhythm		Intraventricular	Ventricular tachycardia	
Accelerated His bundle rhythm				
Parasystole (plus "protection")				

(Kastor JA, Goldreyer BN, Moore EN et al: Cardiovasc Clin 6:111–135, 1974)

TABLE 26-3   ARRHYTHMIAS CLASSIFIED ACCORDING TO MECHANISM

Automaticity	Reentry	Conduction Disturbance
Atrial extrasystole	Atrial extrasystole	Sino-atrial block
Atrial parasystole	Paroxysmal atrial tachycardia	Atrioventricular block
Wandering atrial pacemaker	Atrial flutter	-1st degree
Sinus arrhythmia	Atrial fibrillation	-2nd degree
Sinus tachycardia	Junctional extrasystoles	-3rd degree
Multifocal atrial tachycardia	Junctional tachycardia	Aberrant conduction
Sinus arrest	Ventricular extrasystoles	Intraventricular conduction delay
Sinus bradycardia	Ventricular tachycardia	Bundle branch block
Junctional extrasystoles	Ventricular fibrillation	Hemiblock
Junctional escapes		
Junctional parasystole		
Junctional rhythm		
Accelerated junctional rhythm		
Ventricular extrasystoles		
Ventricular escapes		
Ventricular parasystole		
Idioventricular rhythm		
Accelerated idioventricular rhythm		

increasing rate of impulse formation.[10] With myocardial ischemia, hypoxia, and stretch, the resting transmembrane potential may be reduced so that stimulation at the lower potential will result in a slowly rising phase 0 of the action potential, and this lower amplitude of the action potential results in a delay or a failure of conduction.[7]

Reentrant activity may occur in acute MI because of the alterations in the transmembrane potential of the ischemic cells compared with that of adjacent cells. A change in cell membrane potential leads to slowed conduction, decremental conduction, cell-to-cell depression of conduction velocity,[22] local block, and reentry. Extrasystoles that demonstrate fixed coupling are usually the result of reentrant activity. Figure 26-1A shows normal conduction of a sinus impulse from the Purkinje fibers to the myocardial cells. Figure 26-1B shows altered conduction of a sinus impulse because of ischemia and unidirectional block resulting in reactivation or reentry. The ischemic tissue repolarizes more slowly,

resulting in unidirectional block.[22] By the time the impulse approaches the ischemic area from the opposite direction, it finds the area responsive, and the impulse reenters the circuit, reactivates the myocardium, and propagates a premature impulse. If the circuit is repeated successively, then ventricular tachycardia results.[24]

Some consider enhanced automaticity the major mechanism responsible for arrhythmias in the early hours of acute MI, and reentry to be the major mechanism in the later hours of acute MI (36 to 72 hours after onset). Both mechanisms can occur together.

Eick and co-workers found the following electrophsiologic changes when a coronary artery of a dog was ligated.[5] Within 15 to 20 minutes after ligation, intracellular potassium decreased and intracellular sodium increased because of changes in cell membrane permeability. Within 20 minutes to 2 hours, irreversible cell death occurred. During the next 8 to 10 hours, there was a low incidence of arrhythmias.

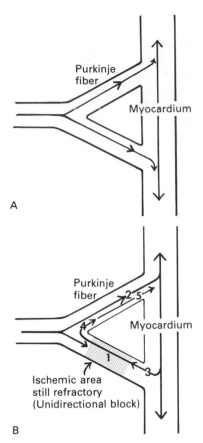

Fig. 26-1. (**A**) Normal activation of the ventricular myocardium. (**B**) Reentrant activation of the ventricular myocardium: (**1**) unidirectional block; (**2**) slow propagation over a parallel route; (**3**) delayed excitation of tissue beyond block; (**4**) reexcitation of the tissues proximal to the block; and (**5**) reexcitation of the myocardium. (After Neasman AR et al: Heart Lung 5(3):498, 1976)

During the next 10 hours, there was a decline (a shift toward zero) of resting membrane potential, a decline in the rate of rise of the action potential, an increase in the slope of phase 4 of the action potential (see Figs. 12-6, 12-7). Consequently, automaticity was increased and conduction velocity slowed. After 3 days, the rate of arrhythmias decreased and the resting membrane potential, upstroke velocity, and automaticity all returned to normal. The action potential duration remained prolonged and the threshold for ventricular fibrillation remained lowered for up to 10 days. After 10 days the action potential normalized.

ARRHYTHMIAS COMMON IN ACUTE MYOCARDIAL INFARCTION AND THEIR TREATMENT

Arrhythmias occurring in acute MI can be caused by altered impulse formation (automaticity) or abnormal impulse conduction, or both. Arrhythmias are presented in three groups: lethal ventricular arrhythmias, bradyarrhythmias, and tachyarrhythmias. See Chapter 17 for the ECG characteristics of these arrhythmias.

Lethal Ventricular Arrhythmias

The lethal ventricular arrhythmias are PVC, ventricular tachycardia and flutter, and ventricular fibrillation.

Premature Ventricular Contraction (PVC). The most common arrhythmia during acute MI is the PVC, occurring in 80% of patients. The occurrence of PVCs is important because it can lead to ventricular tachycardia and ventricular fibrillation, which can result in death. Approximately 90% of PVCs originate in the left ventricle because most infarctions occur in the left ventricle. Malignant PVCs have one or more of the following characteristics:

1. Occurrence in pairs (couplets) or runs
2. Occurrence of six or more per minute
3. Occurrence during the vulnerable period, 0.02 to 0.04 seconds at apex of the T wave (during phase 3 of the action potential)[32]
4. Multiform configuration[8,17]

The ECG characteristics of the PVC are discussed in Chapter 17. The PVC is often confused with a premature supraventricular impulse with aberrant conduction. Both can be premature and have bizarre QRS complexes. Table 26-4 lists criteria that may be helpful in differentiating a PVC from an aberrantly conducted premature supraventricular impulse. Table 26-5 lists criteria that may be useful in this differentiation of a PVC from an aberrantly conducted premature supraventricular impulse, if the patient is in atrial fibrillation.

Most PVCs have complete compensatory pauses. This increased time between the PVC and the next normal impulse allows increased diastolic filling of the heart (increased preload). This increase in preload causes the myocardial muscle fibers to lengthen, resulting in increased contractility and increased stroke volume. Thus, the postextrasystolic impulse (a normal impulse following an ectopic impulse) requires the heart to work harder. Significance of PVCs depends on the patient's ventricular function and the duration of the arrhythmia.[28] In the ischemic heart, malignant PVCs are more likely to lead to ventricular tachycardia, flutter, and fibrillation than they are in the nonischemic heart. Thus, during acute MI, malignant PVCs should be treated in order to prevent ventricular arrhythmias. *Treatment* may include an antiarrhythmic drug to decrease automaticity and to change the effective refractory period.

Drugs such as disopyramide (Norpace), quinidine, procainamide, propranolol, and potassium have a similar antiarrhythmic effect: i.e., they increase the refractory period, slow conduction velocity, and increase threshold potential towards 0. Drugs such as diphenylhydantoin and lidocaine reduce the refractory period and either do not change, or enhance conduction velocity. Both types reduce automaticity by reducing the slope of phase 4 of the action potential, and change the conduction velocity and refractory period of reentrant ectopic impulses.[30] The specific actions of antiarrhythmic drugs can be found in Chapter 34.

Premature ventricular contractions may be caused by such other factors as hypoxia, hypokalemia, myocardial stretch, myocardial irritation because of an intracardiac

TABLE 26-4   CRITERIA FOR DISTINGUISHING A PREMATURE VENTRICULAR IMPULSE FROM A PREMATURE SUPRAVENTRICULAR IMPULSE WITH ABERRANT CONDUCTION

Factors Favoring a Ventricular Impulse	Factors Favoring a Supraventricular Impulse with Aberrant Conduction
1. Complete compensatory pause is common.	1. Complete compensatory pause is uncommon.
2. P wave is usually obliterated by the premature QRS complex, since atrial activity usually continues unrelated to PVC (AV dissociation). Occasionally retrograde conduction occurs, resulting in a P wave after the premature QRS complex.	2. P wave precedes premature QRS complex, but may be hiding in T wave of previous impulse. (No AV dissociation.)
3. In lead V_1 (MCL$_1$), there is a qR'.	3. In lead V_1 (MCL$_1$), there is an RSR'.
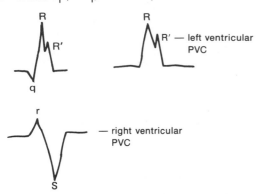	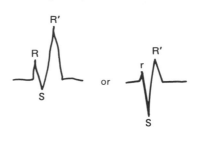
4. In lead V_6 (MCL$_6$), there is a QS, rS, R', or qR.	4. In lead V_6 (MCL$_6$), there is a qR.
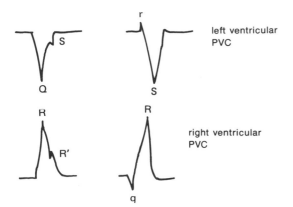	
5. The QRS axis is −90 degrees to −180 degrees. The V leads are all possible or negative. This is termed concordant V leads.	5. The initial QRS axis is identical to normally conducted QRS complexes.
6. The patient has had similar PVCs in the past.	6. The patient has had similar aberrations in the past.
7. Fusion beats may occur.	7. Fusion beats are uncommon.

catheter or pacemaker electrode, or increased circulating catecholamines.

Treatment may include oxygen, potassium, digoxin, an antiarrhythmic drug, repositioning of an intracardiac catheter or pacemaker electrode, or nursing measures to reduce the workload of the heart, thus reducing the myocardial need for oxygen.

Nursing measures may include

• Assisting the patient with activities of daily living and spacing these activities throughout the day to prevent fatigue

• Involving the patient in the planning of his care

• Listening to the patient and allowing him to express his fears and anxieties.

It is important to determine if the arrhythmia occurs in association with, or is related to, any activity. Laboratory tests should be checked to determine the presence of hypokalemia or hypoxemia. Lungs should be auscultated frequently (every 4 hours) to determine the presence of crackling rales, which may indicate congestive heart failure. If the patient has a right heart catheter or electrode, the presence of right PVCs may indicate mechanical irritation to the myocardium. Routine nursing care of the uncomplicated MI patient can be found in Chapter 23.

Ventricular Tachycardia. Ventricular tachycardia occurs in approximately 28% of patients with acute MI and is dangerous because it frequently results in a more lethal arrhythmia, ventricular flutter and fibrillation. The rapid rate compromises cardiac output because the time for diastolic filling of the heart is reduced (decreased preload) and stroke volume is reduced. Coronary artery filling is also

TABLE 26-5 CRITERIA FOR DISTINGUISHING A VENTRICULAR IMPULSE FROM A SUPRAVENTRICULAR IMPULSE WITH ABERRANT CONDUCTION IN ATRIAL FIBRILLATION

Ventricular Impulse	Supraventricular Impulse with Aberrant Conduction
1. Fixed coupling is common.	1. Fixed coupling is rare.
2. Preceding duration between normal QRS complexes is short.	2. Preceding duration between normal QRS complexes is longer.
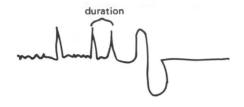	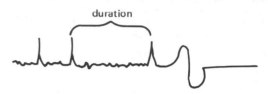
	This lengthened preceding cycle and shortened immediate cycle results in prolonged refractoriness that leads to aberrant conduction (Ashman's phenomenon).
3. There are fewer PVCs when the heart rate is rapid	3. There are more aberrantly conducted impulses when the rate is rapid
4. There is undue prematurity	4. The aberrant impulse is no more premature than other aberrantly conducted impulses

reduced because of the shortened diastolic time. During ventricular tachycardia, atrioventricular dissociation usually occurs. This loss of synchrony between the atria and the ventricles during diastole results in the loss of atrial contraction and active filling of the ventricles. This decreased ventricular filling leads to further reduction in stroke volume, and cardiac output decreases.

The specific *treatment* of ventricular tachycardia and flutter depends on the patient's hemodynamic response to the reduced cardiac output and reduced coronary artery filling. The reduced cardiac output can reduce blood pressure so that the patient exhibits signs of decreased perfusion to vital organs. If unconsciousness occurs, then synchronized defibrillation (cardioversion) is indicated. (Defibrillation and cardioversion are discussed later in this chapter.) If the rhythm converts to normal sinus rhythm or if the patient remains conscious, then treatment is directed toward eliminating the cause in order to prevent recurrence. Treatment would be the same as that for premature ventricular contractions. If the rhythm does not convert to normal sinus rhythm, then cardioversion should be repeated, and if the rhythm does not change, then cardiopulmonary resuscitation (CPR) may be necessary (CPR is discussed later in this chapter.)

Treatment may also include pacemaker overdrive to suppress the ectopic foci. When the diastolic phase is shortened, more uniform depolarization (phase 4 of the action potential) is promoted, and automaticity is reduced.[30]

Ventricular Fibrillation. Ventricular fibrillation occurs in 10% of patients with acute MI. The threshold for ventricular fibrillation is lowered in ischemic tissue.[13] It can occur spontaneously, without any warning arrhythmias. With ventricular fibrillation, many different portions of the myocardium are discharging independently, resulting in uncoordinated and ineffective contractions. The circulation stops completely. The patient has no pulse and very soon loses consciousness. Since there is no cardiac output, *treatment* includes immediate defibrillation, repeated three times if necessary, then cardiopulmonary resuscitation.

Factors that facilitate this arrhythmia are
1. Slow heart rates, because the vulnerable period is increased
2. Prolonged Q–T interval
3. Electrolyte imbalance
4. Hypothermia
5. Use of drugs that increase automaticity
6. Disturbances of nervous regulation
7. Myocardial infarction, because intracellular potassium is reduced in injured cells
8. Metabolic acidosis.[29]

Bradyarrhythmias

Bradyarrhythmias occur in 25% of patients with MI.[8] They are frequently caused by vagal stimulation secondary to stimulation of receptors in the injured myocardium or in the coronary vessels. Vagal stimulation may also be caused by
1. Hypertension
2. Valsalva maneuver
3. Glossopharyngeal or oculocardiac reflex
4. Carotid sinus stimulation
5. Stimulation of receptors in left ventricle or coronary sinus when the heart is distended
6. Fear, despair, isolation, hopelessness
7. Morphine sulfate administration.[32]

Bradyarrhythmias are also caused by ischemia or injury to the various structures of the conduction system. Included in this classification are sinus bradycardia, which occurs in approximately 25% of MI patients; junctional rhythm, which occurs in approximately 19% of MI patients; idioventricular rhythm; and heart block, which occurs in approximately 7% of MI patients.[17]

The slow ventricular rate that accompanies these arrhythmias can cause electrical instability, because of the various recovery periods of the individual's normal and adjacent ischemic ventricular muscle fibers. Thus, reentry

TABLE 26-6 INCIDENCE AND MORTALITY OF HEART BLOCKS

Block	Incidence (%)		Mortality (%)	
	KLEIGER[15]	MULLINS[23]	KLEIGER[15]	MULLINS[23]
RBBB with LAH	—	5	—	45
left bundle branch block (LBBB)	3	5	33	44
RBBB with left posterior hemiblock (LPH)	—	1	—	57

is facilitated and ectopic impulses or rhythms can occur when the ventricular rate is critically low.[14] Bradycardia also reduces the threshold for ventricular fibrillation, because of the heterogeneous electrical fields (varying resting membrane potential of myocardial cells).[8] When heart rate decreases during acute MI with impaired left ventricular function, cardiac output decreases, since stroke volume cannot increase. This reduction in cardiac output can lead to decreased tissue perfusion. With bradyarrhythmias the vulnerable period is longer.

Rather than suppressing automaticity with antiarrhythmic drugs, *treatment* is directed toward acceleration of the sinus rate (or the junctional or ventricular rate in third-degree heart block). Treatment may include a parasympatholytic or sympathomimetic drug (Chap. 35) or a pacemaker (Chap. 40).[32]

Sinus Bradycardia. Sinus bradycardia is usually associated with small MIs, since large MIs usually depress contractility in such a way that stroke volume is reduced and reflex sympathetic discharge has a positive chronotropic effect (increased heart rate). Usually it is not treated unless associated with hypotension.

Junctional Rhythm. Junctional rhythm is usually the result of depressed sinoatrial (SA) node function. There may be a reduction in cardiac output, not only because of the reduced heart rate, but because of the reduced stroke volume. This is due to the loss of effective atrial systole. If both the SA and atrioventricular (AV) nodes are depressed, then an idioventricular rhythm may become the dominant rhythm. If the ventricular rhythm accelerates to 60 to 100 beats per minute, it is usually benign and does not lead to ventricular fibrillation.

First-Degree Heart Block. First-degree heart block occurs in approximately 4% to 13% of patients with MI and usually does not progress to further degrees of block. No treatment is required (Chap. 17).

Second-Degree Heart Block. Second-degree heart block occurs in approximately 6% to 10% of patients with MI, and frequently reverts to normal sinus rhythm. Mobitz I second-degree heart block (Wenckebach) is common and is usually seen with inferior MIs. It is caused by ischemia of the AV node. This ischemia is usually reversible 48 to 72 hours after MI. Mobitz II second-degree heart block is less common and is usually seen with anterior MIs; this usually implies injury to the bundle branches. This injury is usually not reversible (Chap. 17).[12]

Third-Degree Heart Block. Third-degree heart block occurs in 6% to 8% of patients with MI. In patients with inferior MIs, the third-degree heart block is usually due to ischemia and carries a mortality of 25%. In patients with anterior MI, the third-degree heart block is usually due to a large MI and carries a high mortality (75%).[8] These patients usually require permanent pacemakers (Chap. 40). Patients who have fascicular block prior to MI, frequently develop complete heart block during myocardial infarction. Among patients with right-bundle branch block (RBBB) and left anterior hemiblock (LAH), 43% to 67% develop complete heart block. Some revert to RBBB with LAH after MI. Permanent pacing has reduced the mortality in these patients from 65% to 9% (Chap. 17).[23]

Some 18% to 21% of MI patients develop a ventricular conduction block. Bifascicular block occurs in approximately 11% of MI patients and represents 60% to 75% of all conduction blocks. The incidence of the specific blocks and their mortality rates are shown in Table 26-6 (see also Table 26-1).

Unifascicular or Monofascicular Block. This block occurs in 5% to 11% of patients with MI and represents 28% to 36% of all conduction blocks. The incidence of the specific blocks and their mortality rates are shown in Table 26-7 (see also Table 26-1).

The mortality rate for MI patients without block is 15%. The mortality rate for MI patients with block is two to three times greater than if no block exists.[23]

Fascicular block can lead to complete heart block, depending on the anatomic location and size of the MI. For bifascicular block to lead to complete heart block, the septum and a large area of myocardium must be destroyed. The incidence of progression to complete heart block, according to Mullins[23] is shown in Table 26-8.

If first-degree heart block develops with bifascicular block, complete heart block is likely. Patients should be assessed to determine the adequacy of cardiac output. Temporary pacemaker equipment should be available and an isoproterenol drop prepared (1 mg isoproterenol in 1000 ml 5% dextrose in water).

Prophylactic standby pacing is indicated if RBBB, RBBB with LAH, or RBBB with LPH occurs during acute MI, because the mortality is greater than 43%. All MI patients with major ventricular conduction defects have a poor prognosis because of electrical instability, severe coronary disease, and poor left ventricular function. Permanent pacing may prolong life in some of these patients.[23]

TABLE 26-7 INCIDENCE AND MORTALITY OF FASCICULAR BLOCKS

BLOCK	Incidence (%)		Mortality (%)	
	KLEIGER[15]	MULLINS[23]	KLEIGER[15]	MULLINS[23]
LAH	10	5	35	27
RBBB	8	2	47	46
LPH	2	1	14	42

TABLE 26-8 INCIDENCE OF PROGRESSION FROM FASCICULAR TO COMPLETE HEART BLOCK

Block	Incidence (%)
LAH	3
LPH	0
RBBB	43
RBBB with LAH	46
RBBB with LPH	43
LBBB	20

Tachyarrhythmias

Tachyarrhythmias or arrhythmias due to congestive heart failure (CHF) include sinus tachycardia, premature atrial contraction (PAC), paroxysmal atrial tachycardia (PAT), multifocal atrial tachycardia (MAT), atrial flutter and fibrillation, premature junctional contraction (PJC), and junctional tachycardia.

As the left ventricular myocardium is injured, contractility decreases and stroke volume is reduced. Left ventricular end-diastolic pressure increases, resulting in an increase in left atrial pressure and stretching of the atrial myocardium. Myocardial stretch increases automaticity of the atrium. Infarction, injury, and ischemia of the atria also increase automaticity of the atrial cells.[17]

Sinus Tachycardia. Sinus tachycardia occurs in approximately 35% to 43% of patients with acute MI. If the cause of the tachycardia is CHF, the prognosis is poor, since this implies that the infarction is large enough to result in pump failure (or reduced stroke volume). Sinus tachycardia occurs commonly with anterior MI.[8]

Atrial Flutter and Atrial Fibrillation. Atrial flutter occurs in approximately 3% to 5% of patients and atrial fibrillation in approximately 6% to 10% of patients with acute MI. In atrial fibrillation there is loss of effective atrial systole, an inappropriately fast ventricular rate, and irregularity of rhythm that leads to variation in stroke volume. Because of these factors, cardiac output may be reduced. The *immediate treatment* is to increase the AV block and reduce the ventricular rate. Cardioversion may be indicated. If these arrhythmias are due to congestive heart failure (increased left and right atrial pressure causing stretch of the atrial myocardium), then the prognosis is also poor. For CHF to occur, the infarction is usually large.[8]

Paroxysmal Atrial Tachycardia. Paroxysmal atrial tachycardia is seldom seen in patients with acute MI. When it is seen, carotid sinus massage or another form of vagal stimulation should be attempted in order to slow the ventricular rate; this also may prove helpful in diagnosing the arrhythmia. Emotional stress may be the cause and a sedative the treatment. Propranolol may be indicated.

Junctional Tachycardia. Junctional tachycardia is rarely seen in acute MI unless digitalis toxicity coexists.

Premature Atrial Contractions. PACs are common after acute MI, occurring in 37% to 52% of patients. Increasing frequency of PACs may be a warning.[8] Their occurrence is nonspecific but may be caused by increased atrial myocardial

stretch because of CHF or pulmonary embolus, various drugs, or hypokalemia. The aim of treatment is to prevent the occurrence of atrial flutter or fibrillation.

Generally, *treatment* of CHF and subsequent arrhythmias may include oxygen administration, digoxin, diuretics, antiarrhythmic drugs, cardioversion, and nursing measures to reduce the workload of the heart. Thus, myocardial oxygen need is decreased, and the oxygen supply to the heart is improved. The patient must be assessed frequently (every 2 to 4 hours) to determine the effect of the arrhythmia and the treatment of the arrhythmia on the patient's cardiac output.

Signs and symptoms of decreased perfusion pressure may include fatigue; decreased mentation; oliguria; cold, moist, dusky skin; chest pain; decreased blood pressure or decreased pulse pressure; and increased heart rate.

Nursing measures are the same as those for ventricular arrhythmias.

- All patients in the cardiac care unit (CCU) need to be continuously assessed by direct observation, cardiac monitoring, and physical examination, to determine the heart rate and rhythm and its effects on cardiac output.

- Routine nursing care should also include emotional support during this life-threatening period of their illness. The nurse can recognize problems, help the patient solve them, and help the patient cope with his present limitations.

- Not only is it necessary to be able to recognize arrhythmias, but the nurse must also be aware of the threat each poses for the individual patient. This includes knowing which arrhythmias warn of impending lethal arrhythmias and being prepared to treat them—and treat them aggressively.

Other treatment for arrhythmias in patients with MI may include surgical procedures: coronary artery bypass graft, left ventricular aneurysmectomy, infarctectomy, valve replacement or repair of a ruptured interventricular septum. The purpose of surgery is to correct the underlying problem, improve cardiac output, and eliminate the arrhythmia. Prevention or early detection and aggressive management of arrhythmias can thus do much to lower the mortality rate of patients with acute MI.

CARDIOPULMONARY RESUSCITATION

The ABCs of CPR consist of A–airway; B–breathing; C–circulation. Unresponsiveness is established by gently shaking the patient's shoulder and asking him if he is all right.

A—Airway

An airway must be established in order to ensure adequate ventilation.

- If the patient does not respond, call for help.

- Because the tongue is the most common cause of airway obstruction, lifting the jaw forward (chin lift) and tilting the head back (Fig. 26-2A) lifts the tongue away from the back of the throat.

Manual thrust or chest thrust and back blows may be necessary. Chest thrust forces air out of the lungs. In order to clear a completely obstructed airway, the following procedures should be initiated.

If the patient is standing or sitting,[19]

- Stand behind him, place your arms directly under his chest
- Place the thumb side of your fist on his breastbone, but not on the xiphoid process or the margins of the rib cage
- Grasp your fist with your other hand and exert four quick strong compressions.
- Then position yourself at the side and slightly behind the victim;
- Deliver four sharp blows to the back with the heel of your hand over the victim's spine between the shoulder blades
- Place your other hand on the chest to support him.

If the patient is lying down,[19]

- Place him on his back and kneel close beside him, open his airway, and turn his head to one side
- Place hands for chest thrust in the same way as for closed-chest heart compression (heel of hand on lower half of sternum)
- Exert four quick downward thrusts to compress the chest cavity
- Then kneel and roll him onto his side, facing you, with his chest against your thigh
- Deliver four sharp blows to the back, as described.

Whenever possible, the victim's head should be lower than his chest to make use of the effect of gravity.[19]

Back blows produce an instantaneous increase in pressure in the respiratory passages, which may dislodge the foreign body either completely or partly. The manual thrusts produce a more sustained increase in pressure in the respiratory passages and may help to dislodge the foreign body. The combination of the two techniques clears the upper airway better than either one separately.[19]

B—Breathing

If the patient does not begin to breathe spontaneously, artificial ventilation must begin immediately. There are several methods: mouth-to-mouth, mouth-to-nose, mouth-to-stoma, mouth-to-artificial airway, and use of various devices for assisting ventilation.

Mouth-to-Mouth Breathing. This is accomplished as follows:
- Pinch the nose closed with thumb and index finger of one hand while exerting pressure on the forehead to maintain the backward tilt of the head
- Take a deep breath, make a tight seal around the patient's mouth, and blow into the mouth
- Give four quick full breaths without allowing time for full lung deflation between breaths (Fig. 26-3), then two breaths after each cycle of 15 compressions.

If there are two persons doing CPR, one breath every five seconds is needed. Ventilation is adequate if the chest rises and falls and if air can be felt and heard leaving the lungs.[1,8]

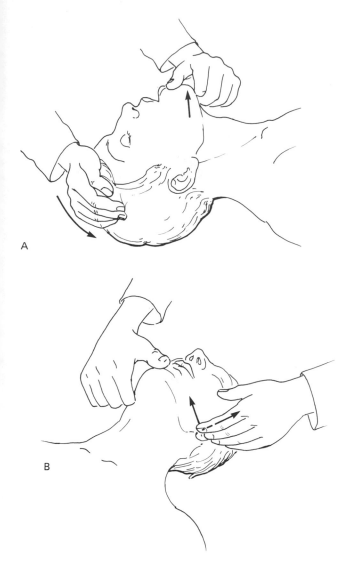

Fig. 26-2. **(A)** Head-tilt method of opening the airway (JAMA 227:843, 1974) **(B)** Chin-lift method of opening the airway. (After *Manual for Instructors in Basic Cardiac Life Support*, p 43. Dallas, American Heart Association, 1977)

- With the jaw-thrust method, the entire jaw is forced forward by placing the fingers of both hands behind the angles of the jaw, or by grasping the jaw (holding the mandible and lower teeth) and tilting the head backward at the same time (Fig. 26-2B).
- In patients with cervical spine injuries the head-tilt method should not be used; instead, the index fingers should be used to displace the mandible forward without moving the head.[1,8]
- If the airway is obstructed, apply suction to the area of obstruction, or roll the patient onto his side and clear his mouth with two fingers.
- While keeping the airway open, place your ear over the victim's mouth and nose and look toward his chest. Look for any rise and fall of the chest, listen for the escape of air during exhalation, and feel for the flow of air on your cheek.

If the airway is completely obstructed by a foreign body, the patient will be unable to speak, breathe, or cough.

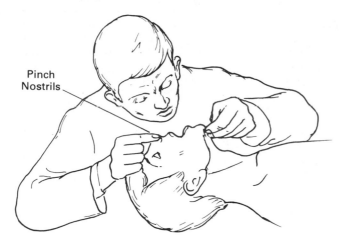

Pinch Nostrils

Fig. 26-3. Mouth-to-mouth resuscitation. (After *Manual for Instructors in Basic Cardiac Life Support*, p 43, Dallas, American Heart Association, 1977)

Artificial ventilation should not be interrupted for more than 5 seconds.

Mouth-to-Nose Breathing. This is accomplished as follows:
* Tilt the head back by placing one hand on the forehead while lifting the lower jaw with the other
* Take a deep breath, and establish a seal between your mouth and the victim's nose
* Blow air into victim's lungs.

Mouth-to-Stoma Breathing. With this technique (for patients with a laryngectomy), the head tilt and jaw thrust maneuvers are unnecessary.
* Establish a seal between your mouth and the victim's stoma
* Blow air directly into the stoma.

Mouth-to-Artificial Airway Breathing and the Use of Devices for Assisting Ventilation. An S-tube artificial airway can be used, but maintaining a tight seal around the mouth is difficult. An oropharyngeal airway should be used whenever a breathing device with a mask is employed. Artificial airways should be lubricated with sterile water-soluble jelly or water prior to insertion. The tip of an upside-down airway is directed toward the palate while the jaw is pulled forward and downward. When the tip of the airway hits the back of the throat, it is rotated so that the tip is in the direction of the trachea and is advanced until the flange is flush with the lips. Ventilation should begin immediately, either by the mouth-to-airway method or by means of a device to assist ventilation.[8]

An *esophageal obturator* airway can be used. This airway consists of a cuffed endotracheal tube mounted through a face mask. An obturator blocks the distal orifice and there are multiple openings in the upper one-third of the tube at the level of the pharynx. The tube is placed into the esophagus and the mask sits on the face. The cuff is then inflated with approximately 25 ml of air. With artificial ventilation (mouth or bag), air is discharged through the pharyngeal openings and passes down the trachea, because

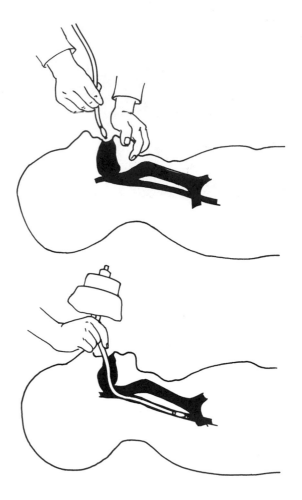

Trachea   Left stem main bronchus

Carina

Right stem main bronchus   Cuff

Fig. 26-4. Insertion of esophageal obturator airway. This airway consists of a cuffed endotracheal tube mounted through a face mask. The tube is placed into the esophagus and the mask sits on the face. The cuff is then inflated with approximately 25 ml of air. With artifical ventilation, air is discharged through the pharyngeal openings and passes down the trachea, because the esophagus is blocked. (After Goldberg AH: Advanced Cardiac Life Support, pp (II):12–13, 1975)

the esophagus is blocked (Fig. 26-4). When this airway is removed, regurgitation usually occurs. Precautions should be taken to prevent aspiration of vomitus.[1]

The trachea may be intubated with an endotracheal tube to create an airway or to improve the existing airway.

Indications for endotracheal intubation include[1]

1. Cardiac arrest
2. Respiratory arrest
3. Inability of rescuer to ventilate the unconscious patient artificially by conventional methods
4. Inability of the patient to protect his own airway (coma, areflexia)
5. Prolonged artificial ventilation.

During artificial ventilation, air can distend the stomach, thereby promoting regurgitation and reducing lung volume by elevating the diaphragm. With the patient's head turned to the side, moderate pressure over the stomach will force air out the mouth.

C—Circulation

If cardiac arrest occurs, the patient will be pulseless. He will have either electrical-mechanical dissociation, marked bradycardia, ventricular fibrillation, or asystole. If the carotid pulse is absent, artificial circulation should be started immediately. For an adult, the precordial thump is worthwhile if the arrest is witnessed, as is generally the case in the monitored CCU patient. A sharp blow is delivered with the fist to the midsternum of the patient from a distance of 8 to 12 inches and may convert the fibrillation or asystole if done within 1 minute of the arrest (Fig. 26-5).[1]

External cardiac compressions are rhythmic applications of pressure over the lower half of the sternum, resulting in compression of the heart between the spine and the sternum and pulsatile artificial circulation. A newer view of CPR holds that chest compression produces a generalized rise in intrathoracic pressure applied to the pulmonary vascular

Fig. 26-5. Precordial thump. (After JAMA 227:847, 1974)

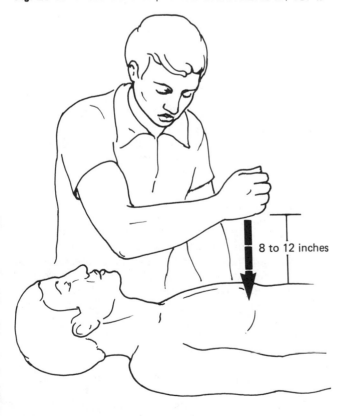

8 to 12 inches

bed and the heart. Thus, the heart acts as a conduit for blood from the lungs. Flow into the extrathoracic vessels depends on the vessels' tendency to remain open or to collapse. Thus, during compression, flow occurs to the head because a pressure gradient is developed between the carotid artery and the compressible jugular vein.[18]

Properly performed cardiac compressions result in a systolic blood pressure of over 100 mm Hg. With the adult patient in a horizontal position (to ensure flow to the brain) on a firm surface, cardiac compression is achieved by exerting 80 lb to 120 lb of pressure over the lower half of the sternum (about 1 inch above the xiphoid process).[1]

- Compress the sternum vertically 1-½ to 2 inches at a regular rate of 60 compressions per minute
- Place the heel of one hand on top of the other (Fig. 26-6).
- Bring shoulders directly over the patient's sternum and keep arms straight.
- Do not remove the heel of the hand from the patient's chest between compressions, but release the pressure that is exerted.

A ratio of five chest compressions to one interposed breath is maintained if two rescuers are present. Interposed breathing prevents a drop in blood flow. If there is only one rescuer, the ratio is 2 breaths to 15 chest compressions (Fig. 26-7, A, and B).

Cardiac arrest lasting 3 to 5 minutes results in irreversible brain damage from anoxia. Fixed, dilated pupils indicate brain anoxia. Effectiveness of CPR is determined by pupils that constrict when exposed to light, because this is an indication of adequate oxygenation and blood flow to the brain and a palpable pulse during cardiac compression.[1]

Complications

Complications of CPR include gastric distention, rib fractures, laceration of the liver, fat emboli and costochondral separation.[1] Supplemental oxygen should be used as soon as possible because the rescuer's exhaled breath will deliver only 16% to 17% oxygen. Bag-mask, or bag tube systems should have supplemental oxygen attached.

Defibrillation

Defibrillation is used immediately after onset of ventricular fibrillation or of ventricular tachycardia without a peripheral pulse. Defibrillation completely depolarizes all the myocardial cells and terminates the chaotic electrical activity, allowing the SA node to regain control of the heart rhythm[16] unless the myocardium is anoxic or acidotic, in which case this may not be possible. As an elective procedure, defibrillation or precordial shock can be synchronized with the ECG so as to avoid discharge during the vulnerable period (T wave). This synchronized precordial shock is called cardioversion.

In defibrillation of an exposed heart, the electrode paddles are directly applied to the myocardium, whereas in the closed-chest procedure, the paddles are usually applied to the anterior chest.

- The standard electrode paddle position for the closed-chest procedure is as follows: one paddle just to the right

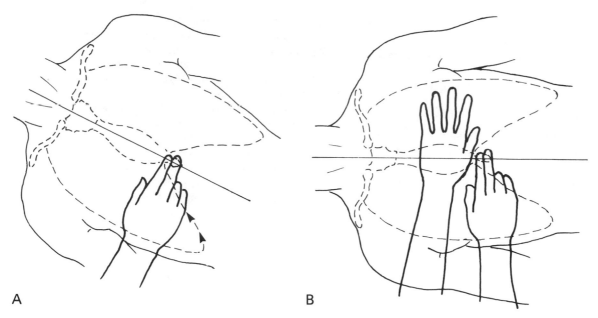

Fig. 26-6. Placement of hands for closed chest cardiac compression: (**A**) With the middle and index fingers of the lower hand, follow the lower edge of the rib cage to the notch where the ribs meet the sternum. (**B**) With the middle finger on the notch and the index finger placed next to it, place the heel of the other hand on the lower half of the sternum, next to the index finger. (After *Manual for Instructors in Basic Cardiac Life Support*, pp 48–49. Dallas, American Heart Association, 1977)

Techniques of CPR, according to American Heart Association Standards,[1] are as follows:

For Witnessed Cardiac Arrest
1. Tilt the patient's head to open the airway and simultaneously palpate the carotid pulse.
2. If the pulse is absent, give a precordial thump.
3. If the victim is not breathing, deliver four quick, full-lung inflations.
4. If pulse and breathing are not immediately restored, begin one-rescuer or two-rescuer CPR.

For Monitored Patient (For use with patients who have sudden ventricular fibrillation, asystole, or ventricular tachycardia without pulse).
1. Give a single precordial thump.
2. Check the monitor quickly for cardiac rhythm, and simultaneously check the carotid pulse. Do not waste time.
3. If there is ventricular fibrillation or ventricular tachycardia without a pulse, apply countershock as soon as possible.
4. If the pulse is absent, tilt the patient's head, deliver four quick, full lung inflations.
5. Check the carotid pulse again.
6. If the pulse is absent, begin one-rescuer or two-rescuer CPR.

---

of the upper sternum below the right clavicle and the other paddle just to the left of the cardiac apex (Fig. 26-8).

In order to reduce skin resistance to current flow and to prevent skin burns, one of the following may be placed between the electrodes and the chest wall: saline-soaked 4-by-4 gauze pads, electrode paste, or defibrillator pads (adhesive pads with electrode gel). Care should be taken to prevent contact between the two areas of conductive material because electrical bridging may occur. If saline-soaked gauze pads are used, cardiac compressions can be resumed after defibrillation without the hands slipping on the chest, a problem that occurs with electrode paste.

- Exert 20 lb to 25 lb of pressure on each paddle in order to ensure good skin contact.
- Do not let anyone touch the patient or the bed when the defibrillator is fired.
- Then discharge the defibrillator at 300 to 400 watt-seconds.[6]

If the patient weighs less than 50 kg, Parker suggests 3.5 to 6.0 watt-seconds per kg. If the patient weighs more than 50 kg, the full output of the defibrillator is suggested.[26] Defibrillation can occur only if the synchronizer switch is off, because a QRS complex is required for synchronized defibrillation and ventricular fibrillation has no QRS complexes. After defibrillation, the cardiac monitor and pulse are checked for signs of restored sinus rhythm.

Cardioversion

Cardioversion is used to terminate arrhythmias that have QRS complexes and is usually an elective procedure. The patient is alert, and informed consent is obtained. The patient is usually given diazepam intravenously prior to cardioversion to promote anesthesia. The amount of voltage used varies from 25 to 400 watt-seconds. Digoxin is usually withheld for 48 hours prior to cardioversion to prevent postcardioversion arrhythmias.

The synchronizer is turned on. The defibrillator is synchronized with a cardiac monitor so that an electrical impulse is discharged during ventricular depolarization (the QRS complex). If the defibrillator were not synchronized, it could discharge during the vulnerable period (T wave)

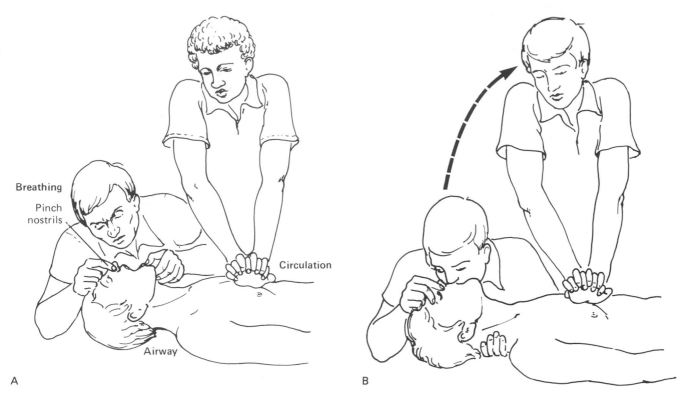

Breathing

Pinch nostrils

Circulation

Airway

A

B

Fig. 26-7. (**A**) Two-rescuer cardiopulmonary resuscitation: five chest compressions at a rate of 60/minute, with no pause for ventilation. One interposed lung inflation after every five chest compressions. (**B**) One-rescuer cardiopulmonary resuscitation: 15 chest compressions, at a rate of 80/minute, after two quick lung inflations. (After JAMA 227:846, 1974)

Fig. 26-8. Paddle placement in defibrillation (Brunner LS, Suddarth DS: Textbook of Medical—Surgical Nursing, p 536. Philadelphia, J B Lippincott, 1980)

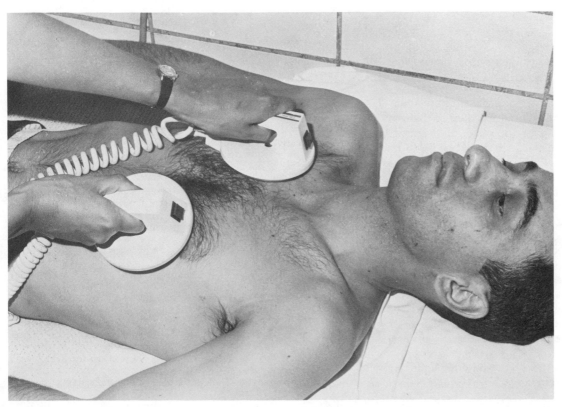

TABLE 26-9 ESSENTIAL DRUGS IN CPR

Drug	Purpose	Dosage	Side Effects and Comments
Oxygen	To correct hypoxia	4 to 10 liters/minute	No lung damage when used for less than 24 hours.
Sodium Bicarbonate (NaHCO₃)	To correct metabolic and respiratory acidosis	1 mg/kg intravenously (IV) initially. One half initial dose (0.5 mg/kg) given IV every 10 minutes. Analysis of arterial blood gases should guide treatment	$HCO_3^- + H^+ \rightleftarrows H_2CO_3 \rightleftarrows CO_2 + H_2O$ Since CO_2 production is increased, adequate ventilation is required. Excessive NaHCO₃ leads to metabolic alkalosis with displacement of oxyhemoglobin-dissociation curve and consequent impairment of oxygen release to tissues. Hyperosomolality may also develop. Catecholamines and calcium salts should not be added to bicarbonate infusions, because inactivation results. Since bicarbonate has a high pH, avoid mixing any drugs with it.
Epinephrine	To increase perfusion pressure during cardiac compressions (Chap. 35).	(See Chap. 35.)	(See Chap. 35.)
Atropine	To accelerate cardiac rate by: Creating a positive chronotrophic effect due to parasympatholytic action (reduces vagal tone); Creating a positive dromotropic effect that accelerates AV conduction	(See Chaps. 34 and 35.)	(See Chap. 34 and 35.)
Lidocaine	(See Chap. 34.)	(See Chap. 34.)	(See Chap. 34.)
Calcium chloride	To stimulate spontaneous or more forceful myocardial contractions by: Creating a positive inotropic effect; enhancing venticular excitability; prolonging systole	2.5–5 ml of 10% calcium chloride solution (3.4–6.8 mEq). May be repeated every 10 minutes. Calcium gluceptate 5 ml (4.5 mEq) Calcium gluconate (less ionized calcium volume) 10 ml of 10% solution (4.8 mEq)	Rapid intravenous injections can produce sinus bradycardia and sinus arrest. Calcium and digoxin are synergistic. Calcium and bicarbonate mixed form a precipitate carbonate; each should be given separately.[29,32]

(White RD: Essential drugs in emergency cardiac care. In American Heart Association Committee on Emergency Cardiac Care VII: 1–13, 1975)

and result in ventricular tachycardia or fibrillation. The synchronizer switch is therefore turned on so that the unit discharges immediately after the onset of the next QRS complex. The "discharge" buttons should be held until the synchronizer fires the defibrillator.

If ventricular fibrillation occurs after cardioversion, the defibrillator must be immediately recharged, the synchronizer turned off, and defibrillation repeated.[26] After use, the defibrillator should be turned off to prevent accidental discharge of the paddles. Oxygen flow should be stopped during precordial shock, if possible, to avoid the hazard of fire.

Indications of a successful response are conversion to sinus rhythm, strong peripheral pulses, and adequate blood pressure. Airway patency should be maintained and the patient's state of consciousness assessed. Vital signs should be obtained at least every 15 minutes for 1 hour, every 30 minutes for 2 hours, then every 4 hours.

Essential drugs used in CPR are outlined in Table 26-9. For an in-depth discussion of each, see Chapters 33 to 37.

REFERENCES

1. American Heart Association Subcommittee on Emergency Cardiac Care. *Standards for Cardiopulmonary Resuscitation (CPR) and Emergency Cardiac Care (ECC)*. JAMA (Suppl) 227:833–868, 1974
2. Brunner LS, Suddarth DS: Textbook of Medical–Surgical Nursing. Philadelphia, JB Lippincott, 1980
3. Col JJ, Weinberg SL: The incidence and mortality of intraventricular conduction defects in acute myocardial infarction. Am J Cardiol 29:344–350, 1972
4. Day HW: Acute coronary care—A five year report. Am J Cardiol 21:252–257, 1968
5. Eick RE, Singer LH, Solberg LE: Coronary occlusion: Effect on cellular electrical activity of the heart. Med Clin North Am 63(1):49–67, 1976
6. Ellis PD, Billings DM: Cardiopulmonary Resuscitation. St. Louis, C.V. Mosby, 1980
7. Fisch C: Self-assessment-aberrant conduction. Heart Lung 2(2):260–264, 1973
8. Foster WT: Principles of Acute Coronary Care. New York, Appleton-Century-Croft, 1976
9. Goldberg AH: Adjuncts for airway and breathing. Advanced

Cardiac Life Support, American Heart Association, II:1–16, 1975

10. Han J: Mechanisms of ventricular tachycardia associated with myocardial infarction. Am J Cardiol 24:800–813, 1969
11. Jacobson LB, Lester RM, Scheinman MM: Management of acute bundle branch block and bradyarrhythmias. Med Clin North Am 63(1):93–112, 1979
12. Julian DG, Valentine MD, Miller GG: Disturbances of rate, rhythm and conduction in acute myocardial infarction. Am J Med 37:915–927, 1964
13. Kastor JA, Goldreyer BN, Moore EN et al: Re-Entry—An important mechanism of cardiac arrhythmias. Cardiovasc Clin 6:111–135, 1974
14. Killip T: Arrhythmias in myocardial infarction. Med Clin North Am 60(2):223–244, 1975
15. Kleiger RE, Martin RF, Miller JP et al: Mortality of myocardial infarction treated in the coronary care unit. Heart Lung 4(2):215–226, 1975
16. Lasry JE, Glassner ML: Precordial Shock: Defibrillation—Cardioversion. San Diego County Heart Association, San Diego May, 1970
17. Lown B, Vassaux C, Hood WB et al: Unresolved problems in coronary care. Am J Cardiol 20:494–508, 1967
18. Luce JM, Cary JM, Ross BK et al: New developments in cardiopulmonary resuscitation. JAMA 244(12):1366–1370, 1980
19. Manual for Instructors of Basic Cardiac Life Support. Dallas, American Heart Association, 1977
20. Marriott HJL: Practical Electrocardiography, 6th ed. Baltimore, Williams & Wilkins Co, 1977
21. Marriott HJL: Workshop in Electrocardiography. Oldsmar, Tampa Tracings, 1972
22. Moe GK: Mechanisms of cardiac dysrhythmias. In Frohlick ED (ed): Pathophysiology: Altered Regulatory Mechanisms in Disease, 2nd ed, pp 83–102. Philadelphia, JB Lippincott, 1976
23. Mullins CB, Atkins JM: Prognosis and management of ventricular conduction blocks in acute myocardial infarction. Mod Concepts Cardiovasc Dis 45(10):129–133, 1976
24. Myerburg RJ, Lazzara R: Electrophysiologic basis of cardiac arrhythmias and conduction disturbance. Cardiovasc Clin 5:2–19, 1973
25. Neasman AR, Schobel RC, Lemberg L: Arrhythmias in the coronary care unit. VI. Physiologic bases for the use of antiarrhythmic drugs. Heart Lung 5:496–501, 1976
26. Parker R: Defibrillation and Synchronized Cardioversion, Advanced Cardiac Life Support, V:1–9. American Heart Association, 1975
27. Shillingford JP, Thomas M: Cardiovascular and pulmonary changes in patients with myocardial infarction treated in an intensive care and research unit. Am J Cardiol 20:484–493, 1967
28. Spence MI, Lemberg L: Arrhythmias in the coronary care unit. I. Physiologic bases of ectopic beats. Heart Lung 4:620–625, 1975
29. Surawicz B, Steffens T: Cardiac vulnerability. Cardiovasc Clin 5:160–181, 1973
30. Vismara LA, Miller RA, DeMaria AM et al: The treatment of ventricular arrhythmias: Evaluation of standard therapy and recent advances. Heart Lung 5(3):485–492, 1976
31. White RD: Essential drugs in emergency cardiac care. American Heart Association Committee on Emergency Cardiac Care, American Heart Association, VII:1–13, 1975
32. Zipes DP: The clinical significance of bradycardic rhythms in acute myocardial infarction. Am J Cardiol 24:814–825, 1969

ADDITIONAL READING

American Heart Association Subcommittee on Emergency Cardiac Care: Standards and guidelines for cardiopulmonary resuscitation (CPR) and emergency cardiac care (ECC). JAMA 244(5):453–509, 1980

Atkins JM, Leshin SJ, Blomquist G et al: Ventricular conduction block and sudden death in acute myocardial infarction. Potential indications for pacing. N Engl J Med 288:281–284, 1973
Col JJ, Weinberg SL: Factors affecting prognosis in acute myocardial infarction. Heart Lung 1:74–79, 1972
Cranefield PF, Wit AL, Hoffman BF: Genesis of cardiac arrhythmias. Circulation 47:190–204, 1973
DeSanctis RW, Block P, Hutter AM: Tachyarrhythmias in myocardial infarction. Circulation 45:681–702, 1972
Fisch C: Electrophysiologic basis of clinical arrhythmias. Heart Lung 3:51–56, 1974
Fisch C: Relation of electrolyte disturbances to cardiac arrhythmias. Circulation 47:408–419, 1973
Fozzard HA, DasGupta DS: Electrophysiology and the electrocardiogram. Mod Concepts Cardiovasc Dis XLIV(6):29–34, 1975
Hamer SS, Lemberg L: Supraventricular tachycardia that mimics ventricular tachycardia: Part I. Heart Lung 6(1):159–163, 1977
Hamer SS, Lemberg L: Supraventricular tachycardia that mimics ventricular tachycardia: Part II. Heart Lung 6(2):344–348, 1977
Hoffman BF, Rosen MR, Wit AL: Electrophysiology and pharmacology of cardiac arrhythmias. III. The causes and treatment cardiac arrhythmias. Part A. Am Heart J 89:115–122, 1975
James T: Pathogenesis of arrhythmias in acute myocardial infarction. Am J Cardiol 24:791–799, 1969
Josephson ME, Horowitz LN: Recurrent ventricular tachycardia: An electrophysiologic approach. Med Clin North Am 63(1):53–71, 1979
Jude JR: Cardiopulmonary resuscitation. In Shibel EM, Moser KM (eds): Respiratory Emergencies, pp 75–84. St Louis, C.V. Mosby, 1977
Lemberg L, Hamer S: Arrhythmias complicating an acute myocardial infarction: A self-teaching program. Heart Lung 5:576–584, 1976
Margolis JR, Wagner GS: Arrhythmias in Acute Myocardial. Dallas, American Heart Association, 1976
Massumi RA, Mason DT, Fabregas RA et al: Intraventricular aberrancy versus ventricular ectopy. Cardiovasc Clin 5:36–86, 1973
Neasman AR, Schobel RC, Lemberg L: Arrhythmias in the coronary care unit. II. Physiological bases of paroxysmal bradycardia-dependent AV block. Heart Lung 4:795–798, 1975
Neasman AR, Schobel RC, Lemberg L: Arrhythmias in the coronary care unit. III. Physiological bases of paroxysmal tachycardia-dependent AV block. Heart Lung 4:964–968, 1975
Neasman AR, Schobel RC, Lemberg L: Arrhythmias in the coronary care unit. IV. Physiologic bases of paroxysmal tachycardia-dependent bundle branch block. Heart Lung 5:139–142, 1976
Neasman AR, Schobel RC, Lemberg L: Arrhythmias in the coronary care unit. V. Physiologic bases of paroxysmal bradycardia-dependent bundle branch block. Heart Lung 5:322–325, 1976
Pelletier GB, Marriott HJ: Atrioventricular block: Incidence in acute myocardial infarction and determinants of its "degrees" Heart Lung 6:327–330, 1977
Peters RW, Scheinman MM: Emergency treatment of supraventricular tachycardia. Med Clin North Am 63(1):73–92, 1979
Resnekov L: Present status of electroversion in management of cardiac dysrhythmias. Circulation 47:1356–1363, 1973
Rosen KM: Junctional tachycardia. Mechanisms, diagnosis, differential diagnosis and management. Circulation 47:654–664, 1973
Rotman M, Wagner GS, Wallace AG: Bradyarrhythmias in acute myocardial infarction. Circulation 45:703–722, 1972
Sweetwood HM, Bloak JG: Aberrant conduction. Heart Lung 6(4):673–684, 1977
Talbot S, Dreifus LS: Characteristics of ventricular extrasystoles and their prognostic importance: A reappraisal of their method of classification. Chest 67(6):665–679, 1975
Vassalle M: Automaticity and automatic rhythms. Am J Cardiol 28:245–252, 1971
Zipes DP, Fisch C: Initiation of ventricular tachycardia. Arch Intern Med 128:988–990, 1971

27

Heart Failure

NANCY A. NILES, R.N., M.A., CCRN

and

ROBERT E. WILLS, M.D.

Heart failure, a serious complication of myocardial infarction (MI), occurs in approximately 60% to 70% of patients with arteriosclerotic disease.[19] Although the mortality rate from arrhythmias after MI has markedly decreased over the last several years, the rate of death due to heart failure has not been appreciably altered and remains close to 33%.[23] Heart failure is defined as a state in which the metabolic needs of the body are not met because of inadequate left ventricular function. After myocardial infarction, heart failure becomes evident with the loss of 20% to 25% of left ventricular mass.[17] If more than 40% of the myocardium is lost, severe heart failure, or cardiogenic shock, develops.[6,17] Congestive heart failure (CHF) occurs when the depressed cardiac output is associated with circulatory congestion, either in the pulmonary system, in the peripheral organs, or both. A series of complex hormonal alterations also occur, resulting in fluid retention.

This chapter will present the effect of an MI on cardiac function, including a discussion of the compensatory mechanisms that maintain cardiac output. As these mechanisms fail, cardiac output falls and heart failure ensues. The pathophysiologic changes, symptoms, physical findings, and nursing and medical therapeutic interventions for patients in left ventricular (LV) failure, pulmonary edema, right ventricular (RV) and biventricular failure, and cardiogenic shock will be presented.

CARDIAC DYSFUNCTION AFTER MYOCARDIAL INFARCTION

Immediately after MI changes in cardiac function take place. Initially, there is a reduction in contractility of the ischemic myocardium, contributing to a reduction in stroke volume.

Paradoxical movement of the central area of the ischemic myocardium also occurs within minutes after infarction. The ischemic myocardium is passively stretched during contraction of surrounding normal myocardium, causing a reduction in stroke volume and an increase in left ventricular end-diastolic volume (LVEDV), or preload (Chap. 2). The ejection fraction is thus reduced (Chap. 19). Ejection fraction can be directly measured by angiography, isotope scans, and in a limited sense, echocardiography.[31] An ejection fraction less than 66% indicates a reduction in contractility, synergy of contraction, or both.

Approximately 6 hours after MI, edema and fibrocellular infiltration results in stiffening of the ischemic myocardial wall. This stiffness helps to reduce paradoxical movement, improving stroke volume and reducing LVEDV. The ejection fraction is thus increased. Figure 27-1 summarizes these events.

Compensatory Mechanisms

The acute fall in cardiac output seen after MI lasts only seconds before several compensatory mechanisms begin to counteract this reduction. Immediately after MI, carotid sinus and aortic arch baroreceptors sense the fall in cardiac output, sending afferent impulses to medullary centers. These centers then increase sympathetic stimulation to the myocardium, while reducing parasympathetic activity. The heart is thus directly stimulated to increase contractility and heart rate, both of which raise cardiac output. These alterations result in increased myocardial oxygen consumption ($M\dot{V}O_2$), and have the potential of increasing myocardial ischemia. Refer to Chapter 2 for a discussion of factors affecting $M\dot{V}O_2$.

The peripheral arterioles constrict to maintain mean aortic pressure and thus coronary perfusion. The skin,

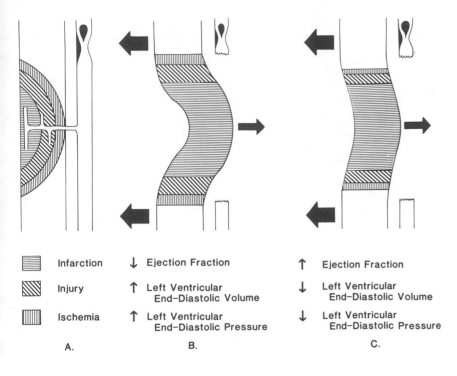

▥ Infarction	↓ Ejection Fraction	↑ Ejection Fraction
▨ Injury	↑ Left Ventricular End–Diastolic Volume	↓ Left Ventricular End–Diastolic Volume
▥ Ischemia	↑ Left Ventricular End–Diastolic Pressure	↓ Left Ventricular End–Diastolic Pressure
	A.	**B.**	**C.**

KEY: ⇆ : Indicate direction and extent of wall motion

↑ : Increased

↓ : Decreased

Fig. 27-1. Hemodynamic responses in acute myocardial infarction. (**A**) Acute spasm or thrombosis resulting in enlarging zones of ischemia, injury, and infarction. (**B**) Paradoxical movement and incomplete ventricular emptying. (**C**) Increased wall "stiffness" and improved ventricular emptying.

viscera, and kidneys are the predominant areas of vasoconstriction. This vasoconstriction shunts blood to the heart and brain, where circulation is crucial. The maintenance of an adequate circulating volume is also affected by peripheral vasoconstriction. Hydrostatic pressure is reduced in these vascular beds, favoring interstitial fluid return into the circulation. Excessive increases in peripheral vascular resistance due to vasoconstriction increase the resistance to LV ejection (afterload), and an increase in $M\dot{V}O_2$ and a decrease in cardiac output result (Fig. 27-2). Constriction in the venous beds also occurs as a result of sympathetic stimulation.

Another compensatory mechanism is an increase in preload, due to a reduction in contractility and an increase in venous return resulting from constriction of the venous vasculature; both of these mechanisms cause an elevation in LVEDV. Through the Frank-Starling mechanism, stroke volume improves as an increase in myocardial fiber stretch occurs from the increased preload (Chap. 2). The increase in intramyocardial tension, however, increases $M\dot{V}O_2$ and predisposes the myocardium to further injury.

An increase in circulating volume through reduced kidney salt and water excretion is a slower adjustment to increase cardiac output.[15,32] Sympathetic stimulation reduces total kidney blood flow. However, selective efferent arteriolar vasoconstriction, which occurs distal to the glomerulus, maintains glomerular filtration pressure and rate. Figure 27-3 shows the anatomic relationship of the glomerulus and

the efferent arteriole.[4] Efferent arteriolar vasoconstriction also reduces hydrostatic pressure in the peritubular capillaries. (Fig. 27-3). This decrease in hydrostatic pressure increases intravascular osmotic pressure, favoring the return of renal interstitial fluid to the capillaries.[8]

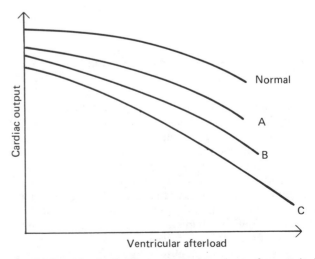

Fig. 27-2. Afterload effects on stroke volume. As ventricular afterload increases, in this case, total peripheral vascular resistance only, cardiac output falls. Increasing depression of contractility (curves **A, B,** & **C**) results in a greater reduction in cardiac output as afterload increases. (Mason DT et al: Hospital Formulary, 641–651, 1979)

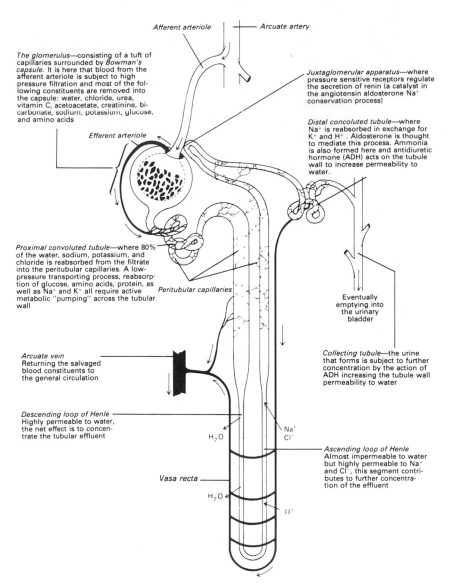

Afferent arteriole — Arcuate artery

The glomerulus—consisting of a tuft of capillaries surrounded by *Bowman's capsule*. It is here that blood from the afferent arteriole is subject to high pressure filtration and most of the following constituents are removed into the capsule: water, chloride, urea, vitamin C, acetoacetate, creatinine, bicarbonate, sodium, potassium, glucose, and amino acids

Juxtaglomerular apparatus—where pressure sensitive receptors regulate the secretion of renin (a catalyst in the angiotensin aldosterone Na⁺ conservation process)

Efferent arteriole

Distal concoluted tubule—where Na⁺ is reabsorbed in exchange for K⁺ and H⁺. Aldosterone is thought to mediate this process. Ammonia is also formed here and antidiuretic hormone (ADH) acts on the tubule wall to increase permeability to water.

Proximal convoluted tubule—where 80% of the water, sodium, potassium, and chloride is reabsorbed from the filtrate into the peritubular capillaries. A low-pressure transporting process, reabsorption of glucose, amino acids, protein, as well as Na⁺ and K⁺ all require active metabolic "pumping" across the tubular wall

Peritubular capillaries

Eventually emptying into the urinary bladder

Arcuate vein Returning the salvaged blood constituents to the general circulation

Collecting tubule—the urine that forms is subject to further concentration by the action of ADH increasing the tubule wall permeability to water

Descending loop of Henle Highly permeable to water, the net effect is to concentrate the tubular effluent

H_2O

Na^+ Cl^-

Ascending loop of Henle Almost impermeable to water but highly permeable to Na⁺ and Cl⁻, this segment contributes to further concentration of the effluent

Vasa recta

H_2O

H^+

Fig. 27-3. The juxtamedullary nephron. (Beland IL et al: *Clinical Nursing: Pathophysiological and Psychosocial Approaches*, 3rd ed, p 478. New York, Macmillan, 1975).

The renin-angiotensin-aldosterone system is the most important mechanism in the development of fluid retention to increase circulating volume. Reduced total kidney blood flow presumably stimulates the juxtaglomerular cells surrounding the afferent arteriole to release renin (Fig. 27-3).[8] Angiotensin II and aldosterone are end-products of renin secretion. Angiotensin II causes peripheral vasoconstriction, whch augments sympathetic nervous system stimulation in maintaining systemic arterial blood pressure; aldosterone causes tubular reabsorption of sodium chloride and water, which increases circulating volume. This system is discussed in greater detail in Chapters 6 and 9. Once circulating volume is sufficient to increase LVEDV, which in turn increases stroke volume and maintains mean arterial pressure, renin secretion declines.[8] If mean arterial pressure is not maintained, renin secretion continues, and volume expansion continues to elevate LVEDV, which increases the cardiac workload and predisposes the patient to pulmonary congestion.

Hypertrophy of the LV myocardium is an adjustment to a prolonged increase in myocardial tension.[18] Myocardial fiber diameter, and hence LV wall thickness, increases, augmenting ventricular contractile force. However, the coronary circulation does not concomitantly increase, and oxygen diffusion to the central area of hypertrophied muscle cells is reduced.

LEFT VENTRICULAR FAILURE

Left ventricular failure is a clinical term describing LV impairment as the primary derangement in cardiac function. Because the right and left ventricles, as well as the pulmonary system, are in circuit with one another, impairments of LV function will eventually affect the entire circuit. Heart failure can therefore be viewed as a continuum in which pathophysiologic changes and associated symptoms can be seen to progress. This progression can be rapid in onset or slow to develop. Because it is more difficult to conceptualize derangements of the entire circuit simultaneously, a categorized discussion of LV, pulmonary, and RV effects, as well as severe pump dysfunction, will be presented.

Pathophysiology of Left Ventricular Failure

When compensatory mechanisms fail to maintain cardiac output after MI, peripheral tissue demands for oxygen and nutrients are not met. Continued catecholamine secretion by the adrenal gland and release of nonepinephrine from myocardial stores attempt to maintain a state of increased contractility, but stroke volume remains depressed. Peripheral vasoconstriction of skin, viscera, and kidneys results in reduced perfusion and the initiation of anaerobic metabolism and lactic acid production.

Vasoconstriction of the renal efferent arterioles results in fluid retention by way of the mechanisms already discussed. Although aldosterone levels may be only slightly increased in mild LV failure, any reduction in systemic mean arterial pressure results in continued renin secretion.[6,13] The peripheral vasconstrictive effects of angiotensin II also continue to operate.

Increasing fluid retention in concert with venoconstriction continues to increase LV preload in an attempt to increase stroke volume via the Frank-Starling mechanism. However, this mechanism no longer adequately compensates for reduced ventricular contractility, so stroke volume falls. Left ventricular end-diastolic volume further increases, causing LV chamber dilation.

As LV function continues to deteriorate, LVEDV becomes increasingly elevated. The rise in LVEDV correlates with an increase in LV end-diastolic pressure (LVEDP), which is transmitted to the pulmonary capillary bed. This increase in hydrostatic pressure causes transudation of sodium and water into the pulmonary interstitium. The precise pressure needed to cause a shift of sodium and water into the interstitial space varies with the rapidity of the pressure rise, the concentration of the serum proteins, which determine osmotic pressure, and the capacity of the lymphatic drainage. With progressive increases in capillary hydrostatic pressure to approximately 18 to 25 mm Hg, salt and water move across the capillary membrane into the interstitial space.[14] Although plasma osmotic pressure (normally 25 mm Hg) may not be exceeded by this range of hydrostatic pressure, it is believed that other forces, one of which is subatmospheric interstitial hydrostatic pressure, tend to draw water into the interstitial space; lymphatic drainage and actual lung motion during respiration are most likely involved in this generation of negative interstitial fluid pressures.[26] Figure 27-4A and B shows the normal alveolar-capillary interface and the accumulation of interstitial fluid, respectively. Initially, the lymphatics transport this additional fluid away from the interstitial space. In addition, the interstitial protein concentration is reduced by dilution, favoring fluid movement back into the capillaries. When these mechanisms are overwhelmed, increased accumulation of interstitial fluid (Fig. 27-4C) leads to reduction in pulmonary compliance.

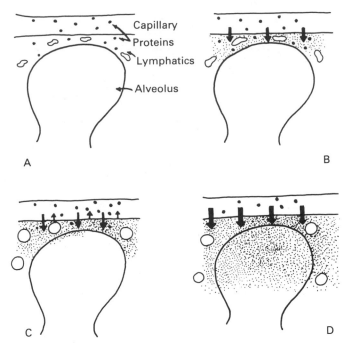

Fig. 27-4. Pulmonary congestion and edema. (**A**) Normal relationship. (**B**) Increased capillary hydrostatic pressure with increased movement of salt and water to the interstitial space. (**C**) Increased lymphatic flow with dilution of interstitial protein, favoring movement of salt and water back into the capillary. (**D**) Failure of compensatory mechanisms with intraalveolar edema. (Robin ED et al: N Engl J Med 288:243, 1973)

As LVEDP continues to rise, accumulation of pulmonary interstitial fluid progresses to intra-alveolar edema (Fig. 27-4D). Oxygen diffusion is retarded by alveolar fluid. Also, the ratio of ventilation to perfusion is sufficiently low that blood flow continues to perfuse underventilated, or gas exchanging, alveoli. Both effects result in a decrease in alveolar-capillary oxygen diffusion.

Assessing Patients in Left Ventricular Failure

Symptoms. Patients in LV failure are characterized by a decreased activity tolerance because of the reduction in stroke volume and peripheral organ perfusion. They frequently complain of fatigue that increases as the day progresses, the cause of which is a reduction in skeletal muscle perfusion and oxygenation. Some patients also complain of skeletal pain. Also contributing to the fatigue are disturbances in sleep patterns (discussed in Chap. 31).

Because coronary perfusion may be reduced, particularly in atherosclerotic vessels, patients may complain of chest pain. This is most likely to occur during exercise, when myocardial demands for oxygen are increased.

Physical Findings. Gradual increases in heart rate (HR) should alert the nurse to a possible progression of LV dysfunction. Observation of the HR response to exercise is also important, since the compromised myocardium is incapable of markedly augmenting stroke volume. Low stroke volume causes an immediate increase in HR as well as a sustained increase after the cessation of activity, resulting in an increased $M\dot{V}O_2$. Assessment of the patient's HR response to activities of daily living provides information about the patient's cardiovascular status, as well as information, with which to plan nursing care activities.

Because stroke volume is reduced, systolic blood pressure falls. Diastolic blood pressure is maintained, however, because of arteriolar vasoconstriction, which causes the pulse pressure to narrow. The maintenance of diastolic pressure helps to prevent a precipitous fall in mean arterial pressure, ensuring adequate coronary perfusion. In some patients diastolic blood pressure is elevated as a result of chronic hypertension, stress, or both. Isometric arm movements will temporarily raise the diastolic pressure, which increases LV afterload. The cardiac workload is thus increased and further reductions in stroke volume occur. Frequent blood pressure assessment, both of absolute values and trends, gives valuable information regarding LV function and the progression of failure.

In addition to a narrowing pulse pressure, a decrease in the strength of peripheral arterial pulsations is found, resulting from a reduced stroke volume. Pulsus alternans, alternating strong and weak pulsations, may also appear. This pattern of pulsations is produced by the alternation of strong and weak contractions of the LV, and results in a variable LVEDV which contributes to the appearance of gallop rhythms (Chap. 14).

Low-frequency vibrations and turbulence occur as blood enters the damaged, dilated ventricle. An S_4 gallop may be heard in the apical area and is caused by turbulence and low-frequency vibrations during atrial contraction which ejects blood into a noncompliant ventricle or ejects it against an area of the LV with reduced compliance. This heart sound alone may not be indicative of LV failure, because it is also associated with other types of cardiovascular damage or mechanical alteration (Chap. 14). An S_3 gallop heart sound, however, is particularly diagnostic of LV failure. It is heard in the apical area as blood passively enters the dilated ventricle during diastole. Frequently premature ventricular contractions (PVCs) are often seen because of the increased myocardial fiber stretch associated with LV dilation. Ventricular dilation can be detected on a chest radiograph and by lateral displacement of the point of maximal impulse on the precordium (Chap. 14).

The signs signaling reduced coronary artery perfusion may include arrhythmias or ECG changes indicating worsening ischemia or extending infarction, as well as the symptom of chest pain. Displacement of the ST segment may be seen on the monitor during episodes of chest pain. However, the ST segment changes seen can serve only as a clue to obtain a standard 12-lead ECG, since a monitoring lead is not standardized.

Skin perfusion is also reduced as a result of adrenergic stimulation. Skin temperature is reduced and the vasoconstriction may cause the patient's general appearance to become dusky.

Reduced peripheral perfusion results in anaerobic metabolism and the production of lactic acid, causing metabolic acidosis (Chap. 9). Arterial blood gases reveal a lowered bicarbonate as the body attempts to buffer the excess hydrogen ions to maintain pH. If the pH begins to fall, the patient may hyperventilate. This hyperventilation compensates for the increased acidity by lowering arterial carbon dioxide tensions, causing a mild respiratory alkalosis which helps to normalize pH.

Because saline and water excess occurs in LV failure, patients frequently show a gradual weight gain. Daily weights should be obtained before breakfast, and the same scale should be used from day to day to increase the reliability of measurement. Fluid intake and output recordings are also necessary to assess fluid balance and to enable the nurse to be aware of intravenous fluid administration associated with intravenous drug therapy, a factor often underestimated. Pitting edema may be seen in dependent areas, such as the sacral area when patients are on bedrest. Because its appearance is most commonly associated with right ventricular failure, it will be more extensively discussed in that section.

Hemodynamic Measurements. Forrester and others have organized changes in hemodynamic function into four subsets which correspond to varying degrees of heart failure.[12,13] Cardiac output is expressed as cardiac index, in $l/min/M^2$, which enables a comparison of output values between patients of different heights by correcting for body surface area; a normal value for cardiac index is 3.5 $l/min/M^2$. Although patients with LV failure have a reduction in cardiac index, values remain above 2.2 $l/min/M^2$. Patients without pulmonary congestion, as may occur in the early stages of disease, have pulmonary artery wedge (PAW) pressures less than 18 mm Hg, and are assigned to Subset I (Chap. 19). These patients usually continue to be hemodynamically stable and usually survive hospitalization.[12]

Symptoms of Pulmonary Congestion. Patients with increasing LVEDV, and therefore LVEDP, complain of dyspnea which is due to pulmonary interstitial fluid accumulation and a resultant decrease in pulmonary compliance. During the initial increase in pulmonary artery hydrostatic pressure, patients may complain of shortness of breath, primarily during exercise when oxygen demands are increased. Others may become dyspneic at rest, while in a supine position, because their ventricles are not adequately able to pump the increased venous return. Since this complaint frequently occurs at night when the patient lies down to sleep, it is called *paroxysmal nocturnal dyspnea*.[29] A more unusual symptom is dyspnea associated with hypotension and reduced myocardial perfusion while the patient assumes a left lateral recumbent position.[23] The physiologic mechanism causing this effect is unknown.

Physical Findings of Pulmonary Congestion. An increase in respiratory rate is associated with complaints of dyspnea in an effort to maintain adequate arterial oxygenation. This mechanism becomes less efficient as alveoli become fluid-filled, however, and is responsible for a lowered arterial carbon dioxide tension, causing respiratory alkalosis (Chap. 9).

Intra-alveolar edema is recognized by crackles in dependent lung fields, as fluid accumulates in areas most affected by gravity. Changes in the patient's position, therefore, affect fluid distribution and must be considered when auscultating lung fields. Using water-soluble ink to mark the level on the patient's back where crackles are first heard is one method of ensuring comparable assessments between nursing personnel on different shifts. Chest radiographs show blood flow redistribution to the upper lung lobes, with perivascular and intra-alveolar edema (Chap. 16).[12]

A dry, hacking cough often accompanies intra-alveolar edema because of irritation of the small airways. Generally, the cough is nonproductive because the distal alveolar fluid is too deep to expectorate. Wheezing may also be heard, and is due to interstitial fluid compression on the small airways. Infrequently, and predominantly in elderly patients, Cheyne-Stokes respiration may be seen.[23] This response may be due to reduced cerebral perfusion, causing an altered neurogenic response.[18,25]

Hemodynamic Measurements. Patients with a reduction in cardiac index as in Subset I, but with pulmonary congestion and intra-alveolar edema as well, are described by Forrester's Clinical Subset II.[12,13] Their PAW pressures are elevated above 18 mm Hg, and the mortality rate for this group of hospitalized patients with MI is approximately 10%.[12]

Therapy for Patients with LV Failure

One of the goals of therapy is the improvement of activity tolerance by the reduction of cardiac work and the increase in stroke volume.

Nursing Interventions. Goals for nursing in caring for the patient with LV dysfunction include: providing a restful environment, preventing fatigue, and reducing stress in order to prevent continuing increases in catecholamine production and release, which raise $M\dot{V}O_2$ by increasing heart rate and blood pressure. Placing patients in private rooms is preferred to placing them in wards, because it reduces stress caused by environmental noise and the activities of nursing personnel attending to other patients. Other nursing interventions to reduce stress are discussed in Chapter 22.

Data obtained from heart rate responses to activities of daily living should be used to develop individualized nursing care plans so that activity modification can be carried out. For instance, if the patient's HR increases during bathing and remains elevated for 10 minutes following delivery of care, other treatments should be deferred until the HR has fallen to preactivity levels. Blood pressure responses to activity should also be used for planning the method of care delivery. Specifically, isometric arm movements should be discouraged so as to prevent increases in blood pressure, and therefore, afterload (Chap. 23).

Because patients with LV failure frequently have generalized fatigue which increases as the day progresses, comfort measures such as bathing should be performed early in the day. Asking patients abut their degree of fatigue following specific procedures of nursing care measures enables pertinent nursing care plan changes.

Medical Interventions. If psychologic supportive measures are insufficient in reducing anxiety as determined by persistently elevated HR or blood pressure, patient complaints,

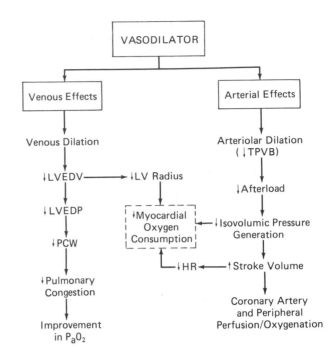

Key: LVEDV = Left ventricular end-diastolic volume
LVEDP = Left ventricular end-diastolic pressure
PCW = Pulmonary capillary wedge pressure
HR = Heart rate
TPVR = Total peripheral vascular resistance

Fig. 27-5. Arterial and venous effects of vasodilators. LVEDV = Left ventricular end-diastolic volume; LVEDP = left ventricular end-diastolic pressure; PCW = pulmonary capillary wedge pressure; HR = heart rate; TPVR = total peripheral vascular resistance.

or family assessments, the periodic use of tranquilizers may be indicated (Chaps. 33, 44).

The use of morphine sulfate or sublingual nitroglycerin to relieve chest pain is necessary to prevent increases in $M\dot{V}O_2$ and the extension of infarction. Hypotension may result from administration of these drugs secondary to a reduction in preload (Chap. 34). However, in patients with heart failure, preload reduction has less effect on stroke volume than in patients with normal myocardial contractility. The effects of preload reduction in hearts with normal and depressed contractility is shown in Figure 27-5. With invasive hemodynamic monitoring by use of a thermodilution pulmonary artery catheter, cardiac function curves can be plotted. Without invasive monitoring, blood pressure response to drug therapy remains the best method of evaluation.

A digitalis glycoside is often used to increase contractility and, therefore, stroke volume. Although increases in myocardial contractility increase $M\dot{V}O_2$, the improved stroke volume and ejection fraction reduce intramyocardial tension and thus increase perfusion and oxygen delivery to the peripheral tissues. A reduction in resting HR and a decreased HR response to exercise indicates improved LV function. Digitalis therapy may be only partially effective in increasing stroke volume, because drug effectiveness declines with increasing LV dysfunction.[13] Drug action, dosages, and side effects of digitalis preparation are discussed in Chapter 34.

Other drug therapy includes the irradication of arrhythmias to prevent decreases in stroke volume (Chap. 34). Chronic or acute hypertension must also be treated to decrease $M\dot{V}O_2$. Several vasodilating agents, such as hydralazine and prazosin, are available (Chap. 37).

Intravenous fluid therapy should be kept to a minimum. Because patients with LV failure have a decreased renal ability to excrete sodium, only 5% Dextrose in water maintenance intravenous solutions should be used. Even more advantageous is the insertion of a herapin lock, which enables periodic drug administration without excessive fluid intake. Dietary sodium restriction is also necessary to prevent increases in circulating volume (Chap. 22).

Pulmonary Congestion

Patients with dyspnea secondary to pulmonary congestion and intra-alveolar edema require interventions to increase the ease of breathing.

Nursing Interventions. Dyspnea may be partially relieved by placing patients in a semi-Fowler's position. Diaphragmatic descent during inspiration is thus facilitated, enabling more effective alveolar ventilation in the basilar lung areas. Frequent determination of respiratory rate, subjective complaints of dyspnea, and the degree of head elevation for comfort are necessary in evaluating the progression of disease, the effectiveness of therapy, or both.

Patients with intra-alveolar edema are likely to develop atalectasis and pneumonia. Frequent turning and the use of incentive spirometry every hour help to prevent these complications.

Medical Interventions. Patients with the clinical evidence of pulmonary congestion and edema, or those with PCW pressures greater than 18 mm Hg, require diuretics. Intravascular volume will then decrease, as will the blood return to the pulmonary system (Chap. 33). The therapeutic benefits include: increased ease of breathing, reduction in crackles, disappearance of gallop rhythm, a reduction in weight, and a reduction in PAW pressure. Although PAW pressure may shortly return to normal, complete disappearance of crackles and chest radiograph changes may take up to 48 hours.[12] Overzealous administration of diuretics can cause intravascular saline deficit that must be monitored by taking postural blood pressure and HR measurements (Chaps. 14, 30, 37). Serum potassium levels may also fall and should be checked daily.

Patients with pulmonary edema, congestion, or both, are frequently hypoxemic from impaired alveolar-capillary oxygen diffusion. With mild arterial hypoxemia, low-flow oxygen administered by nasal cannula may adequately raise arterial oxygen tensions. Humidification is not usually necessary at flow rates of 1–2 l/minute.[35] However, for flow rates of 5–6 l/minute, which cause drying of the mucous membranes and predispose the patient to infection and discomfort, humidification should be used. Arterial blood gas determinations should be made frequently to assess the effects of oxygen therapy on arterial oxygenation; they should also be done after changes are made in delivered oxygen concentrations. The normal values of arterial blood gases and the technique of obtaining blood samples are given in Chapters 15 and 21.

ACUTE PULMONARY EDEMA

Pathophysiology of Acute Pulmonary Edema

Sudden increases in LVEDP, or the delayed treatment of slowly developing intra-alveolar edema, can result in acute, fulminating, pulmonary edema. Accumulation of alveolar fluid becomes more extensive, resulting in a greater lung area with a low ventilation-to-perfusion ratio. As some alveoli become completely fluid-filled, and blood flows by nonventilating alveoli, the degree of shunt increases. Both effects result in further lowering of the arterial oxygen tension.[2,27,29] Because of the extensive fluid accumulation, alveolar hypoventilation with carbon dioxide retention may also occur.

The increased accumulation of pulmonary interstitial fluid can also impair gas exchange by compressing small airways. This fluid accumulation also compresses the pulmonary vasculature, resulting in pulmonary hypertension. In addition, reflex pulmonary arteriolar vasoconstriction of vessels perfusing poorly ventilated, and therefore hypoxic, alveoli also contributes to the development of hypertension. Right ventricular (RV) afterload is thus increased and myocardial oxygen demand elevated. If afterload increases markedly, RV failure may occur.

Sympathetic stimulation of the heart and peripheral vessels continues and may increase if cardiac output begins to fall. Increased stimulation intensifies $M\dot{V}O_2$ by its effect on afterload, further compromising stroke volume. In acute, fulminating pulmonary edema, cardiac output may fall only slightly or may become significantly depressed. This variability in response is dependent on the degree of cardiac reserve following MI and the effectiveness of cardiac compensatory mechanisms. If myocardial infarction is extensive, pulmonary edema may develop rapidly and the compensatory mechanisms may be insufficient to maintain cardiac output.

Assessing Patients with Acute Pulmonary Edema

Symptoms. Patients with acute pulmonary edema are extremely dyspneic and orthopneic. These symptoms are accompanied by extreme anxiety and an impending sense of doom.

Physical Findings. Diffuse rhonchi and crackles are generally heard throughout the lung fields. A productive cough with frothy sputum is often present. Hemoptysis may also occur as blood cells migrate with plasma into the alveoli as a result of markedly elevated arterial pressures.[24] Bronchospasm, due to interstitial fluid compression on small airways, results in wheezing.

Arterial blood gases show worsening hypoxemia. If sufficient hyperventilation occurs in unaffected alveoli, arterial carbon dioxide tension may be lower than normal, causing a respiratory alkalosis; but in most cases, the majority of lung units are affected. Alveolar hypoventilation then causes a rise in arterial carbon dioxide tension and results in a fall in pH.[27] Peripheral hypoperfusion and lactic acid production also changes the pH.

Patients with fulminating pulmonary edema are often markedly tachycardic and hypertensive as a result of intense sympathetic stimulation. If cardiac output falls markedly, hypotension may occur even with intense vasoconstriction. An S_3 gallop is heard and may be accompanied by an S_4 gallop. Because of the persistent tachycardia, the S_3 and S_4 gallops may coincide, resulting in a louder summation gallop (Chap. 14).

Cerebral perfusion may be reduced if stroke volume falls. In any case, oxygen delivery to the cerebrum is impaired because of poor pulmonary gas exchange, resulting in confusion, restlessness, loss of memory, and a decreased attention span. Evaluation of the patient's level of alertness, appropriateness of response, and the presence of extreme restlessness is important in estimating cerebral perfusion and oxygenation, and should be ascertained as frequently as every five minutes, because changes can occur rapidly.

The intense sympathetic-mediated vasoconstriction and decreased cardiac output result in poor peripheral perfusion. The skin is cool and clammy, and often cyanotic. If cardiac output falls significantly, vasoconstriction of the renal afferent arterioles causes a reduction in glomerular filtration rate. Urine output falls and sodium and water are retained. The result is an increase in circulating blood volume with elevated plasma creatinine and blood urea nitrogen (BUN) values. These serum values increase because urinary excretion of these substances is reduced.[8]

Hemodynamic Findings. Patients with acute pulmonary edema are described by Forrester's Clinical Subset II, with PAW pressure frequently exceeding 30 mm Hg.[12] Patients in whom cardiac index falls precipitously to levels below 2.2 l/min/M[2] are described by Forrester's Clinical Subset IV[12,13] and will be discussed in the section on "Cardiogenic Shock."

Therapy for Patients with Acute Pulmonary Edema

The goals of therapy are the immediate relief of dyspnea and the improvement of arterial oxygenation, because this condition constitutes a medical emergency.

Nursing Interventions. A reduction in RV preload and therefore in blood flow to the pulmonary vasculature can be accomplished with the patient sitting on the bed in an upright position with feet dangling, or seated in a chair. A bedside table placed in front of a patient sitting on the edge of the bed imparts a sense of security and prevents a fall.

Assuring patients that specific therapies will ease their breathing may be helpful in partially alleviating anxiety until medical interventions have decreased PAW pressures and improved arterial oxygenation. Because patients suffer from reduced mentation, staying with them at all times is necessary to ensure their safety.

Medical Interventions. Diuretic therapy in the form of an intravenous preparation is necessary to reduce circulating volume and PAW pressures rapidly. Frequently, furosemide is given in this manner. Maximal diuresis occurs in 30 to 60 minutes. An additional benefit is the peripheral venous dilation which occurs within five minutes after administration and which helps to reduce RV preload. The expected result of therapy should be some ease in breathing and a decrease in PAW pressures within minutes.

Morphine sulfate is a particularly useful drug in the treatment of acute pulmonary edema. Anxiety is reduced and peripheral venous dilation occurs. Although morphine sulfate does reduce the rate and depth of respirations, it also directly relaxes the airway smooth muscle and thereby facilitates gas transport.[26] Other dilating drugs that increase venous capacitance and therefore reduce RV preload include nitroglycerin and isosorbide dinitrate (Chap. 36).

The use of rotating tourniquets is an older method of preload reduction. Pressure cuffs applied to the extremities trap the blood in the limbs so that venous return is reduced. Phlebotomy, in which 250 ml to 500 ml of blood is removed, reduces intravascular volume, which in turn affects preload. Both these therapies, however, have been largely replaced by the use of rapid-acting diuretics.

Afterload reduction in normotensive patients with increased total peripheral vascular resistance has been shown to improve cardiac function and increase LV output.[13,21] Hydralazine is one drug that causes arterial vasodilation and results in a reduction of LV afterload. Nitroprusside and prazosin have both arterial and venous vasodilating effects (Chap. 36). The effects of arteriolar and venous dilating agents on the pulmonary and cardiovascular systems are presented in Figure 27-5.

As arterial hypoxemia worsens, high oxygen concentrations become necessary. Warmed humidified oxygen can be delivered in a variety of concentrations with a nebulizer. This method of administration prevents mucous membrane dehydration.[30] The patient must wear a face mask if oxygen is administered in this manner. Because face masks do not fit adequately, room air (21% oxygen concentration) mixes with the delivered oxygen and the oxygen concentration actually received by the patient may not be the same as that for which the nebulizer is set. However, measurement of arterial blood gases is the most accurate method of evaluating arterial oxygenation regardless of exact oxygen concentrations delivered.

Many patients complain of claustrophobia while wearing masks and they frequently remove them, an action which may cause a drop in arterial oxygenation. Face masks must also be removed to cough up secretions and during eating and oral drug administration. The use of low-flow oxygen by way of a nasal cannula, in addition to oxygen administration with a face mask may help to prevent arterial oxygenation from falling precipitously during these times. Non-rebreathing masks can be used to deliver oxygen concentrations higher than those delivered by heated nebulizers; this method most closely approximates 100% oxygen delivery without intubation. If arterial blood gases show worsening hypoxemia in spite of these measures, or if carbon dioxide tensions remain elevated with an acid pH, the patient may require intubation and mechanical ventilation. Patient management during mechanical ventilation will be presented in the section "Cardiogenic Shock."

Bronchodilators are necessary to improve gas transport through the airways and into the distal alveoli. Aminophylline is often used for this purpose. It also increases myocardial contractility and decreases afterload to some degree.[26] However, aminophylline can predispose the patient to the development of arrhythmias and a constant lookout should be kept for this effect. Breathing should be eased, wheezing decreased, and arterial blood gas values improved.

RIGHT VENTRICULAR AND BIVENTRICULAR FAILURE

Pathophysiology of Right Ventricular and Biventricular Failure

In the context of acute MI of the left ventricle, RV dysfunction may follow the progression of LV failure and pulmonary edema, and result in a state of biventricular congestive heart failure. Biventricular failure can also occur in patients with chronic LV dysfunction.

On the other hand, failure of the RV can occur without LV damage. Causative factors include infarction of the RV, chronic obstructive pulmonary disease (Chap. 51), massive pulmonary emboli (Chap. 28), and tricuspid or pulmonary valve dysfunction (Chap. 48).

Regardless of the underlying cause, sustained or sudden, severe increases in pulmonary arterial pressure cause RV dysfunction because of the increased afterload. This increase causes a reduction in the RV ejection fraction, hence an increase in right ventricular end-diastolic volume (RVEDV) and a decrease in RV stroke volume.[18] As RVEDV continues to increase, right atrial and systemic venous pressures rise. Peripheral edema follows, because of this elevation in venous hydrostatic pressure. Hepatomegaly, splenomegaly, and mesenteric venous congestion also occur.

In biventricular failure, fluid retention becomes increasingly severe. Left ventricular dysfunction reduces renal arterial blood flow setting into motion the renin–angiotensin–aldosterone mechanism. Engorgement of the hepatic vein, due to RV failure, retards hepatic blood flow, interfering with the metabolic degradation of aldosterone in the liver; circulating levels of aldosterone are thus increased, favoring continued sodium and water retention.[8,13]

Finally, as RV failure progresses and stroke volume falls, perfusion through the pulmonary vasculature is reduced. This effect alleviates pulmonary congestion through a reduction in pulmonary artery hydrostatic pressure.[21]

Assessment of the Patient with Right Ventricular or Biventricular Failure

Symptoms. Patients with RV failure frequently complain of swelling of the lower extremeties. Shoes become tight and mobility may be impaired. They may gain as much as 10 lb of extracellular fluid before pitting edema becomes readily apparent, however.[15,24]

Hepatic engorgement, due to venostasis, is associated

with right upper quadrant abdominal pain because of stretching of Glisson's capsule, which surrounds the liver. Complaints of poor appetite, nausea, abdominal distention, and a sense of fullness after meals is associated with edema of the bowel, which alters gastrointestinal function.

Patients with biventricular failure may complain less of dyspnea and orthopnea than those with only LV failure, because increasing RV failure reduces RV stroke volume. Pulmonary congestion caused by LV failure is thus reduced as blood flow to the pulmonary system decreases.

Physical Findings. As RVEDV increases, dilation of the RV chamber can be seen on a chest radiograph. Low-frequency vibrations and turbulence may cause a RV S_3 gallop sound, which can best be auscultated along the left sternal border (Chap. 14). Ventricular chamber dilation also produces a sternal heave, which becomes more pronounced as the right ventricle hypertrophies in chronic heart failure (Chap. 14).[18] Arrhythmias associated with RV and right atrial dilation include PVCs, premature atrial contractions, and atrial fibrillation, all of which compromise cardiac output.

As right atrial pressures continue to rise, the jugular veins distend. Central venous pressure (CVP) can be directly measured by assessing jugular vein distention from the phlebostatic level (Chap. 14, Fig. 14-1). Direct CVP measurement is consistently more accurate than neck vein assessment, especially when more than one person does the measurement (Chap. 21).

Hepatic engorgement alters the results of liver function tests; it elevates the serum glutamic-oxaloacetic transaminase (SGOT), bilirubin, and alkaline phosphatase levels. Some patients may also become jaundiced. Hepatojugular reflux is present on physical examination, indicating a persistent rise in jugular venous pressure and is diagnostic of RV failure (Chap. 14).

Interference with the patient's nutritional status due to poor gastrointestinal absorption[16] prolongs myocardial healing. Because of poor appetite and impaired liver function, patients may have low serum albumin levels. This effect, associated with peripheral venostasis, contributes to the development of ascites, an effect generally seen in severe and chronic RV failure.

Fluid extravasation into the pleural space, most commonly on the right side, causes atalectasis of regional alveolar units. Dullness on percussion and reduced breath sounds are heard over the affected area. "Ee" to "ay" changes (an "ay" sound is auscultated while the patient says "ee") are heard directly over the area of pleural effusion when underlying alveoli are compressed. The best method of diagnosing pleural effusion is by comparing upright anteroposterior and lateral chest radiographs to observe for fluid levels. At times, basilar lung infiltrates may make a positive diagnosis of pleural effusion difficult; in this instance, a lateral decubitus radiograph may show the fluid level more clearly. A thorough assessment of breath sounds should be performed at least every four hours, with the patient, if clinically stable, in a sitting position. If respiratory distress, worsening hypoxemia, or an increased body temperature occurs, thoracentesis to remove pleural fluid should be performed to improve alveolar expansion and reduce the chance of infection.

Pericardial effusion may occur and is noted by a fall in blood pressure and the appearance of pulsus paradoxus. As the pericardial constriction increases, RVEDP, mean right atrial pressure, pulmonary diastolic pressure, mean left atrial pressure, and LVEDP approximate each other (Chap. 21).

Although antidiuretic hormone (ADH) secretion is not considered to have a major role in causing edema, patients with severe congestive heart failure or after excessive diuresis, will retain excess water, seen as a lowered serum sodium level.[8] Daily electrolyte measurements are therefore important (Chap. 9).

Patients with biventricular failure have the symptoms and physical findings of LV failure, as well as the findings of RV failure described here.

Therapy for Patients with Right Ventricular or Biventricular Failure

The goals of therapy are the reduction of peripheral edema and organ engorgement through the reduction of RV preload and circulating volume, and the prevention of complications due to venostasis.

Nursing Interventions. Decreased skin and subcutaneous blood flow and edema in the legs predispose patients to the development of decubitus ulcers. Scrupulous skin care and frequent turning are important nursing interventions in preventing this complication. Alternating pressure mattresses, "egg-shell" mattresses, or sheepskins are also helpful.

Because patients are often anorexic, frequent small meals rather than three larger meals may be helpful in ensuring adequate nutrition. Teaching dietary restrictions (Chaps. 22, 43), activity modifications (Chap. 42), and drug actions and side effects (Chaps. 33–39) is particularly important to patients with chronic RV or biventricular failure. The general principles of patient and family teaching are discussed in Chapter 45.

Medical Interventions. Diuretics are used to reduce circulating volume, and therefore edema; dietary sodium restriction is also necessary. Digitalis is used to maximize cardiac output. Medications to eradicate arrhythmias and relieve chest pain are necessary to ensure adequate peripheral perfusion and to lower $M\dot{V}O_2$. Oxygen therapy should be based on the patient's arterial blood gas values. These therapies have all been discussed in previous sections.

Patients with congestive heart failure have an increased risk of developing deep venous thrombosis, which can cause a pulmonary embolus.[33] Because patients with RV or biventricular failure suffer from peripheral venostasis, as well as immobility due to their decreased activity tolerance, prophylactic, low-dose intermittent heparin therapy is indicated to prevent deep venous thrombus formation. Subcutaneous heparin, administered in dosages of 5,000 units every 8 to 12 hours, is generally prescribed.[33] Oral preparation, such as Coumadin, may be indicated for patients with chronic heart failure (Chap. 38).

Patients with biventricular failure also require therapy for LV failure.

CARDIOGENIC SHOCK

Approximately 15% of patients who have an acute MI develop cardiogenic shock.[6,15,28] The mortality rate for patients in cardiogenic shock ranges from 60% to 85%,[6,12,19] and postmortem examinations have shown that often more than 40% of the LV mass is involved.[6,17] A simple, massive MI, or a small MI in an already damaged heart, may precipitate shock.

Pathophysiology of Cardiogenic Shock

Cardiogenic shock represents a state of circulatory failure due to severe depression of myocardial contractility in which cardiac output is markedly depressed. At this time, none of the compensatory mechanisms of increased HR, increased preload, increased sympathetic mediated vasoconstriction, and increased contractility further facilitate cardiac function. However, the deleterious effects of increased $M\dot{V}O_2$ still operate.

Most patients in cardiogenic shock have an elevation of systemic vascular resistance[19] above the normal value: 1130 dynes/sec/cm^{-5} ± 178.[3] Left ventricular afterload becomes increasingly elevated, further compromising LV ejection. The intense vasoconstriction reduces perfusion to the skin and kidneys, and anaerobic glycolysis and lactic acid production is accelerated. The resultant metabolic acidosis further depresses myocardial contractility.[5]

Although the increase in systemic vascular resistance should help coronary arterial perfusion by raising mean aortic pressure, this seldom occurs, because cardiac output is so markedly depressed. Coronary perfusion is also dependent on the pressure gradient, or difference, between right atrial and mean aortic pressures; a wider difference facilitates perfusion. Because right atrial pressure may be elevated because of associated RV failure, this pressure gradient and coronary perfusion are likely to be reduced. Also, increases in HR due to sympathetic stimulation reduce diastolic filling time of the coronary arteries, which further interferes with myocardial perfusion.

As shock continues, intramyocardial norepinephrine stores are reduced and a reduction in adrenal catecholamine secretion interferes with sympathetic stimulation of the heart and the peripheral arterioles.[19] Thus, cardiac output continues to fall and blood pools in the peripheral vasculature, further reducing cardiac output. Unless output is increased by therapeutic measures, a progressive reduction in cellular function occurs in all organs, resulting in irreversible injury and eventual death of the patient.

Assessment of Patients with Cardiogenic Shock

Physical Findings. Patients in cardiogenic shock have systemic arterial systolic pressures of less than 90 mm Hg, or 30 mm Hg below preexisting levels. Reduced perfusion renders measurement by cuff pressures difficult, and often inaccurate because blood flow is markedly reduced and the Korotkoff sounds are faint. Doppler pressures may facilitate auscultation, but invasive arterial pressure monitoring is the most accurate (Chap. 20).

Mean arterial pressures below 65 mm Hg result in a precipitous fall in coronary arterial perfusion; in stenotic arteries, however, perfusion may fall at pressures higher than 65 mm Hg.[19] Increased myocardial damage occurs as perfusion falls. Electrocardiographic changes of ischemia or infarction, chest pain, and arrhythmias may be precipitated at this time as a result of myocardial acidemia.

Heart rate is generally elevated because of sympathetic stimulation. However, the initial HR response to shock may be inappropriately slow, representing an early reflex parasympathetic response to ischemia.[15]

Pulmonary artery and PAW pressures, as well as central venous pressures, are usually elevated because of severe biventricular dysfunction. Occasionally, some patients will have abnormally low PAW pressures and hypoperfusion which are due to hypovolemia.

Thermodilution cardiac output measurement is ideal for monitoring LV function. Mixed venous blood oxygen saturation can also be measured to indicate trends in cardiac output, although exact values of cardiac output are not obtained. A blood sample is obtained from the pulmonary artery to measure oxygen saturation of mixed venous blood and to compare it with oxygen saturation in arterial blood drawn simultaneously. Normal oxygen saturation values of mixed venous blood range from 70% to 75%. Oxygenation values below 65% reflect a decreased cardiac output. This fall in oxygen saturation values in the mixed venous blood occurs because oxygen is increasingly extracted in peripheral tissues to compensate for the reduced blood flow per minute.[1]

Pulmonary congestion and intra-alveolar edema may cause crackles, rhonchi, and wheezing. Evaluation of breath sounds in the posterior bases is difficult in these patients because of hypotension. Placing them in a sitting position during auscultation is contraindicated, since this can precipitate further falls in blood pressure. Turning them from side to side facilitates examination, although the lower most lung will have less alveolar gas exchange because gravity increases intra-alveolar fluid in that lung. Thus, comparisons of breath sound intensity and quality are made more difficult. Upright chest radiographs are also contraindicated.

Arterial blood gases show worsening hypoxemia. Carbon dioxide tensions may be reduced or elevated and are related to alveolar hyperventilation or hypoventilation, respectively. A metabolic acidosis occurs because of reduced peripheral perfusion; this effect is quite pronounced and pH is rarely compensated by effective alveolar hyperventilation.

Reduced kidney perfusion results in oliguria, with less than 30 ml of urine production per hour. Foley catheter placement enables observation of hourly urine output, and changes are associated with altered cardiac function. As cardiac output falls, so does urine output. Serum BUN and creatinine levels are elevated because of reduced glomerular filtration. Daily blood samples should thus be examined.

As cardiac output falls, a reduction in cerebral perfusion occurs and patients become confused, apathetic, and disoriented to time, place, and person. Noting the appropriateness of the patient's response to questions regarding the month, year, and location enables the nurse to assess the presence of cerebral hypoperfusion and the need for safety measures, which will be discussed under "Nursing Interventions."

Reduced skin perfusion is noted by cool, diaphoretic skin, often with a mottled appearance. Symptoms associated with a reduction in liver and gastrointestinal perfusion have been discussed in the section on "Right Ventricular and Biventricular Failure."

Hemodynamic Findings. Patients in cardiogenic shock are described by Forrester's Clinical Subset IV. Their cardiac index falls below 2.2 l/minute/M² and is associated with the clinical signs of hypoperfusion discussed above. Their PAW pressures are elevated above 18 mm Hg, contributing to pulmonary congestion and intra-alveolar edema.[12,13]

Therapy for Patients in Cardiogenic Shock

The goals of therapy for patients in cardiogenic shock are to enhance cardiac output while increasing oxygen supply to the myocardium and reducing LV work, to reduce pulmonary congestion and edema, to improve arterial oxygenation, to provide emotional support, and to provide a safe environment.

Nursing Interventions. Because patients in cardiogenic shock are often confused, safety measures should be instituted. Side rails should be up at all times. The use of soft restraints may be necessary to prevent the patient from removing tubes and other attachments.

These patients may be extremely anxious, even if confused. Sedation is contraindicated, since hypotension is likely to occur. Talking to these patients, preparing them for nursing care procedures in a succinct manner, and assuring them of the nurse's continued presence may be of some help. Family members, in particular, need emotional support during this stressful time. Because the primary nurse is required at the patient's bedside, other personnel should offer their support, as well as communicate changes in the patient's condition.

Patients in cardiogenic shock may also suffer from sleep and sensory deprivation. The symptoms and nursing interventions for these problems are discussed in Chapters 31 and 32.

Because these patients are attached to several pieces of equipment, their movement in bed is severely restricted. Frequent turning prevents alveolar atelectasis as well as skin breakdown. However, frequent vital-sign checks, such as every 5 to 10 minutes, are necessary to ascertain whether turning intensifies hypotension; if this occurs, patients should not be turned.

Medical Interventions. Vasodilator therapy is used to modulate cardiac function by a reduction of afterload and preload. Afterload reduction reduces systemic vascular resistance, which increases cardiac output and coronary perfusion. Preload reduction increases venous capacitance, which decreases LVEDV, LVEDP, and pulmonary congestion, resulting in improved arterial oxygenation.[10,13,21] Because patients in cardiogenic shock have elevated PAW pressure with hypoperfusion, vasodilating agents with venous and arteriolar effects are most beneficial; nitroprusside is often the drug of choice.

A positive inotropic drug, such as dopamine, dobutamine, or norepinephrine (Chap. 35) may be used in combination

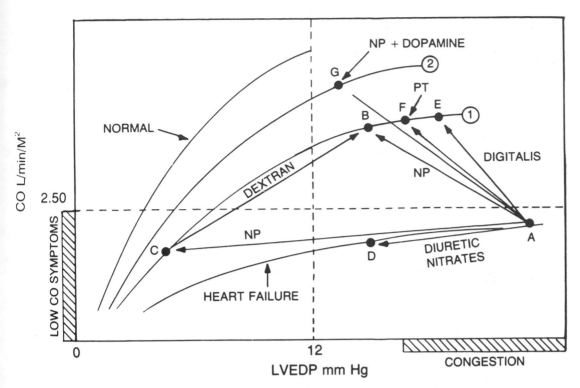

Fig. 27-6. Effects of drug therapy on cardiac function. Representative relationships between cardiac index (CO liter/min/M²) and LVEDP in the normal heart, and a heart with pulmonary congestion and hypoperfusion (*point A*). *Arrows* show variability of cardic output and LVEDP response to drug therapy. *Curves 1 and 2:* Intermediate function curves of improved contractility after drug administration; *point A → B:* nitroprusside therapy; prazosin therapy; hydralazine-nitrate therapy; *point A → C → B:* nitroprusside therapy: hypperfusion with CO increase after dextran administration; *point A → D:* diuretic therapy alone; *point A → E:* digitalis therapy alone; hydralazine therapy alone; *point A → F:* phentolamine therapy; *point A → G:* nitroprusside and dopamine therapy. Mason DT et al: *Hospital Formulary,* p 641–651, 1979)

with nitroprusside to increase cardiac contractility and maintain systolic blood pressure at levels above 90 mm Hg. However, these positive inotropic drugs may increase $M\dot{V}O_2$, further compromising myocardial function. Pulmonary artery wedge pressures should be monitored every 30 to 60 minutes, and reductions below 18 mm Hg with an associated decrease in cardiac output require discontinuance of drug therapy or judicious volume expansion with dextran or saline. The goal of therapy is to obtain a minimum PAW pressure with maximum cardiac output.

Other drugs that produce balanced arteriolar and venous effects are prazosin and combined hydralazine-nitrate administration. Hydralazine or phentolamine therapy without concomitant nitrate administration, raises cardiac output without reducing PCW pressures (Fig. 27-6).

The intra-aortic balloon pump is used to reduce afterload at the time of systolic contraction and to increase myocardial perfusion during diastole.[9,14] It is most frequently used as a short-term measure to partially support cardiovascular hemodynamics during acute decompensation.

A polyurethane, three-chambered balloon is inserted into the descending aorta, distal to the left subclavian artery and proximal to the renal arteries. Carbon dioxide or helium is used to inflate the balloon. Inflation is synchronized to the T-wave of the ECG. This balloon inflation increases coronary artery filling during diastole by increasing aortic root pressure. Deflation of the balloon is synchronized with the

downslope of the P-wave, which reduces LV afterload by decreasing aortic root pressure.[14] The total effects are as follows: a reduction in systolic systemic pressure; increased cardiac index; increased coronary blood flow; and a lowered LVEDP. Perfusion to the kidneys is also increased and pulmonary oxygen exchange improved.[9,14]

Nursing care measures first require the assessment of hemodynamic status. Changes in blood pressure responses, such as diastolic pressures exceeding systolic pressures (Fig. 27-7), a fall in HR, increased urine output, and improvement in mentation are watched for.[22] Pulmonary artery wedge pressure assessment enables evaluation of the intra-aortic balloon pump's effect on LVEDP. The pump must be closely observed during counterpulsation to ensure proper timing with the ECG. As the patient is gradually weaned from this therapy, the signs and symptoms of shock may reappear, and thus constant assessment of cardiovascular function is required.

Patients are usually heparinized before and during the procedure, and bleeding must be watched for. Bleeding may be evidenced by guaiac-positive stools and nasogastric aspirant, petechiae, or oozing from incisions.[14] Recalcification and partial thromboplastin times should also be regularly assessed, and heparin doses adjusted as needed (Chap. 15).

Raising the head of the bed to angles no greater than 30 degrees is important in preventing balloon movement or kinking which would impede circulation to the left subcla-

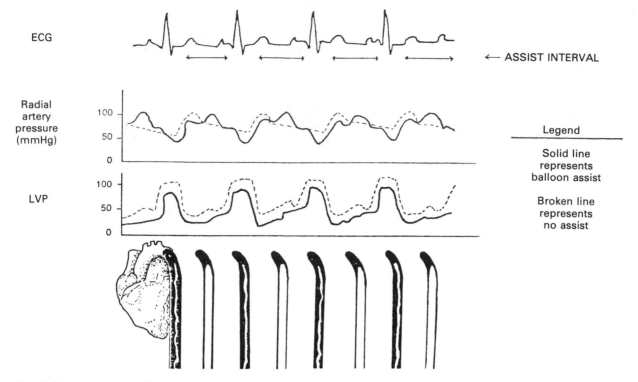

ECG

← ASSIST INTERVAL

Radial artery pressure (mmHg)

LVP

Legend

Solid line represents balloon assist

Broken line represents no assist

Fig. 27-7. Counterpulsation—the intra-aortic balloon pump. The effects of counterpulsation on radial artery and left ventricular pressures. Counterpulsation—the intra-aortic balloon pump (Operator's Manual, Model 10, Avco Intra-Aortic Balloon Pump. Avco Medical Products, Division of Avco Corporation of Roche Medical Electronics, 1976)

vian artery or the lower extremities, respectively.[14] The following signs and symptoms indicate a marked reduction in perfusion: extremity tingling; numbness; pallor and a fall in temperature in both extremities; and the absence of peripheral pulses. The patient should be placed in a supine position immediately, and the physician notified for possible balloon manipulation. Movement of the balloon may also interfere with perfusion to the renal arteries. Kidney function must be closely watched. Hourly urine output and daily serum BUN and creatinine determinations are indicated. Other complications that may occur are perforation or rupture of the aorta causing abdominal or back pain; thromboembolism to kidneys and mesentery; sepsis at the site of catheter insertion in the groin;[9] and thrombocytopenia due to aggregation of platelets around the balloon.[14]

If arterial blood gases show worsening hypoxemia, even with the administration of high oxygen concentrations through a mask, the patient may need to be intubated and a "T-piece" attached to the endotracheal tube, which provides a closed system for oxygen administration. This method may be sufficient to raise arterial oxygenation to an acceptable level. If it is not sufficient, continuous positive airway pressure (CPAP) may be effective in improving oxygenation by preventing alveolar collapse. Continuous positive airway pressure maintains positive intrathoracic pressure at the end of expiration, a technique which keeps alveoli open. If hypoxemia persists, mechanical ventilation is indicated.

The indications for mechanical ventilation are arterial oxygen tensions less than 50 mm Hg while receiving inspired oxygen concentrations of 50%; a vital capacity less than 15 ml/kg of body weight; an inspiratory effort less than −25 cm of water; and an increasing arterial carbon dioxide tension with an arterial pH below 7.25.[7,30] The purpose of mechanical ventilation is to improve arterial oxygenation and to normalize arterial carbon dioxide tensions. The evaluation of therapy is done by frequent assessment of arterial blood gas values.

Positive end-expiratory pressure (PEEP) works on the same principle as CPAP, and is often required for mechanically ventilated patients who have high degrees of shunt. In Chapter 21, the effects of mechanical ventilation and PEEP on cardiovascular hemodynamic measurements are discussed.

Changes in fluid balance may occur when the patient is on mechanical ventilation. Because the positive pressure exerted by mechanical ventilation reduces venous return, low-pressure baroreceptors in the right ventricle, pulmonary vasculature, and the left atrium interpret this effect as a low circulating blood volume; ADH secretion increases and the kidney conserves water.[20] This occurrence may be less likely in patients with cardiogenic shock, because pressures in these chambers are already elevated.

Hourly auscultation of breath sounds is important for detecting rhonchi, which indicate the need for endotracheal suctioning. Suctioning tracheal secretions is important to prevent atelectasis and pulmonary infection. Oxygenation before and after suctioning should be done with an anaesthesia bag, which delivers 100% oxygen, or by increasing the ventilator setting to 100%.[11] This latter method is advocated for patients receiving PEEP. Care must be taken to reduce the oxygen concentration back to presuctioning concentrations when suctioning is completed. Proper oxygenation does not necessarily cause any decrease in arterial oxygenation, however, and continuous ECG monitoring is essential in watching for arrhythmias.

If the patient remains in a metabolic acidotic stage even after vigorous measures to improve cardiac output and arterial oxygenation, sodium bicarbonate should be given. Care should be taken not to overcorrect the acidosis, resulting in a metabolic alkalosis. Alkalosis is associated with a leftward shift of the oxyhemoglobin dissociation curve, resulting in reduced hemoglobin unloading of oxygen in the peripheral tissues.[34] Cardiac arrhythmias may also be precipitated.

SUMMARY

The pathophysiology of heart failure following myocardial infarction is progressive. Left ventricular failure eventually results in pulmonary congestion and edema, unless effectively treated. Likewise, pulmonary edema can precipitate right ventricular failure. Severe pump dysfunction, or cardiogenic shock, occurs as compensatory mechanisms to maintain adequate cardiac output and peripheral perfusion fail. Although this chapter has presented the pathophysiology, symptoms, physical findings, and therapy associated with each portion of the "circuit," the progression of disease may not be so clearly defined in a clinical setting. However, an awareness of symptoms associated with dysfunction of both heart chambers and of the pulmonary and systemic circulations should enable the nurse to assess patients effectively, to institute specific nursing measures, and to evaluate the effects of therapy.

REFERENCES

1. Andreoli KG, Fowkes VH, Zipes PP et al: Comprehensive Cardiac Care, 4th edition. St. Louis, C. V. Mosby, 1979
2. Ayers SM, Mueller H, Gianelli S et al: The lung in shock, alveolar–capillary gas exchange in the shock syndrome. The Am J Cardiol 26:588–594, 1970
3. Barratt-Boyes BG, Wood EH: Cardiac output and related measurements and pressure values in the right heart and associated vessels, together with an analysis of the hemodynamic response to the inhalation of high oxygen mixtures in healthy subjects. J Lab Clin Med 51:72, 1958
4. Beland IL, Passos JY: Clinical Nursing. Pathophysiological Approaches, 3rd edition, New York, Macmillan, 1975
5. Bing OL, Brooks WW, Messer JV: Heart muscle viability following hypoxia: Protective effect of acidosis. Science 180:1297–1298, 1973
6. Bleifeld W, Hanrath P, Mathey D et al: Acute myocardial infarction. V: Left and right ventricular hemodynamics in cardiogenic shock. Br Heart J 36:822–834, 1974
7. Bushnell SS, Bushnell LS, Reichle M et al: Respiratory Intensive Care Nursing. Boston, Little, Brown, & Co, 1973
8. Cannon PJ: The kidney in heart failure. N Engl J Med 296:26–32, 1977
9. Chrzanowski AL: Intra-aortic balloon pumping: Concepts and patient care. Nurs Clin North Am 13:513–529, 1978
10. Cohn JN, Franciosa JA: Vasodilator therapy of cardiac failure (first of two parts). N Engl J Med 297:27–31, 1977
11. Fell T, Cheney FW: Prevention of hypoxia during endotracheal suction. Ann Surg 174:24–28, 1971
12. Forrester JS, Diamond G, Chatterjee K et al: Medical therapy of acute myocardial infarction by application of hemodynamic subsets (first of two parts). N Engl J Med 295:1356–1362, 1976
13. Forrester JS, Diamond G, Chatterjee K et al: Medical therapy of acute myocardial infarction by application of hemodynamic subsets (second of two parts). N Engl J Med 295:1404–1412, 1976
14. Frazee S, Nail L: New challenge in cardiac nursing: The intra-aortic balloon. Heart Lung, 2:526–532, 1973
15. Haddy FJ: Pathophysiology and therapy of the shock of myocardial infarction. Ann Intern Med 73:809–827, 1970
16. Hellerstein HK: Rehabilitation of the postinfarction patient. In Braunwald E (ed): The Myocardium: Failure and Infarction, pp 382–390. New York, HP Publishing Co, 1974
17. Hillis LD, Braunwald E: Myocardial ischemia (first of three parts). N Engl J Med 296:971–977, 1977
18. Hurst JW, Logue RB, Schlant RC et al: The Heart. New York, McGraw-Hill, 1974
19. Kones RJ: Cardiogenic Shock. Mount Kisco, Futura Publishing Co, 1974
20. Kubo WM, Grant MM: The syndrome of inappropriate secretion of antidiuretic hormone. Heart Lung 7:469–476, 1978
21. Mason DT, Awan NA, DeMaria AN: Afterload reduction in the management of congestive heart failure. Hospital Formulary 641–651, 1979
22. Operator's Manual, Model 10, Avco Intra-Aortic Balloon Pump. Avco Medical Products, Division of Avco Corporation of Roche Medical Electronics, 1976
23. Perloff JK: The clinical manifestations of cardiac failure in adults. In Braunwald E (ed): The Myocardium: Failure and Infection, 93–100. New York, HP Publishing Company, 1974
24. Pineo R: Unit I. Congestive Heart Failure. American Heart Association Council on Cardiovascular Nursing. New York, Appleton-Century-Crofts, 1978
25. Plum F, Posner JB: The Diagnosis of Stupor and Coma, 2nd ed. Philadelphia, FA Davis Co 1977
26. Robin ED, Cross CE, Zelis R: Pulmonary edema (first of two parts). N Engl J Med 288:239–246, 1973
27. Robin ED, Cross CE, Zelis R: Pulmonary edema (second of two parts). N Engl J Med 288:292–304, 1973
28. Scheidt S, Ascheim R, Killip T III: Shock after acute myocardial infarction. Am J Cardiol 26:556–564, 1970
29. Schmidt DD, Delany DJ, McLaurin LP: The clinical recognition of congestive heart failure. J Family Practice 5:193–197, 1977
30. Shapiro BA, Harrison RA, Trout CA: Clinical Application of Respiratory Care. Chicago, Year Book Medical Publishers, 1975
31. Sonnenblick EH, Strobeck JE: Current concepts in cardiology. Derived indexes of ventricular and myocardial function. N Engl J Med 296:978–982, 1977
32. Spann JF Jr, Mason DT, Zelis RF: Recent advances in the understanding of congestive heart failure (II). Mod Concepts Cardiovasc Dis 39:79–84, 1970
33. Wessler S, Gitel SN: Low-dose Heparin: Is the risk worth the benefit? Am Heart J 98:94–101, 1979
34. West JB: Respiratory Physiology: The Essentials. Baltimore, Williams & Wilkins Co, 1974
35. Young JA, Crocker D: Principles and Practice of Respiratory Therapy, 2nd ed. Chicago, Year Book Medical Publishers, 1976

ADDITIONAL READING

Afifi AA, Change PC, Lie VY et al: Prognostic indexes in acute myocardial infarction complicated by shock. Am J Cardiol 33:826–832, 1974
Amsterdam E, Massumi RA, Zelis R et al: Evaluation and management of cardiogenic shock. Part III. The roles of cardiac surgery and mechanical assist. Heart Lung 2:122–126, 1973

Arbeit S, Fiedler J, Landau T et al: Recognizing digitalis toxicity. Am J Nurs 77:1936–1945, 1977

Awan NA, Miller, RR, DeMaria AN et al: Efficacy of ambulatory systemic vasodilator therapy with oral prazosin in chronic refractory heart failure. Circulation 56:346–353, 1977

Awan NA, Miller RR, Miller MP et al: Clinical pharmacology and therapeutic application of prazosin in acute and chronic refractory congestive heart failure. Am J Med 65:146–154, 1978

Baden CA: Teaching and the coronary patient and his family. Nurs Clin North Am 7:563–571, 1972

Bates B: A Guide to Physical Examination. Philadelphia, JB Lippincott, 1974

Bleifeld W, Kupper W, Hanrath P et al: New and traditional therapy of congestive heart failure. Am J Med 65:203–207, 1978

Brammell HL, Niccoli A: A physiologic approach to cardiac rehabilitation. Nurs Clin North Am 11:223–236, 1976

Braunwald E: The autonomic nervous system in heart failure. In Braunwald E (ed): The Myocardium: Failure and Infarction, pp 59–69. New York, HP Publishing Co, 1974

Braunwald E: Current concepts in cardiology: Determinants and assessment of cardiac function. N Engl J Med 296:86–89, 1977

Chatterjee K, Parmley WW, Ganz W et al: Hemodynamic and metabolic responses to vasodilator therapy in acute myocardial infarction. Circulation 48:1183–1193, 1973

Chatterjee MB, Swan HJC: Vasodilator therapy in acute myocardial infarction. Mod Concepts Cardiovasc Dis 43:119–124, 1974

Clark NF: Pump failure. Nurs Clin North Am 7:529–539, 1972

Cohn JN, Franciosa JA: Vasodilator therapy of cardiac failure (second of two parts). N Engl J Med 297:254–258, 1977

The Committee on Exercise, American Heart Association: Exercise Testing and Training of Individuals with Heart Disease or at High Risk for its Development: A Handbook for Physicians, 1975

Community Outlook: Asian diet fact sheet. Nursing Times 7:108–110, 1977

Corday E, Meerbaum S, Lang T: Treatment of cardiogenic shock with mechanical circulatory assist: Fact or fiction? Am J Cardiol 30:575–578, 1972

Corday E, Swan HJC, Lang T et al: Physiologic principles in the application of circulating assist for the failing heart. Am J Cardiol 26:595–602, 1970

daLuz PL, Weil MH, Liu VY et al: Plasma volume prior to and following volume loading during shock complicating acute myocardial infarction. Circulation 49:98–105, 1974

daLuz PL, Weil MH, Shubin H: Current concepts on mechanisms and treatment of cardiogenic shock. Am Heart J 92:103–113, 1976

Dodge HA: Hemodynamic aspects of cardiac failure. In Braunwald E (ed): The Myocardium: Failure and Infarction, pp 70–78. New York, HP Publishing Co, 1974

Edelman NH, Gorfinkel HJ, Lluch S et al: Experimental cardiogenic shock: Pulmonary performance after acute myocardial infarction. Am J Physiol 219:1729–1730, 1970

Forrester JS, Swan HJC: Acute myocardial infarction: A physiological basis of therapy. Crit Care Med 2:283–292, 1974

Forrester JS, Water DO: Hospital treatment of congestive heart failure. Management according to hemodynamic profile. Am J Med 65:173–180, 1978

Fox SM: Physical activity and cardiovascular health, III. The exercise prescription: Frequency and type of activity. Mod Concepts Cardiovasc Dis 41:25–30, 1972

Frantz A, Galdys M: Keeping up with automatic rotating tourniquets. Nursing 78 8:31–35, 1978

Gold HK, Leinback RC, Saunders CS: Use of sublingual nitroglycerin in congestive failure following acute myocardial infarction. Circulation 46:839–845, 1972

Goldberg LI, Hsieh Y, Resnekov L: Newer catecholamines for treatment of heart failure and shock. Prog Cardiovasc Dis 29:327–340, 1977

Goodman L, Gilman A: The Pharmacological Basis of Therapeutics, 5th ed. New York, Macmillan, 1975

Gordon EE: Energy costs of activities in health and disease. Am Med Assoc Arch Intern Med 101:701–713, 1958

Gorlin R: Current concepts in cardiology, practical cardiac hemodynamics. N Engl J Med 296:203–208, 1977

Hillis DL, Braunwald E: Myocardial ischemia (second of three parts) N Engl J Med 296:1034–1040, 1977

Hillis DL, Braunwald E: Myocardial ischemia (third of three parts). N Engl J Med 296:1093–1096, 1977

Holzer J, Karline JS, O'Rourke RA et al: Effectiveness of dopamine in patients with cardiogenic shock. Am J Cardiol 32:79–84, 1973

Hudson LD: Diagnosis and management of acute respiratory distress in patients on mechanical ventilators. In Shibel EM, Moser KM (eds): Respiratory Emergencies, pp 207–219. St. Louis, C. V. Mosby, 1977

Jewitt D, Jennings K, Jackson PG: Efficacy of new inotropic drugs in clinical heart failure. Am J Med 65:107–202, 1978

Kirby RR, Perry JC, Calderwood HW et al: Cardiorespiratory effects of high positive end-expiratory pressure. Anesthesiology 43:533–539, 1975

Kostuk W, Barr JW, Simon AL: Correlations between the chest film and hemodynamics in acute myocardial infarction: Help or hazard? Ann Intern Med 82:234–240, 1975

Langer GA: The mechanism of action of digitalis. In Braunwald E (ed): The Myocardium: Failure and Infarction, pp 135–141. New York, HP Publishing Co, 1974

Lawson BN: Clinical assessment of cardiac patients in acute care facilities. Nurs Clin North Am 7:431–444, 1972

Leininger M: Cultural diversities of health and Nursing care. Nurs Clin North Am 12:5–8, 1977

Rahimatoola SH, Gunnar RM: Digitalis in acute myocardial infarction: Help or hazard? Ann of Intern Med 82:234–240, 1975

Rotman M, Chen JTT, Hawley J et al: Pulmonary arterial Diastolic pressure in acute myocardial infarction. Am J Cardiol 33:357–362, 1974

Spann KF Jr, Mason DT, Zelis RF: Recent advances in the understanding of congestive heart failure (I). Mod Concepts of Cardiovasc Dis 39:73–78, 1970

Taylor WR, Forrester JS, Magnusson P et al: Hemodynamic effects of nitroglycerin ointment in congestive heart failure. Am J Cardiol 38:469–473, 1976

Tooker T, Huseby J, Butler J: The effect of Swan–Ganz catheter height on the wedge pressure–left atrial pressure relationship in edema during positive pressure ventilation. Am Rev Respir Dis, 117:721–725, 1978

Waxler R: The patient with congestive heart failure. Nurs Clin North Am 11:297–308, 1976

Webb WR: A Protocol for Managing the Pulmonary Complications of Patients in Shock. Kalamazoo, MI, Upjohn Co, 1975

White EH: Care of minority patients. Nurs Clin North Am 12:27–40, 1977

Willerson JT, Curry GC, Watson JT: Intra-aortic balloon counterpulsation in patients in cardiogenic shock, medically refractory left ventricular failure and/or recurrent ventricular tachycardia. Am J Med 58:183–191, 1975

Williams SR: Nutrition and Diet Therapy. St. Louis, C. V. Mosby, 1977

Winslow EH: The role of the nurse in patient education. Focus: The cardiac patient. Nurs Clin North Am 11:213–222, 1976

Woodbury DM: Physiology of body fluids. In Ruch TC, Patton HD (eds): Physiology and Biophysics, II—Circulation, Respiration and Fluid Balance, pp 450–479. Philadelphia, WB Saunders, 1974.

28

Thromboembolic Complications in Patients with Cardiac Disease

WANDA ROBERTS, R.N., M.N.

A variety of thromboembolic disorders frequently complicate the clinical course and contribute to the mortality of patients with cardiac disease. The incidence of these complications is highest in severely ill patients, such as those with sustained low cardiac output or dissecting aneurysms.[22,53] Large myocardial infarctions and the presence of congestive heart failure are commonly associated factors.[17,51,69] Valvular heart disease, mitral disease in particular, is associated with an increased risk of both pulmonary and systemic emboli.[52] The risk of thromboembolism increases further in patients over 60 years of age and in those with varicose veins, infection, obesity, leg trauma, and previous thromboembolism. Patients subjected to prolonged immobilization, those receiving steroids or oral contraceptives, and those who develop significant arrhythmias also share an increased risk. The severity and duration of illness has been found to be the most important causative factor, rather than the duration of bed rest or any single disease complication. Stroke following myocardial infarction was found to occur more often in patients with major infarctions than in those with less severe damage.[67] The higher incidence of deep vein thrombosis in the aged is thought to be related to anatomic changes in the veins and to the presence of peripheral arterial disease leading to reduced tissue perfusion and to alterations in blood coagulation factors.[47]

Deliberate measures directed toward prophylaxis and early detection of thromboembolic disorders are certainly warranted. An understanding of the pathogenesis, clinical manifestations, medical therapy, methods of prevention, and current research in the area will enable the nurse to participate actively and effectively in all aspects of clinical management.

LEG VEIN THROMBOSIS

Etiology

Although the exact etiology of venous thrombosis remains unclear, three antecedent factors defined by Virchow in 1846 are believed to play a significant role in its development: stasis of blood, injury to the vessel wall, and altered blood coagulation. The coexistence of at least two factors appears to be necessary for local thrombosis to occur.[12]

When cardiac output is low, as after myocardial infarction, surgery, or shock, blood flow to the limbs is retarded, either because perfusion is reduced or because peripheral resistance is increased. Venous dilatation, which may follow drug therapy, recumbency, and congestive heart failure, in addition to reduced calf muscle contractions accompanying immobility, limb paralysis, and anesthesia, can lead to venous stasis. Bed rest has been shown to reduce blood flow in the legs at least 50%. Vein distention following stasis may lead to disruption of the endothelium lining the vessels, thus creating a nidus for thrombus formation.[28]

Intact blood vessel walls have natural antithrombotic properties. Injury or exposure of the collagen underlying the vascular endothelium will cause a rapid and irreversible aggregation of platelets in the area of injury. Some factors identified as causing vessel-wall injury are direct trauma, venous disease, and chemical irritation from intravenous solutions or drugs.

We have no conclusive proof that the blood of cardiac patients is hypercoagulable but positive evidence is strong. Increased stickiness of platelets and increased fibrinogen levels with decreased fibrinolytic activity have been reported in patients suffering an acute myocardial infarction. High plasma fibrinogen levels appear to raise plasma viscosity and can therefore increase the tendency for clotting. Increased prothrombin activity has been observed in patients with congestive heart failure. In addition, abrupt discontinuation of anticoagulants has been implicated as a cause of increased coagulation.[30,33]

Pathophysiology

The saphenous vein is the most common site of superficial vein thrombosis. In deep vein thrombosis (DVT) the ileo-femoral vein, popliteal segments, or small veins of the calf are sites frequently involved.

Venous thrombi are composed primarily of a small white head of platelets attached to the vessel wall and a large red gel-like body and tail containing fibrin, white blood cells, and many red blood cells. Successive layering of the constituents causes propagation or extension of the thrombus along the vessel, usually in the direction of blood flow. In the earliest stages of this process inflammation of the vein wall is not a prominent feature (Fig. 28-1).[68]

The danger associated with a propagating deep vein thrombus is that fragmentation or dislodgment of a part of the thrombus may result in a potentially lethal pulmonary embolus. Thrombi in the iliac or femoral veins most often produce large, fatal pulmonary emboli. Fragmentation of a deep vein thrombus can occur spontaneously during the natural dissolution process, or from mechanical forces that

Fig. 28-1. Propagation of thrombosis. (**A**) Thrombus formation occurs at each entering tributary. This tends to anchor the clot. (**B**) Clotting *en masse* in an extensive length of vein. This occurs when circulation is very sluggish. The long propagated clot can easily become detached and lead to massive pulmonary embolism. (Hadfield G: Ann Coll R Surg Engl, 6:219, 1950)

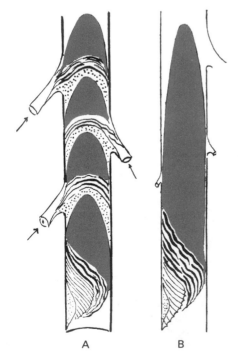

A   B

cause changes in intravascular pressures. Standing, sudden muscle activity after prolonged inactivity, or Valsalva maneuvers during straining are known to increase intravascular pressure and may precipitate an embolic event.[27]

Assessment of the Problem

Clinical Manifestations. The clinical recognition of DVT has proved rather elusive. One-third to two-thirds of patients with DVT have no symptoms, while others manifest only one to two symptoms.[5,41,55,70,72] The classic symptoms of muscle pain, tenderness, swelling and Homans' sign occur as frequently in normal limbs as they do in limbs with DVT.[21] Pulmonary embolism is often the first evidence of a thrombosis of the deep veins.[32] Despite the fact that clinical signs are unreliable for establishing the presence or absence of DVT, they should never be ignored when present, but rather considered as an indication for further investigation.[13]

Obstruction of a deep vein produces sudden edema and swelling of the limb, as venous outflow is inhibited. Swelling can best be demonstrated by careful measurement of limb girth at various levels, using a tape measure or a flexible metal ruler.[45] Minimal ankle circumference and maximal calf circumference should be determined on both limbs and sequentially recorded. At the calf level, differences of more than one centimeter between limbs are considered significant. Thigh swelling should also be investigated since iliac vein obstruction can be revealed only at this level.

Besides swelling, two additional signs may be noted. The skin over the leg and ankle of the affected side may become warmer. Differences in warmth between the limbs is best detected clinically by palpating the skin with the dorsal aspect of the hands. Also, the subcutaneous vein patterns of the affected limb may be prominent.[38]

A somewhat later-occurring and less specific sign than swelling is tenderness over the involved venous segment. Tenderness indicates inflammation of the vein.[47,64] Gentle fingertip palpation should be performed, progressing proximally from the Achilles tendon. Important areas to assess are the midcalf, the medial area above the knee joint, and the medial thigh to the femoral triangle. Applying too much pressure during these maneuvers can lead to misinterpretations of tenderness. Pain in the calf following sharp dorsiflexion of the foot (Homans' sign) is probably the least specific sign of DVT, since pain can be produced with this maneuver in any painful condition of the calf.

Diagnostic Tests. Early detection of DVT by clinical signs alone is unreliable; hence, more definitive diagnostic tests are essential. Some of the more commonly available tests are discussed below.

Ascending Phlebography (Venography). Phlebography is the oldest diagnostic method for examining the venous system and it can demonstrate 90% to 95% of thrombi.[64] It is used as the standard by which the accuracy of newer methods is judged. It is costly and requires injection of radiographic contrast medium into the dorsum of the foot. The injection almost always results in transient, mild phlebitis, making frequent repetition of the test inadvisable.[64] Radiographic diagnosis is based on defining an unfilled segment of vein in an otherwise completely filled or opacified vein with its connecting collaterals.[13]

[125]I Labeled Fibrinogen Scanning. Fibrinogen labeled with radioactive iodine (^{125}I) and injected intravenously has provided a sensitive method for detecting early venous thrombosis in the calf. The test depends on the fact that fibrinogen concentrates in a forming clot and that the radioactivity can be detected by an external counter. Because of the relatively long half-life of this isotope, a portable scanner can be used, and frequent monitoring for the presence or progression of thrombi is possible over a period of several days. Accuracy of the test is greatest when the fibrinogen is given before the clot forms.[13] Fibrinogen will concentrate in hematomas and inflammatory exudates, making diagnosis inaccurate in patients with leg injuries, active arthritis, varicose ulcerations, and edema. The venous system in the legs can also be visualized simultaneously with lung scanning by the injection of radioactive albumin. This technique is called radionuclide or isotope venography.

Ultrasound Flow Detection (Doppler). The theoretic basis for Doppler examination is that, when a beam of ultrasound is reflected from a moving object, the beam will undergo a shift in frequency. This shift is proportional to the rate at which the object is moving and can be detected by a recorder and transcribed onto paper. This test is simple, portable, noninvasive, and relatively inexpensive, and can be rapidly applied to high risk patients.[5]

Placement of the Doppler probe bilaterally over paired veins normally reveals similar Doppler flow readings in each.[6] Augmentation of flow under the probe should be expected when the limb distal to the vein is suddenly compressed. The absence of a venous flow signal at an expected location, or decreased augmentation of flow in response to distal limb compression, characterizes a venous obstruction.[6] The Doppler is not useful in detecting thrombi in the smaller calf veins.[64]

Medical Therapy

Because most patients respond well to treatment, prompt recognition of DVT is important, so that grave complications can be prevented. The goals of therapy are to prevent propagation of the thrombus (and thus the inherent high risk for embolization) and to prevent recurrent thromboemboli. Therapeutic anticoagulation (Chap. 38) with heparin and oral anticoagulant agents accomplishes both these goals.[1,10,19,26,50] In some centers, fibrinolytic agents (for example, streptokinase and urokinase) have been employed experimentally to hasten dissolution of deep vein thrombi (Chap. 38).

Bed rest, elevation of the affected extremity, heat application, elastic stockings, analgesics for pain, and surgery are all adjuncts to anticoagulant therapy. The prescription of bed rest for a patient with DVT varies among physicians and with the severity of the thrombotic process. Many practitioners prefer to keep patients in bed until the inflammatory symptoms subside, indicating that adhesion and organization of the thrombus has occurred. This practice is believed to decrease the risk of embolization by preventing the fluctuations in pressure in the deep venous system that occur with walking.[16,37] The foot of the bed should be elevated to facilitate venous return. Some people believe that mild or passive exercise of the legs in bed may enhance venous return and lessen the likelihood of extension of the clot. Walking is superior to sitting or standing for long periods. When the patient is sitting, the legs should be elevated and not crossed. Straining during defecation can cause marked pressure changes in the deep veins and increase the risk of embolization. Massaging the involved extremity is also contraindicated, because fragmentation and dislodgment of the thrombus can occur.

The use of elastic stockings is usually reserved until after organization of the clot has taken place and ambulation begun. Elastic support facilitates compression of enlarged superficial veins and increases venous flow in deep veins.[39]

Occasionally, a thrombectomy can be performed to remove a recent deep vein thrombus. This surgical procedure is best suited for a fresh, nonadherent thrombus in the femoral or iliac vein, where the risk of embolization is the greatest.[60] A discussion of the prevention of thromboembolism and the nursing care of patients with these disorders can be found later in this chapter.

PULMONARY EMBOLISM

Pulmonary embolism (PE) is a complication, rather than a primary disorder, that can occur in the course of many disease states. Conservative estimates attribute 50,000 deaths annually to PE.[68,20] It is a major factor in the mortality of patients with chronic cardiac or pulmonary diseases, particularly when the PE is preceded by congestive heart failure.[71] Two-thirds of all patients who die from PE do so within the first hour after the event.[11,18] Ileofemoral thrombi carry an increased risk of massive and fatal PE,[11,63] whereas right heart thrombi are usually smaller and not fatal.[7]

Etiology

Of all pulmonary emboli 85% to 95% arise from the dislodgment of thrombi of the deep veins of the legs. The remainder originate from clots in the pelvis or in the right atrium, the latter usually in patients with cardiomyopathy or atrial fibrillation.[32,27]

Pathophysiology

The severity of the hemodynamic and respiratory alterations from PE depends upon the size of the embolus and the previous cardiopulmonary status.[65,66] Generally, obstruction of a small pulmonary artery may be unnoticed, although large emboli cause a sudden rise in pulmonary artery pressure. Because the right ventricle does not tolerate sudden pressure elevations well, acute right heart failure may develop.

Pulmonary infarction following embolic occlusion is relatively rare[24] because of the alternative blood supply to the lungs from the bronchial arterial circulation. Pulmonary infarction is much more likely to occur in the presence of preexisting cardiopulmonary disease and results in alveolar-wall necrosis, hemorrhage into the alveoli, and fibrosis of the affected lung segment.[24,25,46]

The respiratory responses to PE primarily reflect a disturbance of the ventilation-to-perfusion ratio. Lung segments deprived of blood flow can no longer participate in gas exchange, and hypoxia results. Reflex bronchoconstriction follows in order to compensate for the wasted ventilation. Surfactant in the ischemic area of the lung is lost, leading to alveolar collapse. Radiographically, atelectasis can be detected within 24 to 48 hours after blood flow is interrupted.[46,48]

In cases where PE is not fatal, the majority of emboli undergo complete lysis or gradually become organized into small fibrous scars attached to the vessel wall. Pulmonary perfusion is generally restored within 3 or 4 weeks.[62]

Assessment

Clinical Manifestations. Unless a pulmonary embolus is large, the diagnosis cannot be reliably established or ruled out by clinical signs and symptoms alone. Studies have shown that such classic symptoms as cough, pleuritic chest pain, and hemoptysis are often absent. Early manifestations, if any, are subtle, nonspecific, and easily overlooked. Despite these limitations a thorough, ongoing assessment for signs or symptoms of PE is warranted in all high-risk patients.

Sudden, unexplained dyspnea is often an early symptom in patients with PE and is due to the sudden increase in the number of unperfused alveoli. Some form of chest pain, either pleuritic or nonpleuritic, has also been reported. This pain has occasionally been described as a "cold in the back" or as "muscle pain."[28] Substernal discomfort can occur and may, in part, be related to coronary insufficiency when the embolic occlusion of pulmonary vessels is sufficient to cause a reduction in cardiac output.[66]

Apprehension and a nonproductive, annoying cough are present in about one-half of patients with PE. Less frequently, diaphoresis, leg cramps, palpitations, syncope, nausea, vomiting, and chills are reported.[8] In some cases sudden, unexplained changes in the condition of patients with pulmonary or cardiac diseases may be the only indication of an acute pulmonary embolus.

Early signs associated with PE include tachypnea, tachycardia, and rales in the involved area of the lung.[23,68] Hypoxemia is generally seen with large emboli and is accompanied by a reduction in the partial pressure of arterial carbon dioxide ($P_a CO_2$) and an increased pH. An accentuation of the pulmonic component of the second heart sound can be detected in the presence of pulmonary hypertension.[28] Obvious DVT is absent in the majority of patients with PE.

Electrocardiographic (ECG) changes with PE are variable. Often the ECG is normal. The changes reported include right bundle branch block, right heart strain (seen as a S_1, Q_3, T_3 pattern, that is, a prominent S wave in standard lead I and a prominent Q and inverted T in standard lead III), P-pulmonale, and the sudden development of atrial fibrillation or flutter. These changes usually reflect a large embolus and tend to be more pronounced in patients with prior cardiopulmonary disease.[2,3,11,49,63,68]

Hemoptysis (often manifested as blood-streaked sputum rather than frank bleeding), persistent pleuritic chest pain, fever, and the presence of a pleural friction rub usually accompany pulmonary infarction.[4,7] Infarction may also produce leukocytosis, elevated sedimentation rate, elevated LDH and bilirubin and a normal SGOT. This triad of elevated LDH, elevated bilirubin, and a normal SGOT is uncommon, and values are influenced by cardiac or hepatic disorders.[11,63,68]

Radiologic evidence of pulmonary infarction is sometimes manifested as a wedge-shaped density, with its apex toward the hilum and its base on the pleural surface. Pleural effusions and an elevated hemidiaphragm can also be seen.[11,62]

Diagnostic Tests

Because of the unreliability of clinical signs for establishing a diagnosis of PE, confirmation depends upon laboratory findings preceded by a high level of suspicion. Several diagnostic methods currently employed and their specificity for verifying the presence of PE are discussed below.

Chest Radiography. The chest radiograph frequently reveals changes suggestive of PE. These may be classical pleural-based, wedge-shaped opacities of pulmonary infarction. At times there may be an associated small pleural effusion. Less specific changes include atelectasis. Careful inspection of the vascularity may reveal a difference between the two lung fields, with "cutoff" and absence of vessels suggesting embolism.

Lung Perfusion Scanning. Lung scanning is carried out after intravenous injection of radioactively labeled albumin. The presence of radioactivity can then be detected in areas of blood flow. Zones of decreased or absent radioactivity indicate areas of absent or decreased blood flow (Fig. 28-2).[28] As previously mentioned, lower-limb venography can be performed simultaneously with lung scanning.

Perfusion lung scanning is a sensitive method for detecting disturbances in pulmonary blood flow, but it is not specific for PE because the cause of the disturbed flow cannot be directly determined. However, when lung scan is considered along with the chest radiograph or a ventilation scan, the specificity for PE increases.

A ventilation scan involves inhalation of a radioactive gas such as [133]Xenon. The gas will be distributed to ventilated lung areas in amounts proportional to the degree of ventilation. A normal ventilation scan with an abnormal perfusion scan in the presence of a suggestive clinical history should make the examiner suspect PE.[63]

Angiography. Angiography should be used to elucidate the anatomy of the pulmonary vasculature whenever the diagnosis of PE is uncertain from the clinical picture and other diagnostic tests, when anticoagulants are contraindicated, or when surgery is considered.[34] Radiopaque material is injected, preferably through a pulmonary catheter, into the pulmonary arteries and the pulmonary vessels are visualized. Findings characteristic of a pulmonary embolism include an abrupt cutoff or obstruction of a pulmonary artery; or an intraluminal "filling defect" preventing one or more areas

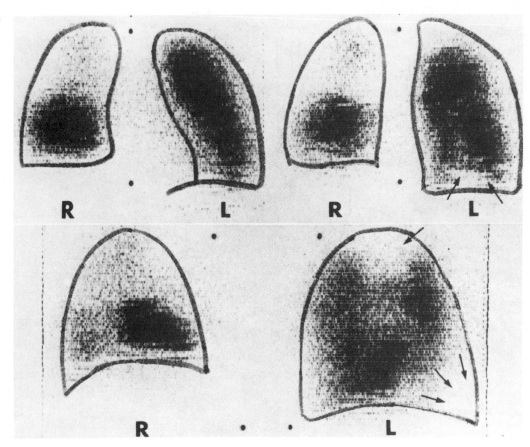

Fig. 28-2. Four-view lung scans in a patient with massive pulmonary embolism. The outline of the lungs was traced from the chest film. The anterior scan (*top left*) shows virtually no radioactivity (absent blood flow) to the upper half of the right lung. The posterior scan (*top right*) shows identical defects on the right lung. The left lung on this posterior view shows a defect at *arrows*). The right lateral scan (*bottom left*) shows that only the inferior anterior portion of the right lung is receiving blood. The left lateral scan (*bottom right*) shows several defects; apex (*arrow*) and base (*arrows*). Pulmonary emboli have blocked blood flow to about 40% of the lungs. (Fitzmaurice J, Sasahara A: Heart Lung 3(2):209–218, 1974)

in the major pulmonary vessels from being visualized as the contrast medium flows around the embolus. The latter is a more common finding, since most emboli do not completely obstruct pulmonary vessels.[11,63,68]

Medical Therapy

The goals of therapy for patients with PE are to sustain life until the embolus is resolved, to stop propagation of the thrombus, to prevent recurrence, and to augment the fibrinolytic removal of the embolus and the thrombotic source of the embolus.[63,68] It is highly probable that patients who are not treated will have recurrent episodes, which are often fatal.

Oxygen, mechanical ventilation, bronchodilators, and circulatory support methods using vasopressors, diuretics, antiarrhythmic agents, and digitalis may be necessary to preserve cardiopulmonary function during the acute phase of PE. Narcotics are used to relieve chest pain.

The use of heparin and, later, oral anticoagulants will arrest the thrombotic process, stop propagation, and prevent recurrence of embolization. An augmentation of fibrinolysis

has been accomplished experimentally with thrombolytic drugs such as streptokinase and urokinase (Chap. 38).

Bed rest is generally prescribed for 5 to 7 days, until organization of the clot has occurred. Ambulation is begun with elastic support applied to the legs and while the patient is on heparin.

In patients in whom anticoagulation for PE is contraindicated or in whom emboli recur despite adequate anticoagulation, surgical intervention may be indicated to prevent lower-limb emboli from reaching the lungs.[11,60] Both complete and partial procedures for vein interruption are employed. With complete interruption, the inferior venae cavae, or lesser veins, are ligated distal to the renal veins. With partial occlusion, sutures or plastic clips are used to create a filter that traps migrating emboli (Fig. 28-3).[60] One of the newest methods of vein interruption is the Mobin–Uddin intracaval "umbrella" filter, which is inserted in a closed position with a catheter through the jugular vein. When the appropriate position has been reached, the "umbrella" is opened and released from the catheter.[11,28] Advantages of this procedure are that it can be performed in critically ill patients without general anesthesia and it does not require laparotomy.

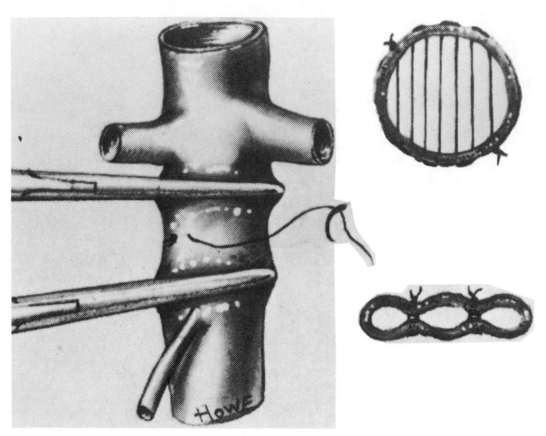

Fig. 28-3. Partial interruption of inferior vena cava; grid and compartmentalization procedures. (Schwartz SG, Shires T, Spencer FC, et al: Principles of Surgery, 3rd ed, p 994. New York, McGraw–Hill, 1979)

No form of venous interruption completely precludes embolic recurrence.[68] Large collaterals can develop around ligated veins and transmit emboli. After partial vein interruption, thrombi can form at the site of the interruption as well as in the right atrium. For these reasons anticoagulants may be continued after surgery.[12]

Pulmonary embolectomy may be indicated in some cases to remove a large embolus from the pulmonary artery. This procedure is usually reserved for patients who remain in shock after conventional therapy. The mortality rate is high.

Prevention of Pulmonary Embolism and Deep Venous Thrombosis

Since most emboli arise from deep venous thrombosis, the prevention of PE is largely accomplished by the prevention of DVT. Efforts should be directed at minimizing or eliminating injury to vessel walls, stasis of blood, and alterations in blood coagulation.

Damage to vein walls can be prevented by avoidance of prolonged pressure or occlusion of veins, by elimination of tight binders, splints, or constricting sutures, and by minimal use of intravenous catheters, needles, and hypertonic or chemically irritating solution. Careful management and prevention of infection and bleeding also contribute to preservation of veins.

Once the thrombus has formed, stasis of blood is believed to accelerate the process.[35] Actions to increase venous flow are thus clearly warranted.[71] In cardiac patients, particularly after myocardial infarction, emphasis should be placed on the development and institution of early mobilization guidelines. Walking rather than standing or sitting is preferred as a means of impeding thrombus formation. When this is not possible, a combination of in-bed exercises, leg elevation, and several physical methods to improve venous flow have been advocated.

While isometric exercises, such as plantar flexion against a footboard and quadriceps setting, have been recommended for surgical patients to increase venous flow, they may be harmful to patients with cardiac disease because of the marked rise in blood pressure that often accompanies these exercises. Isotonic (dynamic) exercises produce a more favorable cardiovascular response and are therefore preferred.[42] Isotonic exercises include active and passive leg exercises, active flexion and extension of the feet, and turning in bed.[49] The effects of in-bed exercises are believed to last for only 1 hour.[39] Exercises should therefore, be performed vigorously, if possible, for at least 5 minutes every hour.[29] When the patient's legs are dangling over the side of the bed, pressure from the edge of the mattress can be imposed on the popliteal space; sitting in this position should therefore be discouraged.

Leg elevation is best accomplished by raising the foot of the bed rather than by propping the legs up with pillows. In this way the entire length of the leg is equally supported

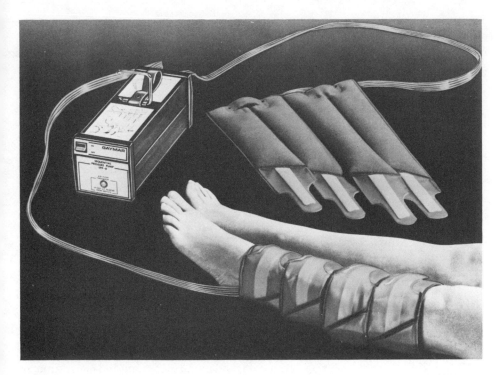

Fig. 28-4. Sequential pressure cuff system for prophylaxis of deep venous thrombosis.

and pressure by pillows on the popliteal space and the calf is eliminated.[14,59]

Elastic compression of the legs reduces venous pooling and enhances venous return by decreasing the total venous pool.[39] In surgical patients it was found that the rate of postoperative formation of deep vein thrombi decreased when elastic stockings were worn during surgery, as well as before and after, because most thrombi began to form in the operating room.[60,61] Also, the fit of the stocking appears to be an important factor in achieving the desired benefit from elastic compression.[13,44] The ideal elastic stocking should provide a decline in pressure from the ankle to the knee or groin and have no constricting garters. Although thrombus formation may not be prevented by elastic stockings, the increase in venous flow velocity they provide inhibit subsequent propagation of thrombi.[56] Recently, more elaborate physical methods such as stimulation of the calf muscles, pneumatic cuffs or boots that intermittently compress the calves and feet (Fig. 28-4) and motor-driven foot pedals to provide passive plantar dorsiflexion have been developed.[18,37,43,64] Although these devices purport to be more efficient in preventing venous stasis, their use has not been shown to reduce the incidence of PE.

The third factor contributing to thromboembolism, intravascular coagulation, is prophylactically altered, mainly by drugs.[9,31] Anticoagulants and drugs affecting platelet function are discussed in Chapter 38.

Nursing Care of Patients With Pulmonary Embolism and Deep Venous Thrombosis

The objectives of nursing care of patients with current or potential thromboembolic disorders include:
1. Prevention or modification of conditions known to be thrombogenic
2. Early detection of thromboembolism
3. Accurate delivery, monitoring, and support of the prescribed medical regimen and the nursing plan of care
4. Provision of pertinent information and instructions that will enable patients or their families to make critical decisions about care
5. Provision of instruction or guidance necessary for patients independently to carry out appropriate preventive or therapeutic measures outside the health care system.

The responsibility of nurses for providing continuous care and the frequent contact they have with patients enable them to make more sensitive evaluations, and give them the opportunity to take methodical and thorough action.

Recognition of conditions under which thromboembolism is likely to occur is the initial step in prevention. Measures aimed at reducing venous stasis and improving venous flow are essential. Stasis can be modified by early ambulation, with emphasis on walking rather than prolonged sitting or standing, or by active and passive bed exercises, as described earlier in this chapter. Activity guidelines for patients with cardiac disease must be established collaboratively with the physician, and modified when changes in the patient's condition occur. The patient's response to exercise should always be evaluated by assessing heart rate and rhythm, blood pressure, respiratory rate and effort, skin color, and temperature, before, during, and after activity. The exercise program should be discontinued when adverse reactions occur.

Points of pressure along the legs should be eliminated by removing pillows or bedrolls from under the knees, keeping the knee gatch of the bed flat, and removing tight-fitting stockings or clothing that produce a garter effect. A high Fowler's position promotes venous stasis and should be avoided.

Elastic stockings are thought to be helpful in reducing venous stasis and may be used in conjunction with other preventive methods. Stockings alone will not protect the patient from thrombus formation. To achieve maximal benefit from elastic stockings, the manufacturer's directions for fit should be strictly followed. Stockings should always be put on while the patient is recumbent, preferably before arising, when venous volume in the legs is minimal. If the patient has been ambulating, lying down with the legs elevated for 15 minutes will help reduce venous volume. Wrinkles and tops that are rolled down create a tourniquet effect. Elastic compression of the legs is generally contraindicated in patients with ischemic vascular disease, leg deformities, gross leg edema and pulmonary edema associated with congestive heart failure.[48] On the other hand, stockings that lose elasticity are ineffective.

Patients can be protected from venous injury by removing environmental obstacles or, in the case of confused or agitated patients, by padding side rails. Insertion of intravenous lines in the lower extremities should be discouraged.

Early detection of thromboembolism requires astute, systematic, and repeated observations by the nurse. Often symptoms and signs of thromboembolism are manifested as subtle changes in a patient's condition, and planned, careful questioning of patients for symptoms may reveal otherwise unnoticed clues. Patients who have been inactive for prolonged periods may develop a pulmonary embolus upon initial ambulation and should thus be closely observed at that time.

When thromboembolism has been identified and medical therapy instituted, monitoring for expected and unexpected effects of therapy becomes a prominent nursing responsibility. Patients and their families need to understand the purpose of therapy, the nature of the disease process, and future plans and expectations. With this information they can begin to make relevant decisions, become more prepared to participate in their therapy, and reduce anxiety stemming from fear of the unknown.

Measures the patient can take to prevent thromboembolism at home should be an integral part of the discharge teaching plan. Positions of stasis, prolonged immobility, and restrictive clothing should be avoided. Ways in which injury can be prevented should be explored with the patient and the proper method and timing for applying stockings should be emphasized. Stockings should be washed every 2 to 4 days and laid flat to dry. At least two pairs of stockings should be sent home with the patient to ensure continued wear.

ARTERIAL EMBOLI

Etiology

Systemic emboli arise most commonly from the heart and are associated with mural thrombi after myocardial infarction, valvular disease (almost exclusively mitral lesions), chronic congestive heart failure, endocarditis, and atrial fibrillation. Other important sources of arterial emboli are aortic aneurysms and the carotid sinuses.[7,58,68]

Pathophysiology

The sequelae of arterial emboli depend primarily on the size of the embolus, the organ involved, and the state of the collateral vessels.[54] The immediate effect of an embolic occlusion is sudden cessation of blood flow distal to the site of the embolus, followed in a few hours by a progression of the clot below and sometimes above the obstruction. Secondary vasospasm contributes further to the ischemia produced by the occlusion. Less tissue ischemia can be expected when collateral circulation is immediately operative. Dangerous fragmentation of the embolus can occur before organization takes place, resulting in occlusion of more distal vessels.

Arterial bifurcations and atherosclerotic narrowings are vulnerable areas in which emboli tend to lodge. Cerebral, mesenteric, renal, and coronary arteries are often involved, in addition to the large arteries of the limbs.

Assessment

Clinical Manifestations. Emboli of the leg arteries with poor collateral flow will produce a fairly characteristic and dramatic clinical picture. Sudden, severe pain occurs in the distal part of the limb and may become excruciating, particularly if oxygen requirements of the limb are increased by exercise. Distal pulses are lost and the limb becomes cool, pale, mottled, and numb. Sensation and motor function gradually decline. Superficial veins may be collapsed because of the decreased blood flow into the extremity.[57] In some patients pain may have a more insidious onset and be preceded by numbness and paresthesia.

As a result of the ischemia, a sharp line of color and temperature demarcation distal to the site of occlusion may be detected. With a femoral embolus, this line may appear in the lower third of the thigh, and with a popliteal embolus, in the midcalf.

Muscle necrosis can develop in 6 to 8 hours after an acute occlusion. Skin breakdown with blister formation and frank gangrene ensue, resulting in loss of the limb.

Symptoms and signs of emboli in arteries will reflect dysfunction of the organ or tissues deprived of blood flow. For example, cerebral emboli will produce a stroke. An occlusion of a coronary artery will result in a myocardial infarction. A renal artery embolus may produce flank pain, fever, hematuria, hypertension, and albuminuria.

Diagnosis of an arterial embolus is made from the history, physical examination, and selected diagnostic tests related to the function or pathologic changes of the organ or tissues involved. Arterial angiography will confirm the extent and location of the embolic occlusion.

Medical Therapy

Early recognition of the problem, prompt restoration of circulation to the organ or extremity affected, and prevention of further emboli are the goals of therapy for patients with systemic arterial emboli. Conservative medical management includes intravenous anticoagulation with heparin, which will prevent propagation of the clot and thus reduce the amount of tissue necrosis. Thrombolytic agents may be used to hasten embolic lysis.

When conservative management fails to improve circulation to an extremity and tissue viability is threatened, or when an embolus lodges at the aortic bifurcation, surgical intervention may be necessary. Emboli elsewhere are often not amenable to surgery.

Embolectomy is the procedure of choice when a major vessel to an extremity is occluded and is most effective if performed within 8 to 10 hours of the incident, prior to the onset of muscle necrosis.[7] Heparin therapy may serve to extend this time limit by preventing propagation. In patients with serious heart disease, surgery must be considered in light of the effects of anesthesia and operation on the heart, particularly if the embolus was formed after a myocardial infarction.[60]

Nursing Care

Since time is crucial in preserving tissue viability, early detection of arterial emboli is essential. High-risk patients should be carefully and frequently monitored for signs and symptoms of reduced organ and limb perfusion. All complaints of pain and altered sensation should be thoroughly evaluated. Meticulous comparisons of the extremities should be made at least every 4 to 8 hours.

If an embolic occlusion of a limb is suspected, measures directed at protecting the extremity, reducing metabolic demands, and improving tissue perfusion should be instituted. Loosely padding the limb or the siderails and bedframe, and placing pillows between the legs will help prevent injury from accidental bumping against hard objects. Bedcradles keep the weight of linen off the affected leg. Frequent changes of position of the limb will avoid prolonged pressure on any single aspect of the extremity.

When heat is applied to an ischemic extremity, the temperature of the heat source should not exceed body temperature. Burn injuries tend to occur at lower temperatures in ischemic limbs than in normal ones. Excess heat to the ischemic limb may accelerate metabolic rate and increase the need for oxygen, which cannot be met by the reduced blood flow through the occluded artery. Muscle work will also require an increased amount of oxygen and should be minimized.

The affected limb should be maintained in a position of 15 degrees of dependency in order to aid arterial flow by gravity. An immoderate amount of dependency, however, will lead to venous stasis and edema which can, if severe, impede blood flow and predispose the limb to thrombus formation.

When anticoagulants are prescribed, nursing responsibilities are the same as those described earlier in this chapter and in Chapter 38. Nursing care of patients with coronary or cerebral emboli is described elsewhere in this text.

REFERENCES

1. Adar R, Salzman EW: Treatment of thrombosis of veins of lower extremities. N Engl J Med 292(7):348–50, 1975
2. Ahonen A: Electrocardiographic changes in massive pulmonary embolism: I analysis of the changes in P wave and QRS complex. Acta Med Scand 201:539–42, 1977
3. Ahonen, A: Electrocardiographic changes in massive pulmonary embolism: II analysis of changes in ST segment and T wave. Acta Med Scand 201:543–45, 1977
4. Alexander J: Differential guide to chest pain. Hosp Med 12(5):6–15, 1976
5. Alexander R, Folse R, Pizzorno J et al: Thromboembolism: Results of a prospective study. Ann Surg 180(6):883–87, 1974
6. Barnes RW, Russell HE, Wu KK et al: Accuracy of doppler ultrasound in clinically suspected venous thrombosis of the calf. Surg Gynecol Obstet 143:425–28, 1976
7. Beeson P, McDermott W (eds): Textbook of Medicine, 14th ed, pp 910–920, 1074–1075. Philadelphia, WB Saunders, 1975
8. Bell WR, Simon TL, DeMets DL: The clinical features of submassive and massive pulmonary embolism. Am J Med 62:355–60, 1977
9. Bergentz SE: Dextran in the prophylaxis of pulmonary embolism. World J Surg, 2(1):19–25, 1978
10. Bjerkland CJ: Anticoagulant therapy in myocardial infarction. Heart Lung, 4(1):61–68, 1974
11. Bloomfield D: The recognition and management of pulmonary embolism. Heart Lung, 3(2):241–46, 1974
12. Britton BJ, Hawkey C, Wood WG et al: Stress—A significant factor in venous thrombosis? Br J Surg 61:814–20, 1974
13. Browse N: Advances in management of deep vein thrombosis. Mod Med September 3, pp 27–32, 1973
14. Burrell ZL, Burrell LO: Critical Care, 3rd ed. St. Louis, C. V. Mosby, 1977
15. Caprini J, Zoellner JL, Weisman M: Heparin therapy—Part I. Cardiovasc Nurs 13(3):13–16, 1977
16. Caprini J, Zoellner JL, Weisman M: Heparin therapy—Part II. Cardiovasc Nurs 13(4):17–20, 1977
17. Chalmers TC, Malta RJ, Smith H et al: Evidence favoring the use of anticoagulants in the hospital phase of acute myocardial infarction. N Engl J Med 297(20):1091–96, 1977
18. Clagett GP, Salzman EW: Prevention of venous thromboembolism in surgical patients. N Engl J Med 290(2):93–96, 1974
19. Coon WW, Willis PW: Recurrence of venous thromboembolism. Surgery 73(6):823–27, 1973
20. Council on Thrombosis of the American Heart Association: Prevention of venous thromboembolism in surgical patients by low dose heparin. Circulation 55(2):423A, 1977
21. Cranley J, Canas AJ, Sull WJ: The diagnosis of deep vein thrombosis: Fallibility of clinical symptoms and signs. Arch Surg iii:34–36, 1976
22. Cristal H, Stern J, Ronen M et al: Identifying patients at risk for thromboembolism: Use of ^{125}I-labeled fibrinogen in patients with acute myocardial infarction. J Am Med Assoc 236(24):2755–57, 1976
23. Cudkowicz L, Sherry S: Current status of thrombolytic therapy. Heart Lung 7(1):97–100, 1978
24. Cudkowicz L, Sherry S: The venous system and the lung. Heart Lung 7(1):91–96, 1978
25. Dalen JE, Haffajee CI, Alpert JS et al: Pulmonary embolism, pulmonary hemorrhage and pulmonary infaction. N Engl J Med 296(25):1431–35, 1977
26. Ebert RV: Use of anticoagulants in acute myocardial infarction. Circulation 45:903–910, 1972
27. Fitzmaurice J: Venous thromboembolic disease: Current thoughts. Cardiovasc Nurs 14(1):1–4, 1978
28. Fitzmaurice J, Sasahara A: Current concepts of pulmonary embolism: Implications for nursing practice. Heart Lung 3(2):209–18, 1974
29. Flanc C, Kakkar VV, Clarke MB: Postoperative deep vein thrombosis: Effect of intensive prophylaxis. Lancet 477–78, 1969
30. Fulton R, Duckett K: Plasma fibrinogen and thromboemboli after myocardial infarction. Lancet ii:1161–64, 1976
31. Gallus AS, Hirsh J, Tuttle RJ et al: Small subcutaneous doses of heparin in the prevention of venous thrombosis. N Engl J Med 288:545, 1973
32. Genton E: Therapeutic aspects of pulmonary embolism. Heart Lung 3(2):233–36, 1974
33. Geske C: Anticoagulant therapy in acute myocardial infarction. Heart Lung 1(5):639–40, 1972
34. Grollman J: Radiological diagnosis of pulmonary thromboembolism. Heart Lung 3(2):219–26, 1974
35. Handley A: Low dose heparin after myocardial infarction. Lancet ii:623–24, 1972

36. Hirsh J: Venous thromboembolism: Diagnosis, treatment, prevention. Hosp Pract, 10(8):53–62, 1975
37. Hirsh J, Gallus AS: ^{125}I-labeled fibrinogen scanning: Use in diagnosis of venous thrombosis. J Am Med Assoc 233(9): 970–73, 1975
38. Hume M, Fremont-Smith P: Role of noninvasive techniques in diagnosing leg thrombosis. Hosp Pract 10(12):57–62, 1975
39. Husni E, Ximenes J, Gayette E: Elastic support of the lower limbs in hospital patients: A critical study. J Am Med Assoc 214(8):1456–62, 1970
40. Kakkar VV: The current status of low-dose heparin in the prophylaxis of thrombophlebitis and pulmonary embolism. World J Surg 2(1):3–18, 1978
41. Kakkar VV, Howe CT, Nicolaides AN et al: Deep venous thrombosis of leg: Is there a high risk group? Am J Surg 120:527–30, 1970
42. Lavin MA: Bed exercises for acute cardiac patients. Am J Nurs 73(7):1226–27, 1973
43. Lee BY, Trainor FS, Kavner D, et al: Noninvasive prevention of deep vein thrombosis. Am Fam Physician 14(5):129–34, 1976
44. Lewis CE, Antoine J, Mueller C et al: Elastic compression in prevention of venous stasis: A critical reevaluation. Am J Surg 132:739–43, 1976
45. Martin JF, Alvarez-Mena SV: Cardiovascular Physical Diagnosis. Chicago, Yearbook Medical Publishers, 1973
46. Mathewson H: Pulmonary thromboembolism: Aspects of critical care. Am Assoc Nurse Anesthetists J 45(2):164–69, 1977
47. Maurer BJ, Wray R, Shillingford JP: Frequency of venous thrombosis after myocardial infarction. Lancet ii:7739–41, 1971
48. McConnell E: Fitting antiembolism stockings. Nursing 78 8(9):67–71, 1978
49. Meltzer L, Abdellah F, Kitchell JR: Concepts and Practices of Intensive Care for Nurse Specialists, 2nd ed. Bowie, MD, Charles Press Publishers, 1976
50. Meltzer LE, Dunning AJ: Textbook of Coronary Care. Philadelphia, Charles Press Publishers, 1972
51. Murray TS, Lorimer AR, Cox FC et al: Leg vein thrombosis following myocardial infarction. Lancet ii:792–93, 1970
52. Neilson GH, Galen EG, Hossack KF: Thromboembolic complications of mitral valve disease. Aust N Z J Med 8(4):372–6, 1978
53. Nicolaides AN, Kakkar VV, Ronney JT et al: Myocardial infarction and deep venous thrombosis. Br Med J i:432–34, 1971
54. Perry TM, Miller FN: Pathology: A Dynamic Introduction to Medicine and Surgery. Boston, Little, Brown & Co, 1961
55. Prevention of fatal postoperative pulmonary embolism by low doses of heparin: an international multicenter trial. Lancet ii:45–51, 1975
56. Prevention of postoperative thromboembolism. Lancet ii(7924):63–64, 1975
57. Price SA, Wilson LM: Pathophysiology: Clinical Concepts of Disease Processes. New York, McGraw-Hill, 1978
58. Roberts B: The acutely ischemic limb. Heart Lung 5(2):273–74, 1976
59. Ryan R: Thrombophlebitis: Assessment and prevention. Am J Nurs 76(10):1634–36, 1976
60. Schwartz S, Shires GT, Spencer FC et al: Principles of Surgery, 3rd ed, pp 913–923. New York, McGraw-Hill, 1979
61. Scurr JH, Ibrahim SZ, Faber RG et al: The efficacy of graduated compression stockings in the prevention of deep venous thrombosis. Br J Surg 64:371–73, 1977
62. Shoop J: Why do a lung scan? J Am Med Assoc 229(5):567–70, 1974
63. Silver D: Pulmonary embolism: Prevention, detection and nonoperative management. Surg Clin North Am 54(5): 1089–1106, 1974
64. Silvergleid A: Thromboembolism diagnosis and treatment. West J Med 120(3):219–25, 1974
65. Simmons AV, Sheppard MA, Cox AF: Deep venous thrombosis after myocardial infarction: Predisposing factors. Br Heart J 35:623–35, 1973
66. Sodeman WA, Sodeman WA: Pathologic Physiology: Mechanisms of Disease, 5th ed. Philadelphia, WB Saunders, 1974

67. Thompson PL, Robinson JS: Stroke after myocardial infarction: Relation to infarct site. Br Med J 2:457–59, 1978
68. Thorn G et al (eds): Harrison's Principles of Internal Medicine, 8th ed, pp 1322–1323; 1327–1329; 1401–1406. New York, McGraw-Hill, 1977
69. Warlow G, Kenmure TG, Beattie ACF et al: A double-blind trial of low doses of subcutaneous heparin in the prevention of deep vein thrombosis after myocardial infarction. Lancet ii:934, 1973
70. Wessler S: Heparin as an antithrombotic agent: Low-dose prophylaxis. J Am Med Assoc 236(4):389–91, 1976
71. Wessler S: Prevention of venous thromboembolism by low-dose heparin: a 1976 status report. Mod Concepts Cardiovasc Dis XLV(6):105–109, 1976
72. Wray R, Maurer B, Shillingford J: Prophylactic anticoagulant therapy in the prevention of calf vein thrombosis after myocardial infarction. N Engl J Med 288(16):815–17, 1973

ADDITIONAL READING

Bergan JJ, Darling RC, deWolfe VG et al: Report intersociety commission for heart disease resources: Medical instrumentation in peripheral vascular disease. Circulation 54(5):1–8, 1976

Corrigan TP, Fossard DP, Spindler J et al: Phlebography in the management of pulmonary embolism. Br J Surg 61:484–88, 1974

deWolfe VG: Assessment of circulation in occlusive arterial disease of the lower extremities. Mod Concepts Cardiovasc Dis XLV(4):91–95, 1976

Deykin D: Indications and techniques for the use of heparin in the treatment of thromboembolism. World J Surg 2(1):39–43, 1978

Dropkin A, Merskey C: Anticoagulant therapy after acute myocardial infarction. J Am Med Assoc 222:541–47, 1972

Emerson P, Marks P: Preventing thromboembolism after myocardial infarction: Effect of low-dose heparin or smoking. Br Med J 1:18–20, 1977

Fratantoni J, Wessler S (eds): Prophylactic therapy of deep vein thrombosis and pulmonary embolism. Department of Health, Education and Welfare, Publication No. (NIH) 76–866

Gifford RH, Feinstein AR: A critique of methodology in studies of anticoagulant therapy for acute myocardial infarction. N Engl J Med 280:351–57, 1969

Glazier RL, Crowell EB: Randomized prospective treatment of continuous versus intermittent heparin therapy. J Am Med Assoc 236:365–67, 1976

Griffith GC, Leak D, Hedge B: Conservative anticoagulation therapy in acute myocardial infarction. Ann Inter Med 57:254–65, 1972

Hayes MJ, Morris GK, Hampton JR: Lack of effect of bedrest and cigarette smoking on the development of deep venous thrombosis after myocardial infarction. Br Med J 38:981–83, 1976

Hinton RC, Kistler JP, Fallon JT et al: Influences of etiology of atrial fibrillation on incidence of systemic emboli. Am J Cardiol 40:509–13, 1977

Hudak CM, Lohr TS, Gallo BM: Critical-Care Nursing, 2nd ed, pp 243–44. New York, JB Lippincott, 1977

Hume M: Examination for venous thromboembolism. Hosp Med 12(7):56–65, 1976

Kakkar VV, Stamatakis VD, Bently PG et al: Prophylaxis for postoperative deep vein thrombosis: Synergistic effect of heparin and dihydroergotamine. J Am Med Assoc 241:39–42, 1979

Levine WG: Anticoagulant, antithrombotic and thrombolytic drugs. In Goodman L, Gilman A (eds): The Pharmacological Basis of Therapeutics, 5th ed. New York, MacMillan Publishing, 1975

McLacklin A: Venous disease of the lower extremities. In Ravitch M et al (eds): Current Problems in Surgery, pp 1–44. Chicago, Yearbook Medical Publishers, 1967

Mobin-Uddin K, Bolooki H, Jude JR: Intravenous caval interruption for pulmonary embolism in cardiac disease. Circulation 41 (II):152, 1970

Richards KL, Armstrong JD, Tikoff G et al: Noninvasive diagnosis of deep venous thrombosis. Arch Inter Med 136:1091, 1976

Salzman EW, Deykin D, Shapiro RM et al: Management of Heparin therapy. N Engl J Med 292:1046–50, 1975

Salzman EW, Harris WH, DeSanctis RW: Reduction in venous thromboembolism by agents affecting platelet function. N Engl J Med 284:1287, 1971

Sharrahan M: Critique of nursing audit of pulmonary embolism and infarction. Qu Rev Bull 21–27, 1976

Szucs M, Brooks H, Grossman W et al: Diagnostic sensitivity of laboratory findings in acute pulmonary embolism. Ann Intern Med 74(2):161–66, 1971

The Urokinase Pulmonary Embolism Trial: A National Cooperative Study. Circulation (suppl 2) 47:1–108, 1973

Wessler S, Gitel SN: Low-dose heparin: Is the risk worth the benefit? Am Heart J 98(1):94–101, 1979

Wilson AF, Surprenant EL, Zucker M: Radioisotopic diagnosis of pulmonary embolism. Heart Lung 3(2):227–32, 1974

ZuWallack RL, Liss JP, Lahiri B: Acquired continuous murmur associated with acute pulmonary thromboembolism. Chest 70(4):557–59, 1976

29

Complications Involving Heart Structures

BRENDA J. SIEWICKI, R.N., M.N.

Each day two thousand people die from one or more complications of myocardial infarction in the United States.[17] This chapter presents a discussion of those complications which involve heart structures: true aneurysms, false aneurysms, papillary muscle rupture, ventricular septal rupture, early pericarditis, and late pericarditis. Of these, a true ventricular aneurysm is the most common, occurring in 20% to 40% of patients with myocardial infarction.[26] Ventricular septal rupture is the least common complication, occurring in 1% of patients with myocardial infarction. The incidence of each of these complications is listed on Table 29-1. Although the incidence of papillary muscle rupture and ventricular septal rupture is relatively low, when it does occur the mortality is exceedingly high. Prompt recognition and proper treatment are therefore mandatory for survival.

To explain the dynamics of these complications, a discussion of the pathophysiology of abnormal wall motions is presented here, followed by discussions of the various complications: true aneurysms, false aneurysms (including cardiac tamponade), papillary muscle rupture, ventricular septal rupture, and early and late pericarditis (Dressler's syndrome).

MYOCARDIAL WALL DYSFUNCTIONS

Regional and global myocardial wall dysfunctions are temporary as a result of ischemia or permanent as a result of infarction. The contraction pattern of the ventricular wall is evaluated during angiography. The normal left ventricle contracts systematically inward toward the center of the chamber (Chap. 10). Abnormal wall motion, or dyssynergy, results in an asymmetric contraction pattern. Dyssynergy is classified into the following types: 1. hypokinesis, the sluggish and incomplete contraction of the entire ventricle; 2. akinesis, the utter motionlessness of a localized area; 3. dyskinesis, the outward or paradoxical bulging of a localized area during systole (Fig. 29-1).[25]

An area of dyssynergy causes the normal left ventricular wall to increase its velocity of contraction, tension generation, and myocardial oxygen consumption to achieve desired total tension. When the area of dyssynergy approaches 20% to 40% of the left ventricular wall, stroke volume and cardiac output are reduced, because of an increase in end-systolic

TABLE 29-1 INCIDENCE OF COMPLICATIONS INVOLVING HEART STRUCTURES IN PATIENTS WITH MYOCARDIAL INFARCTION

Complications	Incidence
True aneurysm	20% to 40%
Early pericarditis	7% to 16%
Late pericarditis (Dressler's syndrome)	1% to 4%
False aneurysm	Rare
Papillary muscle rupture	0.5% to 2%
Ventricular septal rupture	1%

(Schechter D: NY State J Med 74:840–847; 1011–1017; 1439–1444; 1615–1624, 1974; Van Tassel RA, Edwards JE: Chest 61:104–115, 1972)

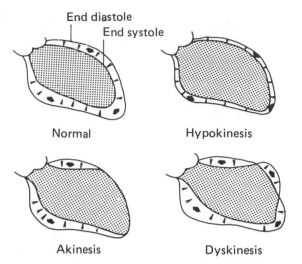

Fig. 29-1. Contraction patterns of ventricular chambers. (Kennedy JW: Cardiovasc Nurs, 12:23–27, 1976)

volume.[14] The reduced stroke volume results in increased end-diastolic volume, left ventricular dilatation, a rightward shift of the Frank–Starling curve, and left-sided congestive heart failure. In addition, ventricular dilatation may stretch an akinetic segment toward a dyskinetic segment. This is not beneficial, since the reduced stroke volume is greater in a dyskinetic area than in an akinetic area.[25]

TRUE ANEURYSMS

A true aneurysm has been defined as an area of akinesis or dyskinesis present 3 months after a myocardial infarction.[26] Usually associated with transmural infarctions, true aneurysms are found in 20% to 40% of patients with myocardial infarctions. Since the left ventricle is the heart chamber with the highest pressures, it is the most common site for infarction and aneurysm formation. However, true aneurysms have been reported to involve the right ventricle, atrial septum, and ventricular septum.[26] The walls of the aneurysm are formed by elements of the infarcted area, as seen in Figure 29-2. During systole, the thin portion of the scarred myocardial wall may bulge as left ventricular pressure increases. Thus, the area of akinesis or dyskinesis results in an increased end-diastolic volume and a reduced ejection fraction. If the aneurysmal wall ruptures, which is rare, a massive hemopericardium results.

The majority of true aneurysms are discovered 3 months after a myocardial infarction. Physical findings are inconsistent and must be correlated with diagnostic tests to verify the diagnosis. The physical findings include signs of congestive heart failure due to reduced cardiac output and increased left ventricular end-systolic volume, mitral and aortic regurgitation due to traction on the valves by the aneurysmal sac, and idiosyncratic findings due to unknown causes. Some of the common physical findings are a high, sustained ventricular impulse that is separate from the apical impulse, atrial (S_4) and ventricular (S_3) gallops, muted heart sounds, accentuated first heart sounds, systolic murmurs, and diastolic murmurs.[26]

In order of prevalence, the complications that occur as a result of a true aneurysm are recurrent severe angina pectoris, progressive congestive heart failure that is difficult to manage medically, a variety of paroxysmal atrial and ventricular arrhythmias, and multiple systemic emboli. Angina pectoris may result from the increased myocardial oxygen consumption caused by dyssynergy in the presence of coronary artery disease. Congestive heart failure is present in 75% of these patients and causes the death of half its population. Ventricular arrhythmias, such as ventricular tachycardia, are present 40% to 70% of the time and are thought to result from increased automaticity of the myocardium at the border of the aneurysm and normal tissue. Although ventricular arrhythmias are the most prevalent, a variety of atrial arrhythmias, such as paroxysmal atrial tachycardia, may occur. It should be noted that the paroxysmal arrhythmias potentiate congestive heart failure in the presence of true aneurysms. Multiple systemic emboli originate from thrombus formation inside the aneurysmal sac and can affect any area of the body.

Some of the diagnostic procedures used to assess true aneurysms are electrocardiography, chest radiography, scintiphotography, and left ventriculography. Results of the noninvasive procedures are only suggestive of a true aneurysm, but diagnosis can be made unequivocally with a left ventriculogram, since true aneurysms are easily visualized. After the acute phase of an infarction, the electrocardiogram (ECG) may suggest an aneurysm when the QRS exceeds 0.08 seconds and there is a persistent elevation of the ST segment in I, aVL and one or more precordial leads, usually between V_1 and V_4.[26] The chest radiograph reveals an enlarged left ventricle. Scintiphotograms, such as gated blood pool images, are also effective in localizing dyssynergy.[1]

During medical management, intermittent Holter monitoring is useful in evaluating the presence and frequency of arrhythmias. After the arrhythmias have been evaluated, antiarrhythmic medications such as quinidine sulphate or propranolol may be prescribed. When present, congestive heart failure is treated with digoxin, furosemide, and potassium chloride. Also, prophylactic anticoagulation may be prescribed to prevent systemic emboli.

Patients are medically managed until one or more of the following complications indicates the necessity for surgical intervention: refractory angina pectoris, intractable or recurrent congestive heart failure, systemic emboli, or recurrent atrial or ventricular arrhythmias. Surgery may be withheld for 3 months after a myocardial infarction to reduce

Fig. 29-2. True left ventricular aneurysm.

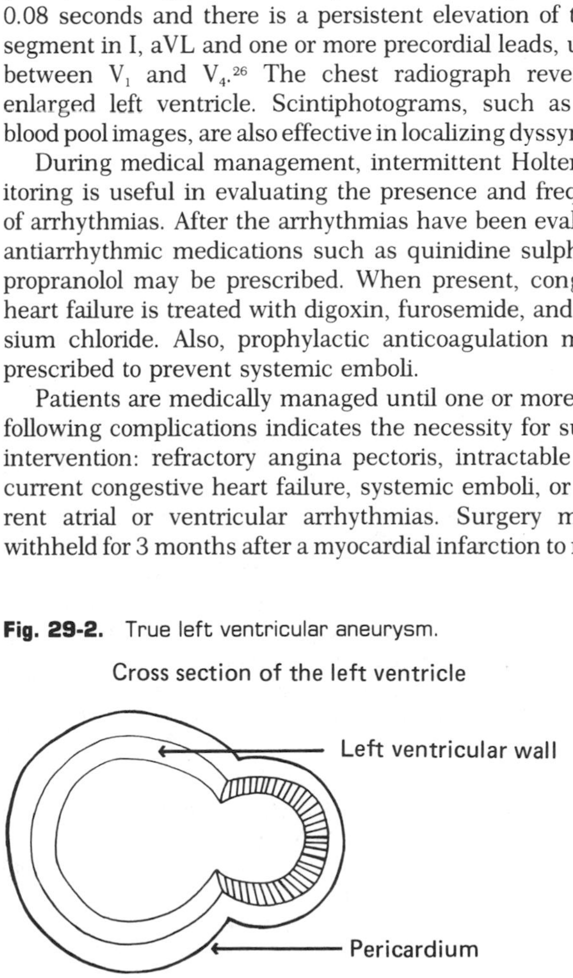

Cross section of the left ventricle

Left ventricular wall

Pericardium

the chances of perioperative mortality and morbidity. The aneurysm is usually clearly demarcated from the normal myocardial wall. The types of surgery that may be done are aneurysmectomy, coronary artery bypass grafting or mitral valve replacement. Aneurysmectomy reduces the ventricular volume, wall tension, and oxygen consumption. Coronary artery bypass grafting may be performed in the presence of significant lesions visualized during coronary angiography. This is done in an attempt to reduce the recurrence of acute myocardial infarction (MI). Replacement of the mitral valve may be necessary if papillary muscle dysfunction has produced severe mitral incompetence.[22]

In 1978, the 2½-year survival rate for patients after ventricular aneurysmectomy was reported to be 82%. Coronary artery bypass grafting did not affect the mortality from aneurysmectomy. Since an ejection fraction above 45% has been reported to result in a lower operative mortality, the outcome of the surgery may be associated with the function of the contractile segment of the ventricle.[20]

Nursing Management

The nursing management of a patient with a true aneurysm includes a comprehensive assessment of:

1. Recurrent severe angina pectoris (Chap. 22)
2. Progressive congestive heart failure that is difficult to manage medically (see Chap. 27)
3. Paroxysmal ventricular arrhythmias (i.e., ventricular tachycardia) which potentiates the congestive heart failure (see Chap. 26)
4. Multiple systemic emboli (see Chap. 28).

One physical finding specific for a true aneurysm is a high, sustained ventricular impulse separate from the apical impulse. The nurse should place her fingertips over the apex of the heart while feeling the carotid artery pulsation. This allows timing of the ventricular impulse with ventricular systole. In addition, the nurse should listen for the murmurs of mitral and aortic regurgitation (Chaps. 14 and 48). The ECG findings specific for true aneurysms should be assessed and documented.

Since medical management is based on the presenting complications, the nursing interventions should be correlated with these complications. Drug education is needed if propranolol is prescribed for recurrent severe angina pectoris or ventricular arrhythmias. Heart rate monitoring for activity progression is necessary for patients with congestive heart failure. If a patient is taking anticoagulants to prevent recurrent systemic emboli, instruction regarding avoidance of aspirin must be given. (See Chapter 38 regarding specific nursing interventions for these complications.) When complications occur, the symptoms are dramatic, and maximum effort is required to stabilize the patient.

Cardiac catheterization and possible open heart surgery should be anticipated. (See Chaps. 19 and 24 for nursing interventions.) Whenever possible, patient and family teaching should be done in several sessions to promote optimal learning. The spouse should be involved in the teaching/learning process. In general, a cardiac catheterization teaching plan should include sensory information about the catheterization laboratory (what the patient will see, hear, and feel) and procedural information (precatheterization preparation, operative procedures, and postcatheterization routines). An open-heart surgery teaching plan should include information on procedures carried out on the day before surgery (skin preparation, coughing, and deep breathing exercises), the duration of surgery, location of incisions, and postoperative phase (time in the intensive care unit, diet, and activity progression).

FALSE ANEURYSMS

The false (pseudo) aneurysm is a rare phenomenon. Theoretically, its formation is due to an initial rupture and a slow leak of blood through the myocardial wall. A reaction occurs over the initial rupture, creating adhesions that prevent a free escape of blood into the pericardial space. An extracardiac fibrous sac is formed, the walls of which do not contain any myocardial muscle cells. As seen in Figure 29-3, the aneurysm has a small mouth with a wide diameter. This aneurysmal sac is often filled by a clot.

Stroke volume is partly diverted into the aneurysmal cavity, reducing the cardiac output. Since aneurysmal sacs differ in size and distensibility, the amount of reduction in cardiac output and increase in myocardial oxygen consumption is variable.[27]

The diagnosis of a false aneurysm is usually made 2 months after a myocardial infarction. The physical findings are nonspecific and the complications are similar to those of true aneurysms. The complications that may occur are angina pectoris, congestive heart failure, arrhythmias, and cardiac tamponade.[27] Cardiac tamponade is the main complication that differentiates the two types of aneurysms. Thromboembolism is frequently seen with true aneurysm, but is rarely seen with false aneurysm.

In an attempt to diagnose false aneurysms before cardiac tamponade occurs, the following tests are used: left ventriculography, echocardiography, and radionuclide gated blood pool imaging. The small opening of the sac may make false aneurysms difficult to visualize with left ventriculography. Echocardiography has been effective for the detection of soft tissue structures such as false aneurysms, and of cardiac tamponade.[5,23] In addition, radionuclide gated

Fig. 29-3. False left ventricular aneurysm.

Cross section of the left ventricle

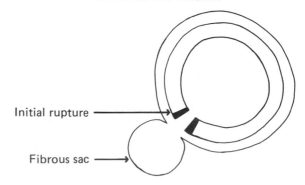

Initial rupture ⟶

Fibrous sac ⟶

blood pool imaging makes it possible to identify the large lateral or posterior chamber of the false aneurysm attached by a small neck to the left ventricular cavity.[4] Because of the threat of rupture, a false aneurysm should be resected. If rupture occurs, emergency pericardiocentesis is a life-saving procedure. A drain may be left in the pericardial sac to provide continued relief of the tamponade while the patient is transported to the operating room.[13]

Excluding cardiac tamponade, the nursing management of a patient with a false aneurysm is the same as that for a true aneurysm. A discussion of cardiac tamponade follows.

CARDIAC TAMPONADE

Cardiac tamponade is an acute compression of the heart due to rapid accumulation of fluid in the pericardium. In an acute state, the amount of fluid that will cause symptoms to occur may be as little as 250 ml, but, when the bleeding occurs more slowly, it may take as much as 1 liter. The signs, symptoms and ECG findings are listed in Table 29-2. A pericardiocentesis will relieve these symptoms in a characteristic manner, decrease neck vein distention and increase systolic blood pressure (Chap. 14).

Pulsus paradoxus is a classical sign of tamponade (Chap. 14). The mechanism behind it is as follows: the escape of fluid from the left ventricle into the pericardium increases the intrapericardial pressure and impedes left ventricular inflow. Traction is exerted on the taut pericardium by the movement of the diaphragm. During inspiration, the diaphragm descends and restricts filling of the left ventricle, causing a corresponding decrease in stroke volume and the decreased systolic pressure of pulsus paradoxus. Right ventricular filling is also restricted, creating either no change or an increase in venous pressure.[9]

Cardiac tamponade is only one of the many causes of pulsus paradoxus. It may also occur with pericardial effusion, adhesive pericarditis, pulmonary emphysema, severe asthma, endocardial fibrosis, scleroderma, mitral stenosis with right-sided cardiac failure, tricuspid stenosis, hypovolemia, and massive pulmonary embolism.

The nursing management of a patient with cardiac tamponade is shown in Table 29-3.

TABLE 29-2 CARDIAC TAMPONADE: SYMPTOMS AND SIGNS

Symptoms	Signs
Pulsus paradoxus	Decreased systolic pressure
Kussmaul respiratory sign	
Increased neck vein distention	feeble heart tones
	Pericardial friction rub
Narrowing pulse pressure	
Chest pain	Electrical alteration, low amplitude QRS complexes
Stupor	

(Schechter D: NY State J Med 74:1011–1017, 1974; Spodick DH: Am J Cardiol 10:155–165, 1962; Spodick DH: Prog Cardiovasc Dis 10:64–96, 1967; Van Tassel RA, Edwards JE: Chest 61:104–115, 1972)

TABLE 29-3 CARDIAC TAMPONADE: NURSING MANAGEMENT

Goals of Care

A. Identify the problem early by:
  1. Recognizing this emergency situation from the clinical findings.
  2. Simultaneously monitoring and preparing the patient for a pericardiocentesis and possible surgery.
B. Reduce anxiety through emotional support to the patient and family.

Interventions

Obtain a pericardiocentesis tray and set up for the procedure.
If indicated, prepare to take the patient to surgery.
Monitor the blood pressure every 5 to 10 minutes. Note changes in pulse pressure as well as in systolic and diastolic fluctuations during inspiration and expiration. Note the ECG for arrhythmias and electrical alterations, every 5 to 10 minutes.
Administer pain medications and assess their effectiveness.
Watch for signs of shock and cardiac arrest.
Support the family during this crisis. Explain events to be expected, *i.e.,* duration of pericardiocentesis or surgery.

Evaluation

After pericardiocentesis, watch for relief of symptoms of cardiac tamponade, *i.e.,* less neck vein distention and increased systolic blood pressure.
Assess the coping mechanisms of the family.

PAPILLARY MUSCLE DYSFUNCTION

The two left ventricular papillary muscles (anterolateral and posteromedial) have a higher oxygen consumption than the oxygen consumption per unit volume of tissue of the rest of the myocardium. This increased oxygen requirement is due to generation of an increased tension during traction on the mitral valve. In addition, the blood supply to the papillary muscles is at the termination of the coronary arterial system, rendering them highly susceptible to ischemia.

Papillary muscle dysfunction can result from infarction of the myocardium at the base of the papillary muscle or from ventricular dilatation even when the papillary muscles are normal. Each papillary muscle is supplied by more than one coronary artery. Thus, a papillary muscle infarct suggests multivessel disease.[29] When a papillary muscle is infarcted, valve closure is not synchronized and regurgitation occurs during systole. Papillary muscle dysfunction may result from ventricular dilatation when the closure of the mitral leaflets is hindered by lateral displacement of the papillary muscles.

The clinical picture of papillary muscle dysfunction includes increased heart size, atrial (S_4) gallop, ventricular (S_3) gallop, and a murmur of mitral insufficiency heard best at the apex. It is a soft, blowing crescendo-decrescendo systolic murmur, ending before the second heart sound.[29] If the papillary muscle ruptures, precipitous left-sided

TABLE 29-4 PAPILLARY MUSCLE RUPTURE: SYMPTOMS AND SIGNS

Symptoms	Signs
Syncope	Increased heart size
Dyspnea	Tachycardia
Angina pectoris	Atrial (S$_4$) gallop
Hemoptysis	Tall jugular A-wave
	Hypotension and signs of hypoperfusion
	Crackles
	Grade III–IV/VI, pansystolic murmur, with wide radiation

(Schechter D: NY State J Med 74:1615–1624, 1974)

congestive heart failure is evident. The signs and symptoms of papillary muscle rupture are listed in Table 29-4.

A chest radiograph initially shows a normal heart with extensive pulmonary congestion. During cardiac catheterization, the findings are of mitral regurgitation: left atrial enlargement and regurgitation of blood from the left ventricle to the left atrium during systole. An echocardiogram demonstrates increased septal motion, decreased systolic posterior wall motion, increased left ventricular size, and bizarre motion of the mitral valve leaflets.[2] A prominent V wave of mitral insufficieny is seen on the pulmonary artery wedge pressure tracing.

During the acute period of papillary muscle rupture, unloading therapy such as intravenous diuretics is a lifesaving intervention. When rupture of the muscle trunk occurs and is managed medically, 50% of patients die within 24 hours and 80% die within 2 weeks. The treatment of choice for papillary muscle rupture is mitral valve replacement, despite the 50% operative mortality.

Nursing management of patients with papillary muscle rupture begins with careful assessment and documentation of the signs and symptoms listed in Table 29-4. Other nursing interventions are listed in Table 29-5.

VENTRICULAR SEPTAL RUPTURE

Ventricular septal rupture occurs in less than 1% of postmyocardial infarction patients. Dyskinesis of the septum results in protrusion of the septum into the right ventricle. Frequently, the rupture involves the adjacent wall of the myocardium; it may also be the site of an acute left-to-right shunt. Centrally located to the infarct, the rupture is usually ragged and ranges in size from a few millimeters to more than 4 cm.[28]

Ventricular septal ruptures usually occur during the first week after an acute myocardial infarction, with 35% occurring on the first day of the infarction. There is an abrupt and dramatic overloading of the right ventricle, resulting in signs and symptoms of right-sided or biventricular congestive heart failure. These conditions are discussed in Chapter 27 (See Table 29-6). Refer also to Chap. 14 for assessment of these findings.

Diagnostic tests used to detect ventricular septal rupture are chest radiograph, cardiac catheterization, and bedside pulmonary artery monitoring. The chest radiograph may show an enlarged heart with a prominent right ventricular outflow tract and pulmonary congestion. The cardiac catheterization and bedside pulmonary artery monitoring show an increased oxygen saturation in the right ventricle and elevated pulmonary artery pressures.[28]

TABLE 29-5 PAPILLARY MUSCLE RUPTURE: NURSING MANAGEMENT

Goals of Care

A. Identify the problem early:
1. Recognize this event as catastrophic from the clinical findings.
2. Simultaneously monitor and prepare the patient for surgery.

B. Increase coping mechanisms of patient and family by offering emotional support.

Interventions

Preoperative Phase

Notify the physician immediately if symptoms and signs of papillary muscle rupture occur.

If the patient is not in an intensive care unit, prepare for a move to one. Temporary measures such as an intra-aortic balloon assist device may be used. Monitor the patient's blood pressure, heart rate, and rhythm.

Administer pain medications and diuretics, and assess their effectiveness.

Place the patient in a high Fowler's position to promote optimal pulmonary ventilation.

Postoperative Phase (see Chap. 24)

Encourage coughing and deep breathing.

Listen for reoccurrence of an atrial gallop or a systolic murmur.

Watch for signs of reduced cardiac output (*i.e.*, reduced blood pressure, increased heart rate, reduced urinary output, etc.) or increased heart failure (*i.e.* crackles).

After a mitral valve replacement, be aware of possible early and late complications. Early complications are: bleeding, arrhythmias, pneumonia, and atelectasis. The late complications are: anemia, thromboembolic events, infections, and side effects of anticoagulation.

Evaluation

Assess the coping mechnism and support systems of the family.

Auscultate the lungs (every 4 to 8 hr) for early recognition of impending heart failure.

TABLE 29-6   VENTRICULAR SEPTAL RUPTURE:
SYMPTOMS AND SIGNS

Symptoms	Signs
Severe chest pain	Hypotension and hypoperfusion
Orthopnea	Bradycardia
Syncope	Atrial (S_4) gallop
	Ventricular (S_3) gallop
	Atrial–ventricular conduction
	disturbances
	A loud holosystolic murmur
	along the lower left sternal
	margin

(Schechter D: NY State J Med 74:1439–1444, 1974)

Ventricular septal rupture is usually treated by surgical repair. In the presence of an acute myocardial infarction, the operation may be postponed for several weeks. The patient may be maintained on the intra-aortic balloon pump while an attempt is made to reduce afterload by administering nitroprusside intravenously or isosorbide dinitrate (Isordil) by mouth. The beneficial effects of nitroprusside include a reduced left ventricular filling pressure, an increased stroke volume into the aorta with a reduced left-to-right shunt and an increased cardiac index.

When surgery becomes a necessity, an incision is made through the left ventricular infarct and a Dacron patch is placed over the septal perforation.[7,8,12] Additional surgical procedures may include coronary artery bypass grafting for stenosis of the coronary arteries, with or without valve replacements for valvular deficiencies.

The nursing management begins with careful assessment and documentation of the findings listed in Table 29-6. (Refer to Chap. 14.) As stated earlier, the clinical picture is that of an abrupt right-sided or biventricular congestive heart failure. See Table 29-7 for goals and nursing interventions for a patient with a ventricular septal rupture.

EARLY PERICARDITIS

The incidence of early pericarditis after MI is reported to be 14.9%.[20] Transient and benign pericarditis usually occurs on the second or third day after myocardial infarction. The presence of an early pericardial friction rub is the typical finding of pericarditis. The friction rub occurs when an inflamed area over a transmural infarction causes the pericardial surface to lose its lubricating fluid, a possible result of dyskinesis. Since the infarction is transmural and therefore more extensive than nontransmural infarctions, many patients with early pericarditis have a higher incidence of arrhythmias, congestive heart failure, and shock than do patients without pericarditis. In addition, the intitial ST segment `elevation is not localized and cardiac enzyme changes are typically higher in patients with pericarditis.[12] Persistence of a friction rub beyond 3 days may indicate a poor prognosis. Patients may or may not experience chest pain. If present, it may be dull and may resemble the pain of a myocardial infarction. Hemopericardium has been reported as a possible complication of anticoagulant therapy during pericarditis, especially when sodium heparin is used. Therefore many physicians discontinue anticoagulant therapy after pericarditis develops.

The goal of treatment for early pericarditis is to relieve the chest pain by administering analgesics such as acetaminophen (Tylenol). On occasion, anti-inflammatory agents such as indomethacin (Indocin) or steroids, and narcotics such as methylmorphine (codeine) or meperidine (Demerol)

TABLE 29-7   VENTRICULAR SEPTAL RUPTURE: NURSING MANAGEMENT

Goals of Care

  A. Early identification of the problem
    1. Recognize the clinical findings as those of a ventricular septal rupture.
    2. Simultaneously monitor and prepare the patient for surgery.
  B. Increase coping mechanisms of patient and family by offering emotional support.

Interventions

Preoperative Phase

  During intra-aortic monitoring, palpate pedal pulses every two hours. Be alert for inadequate urinary output and check the timing of the diastolic inflation with an arterial tracing. While administering nitroprusside intravenously, check urinary output, right atrial pressure and cardiac output every 2 to 4 hours.

  Administer and assess the efficacy of pain medications.

  Prevent the hazards of immobility (Chap. 30).

  Before surgery, prepare patient and family for length of surgery, intensive care environment, location of the incision, and answer any questions they may have.

Postoperative Phase (see Chap. 24)

  Encourage coughing and deep breathing.

  Watch for signs of reduced cardiac output (*i.e.*, reduced blood pressure, increased heart rate, reduced urinary output) or increased heart failure (*i.e.*, crackles).

Evaluation

  Assess the patient for side effects of intra-aortic balloon monitoring and nitroprusside administration, *i.e.*, decreased pedal pulses and decreased urinary output (less than 30 ml/hr).

  Be alert for recurrences of right-sided or biventricular failure, (*i.e.*, peripheral edema and crackles).

TABLE 29-8 EARLY OR LATE PERICARDITIS: NURSING MANAGEMENT

Goals of Care

A. Reduce the patient's anxiety by distinguishing between the pain of pericarditis and that of recurrent myocardial infarction.

B. Establish a pain management program for the dull chest pain of pericarditis.

C. Develop a drug teaching plan for the prescribed medication(s).

Interventions

If the patient is receiving heparin, expect it to be discontinued.

Educate the patient and family regarding a definition of pericarditis and probable etiology of the chest pain. Stress that this is a benign, self-limiting phenomenon and does not indicate further heart damage.

Assess the effectiveness of the indomethacin (Indocin), methylmorphine (codeine), or meperidine (Demerol). Document the frequency of occurrence, duration, and intensity of pain.

When the drug is chosen for pain management, educate the patient regarding side effects, frequency of administration, and importance of continuing with the medication for a prolonged time.

Evaluation

To evaluate the learning process, ask the patient to define pericarditis, to describe the purpose of the medications, and to list the possible side effects of these medications.

---

are prescribed. The nursing management of a patient with early pericarditis is listed in Table 29-8.

LATE PERICARDITIS (DRESSLER'S SYNDROME)

Late pericarditis is also referred to as Dressler's syndrome or the postmyocardial infarction syndrome (PMIS). The onset can be as early as 1 day after an infarction, or as late as 28 months after an infarction.[6,24] The etiology is unknown, but current research suggests an autoimmune response. Animal research has shown that an allergy may produce pericarditis, pleurisy, and pneumonitis. The presence of circulating heart-specific antibodies that respond to corticosteroids and antimetabolites has been documented. It may be that an antigen is produced by myocardial necrosis which in turn leads to the formation of autoantibodies that cause this syndrome.

This syndrome is characterized by a dull pain, either mild or crushing, that resembles the pain of a myocardial infarction in its quality and location.

The pain may radiate to the neck, shoulders, or arms. It can be intensified by deep inspiration, turning in bed, yawning, coughing, or swallowing. To effect a splinting action, the patient may lean forward in an attempt to obtain relief.[12] The pain is accompanied by a prolonged (longer than 1 week) and recurrent fever between 101°F (38.3°C) and 102°F (38.9°C). A pericardial friction rub occurs and lasts from 3 days to several weeks. A resulting pleuritis, pneumonitis, or both, will respond better to prednisone instead of antibiotics.

Cardiac tamponade may occur during anticoagulation therapy in patients with late pericarditis.[6,11] Since anticoagulants may be ordered when reinfarction is suspected (e.g., the dull pain of late pericarditis), definitive diagnosis is very important. Treatment may include acetlysalicylic acid (aspirin), methylmorphine (codeine), and prednisone. This is a prolonged but self-limiting phenomenon that may not require any medical intervention. Since procainamide hydrochloride (Pronestyl) and diphenylhydantoin sodium (Dilantin) have been reported to induce a lupus-like syndrome with occasional pericarditis, the nurse should be alert for signs of pericarditis when these drugs are administered. The nursing management is listed in Table 29-8.

There are many complications that affect the structure of the heart after a myocardial infarction and may lead to dyssynergy and cardiorrhexis (rupture of the heart). It is estimated that more than 25,000 Americans die every year from this unexpected complication.[13] Early diagnosis and the combined efforts of medical and nursing interventions are crucial.

REFERENCES

1. Ahmad S, Kleiger RE, Connors J et al: The echocardiographic diagnosis of rupture of a papillary muscle. Chest 73:232–234, 1978
2. Bates R, Beutler S, Resnekov L et al: Cardiac rupture—Challenge in diagnosis and management. Am J Cardiol 40:429–437, 1977
3. Blau N, Shen BA, Pittman DE et al: Massive hemopericardium in a patient with postmyocardial infarction syndrome. Chest 71:549–552, 1977
4. Daggett WM, Guyton RA, Mundth ED et al: Surgery for postmyocardial infarct ventricular septal defect. Ann Surg 186:260–271, 1977
5. Davidson KG, Wallwork J, Miller HC et al: Early closure of ventricular septal defect complicating myocardial infarction. Br Heart J 38:874–875, 1976
6. D'Cruz IA, Cohen HC, Prabhu R et al: Diagnosis of cardiac tamponade by echocardiography. Circulation 52:460–465, 1975
7. Dock W: Inspiratory traction on the pericardium. Arch Intern Med 108:81–84, 1961
8. Donaldson RM, Honey M, Balcon R et al: Surgical treatment of postinfarction left ventricular aneurysm in 32 patients. Br Heart J 38:1223–1228, 1976
9. Dressler W: The post-myocardial infarction syndrome. Arch Intern Med 103:28–42, 1959
10. Kahn, JC, Rigaud M, Gandjbakhch I et al: Posterior rupture of the interventricular septum after acute myocardial infarction: Successful early surgical repair. Ann Thorac Surg 23:483–486, 1977
11. Kendall RW, DeWood MA: Postinfarction cardiac rupture: Surgical success and review of the literature. Ann Thorac Surg 25:311–315, 1978
12. Kennedy JW: Myocardial function in coronary artery disease. Cardiovasc, Nurs 12:23–27, 1976
13. Khan AH: Pericarditis of myocardial infarction: Review of the literature with case presentation. Am Heart J 90:788–793, 1975
14. Kleiger R, Shaw R: (Discussants); Avioli LV (ed): Postmyocardial infarction complications requiring surgery. Arch Intern Med 137:1580–1586, 1977
15. Koopot R, Diethrich EB: A review of the surgical treatment of complications of myocardial infarction. Heart Lung 6:487–492, 1977

16. Kossowsky W, Epstein PJ, Levine RS: Postmyocardial infarction syndrome: An early complication of acute myocardial infarction. Chest 63:35–40, 1973

17. Krumbhar EB, Crowell C: Spontaneous rupture of the heart. Am J Med Sci 170:828–856, 1925

18. McLean KH, Bett JHN, Saltups A: Pericarditis in acute myocardial infarction. Aust NZ J Med 5:1–2, 1975

19. Piessens J, DeGust H, Kesteloot H: Indications for surgical treatment of left ventricular aneurysm. J Cardiovasc Surg 15:91–94, 1974

20. Roelandt J, van den Brand M, Vletter WB et al: Echocardiographic diagnosis of pseudoaneurysm of the left ventricle. Circulation 52:466–472, 1975

21. Sawaya MP, Favrot LK, Smith SC Jr: Hemorrhage cardiac tamponade complicating the postmyocardial infarction syndrome in the absence of anticoagulation. Heart Lung 4:770–774, 1975

22. Schechter D: Cardiac structural and functional changes after myocardial infarction—I. Dyssynergy. NY State J Med 74:666–673, 1974

23. Schechter D: Cardiac structural and functional changes after myocardial infarction—II. True parietal aneurysm. NY State J Med 74:840–847, 1974

24. Schechter D: Cardiac structural and functional changes after myocardial infarction—III. Parietal rupture and pseudoaneurysm. NY State J Med 74:1011–1017, 1974

25. Schechter D: Cardiac structural and functional changes after myocardial infarction—IV. Ventricular septal dysfunction and rupture. NY State J Med 74:1439–1444, 1974

26. Schechter D: Cardiac structural and functional changes after myocardial infarction—V. Papillary muscle dysfunction and rupture. NY State J Med 74:1615–1624, 1974

27. Shaw R, Ferguson TB, Weldon CS et al: Left ventricular aneurysm resection: Indications and long-term follow-up. Ann Thorac Surg 25:336–339, 1978

28. Spodick DH: Electric alternation of the heart—Its relation to the kinetics and physiology of the heart during cardiac tamponade. Am J Cardiol 10:155–165, 1962

29. Spodick DH: Acute cardiac tamponade—Pathologic physiology, diagnosis and management. Prog Cardiovasc Dis 10:64–96, 1967

30. Techlenberg PL, Fitzgerald J, Allaire BI et al: Afterload reduction in the management of postinfarction ventricular septal defect. Am J Cardiol 38:956–958, 1976

31. Van Tassel RA, Edwards JE: Rupture of heart complicating myocardial infarction. Chest 61:104–115, 1972

30

Physical Immobility and Recumbency

SANDRA L. UNDERHILL, R.N. M.N.

Extended bed rest is no longer recommended therapy for the patient with an acute, uncomplicated myocardial infarction (MI), but for the patient with a complicated MI, for instance with cardiogenic shock, physical immobility may result from the complication or may be prescribed by the physician or nurse. In this chapter, bed rest, unless otherwise stated, is assumed to be the flat supine or recumbent position (Fig. 30-1). Prolonged bed rest, defined as bed rest lasting 3 days or longer, detrimentally affects the functioning of most body systems: cardiovascular, respiratory, renal, gastrointestinal, musculoskeletal and integumentary. Psychologic well-being is also adversely affected.

In acute care, prevention of many of the effects of physical immobility is delegated to nurses. Nurses must, therefore, understand the dangers to the patient of prolonged bed rest in order to prescribe appropriate nursing interventions. Although physical immobility occurs in a wide variety of situations, its discussion in this chapter centers on prolonged bed rest as it affects the patient with acute MI. Most of the research in this area has been done with young, healthy individuals. It has therefore been assumed that these physiological effects apply as well to older patients with MIs. Emphasis is placed on effects on the cardiovascular system, although it must be understood that all systems interrelate and that what affects one will influence the others. Taking a systems approach, this chapter discusses pathophysiology, awareness of potential problems, and prevention of these problems by the nurse, as well as recognition of existing problems and of nursing and medical management.

CARDIOVASCULAR EFFECTS

Prolonged bed rest influences the cardiovascular system in four major ways: it promotes thrombus formation (see Chaps. 8 and 28), increases the workload of the heart, decreases the cardiac reserve, and causes postural hypotension.

Increased Myocardial Work

Myocardial work can be estimated indirectly by calculating pressure–rate product, the product of systolic blood pressure (BP) and heart rate (HR). Stroke volume (SV) and cardiac output (CO) are considered minor determinants of work. When myocardial work is increased, myocardial oxygen consumption ($M\dot{V}O_2$) is also increased. When the patient is in the flat supine position, CO is 30% greater than when he is sitting.[4] The increased myocardial work may be the result of several factors: increased pressure–rate product during prolonged bed rest, increased heart and stroke volume, increased CO, and the Valsalva maneuver (Chap. 23), which may be performed as many as 10 to 20 times per hour in the bedfast patient.[1,9]

Pressure–Rate Product. Changes in pressure–rate product depend on the duration of bed rest. Mean arterial pressure is slightly reduced or remains unchanged during supine bed rest. Changes in HR vary with the amount of time spent at bed rest. In normal subjects, an initial HR

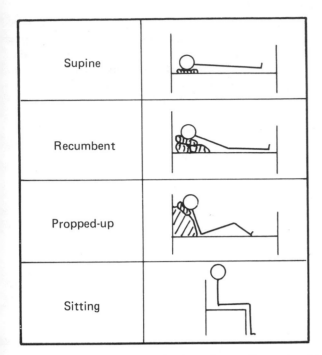

Fig. 30-1. Posture in bed. Supine refers to flat supine. Note that "sitting up" in bed is quite different from sitting in a chair. "Propped-up" is a more exact description. (Browse NL: The Physiology and Pathophysiology of Bed Rest, p 43. Springfield IL: Charles C Thomas, 1965)

drop of 10 to 15 beats per minute occurs when the supine position is assumed.[7] However, when normal subjects were confined to bed for 3 weeks, an HR increase of one-half beat per minute per day occurred, accounting for a 20% to 56% increase.[*][16] Thus, pressure–rate product may be reduced or unchanged initially, but increased during more prolonged bed rest. In the patient with an MI on prolonged bed rest, the increase in pressure–rate product and $M\dot{V}O_2$ may cause further myocardial ischemia.

Increased Heart and Stroke Volume. Assumption of the supine position causes peripheral arterial and venous dilation and redistribution of blood flow. In the supine position, according to Sjöstrand, 11% of the total blood volume leaves the legs for redistribution to other parts of the body. Most of this amount (78%) enters the thorax, three-fourths of it to the lungs and one-fourth to the heart and great vessels.[13,14] When the patient is supine, SV increases, in accordance with Starling's law, from 41%[2] to 62%.[19]

In the normal heart, these changes in blood flow are well tolerated. However, in the patient with congestive heart failure (CHF), this sudden increase in venous return may promote further left and right heart failure. If the legs of the patient in CHF are elevated above heart level, cardiac arrest can ensue.[1]

Increased Cardiac Output. Changes in CO also depend on the amount of time spent at bed rest. SV has already been shown to increase with recumbency, as has HR with

---

* It should be noted that a moderate increase in HR in healthy individuals is not detrimental, but in the cardiac patient, tachycardia, with its reduced diastolic filling time and subsequent decrease in SV, may reduce coronary artery perfusion and precipitate an ischemic episode.

prolonged bed rest. This increase in SV and HR, together with reduced peripheral vascular resistance (PVR), increases CO from 4 to 7 l/minute (erect) to 5 to 9 l/minute (supine), or by 20% to 30%.[1]

Decreased Cardiac Reserve

Taylor's study of normal subjects demonstrates that cardiac deconditioning occurs during immobilization. During physical work immediately after a 3-week bed rest period, HRs averaged 40 beats per minute faster than during the same physical work before the bed rest. Five to ten weeks of reconditioning were required for these healthy men to regain their prestudy level of cardiac function.[16]

Saltin and associates studied five healthy young men (three sedentary, two active) during 20 days of bed rest and 53 to 55 days of physical training. During the period of bed rest, mean maximal oxygen uptake fell by 28% and did not return to baseline for 8 to 12 days after bed rest in the sedentary subjects and 29 to 43 days after bed rest in the active subjects.[11] It should be emphasized that the subjects of Taylor and of Saltin were young and healthy. This has implications for patients who experience physical immobilization and have losses in cardiac reserve so that the heart is unable to adapt itself to increasing physiological demands. Older, sedentary individuals, such as many of those with acute MIs, may experience even greater losses in cardiac reserve than those reported in younger individuals without coronary artery disease. The deconditioning associated with bed rest may not result entirely from decreased cardiac reserve. Further investigation is needed to determine whether increased peripheral compliance and reduced blood volume are contributing factors.

Postural Hypotension

Postural hypotension is a fall in BP that accompanies a change in posture, such as from lying to sitting or from lying to standing (Chap. 14). In addition to loss of sense of balance, other factors may contribute to postural hypotension secondary to bed rest, among them a loss of general muscle tone and a decrease in intravascular and extracellular fluid (ECF) volume.

In a study by Chobanian and associates, 4 healthy males were kept on bed rest for 3 weeks and then subjected to a 15 minute 70-degree tilt. Table 30-1 summarizes the responses to tilt during the bed-rest period and compares them with those of the control (ambulatory) period. In all instances

TABLE 30-1 DEVELOPMENT OF POSTURAL HYPOTENSION IN NORMAL SUBJECTS DURING A 15-MINUTE 70-DEGREE TILT

Investigators	Variable Studied	Control (Ambulatory) Period	Bed Rest Period
Chobanian, Little, Tercyak et al 1974	CI	↓ 17%	↓ 39%
	SV	↓ 33%	↓ 57%
	HR	↓ 20%	↓ 44%
	PVR	↑ 18%	↑ 36%

CI = cardiac index

TABLE 30-2 CHANGES IN TOTAL BLOOD VOLUME, PLASMA VOLUME, EXTRACELLULAR FLUID VOLUME, AND RED-CELL MASS

Investigators	Variable Studied		
Miller, Johnson, Lamb 1964 (normal subjects)		28-DAY BED REST PERIOD	15 DAYS AFTER THE END OF BED REST
	TBV	↓ 11% (655 ml)	further ↓ to 15%
	Plasma volume	↓ 15% (500 ml)	↓ 11%
	Red-cell mass	↓ 6.5% (160 ml)	further ↓ to 22.5%
Vogt, Johnson 1967 (normal subjects)		1–4 DAYS OF BED REST	4–10 DAYS OF BED REST
	Plasma volume	rapid ↓	stabilized
	ECF volume	↓ 6.7%	↓ 13.4%

bed rest exaggerated the normal, physiologic effects.[3] (Note that an increase in PVR after bed rest is in direct opposition to the long-held belief that there is a diminished vasoconstriction reflex after bed rest.)[14] In another study, after 3 weeks of bed rest, healthy young men required 7 weeks to regain fully their cardiovascular response to assumption of the erect position.[16] Chobanian and associates suggest that a decrease in myocardial function per se, as demonstrated by a reduction in left ventricular ejection time index, may be a factor in the cardiovascular changes occurring with bed rest.[3] Increased compliance of peripheral veins can have equally important consequences.

Since mean BP does not change over prolonged periods of bed rest,[3] hypotension does not become a problem until the patient with an MI is beginning to be mobilized from the supine to the sitting position. Symptoms accompanying postural hypotension are those of decreased cerebral perfusion (weakness, dizziness, ataxia, blurring of vision, dysarthria, and syncope). All of these symptoms disappear as soon as the supine position is resumed. Decreased coronary artery perfusion, which can precipitate myocardial ischemia or extend infarction, is of particular concern in the cardiac patient.

Loss of General Muscle Tone. The "muscle pump" or "venopressor mechanism" (compression of the lower leg veins by contraction of the calf muscles) contributes to venous return to the heart. It is estimated that the loss of muscle tone from complete disuse is 10% to 15% of strength per week.[9] Because of reduction in muscle tone, patients on prolonged bed rest have a diminished venopressor mechanism and, therefore, a decrease in venous return.

Decrease in Intravascular and Extracellular Fluid Volume. Total blood volume (TBV), plasma volume, ECF volume, and red-cell mass are known to decrease with prolonged bed rest.[8,15,18] The results of two studies on normal subjects are summarized in Table 30-2. Reductions in TBV and plasma volume are large and occur early during the period of bed rest (after 2 days), whereas reductions in red-cell mass are smaller and occur more slowly.[8] This results in increased blood viscosity early in bed rest.

Reductions in plasma volume may contribute to postural hypotension but may be insufficient to cause a drop in BP. Plasma reduction by diuresis caused no postural intolerance in an ambulatory control group of normal subjects. With the same plasma reduction induced by recumbency, the bed-rest group suffered subsequent postural hypotension. Reduced ECF volume may reduce tissue pressure, decrease resistance to capillary filling, and increase pooling in the lower extremities upon assuming the upright position.[3]

In the cardiac patient, losses of ECF and intravascular fluid volume may cause a reduction in CO, which may contribute to reduced coronary artery perfusion. In addition, loss of red-cell mass and reduced O_2-carrying capacity of the blood may contribute to myocardial ischemia.

Nursing Intervention

Nursing interventions for prevention of cardiovascular complications can generally be divided into two areas: effects of recumbency and effects of physical immobility. Nursing measures to prevent thrombus formation and pulmonary embolism are discussed in Chapter 28.

Recumbency. As soon as the patient's condition permits, the head of the bed should be raised. The patient should be observed closely for any symptoms of reduced cerebral blood flow or coronary perfusion, such as chest pain. BP, HR, and when possible, electrocardiographic changes and CO, must also be assessed. During the day, the head of the patient's bed should be raised every 2 hours for 15 to 30 minutes in increments of 15 to 20 degrees, using the patient's symptoms and signs as a guide.

Once the patient tolerates being propped up in bed, he should be allowed to dangle his legs over the side of the bed. A minimum of two nurses should be present at the bedside, because many patients who do well as long as their legs remain elevated become quite symptomatic when their legs are in the dependent position. Again, physiologic variables must be assessed. When a patient is first permitted to sit on the edge of the bed, other activities, such as eating or using the urinal, should be avoided. Eating and digesting further increase O_2 consumption, and urinating is associated with vagal stimulation, decreasing both HR and CO.

For the patient with reduced cardiac function, care must be taken when applying antiembolic stockings or performing range-of-motion exercises not to elevate legs any higher off the bed than is absolutely necessary. Only one leg at a time should be raised. During these procedures the patient should be watched for any signs or symptoms of increasing CHF, such as increased respiratory rate, increased HR, or shortness of breath.

Physical Immobility. Range-of-motion exercises can help prevent joint stiffness, loss of muscle tone, and cardiac deconditioning. Teaching patients how to move properly in bed (breathing out when moving) helps to decrease the number of Valsalva maneuvers performed, and the associated O_2 cost. Offering assistance in repositioning every 1 to 2 hours may deter the alert patient from trying to move himself and decrease the frequency of Valsalva maneuvers.

Preventing constipation and positioning the patient as upright as possible when using the bedpan or urinal reduces straining and the incidence of Valsalva maneuver. Sitting on the edge of the bed may be the only position in which a male patient who has received atropine sulfate or has benign prostatic hypertrophy can urinate. Even so, a great deal of straining may occur. If concern of increased MVO_2 outweighs the dangers of urinary catheterization, a Foley catheter may be inserted. Because HR and BP changes are greater using a bedpan than a commode,[6] use of the bedside commode should be permitted as soon as possible.

RESPIRATORY EFFECTS

It is more difficult to breathe when lying down.[1] The major effects on the respiratory system secondary to recumbency and physical immobility are hypoventilation, atelectasis, and stasis of secretions, all of which can alter O_2 and CO_2 balance. Hypostatic pneumonia is the important clinical finding, although, for the cardiac patient, a decrease in P_aO_2 for any reason must be prevented. In the patient with CHF, increased venous return can cause pulmonary edema (Chap. 27).

Hypoventilation and Atelectasis

Movement of the diaphragm downward is made more difficult in the flat supine or recumbent position. Abdominal obesity or distention, for instance from constipation, adds to this effect. Outward movement of the chest wall is inhibited by chest wall contact with a firm surface, such as a bed. Respiratory muscle weakness and loss of reserve demand of the patient more energy expenditure to breathe. Although O_2 consumption is thereby increased, some patients are capable of continuing to meet their ventilatory needs, whereas in others fatigue and hypoventilation ensues.

Splinting to prevent respiratory movement because of chest pain also promotes hypoventilation and atelectasis. Such medications as morphine sulfate or diazepam (Valium), commonly administered to patients with an acute MI, reduce the rate and depth of respirations by depressing the central nervous system (CNS). Hypoventilation causes a decrease in P_aO_2 and an increase in P_aCO_2, the extent of which depends on the rate and depth of respirations. Although rare in the individual without primary respiratory disease, hypoventilation from immobility alone, if severe enough, can cause respiratory acidosis (Chap. 9).

Stasis of Secretions and Hypostatic Pneumonia

In the healthy individual, stasis of secretions is prevented by coughing and frequent movement, even during rest and sleep. Normally, mucus is spread evenly around the bronchioles, but during recumbency mucus secretions pool on the dependent side of the bronchiole. As a result of this pooling, blood is shunted past unventilated alveoli and hypostatic pneumonia develops. The small number of bacteria normally found in the tracheobronchial tree proliferate because they are no longer in contact with the bronchial mucous membrane with its phagocytic action.[1]

Coughing can prevent pooling of mucus. In the immobilized patient the respiratory muscles may be too weak to produce an effective cough. Drugs affecting the CNS can depress the cough reflex. The patient in pain may supress the cough because of fear of causing even more discomfort. Inadequate fluid intake, excessive fluid loss, lack of humidity in the ambient air or in the compressed air and oxygen, and such anticholinergic drugs as atropine sulfate thicken the mucus, making it even more difficult to expectorate.

Nursing Intervention

The alert patient must be encouraged to turn, cough, and breathe deeply every hour during waking hours and during routine vital-sign checks (every 4 hours) at night. An incentive spirometer may be useful and may provide a rough estimate of increasing or decreasing respiratory function. Adequate fluid intake (2 to 3 liters daily) must be maintained. If the patient is on fluid restriction, a room humidifier can be used, or moisture can be added to the respiratory equipment. In the alert but uncooperative patient, yawning by the nurse frequently precipitates yawning by the patient, an excellent way of promoting deep inspiration. Intermittent positive-pressure breathing (IPPB) treatments or hyperinflation using an anesthesia bag may be necessary to prevent atelectasis in the heavily sedated or comatose patient.

The patient unable to move in bed by himself should have his position changed at least every 2 hours and, ideally, even more frequently. For the comatose or heavily sedated patient, care must be taken to keep the patient turned off his back so that he does not aspirate his oral secretions, or vomit and aspirate stomach contents. When administering sedatives or pain medication, the nurse must first assess the patient's respiratory status. If excessive hypoventilation results from the medication, the drug should be held and the order questioned.

Patients with a decreased P_aO_2 and experiencing symptoms of myocardial ischemia should have an order for O_2 administration. Hypoxemia as a result of a shunt cannot be abolished by having the patient breathe 100% O_2,[20] although the P_aO_2 of unshunted blood will be increased. In that event, atelectatic areas must be reexpanded and chest physiotherapy and postural drainage instituted to break up and drain the mucus pools. Nebulized mucolytic drugs, such as acetylcysteine (Mucomyst), are useful for liquifying mucus secretions. Patients with hypostatic pneumonia should have appropriate antibiotic therapy.

RENAL EFFECTS

For the cardiac patient, immobility may have important effects on the kidney and urinary system: diuresis, kidney-stone formation, difficulty in voiding, urinary retention, and urinary-tract infection.

Diuresis

Effective renal blood flow (RBF) increases 54% and renal plasma flow rises 71% when a person goes from the erect to the supine position.[1] The greatest diuresis occurs during the first 4 days of bed rest. The major reason for the increased RBF and subsequent diuretic effect is an increase in thoracic blood volume that stimulates cardiopulmonary stretch-receptors, resulting in suppression of antidiuretic hormone. During the first few days of immobilization, the patient with CHF may benefit from this natural diuresis. However, care must be taken that the cardiac patient with low CO does not become volume-depleted.

Kidney-Stone Formation

Development of renal stones may depend upon the length of immobilization. Although it seems unlikely that a patient in bed fewer than 1 or 2 weeks would develop renal calculi, the patient with an acute MI who does develop calculi may not be able to tolerate the pain and stress of passing a kidney stone.

Changes in the Characteristic of Urine During Bed Rest. The concentrations of calcium (Ca^{2+}) and phosphorous increase because of disuse osteoporosis. After 2 weeks of bed rest the concentration of urinary Ca^{2+} increases three fold. The amount of citric acid, which is responsible for keeping Ca^{2+} in solution, remains unchanged, so that the ratio of Ca^{2+} to citric acid increases.[1] After the diuretic phase, the volume of urine returns to normal or may be reduced.[10]

Urine drainage from the kidneys is facilitated in the upright position. Lying supine or recumbent causes pooling of urine in the renal pelvis (Fig. 30-2). Precipitation of Ca^{2+} occurs in the stagnant areas.

Difficulty in Voiding, Urinary Retention, and Urinary-Tract Infection

Micturition depends on the integrated action of the external and internal sphincters and the detrusor muscle of the bladder wall. By consciously relaxing the perineal muscles, the external sphincter is also relaxed. The voiding reflex is initiated, causing the detrusor muscle to contract and the internal sphincter to relax.

Fig. 30-2. Effect of posture on drainage of urine from the renal pelvis. (Browse NL: The Physiology and Pathophysiology of Bed Rest, p 83. Springfield, IL: Charles C Thomas, 1965)

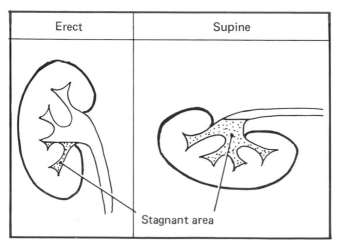

Erect	Supine
	Stagnant area

It is difficult to relax the perineal muscles in the supine position, thereby interfering with initiation of the voiding reflex. Retention of urine can develop, sometimes causing overflow incontinence. The cardiac patient receiving atropine sulfate may experience even further difficulty in voiding and increased likelihood of urinary retention.

Stasis of urine in the bladder promotes urinary tract infections. In addition, bacteria are more likely to proliferate in a less acidic environment. Insertion of a Foley catheter, either to relieve retention or for assessment of urine output, also increases the risk of urinary tract infections.

Nursing Intervention

The effects on the patient of volume loss, for example increased HR, decreased BP with postural changes, and decreased CO, must be assessed. Using the guidelines discussed under cardiovascular effects, the head of the bed should be raised to permit drainage of urine from the renal pelvis. When possible, the patient should be allowed to sit up to urinate. Privacy should be ensured. Running tap water may help the patient to initiate urination. Straining should be prevented. If overflow incontinence develops, the skin should be kept clean and dry. Routine checks should be made for bladder distention (Chap. 14). Care of the patient with a Foley catheter can be found in a standard nursing textbook.

If the patient is not on fluid restriction, fluid intake should be 2 to 3 liters daily. Urine output and signs of fluid retention, such as edema and weight gain, will need careful observation. Foods or fluids with an acid ash, such as cereal, meat, fish, and cranberry juice, should be encouraged.

GASTROINTESTINAL EFFECTS

For the cardiac patient, the major effects of immobility are constipation and increased catabolism with its subsequent negative nitrogen balance. Constipation can be caused by a change in (or absence of) diet, activity, or routine habits, weakened abdominal muscles, or suppression of the defecation reflex because of lack of privacy or the embarrassment and discomfort of using a bedpan. The degree of immobilization affects the amount of protein catabolism. Positive nitrogen balance is maintained for 4 days after initiation of bed rest, but by the 7th day negative nitrogen balance occurs, peaking by the 10th day.[5]

Nursing Intervention

Constipation must be prevented because of the increase in $M\dot{V}O_2$ associated with straining. Privacy must be provided. If tolerated, the head of the bed should be raised for the patient during attempts to use the bedpan and the use of the bedside commode should be permitted as soon as possible. Unless contraindicated by fluid restriction, fluid intake should be at least 2 to 3 liters per day. For patients receiving regular diets, bulk-forming foods should be offered and gas-forming foods avoided. Stool softeners and laxatives (Chap. 33) should be given routinely. Adequate protein intake should be maintained. Consultation between the patient, nurse, and dietician is helpful in finding satisfactory ways to meet the need for increased proteins.

MUSCULOSKELETAL AND INTEGUMENTARY EFFECTS

Development of joint stiffness, muscle weakness, atrophy, contractures, pressure sores, and disuse osteoporosis are of concern in any patient on prolonged bed rest. The process of muscle weakening and atrophy begins after only a few days in bed. The recovery period depends on the length of immobilization.[1] Muscle contractures can develop in patients unable to carry out routine activities of daily living (ADLs), which provide full joint range of motion. Pressure sores develop because of decreased blood flow to an area, or because of negative nitrogen balance.

Disuse osteoporosis develops during immobility when the stresses of weight-bearing on the bones are eliminated. An imbalance of bone formation and bone destruction is created. Calcium and phosphorous are released from the bone matrix into the blood stream and are eliminated by the kidneys.

Nursing Intervention

Joint stiffness is quick to develop after disuse or improper positioning. Range-of-motion exercises should be carried out every 2 to four hours while awake. Range-of-motion exercises can also help to prevent disuse osteoporosis.[17] Proper positioning and position changes should be provided at least every 2 hours, or as needed. Close observation of the skin, at least every 8 hours, can detect reddened areas that may break down. Fade time, or the amount of time necessary for the reddened area to return to normal color, should be 15 minutes or less. This red color is a result of reactive hyperemia from ischemia. Physical management of the bedfast patient can be found in standard nursing textbooks.

PSYCHOLOGIC EFFECTS

Any patient on prolonged bed rest may experience changes in psychological well-being. Increases in anxiety, hostility, and depression have been noted in persons subjected to bed rest.[10] The recumbent position alone may result in complex dreams, restlessness, hunger, worry, and fright.[21] Sensory deprivation (Chap. 32) may be caused by immobility. Sleep deprivation (Chap. 31) can occur because of the anxiety and fear of the condition requiring bed rest. It should be noted that most studies of psychologic effects of bed rest have been done on healthy volunteers. The psychologic reactions of patients with acute MIs may become even more intense because bed rest has been enforced as a life-saving intervention. Perception of body image may change because of immobility, the MI, or both.[9] Physical immobility may underscore the patient's new role, that of being ill and dependent.

Nursing Intervention

Purposes of bed rest should be explained to the patient and his family. Psychologic support of both patient and family is necessary throughout the period of bed rest. There may be as many implications of the new invalid role for the family as for the patient. The anger, fright, and depression that may be displayed should be anticipated and dealt with as a normal occurrence. Drawing attention to even slight improvements in the patient's condition may be beneficial. The patient should be ambulated as soon as the physical condition permits. Specific nursing measures for sensory and sleep deprivations are discussed in Chapters 32 and 31, respectively.

REFERENCES

1. Browse NL: The Physiology and Pathology of Bed Rest. Springfield, Charles C Thomas, 1965
2. Chapman CB, Fisher JN, Sproule BJ: Behavior of stroke volume at rest and during exercise in human beings. J Clin Invest 39:1208–1213, 1960
3. Chobanian AV, Little RD, Tercyak MA et al: The metabolic and hemodynamic effects of prolonged bed rest in normal subjects. Circulation 49(3):551–559, 1974
4. Coe SW: Cardiac work and the chair treatment of acute coronary thrombosis. Ann Intern Med 40(1):42–48, 1954
5. Deitrick JE, Whedon GD, Shorr E: Effects of immobilization upon various metabolic and physiologic functions of normal men. Am J Med 4(1):3–36, 1948
6. Dock W: The therapeutic use and hazards of bed rest. Conn State Med J 11(8):606–608, 1947
7. Holmgren A, Ovenfors CO: Heart volume at rest and during muscular work in the supine and sitting position. Acta Med Scand 167(4):267–277, 1960
8. Miller PB, Johnson RL, Lamb LE: Effects of four weeks of absolute bed rest on circulatory functions in man. Aerospace Med 35(12):1194–1200, 1964
9. Olson EV, Thompson LF, McCarthy J et al: Immobility. Am J Nurs 67(4):781–796, 1967
10. Ryback RS, Lewis OF, Lessard CS: Psychologic effects of prolonged bed rest (weightless) in young, healthy volunteers (Study II). Aerospace Med 42(5):529–535, 1971
11. Saltin B, Blomqvist G, Mitchell JH et al: Response to exercise after bed rest and training. Circulation (Suppl 7)38:1–55, 1968
12. Sjöstrand T: The regulation of the blood distribution in man. Acta Physiol Scand 26(4):312–327, 1952
13. Sjöstrand T: The volume and distribution of the blood. Physiol Rev 33(2):202–228, 1953
14. Tarazi RC, Gifford RW Jr: Systemic arterial pressure. In Sodeman WA Jr, Sodeman WA (eds). Pathologic Physiology, 5th ed, pp 177–205. Philadelphia, WB Saunders, 1974
15. Taylor HL, Erickson L, Henschel A: Effect of bed rest on the blood volume of normal young men. Am J Physiol 144(2):227–232, 1945
16. Taylor HL, Henschel A, Brožek J et al: Effects of bed rest on cardiovascular function and work performance. J Appl Physiol 2(5):223–239, 1949
17. Toohey P, Larson CW: Range of motion exercise: Key to joint mobility. Minneapolis, Sister Kenny Institute, 1968
18. Vogt FB, Johnson PC: Plasma volume and extracellular fluid volume changes associated with 10 days bed recumbency. Aerospace Med 38(1):21–25, 1967
19. Wang Y, Marshall RJ, Shephard JT: The effects of changes in posture and of graded exercise on stroke volume in man. J Clin Invest 39(7):1051–1061, 1960
20. West JB: Respiratory Physiology—The Essentials. Baltimore, Williams and Wilkens, 1974

21. Zubek JP, MacNeil M: Perceptual deprivation phenomena: Role of the recumbent position. J Abnorm Psychol 72(2): 147–150, 1967

ADDITIONAL READING

Asher RAJ: The dangers of going to bed. Br Med J p. 967, 1947

Asmussen E, Nielson M: Cardiac output in rest and work determined simultaneously by acetylene and the dye injection methods. Acta Physiol Scand 27(2–3):217–230, 1952

Bergstrom D, Coles CH: Basic Positioning Procedures. Minneapolis, Sister Kenney Institute, 1971

Bergstrom WH: Hypercalciuria and hypercalcemia complicating immobilization. Am J Dis Chil 132(6):553–554, 1978

Booth FW: Time course of muscular atrophy during immobilization of hindlimbs in rats. J Appl Physiol 43(4):656–661, 1977

Carnevali D, Bruekner S: Immobilization—Reassessment of a concept. Am J Nurs 70(7):1502–1507, 1970

Conrad L: The valsalva maneuver: A clinical inquiry. Am J Nurs 71(3):553–554, 1971

Cuthberton DP: Influence of prolonged muscular rest on metabolism. Biochem J 23:1328–1345, 1929

Donaldson CL, Hulley SB, Vogel JM et al: Effect of prolonged bed rest on bone material. Metabolism 19(12):1071–1084, 1970

Downs FS: Bed rest and sensory disturbances. Am J Nurs 74(3): 434–438, 1974

Goldstrom DK: Cardiac rest: Bed or chair? Am J Nurs 72(10): 1812–1816, 1972

Holmgren A, Jonsson B, Sjöstrand T: Circulatory data in normal subjects at rest and during exercise in the recumbent position, with special reference to the stroke volume at different work intensities. Acta Physiol Scand 49:343–363, 1960

Issekutz B Jr, Blizzard BJ, Birkhard NC et al: Effect of prolonged bed rest on urinary calcium output. J Appl Physiol 21(3):1013–1020, 1966

Kelly MM: Exercises for bedfast patients. Am J Nurs 66(10):2209–2213, 1966

Larsson H, Kjellberg SR: Roentgenological heart volume determination with special regard to pulse rate and position of the body. Acta Radiol 29(2):159–177, 1948

Lavine MA: Bed exercises for acute cardiac patients. Am J Nurs 73(7):1226–1227, 1973

Lerman S, Canterbury JM, Reiss E: Parathyroid hormone and the hypercalcemia of immobilization. J Clin Endocrinol Metabol 43(3):425–428, 1977

Levine SA, Lown B: 'Armchair' treatment of acute coronary thrombosis. JAMA 148(6):1365–1369, 1952

Lindgren JU: Studies of the calcium accretion rate of bone during immobilization in intact and thyroparathyroidectomized adult rats. Calcif Tissue Res 22(1):41–47, 1976

Mayer RF, Burke RE, Kanda K: Immobilization and muscle atrophy. Trans Am Neurol Assoc 101:145–150, 1976

Mead S: A century of the abuse of rest. JAMA 182(4):344–345, 1962

Michelsson J-EL, Videman T, Langenskiold A: Changes in bone formation during immobilization and development of experimental osteoarthritis. Acta Orthop Scand 48(3):443–449, 1977

Miller PB, Johnson RL, Lamb LE: Effects of moderate physical exercise during four weeks of bed rest on circulatory functions in man. Aerospace Med 36(11):1077–1082, 1965

Müller EA: Influence of training and inactivity on muscle strength. Arch Phys Med Rehab 51(8):449–462, 1970

Nursing Care of the Skin, revised ed. Minneapolis, Sister Kenny Institute, 1975

Petukhov BN, Purakhin YN: Effect of prolonged bed rest on cerebral biopotentials of healthy subjects. Space Biol Med 2:56–61, 1968

Sharp JT, Rakowski D, Keefer YD: Effect of position change on lung compliance in normal subjects and in patients with congestive heart failure. J Clin Invest 38(4):659–667, 1959

Stryker R: Rehabilitation Aspects of Acute and Chronic Nursing Care, 2nd ed. Philadelphia, WB Saunders, 1977

Vogt FB, Mark PB, Johnson PC: Tilt table response and blood volume changes associated with thirty days of recumbency. Aerospace Med 37(8):771–777, 1966

Whedon GD: Metabolic effects of immobilization. In Milhorat AT (ed): Proceedings of the First and Second Medical Conferences of the Muscular Dystrophy Association of America, pp 39–45. New York, Muscular Dystrophy Association of America, 1952

Wishnie HA, Hackett TP, Cassem NH: Psychological hazards of convalescence following myocardial infarction. JAMA 215(8): 1292–1296, 1971

Zohman LR, Tobis JS: Cardiac Rehabilitation. New York, Grune and Stratton, 1970

Zubel JP, Wilgosh L: Prolonged immobilization of the body: Changes in performance and in the electroencephalogram. Science 140:306–308, 1963

31

Sleep Disruption in Cardiac Patients

SARAH J. SANFORD, R.N., M.A., CCRN

Patients with possible or true compromise in cardiac function are admitted to cardiac care units for the purpose of preserving and maximizing myocardial performance. One of the most basic principles in the care of patients with such compromise is reduction in cardiac work, that is, allowing the patient to rest. Physical activity and sources of noise and disturbances, such as telephones and visitors, are limited in the hope of reducing both physiological and psychologic demands upon the body. Patients are treated with sedative and analgesic medications in the hope of promoting rest. Under such conditions, sleep disruption is highly unlikely. However, despite the fact that patients frequently spend many hours with their eyes closed, apparently asleep, they rarely report feeling rested. Persistent fatigue is frequently explained on the basis of decreased myocardial function, a possible contributing factor to be sure, but ineffective sleep must also be considered. In order to achieve a subjective feeling of rest, sleep not only must be quantitatively adequate, but, in addition, must have certain qualitative characteristics. The discussion that follows includes information about the nature of sleep activity, qualitative and quantitative aspects of sleep, disruptive influences inherent in cardiac care units, and finally, the nursing process in relation to minimizing those disruptions.

NATURE OF SLEEP ACTIVITY

Sleep has been viewed historically as a quiet, uniform state of unresponsiveness and relaxation. However, simultaneous recording of electroencephalograms (EEGs), electromyograms (EMGs), and electrooculograms (EOGs) has re-vealed that the process of sleep is composed of two distinct types of sleep activity: REM sleep and NREM sleep.

REM Sleep

REM, or rapid eye movement sleep, is characterized by a high degree of both cerebral and physiologic activation.[9,39] The EEG of REM resembles that seen in waking states, the EOG reflects extremely rapid, conjugate eye movements (the basis for its name), and the EMG is almost flat.[39] The extremely low EMG seen in REM reflects immobility of the large postural and skeletal muscles due to hyperpolarization of alpha motor neurons in the brainstem.[12]

Physiologically, REM is characterized by increases in body temperature, cerebral blood flow, and oxygen consumption; clinically, heart rate, blood pressure, and cardiac output approach or surpass waking values and frequently become erratic.[39] Respiratory rates vary between fast and slow, and apneic periods have been noted.[2] In cardiac patients, REM has been associated with both premature ventricular contractions and nocturnal angina.[21,30] Thus, REM sleep is hardly a relaxed state; synonyms given to this type of sleep activity include active and paradoxic.[9,12]

NREM Sleep

NREM, or non-REM sleep, is further classified into four stages. To the sleeper, stage 1 NREM is the lightest of all sleep stages; it most commonly initiates the sleep cycle and is considered by many researchers to be a transition state. Stage 2 NREM is often referred to as the "door" stage because it both precedes and follows REM in the characteristic cycle of sleep stages.[39] This sleep-stage cycle is important, and will be discussed further. Stages 3 and 4 NREM are referred to as slow-wave, delta, and quiet sleep; these two stages differ from each other only on the basis of the percentage of very large, low-frequency (delta) waves seen in the EEG.[39]

Physiologically, NREM is consistent with the historic view of sleep. As the individual progresses through the four NREM stages, cardiac and respiratory rates, blood pressure, metabolic rate, and body temperature decrease to basal levels.[39] Clinically, there is progressive muscle relaxation; snoring is common in stages 3 and 4, and is due to reduced tone in the oral pharyngeal and laryngeal musculature.[9] Although profound muscle relaxation is present in NREM, it should not be compared to the immobility of large muscle seen in REM; in REM the immobility more closely resembles paralysis; reflexes are absent.[12] They are present in NREM.[12]

THEORIES OF SLEEP FUNCTION

Beyond prevention of the syndrome associated with sleep deprivation, researchers have only theories as to the function of sleep.[12] That it is generally both physically and mentally refreshing is, however, widely accepted.

Restorative Role

One of the major findings supporting a restorative purpose for sleep is that increased secretion of growth hormone occurs during stages 3 and 4 NREM.[4] Stimuli for the secretion of growth hormone include a reduction in energy substrate availability, or an increased energy demand, or both.[13] Since this hormone acts to promote protein synthesis and protect protein from breakdown, its elevated secretion during slow-wave sleep is consistent with an anabolic role, particularly for tissues with high protein content, such as muscle. Physical exercise during the afternoon has been found to produce increases in stages 3 and 4 NREM during the subsequent night's sleep, implying that energy substrate use or depletion, or both, during exercise increases the need for anabolic periods during sleep.[3] Similar increases in slow-wave sleep have been found to occur with starvation.[22]

Sleep also plays a restorative role in cerebral neurochemistry.[33] Compared with animals allowed to sleep normally, sleep-deprived animals have been found to demonstrate depletion of cerebral levels of glucose, adenosine triphosphate (ATP), and other high-energy phosphate compounds.[12] Seizure activity, with its associated excessive cerebral and physiologic metabolic expenditure, has been found to result in marked depletion of high-energy phosphate levels; the postictal drowsiness and sleep that follow such activity is thought to represent the time in which these compounds are restored to preseizure levels.[10] Incorporation of phosphorus into phosphoproteins and phosphopeptides does, indeed, increase during sleep.[12]

Psychologic Role

Evidence that effective sleep is a prerequisite for the maintenance of mental and emotional well-being is based largely on the discovery that disorientation, paranoia, and inappropriate categorization of perceptions are common findings in sleep deprivation.[26,27] Sleep is thought to be the period during which the day's information is categorized and rehearsed; there is selective storing of some information and clearing of the remainder to make room for the following day's input.[9,14]

Some researchers hypothesize that REM is the actual sleep activity in which these storing and clearing activities occur.[33] Investigators have found that healthy subjects, when selectively deprived of REM sleep, report feelings of increased suspiciousness, and tendencies toward withdrawal and introversion; inappropriate interpretation of reality has also been observed.[12,36]

QUALITATIVE ASPECTS OF SLEEP

Sleep is a phenomenon of cycles. The bulk of sleep activity most commonly occurs rhythmically, once a day, and that activity is composed of specific cycles of sleep stages.

Circadian Rhythm

The circadian rhythm is the name given to man's biologic clock or pattern of endogenous oscillations in both physiological (body temperature, hormone secretion levels) and mental (efficiency and concentration) parameters of function, a pattern that repeats roughly every 24 hours.[8] It is this circadian pattern of oscillation that dictates the periods within any 24-hour block of time when high and low phases of physical and mental function occur. Early man's need to function at optimum levels when his visual capabilities were at their greatest, that is, during daylight hours, and to sleep during darkness when his vision was severely decreased, may have been instrumental in the original setting of his biologic clock to a day–night pattern.[8] Once set to a particular cycle, however, circadian oscillations are self-sustaining and continue even when environmental input regarding time of day, light, or darkness is totally lacking.[8]

For sleep to be of optimum benefit, it must occur during the low phase of these inherent circadian oscillations; in other words, it must be synchronized with the biologic clock.[34,35] Sleep is qualitatively rated poorest when it is obtained during an inappropriate phase of the circadian cycle, or, in other words, when it constitutes a phase shift.[34,35] In this situation sleep is desynchronized. When the sleep–wakefulness schedule involves such a phase shift, resynchronization is necessary.[34,35] However, this process of establishing a circadian-appropriate pattern of sleep requires 3 to 5 days and is associated with chronic fatigue and restlessness.[34,35]

Sleep Stage Cycling

The sleep period itself consists of specific, ordered progressions, or cycles, of sleep stages. The length of a complete cycle varies from 60 to 120 minutes, but averages 90 minutes.[25] This 90-minute period between the occurrence

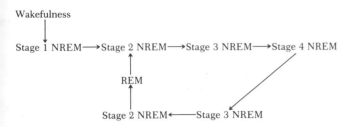

Fig. 31-1. The sleep-stage cycle.

of a given sleep stage corresponds to and reflects an inherent, basic rest-activity cycle (BRAC) of the nervous system. Every 90 minutes, a REM or active stage of sleep occurs.[24,34,35]

With the onset of sleep there is first a general descending pattern through the NREM stages (from 1 to 4).[20] The pattern then reverses itself, the sleeper ascends to stage 2 NREM, or the "door" stage and from this stage enters REM.[20] Upon completion of REM, the sleeper once again enters stage 2 NREM to restart the initial descending pattern.[20] The sleep-stage cycle is schematically illustrated in Figure 31-1.

Although progression of sleep stages can occur in almost any order, sleep is much less effective when it does not involve the specific pattern of stage progression described. If the sleeper is aroused or awakened at any point during the progression, he does not return to the stage from which he was aroused, but instead, starts the initial descending pattern from the beginning.[20,34,35] Thus, frequent sleep interruptions can lead to a predominance of the qualitatively lighter stages of sleep; occurrence of NREM stages 3 and 4 and of REM decrease both in frequency and length whenever such interruptions necessitate repeated sleep cycle initiation.[20,34,35]

The percentage of the 90-minute cycle occupied by each of the respective sleep stages depends on the point during the total sleep period in which the cycle occurs. During the early part of the sleep period, the 90-minute cycles are dominated by stages 3 and 4 NREM, with only brief REM periods.[1,38] During the later portions of the period, however, REM dominates, with proportionate shortening of NREM 3 and 4.[1,34] Thus, NREM is experienced chiefly during the early hours of the sleep period, while REM occurs mainly during the later hours. When an individual does not obtain several complete sleep cycles during a total sleep period, the relative proportion of time occupied by NREM and REM is altered.[34,37] The result is that time spent in REM is reduced and sleep is less effective.[35,36]

Cycling of sleep stages also occurs during daytime naps. The relative quantities of NREM and REM depend on the time of day in which naps are taken. Morning naps, as if a continuation of the second half of the night, are composed of large proportions of REM sleep.[37] Afternoon naps on the other hand, are proportionately higher in slow-wave sleep. Because of this relatively greater content of NREM, afternoon naps can result in reduced amounts of NREM 3 and 4 during the early part of the night sleep.[37]

Because of the critical or potentially critical nature of illness of the patients admitted to cardiac care units, vital signs and treatment procedures must often be performed not only at frequent intervals but on a 24-hour basis as well.

Because of these sleep disruptions patients are likely to suffer in relation to the quality of sleep obtained. Circadian-phase shifts result in less effective sleep. Desynchronization occurs despite the fact that sleep may be obtained during the customary hours of the day or night, simply because sleep is also obtained during hours other than those to which the patient is accustomed. Continual attempts at resynchronization are therefore necessary but generally unsuccessful, because napping interferes with sleep in subsequent sleep periods, and also because daily schedules are rarely constant over a consecutive three-day period. In addition, because of frequent interruptions, sleep-stage cycling lacks full progression and cycles are dominated by the lighter sleep stages. The result, all too frequently, is that the patient is chronically fatigued and restless at a time when optimum sleep is important to compensate for physiologic stress.

QUANTITATIVE ASPECTS OF SLEEP

Individuals develop characteristic quantities of bulk sleep time from night to night.[1,21,38] Gender plays a role in determining characteristic sleep durations; females sleep longer and have slightly more sleep in NREM stage 4 than do males.[39] Age is also a factor.[11] Generally, as age increases, total sleep time decreases, primarily as a function of decreasing percentages of time in NREM 3 and 4, but to a lesser extent REM as well. Stages 1 and 2 NREM both increase, as do the number of arousals.[1,11,39]

General Guidelines

Research has provided quantitative guidelines for sleep activity. Those reported here refer to adults between the ages of 40 and 59 years. The mean number of hours slept per night is roughly seven, with men falling slightly below and women slightly above this mean.[39] Percentages of the sleep period occupied by each of the stages are as follows: stage 1, NREM 3–7.5; stage 2, NREM 54–68; stage 3, NREM 3–7; stage 4, NREM 2–4.5, and REM 22–27.[39] In women, percentages generally approach the upper end of the ranges listed; in men they characteristically approach the lower end.[39] While these guidelines provide a general framework for quantification of sleep, the degree of individual variation is wide.[12] For exact figures, as well as figures for other groups, see references cited in this paragraph.

Sleep Environment

The physical setting in which a person sleeps can be a variable in determining the quantity of sleep obtained. Quantitative alterations occur when one sleeps in an unfamiliar bed, in a different room, or in the presence of unfamiliar or frightening noises or a change in light intensity.[7] Characteristically, there is a decrease in overall sleep time due to a decrease in REM, and also a prolonged time in bed before the onset of sleep.[7] Fortunately, these alterations subside after 2 days' acclimatization to the new setting.[7]

TABLE 31-1   SUMMARY OF NREM vs REM ACTIVITY

Feature	NREM	REM
Synonyms	Stage 1: transition Stage 2: door Stage 3&4: slow-wave, quiet, delta sleep	Active, paradoxic sleep
Physiologic correlates	Fall to basal levels of cardiac, respiratory, metabolic rates and temperature	Increases in heart rate, cardiac output, blood pressure, cerebral blood flow, and oxygen consumption
Clinical correlates	Progressive muscle relaxation, snoring	Rapid, darting eye movements; large-muscle immobility; vital signs at waking levels or above can be erratic; respiratory rate irregular, with apneic periods
Postulated function	Energy substrate restoration, anabolism	Psychologic equilibrium
Percentages of sleep time (adults, 40–59 years)	Stage 1: 3–7.5 Stage 2: 54–68 Stage 3: 3–7 Stage 4: 2–4.5	22–27
Rebounds	Stages 1,2,&3: no Stage 4: Yes*	Yes

*Preferentially rebounded when selective loss of both NREM 4 and REM occurs.

Rebounds

Two sleep stages, REM and stage 4 NREM, display consistent compensatory increases on nights following their selective loss.[12] These compensatory increases are termed rebounds; they are believed to occur because loss of these stages results in development of a debt-like phenomenon. When rebounds occur, the sleeper enters the stage for which the debt has been developed both more often and from stages which normally do not precede the deficient stage.[12] The result is a relative percentage increase in REM or NREM, or both, during recovery sleep periods.

Because REM sleep places a relatively high degree of physiologic demand on the cardiovascular system, rebounds of this stage can produce clinically significant problems in patients with coronary disease. Increased vulnerability to ventricular arrhythmias, extension of infarction and development of new infarctions are especially dangerous possibilities.

Stage 4 NREM rebounds are thought to reflect restorative compensation for increased wakefulness and, consequently, for depletion of energy stores. This apparently represents a high priority, since, when both stage 4 NREM and REM losses occur, NREM stage 4 is preferentially rebounded.[4,29]

Growth hormone secretion does increase during stage 4 rebounds.[4] A summary of NREM versus REM activity can be found in Table 31-1.

Clinically, selective loss of both these types of sleep can and does occur. As mentioned, REM time is initially reduced by sleeping in a new environment, for example, a cardiac care unit. Then, just about the time that the impact of a strange environment may be overcome, REM again suffers, because sleep is difficult to obtain in bulk periods of adequate duration. Also, stage 4 NREM and REM can be selectively lost in conjunction with the use of certain medications.

MEDICATIONS AND SLEEP

Since it is hoped that patients in the cardiac care unit will rest, sedative, hypnotic, or analgesic medications are used frequently.

Barbiturates

Barbiturates are known to alter sleep. Amobarbital, secobarbital (Seconal, Tuinal) and pentobarbital (Nembutal) markedly reduce REM, simultaneously increasing the amount of stage 2 NREM sleep.[23] Their use to aid effective sleep is thus somewhat self-defeating. Phenobarbital (Luminal), on the other hand, increases stage 4 NREM, and in large doses (greater than 200 mg) also decreases REM sleep.[23] If given in small amounts, this drug may serve to promote sleep (Chap. 33).

Diazepam (Valium)

Although diazepam is considered a sedative, it increases time spent awake during the sleep period, increases stage 1 NREM, and reduces both REM and slow-wave sleep.[18] The degree of REM suppression is dose-dependent: the greater the dose administered, the greater the reduction in REM.[18] Slow-wave sleep suppression, on the other hand, occurs to the same extent at all doses within the therapeutic range.[18] Its overall effect is to reduce deep sleep while simultaneously increasing light sleep (Chap. 33).[18]

Morphine Sulfate

Morphine sulfate increases drowsiness, but at the same time increases time spent awake during the sleep period.[23] It also shortens total sleep time by reducing both REM and NREM stages 3 and 4, thus resulting in relative increases in the lighter stages of sleep.[23] Its effectiveness as an analgesic is unquestioned in the acute phase of illness, and by reducing REM, it may reduce the physiological demand on a vulnerable myocardium. However, its use can lead to psychologic disruption from REM deprivation and, when withdrawn, creates the potential for REM rebounds, with associated increased physiological stress (Chap. 33).

In light of their effect on sleep, it is no surprise that patients receiving both morphine sulfate and diazepam frequently display inappropriate or confused behavior, or both. Because both drugs decrease NREM stage 4 sleep and REM sleep and because in cases of loss of both, stage 4 NREM is preferentially rebounded, development of a chronic REM debt is likely. Continued loss of REM sleep cannot realistically be ruled out as at least a contributing factor in these psychologic disturbances.

Chloral Hydrate (Noctec) and Flurazepam (Dalmane)

Chloral hydrate (Noctec) and flurazepam (Dalmane) are thought to be two effective hypnotics that do not result in simultaneous disruption of sleep activity. In research settings, chloral hydrate has been administered for as long as a month with resultant increased effectiveness of sleep and no associated disruption of the sleep pattern.[16,23] This has been found true also of flurazepam if not administered in doses greater than 60 mg per day,[16,23] but this does not occur in all cases (Chap. 33).[20]

Tryptophan

An essential amino acid, tryptophan is not generally considered a hypnotic medication, but perhaps it should be. It is present in dairy products, meats, and legumes. Ingestion of this substance is associated with an increased level of cerebral serotonin, a neurotransmitter implicated in the production of NREM sleep.[17,19] Thus, the old adage that warm milk before bedtime aids sleep seems to have scientific basis. Ingestion of milk, which abounds in tryptophan, has been found to increase total sleep time by increasing stages 3 and 4 NREM and reducing time spend awake during the sleep period.[6,17]

APPLICATION OF THE NURSING PROCESS TO THE PROMOTION OF SLEEP

It should be clear that normal sleep in the setting afforded by the cardiac care unit is impossible. Both qualitative and quantitative alterations in sleep activity occur because of the unfamiliar nature of the environment, circadian phase shifts, disrupted sleep stage cycles, and medications. Perhaps one of the biggest challenges to nurses caring for patients in such a setting is to minimize disruptions in sleep within the framework necessary to manage severe cardiovascular compromise, real or potential.

Sleep Assessment

The first step in assessing the patient's ability to obtain effective sleep is to obtain a sleep history. Key information includes number of hours customarily slept per night; the time frame in which these hours usually occur; the number of naps and the time they are customarily taken; a description of the usual sleep environment, including number of pillows, blankets, and the presence of light and noise; the usual bedtime routine, if any; and finally, any sleep aids customarily used. Either the patient or his family can supply this information, and it should be gathered as soon as is feasible

---

TABLE 31-2 SLEEP HISTORY

1. Number of hours per night
2. Time frames for bulk sleep activity
3. Number and time frames of naps
4. Description of sleep environment
   a. Pillows
   b. Blankets
   c. Degree of light, if any
   d. Type of noise, if any
5. Usual bedtime routine, if any
   a. Bath, shower
   b. Snack; if so, what?
6. Sleep aids used, if any

---

after the patient's admission to the cardiac care unit. Information to be gathered in the sleep history is summarized in Table 31-2.

Assessment should also include the medications the patient will be receiving, the time interval between doses, and the manner of administration. During the course of admission of the patient to the cardiac care unit, a thorough evaluation of cardiovascular function is performed; this information should be used as the framework for gauging the approximate time interval between nursing procedures and on-going diagnostic procedures. The information gathered in the assessment phase allows a plan to be formulated that not only recognizes individual sleep patterns from the outset, but also allows their inclusion into the initial framework of intervention to be used in case of acute and severe distress.

Planning Care to Minimize Sleep Disruption

By referring to the sleep history, nursing procedures can be scheduled so that usual hours for the bulk sleep period are either protected or minimally interrupted. Since the majority of the population is synchronized to sleeping at night, no routine procedures should be planned during these hours. If the patient's condition preempts uninterrupted sleep during the customary bulk period, the plan should reflect the fact that the average sleep cycle is 90 minutes long. With the development and availability of sophisticated hemodynamic monitoring equipment, evaluation of many physiological parameters does not always require that the patient be awakened. Extensive nursing evaluations of physiological status should be planned in conjunction with procedures that invariably waken the patient, for example, laboratory work and x-ray examination, rather than with such procedures as obtaining serial one-lead ECG samples that do not necessarily require the patient's being awake. The plan also needs to stress the importance of full use of the times that the patient is already awake for procedures such as obtaining 12-lead electrocardiograms, obtaining vital signs, auscultation of the heart and of the lung fields, and recording of intake and output.

Customary bedtime routines, if any, should be planned to precede the bulk sleep period. For instance, if the patient customarily takes a shower or bath prior to retiring, daily hygiene needs should be planned to precede the bulk sleep period. Likewise, if the patient customarily has a bedtime snack, planning with the dietary department will allow continuation of this practice. If diet restrictions preclude the usual snack, a replacement containing tryptophan, such as milk, may be considered.

For patients on a graduated exercise regime, this activity should be planned to take place during the afternoon, the rationale being that afternoon exercise facilitates slow-wave sleep during subsequent sleep periods. If the patient customarily naps at certain times of the day, scheduling of activities should allow this practice to continue. However, naps should always be encouraged in the morning, because during this period they tend to have high REM proportions, a kind of sleep in which this population is likely to be deficient.

To keep potential sources of noise and disturbance to a minimum, it is sometimes possible to plan unit quiet periods. By informing personnel from such other departments as housekeeping, dietary, and radiology that routine duties should not be performed during these periods, unnecessary arousals can be minimized. Unit doors can have signs posted on them as reminders. Patients' physicians and visitors should be similarly informed; providing the rationale behind scheduling of these quiet periods is important to ensure cooperation.

Finally, as obvious as it seems, plans must be available if success is to be achieved. Both verbal and written communication of the plan and its rationale are critical. Without such communication, inadvertent awakenings or interruptions may occur; the last thing that patients with physiologic compromise need is added compromise due to interruptions of sleep.

Implementation of the Plan

As closely as possible, the customary sleep environment needs to be duplicated. Extra pillows or blankets may be needed; likewise, if the patient is accustomed to sleeping with a night light or a ticking clock, these should be obtained or duplicated to the extent that electrical safety allows.

Even with familiar characteristics in the physical environment, the setting is rampant with strange and frequently frightening noises. Monitors need to be explained and to be as muted as much as possible; alarms should be tested and explained to the patient; and false alarms should be explained as frequent culprits. Similar explanations should be provided for any other patient-care equipment, for example, ventilators or suction apparatus.

In the process of deciding upon the use of medications, the nurse must be continually aware of the effects they can have on sleep. Drugs that are REM blockers can contribute to the preexisting REM debt resulting from shortened bulk sleep periods and the effect of the strange nature of the environment. Their use can result in psychological disequilibrium, in addition to adding to the potential for a physiologically stressful rebound. This is not meant to imply that such drugs as morphine sulfate should be withheld; effective analgesia is critical in cardiac patients, and in fact, blocking REM in the acute phase of myocardial compromise may be physiologically helpful. However, the dosage should be reduced gradually. In this way, the chance of pronounced and clinically dangerous rebounds is lessened.

Ensuring that beds are dry and wrinkle-free, and providing back rubs and proper positioning can promote relaxation and reduce the need for sedatives. Frequent reassurances, explanations, and availability to listen to the patient's fears can all be of immeasurable value in reducing stress and anxiety. If sedation is necessary, phenobarbital in small doses, or chloral hydrate, with or without flurazepam, should be considered. Administration of these drugs is thought to result in minimal, if any, disruption in sleep activity. As mentioned, tryptophan-containing substances may also be considered.

Despite nursing efforts at implementation, even the best-laid plans may be rendered unworkable by alterations in patient status. Thus, continual review and updating of the patient's overall plan, nursing care needs, and priorities is necessary if sleep disruption is to be minimized.

Evaluation

Short of simultaneous EEG, EOG, and EMG recording, one of the best evaluations of sleep activity is the patient's own report of its effectiveness.[28] Thus, an easy and effective evaluation criterion for measuring the success of the prescribed sleep plan is to ask the patient how his sleep in the hospital compares in effectiveness with that at home. If the patient reports it to be consistently less effective than that at home, questions should be asked to discover the reason. More than likely the patient's responses will provide helpful information for revising and updating the plan, as well as revealing possible ways of implementing the revisions. Unavoidable deterrents to sleep should be explained; even though explanations do not remove them, they can lessen their impact considerably.

Less direct evaluation criteria can also be used. Inappropriate or confused behavior may implicate the presence of a severe REM sleep debt. Restlessness can be a function of desynchronization and phase shifts. Obviously, these phenomena can be the result of poor myocardial function or hypoxemia, as well as idiosyncratic or toxic reactions to various drugs. Nonetheless, their presence indicates the need for review of the nursing process, both to determine their cause and to eliminate avoidable sleep distortion.

REFERENCES

1. Agnew HW, Wilse MA, Webb WW et al: Sleep patterns in late middle age males: An EEG study. Electroencephalogr Clin Neurophysiol 23:168–171, 1967
2. Aserinsky E: Periodic respiratory pattern occurring in conjunction with eye movement during sleep. Science 150:763–766, 1965
3. Baekland F, Lasky R: Exercise and sleep patterns in college athletes. Percept Mot Skills 23:1203–1207, 1966
4. Beck U, Brezinova V, Hunter W et al: Plasma growth hormone and slow wave sleep increase after interruption of sleep. J Clin Endocrinol Metabol 40(5):812–815, 1975

5. Berger RJ: The sleep and dream cycle. In Kales A (ed): Sleep Physiology and Pathology, pp 17–32. Philadelphia, JB Lippincott, 1969

6. Brezinova V, Oswald I: Sleep after a bedtime beverage. Br Med J 2:431–433, 1972

7. Coble P, McPartland R, Silva W et al: Is there a first night effect? (a revisit). Biol Psychiatry 9(2):215–219, 1974

8. Conroy RT, Miles WL, Miles JN: Human Circadian Rhythms. London, J & A Churchill, 1970

9. Dement WC: Some Must Watch While Some Must Sleep. San Francisco, WH Freemon, 1974

10. Dement WC, Mitler MM: New developments in the basic mechanisms of sleep. In Usdin G (ed): Sleep Research and Clinical Practice, New York, Brunner/Mazel Co, 1973

11. Feinberg I: Effects of age on human sleep pattern. In Kales A (ed): Sleep Physiology and Pathology, pp 39–52. Philadelphia, JB Lippincott, 1969

12. Freemon FR: Sleep Research: A Critical Review, 2nd ed. Springfield, Charles C Thomas, 1974

13. Ganong WF: Review of Medical Physiology, 8th ed. Los Altos, Lange Medical Publications, 1977

14. Hartmann E: The Functions of Sleep. New Haven, Yale University Press, 1973

15. Hartmann E: Sleep requirements: Long sleepers, short sleepers, variable sleepers and insomniacs. Psychosomatics 14:95–103, 1975

16. Hartmann E, Cravens J: The effects of long-term administration of psychotropic drugs on human sleep: I–IV. Psychopharmacologia 33(2):153–202, 1973

17. Hartmann E, Cravens J, List S: Hypnotic effects of L-tryptophan. Arch Gen Psychiatry 31:394–397, 1974

18. Itel TM: Discrimination between some hypnotic and anxiolytic drugs by computer-analyzed sleep. In Williams RL, Karacan I (eds): Pharmacology of Sleep, pp 225–238. New York, John Wiley & Sons, 1976

19. Jouvet M: Biogenic amines and the states of sleep. Science 163:32–38, 1969

20. Kales A, Kales J: Sleep disorders. N Engl J Med 290(9):487–499, 1974

21. Karacan I, Eliot RS, Williams RS et al: Sleep in post-myocardial infarction patients. In Eliot RS (ed): Stress and the Heart, Vol I. Mount Kisco, Futura Publishing Co, 1974

22. Karacan I, Rosenbloom AL, Londono JH et al: Effect of acute fasting on sleep and the sleep-growth hormone response. Psychosomatics 14:33–37, 1973

23. Kay DC, Blackburn AB, Buckingham JA et al: Human pharmacology of sleep. In Williams R, Karacan I (eds): Pharmacology of Sleep, pp 83–210. New York, John Wiley & Sons, 1976

24. Kleitman N: Basic rest–activity cycle in relation to sleep and wakefulness. In Kales A (ed): Sleep Physiology and Pathology, pp 33–38. Philadelphia, JB Lippincott, 1969

25. Kleitman N: Sleep and Wakefulness. Chicago, University of Chicago Press, 1963

26. Kollar, EJ, Namerow N, Pasnau RO et al: Neurological findings during prolonged sleep deprivation. Neurology 18:836–840, 1968

27. Kollar EJ, Pasnau RO, Rubin RT et al: Psychologic, psychophysiologic, and biochemical correlates of prolonged sleep deprivation. Am J Psychiatry 126(4):488–500, 1969

28. McGhie A, Russell S: The subjective assessment of normal sleep patterns. J Mental Sci 108:642–654, 1962

29. Moses JM, Johnson LC, Naitoh P et al: Sleep stage deprivation and total sleep loss: Effects on sleep behavior. Psychophysiology 12(2):141–146, 1975

30. Nowlin JB, Troyer WG, Collins WS: The association of nocturnal angina pectoris with dreaming. Ann Intern Med 63:1040–1042, 1965

31. Oswald I: Drug research and human sleep. Ann Rev Pharmacol 13:243–253, 1973

32. Rechtschaffen A, Monroe LJ: Laboratory studies of insomnia. In Kales A (ed): Sleep Physiology and Pathology, pp 158–169. Philadelphia, JB Lippincott, 1969

33. Salamy JG: Sleep: Some concepts and constructs. In Williams RL, Karacan I (eds): Pharmacology and Sleep, 53–82. New York, John Wiley & Sons, 1976

34. Taub J, Berger RJ: Acute shifts in the sleep–wakefulness: Effects on performance and mood. Psychosom Med 36(2):164–173, 1974

35. Taub J, Berger RJ: The effects of changing phase and duration of sleep. J Exp Psychol 2(1):30–41, 1975

36. Vogel GW: REM deprivation III: Dreaming and psychosis. Arch Gen Psychiatry 18:312–316, 1968

37. Webb W: Sleep: An Experimental Approach. New York, Macmillan Co, 1968

38. Williams RL, Agnew HW, Webb WG: Sleep patterns in young adults: An EEG study. Electroencephalogr Clin Neurophysiol 20:376–385, 1964

39. Williams RL, Karacan I, Hursch CJ: EEG of Human Sleep—Clinical Applications. New York, John Wiley & Sons, 1974

ADDITIONAL READING

Albert IB, Albert SE: Penetrating the mysteries of sleep and sleep disorders. RN 31:36–39, 1974

Buquet A et al: Heart blocks during sleep: a case report in a healthy subject. Sleep 4(1):99–104, 1981

Cirignotta F, Lugaresi E: Some cineradiographic aspects of snoring and obstructive apneas. Sleep 3(3/4):225–226, 1980

Dement WC, Mitler MM, Zarcone VP: Some fundamental considerations in the study of sleep. Psychosomatics 14:89–94, 1973

Eliot RS (ed): Stress and the Heart, Vol I. Mount Kisco, Futura Publishing Company, 1974

Fink RD, Knott DH, Beard JD: Sedative–hypnotic dependence. Am Family Physician 10(3):116–122, 1974

Freeman FR: Sleep Research: A Critical Review, 2nd ed. Springfield, Charles C Thomas, 1974

Guilleminault C: Sleep apnea syndromes: impact of sleep and sleep states. Sleep 3(3/4):227–234, 1980

Hartmann E, Blakeland F, Zwilling G et al: Sleep need; How much sleep and what kind? Am J Psychiatry 127:1001–1008, 1971

Kales A: To sleep, perchance . . . , Emergency Medicine 6(12):23–28, 1974

Kales A, Bixler E, Tjiauw-Ling T et al: Chronic hypnotic-drug use—Ineffectiveness, drug-withdrawal insomnia and dependence. JAMA 227(5):513–517, 1974

Kales A, Kales J: Evaluation, diagnosis, and treatment of clinical conditions related to sleep. JAMA 213(3):2229–2235, 1970

Lugaresi E et al: Snoring. Electroencephalogr Clin Neurophysiol 39:59–64, 1975

Rosenblatt G et al: Cardiac irritability during sleep and dreaming. J Psychosomat Res 17:129–134, 1973

Sanford SJ: Sleep in the critical care setting. In Current Practice in Critical Care, Vol. 1. St. Louis, C.V. Mosby, 1979

Tilkian AG et al: Sleep-induced apnea syndrome. Prevalence of cardiac arrhythmias and their reversal after tracheostomy. Am J Med 63:348–358, 1977

32

Sensory Deprivation in Cardiac Patients

ROSE HOMAN, R.N., M.A., D.D.S.

When the patient who has experienced a myocardial infarction enters the hospital, he is usually frightened, anxious, and in pain. From the time of his admission, via the emergency room, he is bombarded by numerous sensory stimuli, deprived of his supportive relationships, and placed into a foreign environment where a group of strangers is responsible for his care. The acutely ill person is often anxious and apprehensive; he may have a narrowed perception, and his ability to cope with a foreign environment may be limited. The nurse who is aware of a patient's sensory status will be better able to aid the patient in adjusting to his new environment and to detect, minimize, and perhaps prevent the effects of sensory overload or restriction.

The Sensory Process

Normally, an individual is able to adapt to a wide range of sensory input from his environment. Sensations are the feeling or awareness of stimuli from inside or outside the body that are received from sensory receptors and transmitted to the brain. Sensations include such external stimuli as sight, hearing, taste, smell, and touch and the internal sensations of hunger, thirst, fatigue, and pain. Perception is the complex process through which sensations are integrated and organized into meaningful patterns. A person does not respond equally to all sensations; some are focused upon while others are deemphasized or ignored. This selectivity in perception is called attention. The intensity, size, change, and repetition of stimuli influence the amount of attention that a person gives to selected parts of his environment.[11,16] For example, the larger of two visual stimuli will attract more attention in an environment where other factors are equal. A stimulus that is repeated is more likely to receive attention (although to a limited extent only), than one that is less frequent. After a time, a change in the stimulus is likely to receive more attention than repetition of the stimulus.[4]

The reticular activating system (RAS) appears to be the mechanism through which we receive and organize stimuli. Anatomically the RAS is composed of a diffuse set of neurons that begins in the lower brain stem and extends upward through the mesencephalon and thalamus to be distributed throughout the cerebral cortex.[7] One segment of the RAS receives stimuli from sensory receptors of the body; these impulses are then transmitted to the cerebral cortex, where they exert an arousal or alerting effect. The cerebral cortex may also activate the RAS. These impulses may then influence the body musculature and the autonomic nervous system. Thus, the RAS may be viewed as a relay station sending and receiving impulses between the cortex and the sensory receptors of the body. Numerous feedback systems within the RAS control wakefulness and sleep, and influence, at least in part, our ability to direct attention toward specific parts of our environment.

Two authors, D.O. Hebb and D.P. Schultz, have suggested that the arousal state of the RAS is synonymous with a general drive state, meaning that we behave in such a way as to maintain an optimal arousal level.[10,15] Behavior which increases or reduces sensory input to bring it to an optimal level will be reinforced. We are thus sometimes motivated to seek stimulation and sometimes to reduce it.

Our specific response to an altered sensory environment is influenced by individual differences and the variables in the environment. Schultz proposes that in addition to the level of stimulation, the quality of stimulation, as reflected in stimulus variation and meaningful contact with the outside world, is important for cortical arousal and behavioral efficiency.[15]

An altered sensory environment upsets the balance of the RAS.[3] Under conditions of reduced sensory input, for example, the RAS is no longer able to project a normal level of activation to the cortex. The stimulus-deprived person becomes more sensitive to any remaining stimulation and, as a consequence, his thoughts and perceptions become dominated by residual stimuli. He may even begin to hallucinate in an attempt to maintain an optimal level of arousal. These changes may be stressful to him, resulting in changes in his affect. Conditions of sensory distortion (lack of stimulus relevance) or sensory overload may also interfere with the delicate functions of the RAS.

Sensory Deprivation as a Clinical Concept

Sensory deprivation has been the subject of much research and attention since the early 1950s. At that time the Canadian government, prompted by reports of "brainwashing" in Chinese and Russian prisons by the use of restricted sensory conditions, funded the first sensory deprivation experiments.[1] Healthy volunteers were placed in environments where they were deprived of auditory, visual, and tactile stimulation. These laboratory studies demonstrated that restricted sensory environments can produce a wide variety of behavioral disturbances. These disturbances include inability to think and reason; disorientation as to time, place, and person; disturbances in feeling states; and occurrences of bizarre hallucinations and delusions.

Settings that have been shown to produce sensory deprivation include environments in which there is sensory restriction or perceptual deprivation, with or without sensory overload. Sensory restriction is a term used to describe a decrease in the amount or intensity of sensory input. Clinical examples of sensory restriction include the restriction of mobility produced by bedrest and of visual input by an eye patch. Sensory restriction can also be a result of the reduced perception which occurs when a high anxiety level interferes with the body's ability to attend to normal stimuli that are being received by the receptors.[16] Perceptual deprivation refers to a reduction in the patterning or meaning of stimulation. The beeping sound of the cardiac monitor, rooms without windows, and a constant overhead light which makes discrimination of night and day difficult, and the isolation from family in the hospital, are typical contributors to perceptual deprivation. On the other hand, sensory overload is the presence of multi-sensory experiences in action simultaneously and at a higher intensity than normal. This can produce a type of sensory deprivation due to the reduction or absence of meaningful stimuli in the presence of stimuli of greater intensity. Pain and a constant high noise level are types of sensory overload.

All hospitalized patients are exposed to altered sensory conditions to a greater or lesser degree. Cardiac patients who require surgery or a respirator, intra-aortic balloon pump or other mechanical-assist devices are subjected to all three elements of sensory deprivation and are likely to experience its effects. For this reason the behavioral disturbances of cardiac surgery patients, sometimes referred to as "cardiac psychosis" or "cardiac delirium," have been studied by many different investigators.[6,9,12] Reports of the incidence of "delirium" after open heart surgery have ranged from 39%–60%.[12] Typically, "delirium" develops after a lucid interval during the postoperative period. The patient may experience an illusion; for example, the hum from an air conditioner sounds like someone is calling him. This may progress to auditory and visual hallucinations and even to frank paranoid delusions. Patients who experience these recurring sensory hallucinations and delusions may or may not be oriented as to time, place, and person. Usually these psychotic symptoms resolve completely in a relatively short time. Although the experiences are generally transitory, they can be very frightening to the patient.

Ellis found that 20 out of 43 cardiac surgery patients (67%) experienced one or more unusual sensory or thought disturbance in the postoperative period.[6,11] The type of experiences reported by these patients included altered hearing, smell, taste, and visual sensations, plus disturbances in orientation and other thought processes. The disturbances were not a misinterpretation or misperception of something in the environment that the patient could see, hear, or feel. Rather, the patient actually felt, heard, or saw something, such as a black, menacing bear, for which there was no appropriate stimulus. Patients' experiences which could be attributed to physical problems or postoperative neurologic changes were not included in this study.

Possible explanations for these behavioral disturbances include hypotension and cerebral ischemia during bypass, metabolic causes, and embolization due to air, fat, silicone particles, and platelet and leukocyte aggregates.[13] However, physiologic factors alone do not seem to adequately account for the problems experienced by these acutely ill cardiac patients. Pain, stress, preoperative psychosis or neurosis, and alterations in the patient's usual pattern and environment of sleep are also probable contributory factors. Although it is difficult to quantify the amount of dysfunction caused by sensory disruption, laboratory and clinical studies strongly suggest that an altered sensory environment can interfere with one's adaptive abilities. The hospitalized patient who is already physically and emotionally stressed may have particular difficulty in coping with his unfamiliar environment.

APPROACH OF THE NURSING PROCESS TO PROMOTE NORMAL SENSORY STATUS

Nursing Assessment

When assessing the patient's sensory status, it is helpful to be aware of the patient's past experiences, knowledge level, and attitudes. Is the patient accustomed to an environment that produces a high level of stimulation or does he prefer a quiet environment with minimal sensory input? What does he like to do when he is alone? Individuals vary in what they consider normal. For example, patients who are required to wear eye patches postoperatively may not benefit from the often prescribed remedy of a light at night.[5] Is the patient knowledgeable about the mechanical devices in his environment? A patient may consider a monitor strange until its purpose is explained, after which he may find its presence reassuring.[8]

The following guidelines may be offered to assess the patient who is experiencing the sensory or thought disturbances associated with sensory deprivation.[3] First of all, the nurse should be aware of the patient's tendency to conceal such experiences. A patient may think that his perceptions, thoughts, or feelings are abnormal and indicate an underlying mental disturbance. Skillful questioning may be necessary before a patient can reveal his experiences. The patient may offer cues about his experience in the use of words such as "daydream," "nightmare," or "dream." Since some patients may not wish to discuss their experiences, the nurse must then rely on her observations of sensory deprivation. Worrell suggests several ways in which the nurse can determine whether the patient is experiencing a perceptual disturbance.[20] Does he seem indifferent to people and events surrounding him? Does the nurse encounter difficulty in getting the patient's attention? Is he fully oriented to time, place, and person? The patient's sleeping patterns, appetite, reaction to visitors, and attention to personal hygiene may also provide valuable information.

Nursing Actions to Prevent Sensory Deprivation

The nurse can prevent, or at least minimize, the severity of sensory or thought disturbances through skillful manipulation of the patient's environment. Providing an optimal sensory environment for the patient in an acute care unit, with all its electronic equipment, multiple alarm systems, and large number of personnel, is perhaps one of the most difficult tasks confronting nurses working in that environment. The patient whose mobility is restricted by pain, cardiac monitoring cables, and various types of tubes may experience a sensory restriction. At the same time, the noise level and activity of the unit may be producing a sensory overload. Hospital routines and the technical language used by those who care for him may have little meaning for the patient and may be misleading. Monotony and boredom may result from confinement to the same room. The patient's overhead light may be on constantly. There are frequent interruptions of his sleep, producing perceptual as well as sleep deprivation.

Noise levels in an acute care environment should be continuously monitored to prevent sensory overload. Nurses sometimes become so accustomed to the sound of the mechanical devices depended upon to provide safe patient care that they forget how noisy these devices must sound to patients. Noise levels of acute care units have been found to be comparable to a hospital cafeteria at noon, and only somewhat less noisy than the hospital boiler room.[14]

The nurse can reduce the decibel level in the cardiac unit by limiting conversation at the bedside to that essential for patient care, and by using tactile rather than loud auditory stimulation to arouse a patient from sleep.[19] Patients who are likely to cry out in pain, cough, or require frequent suctioning will probably disturb other patients' rest if they are placed in close proximity to one another. When possible, patients should be placed away from work areas and, if all beds are not occupied, a newly admitted patient should not be placed in a bed immediately adjacent to that of another patient. Nursing measures to reduce noise from mechanical devices include positioning respirators with the bellows away from a patient's ear, turning off suction equipment that is not in use, and insulating noisy machinery, when possible.

The architectural design of the cardiac unit is another important consideration in providing orientation for the patients. Wilson found that the incidence of postoperative behavioral disturbances in surgical patients was significantly higher in patients in an acute care unit without windows than in a similar unit with windows.[18] He recommended that outside windows be visible to each patient in the acute care unit to assist the patient in maintaining orientation to his environment. This stresses the need for nurses to have input concerning the architectural design of acute care units.

Acute Sensory Deprivation

Special consideration needs to be given to the patient who experiences perceptual and thought disturbances. When caring for these patients the nurse should be aware that for some patients an opportunity to simply relate their experiences may provide great emotional relief.[5] The patient should be assured that such experiences are not unusual, under the circumstances, and are usually transitory. The nurse should avoid telling the patient either that the experience did not occur or that it should be forgotten. Such an approach can reinforce the idea that the experience was "bad." In addition, it may create a barrier to further sharing of the patient's experiences.

Sensory and thought disturbances may occur with or without orientation to time, place, and person. A patient may be keenly aware of reality and talk rationally about his experiences; that is, he knows that the things being "seen" or "heard" are not there. Terms such as "psychosis" and "delirium" should be avoided because they connote more serious disturbance than what the patient is experiencing and, for some, may bear a stigma.[6]

The nurse can further assist the patient by teaching him in a matter-of-fact fashion about the various aspects of his care. If a patient understands his environment, he is less likely to be frightened of it. When possible, a visit to the acute care unit before surgery should be arranged for the surgical patient, to allow him to ask questions and establish rapport with the staff who will provide his postoperative nursing care.

During the postoperative period, useful orientation can be provided by encouraging the patient's family to keep him up to date on events at home. Though visiting hours are restricted in acute care areas, the family can be helped to use their time with the patient more effectively. The nurse can make the hospital environment appear more personal to some patients by encouraging them to use personal belongings such as toilet articles, clocks, calendars and sleepwear.

Chronic Sensory Deprivation

After the acute phase of care is over for the myocardial infarction or surgical patient, he enters a prolonged period of convalescence. During this time he may experience perceptual monotony and boredom. Some individuals have a low tolerance for experiences that are repetitious or constant.[22] Such "boredom-susceptible" persons may become extremely restless during the convalescent period. The nurse should use the appropriate measures mentioned above to provide an optimal sensory environment for the patient. In addition, diversion can be provided by positioning the patient near a window, or elsewhere where he can observe activity. The use of a clock, calendar, or colorful posters may provide orientation and stimulation. If a patient is in isolation, a special attempt should be made to prevent him from feeling separated from family and hospital staff and to increase his social contacts.

If sensory restriction is present, additional stimulation can be provided by a telephone, radio, television, or occupational therapy. Patients on bedrest should be encouraged to participate in as much self-care and exercise as their medical condition allows.[2] Adherence to an exercise program by individuals who are immobilized has been associated with improved mental status and intellectual abilities.[17,21]

Evaluation

When caring for patients experiencing sensory deprivation, the nurse should be aware that there are individual differences in the range of stimulation considered normal, and that a variety of factors—physiologic, psychologic, and environmental—contribute to the patient's behavior. When assessing the patient in the acute care unit, the nurse should therefore be particularly attuned to individual needs. Each patient's situation must be carefully analyzed to determine the effectiveness of nursing actions.

REFERENCES

1. Bexton WH, Heron W, Scott TH: Effects of decreased variation in the sensory environment. Can J Psychol 8:7076, 1954
2. Bolin RH: An Investigation of Sensory Deprivation in Immobilized Orthopedic Patients. Unpublished Master's Thesis, University of Iowa, 1972
3. Bolin RH: Sensory deprivation: An overview. Nursing Forum 13(3):240–258, 1974
4. Chodil J, Williams B: The concept of sensory deprivation. Nurs Clin North Am 5:454–465, 1970
5. Ellis R: Suggestions for the Care of Eye Surgery Patients Who Experienced Reduced Sensory Input. ANA Regional Clinical Session, 1967, pp 131–136. New York: Appleton-Century-Crofts, 1968
6. Ellis R; Unusual sensory and thought disturbances in cardiac surgery. Am J Nurs 72:2021–2025, 1972
7. Guyton AC: Textbook of Medical Physiology, p 705. Philadelphia: WB Saunders, 1971
8. Hackett TP, Cassem NH: Coronary Care: Patient Psychology. Dallas, American Heart Association, 1975
9. Hazan SJ: Psychiatric complications following cardiac surgery: A review. J Thorac Cardiovasc Surg 51:307–318, 1966
10. Hebb DO: Drives and the C.N.S. (Conceptual Nervous System). Psychol Rev 62:243–254, 1955
11. Jackson CW, Ellis R: Sensory deprivation as a field of study. Nurs Res 20:46–54, 1971
12. Kornfield DS: The hospital environment: Its impact on the patient. Ad Psychosom Med 8:252–270, 1972
13. Mossing KA: Post Cardiotomy Delirium and Microfiltration. Unpublished Master's Thesis, University of Washington, 1975
14. Redding JS, Hargest TS, Minsky SH: How noisy is intensive care? Crit Care Med 5:275–276, 1977
15. Schultz DP: Sensory Restriction. New York, Academic Press, 1965
16. Shelby JP: Sensory deprivation. Image 10:49–55, 1978
17. Sorokin PA, Simonenko VV, Korolev BA: Clinical observations on prolonged hypodynamia. In Genin AM, Sorokin PA (eds): Problems of Space Biology, NASA Technical Translation, NASA TT F-639. Washington DC, National Aeronautics and Space Administration 13:15–20, 1970
18. Wilson LM: Intensive care delirium: The effects of outside deprivation in a windowless unit. Arch Intern Med 130:255–256, 1972
19. Woods NF, Falk SA: Noise stimuli in the acute care area. Nurs Res 23:144–150, 1974
20. Worrell JD: Nursing implications in the care of the patient experiencing sensory deprivation. In Kintzel KC (ed): Advanced Concepts in Clinical Nursing, p 130. Philadelphia: JB Lippincott, 1971
21. Zubek JP: Counteracting effect of physical exercises performed during prolonged perceptual deprivation. Science 142:504–506, 1963
22. Zuckerman M: The search for high stimulation. Psychology Today 11:38–40, 43, 46, 96, 99, 1978

ADDITIONAL READING

Abram HS: Psychological reactions to cardiac operations: An historical perspective. Psychiatry in Medicine 1:277–294, 1970
Brownfield CA: Isolation: Clinical and Experimental Approaches. New York, Random House, 1965
Corso JF: The Experimental Psychology of Sensory Behavior. New York, Holt, Rinehart & Winstons, 1967
Downs FS: Bedrest and sensory disturbances. Am J Nurs 74:435–438, 1974
Ellis R: Theory–Research–Theory–Cycle. In Norris CM (ed): Proceedings of Third Nursing Theory Conference. Kansas City, University of Kansas Medical Center, Department of Nursing Education, January 29–30, 1970
Jackson CW, O'Neil M: Experiences associated with sensory deprivation reported for patients having eye surgery. In Ross Roundtable on Maternal and Child Nursing: Patients with Sensory Disturbances: Implications for Nursing Practice and Research. Columbus, Ross Laboratories, 1966
Madow L, Snow L (eds): The Psychodynamic Implications of Physiological Studies on Sensory Deprivation. Springfield, Charles C Thomas, 1970
Mitchell PH: Concepts Basic to Nursing. New York, McGraw-Hill, 1973
Roberts S: Behavioral Concepts and the Critically Ill Patient. Englewood Cliffs, Prentice-Hall, 1976
Solomon P, Rossi AM: Sensory deprivation. In Howells JG (ed): Modern Perspectives in World Psychiatry. New York, Brunner/Mazel, 1971
Woodward JA: An ICU is a place to live—Not just survive. RN 41:62, 1978
Zubek JP (ed): Sensory Deprivation: Fifteen Years of Research. New York, Appleton-Century-Crofts, 1969

SECTION E
CARDIOVASCULAR DRUGS

33

Common Noncardiac Drugs Used in the Cardiac Care Unit

LORA E. BURKE, R.N., M.N.

Certain drugs are routinely administered to the patient with acute, uncomplicated myocardial infarction and are frequently included as a part of standing orders. For each category of these drugs, actions, indications, contraindications, and nursing implications are presented in text. Dosage, administration, and side- and toxic-effects are summarized in Tables 33-1 through 33-4.

NARCOTIC ANALGESICS

The extract of the opium poppy is among the oldest medicinals, and the study of the major alkaloid in this extract, morphine, is one of the oldest areas of biologic research. A discussion of the actions and use of the opiates would not be complete without initially reviewing the most significant advance in neuropharmacology in the past decade. It had long been postulated that the mechanism of action of the opiates was related to their initial binding to a specific receptor site on the surface of or within nerve cells. In 1973 three independent laboratories reported specific opiate binding in rat brain.[32,36,39] Subsequently, these results have been confirmed in many laboratories and much evidence has accumulated suggesting that these specific binding sites indeed represent the receptors to which opiates must bind in order to produce their pharmacologic responses. They have been found in man[18] and in all vertebrates so far studied.[33] The regional distribution of specific opiate binding

in the central nervous system (CNS) is of considerable interest because it may reveal a relationship between opiate receptor localization and regional brain function. Studies in human brain[18,37] have indicated that many areas demonstrating high levels of opiate binding are located in, or associated with, the limbic system. This system has frequently been suggested as a possible region of opiate action on the basis of ablation and electrical stimulation experiments.[8,25] Electrical stimulation of the brain in the region where morphine was found to act selectively resulted in analgesia that outlasted the period of stimulation[27,28] and was reversed by the specific opiate antagonist naloxone.[2] This implies the existence of a native substance in the brain with opiate-like properties. The discovery of an endogenous factor in brain extracts which had opiate-like properties was first reported in 1975[20] and, subsequently, a number of other peptides with similar activity were isolated, leading to the creation of the generic term for these substances *endorphin* (for *endo*genous mor*phine*-like material). The physiologic functions of the various endorphins remain unknown. Their discovery has added a new dimension to investigations of the opiate receptor by increasing the likelihood that this receptor is an important functional constituent of the CNS of all vertebrates. The advances in this field are occurring at a rapid pace. There is every reason to believe that future studies in this area will shed light on the mode of action of the opiates and will provide insight into the biochemistry underlying analgesia, euphoria, and addiction. Refer to Table 33-1 for dosage, administration, side and toxic effects of narcotic analgesics.

TABLE 33-1 NARCOTIC ANALGESICS

Agent	Dosage/Administration	Side and Toxic Effects
Morphine sulfate, U.S.P.	Usual IV dose is 4–10 mg. The analgesic effect starts immediately, reaches its peak in 20 minutes. The relief of the acute pain of an MI may require larger doses. It should not be administered SC into chilled skin areas of patients with low BP and in shock. It should not be administered IM to the CCU patient, because it will cause an elevation of enzymes.	Nausea and vomiting, orthostatic hypotension, constipation Increase in biliary-tract pressure, which may be accompanied by epigastric distress or biliary colic Urinary-bladder distention Hypersensitivity phenomena (urticaria, rash, and rarely anaphylactic reactions). This may be due to histamine release and not an allergic reaction. Frequent repeated use produces psychic and physical dependence. Respiratory depression (can be antagonized by naloxone or nalorphine). Elevated cerebrospinal fluid pressure because of an accumulation of CO_2 secondary to the respiratory depression.
Meperidine hydrochloride (Demerol, Dolaxtin, Dolosal, Pethoid)	Varies with the clinical situation. Most patients with moderate-to-severe pain are relieved by 100 mg parenterally. Duration of action is considerably shorter than that of morphine. Continuous depression of the CNS is attained only when the drug is used at less than 4 hr intervals. 80–100 mg of meperidine is approximately equivalent to 10 mg of morphine. After IV administration, plasma values decline rapidly for the first 1–2 hrs, and more slowly thereafter.	Dizziness, sweating, euphoria, dry mouth, nausea, vomiting, weakness, visual disturbances, palpitation, dysphoria, syncope, and sedation. In equianalgesic doses it depresses respirations to the same degree as morphine. Peak respiratory depression is observed within 1 hr after IM administration. After usual therapeutic doses there is a return toward normal, starting at about 2 hrs, although minute volume is usually measurably depressed for as long as 4 hrs. Respiratory depression (can be antagonized by naloxone or nalorphine). Toxic doses sometimes cause CNS excitation (tremors, muscle twitches, seizure). Constipation and urinary retention occur less frequently with meperidine than with morphine. IV administration frequently produces an increased heart rate. Elevated cerebrospinal fluid pressure because of an accumulation of CO_2 secondary to the respiratory depression. Subcutaneous administration causes local irritation and tissue induration.

Morphine Sulfate, U.S.P.

Actions. Morphine and other opiates produce their major effects on the CNS and the bowel.

The mechanisms by which the opiates exert their effects remain unexplained (see above). The relief of pain by these agents is selective, since other sensations (touch, vibration, vision, and hearing) are not affected. With therapeutic doses the painful stimulus itself may be recognized but it may not be perceived as painful. The opiates more effectively relieve continuous, dull pain than sharp, intermittent pain, but with sufficient amounts of morphine it is possible to relieve even the severe pain associated with renal or biliary colic.[22,43]

All types of painful experiences are combinations of the original sensation and the reaction to that sensation.[23] Administration of typical therapeutic doses causes the opiates to act primarily on the systems responsible for the affective responses to noxious stimuli. When pain does not evoke its usual responses (anxiety, fear, panic, and suffering), a patient's ability to tolerate the pain can be markedly increased even when the capacity to perceive the sensation is virtually unaltered.[4]

While producing analgesia in patients, morphine may also cause such changes in mood as apathy or euphoria. Lethargy, drowsiness, or mental confusion may also occur. The mental clouding is characterized by drowsiness, inability to concentrate, and difficulty in mentation. The sedation and alteration in mood observed may simply result from the relief of pain.[43] Sleep may ensue if the environment is conducive.

Morphine directly affects the respiratory centers in the brainstem, resulting in a depression of respiratory ability. All phases of respiratory activity (rate, minute volume, and tidal exchange) are depressed by therapeutic doses of morphine. Maximal respiratory depression occurs within approximately seven minutes after intravenous (IV) administration of morphine, 30 minutes after intramuscular (IM) administration, and 90 minutes after subcutaneous (SC) administration. Within two or three hours, the sensitivity of the respiratory center begins to return toward normal but minute volume remains considerably below normal for as long as four or five hours after a therapeutic dose is administered. These effects seem to be a result of diminished sensitivity of respiratory chemoreceptors to this stimulus of carbon dioxide. Natural sleep also reduces the sensitivity of the medullary center to carbon dioxide tension (P_aCO_2), and the effects of morphine and sleep are additive. For these reasons it is dangerous to administer opiates to a patient with respiratory insufficiency. In addition to markedly depressing the automatic regulation of respiration, morphine can alter voluntary control of respiration. After large doses of morphine or synthetic narcotics, patients will breathe if instructed to do so, but without such instruction they may remain relatively apneic. This indifference to respiration may account in part for the usefulness of these agents in pulmonary edema and other situations in which the patient's struggle to breathe aggravates the basic pathologic condition.[22,31,43]

The mechanism responsible for the circulatory effects of morphine administered in significant doses is still being studied and disputed. Studies to date have not excluded an effect on respiration or the heart. The IV administration of large doses of morphine (1–3 mg/kg body weight) to cardiac surgical patients resulted in an increase in cardiac index and stroke index and a decreased systemic vascular resistance. In addition, there was an increase in central venous and pulmonary artery pressure. The results of this study led to the more extensive use of morphine as an analgesic and anesthetic agent in patients undergoing cardiovascular operations. The elevated central venous and pulmonary artery pressures which result from large intravenous doses of morphine may be explained by increased venous tone in the pulmonary artery or the effect of an increased carbon dioxide tension on the pulmonary vasculature.[4,17,19,38]

Therapeutic doses administered to the supine patient have no major effect on blood pressure (BP), or on heart rate (HR) and rhythm. Effects on the myocardium are not important. In normal men the heart rate is either unaffected or slightly increased, and there is no consistent effect on cardiac output (CO). No alterations occur in the electrocardiogram (ECG). Morphine decreases the capacity of the cardiovascular system to respond to gravitational shifts. This is primarily due to peripheral vasodilation and causes orthostatic hypotension. The peripheral vasodilation that results is due to a direct effect on the smooth muscle of peripheral vessels, possibly caused by histamine release. In patients with acute myocardial infarction (MI), the cardiovascular response to morphine can be more variable than in normal subjects, and the magnitude of changes can be more pronounced. In patients with coronary artery disease (CAD) but with no acute medical problems, 8 mg of morphine IV produces a decrease in oxygen consumption, cardiac index, left ventricular end-diastolic pressure, and cardiac work.[3,35,40,44,45]

A combination of actions by morphine results in nausea and vomiting, which occurs much more frequently in the ambulatory than in the recumbent patient. The primary cause is a stimulation of the emetic chemoreceptors in the medulla. An increase in vestibular sensitivity causes symptoms of motion sickness compounded by an increase in labyrinthine sensitivity. The administration of a therapeutic dose of morphine eventually leads to depresssion of the vomiting center, so that subsequent doses may not induce vomiting.[22,43]

Because of the effect opiates exert on the gastrointestinal tract, they were used for several years in the treatment of diarrhea prior to their use as analgesics. In the stomach there is diminished secretion of hydrochloric acid and an increased tone of the duodenum which significantly delays the passage of gastric contents and is an important contributing factor to the constipation which results from morphine usage. Biliary and pancreatic secretions are also reduced, leading to a delay in the digestive process, and the propulsive contractions of the small and large intestines are markedly decreased. Increased anal sphincter tone and reduced awareness of sensory stimuli and the urge to defecate complete the list of major causes for the constipation so frequently

encountered in the patient receiving these agents. Effects similar to those in the gastrointestinal tract are seen in the urinary tract. Increased tone of the detrusor muscle and of the sphincter frequently results in urinary retention.[22,26,43]

Some miscellaneous effects which may be seen after the administration of morphine are constriction of the pupils, dry mouth and hyperglycemia. Flushed skin, sweating, pruritus and urticaria at the site of injection are effects which are probably accounted for by histamine release.[22,31,43]

Indications and Contraindications. The most frequently encountered clinical situation in the cardiac care unit (CCU) for which the use of morphine is indicated is in the treatment of severe chest pain of an acute MI. The euphoria caused by morphine and the alterations in the patient's perception of the pain make this a valuable drug. Morphine may also provide relief from the dyspnea of pulmonary edema secondary to acute left-sided heart failure. It allays the anxiety caused by hypoxemia and causes peripheral pooling of blood, which leads to a reduction of the heart's workload. Ventilation must be adequately controlled when morphine is given in this clinical situation.[4,19,26,31]

Since respiratory depression and CO_2 retention result in vasodilation of the cerebral vessels and a consequent increase in cerebrospinal fluid pressure, morphine is contraindicated or used cautiously in patients with head injuries or postoperative neurologic surgery. Pupillary constriction, nausea and mental clouding are important signs in following the clinical course of neurologic patients. These symptoms may be caused by the administration of narcotics, making evaluation difficult. Morphine must be used with extreme caution in a patient with a reduced respiratory reserve such as that caused by emphysema or cor pulmonale. These patients are already using compensatory mechanisms and may have chronically elevated P_aCO_2 levels. The respiratory-depressant effects of morphine can seriously compromise these patients. Because morphine depresses ciliary activity and cough reflex, and increases bronchomotor tone, it should be used cautiously in patients who have excessive pulmonary secretion, for example those with chronic lung disease.

Nursing Implications. The nurse needs to know that pain may act as a physiologic antidote to the depressant effects of morphine sulfate. The patient may initially require more than a therapeutic dose to obtain relief from the pain but show no signs of respiratory or general depression until the pain subsides. Once the pain and its associated fear and anxiety are overcome, the patient relaxes and depressant effects of the analgesic become evident.

The individual's response to morphine is influenced by factors which the nurse needs to be aware of when administering this drug, for example the patient's age and general state of health. Older patients, in particular those over 60, seem to be less sensitive to pain and more sensitive to the analgesic effects of morphine. Therefore, smaller doses would be appropriate for patients in the older age group. Morphine is metabolized by the liver. Precautions should be taken when administering this drug to individuals with any hepatic insufficiency, because the duration of action may be prolonged. Because of its depressant effects on the respiratory center and cough reflex, the patients who are receiving morphine, particularly for longer periods, should be encouraged to cough and deep breathe at regular intervals of two hours.

All patients may experience postural hypotension after receiving morphine because of its vasodilating effects. The patient who is hypovolemic, which may be secondary to blood loss or excessive diuresis, is more susceptible to the hypotensive effects of morphine. If it is necessary for the patient who has received morphine to get out of bed, for example to void, a bedside commode should be used and the nurse should remain in attendance while the patient is out of bed. When the patient is getting up, he should sit up slowly and sit on the edge of bed for a minute, or until he feels he has adjusted to the change in position, before he is allowed to stand. Vital signs should be closely monitored during this time and the patient should be returned to bed immediately if the blood pressure falls below 90 mm Hg systolic, or if other symptoms develop.

The nurse caring for these patients should be aware that the nausea and vomiting caused by morphine occurs less frequently in the recumbent patient. If nausea and vomiting occur, the effects may be counteracted by a phenothiazine derivative.

Morphine relieves suffering, primarily by altering the emotional component of the painful experience. The patient who receives psychologic support from the health team may need less analgesic medication. In addition to providing emotional support, the physician should also take into account the substantial variability in both the capacity to tolerate pain and the individual response to narcotics and analgesics. Patients should be reassured that they will not become addicted with short-term use of the drug and should be reminded of the importance of informing the nurse whenever chest discomfort occurs.

Meperidine Hydrochloride, U.S.P. (Demerol, Dolantin, Dolosal, Pethoid)

Like morphine sulfate, the chief pharmacologic actions of meperidine are exerted on the CNS. Meperidine is also used in the treatment of pain of an MI, but it is much less effective in relieving this severe pain than morphine. It also has the disadvantage of having a vagolytic effect, which may exaggerate the tachycardia in patients with sympathetic imbalance. This may, however, be an advantage to the patients with inferior or posterior infarction and sinus bradycardia.[1,15,16,34]

Indications and Contraindications. The indications and contraindications for meperidine are the same as those for morphine.

Nursing Implications. The nurse should be aware that meperidine has a more rapid onset of action than morphine; usually within 10 minutes after SC or IM injection. The duration of analgesic action is also shorter for meperidine, lasting 2–4 hours as compared to the 4–5 hour analgesic effect of morphine. Meperidine, in doses equianalgesic to morphine, results in the same amount of respiratory depression produced by morphine. Doses of 75–100 mg of meperidine are considered equivalent to 10 mg of morphine. Constipation and urinary retention occur less often in the patient receiving meperidine. The nursing implications discussed for the patient treated with morphine also apply to meperidine.

OXYGEN

Since its discovery two hundred years ago, oxygen has been used as a drug to treat hypoxemia. For many years it has been part of the treatment for patients with myocardial ischemia. The utilization of oxygen in this situation is justified by the frequent presence of arterial hypoxemia[7,9,10,42] and supported by recent studies which suggest that oxygen therapy may have a beneficial effect in limiting infarct size.[13] The nursing implications and harmful effects of oxygen therapy are discussed in the text. The various modes used for the delivery of oxygen, liter flow and percent of oxygen delivered, as well as the advantages of each type, are summarized in Table 33-2.

Monitoring Dosage Levels

A study done by Gibson et al suggested that the actual inspired percentage of oxygen reaching the trachea in spontaneously breathing patients is never as high as that measured in the masks or tubing.[14] The importance of monitoring serial arterial blood gases is underscored by this study, in addition to the fact that variables such as respiratory rate, tidal volume, and technique of applying the equipment influence the delivered concentration of gas by any mode.[9,14,46] The objective of oxygen therapy is to maintain the P_aO_2 between 60 to 100 mm Hg, which provides for a 90%–98% saturation of the hemoglobin.

Hazards in the Use of Oxygen

Although oxygen is not explosive, it does support combustion. Smoking in a room where oxygen is in use should be prohibited. Caution must be used in administering oxygen to the patient who is dependent upon a hypoxic drive as the respiratory stimulus, for example, the patient with chronic obstructive airway disease. The administration of oxygen above a low flow rate ($\leq$ 3 liters/min) will suppress the chemoreceptors and result in an oxygen-induced hypoventilation.

Oxygen Toxicity. The development of symptoms of oxygen toxicity tends to be a function of both the fraction of inspired oxygen (FIO_2) and length of exposure. The only clinical criterion is a decrease in vital capacity leading to progressive hypoxemia. This usually occurs when an individual is exposed to an FIO_2 of greater than 60% and may occur within hours, or not occur until after 16–36 hours of administration. The spectrum of O_2-induced injury includes pulmonary edema and atelectasis, congestion, fibrosis, impaired ciliary function leading to increased sensitivity to infection, and damaged capillary endothelium. This damage can be prevented only by reducing the duration of exposure to a high FIO_2, which may be achieved by utilizing other supportive measures such as intermittent positive pressure breathing (IPPB) treatments, vigorous pulmonary toilet, and

TABLE 33-2   OXYGEN

Mode of Delivery	Liter Flow	O₂ Concentration Delivered (%)	Advantages	Disadvantages
Nasal cannula or prongs	2–3 liters/min 3–5 liters/min	24%–28% 28%	Allows for uninterrupted flow Is most comfortable Directs O₂ through turbinates to allow for greater humidification Inexpensive	Final FIO₂ is determined by the proportionate mixing of O₂ flow and amount of ambient air (21% O₂) moved in and out of lungs. Flow >6 liters/min causes drying and irritation of nasal mucosa. May become displaced.
Nasal catheter	4–6 liters/min	30%–40%	Allows for continuous flow Easily inserted if well lubricated with water soluble jelly (measure from nose tip to tip of earlobe; insert with O₂ on; should end at uvula) Inexpensive	Requires changing q8h and alternating nares. May cause drying of nasal-pharyngeal mucosa, increasing the risk of infection Is less well tolerated than cannula Cannot deliver O₂ within a narrow fixed range of FIO₂ Complications include gastric distention and rupture, and nasal necrosis
Oxygen mask	6–8 liters/min 10 liters/min	35%–45% 45%–55%	Allows for slightly higher O₂ concentrations without causing drying of the nasal mucosa	Interferes with talking, eating, drinking, expectorating. One size only. Are often hot and may have an unpleasant odor May cause panic in a patient because of a closed-in feeling Can create pressure sores on face Are dangerous in patients who tends to vomit, especially in those with a decreased level of consciousness, or whose arms are in restraints or secured on armboards. Adds dead space to the patient's airway, which may be considerable with some appliances. Difficult to deliver exact amount of O₂ to patient
Partial rebreathing mask	8–10 liter/min; oxygen flow should be sufficient to keep reservoir bag partially inflated during inspiration	60%	Able to deliver high concentrations of O₂	There are no adequate means of humidifying the gas. Dangerous if liter flow decreased—the patient may rebreathe CO₂
Non-rebreathing mask	10–12 liter/min	80%–90%	No exhaled air is rebreathed because of the one-way valve It is the most precise method of administering a specific gas concentration because the patient inhales the gas present in the bag only. Allows for humidification of the gas Some reservoir bags have drain plugs for removal of accumulated moisture	Tight seal needed Often hot May cause panic in a patient because of a closed-in feeling Can create pressure sores on the face. Are dangerous in a patient who tends to vomit. Interferes with talking, eating, drinking, expectorating

TABLE 33-2   OXYGEN (Cont.)

Mode of Delivery	Liter Flow	O₂ Concentration Delivered (%)	Advantages	Disadvantages
Venturi mask (Venti-mask, air-mix or dilution mask)	4–6 liters/min 4–6 liters/min 8–10 liters/min 8–10 liters/min	24% 28% 35% 40%	Allows for precise concentration of O₂ at low flow The FIO₂ is relatively independent of the O₂ flow rate as long as it exceeds the stated minimum	Uncomfortable and inconvenient. Same as above Not always as reliable as claimed Relatively expensive
Face tent or trach mask	6–10 liters/min	30%–65%	Provides high humidity, allowing for wetting of secretions	The appliance attached to the face may be a nuisance Heat is retained about the face by the plastic
Mechanical ventilators	21–100 liters/min	21%–100%	Allows for precise FIO₂ Allows for the addition of other techniques, such as increased tidal volume or positive end expiratory pressure (PEEP) to increase oxygenation	Over-oxygenation can occur.
Intermittent positive pressure breathing (IPPB)	"Airmix" 100%	40%–90% 100%	Valuable treatment for acute pulmonary edema Allows for administration of medications through nebulizer	Over-oxygenation can readily occur. Forced inspiration may be uncomfortable for patient.

specific therapeutics directed to the remedial causes of respiratory distress, for example, antibiotic therapy.[13,41]

Nursing Implications

Most CCUs have standing orders for admission of oxygen to newly admitted patients suspected of having an acute myocardial infarction, for example, 5 liters of O₂ per minute via nasal prongs. However, if the nurse has any reason to suspect the patient of having chronic obstructive airway disease, such as a lengthy history of smoking or a barrel-chested appearance, she should administer only low-flow oxygen until the physician can be contacted or arterial blood gases drawn.

All the devices utilized in the administration of oxygen may be uncomfortable to the patient and also have the potential for causing pressure sores in such areas as the bridge of the nose, cheeks, nares, and over the ears. The nurse can take measures to prevent the development of tissue damage, and also make the patient more comfortable, by such measures as keeping the face dry under a mask or padding areas under the head strap. Since the nurse is in almost constant attendance of the patient, she can see that the device being used fits properly and is being kept in place by the patient. Changing the mask as needed provides additional comfort. Also, oxygen is very drying to the mucuous membranes. A humidifier should be routinely added to all oxygen administered.

Carrying out efforts for good pulmonary toilet and observing for signs of hypoventilation or oxygen intolerance are important for the nurse to remember when caring for patients receiving oxygen therapy. Since suctioning a patient may cause a severe fall in P_aO_2 increasing the oxygen flow or the oxygen percentage for a few minutes prior to suctioning is a recommended preventive measure.

ANTIANXIETY DRUGS, SEDATIVES AND HYPNOTICS

There are many reasons why patients in a CCU have difficulty in obtaining rest and sleep (Chap. 31). The surroundings are unfamiliar and the patient may find himself amid equipment that is comforting but at the same time threatening. It may reassure the patient that every heart beat is being monitored, but the triggered alarm system may induce increased levels of anxiety. The electronic equipment and the simultaneous isolation subjects the patient to both sensory overload and sensory deprivation (Chap. 32). This is compounded by the patient's internal stimuli, such as fears regarding the diagnosis of an MI, anxieties associated with the strange environment, and concerns regarding the implications and significance of the illness in terms of his future, job, and family. The high level of anxiety in the cardiac patient may be very costly in terms of workload on the myocardium because the patient may suffer from restlessness, insomnia, or resting tachycardia. The judicious use of sedatives can diminish this anxiety and allow the patient much more effective rest.[15,24,29]

The sleep induced by these drugs differs in physiologic parameters from normal sleep, but the clinical significance of this is unknown. Sleep studies in laboratories have demonstrated that hypnotic doses of most of these agents reduce the amount of time spent in rapid eye movement (REM) sleep, and a number of hypnotics, especially the benzodiazepines, reduce stage IV sleep, which is the deepest stage. Such changes in sleep stage have not been linked to alterations in human behavior.[1,5] Refer to Chapter 31 for a complete discussion of sleep and the effects of sleep deprivation in these patients.

Diazepam, the prototype of the benzodiazepines, is the only antianxiety drug that will be described, and while a large number of hypnotic agents is available, this discussion will be limited to flurazepam and chloral hydrate. Barbiturates are not included because they are rarely used for cardiac patients. Barbiturates increase the risk of dependence and the rate of hepatic metabolism of many drugs, particularly anticoagulants. Actions, indications, contraindications and nursing implications are discussed in text. Table 33-3 summarizes dosage, administration, toxic effects, and side-effects.

Diazepam (Valium)

Actions. The site of antianxiety activity appears to be the limbic system. Electrical discharges and transmission in the limbic system are inhibited by low doses of benzodiazepines. The administration of diazepam results in CNS depression and an alleviation of anxiety. Mild sedation results, without impairing psychomotor performance. An overall muscle relaxant effect follows the administration of the drug. Their mechanism of action remains speculative.[6,21]

Indications and Contraindications. Diazepam is useful in the symptomatic relief of tension and anxiety states resulting from stressful circumstances, or whenever somatic complaints are concomitant with emotional factors. It has been shown to safely control the serious anxiety reactions often seen during the initial phase of acute myocardial infarction. Diazepam is also useful prior to cardioversion for diminishing anxiety, tension, and the patient's recall of the procedure.[1,12,29]

The use of diazepam is contraindicated in patients with a known hypersensitivity to the drug. It is also contraindi-

cated in patients suffering from acute narrow-angle glaucoma or open-angle glaucoma, unless patients are receiving appropriate therapy. Diazepam should not be administered to patients in shock, coma, or in a state of acute alcoholic intoxication with depression of vital signs.

Nursing Implications. Admission to a CCU, especially with a life-threatening problem, causes severe anxiety. Often the basic personality further increases the baseline anxiety level of the individual with cardiac disease when confined to a hospital. This individual may be afraid he will no longer be in control if he begins taking antianxiety drugs, and may refuse administration. The nurse can inform the patient that he has control over ingestion of the medication and that it will be withheld if the patient's alertness and arousability are impaired. She should emphasize the benefits of taking the medication; that he, and therefore his heart, will rest much better, an essential element during the acute phase, and that he will probably sleep better at night, experiencing a less anxious state.[29]

When diazepam is administered IV it may cause respiratory depression. The nurse should closely observe the patient's respiratory function, particularly after a cardioversion procedure when the patient may have received a larger dose. Caution must be used when administering the drug IV to patients who are elderly, very ill, and to those with limited pulmonary reserve, since there is increased risk for apnea, cardiac arrest, or both. This also applies particularly to the patient who is receiving other CNS depressants. The dose of diazepam has to be adjusted when administered to older patients, because they often show a reduced tolerance to this agent. Due to a possible accumulation of active

TABLE 33-3 SEDATIVES AND HYPNOTICS

Agents	Dose/Administration	Side and Toxic Effects
SEDATIVES Diazepam (Valium)	Usual dose 5 mg Low dose (2–5 mg) for elderly and debilitated patients Oral administration is generally preferred; is absorbed more rapidly after oral than IM administration IV administration should be done slowly, taking at least one minute for each 5 mg (1 ml) Optimal dose varies widely. In general, therapy should be initiated with the smallest dose, and amount increased as required. It may be given once daily at h.s. because of its long half-life. After the first week of therapy, when divided doses are given, the primary dose should be taken at h.s. with smaller doses during the day. May be given IM (irregular absorption may occur) to allay preoperative apprehension or IV to diminish recall of procedures. If countershock is performed within 5 min, patient will be in a state of light sleep and will not recall the shock.	Drowsiness Ataxia, dizziness, headache. Venous thrombosis and phlebitis at the site of injection. Other reactions include fatigue, dysarthria, and muscle weakness. GI discomfort, dryness of the mouth, nausea, and vomiting Rash, chills, fever have been noted. Blood dyscrasias and a paradoxical aggravation of the symptoms of anxiety have been reported rarely. Parenteral administration has caused hypotension or muscular weakness in some patients, particularly when used with CNS depressants. Rapid IV injection can cause transient bradycardia, hypotension, and apnea. Cumulative effects may occur until steady state concentrations are reached (several days to one week). Excess accumulation may occur in patients with compromised kidney function. Long-term use may result in psychic and physical dependence.
HYPNOTICS Flurazepam (Dalmane)	Usual adult dose is 30 mg. In elderly or debilitated patients, begin with 15 mg.	There is a 7% incidence of side effects; dizziness, drowsiness, lightheadedness, staggering, ataxia and falling, particularly with impaired renal or hepatic function Paradoxical reactions are rare Severe sedation, lethargy, disorientation and coma
Chloral hydrate (Noctec, Somnos, Aquachloral)	500 mg to 1 g orally, h.s.	Unpleasant taste, epigastric distress, nausea, vomiting. Lightheadedness, malaise, ataxia, and nightmares. "Hangover" may also occur; rarely, idiosyncratic reactions.

metabolities with a long half-life, there is increased likelihood of adverse reactions in the elderly and in individuals with diminished kidney function.[1,29]

To reduce the chance of venous thrombosis, phlebitis, local irritation or swelling occurring after IV injection, the drug should be administered slowly (1 ml/min) and the small veins should be avoided. The drug should not be mixed with other solutions or drugs in the syringe and should be administered as close to the IV injection site as possible. Diazepam burns when administered IV, so it is often beneficial to tell the patient in advance that it will burn or sting and then increase the rate of fluid infusion to further dilute the drug solution. Recent studies show considerable loss of the drug when it is administered in plastic intravenous-fluid bags and also through plastic tubing from glass containers. Consequently, it is recommended that the IV administration of diazepam be restricted to direct venous injection and that the drug not be left in plastic syringes at the bedside.[30] Intramuscular administration should be avoided because of irregular absorption.

If diazepam has been prescribed for the patient being discharged, its use should be explained. The patient must be instructed about the use of diazepam, its effect in terms of driving a motor vehicle, and the dangers of combining diazepam with any other depressant medication or with alcohol. The patient should be informed that if he is going to experience a particulary stressful situation which may precipitate angina, then taking a diazepam tablet a few hours prior to the anticipated experience may lessen the anxiety response. However, limiting the use of diazepam may be advisable in order to prevent tolerance.

Flurazepam Hydrochloride (Dalmane)

Action. This drug effectively reduces sleep-induction time, number of awakenings, and time spent awake, and increases sleep duration. Within 20–45 minutes of oral administration, satisfactory hypnotic effects begin to occur. Rapid eye movement (REM) sleep may be reduced by flurazepam, but it does not produce REM rebound and associated sleep disturbances when withdrawn. It also causes suppression of Stage IV sleep and increases Stage II sleep. The sleep pattern reverts to normal when the drug is withdrawn. Other advantageous properties of this medication are that "drug hangover" occurs infrequently and that rebound insomnia is not observed as it is with shorter-acting benzodiazepines. Flurazepam has also been reported to maintain its effectiveness for inducing and maintaining sleep patterns for long periods. An additional property is that it does not increase the metabolism of oral anticoagulants.

Indications and Contraindications. The use of flurazepam is indicated in acute or chronic medical situations requiring restful sleep. It is useful for treating all types of insomnia characterized by difficulty in falling asleep, frequent nocturnal awakenings or early morning awakening, or both. A history of known hypersensitivity to the drug provides the major contraindication for administration of flurazepam.

Nursing Implications. Nurses have two major responsibilities in relation to the administration and use of hypnotics.

First, the nurse should educate the patient about the use of these agents so that he will feel more comfortable taking them. Many individuals fear dependency and therefore refuse sleeping medications. Patients may also find themselves having bizarre dreams or nightmares and become concerned that these will become more severe with sleeping pills. The nurse can instruct patients that these dreams may lessen when they are sleeping better and that sleeping agents themselves do not cause nightmares. If the patient is clearly having difficulty in sleeping the nurse should encourage the patient to make use of these agents and remind him that this is a short-term requirement. Second, after the nurse identifies the patient who needs a sleeping agent and administers the agent, she should then optimize its potential effect by quieting the surrounding environment and not disturbing the patient more frequently than necessary.[8]

Chloral Hydrate
(Noctec, Somnos, Aquachloral)

Action. The effect of chloral hydrate on REM sleep is not established. It has little analgesic activity and, in doses of one gram, it is only slightly effective as a hypnotic. In therapeutic doses, respiration and BP are affected little more than by ordinary sleep, and there is no evidence of deleterious effects on the heart. In large doses it depresses myocardial contractility and shortens the refractory period. In the body, chloral hydrate is very rapidly reduced to trichlorethanol, which is believed to cause the CNS depressant effects.[1,16]

It is relatively safe, reliable, and rapidly effective as a sedative. With continued administration it may lose its effectiveness by the second week.

Indications and Contraindications. Chloral hydrate is indicated in situations requiring short-term use of a hypnotic. This drug may be especially useful in elderly patients who tend to become agitated with barbiturates, although paradoxical responses are common.

The use of chloral hydrate is contraindicated in patients with marked hepatic or renal impairment, and should probably be avoided in patients with severe cardiac disease. It should not be administered to a patient receiving oral anticoagulant therapy, since it alters the metabolism of these agents.

Nursing Implications. The nursing implications are the same as those for flurazepam.

STOOL SOFTENERS AND LAXATIVES

Many conditions exist in the CCU which may lead to a patient's constipation, for example, a decrease in physical activity, change in diet or appetite which may result in a decreased intake of food, or a decreased fluid intake. The administration of narcotic analgesics may further contribute to this potential problem for the acutely ill cardiac patient. Since it is essential that the MI patient avoid straining to have a stool, the administration of stool softeners or a mild laxative may be required.

TABLE 33-4 STOOL SOFTENERS AND LAXATIVES

Agents	Dosage/Administration	Side and Toxic Effects
FECAL SOFTENERS		
Dioctyl sodium sulfosuccinate (Colace, Doxinate)	50–200 mg Higher doses are recommended for initial therapy. Mix liquid in ½ glass of milk or juice.	Bitter taste, sore throat, nausea (associated with use of syrup and liquid)
Casanthranol and dioctyl sodium sulfosuccinate (Peri-Colace)	1–2 capsules 1–2 tbsp. syrup May be administered b.i.d. in severe cases	Nausea, abdominal cramping, diarrhea, rash
Dioctyl calcium sulfosuccinate N.F. (Surfak)	240 mg daily Take daily for several days until bowel movements are normal	None except the unusual occurrence of mild, transitory, cramping pains
Dioctyl sodium sulfosuccinate, sodium carboxymethylcellulose (Dialose)	1 capsule t.i.d. Increase daily fluid by drinking a large glass of water with each dose.	None
Casanthranol dioctyl sodium sulfosuccinate sodium carboxymethylcellulose (Dialose Plus)	1 capsule b.i.d. Increase daily fluid intake by drinking a large glass of water with each dose.	Abdominal cramping
EMOLLIENT LAXATIVES		
Mineral oil	15–45 ml, usually h.s. Best given between meals or at h.s. Should not be given with or immediately after meals. May be given with fruit juice	Occasionally pruritus ani, due to leakage of oil past anal sphincter. May produce a lipid pneumonitis if aspirated into the lungs.
BULK-FORMING LAXATIVES		
Methylcellulose, U.S.P.	500 mg tablets or 200 mg/ml syrup. Dose of 1–1.5 g 2–4 times daily. Each dose should be accompanied by 1–2 glasses of water. Tablets should *not* be chewed.	No systemic effects. Flatulence may occur. Intestinal obstruction has been reported. Impaction may result when there are gross intestinal changes. Esophageal obstruction has occurred when agents have been swallowed dry or the tablets are chewed.
Carboxymethylcellulose, U.S.P.	225 and 500 mg tablets, 4–6 g daily with 1–2 glasses of water	Same as methylcellulose
Psyllium hydrophyllic mucilloid (Metamucil)	4–10 grams q.d. to t.i.d., stirred in a glassful of water	Same as methylcellulose
SALINE CATHARTICS		
Magnesium hydroxide (milk of magnesia, U.S.P.)	15–30 ml	May cause gaseous distention and abdominal cramping
Magnesium citrate solution, N.F.	200 ml	May cause gaseous distention and abdominal cramping

Stool Softeners

The use of fecal moistening agents has become accepted as routine therapy in CCUs and has resulted in a decrease in the use of cathartics. Actions, indications, contraindications, and nursing implications of stool softeners and laxatives are discussed in text. Table 33-4 summarizes dosage, administration, side-effects, and toxic-effects.

Action. Dioctyl sodium sulfosuccinate (DSS), probably the most widely used preparation, softens stool by lowering the surface tension so that the fecal material may be penetrated by water and fatty substance. The use of this agent results in soft stool within one to two days after its administration. Several compounds with different actions are available.[11] Dioctyl sodium sulfosuccinate is combined with casantranol to form the agent known as Peri-Colace which provides mild peristaltic stimulation, in addition to softening the stool. It produces a soft formed stool within 8 to 12 hours. Dioctyl calcium sulfosuccinate (Surfak) is claimed to provide superior surfactant activity.[4] This agent provides homogenization and formation of soft, easily evacuated stool without a disturbance of body physiology or the discomfort of bowel distention. Because of this safety, it may be effectively used in patients with heart conditions. Dioctyl sulfosuccinate and sodium carboxymethylcellulose combine to form Dialose, a fecal-moistening and bulk producing agent. Dialose Plus has an added ingredient, casanthranol, which stimulates peristalsis.

Indications and Contraindications. The clinical usefulness of these agents is mainly in situations when straining at stool should be avoided. They are particularly useful in bedridden patients. Agents which stimulate peristalsis should not be used in the presence of abdominal pain, nausea, or vomiting.[34] Mixtures of surface-active agents with mineral oil are contraindicated because the surface-active agent may enhance absorption of the oil.

Nursing Implications. Since frequent and prolonged use of the agents which stimulate peristalsis may result in dependence on laxatives, it is beneficial to return to the use of other measures to promote stool regularity as soon as possible.

Laxatives

Action. Laxatives produce evacuation of the bowel by different mechanisms. Mineral oil is an emollient which softens the fecal contents by retarding the reabsorption of water. The bulk-forming laxatives (methyl cellulose, U.S.P., carboxymethylcellulose sodium, U.S.P., and psyllium hydrophyllic mucilloid) swell in water to form a substance which results in keeping the fecal material soft and hydrated. The resultant increased bulk promotes peristalsis. This is one of the most natural mechanisms for catharsis and thus one of the least harmful. The chronic administration of psyllium hydrophyllic mucilloid (Metamucil) may cause a modest reduction in serum cholesterol by interfering with absorption of bile acids. The saline cathartics, (magnesium hydroxide, magnesium citrate) utilize osmotic forces to retain water in the intestinal lumen, and indirectly increase peristalsis. A semifluid or watery evacuation results within 3 to 6 hours after administering this agent.

Indications and Contraindications. Mineral oil is useful in clinical situations when straining at stool should be avoided, and thus a soft stool is desired. It may also be useful for patients who have a chronic type of constipation because of prolonged inactivity. The bulk-forming laxatives may be useful in the same clinical situations. They may also be useful when a low-residue diet is necessary. The saline cathartics are indicated when defecation needs to be promoted, either because of constipation or in preparation for an examination of the lower gastrointestinal tract. Agents which stimulate peristalsis should not be administered in the presence of abdominal pain, nausea, or vomiting.

Nursing Implications. The regular use of laxatives should be discouraged, and information should be provided for the patient on natural means to maintain regular bowel habits. As assessment should be made of the patient's dietary practices and his past bowel habits. The nurse may then direct her teaching to the individual's specific problem and how he may decrease his dependency on laxatives. For the elderly patient who may not be willing to change his habits and who may not be able to eat foods high in roughage, the nurse can recommend that he have his physician prescribe a stool softener rather than taking harsh over-the-counter laxatives.

REFERENCES

1. AMA Department of Drugs, In cooperation with the American Society for Clinical Pharmacology and Therapeutics: AMA Drug Evaluations, 4th ed. New York, John Wiley & Sons, 1980
2. Akil H, Mayer DJ, Liebeskind JC: Antagonism of stimulation-produced analgesia by naloxone, a narcotic antagonist. Science 191:961–962, 1976
3. Alderman EL, Barry WH, Graham AF et al: Hemodynamic effects of morphine and pentazocine differ in cardiac patients. N Engl J Med 287:623–627, 1972
4. Beecher HK: The Measurement of Subjective Responses: Quantitative Effects of Drugs. New York, Oxford University Press, 1959
5. Bergersen BS: Pharmacology in Nursing. St. Louis, CV Mosby, 1979
6. Byck R: Drugs and the treatment of psychiatric disorders, In Goodman LS, Gilman A (eds): The Pharmacological Basis of Therapeutics, 5th ed, pp 152–200. New York, Macmillan, 1975
7. Coglman MM: Effects of oxygen on ischemic myocardium. Heart Lung 7:635–639, 1978
8. Dement WC, Guilleminault C, Kramer M et al: Round table discussion: Sleep and cardiovascular disease. Behav Med 5:24–31, 1978
9. Egan DF: Gas therapy. In Fundamentals of Respiratory Therapy, pp 269–321. St. Louis, CV Mosby, 1977
10. Fillmore SJ, Guymaraes AC, Scheidt SS et al: Blood gas changes and pulmonary hemodynamics following acute myocardial infarction. Circulation 45:583, 1972
11. Fingl E: Laxatives and cathartics. In Goodman LS, Gilman A (eds): The Pharmacological Basis of Therapeutics, 5th ed, pp 245–283. New York, Macmillan, 1975
12. Fowler AW: Diazepam for distressing procedures. Br Med J 2:1073, 1979
13. Frank L, Massaro D: The lung and oxygen toxicity. Arch Intern Med 139:347–350, 1979
14. Gibson RL, Comer PB, Beckham RW et al: Actual tracheal oxygen concentrations with commonly used oxygen equipment. Anesthesiology 44:71–73, 1975
15. Gunnar RM, Leob HS, Scanlon PJ et al: Management of acute myocardial infarction and accelerating angina. Prog Cardiovasc Dis 42:1–30, 1979
16. Harby SC: Hypnotics and sedatives. In Goodman LS, Gilman A (eds) The Pharmacological Basis of Therapeutics, 5th ed, pp 124–136. New York, Macmillan, 1975
17. Henney RP, Vasko JS, Brawley RK et al: The effects of morphine on the resistance and capacitance vessels of the peripheral circulation. Am Heart J 72:242–250, 1966
18. Hiller JM, Pearson J, Simon EJ: Distribution of stereospecific binding of the potent narcotic analgesic etorphine in the human brain: Predominance in the limbic system. Research Commun Chem Pathol Pharmacol 6:1052–1062, 1973
19. Hsu HS, Hickey RF, Forbes AR: Morphine decreases peripheral vascular resistance and increases capacitance in man. Anesthesiology 50:98–102, 1979
20. Hughes J: Isolation of an endogenous compound from the brain with properties similar to morphine. Brain Res 88:295–308, 1975
21. Iversen LL: GABA and benzodiazepine receptors. Nature 275:477, 1978
22. Jaffe JH, Martin WR: Opiod analgesics and antagonists. In Goodman LS, Gilman A (eds) The Pharmacological Basis of Therapeutics, 6th ed pp 494–534. New York, Macmillan, 1980
23. Johnson M: Pain—How do you know its there and what do you do? Nursing '76, 6:48–50, 1976
24. Kales A, Kalu JD: Sleep disorders—Recent findings in the diagnosis and treatment of disturbed sleep. N Engl J Med 290:487–499, 1974
25. Kerr FWL, Pozuelo J: Suppression of physical dependence and induction of hypersensitivity to morphine by stereotaxic hypothalamic lesions in addicted rats. Proc Mayo Clin 46:653–655, 1971
26. Lasagna L: The clinical evaluation of morphine and its substitutes as analgesics. Pharmacol Rev 16:47–83, 1964
27. Liebeskind JC, Mayer DJ, Akil H: Central mechanisms of pain inhibition studies of analgesia from focal brain stimulation. Adv Neurol 4:261–268, 1974
28. Mayer DJ, Liebeskind JC: Pain reduction by focal electrical stimulation of the brain: An anatomical and behavioural analysis. Brain Res 68:73–93, 1974
29. Melsom M, Andreassen P, Melson H et al: Diazepam in acute myocardial infarction—Clinical effects and effects on catecholamines, free fatty acids, and cortisol. Br Heart J 38:804–810, 1976
30. MacKickan J, Duffner PK, Cohen ME: Absorption of diazepam to plastic tubing. New Engl J Med 30:332–333, 1979
31. McCaffery M, Hart LL: Undertreatment of acute pain and narcotics. Am J Nurs 76:1586–1591, 1976
32. Pert CB, Snyder SH: Opiate receptor: Demonstration in nervous tissue. Science 179:1011–1014, 1973
33. Pert CB, Aposkian D, Snyder SH: Phylogenetic distribution of opiate receptor binding. Brain Res 75:356–361, 1974
34. Physicians Desk Reference. Oradell NJ, Medical Economics Company, 1980
35. Samuel IO, Dunder JW: Circulatory effects of morphine. Br J Anesth 47:1025–1026, 1975

36. Simon EJ, Hiller JM, Edelman I: Stereospecific binding of the potent narcotic analgesia H-etorphine to rat brain hemogenate. Proc Nat Acad Sci USA 70:1947–1949, 1973

37. Simon EJ: Opiate receptor binding with ^{3}H-etorpine. Neurosci Res Prog Bull 13:43–50, 1975

38. Stoelting RK, Gibbs PS: Hemodynamic effects of morphine and morphine-nitrous oxide in valvular heart disease and coronary artery disease. Anesthesiology 38:45–52, 1973

39. Terenius L: Stereospecific interaction between narcotic analgesics and a symoptic plasma membrane fraction of rat cerebral cortex. Acta Pharmacol Toxicol 32:317–320, 1973

40. Thomas M, Malmcrona R, Fillmore S et al: Haemodynamic effects of morphine in patients with acute myocardial infarction. Br Heart J 27:863–875, 1965

41. Tierney DF. Oxygen toxicity. West J Med 130:227–229, 1979

42. Valencia A, Burgess JH: Arterial hypoxemia following acute myocardial infarction. Circulation 40:641–652, 1969

43. Vandam LD: Analgetic drugs—The potent analgetics. N Engl J Med 286:249–253, 1972

44. Ward JM, McGrath RL, Weil JV: Effects of morphine on the peripheral vascular response to sympathetic stimulation. Am J Cardiol 29:659–666, 1972

45. Zelis R, Mansour EJ, Capone RJ et al: The cardiovascular effects of morphine: The peripheral capacitance and resistance vessels in human subjects. J Clin Invest 54:1247–1258, 1974

46. Ziment I: Respiratory gases. In Respiratory Pharmacology and Therapeutics, pp 442–478. Philadelphia, WB Saunders, 1978

ADDITIONAL READING

Bellville JW, Forrest WH Jr, Miller E et al: Influence of age on pain relief from analgesics. JAMA 217:1835–1841, 1971

Guillemin R: Beta-lipotropin and endorphins: Implications of current knowledge. Hosp Prac 13:53–60, 1978

Hackett TP, Cassem NH, Wishnil H: Detection and treatment of anxiety in the coronary care unit. Am Heart J 78:727, 1969

Sellers, EM: Clinical pharmacology and therapeutics of benzodiazepines. Can Med Assoc J 118:1533–1538, 1978

Simon EJ, Miller JM: The opiate receptors. Ann Rev Pharmacol Toxicol 18:371–394, 1978

Warnica JW, White AVM, Burgess JH: Cardiorespiratory function and extravascular lung water following acute myocardial infarction. Am Heart J 79:469–476, 1979

Woy EL, Glasgow CE: The endorphins: Possible physiologic roles and therapeutic applications. Clin Ther 1:371–386, 1978

34

Antiarrhythmic and Cardiotonic Drugs

ELEANOR F. BOND, R.N., M.A.

and

SANDRA L. UNDERHILL, R.N., M.N.

ANTIARRHYTHMIC DRUGS

Arrhythmias are cardiac firing patterns other than normal sinus rhythm.[132] They are the result of abnormalities in impulse generation, conduction, or both, and may be associated with such problems as myocardial ischemia, acid–base or electrolyte disturbances, hypoxemia, hypothermia, and altered autonomic or thyroid outflow. To some extent, errors of rhythm are observed in apparently normal subjects. In the situation in which arrhythmia causes the patient to be symptomatic or constitutes a danger to the person experiencing it, the abnormal rhythm should be eliminated. Many arrhythmias, for example frequent or multifocal premature ventricular contractions (PVCs), are considered more dangerous in the patient with myocardial ischemia and infarction than in asymptomatic people in the general population; for this reason, these arrhythmias, when they occur in patients with acute myocardial infarction (MI), are treated very aggressively. Whenever possible, elimination of the abnormal rhythm should involve correction of the original cause of the arrhythmia (for example, correction of an abnormal serum K+ concentration).

Current theories of arrhythmogenesis are expressed in terms of errors of impulse generation (automaticity) or conduction, or both. Automaticity and a conduction abnormality known as reentrant excitation have been presented in detail in Chapter 11. Chapters 3 and 26 provide background material concerning the electrophysiology of cardiac cells and the genesis of arrhythmias.

Many therapies are designed to suppress abnormal or increased normal automaticity. Drugs can alter automaticity by changing the maximum diastolic potential, slope of phase-4 depolarization, or threshold (Fig. 34-1).

Reentrant excitation occurs when "a cardiac impulse enters a circuit and returns to or toward its area of origin" (Fig. 26-2).[132] Both normally initiated and ectopic impulses can also travel in reentrant circuits. Drugs can abolish reentrant circuits by changing refractoriness or by increasing or further decreasing the impeded conduction. Drugs which reduce membrane responsiveness slow conduction. Similarly, drugs which reduce the potential difference across the cardiac membranes also slow conduction, while drugs which make the membrane potential more negative speed conduction velocity. Each of these mechanisms favors the abolition of reentrant arrhythmias. Perhaps the most important way in which reentrant arrhythmias can be suppressed is by increasing the refractory period during which tissue is unresponsive to a reentering impulse (see Fig. 34-2).

Actions, elimination, indications, contraindications, and nursing implications specific to each antiarrhythmic agent discussed are described in text. Table 34-1 presents dosage, administration, peak plasma concentration time, therapeutic and toxic plasma levels, drug interactions, and side and toxic effects for each antiarrhythmic drug. The use of propranolol (Inderal) as an antiarrhythmic agent is discussed in Chapter 35. (Refer to Fig. 35-1 for an illustration for its effects on the action potential.)

General Nursing Implications of Antiarrhythmic Therapy

Extreme caution should be exercised when administering any antiarrhythmic agent in the face of atrioventricular (AV) block with recent MI or digitalis toxicity. The antiarrhythmic drug may suppress lower pacemaker foci which are necessary if the AV block becomes more advanced, whether or

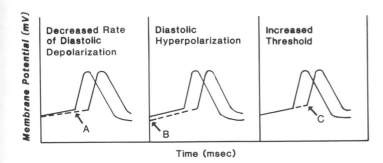

Fig. 34-1. Three mechanisms which decrease the firing rate of pacemaker cells. (The *dashed line* illustrates the slowed firing.) The opposite changes increase the rate of pacemaker discharge. (**A**) Slope of phase 4 depolarization is slowed. (**B**) Maximum diastolic potential is more negative. (**C**) Threshold potential is less negative. (From Katz AM: Physiology of the Heart, p. 253. New York, Raven Press, 1977)

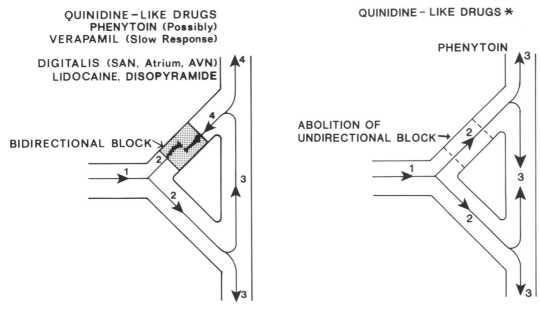

Fig. 34-2. Possible mechanisms for correction of reentrant arrhythmias. *Numbers* refer to the sequence of impulse arrival; *jagged lines* refer to slowed conduction. (**A**) Elimination of reentrant disturbance by further decrease in conduction through the diseased tissue. Drugs that may have this mechanism of action are listed. (**B**) Elimination of the reentrant disturbance by improving conduction through the diseased tissue. Drugs that may have this mechanism of action are listed. (*Quinidine-like drugs have this action only under special conditions—see text) (Adapted from Hsieh Y-Y, Arnsdorf MF, Goldberg LI: The Heart, 4th ed., p. 1947. New York, McGraw-Hill, 1978)

not the worsening of the AV block is related to the drug administered.

Patients and their families need to have an understanding of the antiarrhythmic drug(s) and the importance of adhering to the therapy as prescribed by the physician. A dosage schedule should be implemented that will provide optimal antiarrhythmic protection for the patient without interfering with his lifestyle or disturbing his sleep anymore than necessary. A patient who states his unwillingness to take a drug every four hours around the clock should discuss the possibility with his physician of switching to a long-acting (and usually more expensive) preparation. (Long-acting preparations are not available for all antiarrhythmic drugs.) Patients who are able to detect the symptoms of arrhythmia (*e.g.,* palpitations, dizziness, lightheadedness, fatigue) should be advised to notify the nurse or physician when arrhythmias increase.

Evaluation of Antiarrhythmic Therapy. In addition to noting the patient's subjective opinion, the nurse in a monitored cardiac care unit (CCU) or telemetry unit should record apical–radial heart rates (HR), a blood pressure (BP) (Chap. 14 describes changes in BP with arrhythmias) and an electrocardiographic rhythm strip (with intervals counted) every four hours, or more frequently if symptoms or changes in rhythm occur. The nurse working in a general medical–surgical unit or in the outpatient setting should also record apical–radial HRs and a BP, either before each dose of medication or with each clinic visit. If the HR or rhythm has changed and if arrhythmia is suspected, an electrocardiographic rhythm strip should be obtained and a full 12-lead electrocardiogram (ECG) should be done. Exercise tolerance testing or 24-hour ECG recordings during the patient's normal activities may help document the

(Text continues on p. 448.)

TABLE 34-1 ANTIARRHYTHMIC AGENTS

Agent	Dosage/Administration	Peak Plasma Concentration Time	Therapeutic Plasma Level	Toxic Plasma Level
Lidocaine Hydrochloride, U.S.P.	IV loading dose: 1 mg/kg body weight IV at rate of 25–50 mg/minute; may repeat in 3–5 minutes; not to exceed 300 mg in 1-hour period. IV maintenance dose: 20–50 μg/kg body weight per minute (usually 1–4 mg/minute); to mix infusion, add 1–2 g lidocaine to 500–1000 ml D_5W; solution of 2 g lidocaine to 500 ml D_5W provides 4 mg lidocaine/1 ml; using mini-drip IV chamber: 15 gtts = 1 mg 30 gtts = 2 mg 45 gtts = 3 mg 60 gtts = 4 mg Do not change drip rate more than 1 mg/minute every shift because of prolonged t½; repeat bolus with ½ initial dose if necessary. IM dose: 250 mg q. 2h. until IV infusion can be initiated.	Rapid	1.6–5.0 μg/ml	>5–10μg/ml
Quinidine Sulfate, U.S.P. Long-acting (Quinidine Extentabs)	200–300 mg PO q. 6–8h. 600 mg PO q. 8–12 hours	60–120 minutes	2.3–5.0 μg/ml when measured by double extraction method[58]	>5.0 μg/ml
Quinidine Gluconate (Quinaglute Duratabs)	1–2 tablets (324 mg each) PO q. 8–12 h.	240 minutes	As above	As above
Quinidine Gluconate injection, U.S.P.	IM dose: 600 mg initially followed by 400 mg as often as q. 2h. IV dose: usually 330 mg or less, but occasionally 500–750 mg; dilute 10 ml (80 mg) to 50 ml with D_5W; administer at rate not exceeding 1 ml/minute	Within minutes	As above	As above
Quinidine Polygalucturonate (Cardioquin)	275 mg tablets PO loading dose: 1–3 tablets to terminate arrhythmia, repeated in 3–4 hours; if NSR not restored after 3 or 4 equal doses, increase dose by ½–1 tablet administered 3–4 times before any further increase PO maintenance dose: 1 tablet b.i.d.-t.i.d.: usually 1 tablet q. 12h.	—	As above	As above
Procainamide Hydrochloride (Pronestyl)	PO dose: 100–600 mg q.d. in 4, 6, or 8 divided doses; never allow more than 6 hours to lapse between doses. IV loading dose: 100 mg q. 5 minutes until arrhythmia controlled or toxic signs appear, or 1 g has been given;[38] or 275 μg/kg body weight/minute for 25 minutes IV maintenance dose: 20–80 μg per kg body weight per minute[38,139]	60–120 minutes Within minutes	4–8 μg/ml[139] NAPA: 2–22 μg/ml [2]	>8 μg/ml >22 μg/ml As above
Disopyramide Phosphate (Norpace)	Loading dose: 200–300 mg PO Maintenance dose: 100–200 mg PO q. 6h.	½–3 hours	2–4 μg/ml	Not established

TABLE 34-1 ANTIARRHYTHMIC AGENTS

Drug Interactions	Side and Toxic Effects
Drugs which alter hepatic perfusion change the rate of elimination of lidocaine from the body. Propranolol (Inderol) may decrease elimination of lidocaine by this mechanism and thus require smaller maintenance doses to achieve the same plasma levels. Glucagon, U.S.P., and isoproterenol (Isuprel) may increase hepatic blood flow and elimination of lidocaine; larger maintenance doses may be required.	CNS: lightheadedness; drowsiness; dizziness; apprehension, agitation, disorientation, euphoria; tinnitus; blurred or double vision; dysarthria; vomiting; sensation of heat or cold, or numbness; twitching; tremors; convulsions; unconsciousness; respiratory depression and arrest. Cardiovascular: hypotension, cardiovascular collapse; bradycardia, which may lead to cardiac arrest.
Concurrent oral anticoagulants cause increased bleeding[49]; concurrent diphenylhydantoin or phenobarbital increases elimination of quinidine, causing a dose which has been effective to become inadequate[25]; quinidine and propranolol have additive electrophysiological effects (depressing automaticity, upstroke velocity and membrane responsiveness)[127]; effects are exaggerated when serum K^+ level is high and depressed when serum K^+ level is low. Quinidine diminishes the renal excretion of digoxin: maintenance doses of digoxin should be reduced by 30–50% when quinidine is added to a therapeutic regimen.[28,45]	Cardiovascular: with excessive doses, high-grade AV blocks, bundle branch blocks, asystole, premature depolarizations, fibrillation, tachycardia, excessive QT prolongation; >35% increase in QRS duration is ominous and is soon followed by dangerous arrhythmias and conduction disturbances[50]; negative inotropic effects can lead to cardiovascular collapse; hypotension after IV dosage; idiosyncratic episodes of ventricular tachycardia and fibrillation may occur, especially with hypokalemia. Gastrointestinal: nausea, vomiting, abdominal pain, diarrhea Hematologic: acute hemolytic anemia, hypoprothrombinemia, thrombocytopenia purpura, agranulocytosis CNS: headache, fever, vertigo, apprehension, excitement, confusion, delirium, syncope, disturbed hearing, disturbed vision, optic neuritis Dermatologic: cutaneous flushing with intense pruritus Hypersensitivity: angioedema, acute asthmatic episode, vascular collapse, respiratory arrest Symptoms of toxicity (cinchonism): nausea, vomiting, anorexia, abdominal pain, diarrhea, and neurologic problems such as tinnitus, hearing loss, visual disturbances (blurring diplopia, photophobia, altered color vision), severe headache, confusion, delirium, psychosis
Procainamide and propranolol have additive electrophysiological effects (depressing automaticity, upstroke velocity, and membrane responsiveness), resulting in the appearance of conduction blocks at lower plasma levels.[127] The effects of procainamide when serum K^+ is elevated or lowered are the same as with quinidine.	Cardiovascular: Hypotension following PO administration is rare, following IV administration, transient, but severe hypotension may occur, particularly in conscious patients. Serious disturbances of cardiac rhythm (ventricular asystole or ventricular fibrillation) may occur but are more common with IV administration. Gastrointestinal: nausea, vomiting, diarrhea, bitter taste, chills, fever, abdominal pain, acute hepatomegaly, rise in SGOT. Hematologic: agranulocytosis. CNS: neurologic disturbances (depression, giddiness, convulsions, psychoses) have all been reported. Immunologic: as many as 40% of the patients receiving PO procainamide develop a syndrome resembling systemic lupus erythematosus (SLE),[49] although this may also occur following parenteral therapy. Hypersensitivity: angioneurotic edema and maculopapular rash have also occurred.
Effects of K^+ are same as those of quinidine. Potentiates warfarin.[46] Because this drug is relatively new, much remains to be learned about its drug interactions; caution is advised.	Anticholinergic: dry mouth, eyes and throat, urinary hesitancy and retention, constipation, blurred vision Genitourinary: urinary frequency and urgency Gastrointestinal: nausea, pain, bloating, gas, anorexia, diarrhea, vomiting General: dizziness, fatigue, muscle weakness, headache, malaise Cardiovascular: edema, weight gain, cardiac conduction disturbances, shortness of breath, syncope, chest pain, hypotension, CHF;[97] sudden cardiac death has been reported.[93] CNS: nervousness. Rare (<1%): impotence, depression, insomnia, dysuria, acute psychosis

TABLE 34-1 ANTIARRHYTHMIC AGENTS (Cont.)

Agent	Dosage/Administration	Peak Plasma Concentration Time	Therapeutic Plasma Level	Toxic Plasma Level
Phenytoin Sodium (Dilantin)	IV: use only if solution clear; faint yellow coloration may develop and does not effect potency of solution IV loading dose: 750–1000 mg in small increments (not exceeding 25–50 mg/minute); stop when arrhythmia is abolished or when toxicity (nystagmus) occurs; plasma levels remain in therapeutic range for about 24 hours IV maintenance dose: 300 to 400 mg q.d. PO loading dose: 300 mg; then 200 mg q. 2–3h. until toxic symptoms (nystagmus) occur, or until 900–1100 mg given PO maintenance dose: 300–400 mg PO q.d. in single or divided doses	Immediate	10–20μg/ml	>30 μg/ml (toxic symptoms appear at lower plasma levels in uremia; hypoalbuminemia, some forms of liver disease and hyperkalemia)[136,139]
Bretylium Tosylate (Bretylol, Bretylan)	IV dose in ventricular fibrillation: administer undiluted solution (500 mg/10 ml at dosage of 5 mg/kg by rapid injection; if ventricular fibrillation persists, increase dose to 10 mg/kg and repeat at 15–30 minute intervals until a total dose of not more than 30 mg/kg has been given. IV dose for other ventricular arrhythmias: dilute the solution (500 mg/10 ml) to a minimum of 50 ml with dextrose injection or sodium chloride injection; administer diluted solution at dosage of 5–10 mg/kg by IV infusion over a period longer than 8 minutes; repeat dose in 1–2 hours if arrhythmia persists IV maintenance dose: intermittent bolus—infuse diluted solution at dosage of 5–10 mg/kg over a period longer than 8 minutes q. 6h. constant infusion—infuse diluted solution at a dosage of 1–2 mg/minute. IM dose: 5–10 mg/kg, repeat in 1–2 hours if arrhythmia persists; thereafter, maintain with same dose q. 6–8h. According to package insert, reduce and discontinue bretylium in 3–5 days under ECG monitoring; however, bretylium has been reported to be well tolerated for more than 3 days in 70% of patients and for more than 5 days in 50% of patients[8]	Within minutes 20–60 minutes	Plasma levels have not been correlated with intensity of antiarrhythmic effects, and therefore cannot be used as a guide for dosage determination[63]	—
Verapamil (Isoptin, Cordilox) (not currently approved by FDA for use in U.S.)	IV bolus: for reversal of supraventricular tachycardia, atrial fibrillation or atrial flutter, give 10 mg IV push at 1 mg/minute; if no response in 30 minutes repeat 10 mg IV push (this has been given as fast as over 15 seconds without complications).[48,69,116] IV maintenance: infuse at rate of 0.005 mg/kg/min.[119] PO: for angina, administer 120 mg t.i.d.[80,112]	3–12 minutes	Unknown	Unknown
Atropine Sulfate, U.S.P.	IV: 0.5 mg direct IV push, repeated at 5-minute intervals until desired HR (usually about 60 beats per minute) achieved; total dose should generally not exceed 2.0 mg.[131]	1–5 minutes (effective for 2–6 hours)	—	—

TABLE 34-1 ANTIARRHYTHMIC AGENTS (Cont.)

Drug Interactions	Side and Toxic Effects
Drugs that inhibit metabolism of phenytoin (lengthen t ½): isoniazid, chloramphenicol, bishydroxycoumarin (Dicumarol), phenothiazines, diazepam (Valium), methylphenidate (Ritalin), disulfiram (Antabuse), phenylbutazone (Butazolidin), chlordiazepoxide (Librium, Libritabs).[64,139] Drugs that increase rate of phenytoin elimination (shorten t ½): phenobarbitol, carbamazepine (Tegretol).[139] Accelerates metabolism of coumarin.[65] The transient impairment of hepatic function following halothane anesthesia is associated with diminished elimination.[56]	Cardiovascular (with IV administration): cardiovascular collapse, hypotension with rapid administration; atrial and ventricular conduction depression; ventricular fibrillation CNS (most commonly): nystagmus, ataxia, slurred speech, drowsiness, mental confusion, dizziness, blurred vision, vertigo, insomnia, transient nervousness, motor twitchings, circumoral tingling, headache (these may disappear with continuing therapy or reduced dosage); convulsions; respiratory arrest Gastrointestinal: nausea, vomiting, constipation Integumentary (sometimes accompanied by fever): scarlatiniform or measleslike rash (common); bullous, exfoliative, or purpuric dermatitis, SLE, Stevens–Johnson syndrome (can be fatal.) Hemopoietic: thrombocytopenia, leukopenia, granulocytopenia, agranulocytosis, and pancytopenia; megaloblastic anemia and macrocytosis usually respond to folic acid therapy; lymph adenopathy Other: gingival hyperplasia, polyarthropathy, hirsutism, hyperglycemia; toxic hepatitis, liver damage, and periarteritis nodosa may be fatal; teratogenesis
These drugs block, in varying degrees, the action of bretylium (in animals): quinidine, guanethidine, and large doses of phenytoin.[4] Previous administration of antiarrhythmic agents may decrease the effectiveness of bretylium, but this is not well documented.	Cardiovascular: hypotension and postural hypotension (most frequent); occasionally bradycardia, increased frequency of PVCs, transitory hypertension, initial increase in arrhythmias, precipitation of angina, sensation of substernal pressure Other: nausea and vomiting (3%); vertigo, dizziness, lightheadedness, syncope, rarely, renal dysfunction, diarrhea, abdominal pain, hiccups, erythematous macular rash, flushing, hyperthermia, confusion, paranoid psychosis, emotional lability, lethargy, generalized tenderness, anxiety, shortness of breath, diaphoresis, nasal stuffiness, mild conjunctivitis
Concurrent administration with β-blocking agents results in CHF, sinus arrest, or both. β-blocking drugs must be discontinued 48 hours prior to verapamil administration.	Cardiovascular: mild, transient hypotension after IV administration;[48,115,116] severe hypotension, bradycardia and asystole if given in the presence of pre-existing hypotension or with β-blocking agents.[7,126] CNS (minimal): dizziness, headache, lassitude, drowsiness, fatigue after PO administration.[90,119] GI (infrequent): nausea, diarrhea, constipation, flatulence.[90] Liver: transient increase in SGOT, SGPT after PO administration without evidence of hepatotoxicity.
Phenothiazines have additive effects; concurrent use may result in toxic symptoms of atropine at lower doses.[53]	Dryness of mouth, nose and throat; thirst; urinary retention; varying degrees of mydriasis; palpitations; blurring of near vision; photophobia; hot, flushed, dry skin; disturbance of speech; difficulty swallowing; headache; restlessness with asthenia; ataxia; excitement; disorientation; hallucinations; delirium; coma; scarlatinoform rash; fever

TABLE 34-1   ANTIARRHYTHMIC AGENTS (Cont.)

Agent	Dosage/Administration	Peak Plasma Concentration Time	Therapeutic Plasma Level	Toxic Plasma Level
Edrophonium Chloride (Tensilon)	IV: give 2 mg test doses; increase 2 mg/minute until 10 mg has been infused or a response seen.[36]	30—60 seconds (effective for 10 minutes)	—	—

presence or absence of arrhythmias. In addition, His bundle electrocardiography, may help evaluate the effectiveness of antiarrhythmic therapy (Chap. 17).

Lidocaine Hydrochloride, U.S.P.

Action. Lidocaine appears to be effective in abolishing both automatic and reentrant arrhythmias. In general, it appears to have a depressant effect on myocardial cells: action potential amplitude, velocity of phase 0 (upstroke) depolarization, V_{max}* and membrane responsiveness are all reduced (Fig. 34-3). Some clinical studies suggest that lidocaine at low therapeutic levels increases the velocity of phase 0; this property is used to differentiate lidocaine from quinidine-like drugs. However, some experimental results are not in agreement with this observation; a depressant effect appears to be more likely.[106] Thus, a likely mechanism by which lidocaine may oppose reentrant arrhythmias is the conversion of a unidirectional block into a bidirectional block.

Lidocaine shortens the action potential duration and refractoriness in some cardiac tissues. In the His–Purkinje system, it shortens these parameters most markedly at the gate region.** The net result is a more homogeneous response in this tissue. This may oppose reentrant arrhythmias even though the effective refractory period of the His–Purkinje system may be shortened.[106]

Lidocaine tends to suppress ventricular automatic arrhythmias. It may increase the outward membrane K+ current (i_{k_2}), and by so doing, slow spontaneous rates of membrane depolarization in some automatic cells, such as in the ventricular Purkinje fibers. It appears that the atrial and sinoatrial (SA) nodal fibers are less sensitive to this effect than ventricular Purkinje fibers; it is well known that atrial arrhythmias are more refractory to lidocaine treatment. This is also consistent with the observaton that sinus rate does not normally change with lidocaine therapy.

Another mechanism for initiation of abnormal automatic impulses is the so-called slow wave or slow-frequency oscillation in membrane voltage. There is no evidence that lidocaine can improve arrhythmias caused by this mecha-

nism. This may explain the resistance of some ventricular arrhythmias to lidocaine.

Lidocaine has no effect on, or may shorten the AV nodal refractory period.[55] However, in some patients with pre-excitation, the effective refractory period of the anomalous pathway is prolonged.[103]

Elimination. Lidocaine is rapidly degraded in the liver and the degradation products are excreted in the urine. The half-

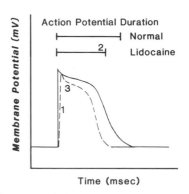

Fig. 34-3. Summary of electrophysiologic actions of lidocaine. (*Dashed line* indicates lidocaine effect.) **(1)** Slow velocity of phase 0 (upstroke) depolarization. **(2)** Decreased action potential duration. **(3)** Decreased action potential amplitude.

Fig. 34-4. Estimated blood levels of lidocaine in a man of average weight after receiving a 100-mg IV bolus of the drug. (White RD: Advanced Cardiac Life Support, pp VII—13. Dallas, American Heart Association, 1975. By permission from the American Heart Association, Inc.)

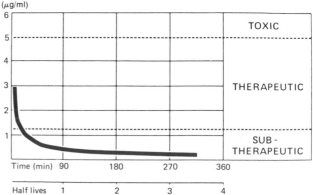

---

* V_{max} = maximum velocity of depolarization during phase 0 (upstroke) of the cardiac action potential

** Gate region: normally, ventricular Purkinje fibers which are located progressively more distally have gradually increasing action potential durations and refractory periods until a peak value is reached. This region of longest action potential duration and refractory period is sometimes referred to as the "gate" region. Beyond the gate, action potential duration and refractory periods progressively decrease.

TABLE 34-1   ANTIARRHYTHMIC AGENTS (Cont.)

Drug Interactions	Side and Toxic Effects
Additive effect if given with other anticholinesterase drugs. Contraindicated when digitalis toxicity is suspected.	Eye: increased lacrimation, pupillary constriction, spasm of accommodation, diplopia, conjunctival hyperemia CNS: convulsions, dysarthria, dysphonia, dysphagia Respiratory: increased tracheobronchial secretions, laryngospasm, bronchiolar constriction, paralysis of respiratory muscles, central respiratory paralysis Cardiac: arrhythmias (esp. bradycardia), fall in CO resulting in hypotension Gastrointestinal: increased salivary, gastric, and intestinal secretion; nausea; vomiting; increased peristalsis; diarrhea; abdominal cramps Skeletal muscle: weakness, fasciculations Miscellaneous: increased urinary frequency and incontinence, diaphoresis

life (t½) is variable, depending upon the manner and duration of administration: 30 minutes after an intravenous bolus (Fig. 34-4), 100 minutes when equilibrated with body tissues, 240 minutes after 48 hours of continuous infusion (Fig. 34-5).[76] The rate of elimination of lidocaine is decreased with liver disease or dysfunction (such as may occur in congestive heart failure), but not with renal disease (Fig. 34-6).[139]

Indications and Contraindications. Lidocaine is a local anesthetic that was first administered as a cardiac antiarrhythmic agent in 1950. It is indicated in the treatment of PVCs and ventricular tachyarrhythmias that are caused by heart disease or digitalis toxicity. It may have greater efficacy against unifocal than against multifocal PVCs or than against PVCs occurring close to the T wave (R-on-T phenomenon).[18] It has some antifibrillatory effect in patients with acute MI.[78] Prophylactic administration of lidocaine after acute MI may be useful in preventing primary ventricular fibrillation.

Lidocaine can be used in atrial or AV junctional premature depolarizations and paroxysmal supraventricular tachycardias, although it is less successful in the treatment of these conditions than of ventricular arrhythmias (40%–50% improvement in the former; 70%–90% improvement in the latter). It is almost totally ineffective (0%–15% improvement) as therapy against other supraventricular arrhythmias.[9] Li-

docaine may be useful in the management of the patient with anomalous AV conduction paths, such as are encountered in the Wolff–Parkinson–White (W–P–W) syndrome. The rapid arrhythmias in this syndrome are often initiated by premature atrial and ventricular impulses.

Lidocaine is contraindicated in patients with a known hypersensitivity to local anesthetics of the amide type, or with Stokes–Adams syndrome, or severe SA, AV, or intraventricular heart block.

Nursing Implications. Because lidocaine, as an antiarrhythmic agent, is administered in life-threatening situations, certain baseline information should be obtained from the patient on admission before the emergency occurs, and recorded on the chart or nursing care plan for later use. Ask the patient if he has an allergy to lidocaine. Most patients' experiences with lidocaine are limited to its use as a local anesthetic, for instance during dental work. The preparation of lidocaine used at that time probably contained the vasoconstrictor epinephrine (to prolong the anesthetic effect). If the patient replies that he is allergic to lidocaine, care must be taken to discover whether he has a true allergy (cutaneous lesions of delayed onset, urticaria, or edema) or

Fig. 34-5. Estimated blood levels of lidocaine in a man of average weight, after receiving a 100-mg IV bolus and a 2-mg/minute infusion of the drug. (White RD: Advanced Cardiac Life Support, pp VII–13. Dallas, American Heart Association, 1975. By permission from the American Heart Association, Inc.)

Fig. 34-6. Illustration of the difference in plasma-level response to infused lidocaine in a normal subject and in a patient of the same size who had heart failure. Within 2 hours, concentrations of lidocaine approached toxic levels in the patient with advanced heart failure, even though the infusion rate was near the minimum recommended dose. (White RD: Advanced Cardiac Life Support, pp VII–14. Dallas, American Heart Association. 1975. By permission from the American Heart Association, Inc.)

LIDOCAINE BLOOD LEVEL (μg/ml)

6				TOXIC
5				
4				THERAPEUTIC
3				
2				
1				SUB-THERAPEUTIC

Time (min)   90   180   270   360
Half lives   1   2   3   4

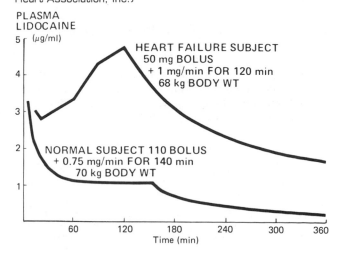

PLASMA LIDOCAINE (μg/ml)

HEART FAILURE SUBJECT
50 mg BOLUS
+ 1 mg/min FOR 120 min
68 kg BODY WT

NORMAL SUBJECT 110 BOLUS
+ 0.75 mg/min FOR 140 min
70 kg BODY WT

60   120   180   240   300   360
Time (min)

whether his symptoms were side effects of the epinephrine (anxiety, headache, fear, or palpitations); the latter are more common in hyperthyroid individuals. Because the dosage of lidocaine is weight-related, an initial admission weight should be obtained as soon as possible, and daily thereafter. Weights should be recorded (in kilograms) and kept in an easily accessible location. This eliminates guessing the patient's weight during an emergency.

Lidocaine can be administered IV or intramuscularly (IM); studies to find a lidocaine-like preparation for oral administration are currently under way.* Lidocaine is most commonly administered IV, and lidocaine hydrochloride injection, U.S.P., is the only preparation that should be given. It contains no preservatives or vasoconstrictive agents. Rapid achievement and maintenance of a therapeutic plasma level requires that a bolus injection be given and followed immediately by a continuous infusion. Dosage of lidocaine should be reduced in patients with liver disease and in those over 70 years of age. Up to 40% reduction of the maintenance dose is required in patients with congestive heart failure (CHF), depending on the degree of failure.

Intramuscular lidocaine is administered less frequently, usually to patients living in rural areas with long transport times to the hospital. As with any IM injection, serum enzymes can be elevated and, unless isoenzyme tests are performed, may make accurate diagnosis of MI difficult.

If an infusion pump is not available, use a minidrip IV set for IV lidocaine administration. Choose an appropriate solution concentration. For example, in patients with an MI who have compromised cardiac function, a concentrated solution (4 mg/ml) provides maximum protection from fluid overload. Obtain baseline BP, HR, and ECG intervals, and assess the patient's neurologic status. During the IV infusion, continuously monitor the ECG, and every 2 to 4 hours (more often if indicated) record duration of the PR interval and QRS segment on the rhythm strip, and record the BP and neurologic status on the nursing notes.

Lidocaine has a differential response in diseased and healthy tissue. Although normally it does not affect the firing of the SA node or atrial conduction there are occasional reports in the literature of sinus arrest following administration of the drug. It is possible that this response is related to underlying SA node disease or abnormality, and its use in such conditions may be associated with increased hazard.[17] Before administering lidocaine to patients in sinus bradycardia, it may be advisable first to increase the HR (with atropine, isoproterenol, or artificial pacing). This may prevent the occurrence of more frequent and serious ventricular arrhythmias, or may abolish the necessity for escape ventricular arrhythmias to improve cardiac output.

Similarly, there appears to be no change in AV nodal or His–Purkinje conduction times in normal tissue during lidocaine administration.[102] However, a number of literature reports document cases of third-degree AV block or cardiac arrest following administration to patients with diseased AV conduction systems.[37,44,55,77] If cardiac conductivity is excessively depressed* (prolongation of PR and QRS intervals), promptly discontinue the infusion and notify the physician. If arrhythmias are not abolished and become worse (after another bolus is injected and the drip rate is increased as prescribed under standing orders), notify the physician so that another antiarrhythmic regimen can be ordered. Because AV nodal refractory times may be decreased with lidocaine, use of the drug in atrial fibrillation or atrial flutter may occasionally be associated with increased ventricular response rate.[23,83] When lidocaine is used as a local anesthetic, for example during the insertion of permanent pacemakers, it is gradually absorbed into the systemic circulation and may contribute to therapeutic or toxic blood levels. Have emergency life support equipment and drugs readily available during administration of lidocaine.

Quinidine and Procainamide

Quinidine and procainamide are similar in actions, elimination, indications, and contraindications, and are presented together. The term "quinidinelike drug" is used to refer to both. The specific nursing implications for each drug are presented separately and are also described for quinidinelike drugs in more general terms.

Action. In general, the effects of quinidine and procainamide are depressant on cardiac cells of all types. These drugs depress membrane responsiveness by depressing the voltage-dependent Na^+ current, slowing the velocity of the upstroke phase 0. A related effect is to make the threshold for firing less negative; thus, a greater amount of depolarizing current is necessary to fire the cell. Together, these two effects slow conduction velocity in cardiac cells, and may abolish reentrant arrhythmias by changing an area of unidirectional block into bidirectional block (Chap. 26). An exception to this is in Purkinje fibers, where low doses of quinidinelike drugs can slow the rate of phase-4 (diastolic) depolarization and increase conduction velocity indirectly, since the membrane potential is more negative when the cell is fired.[118] This can counter reentrant arrhythmias by abolishing unidirectional blocks.

Quinidinelike drugs depress the rate of phase-4 depolarization in spontaneously depolarizing cells. This effect, in combination with the change in threshold to less negative values, suppresses enhanced automaticity.

A fourth effect of these drugs is to delay repolarization, thereby prolonging the action potential. This, in conjunction with decreased membrane responsiveness, prolongs the refractory period. Although the action potential is prolonged in all cardiac cells, the degree of prolongation in the His–Purkinje system varies with anatomic location. Fibers that normally have the shortest action potentials are affected to a much greater degree than are fibers at the gate region.[104] As a result, action potential duration becomes more uniform throughout the His–Purkinje network. This may oppose the establishment of reentrant circuits in this tissue.[135] The prolonged refractory period counters reentrant arrhythmias in all tissues.

Quinidinelike drugs also may attenuate the effects on

---

* Oral lidocaine is poorly absorbed from the gastrointestinal tract; the small amount which is absorbed passes immediately into the hepatic portal circulation and is largely degraded. The results of investigations of whether therapeutic plasma levels can be achieved with oral lidocaine are not consistent. Dizziness has been reported following oral lidocaine in normal humans, despite the fact that plasma levels remained below the minimum effective concentration. Dizziness is probably due to the very high level of metabolites from the rapid hepatic degradation. Tocainide and mexilitene are congeners of lidocaine and are less efficiently extracted by the liver, and thus are effective orally; they are not currently approved for clinical use.

* Lidocaine can depress cardiac cells sufficiently to prevent an artificial pacemaker from initiating myocardial depolarization.

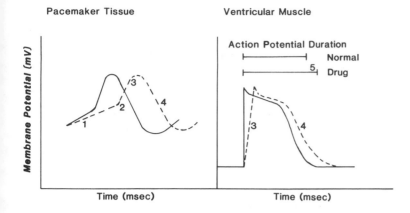

Fig. 34-7. Summary of electrophysiologic actions of quinidine-like drugs (*dashed line* indicates quinidine-like drug effect). **(1)** Slow velocity of phase 4 resting depolarization; **(2)** less negative threshold; **(3)** slow velocity of phase 0 (upstroke) depolarization; **(4)** delay repolarization; **(5)** prolonged action-potential duration.

the heart of catecholamines and acetylcholine, the parasympathetic vagal transmitter. Antivagal effects may account for the observed increase in HR with quinidine administration, despite the drug's direct depressant effect on the SA node.

Electrophysiologic effects of quinidine and procainamide are summarized in Figure 34-7. Chapter 17 describes electrocardiographic changes associated with the quinidinelike drugs. Refer to Figure 17-31 for illustrations of these changes.

Elimination. Quinidine is metabolized in the liver; 17% is excreted unchanged in the urine.[123] Normally, t½ is 6 to 7 hours. Liver disease can slow elimination of the drug; hence lower doses will achieve the same plasma level. Some metabolites may be active and accumulate with renal disease; dosage may require adjustment.[30]

Procainamide is also metabolized in the liver. Because 30% to 60% of the drug is excreted unchanged in the urine, both liver and renal dysfunction can change t ½ of elimination (normally 3 to 4 hours). Congestive heart failure (CHF) commonly prolongs t½. Alkalinization of the urine or decreased renal perfusion can impair elimination of the drug and its active metabolites.

Indications and Contraindications. Atrial fibrillation or flutter may be converted to normal sinus rhythm (NSR) either with electrical countershock or with the combined use of a digitalis derivative and quinidine or procainamide. Quinidinelike drugs are sometimes used prophylactically in patients likely to develop atrial fibrillation or atrial flutter, but are less useful in paroxysmal or nonparoxysmal atrial tachycardias.

Quinidinelike drugs are useful in the suppression of premature atrial, AV junctional, and ventricular contractions, and in the prevention of ventricular tachycardia or fibrillation. One study shows procainamide successful in treating 70% to 80% of the cases of AV junctional arrhythmias, and effective in suppressing 80% of the PVCs caused by a variety of factors.[11] Quinidinelike drugs may be used for suppression of PVCs caused by recent MI or digitalis toxicity, as long as conduction blocks are not present.

Quinidinelike drugs are also used in the management of the patient with the W–P–W syndrome. These drugs suppress premature impulses likely to precipitate tachyarrhythmias and also selectively increase the effective refractory period in the anomalous pathway, thus suppressing conduction.[130]

Contraindications to the use of quinidine include hypersensitivity or idiosyncracy to the drug, history of thrombocytopenia purpura associated with previous quinidine administration, and AV conduction disorders, complete AV block with AV nodal or idioventricular pacemaker, and ectopic impulses and rhythms due to escape mechanisms; all of these conduction disorders may result from digitalis toxicity.

Because it can cause or potentiate the arrhythmia, quinidine is absolutely contraindicated in *torsade de pointes*. The hallmarks of this arrhythmia are bursts of ventricular tachycardia, undulation of the QRS axis, and failure of conventional antiarrhythmic therapy.[70] Episodes usually occur in association with bradycardia and prolongation of the QT interval, and often with hypokalemia. Progression to ventricular fibrillation is common. When therapy with quinidine is associated with an idiosyncratic increase in ventricular tachycardia, *torsade de pointes* should be suspected and the drug discontinued immediately.

Contraindications to the use of procainamide are known hypersensitivity to the drug (cross-sensitivity to procaine and related drugs) and those same conduction abnormalities and rhythm disturbances for which quinidine is contraindicated. It has been suggested that procainamide should be contraindicated in patients with myasthenia gravis.

Nursing Implications of Quinidine Therapy. Quinidine is most commonly administered orally as quinidine sulfate. Slow-release oral preparations of quinidine sulfate (Quinidex Extentabs), quinidine gluconate (Quinaglute Dura-Tabs), and quinidine polygalacturonate (Cardioquin) are available. (Comparable dosage of the long-acting preparations can be calculated from the amount of quinidine base in the tablets.) Because they need to be taken only two or three times daily, the slow-release preparations may be particularly helpful for patients who have difficulty in adhering to the dose regimen. However, these preparations given two or three times daily may not control arrhythmias as well as the other preparations given at more frequent intervals. Quinidine gluconate and polygalacturonate are not so frequently associated with gastrointestinal symptoms as is quinidine sulfate.

Parenteral quinidine (quinidine gluconate injection, U.S.P.) is rarely given IM or IV. Intramuscular administration is painful and requires a dose larger than the oral dose to achieve the same plasma level.[49] Extreme caution is advised when administering quinidine intravenously. Because of vasodilation and, to a lesser extent, depressed cardiac contractility, IV quinidine can cause cardiovascular collapse or profound shock.

Quinidine tends to increase markedly the QT interval. Its use in suppression of PVCs that occur early in the cycle may be associated with an increased risk of occurrence of the R-on-T phenomenon.[96] Continuously monitor both the ECG and the systemic arterial BP during and immediately after parenteral administration.

An oral test dose of 100 mg to 200 mg of quinidine should be administered under professional surveillance to determine if the patient has an idiosyncrasy to it. Idiosyncratic reactions include nausea, diarrhea, hypotension, or arrhythmias, such as *torsade de pointes*. This needs to be done only the *first* time quinidine is ever administered.

Quinidine dosage should be determined by plasma quinidine levels. There is a wide range of individual variation (40% to 93%) in quinidine absorption.[42] Quinidine gluconate is more slowly and less completely absorbed than is the sulfate salt of the drug.

There is some evidence that the volume of distribution of quinidine is reduced with CHF.[22] This would mean that the same dose would result in higher drug levels in the plasma and active tissues, while less active and more poorly perfused areas would have a lower drug level.

Metabolic and respiratory disorders that raise the pH of plasma increase the binding of quinidine to albumin. Because only the unbound (free) portion of the drug is physiologically active, this reduces the effect of the drug. Generally, higher plasma levels within the therapeutic range are required to suppress atrial arrhythmias. Plasma levels do not show the wide excursions seen with procainamide. (Refer to section on additional nursing implications of therapy with quinidinelike drugs for description of precautions and treatment of their toxicity.)

Nursing Implications of Procainamide Therapy. Procainamide is most commonly administered orally; it must be given at least every 6 hours. Peak drug levels may rise into the toxic range, yet plummet to levels below the minimum effective plasma concentration before administration of the next dose. Periodic recurrence of an arrhythmia or of toxic ECG changes may indicate that this is happening and be an indication to give smaller amounts of the drug more frequently.

Procainamide can also be given parenterally. Intravenous administration is associated with danger of life-threatening arrhythmias or severe hypotension. It is essential to monitor the ECG continuously during IV administration. Arterial BP should also be monitored closely; during administration of the loading dose, BP should be measured at least every 5 minutes. If a constant infusion is begun without a loading dose, achievement of a minimum effective concentration may take more than 6 hours.[49] Intramuscular procainamide is available but rarely used because of the need for repeated injections.

Initial doses of procainamide should be reduced by 30% to 50% in patients with severe CHF because the drug is cleared more slowly than in patients with normal liver and renal perfusion. Doses should also be decreased with liver and renal dysfunction.[139] A metabolite of procainamide, N-acetylprocainamide (NAPA or acecainide) has antiarrhythmic activity[2] and may have toxic effects. Unlike procainamide, NAPA is 85% cleared by the kidneys. In patients with severe renal disease, plasma levels of NAPA can greatly exceed the therapeutic range; thus procainamide should be used in such patients only if it cannot be avoided. If it is used, monitor plasma levels of both procainamide and NAPA and observe for QRS-complex prolongation.[139]

Routine blood counts should be monitored because of the possibility of development of agranulocytosis. For the same reason, patients should be instructed to report any soreness of the mouth, throat, or gums, and any unexplained fever or symptoms of upper respiratory infection. Patients who develop a systemic lupus erythematosus (SLE)-like syndrome (arthralgia, fever, hepatosplenomegaly, pleural and lung changes) should be told that these symptoms will disappear—often dramatically—as soon as the drug is stopped.

Additional Nursing Implications of Therapy with the Quinidinelike Drugs. Before quinidinelike drugs are used in the conversion attempts of atrial fibrillation or atrial flutter, it is essential that the patient have cardiac glycoside levels sufficient to increase the effective refractory period of the AV junction. Used alone, quinidinelike drugs tend to increase the response rate of the ventricles, possibly to dangerously high rates. For example, by reducing the rate of atrial depolarization in atrial flutter from 350 to 275 per minute, the AV junction is bombarded at a slower rate, which allows one-to-one conduction. This permits more impulses to be conducted to the ventricles.

Quinidinelike drugs have a negative inotropic effect which may lead to severe hypotension. Hypotension is extremely common with intravenous administration. The arterial blood pressure should be monitored closely if this route must be used.

It is interesting that at high concentrations, quinidine and, to a lesser extent, procainamide increase the slope of phase-4 depolarization and increase spontaneous firing rates. These changes are probably not, however, clinically important. High concentrations of the drugs also make the maximum diastolic potential less negative, again increasing spontaneous firing rates.[50] Thus these drugs can cause the very arrhythmias, such as atrial or ventricular tachycardia, flutter, or fibrillation, that they were given to treat. Monitoring of plasma drug levels is often helpful.

If toxicity is suspected (prolongation of QT interval or advanced AV block),[72] withhold the next dose of quinidine or procainamide and notify the physician. Toxicity may be treated adequately by stopping the drug. Because both drugs are rapidly degraded, this may be the only measure necessary. Monitor the serum K+ level closely. Low serum K+ levels diminish the effects of both procainamide and quinidine on cardiac electrical activity; measures such as sodium lactate infusion, or insulin and glucose administration, may force K+ into the intracellular space and improve electrical activity. A final measure used to counteract toxic effects of quinidinelike drugs is the administration of β-adrenergic drugs and agonists, such as isoproterenol (Isuprel). These drugs may improve electrical activity and counter the negative inotropic effects on the heart (Chap. 35).

Disopyramide Phosphate (Norpace)

Action. Disopyramide decreases conduction velocity and increases action potential duration in myocardial tissue. The

P wave, QRS complex, or PR interval may be prolonged.[24] Reentrant arrhythmias are possibly abolished by conversion of unidirectional into bidirectional conduction block.[31] Disopyramide also appears to reduce automaticity.[24] Some of its actions are due to anticholinergic properties of the drug. In animal studies disopyramide decreases myocardial contractility, cardiac output (CO), and coronary blood flow.[87] It has a profound negative inotropic effect in man, a situation unique among current antiarrhythmic agents.[97]

Elimination. Disopyramide is metabolized in the liver, but 40% to 60% is excreted unchanged in the urine. Its t½ is 5 to 6 hours.

Indications and Contraindications. Disopyramide is indicated for treatment of ventricular arrhythmias, including PVCs (unifocal and multifocal), and in ventricular tachycardia. It is not indicated for treatment of digitalis toxicity; however, it may be used for treatment of ventricular arrhythmias in the appropriately digitalized patient. Disopyramide has also been used successfully in treatment of premature atrial contractions (PACs) and paroxysmal atrial tachycardia (PAT).[121] It appears to be a useful alternative to procainamide and quinidine in cases where the arrhythmias are unresponsive to these drugs or when side effects make the drugs unacceptable.

Disopyramide is contraindicated in the presence of cardiogenic shock, preexisting second- or third-degree AV block (unless a pacemaker is in place and functioning), or known hypersensitivity to the drug. It should be administered with caution to patients with cardiomyopathy, uncorrected CHF (unless the failure is due to an arrhythmia), W–P–W, or bundle branch block.

Nursing Implications. Be observant for signs and symptoms of impending CHF. Disopyramide given to patients with a history of congestive failure may precipitate recurrent episodes of CHF in as many as 50% of patients. In patients without a prior history of congestive failure, CHF as a complication of disopyramide occurs in less than 5%.[97] Failure may result because of a combination of both depressed left ventricular function as well as some nonspecific effects which have not been well explained, such as possible changes in capillary permeability. If failure occurs, digitalis or diuretics can be ordered to improve the CHF, or the drug may be discontinued and a different antiarrhythmic agent substituted. Monitor the BP carefully after disopyramide administration. If severe hypotension develops, discontinue the drug. Carefully observe the ECG intervals: QRS widening (>25%) indicates that disopyramide should be discontinued; Q–T$_c$ prolongation (>25%) requires consideration of a different antiarrhythmic drug; PR interval prolongation indicates that the dose should be reduced. As with the quinidinelike drugs, patients with atrial fibrillation or atrial flutter should be digitalized before initiation of disopyramide therapy.

Because of its anticholinergic activity, disopyramide should be avoided in patients with glaucoma or urinary retention. If this drug must be used, a topical miotic should be given to patients with glaucoma. Urinary retention must be carefully assessed; a urethal catheter may be required.

Be aware that dosages should be reduced in patients with renal and hepatic impairment. As with most antiarrhythmic drugs, the serum K$^+$ level should be corrected to achieve optimum antiarrhythmic effect. Well-controlled studies of the use of disopyramide have not been performed on pregnant women and the use of disopyramide should be avoided in such patients when possible. It is not known whether this drug is excreted in human milk. Its effectiveness and safety for children has not been established.

Phenytoin Sodium (Dilantin)

Action. The electrophysiologic effects of phenytoin are highly dependent on the K$^+$ concentration in the extracellular fluid, the preexisting electrophysiologic characteristics of the cells, and the level of the drug itself.[137] If resting membrane potenial, action potential amplitude, V$_{max}$, membrane responsiveness, and conduction velocity are depressed (as may be seen with anesthesia, hypothermia, cardiac disease, or digitalis toxicity), low concentrations of phenytoin may restore these values toward normal. This effect is especially marked if the K$^+$ concentration is low. Low doses of phenytoin can improve conduction through or abolish regions of unidirectional block and oppose reentrant arrhythmias. Higher concentrations of phenytoin (still within the therapeutic range) tend to depress membrane responsiveness and V$_{max}$, make the resting membrane potential less negative, and decrease action potential amplitude. The depressant effect is less than that caused by quinidine and procainamide; it is unclear whether phenytoin can convert unidirectional block into bidirectional block and abolish a reentrant circuit.

Independent of K$^+$ concentration and drug level, phenytoin shortens the action potential duration and effective refractory period of Purkinje cells. This means that premature impulses are more likely to arrive when the membrane is at a more negative level. Such premature impulses have a greater V$_{max}$ and a greater amplitude, and are less likely to become established in reentrant circuits caused by unidirectional blocks.

Phenytoin depresses the slope of phase-4 (diastolic) depolarization of Purkinje fibers; it opposes the increase in slope caused by catecholamines and digitalis. Such an action may lessen the numbers of premature impulses, and tend to delay those that do occur (threshold is approached more slowly). It may also improve conduction, because impulses arrive when the membrane potential is at a more negative value (Fig. 34-8).

The exact ionic nature of the action of phenytoin on cardiac cells is unknown. It may directly affect ionic movements across membranes; it is also possible that major effects of the drug are the result of the drug's ability to mediate autonomic outflow. Phenytoin decreases activity in sympathetic nerves to the heart.[39] The activity in these nerves is known to be increased in MI and digitalis toxicity. Phenytoin does not appear to modify vagal outflow.

Elimination. Phenytoin is metabolized by the liver and the products are excreted in the urine. The metabolism of phenytoin can be saturated at levels close to the therapeutic range, such that beyond the saturation level addition of more drug results in no increase in drug breakdown. Plasma levels increase dramatically beyond this level; small increments in dosage may result in toxicity. This characteristic,

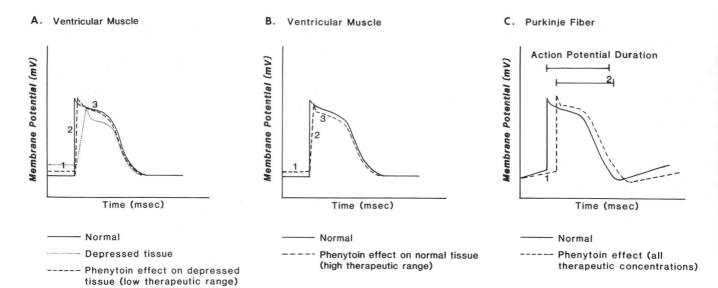

Fig. 34-8. Summary of electrophysiologic effects of phenytoin. (**A**) Low therapeutic drug level may correct preexisting problems in depressed cells: (1) Repolarizes membrane with depolarized resting potential. (2) Increases velocity of phrase 0 (upstroke) when it has been diminished. (3) Increases action potential amplitude when it is abnormally low. (**B**) Higher therapeutic drug level. (1) Depolarizes resting membrane potential. (2) Decreases velocity of phase 0 (upstroke). (3) Decreases action potential amplitude. (**C**) Purkinje fibers. (1) Decreased velocity of phase-4 resting depolarization. (2) Decreased action potential duration.

plus the wide range of variation in t½ between individuals and in the same individual (mean t½ 22 hours; range of t½ 7–42 hours) at different plasma concentrations, makes monitoring of plasma levels essential to good patient care.[139]

Indications and Contraindications. The major antiarrhythmic use for phenytoin is in treatment of arrhythmias caused by digitalis toxicity. Reports of the efficacy of phenytoin in the management of digitalis-toxic supraventricular tachycardia and paroxysmal atrial arrhythmias are contradictory. Some investigators indicate good response to phenytoin therapy,[47,88,105] while others report less successful treatment (H. L. Greene, personal communication). Junctional digitalis-toxic arrhythmias may also respond, although less well. Phenytoin therapy for ventricular arrhythmias resulting from digitalis toxicity, such as bigeminy, PVCs, and ventricular tachycardia, may be successful in as many as 92% of cases[105] but again, opinions about its effectiveness are contradictory (H. L. Greene, personal communication). Because of conflicting reports and the difficulties of intravenous administration, lidocaine is often preferred. Phenytoin is sometimes effective in treatment of ventricular arrhythmias associated with acute MI,[32,88] general anesthesia, open-heart surgery, cardiac catheterization studies and radiopaque dye injection.[88] It is ineffective in almost all cases of atrial arrhythmias of origin other than digitalis toxicity.[47,88,105] It may relieve heart block.[110] Phenytoin may also be given orally to patients for suppression of arrhythmias of a more chronic nature.

Phenytoin is contraindicated in patients with known hypersensitivity to the drug, and with sinus bradycardia, SA block, second- and third-degree AV block, and Stokes–Adams syndrome. Fetal abnormalities may occur if phenytoin is used during pregnancy.[85]

Nursing Implications. Phenytoin can be administered effectively IV or orally; it cannot be given IM because absorption is inconsistent and unpredictable, and tissue necrosis and abscesses commonly occur.[133] Because absorption of oral phenytoin is slow, IV administration is indicated in the case of acute arrhythmia. Loading doses for both the IV and oral routes are necessary.

Before administering IV phenytoin, obtain baseline BP, HR, and ECG intervals. In the cardiac patient, continuous monitoring of the ECG is mandatory. When starting the IV line for administration of phenytoin, avoid selection of very small veins, such as hand veins. If the IV line is already in place, ascertain that it is completely in the vein and that there is no phlebitis before administering this drug. Because of its alkalinity (pH 12.0),[41] phenytoin is extremely irritating to the veins (and also to the surrounding tissue, should extravasation occur); phlebitis should be anticipated, and the IV site changed every 24 to 48 hours to prevent its occurrence.

The injection should be given as close to the IV catheter hub as possible; a stopcock connecting the IV catheter and tubing provides easy access. (Always protect the sterility of its open port by covering it with a sterile injection cap.) Because phenytoin precipitates in dextrose-containing solutions, the IV tubing should only be filled with normal saline. Never mix phenytoin with any other drug. Administer phenytoin as a direct IV push very slowly, not exceeding 25 mg to 50 mg per minute. Phenytoin equilibrates slowly between tissues and plasma; rapid IV administration may result in toxic plasma concentrations and hypotensive crises. Even at a slow rate of injection, pain can result, and the speed of the injection needs to be reduced. After each 25 mg to 50 mg is injected, flush the IV line completely with normal saline (at the same injection rate as the drug), and record the BP and HR. If the BP falls more than 10 to 15 mm Hg, wait until it stabilizes before continuing to administer the phenytoin. (Reduce the rate of injection to prevent a further drop in BP.) Continue monitoring the vital signs frequently (every 5–10 minutes, depending upon their stability). Continuous infusion of phenytoin causes pain and thrombosis, and should be avoided.

Absorption of oral phenytoin is nearly complete, but slow. As with IV use, loading doses are required. Initiation of maintenance therapy without a loading dose will not result in steady therapeutic plasma levels for 5 to 15 days.[74] Lower dosages are required for patients with some liver diseases (cirrhosis, infectious hepatitis) because they metabolize phenytoin more slowly.[74] The transient impairment of hepatic function following halothane anesthesia is also associated with diminished phenytoin elimination.[56]

Phenytoin has a varying effect on firing rate of the SA node. It may increase, decrease, or not change the rate. Sinus tachycardia, bradycardia, or arrest have been rarely reported.[14,124] This same variability characterizes the AV nodal response to phenytoin. It often accelerates AV nodal conduction; however, it may slow conduction.[14] This ability to accelerate AV nodal conduction dictates a need for caution when using the drug in patients with atrial fibrillation or atrial flutter, because faster ventricular responses may result. There are also reports of worsening of already depressed AV nodal conduction when phenytoin is used. Complete AV block may result.[114] The most severe effects on the cardiovascular system occur more frequently in the elderly or in debilitated patients. When using intravenous phenytoin, emergency life-support equipment and drugs should be readily available.

Because of the effects on the hematopoietic system, complete blood counts (CBCs) should be obtained routinely. All patients taking phenytoin should also have their blood glucose level monitored, because phenytoin inhibits insulin release. Both CBC and blood glucose should be obtained, ideally prior to phenytoin therapy, soon after initiation of treatment, and periodically during its course.

Many patients taking oral phenytoin are able to take a single, daily dose of 300 mg (rather than 100 mg three times daily) and maintain therapeutic plasma drug levels; there is no reported evidence of increased toxicity with a single daily dose. This method may assist the nonadherent patient in adhering to his drug regimen.

The gastrointestinal upsets which may accompany phenytoin ingestion can be minimized by taking the drug with meals. Good oral hygiene (gum massage, frequent brushing and flossing, and regular dental visits) may reduce or prevent gingival hyperplasia. Patients should be instructed to call the physician if a rash appears; the physician will discontinue phenytoin at this time. If the rash is exfoliative, purpuric, or bullous, the drug should not be restarted; if the rash is of a milder type (measleslike or scarlatiniform), the drug may be restarted after the rash completely disappears. Phenytoin is teratogenic and to be avoided if possible during pregnancy.[85]

Bretylium Tosylate (Bretylol, Bretylan)

Action. Bretylium, a postganglionic adrenergic blocking agent, which was originally used in the treatment of hyper-

tension, is unique among antiarrhythmic drugs in that it has a positive inotropic effect on the myocardium.[20] Its antiarrhythmic properties are due to two different sites of action: the adrenergic neurons and the myocardium. Bretylium alters adrenergic function in three ways.[63] Initially, high concentrations of bretylium release norepinephrine from adrenergic nerve endings.[63,82] (Refer to Fig. 3-24 for effects of catecholamines on the action potential.) This raises BP in 16%–17% of patients, but is usually not clinically important)[8] and increases inotropism, sinus rate, and automaticity, resulting in more frequent PVCs (in 10%–20% of patients).[63] Subsequently, and with lowered concentrations, the release of norepinephrine from these nerve endings is inhibited.[63,82] This reduces peripheral vascular resistance (PVR) and may cause postural hypotension. The reuptake of both epinephrine and norepinephrine into the adrenergic nerve endings is also subsequently blocked.[59,63] This potentiates the actions of both endogenous and exogenous catecholamines, and may maintain the positive inotropic effects, increasing the CO. The importance of these effects depends on the dose of bretylium, how long it has been acting, its concentration at the nerve endings, the preexisting rate of adrenergic discharge on the myocardium, and the levels of circulating catecholamines.[63]

Direct electrophysiologic effects on the heart include increased action potential duration and increased effective refractory period without a change in the ratio between the two (reduces reentry),[10,15,63,128,138] and increased ventricular fibrillation threshold (up to three times) in experimental animals,[3,5,6,60] more effectively than do lidocaine, phenytoin, procainamide, propranolol, or quinidine.[4,13]

Elimination. Bretylium is not detoxified or metabolized to any important extent in the body. During the first 24 hours, 70% to 80% of the administered drug is excreted unchanged in the urine,[54] and an additional 10% is excreted unchanged during the next three days.[73] The t½ of bretylium is approximately 5 to 10 hours (range 4–17 hours).[101]

Indications and Contraindications. Bretylium is indicated as a second-line drug for life-threatening ventricular tachyarrhythmias which are refractory to other antiarrhythmic drugs, such as lidocaine and procainamide; it should be used in conjunction with appropriate electrical cardioversion.[8,19,27,101,113]

There are no absolute contraindications to bretylium. However, because of the initial release and subsequent potentiation of catecholamines, it should be used with extreme caution, if at all, in patients with ventricular tachyarrhythmias resulting from a pheochromocytoma. Bretylium exacerbates digitalis-toxic arrhythmias; it is contraindicated if the arrhythmia to be treated is possibly related to digitalis toxicity.

Nursing Implications. Bretylium is generally administered IV or IM. Oral bretylium is absorbed erratically and is not recommended; oral bretylium is not currently approved by the Food and Drug Administration for use in the U.S. Although suppression of ventricular fibrillation may be rapid, other ventricular arrhythmias may not be suppressed for 20 to 60 minutes after IV administration.[27,113] In nonemergency situations, IV infusions should be given slowly to prevent nausea and vomiting. When administering IM bretylium, do not inject more than 5 ml in one site.[63] Rotate the injection sites, because repeated IM injections at the same site cause necrosis and fibrosis.

Because of the initial sympathomimetic effect, bretylium may cause an *increase* in ventricular arrhythmias, HR, and BP. This effect usually lasts about 30 minutes. During this time the patient should be closely observed for increased myocardial ischemia or extension of infarction. Because of its hypotensive effects, especially posturally, the patient must remain supine and as flat as possible until tolerance to the hypotension develops, often within a few days.[63] Patients with fixed CO, such as those with aortic or mitral stenosis, or with severe pulmonary hypertension, are particularly susceptible to the drug's hypotensive effects because the decrease in PVR cannot be opposed by increases in CO. Excessive hypotension (<75 mm Hg systolic or with symptoms) can be treated with IV fluids (unless contraindicated) or with vasopressors. However, because of associated catecholamine potentiation, vasopressors should be administered with caution. Maintenance doses should probably be decreased in patients with renal disease.

Verapamil (Isoptin, Cordilox)

Verapamil is not currently approved for use in the U.S. However, because it is highly effective in the treatment of some arrhythmias and its mechanism of action is unique, it merits discussion. The experimental drug D600 has a similar mechanism of action.

Action. Verapamil appears to block the slow inward current (i_{s_i}) which is carried primarily by Ca^{2+}. This current generates the "slow response" action potential seen in diseased tissue and the delayed afterdepolarizations following the action potential in some cardiac tissues when exposed to catecholamines or toxic levels of digitalis. Both of these mechanisms may contribute to the genesis of arrhythmias.[134,135] Verapamil's ability to block this current may account for its antiarrhythmic action. Verapamil depresses the SA and AV nodes, which probably accounts for its great efficacy in slowing ventricular response in atrial fibrillation or flutter. Because verapamil reduces the Ca^{2+} current into the heart, it has a negative inotropic effect on the myocardium (Chap. 2). It may limit the area of cardiac necrosis following a coronary occlusion.[98]

Elimination. Verapamil is metabolized in the liver. Oral verapamil undergoes extensive (approximately 70%) "first pass" metabolism (the drug is metabolized during absorption in the liver or gut wall). About 50% of verapamil is excreted by the kidney within the first 24 hours; 9% to 16% is excreted in the stool. For both IV and oral administration, the t½ of the initial α-phase (rapid rise in blood level after administration) is 18 to 35 minutes;[51] the t½ of the slower β-phase (sustained rise in blood level immediately following the α-phase) is 170 to 440 minutes.[51,117]

Indications and Contraindications. Verapamil is highly effective in the treatment of supraventricular tachycardia. Ventricular response rate is slowed in both atrial fibrillation and atrial flutter. In addition, NSR may be achieved in patients with atrial flutter, or supraventricular or junctional tachycardia.[116] Verapamil is less effective in treating ventricular arrhythmias.

Verapamil is contraindicated in patients who have received β-blocking agents within the preceding 48 hours. It is contraindicated in high degree SA and AV blocks, advanced heart failure, cardiogenic shock, SA node disease, and severe hypotension; complete AV conduction block, asystole, or severe hypotension may result.[69,111] Verapamil is also contraindicated in patients with known hypersensitivity to the drug.

Nursing Implications. Extreme caution must be exercised if verapamil is used in patients with SA and AV nodal dysfunction.[1] Verapamil may cause hypotension.[69,116] The therapy for verapamil overdose can be β-adrenergic amines, glucagon, IV Ca^{2+}, or pacing.[16,69,108,119] As clinical experience with verapamil increases, more detailed information regarding the use of this drug will become available; the nurse should update her information regarding this drug frequently until it is better understood.

Atropine Sulfate, U.S.P.

Action. Atropine is a vagolytic or parasympatholytic agent. It blocks the muscarinic type of acetylcholine receptors, which include parasympathetic receptors in the heart (vagus), some glands, and smooth muscle, and in some non-parasympathetic muscarinic receptors, such as in sweat glands and in the central nervous system (CNS). Atropine does not block nicotinic acetylcholine receptors; neuromuscular transmission and transmission in autonomic ganglia are spared.

Vagal innervation of the heart is primarily to the SA and AV nodal regions and the atrial muscle. Vagal stimulation appears to increase the K^+ permeability of tissue and decrease the slow inward (i_{s_i}) Ca^{2+}/Na^+ current. Cells repolarize faster and seek a more negative maximum diastolic potential (Fig. 3-25). Pacemaker cells may approach threshold more slowly (decreased slope of phase-4 depolarization). Action potential duration is reduced, making reentrant arrhythmias such as atrial fibrillation more common. Atropine opposes the most common effects of vagal outflow, bradycardia (which may be profound), and slowing of AV nodal conduction.

Methscopolamine has been recommended by some as a substitute for atropine. Because it does not appear to cross the blood-brain barrier, it has fewer CNS side effects; it has been reported to be more consistent in its acceleration of the HR. However, it may produce more junctional arrhythmias and conduction disturbances than atropine.[92]

Elimination. Of the administered atropine, 13% to 50% is eliminated unchanged in the urine. The remainder of the atropine is metabolized by the liver.

Indications and Contraindications. Atropine is indicated in instances of excessive, vagus-induced bradycardia, which is associated with such rate-related complications as severe hypotension and escape rhythms. Such bradycardia may be seen with MI, particularly of the inferior myocardium.

Atropine can also improve AV nodal conduction, which is impaired as a result of excessive vagal outflow. First-degree AV block and Mobitz type I block are frequently related to increased vagal outflow and, if treatment is necessary, atropine may be successful. Mobitz type II block is not usually related to vagal outflow, and therefore atropine would not be indicated.[26] Use of the drug in complete AV block if a junctional pacemaker is present, may be successful. However, its success is variable and artificial pacing is often required.

Several less common uses in cardiac patients are also related to the parasympathetic (vagal) blocking properties of atropine. It is an antidote for the effects of edrophonium chloride (Tensilon) and choline esters, and should be given in the event that these drugs evoke cardiovascular collapse. It may be given to counteract the bradycardia and the gastrointestinal effects associated with morphine sulfate. Atropine is not indicated for bradycardia associated with sick sinus syndrome because of the rebound tachycardia which may occur.[26] Contraindications include narrow-angle glaucoma and adhesions (synechiae) between the iris and the lens of the eye. Atropine forces the iris back and into a position which may interfere with drainage of the aqueous humor and precipitate a dangerous and dramatic rise in intraocular pressure. Use of atropine in wide-angle glaucoma is usually safe; however, monitoring of intraocular pressure may be a wise precaution in these patients.[33]

Nursing Implications. Atropine 0.5 mg should be administered by direct IV push. Smaller doses (0.4 mg) may cause at least a transient further reduction in HR (4–8 beats per minute) because of a vagomimetic effect. This can be avoided by rapidly administering the IV dose so that the blood level rises quickly. If slowing of the HR does occur, a repeat dose should be given. Atropine may be associated with increased myocardial ischemia[100] and with increased incidence of arrhythmia in the patient with acute MI.[61] Recent literature recommends that atropine be used with extreme caution in acutely infarcted patients and only when rate-related complications, such as hypotension and escape rhythms, require correction.[21,26,40] This may occur more frequently when larger doses (>1.0 mg) are given. Ventricular tachycardia and fibrillation have been reported after IV administration.[86] Table 34-2 summarizes the effects of atropine in relation to dosage.

The effects of atropine are greater in younger patients. Vagal tone diminishes with age. Older patients (70 or more years of age) may not experience acceleration of HR after administration of atropine because they no longer have vagal tone to inhibit.

Administration of atropine may result in acute urinary retention, especially in men with benign prostatic hypertrophy. If the patient's condition permits, allowing the male patient to stand to use the urinal, or the female patient to use the bedside commode may facilitate urination. If those approaches are contraindicated or do not succeed, urethral catheterization may be required.

Patients who experience untoward symptoms (hot, dry, flushed skin and extreme anxiety, restlessness, and hallucinations) should be reassured that these symptoms will soon disappear (phenothiazines are contraindicated in suppression of CNS stimulation). Physostigmine, U.S.P., an

TABLE 34-2   EFFECTS OF ATROPINE IN RELATION TO DOSAGE

Dose	Effects
0.5 mg	Slight cardiac slowing; some dryness of mouth; inhibition of sweating
1.0 mg	Definite dryness of mouth; thirst; acceleration of heart, sometimes preceded by slowing; mild dilatation of pupil
2.0 mg	Rapid heart rate; palpitation; marked dryness of mouth; dilated pupils; some blurring of near vision
5.0 mg	All the above symptoms marked; speech disturbed; difficulty in swallowing; restlessness and fatigue; headache; dry, hot skin; difficulty in micturition; reduced intestinal peristalsis
10.0 mg and more	Above symptoms more marked; pulse rapid and weak; iris practically obliterated; vision very blurred; skin flushed, hot, dry, and scarlet; ataxia, restlessness, and excitement; hallucinations and delirium; coma

(Innes IR, Nickerson M: Atropine, scopalamine and related antimuscarinic drugs. In Goodman LS, Gilman A (eds): The Pharmacological Basis of Therapeutics, 5th ed, pp 514–532. New York, Macmillan. Copyright © 1975 by Macmillan Publishing Co., Inc.)

anticholinesterase, is an antidote for atropine toxicity and should be readily available.

Edrophonium Chloride (Tensilon)

Action. Edrophonium is a cholinesterase inhibitor. It thus has vagomimetic action and causes slowing of the sinus rate and of AV nodal conduction.

Elimination. The exact fate of edrophonium is unknown. It is probably both destroyed by cholinesterases and excreted in the urine.

Indications and Contraindications. In the cardiac patient edrophonium may occasionally be used to treat supraventricular arrhythmias. Its most common use is as a test for myasthenia gravis and to evaluate the treatment requirements of that disease. It is contraindicated in patients in which digitalis toxicity is suspected,[109] and in those with known hypersensitivity to anticholinesterase agents, or with intestinal or urinary obstructions of a mechanical type.

Nursing Implications. Administer edrophonium, using a tuberculin syringe, by injecting 0.2 ml (2 mg) in 15 to 30 seconds. Because it may cause serious bradycardias and ventricular tachycardia, it has not gained widespread use. Weakness and muscle fasciculations may ensue. Facilities for endotracheal intubation and assisted ventilation must be immediately available when the drug is used. Atropine is the antidote for edrophonium toxicity and should be immediately available.

CARDIOTONIC DRUGS

Digitalis

Digitalis and its congeners (digoxin, digitoxin, deslanoside, ouabain) belong to a class of drugs known as cardiac glycosides, cardiotonic steroids, or simply digitalis. There are significant pharmacokinetic differences among the var-

TABLE 34-3 CARDIOTONIC DRUGS

Agent	Dosage/ Administration	Onset of Action	Peak Plasma Concentration Time	Plateau Plasma Concentration Time	Therapeutic Plasma Level	Toxic Plasma Level	Drug Interactions	Side and Toxic Effects
DIGITALIS PREPARATIONS Digitoxin, U.S.P. (Crystodigin)	IV digitalizing dose: Rapid—1.2–1.6 mg IV in a single dose. Slow (usual method)—0.6 mg initially, followed by 0.4 mg 4–6 hours later, and by 0.2 mg q. 4–6 hours thereafter until digitalization achieved (usually 8–12 hours). IV maintenance dose: 0.05–0.3 mg daily. PO digitalizing dose: Rapid—0.6 mg initially, followed by 0.4 mg 4–6 hours later, and by 0.2 mg q. 2h. thereafter until digitalization achieved. Slow—0.2 mg b.i.d. for 7 days, following by maintenance dose. PO maintenance: 0.05–0.3 mg q.d.; most commonly, 0.15 mg q.d.	$\frac{1}{2}$–2 hours	4–12 hours	6–8 hours	14–26 ng/ml	>34 ng/ml	Drugs that alter myocardial sensitivity to digitalis preparations: A. K^+-depleting diuretics—↑ toxicity with a given dose B. Mg^{2+}-depleting diuretics—↑ toxicity with a given dose C. Thiazide diuretics may ↑ extracellular Ca^{2+}—↑ toxicity with a given dose D. Ca^{2+} salt IV administration—↑ toxicity with a given dose. E. Ca^{2+} chelators—↑ toxicity with a given dose	Side effect: Gynecomastia can occur, but is uncommon. Overdosage and toxic effects: GI: anorexia, nausea, vomiting, diarrhea (those same symptoms can be produced by uncontrolled CHF for which the drug is prescribed). CNS: headache, weakness, apathy, visual disturbances (blurred vision, yellow vision); mental depression and confusion, disorientation, delirium. Cardiovascular: refer to Table 34-4.
Digoxin, U.S.P. (Lanoxin, SK-Digoxin)	IV digitalizing dose: Rapid—0.5–1.0 mg initially, followed by 0.25–0.5 mg q. 6 h. until digitalization achieved Slow—0.25–0.5 mg initially, followed by 0.25 mg q. 4–6 h. until digitalization achieved (usually at total 1.0 mg) IV maintenance dose: 0.125–0.5 mg (usually 0.25 mg) q.d. IM digitalizing dose: 0.25–0.5 mg initially, followed by 0.25 mg q. 4–6 h. until digitalization achieved (usually at total of 1.0 mg) IM maintenance dose:	15–30 min.	1–5 hours	2–4 hours 10–12 hours	0.8–1.6 ng/ml	>2.4 ng/ml	Pharmacokinetic interactions: A. Drugs which ↓ GI motility—propantheline bromide (Pro-Banthine), morphine sulfate—↑ uptake of PO digoxin B. Drugs which ↑ GI motility—cathartics, metoclopramide—↓ uptake of PO digoxin C. Anion exchange resins—cholestyramine (Cuemid, Questran) and colestipol (Colestid)—↓ absorbability of PO digoxin and digitoxin D. Antacids, charcoal, antidiarrhea medications—↓ absorbability of PO digoxin and digitoxin	

Drug	Dose			Interactions	Side effects
	0.25–0.5 mg q. 6–8 h. until digitalization achieved (usually at total of 1.0–1.5 mg) Slow—0.125–0.5 mg q.d. usually results in digitalization in 7 days. PO maintenance dose: 0.125–0.5 mg (usually 0.25 mg) q.d.			(Dilantin), phenylbutazone (Butazolidin)—↑ hepatic breakdown rate of digitoxin F. Antiarrhythmic drugs: quinidine—quinidine decreases renal clearance of digoxin; digoxin level may increase to toxic when quinidine is added to digitalized patient.[28,34] Decrease maintenance digoxin doses by 30%–50% and monitor serum digoxin levels when quinidine is added.[45] Increase maintenance digoxin dose and monitor serum digoxin levels when quinidine is discontinued.	
Deslanoside, U.S.P. (Cedilanid-D)	IV or IM digitalizing dose: 1.2–1.6 mg as single dose or divided dose	10–30 min.	1–2 hours	—	—
Ouabain injection, U.S.P.	IV digitalizing dose: 0.25–0.5 mg	5–10 min.	½–2 hours	—	—
				Autonomic drugs: A. β-sympathomimetic amines—epinephrine—↑ ectopic activity B. β-sympathomimetic blocking agents—propranolol (Inderol)—↓ blocking of AV node conduction	
GLUCAGON, U.S.P.	IV, IM, or SC: dissolve lyophilized glucagon in accompanying solvent; administer single dose of 1–5 mg[92,95] (1 unit glucagon = 1 mg) Must be mixed only with diluent provided[40]	IV: 1–3 min.[94]	IV: 5–7 min.[94] 10–15 min. duration[94]	—	Glucagon increases hepatic blood flow in man.[62] This may change the rate of metabolism of some drugs: lidocaine breakdown is notably influenced by changes in hepatic blood flow. Glucagon potentiates warfarin anticoagulants, especially when more than 50 mg glucagon is given within a 24-hour period.[66] Glucagon is incompatible with infusion vehicles that are acidic in nature (pH 4-5).[41]

Hyperglycemia; nausea and vomiting

ious preparations. The basic mechanisms of action are, however, the same for the various derivatives and are described generally with the term "digitalis" used in a broad sense. Table 34-3 lists dosage, administration, onset of action, peak plasma level, plateau plasma time, therapeutic and toxic plasma levels, drug interactions, and side and toxic effects.

Action. The action for which digitalis is most frequently used is its positive inotropic effect. It increases the contractility of the normal and failing myocardium.[12] In the distended, failing heart, increased contractility results in more complete systolic emptying of the ventricles; end-diastolic ventricular volumes are reduced, and ventricular distention is diminished. Additionally, filling pressures of the heart (such as central venous pressure and pulmonary artery wedge pressure) fall and venous congestion is diminished. The CO also increases, renal blood flow improves, allowing retained water and salt to be eliminated via the kidneys.

The increase in contractility with digitalis is associated with increased myocardial oxygen consumption. This increase may, however, be offset by the decreased demand for oxygen which accompanies the reduction in cardiac size. Reduced chamber size results in reduced intramyocardial tension (the law of Laplace). Intramyocardial tension is a major determinant of myocardial oxygen consumption. Furthermore, oxygen delivery to myocardial tissue may increase, further improving the myocardial energy balance.

The mechanism which accounts for the improved contractility is not understood. Digitalis does not reverse the underlying cause of failure and cure the patient, but only opposes some of the manifestations of the basic problem. Thus, therapy is usually long term.

Digitalis is also an antiarrhythmic at therapeutic plasma levels, but becomes very arrhythmogenic at toxic plasma levels. The four major therapeutic electrophysiologic effects of digitalis on the myocardium are a slowing of the firing rate of the SA node, improved intra-atrial conduction, depressed AV nodal conduction, and prolonged effective refractory period in the AV node.[107] A nontherapeutic effect is the increase in pacemaker automaticity in the Purkinje fibers, resulting in development or increase of PVCs.[89] The depressant actions on sinus firing rate and AV nodal conduction are largely mediated by increases in vagal tone (there is little or no slowing in the transplanted heart). However, large doses of digitalis are associated with a slowing of the sinus mechanisms which atropine does not block, which must, therefore, be nonvagal.

The effects of digitalis on a spontaneously depolarizing conducting cell are illustrated in Figure 34-9. The hemodynamic and electrophysiologic effects of digitalis are summarized in Table 34-4. Chapter 17 describes electrocardiographic changes seen with digitalis therapy and toxicity. Figures 17-30 A and B illustrate some of these changes.

Elimination. Elimination of cardiac glycosides is variable, depending on the preparation of digitalis administered. Digoxin, deslanoside, and ouabain are excreted by the kidneys, with t½s of 36 hours, 36 hours, and 21 hours, respectively. Digitoxin is degraded by the liver before it is excreted by the kidneys. Its t½ is 5 to 7 days.[89] Neither

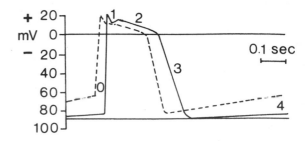

Fig. 34-9. Summary of electrophysiologic actions of digitalis on a spontaneously depolarizing conductive fiber in the atrial, junctional, or ventricular myocardium. (*Dashed line* indicates effect of digitalis.) Phase 0 is less steep, decreasing the conduction velocity. The increase in the slope of phase 4 results in a more rapid depolarization. (Mason DT Zelis R, Lee G et al: Am J Cardiol 27:547, 1971)

peritoneal dialysis nor hemodialysis removes significant amounts of these drugs.[29]

Indications and Contraindications. Digitalis has both cardiotonic and electrophysiologic activity. As a cardiotonic drug, it is used to increase myocardial contractility and CO in patients with acute and chronic CHF. It is useful in CHF associated with low CO, such as that caused by ischemic, hypertensive, rheumatic, or congenital heart disease. It is usually not indicated in cases of CHF associated with high cardiac output states, such as that caused by thyrotoxicosis or anemia, nor in CHF due to obstructive lesions, such as subvalvular stenosis. Digitalis may be helpful in CHF associated with acute MI, but its use in this instance requires great caution.

As an antiarrhythmic drug, digitalis is indicated in cases of atrial and junctional arrhythmias. It slows the SA-nodal firing rate in sinus tachycardia. The ventricular response to atrial fibrillation or atrial flutter is slowed by digitalis and may be converted to NSR. (It is imperative that digitalis be administered before quinidinelike drugs are given in these rhythms.) Because of reduction in atrial size and, therefore, stretch, atrial arrhythmias may be abolished when CHF is improved.

TABLE 34-4 EFFECTS OF DIGITALIS

Hemodynamic

Venae cavae, pulmonary veins, atria: lowers filling pressures

Ventricular muscle: positive inotropic effect → increased O_2 consumption and reduced distention → improved O_2 delivery and reduced O_2 consumption

Arteries: transient increase in PVR if infused rapidly → increased BP

Electrophysiologic

SA node: slows firing rate

Atrial tissue: improves conduction

AV node: depresses conduction; prolongs effective refractory period

Purkinje fibers: enhances automaticity

Ventricular muscle: may abolish arrhythmias by improving myocardial size, perfusion, and electrolyte imbalance

---

(From Mason DT, Zelis R, Lee G et al: Current concepts and treatment of digitalis toxicity. Am J Cardiol 27:546–559, 1971)

Although digitalis is not thought to have any direct antiarrhythmic actions on the ventricle, it may act indirectly to abolish arrhythmias in this part of the heart by reduction in cardiac size and improvement in cardiac perfusion and electrolyte balance.

Contraindications to digitalis therapy include the presence of digitalis toxicity (suspected or confirmed by plasma levels), AV block with a history of Stokes–Adams attacks, or uncomplicated idiopathic hypertrophic subaortic stenosis (IHSS). Hypersensitivity to the drug is extremely uncommon; when present, digitalis is contraindicated.

Nursing Implications. There are many preparations of digitalis-related drugs. If "digitalis" is prescribed, the nurse or pharmacist is legally required to use the digitalis leaf preparation, Digitalis, U.S.P. (primarily digitoxin), which is rarely used today.

Digoxin is the most commonly prescribed form of glycoside. It may be administered IV, IM, or orally. In the CCU setting it is commonly given IV to digitalize* the patient. Administer undiluted digoxin (0.25 mg/ml) no faster than 0.25 mg per minute. Faster IV administration may result in a transient increase in PVR, and consequently, an increased afterload and elevated myocardial O_2 consumption; pulmonary edema can be precipitated or exacerbated. If the patient is well enough to receive a diet, oral maintenance doses will probably be given. If the patient cannot tolerate oral medications, IV injections are required to maintain plasma digoxin levels. Absorption of oral digoxin varies widely and makes monitoring of digoxin levels nearly essential. Although IM injection of digoxin may be given, it is not recommended because absorption of the drug is somewhat erratic and tissue necrosis at the injection site is common. This is particularly true in patients with advanced CHF or shock who have decreased peripheral perfusion. Digoxin is distributed primarily in the lean tissue, and calculations of doses in the obese should be based only on lean body mass.[35] Similarly, doses should be decreased in the elderly, because they usually have decreased lean body mass.[29]

Digoxin is safe to use in patients with liver disease, because it is excreted unchanged by the kidneys. However, it must be used with caution in patients with renal dysfunction. The dose should be reduced according to the degree of renal-function impairment. In patients with normal renal function who develop digoxin toxicity, the toxic symptoms should subside when the t½ (36 hours) is reached. However, in digoxin-toxic patients with renal dysfunction, the t½ is prolonged because elimination is reduced.

Digitoxin is used infrequently. It may be administered either IV or orally. Like digoxin, rapid IV administration of digitoxin can increase PVR. Administer undiluted digitoxin (0.2 mg/ml) no faster than 0.2 mg per minute. Oral digitoxin is more consistently absorbed than is oral digoxin. An advantage of digitoxin therapy is that it is safer to use in patients with renal disease than are other digitalis preparations, because it is degraded by the liver prior to elimination. However, renal dysfunction still delays excretion of the digitoxin metabolites, and dosage adjustments should

be made accordingly. A major disadvantage is that the t½ of digitoxin is very long, and should the patient develop digitalis toxicity, the toxic symptoms will remain for a long time. Presence of a biliary fistula may result in increased elimination of the drug and require larger dosages. A decrease in dosage is required in patients with hepatic insufficiency.

Deslanoside and ouabain are administered only IV. They are used when rapid digitalization is required.

The nurse's role in the treatment of the patient on digitalis is not only to provide symptomatic relief to the patient and administer the digitalis as ordered, but to be extremely watchful for signs and symptoms of digitalis toxicity. It is commonly seen because the toxic plasma level is only slightly greater than the therapeutic level, and in some cases, therapeutic levels can be associated with toxic symptomatology. Digitalis toxicity is estimated to occur in 8% to 35% of all hospitalized patients receiving digitalis.[84,120] This is an extremely dangerous adverse drug reaction. Mortality rates with this complication have been estimated at 7% to 50%.[29] Digitalis intoxication can be potentiated by a low serum K+ level. (Many patients taking digitalis also receive diuretics, which increase urinary K+ excretion and lower serum K+. Fig. 17-25 illustrates the electrocardiographic effects of hypokalemia.) Therapy for digitalis intoxication includes discontinuation of the drug, administration of potassium chloride supplement, with or without concomitant hypokalemia (unless conduction disturbances or renal failure are present), and correction of other factors which may contribute to arrhythmias, such as hypoxemia and acid–base and electrolyte disturbances. The ventricular arrhythmias seen in isolation with digitalis toxicity can sometimes be treated successfully with propranolol. Magnesium infusion may also be indicated. Cholestyramine may be used to eliminate digitoxin. Arrhythmias may be treated with phenytoin, lidocaine, atropine, or pacing, as appropriate. Bretylium is contraindicated.

Almost any arrhythmia or conduction disturbance can be caused by digitalis toxicity. Prior to administration of each dose of digitalis, the apical HR and rhythm should be assessed (with the patient at rest), recorded, and compared with the resting HR and rhythm before the previous dose. If the patient's rhythm is being observed on a cardiac monitor, record the duration of the PR, QRS, and QT intervals on the rhythm strip every 4 hours, or as indicated. As a general rule, the drug should be held if the apical HR is less than 60 beats per minute, or if there is an important change in either HR or, if on ECG, the conduction is prolonged. (Digitalis toxicity is frequently present even when the HR is greater than 60.) For example, if the apical HR was 75 beats per minute and regular before the previous dose and is currently 72 beats per minute and irregular, with an apical–radial difference of 8, the patient may be having digitalis-induced PVCs. If the HR was 65 beats per minute and regular before the previous dose and is currently 90 beats per minute and regular, the patient may have PAT with block, a digitalis-toxic rhythm. Likewise, if the HR was 90 and irregularly irregular (atrial fibrillation) and is currently 64 and regular, rather than having converted to NSR as the regularity and rate indicate, the patient may still be in atrial fibrillation, but with complete AV block and a

---

*Digitalization implies that a sufficient amount of digitalis has accumulated in the body to sustain a therapeutic level, and therefore, a therapeutic effect.

junctional pacemaker. This is another example of a digitalis-toxic rhythm. If the HR is less than 60 beats per minute, or if important changes in HR, rhythm, or conduction have occurred, always hold the drug until a complete 12-lead ECG can be taken, the physician consulted, and the diagnosis confirmed.

To ensure that therapeutic rather than toxic plasma levels of digitalis will be attained, several routine laboratory tests require close monitoring. The serum K^+ level should be kept in the upper limits of the normal range. As with any drug, know how it is eliminated from the body and monitor the laboratory tests reflecting that mechanism. For patients receiving digoxin, deslanoside, or ouabain, monitor the renal function tests (BUN, creatinine). In addition, liver function tests (SGOT, SGPT) should be monitored in patients receiving digitoxin. Patients in severe CHF or cardiogenic shock have decreased renal and hepatic blood flow. Watch carefully for development of hepatic impairment or prerenal azotemia in order to prevent digitalis toxicity from occurring. Monitor plasma digitalis levels when possible (Chap. 15).

Digitalized patients may have a decreased threshold for ventricular tachycardia, especially if hypokalemia is present. If electrical cardioversion is required, discontinue digoxin for 1 day, or digitoxin for 2 days, prior to the elective procedure. If this is impossible, it may be beneficial to precede the cardioversion with prophylactic lidocaine, phenytoin, or procainamide.[99] The serum K^+ should be carefully monitored and maintained at normal levels. For cardioversion of digitalized patients, current recommendations are to begin with 10 watt seconds and increase by increments of 5 to 10 watt-seconds to a maximum of 200 watt-seconds.[52]

The decision to use digitalis in the patient with acute MI is difficult. It frequently has little benefit in acute MI because the remaining healthy tissue is already maximally stimulated by catecholamines. Digitalis may be unevenly distributed in infarcted tissue. In animals with infarction, smaller than normal doses are required to produce ventricular fibrillation.[122] A compromised coronary circulation may be unable to provide the additional oxygen the digitalized myocardium may require. Furthermore, increased afterload may transiently follow rapid digitalization, putting additional strain on the damaged heart. However, in cases of cardiogenic shock, digitalis may be indicated.

Digitalis must be used with great caution in many cardiac conditions. In W–P–W syndrome, the effective refractory period of the anomolous AV bundle is decreased by digitalis although the drug increases the effective refractory period in the AV node. This may favor conduction in the anomolous tissue and, in the presence of atrial fibrillation, may result in a dangerously rapid ventricular response.[129]

In IHSS, digitalis may be used to treat CHF due to atrial fibrillation with rapid ventricular response. However, the obstructive gradient can be increased with digitalis and the hemodynamic problems exacerbated.

The use of digitalis in AV block or sick sinus syndrome may increase the block or cause asystole. Hypothyroid individuals require less digoxin because the excretion rate is reduced and blood levels are higher.

Before discharge, patients should understand that digitalis will be a long-term therapy. They must know the need for daily administration, but may choose the time of day most suitable to them for taking it. The patient (or a family member) should be taught to count the pulse rate for a full minute, and must understand the importance of notifying the physician or nurse if the pulse rate is less than 60 beats per minute or if there is an important change in rate or rhythm. To prevent the hypokalemia and resultant digitalis toxicity, encourage patients (without renal disease) to maintain high K^+ food intake. Table 37-6 lists foods high in K^+

Glucagon, U.S.P.

Glucagon, a naturally occuring peptide hormone produced by the pancreas, is a hormone of starvation. It promotes fuel mobilization: glycogen, amino acids, and fat breakdown is increased, as are blood glucose levels. It stimulates release of insulin, thyroid hormone, catecholamines, and other hormones. It is not clearly understood which effects of the drug are direct and which are secondary to the altered hormonal state.

Action. Glucagon increases the HR and force of contraction in the normal and acutely failing myocardium; it is ineffective in the chronically failing heart. Myocardial oxygen consumption is not inordinately increased with glucagon. Systemic vascular resistance is decreased and, fortuitously, renal blood flow is increased.[67]

Glucagon is not arrhythmogenic; in some cases it appears to have antiarrhythmic activity. It increases sinus discharge rate, and decreases the number of ectopic impulses by driving the heart at a faster rate. It increases AV nodal conduction velocity.[79]

Elimination. Glucagon undergoes degradation in the liver and kidney and in the plasma at its receptor sites. It is also destroyed by enzymes.[75]

Indications and Contraindications. Glucagon is a cardiotonic agent which is currently used infrequently. It may be indicated in low cardiac output states of acute onset.[94] Its most important therapeutic uses in the cardiac patient are in acute CHF and in low cardiac output states following open heart surgery.[95,125] It is useful in treatment of the low CO which is associated with toxic β-adrenergic blockade (propranolol or practolol).[81] Glucagon is recommended in therapy of cardiogenic shock if additional positive inotropic action is required following volume replacement and catecholamine and digitalis administration.[43] It can be effectively used in conjunction with counterpulsation devices. Glucagon is ineffective in, and not recommended for, chronic CHF. Its primary uses, unrelated to cardiac patients, are to counteract severe hypoglycemic reactions in diabetics and to reverse the insulin shock used in treatment of psychiatric patients. Glucagon is contraindicated in patients with known hypersensitivity.

Nursing Implications. Make certain that the glucagon is completely dissolved before administering it. If giving an IV injection, administer the drug slowly (1 ml/minute). Glucagon is very acidic (pH 2.5–3.0)[41] and is, therefore, very irritating to tissues; care must be taken that extravasation does not occur. Record baseline vital signs and a rhythm strip before beginning. Monitor the ECG continuously during the infusion, particularly for signs of ischemia.

Although the increase in myocardial O_2 consumption is not inordinate with glucagon, even the small increases associated with its positive inotropic and chronotropic action may be intolerable to the critically ill heart patient. One study reports evidence of ischemia (angina, depressed ST segment, T-wave inversion) associated with administration of this drug.[68]

Glucagon alters electrolyte distribution. It significantly lowers serum K^+ concentration; this may be arrhythmogenic or may alter the response of the heart to antiarrhythmic drugs. Hypocalcemia also has been reported. Draw baseline electrolytes before giving glucagon and again within several hours of administration.

Hyperglycemia commonly follows glucagon administration. It should be given with caution in known diabetics or in those patients whose blood glucose is elevated as a response to the stress of illness and hospitalization. Baseline blood glucose should be obtained before giving the drug, and periodically as indicated thereafter. Urine tests for sugar and acetone should be done every 6 hours daily. Glucagon decreases gastrointestinal motility. Reports of nausea and vomiting are common. A clear or full liquid diet may be tolerated better than a regular meal and should be ordered, if indicated.

REFERENCES

1. Arnsdorf, MF, Hsieh Y–Y: Antiarrhythmic agents. In Hurst JW, Logue RB, Schlant RC et al (eds): The Heart, 4th ed, pp 1943–1963. New York, McGraw-Hill, 1978
2. Atkinson AJ, Lee WK, Quinn ML et al: Dose-ranging of N-acetylprocaine amide in patients with premature ventricular contractions. Clin Pharmacol Ther 21:575–587, 1977
3. Bacaner MB: Bretylium tosylate for suppression of induced ventricular fibrillation. Am J Cardiol 17:528–534, 1966
4. Bacaner MB: Quantitative comparison of bretylium with other antifibrillatory drugs. Am J Cardiol 21:504–512, 1968
5. Bacaner MB, Schrienemachers D: Bretylium tosylate for suppression of ventricular fibrillation after experimental myocardial infarction. Nature 220:494–496, 1968
6. Bacaner MB, Schrienemachers D, Visscher MB: Effect of bretylium tosylate on ventricular fibrillation threshold. Arch Intern Med 124:95–100, 1969
7. Benaim ME. Letter to the Editor: Asystole after verapamil. Br Med J 2:169–170, 1972
8. Bernstein JC, Koch-Weser J: Effectiveness of bretylium tosylate against refractory ventricular arrhythmias. Circulation 45:1024–1034, 1972
9. Bigger JT Jr, Heissenbuttal RH: The use of procaine amide and lidocaine in the treatment of cardiac arrhythmias. In Friedberg CK (ed): Current Status of Drugs in Cardiovascular Disease, pp 125–144. New York: Grune & Stratton, 1969
10. Bigger JT Jr, Jaffe CC: The effect of bretylium tosylate on the electrophysiologic properties of ventricular muscle and Purkinje fibers. Am J Cardiol 27:82–92, 1971
11. Bigger, JT Jr, Giardina EGV: The pharmacology and clinical use of lidocaine and procaine amide. Medical College of Virginia Q 9:65–76, 1973
12. Braunwald E, Bloodwell RD, Goldberg LI et al: Studies on digitalis preparations on the contractility of the nonfailing heart and on total vascular resistance. J Clin Invest 40:52–59, 1961
13. Buckley JJ, Bosch OK, Bacaner MB: Prevention of ventricular fibrillation during hypothermia with bretylium tosylate. Anesth Anal 50:587–593, 1971
14. Caracta, AR, Damato AN, Josephson ME et al: Electrophysiologic properties of diphenylhydantoin. Circulation 47:1234–1241, 1973
15. Cardinal R Sasyniuk BI: Electrophysiologic effects of bretylium tosylate on subendocardial Purkinje fibers from infarcted canine hearts. J Pharmacol Exper Ther 204:159–174, 1978
16. Carrasco HA, Fuenmayor A, Barboza JS et al: Effect of verapamil on sinoatrial function and on sick sinus syndrome. Am Heart J 96:760–771, 1978
17. Chang TO, Wadhwa K: Sinus standstill following intravenous lidocaine administration. JAMA 223:790–792,1973
18. Chopra MP, Thadani U, Portal RW et al: Lidocaine therapy for ventricular ectopic activity after acute myocardial infarction: A double-blind trial. Br Med J 3:668–670, 1971
19. Cohen HC, Gozo EG, Langendorf R et al: Response of resistant ventricular tachycardia to bretylium. Circulation 47:331–340, 1973
20. Cooper JA, Frieden J: Bretylium tosylate. Am Heart J 32:703–706, 1971
21. Cooper MJ, Abinader EG: Atropine-induced ventricular fibrillation: Case report and review of the literature. Am Heart J 97:225–228, 1979
22. Couthamel WG: The effect of congestive heart failure on quinidine pharmacokinetics. Am Heart J 90:335–339, 1975
23. Danahy DT, Aronow WS: Lidocaine-induced cardiac rate changes in atrial fibrillation and atrial flutter. Am Heart J 95:474–482, 1978
24. Danilo P Jr, Rosen MR: Cardiac effects of disopyramide. Am Heart J 92:532–536, 1976
25. Data JL Jr, Wilkinson GR, Nies AS: Interaction of quinidine with anticonvulsive drugs. N Engl J Med 294:699–702, 1976
26. Dauchot P, Gravenstein JS: Bradycardia after myocardial infarction and its treatment with atropine. Anesthesiology 44:501–518, 1976
27. Day HW, Bacaner M: Use of bretylium tosylate in the management of acute myocardial infarction, Am J Cardiol 27:177–189, 1971
28. Doering W: Quinidine-digoxin interactions. N Engl J Med 301:400–404, 1979
29. Doherty JE, Kane JJ: Clinical pharmacology of digitalis glycosides. Ann Rev Med 26:159–171, 1975
30. Drayer DE, Lowenthal DT, Restivo KM et al: Steady-state serum levels of quinidine and active metabolites in cardiac patients with varying degrees of renal function. Clin Pharmacol Ther 24:31–39, 1978
31. Dreifus LS, Filip Z, Sexton DM et al: Electrophysiological and clinical effects of a new antiarrhythmic agent: Disopyramide (abstr). Am J Cardiol 31:129, 1973
32. Eddy JD, Singh SP: Treatment of cardiac arrhythmias with phenytoin. Br Med J 4:270–273, 1976
33. Effects of systemic drugs with anticholinergic properties on glaucoma. Med Lett Drugs Ther 16:28, 1974
34. Ejvinsson G: Effect of quinidine on plasma concentrations of digoxin. Br Med J 1:279–280, 1978
35. Ewy GA, Groves BM, Ball NF et al: Digoxin metabolism in obesity. Circulation 44:810–814, 1971
36. Frieden H, Cooper JA, Grossman JI: Continuous infusion of edrophonium (Tensilon) in treating ventricular arrhythmias. Am J Cardiol 27:294–297, 1971
37. Gianelly R, Von der Groeben JD, Spivack AP et al: Effect of lidocaine on ventricular arrhythmias in patients with coronary heart disease. N Engl J Med 277:1215–1219, 1967
38. Giardina EV, Heissenbuttal RH, Bigger JT Jr: Intermittent intravenous procainamide to treat ventricular arrhythmias. Ann Intern Med 78:183–193, 1973
39. Gillis RA, McClellan JR, Sauer TS et al: Depression of the cardiac sympathetic nerve activity in diphenylhydantoin. J Pharmacol Exper Ther 179:599–610, 1971
40. Goldberg LI, Hsieh Y-Y: Drugs acting on the autonomic nervous system. In Hurst JW, Logue RB, Schlant RC et al (eds): The Heart, 4th ed, pp 1981–1987 New York, McGraw-Hill, 1978
41. Goldstein B: Guidelines to drug incompatibilities in large volume parenterals. Nurses' Drug Alert 4(8):57–60, 1980

42. Greenblatt DJ, Pfeifer HS, Rochs H et al: Pharmacokinetics of quinidine in humans after intravenous, intramuscular and oral administration. J Pharmacol Exper Ther 202:365–378, 1977

43. Gunnar RM, Loeb HS: Use of drugs in cardiogenic shock due to myocardial infarction. Circulation 45:1111–1124, 1972

44. Gupta PK, Lichstein, E, Chadda KD: "Lidocaine-induced heart block in patients with bundle branch block. Am J Cardiol 33:487–492, 1974

45. Hager WD, Fenster P, Mayersohn M et al: Digoxin-quinidine interaction. N Engl J Med 300:1238–1240, 1979

46. Haworth E, Burroughs AK: Disopyramide and warfarin interaction. Br Med J 2:866–867, 1977

47. Helfant RH, Seuffert GW, Patton RD et al: The clinical use of diphenylhydantoin (Dilantin) in the treatment and prevention of cardiac arrhythmias. Am Heart J 77:315–323, 1969

48. Heng MK, Singh BN, Roche AHB et al: Effects of intravenous verapamil on the electrocardiogram. Am Heart J 90 (4): 487–498, 1975

49. Hoffman BF, Rosen MR, Wit AL: Electrophysiology and pharmacology of cardiac arrhythmias VII. Cardiac effects of quinidine and procaine amide. A. Am Heart J 89:804–808, 1975

50. Hoffman BF, Rosen MR, Wit AL: Electrophysiology and pharmacology of cardiac arrhythmias VII. Cardiac effects of quinidine and procaine amide. B. Am Heart J 90:117–122, 1975

51. Hsieh Y–Y, Arnsdorf MF, Goldberg LI: Pharmacology of cardiovascular drugs: Antiarrhythmic agents. In Hurst JW, Logue RB, Schlant RC et al (eds): The Heart, 4th ed, p 1942. New York, McGraw-Hill 1978

52. Hsieh YY, Goldberg LI, Arnsdorf MF: Pharmacology of cardiovascular drugs: Cardiac glycosides, theophylline, morphine, and vasodilators, Hurst JW, Logue RB, Schlant RC et al (eds): The Heart, 4th ed, pp 1964–1980. New York, McGraw-Hill 1978

53. Innes IR, Nickerson M: Atropine, scopalamine and related antimuscarinic drugs. Goodman LS, Gilman A. (eds): The Pharmacological Basis of Therapeutics, 5th ed, pp 514–532. New York, Macmillan, 1975

54. Jewitt DE: Limitations of present drug therapy of cardiac arrhythmias: A review. Postgrad Med J (Suppl 1) 53:12–21, 1977

55. Josephson ME, Caracta AR, Lau SH et al: Effects of lidocaine on refractory periods in man. Am Heart J 84:778–786, 1972

56. Karlin JM, Kutt H: Acute diphenylhydantoin intoxication following halothane anesthesia. J Pediatr 76:941–944, 1970

57. Katz AM: Cardiac action potential. Physiology of the Heart, pp. 229–256. New York, Raven Press, 1977

58. Kessler KM, Lowenthal DT, Warner H et al: Quinidine elimination in patients with congestive heart failure or poor renal function. N Engl J Med 290:706–709, 1974

59. Kirpekar SM, Furchgott RF: The sympathomimetic action of bretylium on isolated atria and aortic smooth muscle. J Pharmacol Exper Ther 143:64–76, 1964

60. Knifien FJ, Lomas TE, Counsell RE et al: The antiarrhythmic and antifibrillatory actions of bretylium and its o-iodobenzyl trimethyl-ammonium analog UM-360. J Pharmacol Exper Ther 192 : 120–128, 1975

61. Knoebel SB, McHenry PL, Phillips JF et al: Atropine-induced cardioacceleration and myocardial blood flow in subjects with and without coronary artery disease. Am J Cardiol 33:327–332, 1974

62. Koch NG, Roding B, Hahnloser P et al: The effect of glucagon on hepatic blood flow. Arch Surg 100:147–149, 1970

63. Koch-Weser J: Drug therapy: Bretylium. N Engl J Med 300(9):473–477, 1979

64. Koch-Weser J: Drug interactions in cardiovascular therapy. Am Heart J 90:93–116, 1975

65. Koch-Weser J: Hemorrhagic reactions and drug interactions in 500 warfarin-treated patients. Clin Pharmacol Ther 14:139, 1973

66. Koch-Weser J: Potentiation by glucagon of the hypoprothrombinemic action of warfarin. Ann Intern Med 72:331–335, 1970

67. Kones RJ: Cardiogenic Shock, Mt. Kisco, Futura Publishing Co, 1974

68. Kones RJ, Phillips JH: Glucagon in congestive heart failure. Chest 59:392–397, 1971

69. Krikler D: Verapamil in cardiology. Eur J Cardiol 2(1):3–10, 1974

70. Krikler DM, Curry PVL: Torsade de pointes, an atypical ventricular tachycardia. Br Heart J 38:117–120, 1976

71. Krikler DM, Spurrell RAJ: Verapamil in treatment of paroxysmal supraventricular tachycardia. Postgrad Med J 50:447–453, 1974

72. Kuman C, Hamer J: Anti-arrhythmic drugs. In Hamer J (ed) Drugs for Heart Disease, pp 44 –147. Chicago, Yearbook Medical Publishers, 1979

73. Kuntzman R, Tsai I, Chang R et al: Disposition of bretylium in man and rat: A sensitive chemical method for its estimation in plasma and urine. Clin Pharmacol Ther 11:829–837, 1970

74. Kutt H: Biochemical and genetic factors regulating Dilantin metabolism in man. Ann N Y Acad Sci 179:704–722, 1971

75. Larner J, Haynes RC Jr: Insulin and oral hypoglycemic drugs: Glucagon. In Goodman LS, Gilman A (eds): Pharmacological Basis of Therapeutics, 5th ed, pp 1507–1533. New York, Macmillan, 1975

76. LeLoner J, Gremon D, Labon Y et al: Pharmacokinetics of lidocaine following prolonged intravenous infusion in uncomplicated myocardial infarction. Ann Intern Med 87:700–702, 1977

77. Less JP Jr, Jenesaty RM, Nakhoul J: Letter to Editor: Lidocaine in ventricular arrhythmia. Am Heart J 86:143, 1973

78. Lie KI, Wellens HS, Capelle FJV et al: Lidocaine in the prevention of primary ventricular fibrillation. N Engl J Med 291:1324–1326, 1974

79. Lipski JI, Kaminsky DM, Donoso E et al: The electrophysiological effects of glucagon on the normal canine heart. Am J Physiol 222:1107–1112, 1972

80. Livesley B, Catley PF, Campbell RC et al: Double-blind evaluation of verapamil, propranolol, and isorbide dinitrate against a placebo in the treatment of angina pectoris. Br Med J 1:375–378, 1973

81. Lvoff R, Wilkin DEL: Glucagon in heart failure and in cardiogenic shock. Circulation 45:534–542, 1972

82. Markis JE, Koch-Weser J: Characteristics and mechanisms of inotropic and chronotropic actions of bretylium tosylate. J Pharmacol Exper Ther 178:94–102, 1971

83. Marriott HJL, Bieza CF: Alarming ventricular acceleration after lidocaine administration. Chest 61:682–683, 1972

84. Mason DT, Zelis R, Lee G et al: Current concepts and treatment of digitalis toxicity. Am J Cardiol 27:546–559, 1971

85. Massey K: Teratogenic effects of diphenylhydantoin sodium. J Oral Ther Pharmacol 2:380–385, 1966

86. Massumi RA: Ventricular fibrillation and tachycardia after intravenous atropine for treatment of bradycardias. N Engl J Med 287:336–338, 1972

87. Mathur PP: Cardiovascular effects of a newer antiarrhythmic agent, disopyramide phosphate. Am Heart J 84:764–770, 1972

88. Mercer EN, Osborn JA: The current status of diphenylhydantoin in heart disease. Ann Intern Med 67:1084–1107, 1967

89. Moe GK, Farah AE: Digitalis and allied cardiac glycosides. In Goodman LS, Gilman A (eds): Pharmacological Basis of Therapeutics, 5th ed, pp 653–682. New York, Macmillan, 1975

90. Moyer RR: Verapamil: An antianginal agent. Minn Medicine 55:1043–1045, 1972

91. Murtagh JG, Binnion PF, Lal S: Haemodynamic effects of glucagon. Br Heart J 32:307–315, 1970

92. Neeld JB, Allen AT, Coleman E et al: Cardiac rate and rhythm changes with atropine and methscopalamine. Clin Pharmacol Ther 17:290–295, 1975

93. Nicholson WJ, Martin CE, Gracey JG et al: Disopyramide induced ventricular fibrillation. Am J Cardiol 43(5):1053–1055, 1979

94. Parmley WW, Glick G, Sonnenblick EH: Cardiovascular effects of glucagon in man. N Engl J Med 279:12–17, 1968

95. Parmley WW, Matloff JM, Sonnenblick EH: Hemodynamic

effects of glucagon in patients following prosthetic valve replacement. Circulation (Suppl 1)39:163–176, 1969

96. Pick A: Manifestations of a vulnerable phase in human heart. In Surawicz B, Pellegrino ED (eds): Sudden Cardiac Death, pp 44–49. New York, Grune & Stratton, 1964

97. Podrid PJ, Schoeneberger A, Lown B: Congestive heart failure caused by oral disopyramide. N Engl J Med 302(11):614–617, 1980

98. Reimer KA, Lower JE, Jennings RB: Effect of the calcium antagonist verapamil on necrosis following temporary coronary artery occlusion in dogs. Circulation 55:581–584, 1977

99. Resnekov L: Drug therapy before and after the electroversion of cardiac dysrhythmias. Prog Cardiovasc Dis 16:531–538, 1974

100. Richman S: Adverse effect of atropine during myocardial infarction. Enhancement of ischemia following intravenously administered atropine. JAMA 228:1414–1416, 1974

101. Romhilt DW, Bloomfield SS, Lipicky RJ et al: Evaluation of bretylium tosylate for the treatment of premature ventricular contractions. Circulation 45:800–807, 1972

102. Rosen KM, Lau SH, Weiss MB et al: The effect of lidocaine on atrioventricular and intraventricular conduction in man. Am J Cardiol 25:1–5, 1970

103. Rosen KM, Barwolf C, Ehsani A et al: Effects of lidocaine and propranolol on the normal and anomalous pathways in patients with preexcitation. Am J Cardiol 30:801–809, 1972

104. Rosen M, Gelband H, Merker C et al: Effects of procaine amide on the electrophysiologic properties of the canine ventricular conducting system. J Pharmacol Exper Ther 185:438–446, 1973

105. Rosen M, Lisak R, Rubin JL: Diphenylhydantoin in cardiac arrhythmias. Am J Cardiol 20:674–678, 1967

106. Rosen MR, Hoffman BF, Wit AL: Electrophysiology and pharmacology of cardiac arrhythmias V: Cardiac antiarrhythmic effects of lidocaine. Am Heart J 89:526–536, 1975

107. Rosen M, Wit AL, Hoffman BF: Electrophysiology and pharmacology of cardiac arrhythmias IV: Cardiac antiarrhythmic and toxic effects of digitalis. Am Heart J 89:391–399, 1975

108. Rosen M, Wit AL, Hoffman BF: Electrophysiology and pharmacology of cardiac arrhythmias, VI: Cardiac effects of verapamil. Am Heart J 89:665–673, 1975

109. Rossen RM, Krikorian J, Hancock EW: Ventricular asystole after edrophonium chloride administration. JAMA 235(10): 1041–1042, 1976

110. Rumack BH, Wolfe R, Gelfrich H: Phenytoin (diphenylhydantoin) treatment of massive digoxin overdose. Br Heart J 36:405, 1974

111. Sacks H, Kennelly BM: Verapamil in cardiac arrhythmias. Br Med J 2:716, 1972

112. Sandler G, Clayton GA, Thornicroft SC: Clinical evaluation of angina pectoris. Br Med J 3:224–227, 1968

113. Sanna G, Ancidiacono R: Chemical ventricular defibrillation of the human heart with bretylium tosylate. Am J Cardiol 32:982–987, 1973

114. Sasyniuk BI, Dresel PE: The effects of diphenylhydantoin on conduction in isolated blood-perfused dog hearts. J Pharmacol Exper Ther 161:191–196, 1968

115. Schamroth L: Immediate effects of intravenous verapamil on atrial fibrillation. Cardiovasc Res 5(4):419–424, 1971

116. Schamroth L, Krikler DM, Garrett C: Immediate effects of intravenous verapamil in cardiac arrhythmias. Br Med J 1:660–662, 1972

117. Schomerus M, Spiegelhalder B, Stieren B et al: Physiological disposition of verapamil in man, Cardiovasc Res 10:605–612, 1976

118. Singer DH, TenEick RE: Pharmacology of cardiac arrhythmias. Prog Cardiovasc Dis 11:488–514, 1969

119. Singh A, Singh P, Singh P: Oral use of low dosage schedule of Isoptin (verapamil) in cardiac arrhythmias. Indian J Med Sci 30:7–11, 1976

120. Smith TW, Hager T: Digitalis, Part 3. N Engl J Med 289:1063–1072, 1973

121. Smith WS: Clinical studies of Norpace, Part I. Angiology 26:124–131, 1975

122. Thompson AJ, Hargix J, Murphy ML et al: Tritiated digoxin: XX. Tissue distribution in experimental myocardial infarction. Am Heart J 88:319–324, 1974

123. Ueda CT, Hirschfield DS, Scheinman MM et al: Disposition kinetics of quinidine. Clin Pharmacol Ther 19:30–36, 1976

124. Unger AH, Sklaroff HJ: Fatalities following intravenous use of sodium diphenylhydantoin for cardiac arrhythmias: Report of 2 cases. JAMA 200:335–336, 1967

125. Vaughn CC, Warner HR, Nelson RM: Cardiovascular effects of glucagon following cardiac surgery. Surgery 67:204–211, 1970

126. Vaughnan-Neil EF, Snell NJC, Bevan G: Letter: Hypotension after verapamil. Br Med J 2:529, 1972

127. Watanabe L, Dreifus LS: Cardiac Arrhythmias: Electrophysiologic Basis for Clinical Interpretation, New York, Grune & Stratton, 1977

128. Waxman MB, Wallace AG: Electrophysiologic effects of bretylium tosylate on the heart. J Pharmacol Exper Ther 183:264–274, 1972

129. Wellens HJ, Durrer D: Effect of digitalis on atrioventricular conduction and circus movement tachycardias in patients with Wolff–Parkinson–White Syndrome. Circulation 47:1229–1233, 1973

130. Wellens HJ, Durrer D: Effect of procaine amide, quinidine, and ajamaline in the Wolff–Parkinson–White Syndrome. Circulation 50:114–120, 1974

131. White RD: Essential drugs in emergency cardiac care. Advanced Cardiac Life Support. Dallas, American Heart Association, 1975

132. WHO/ICS Task Force: Definitions of terms related to cardiac rhythm. Am Heart J 95:796–806, 1978

133. Wilensky AJ, Lowden JA: Inadequate serum levels after intramuscular administration of diphenylhydantoin. Neurology 23:318–324, 1973

134. Wit AL, Rosen MR, Hoffman BF: Electrophysiology and pharmacology of cardiac arrhythmias. II. Relationship of normal and abnormal electrical activity of cardiac fibers to the genesis of arrhythmias. A. Automaticity. Am Heart J 88:515–524, 1974

135. Wit AL, Rosen MR, Hoffman BF: Electrophysiology and pharmacology of cardiac arrhythmias. II. Relationship of normal and abnormal electrical activity of cardiac fibers to the genesis of arrhythmias. B. Reentry. Section I; B. Reentry. Section II. Am Heart J 88:664–670, 798–806, 1974

136. Wit AL, Rosen MR, Hoffman BF: Electrophysiology and pharmacology of cardiac arrhythmias. VIII. Cardiac effects of diphenylhydantoin. A. Am Heart J 90:265–272, 1975

137. Wit AL, Rosen MR, Hoffman BF: Electrophysiology and pharmacology of cardiac arrhythmias. VIII. Cardiac effects of diphenylhydantoin. B. Am Heart J 90:397–404, 1975

138. Wit AL, Steiner C, Damato AN: Electrophysiologic effects of bretylium tosylate on single fibers of the canine specialized conducting system and ventricle. J Pharmacol Exper Ther 173:344–356, 1970

139. Woosley RL, Shand DG: Pharmacokinetics of antiarrhythmic drugs. Am J Cardiol 41:986–995, 1978

ADDITIONAL READING

Befeler B, Casellanos A, Wells DE et al: Electrophysiologic effects of the antiarrhythmic agent disopyramide phosphate. Am J Cardiol 35:282–287, 1975

Holder DA, Sniderman AD, Fraser G et al: Experience with bretylium tosylate by a hospital cardiac arrest team. Circulation 55:541–544, 1977

Kutt H, Winters W, Scherman R et al: Diphenylhydantoin and phenobarbital toxicity: The role of liver disease. Arch Neurol 11:649–656, 1964

Naylor WG, Krikler D: Verapamil and the myocardium. Postgrad Med J 50:441–446, 1974

Sacks H, Kennelly BM: Letter. Verapamil in cardiac arrhythmias. Br Med J 2:716, 1972

35

Drugs that Affect the Sympathetic Nervous System

LINDA ANN FELTHOUS, B.S. in Pharm.

and

SANDRA L. UNDERHILL, R.N., M.N.

The drugs affecting the sympathetic nervous system are divided into two categories: the sympathomimetic amines, or those that stimulate the adrenergic receptor sites, and the sympatholytic agents, or those that block the adrenergic receptor sites. The term catecholamine refers to any amine (such as epinephrine, norepinephrine, dopamine, or serotonin) that functions as a hormone or neurotransmitter.

SYMPATHOMIMETIC AMINES

Sympathomimetic amines simulate the effects of sympathetic nerve stimulation. Their effects depend upon the action of the adrenergic receptor sites stimulated. There are three types of receptors: alpha (α) adrenergic, beta (β) adrenergic, and dopaminergic. Alpha adrenergic receptors reside primarily in the resistance vessels of the skin, mucosa, intestine, and kidney. Drugs that stimulate α receptors produce vasoconstriction of these vascular beds. There appear to be two types of beta adrenergic receptors: β_1 and β_2. Stimulation of β_1 receptors increases cardiac contractility and heart rate (HR), and accelerates atrioventricular (AV) conduction. Beta$_2$ effects include bronchial relaxation and vasodilation in peripheral arterioles, especially in skeletal muscle. Dopamine receptors promote vasodilation in the renal and mesenteric vascular beds.

Sympathomimetic amines administered for their cardiovascular effects include epinephrine hydrochloride, levarterenol bitartrate (norepinephrine), isoproterenol hydrochloride, dopamine hydrochloride, epinephrine sulfate, mephentermine sulfate, metaraminol bitartrate, phenylephrine hydrochloride, methoxamine hydrochloride, and dobutamine hydrochloride. These agents act directly or indirectly to release norepinephrine from tissue stores (see Table 35-1).

Sympathomimetic amines are sold as over-the-counter preparations as cold and allergy products, including topical decongestants, and as allergy products. Table 37-3 lists some commonly used over-the-counter drugs containing sympathomimetic amines.

Sympathomimetic amines also affect the central nervous system (CNS). They have been used as appetite depressants, in conjunction with calorie restricted diets, for the treatment of obesity. However, the most commonly used agents, dextroamphetamine sulfate (Dexedrine) and methamphetamine hydrochloride (Desoxyn) have a high potential for drug abuse and are less frequently prescribed. Other uses of the CNS effects of sympathomimetic amines include the treatment of narcolepsy, parkinsonism, depressant-drug poisoning, psychogenic disorders, hyperkinetic syndrome, epilepsy, and fatigue. Although the CNS effects of sympathomimetic amines will not be discussed further, nurses should be aware of the cardiovascular effects that can be demonstrated by users or abusers of these drugs.[17] Actions, indications, contraindications, and nursing implications are described for each sympathomimetic amine. See Table 35-2 for specific information about dosage, administration, and toxic effects of each.

Epinephrine Hydrochloride (Adrenalin)

Epinephrine stimulates the β_1 receptors of the heart and both α and β_2 receptors in the peripheral vessels. In small doses, the primary effect is on the β_2 receptors, producing dilation of arterial vessels in skeletal muscle and the mesentery, which may lower blood pressure (BP). However, large doses stimulate the α receptors, producing an elevated BP.

Epinephrine increases BP because of vasoconstriction and a positive inotropic effect. A powerful cardiac stimulant, epinephrine acts directly on the β_1 receptors of the myocardium and on pacemaker and conduction tissues. The result is increased HR, cardiac output (CO), heart work and myocardial oxygen consumption ($\dot{M}VO_2$), and a decreased cardiac efficiency (work done relative to oxygen consumption). Epinephrine relaxes bronchial smooth muscle to produce bronchial dilation. Total peripheral vascular resistance (PVR) decreases by action of epinephrine on β receptors of the skeletal muscles, and blood flow is therefore enhanced.

The pharmacologic actions of epinephrine are terminated primarily by reuptake and metabolism in the sympathetic nerve endings. The circulating drug is metabolized in the liver and other tissues. Only a small amount is excreted unchanged.

Indications and Contraindications. Epinephrine is used to relieve bronchospasm associated with anaphylaxis, asthma, and hypersensitivity reactions. Its cardiac effects are useful in restoring cardiac rhythm and enhancing cardiac tone. An increase in cardiac tone is useful for converting "fine" ventricular fibrillation into "coarse" ventricular fibrillation prior to an attempt at defibrillation. Epinephrine is also used to treat asystole and complete heart block, although if indications are of the latter, isoproterenol is preferred.[10]

Epinephrine is a topical hemostatic on bleeding surfaces. When added to solutions of local anesthetics used for infiltration, epinephrine decreases the potential for systemic toxicity and increases the duration of action of the anesthetic through its vasoconstrictor effect. Contraindications to the use of epinephrine include narrow angle glaucoma, general anesthesia with halogenated hydrocarbons or cyclopropane, organic brain disease, cardiogenic hemorrhage, and traumatic shock.

Nursing Implications. Always correct acidosis with sodium bicarbonate, ventilation or both, prior to giving epinephrine, because epinephrine is less effective in an acidic milieu. Epinephrine is chemically and physically incompatible with many drugs, including, but not limited to, aminophylline, phenytoin, sodium bicarbonate, and calcium. Administer it with caution to elderly people and to patients with high blood pressure, diabetes mellitus, hyperthyroidism, psychoneurosis, or long-standing bronchial asthma and emphysema who have developed cor pulmonale.

During a cardiac arrest, epinephrine may be administered intravenously, directly into the tracheobronchial tree, or as an intracardiac (IC) injection. There are many hazards associated with any drug given as an IC injection: interruption of cardiopulmonary resuscitation, cardiac tamponade, coronary artery laceration, pneumothorax, and intramy-

TABLE 35-1 CLASSIFICATION OF SYMPATHOMIMETIC AMINES

Agent	Receptor Site Stimulated
Epinephrine hydrochloride (Adrenalin)	β_1 β_2 (small doses) α (large doses)
Levarterenol bitartrate (Norepinephrine; Levophed)	α β_1
Isoproterenol hydrochloride (Isuprel)	β_1 β_2
Dopamine hydrochloride (Intropin)	β_1 (small doses) α (large doses) dopaminergic
Ephedrine sulfate, U.S.P.	α β_1 β_2
Mephentermine sulfate (Wyamine)	α β_1
Metaraminol bitartrate (Aramine)	α β_1
Phenylephrine hydrochloride (Neo-Synephrine)	α
Methoxamine hydrochloride (Vasoxyl)	α
Dobutamine hydrochloride (Dobutrex)	β_1 β_2 (slight) α (slight)

ocardial injection. Intramyocardial epinephrine may produce intractable ventricular fibrillation. Therefore, IC epinephrine should be avoided.

Intravenous epinephrine must be used with extreme caution in the presence of ventricular arrhythmias because of its excitatory action on the heart. Potentially fatal ventricular arrhythmias including fibrillation can occur, especially in patients with organic heart disease or those receiving drugs that sensitize the heart to arrhythmias, such as digitalis. Do not administer epinephrine simultaneously with isoproterenol because their combined action may cause serious cardiac arrhythmias. The two drugs may, however, be administered alternately when the preceding effect of either drug has subsided. Epinephrine may precipitate or aggravate angina pectoris in patients with ischemic heart disease by increasing myocardial oxygen consumption.

The effects of epinephrine can be potentiated by tricyclic antidepressants, such as amitriptyline and imipramine, by certain antihistamines, such as diphenhydramine and tripelennamine, and by sodium 1-thyroxin. The pressor effect of epinephrine may be markedly potentiated in patients receiving monoamine oxidase (MAO) inhibitors. In patients who receive repeated intramuscular (IM) injections, observe the infusion site for necrosis from vascular constriction. Absorption of epinephrine from subcutaneous sites can be increased by briskly massaging the injection site. Forewarn the alert patient that he may experience some uncomfortable side effects.

Levarterenol Bitartrate (Norepinephrine; Levophed)

Levarterenol has both α and β_1 effects. The α effect, which is less potent than that of epinephrine, produces vasoconstriction, resulting in decreased blood flow to the skin, skeletal muscle, and all vital organs except the heart and

(Text continues on p. 470.)

TABLE 35-2 SYMPATHOMIMETIC AMINES

Agent	Dosage and Administration	Side and Toxic Effects
Epinephrine hydrochloride (Adrenalin)	Not effective orally as it is destroyed in the GI tract. Deteriorates in a few hours when diluted. Should be clear; discard if colored. During a cardiac arrest, give IV, directly into the tracheobronchial tree, or as an IC injection. However, because of the hazards associated with IC use, either the IV or tracheobronchial routes are preferred. Adult dose: 0.5 mg (5 ml of a 1:10,000 solution), which may be repeated at 5-minute intervals, if necessary. In children: maximum dose is 0.1 ml per kg of a 1:10,000 solution.[30] Peak effect in 1–2 minutes; duration 3–5 minutes. SC or IM in adults: 0.2–1.0 ml of 1:1000 aqueous solution. In children, 10 μg, or 0.01 ml of 1:1000 solution, per kg body weight SC. Start with small doses and increase if required. IM absorption is more rapid than SC. SC produces bronchodilation in 5–10 minutes, with maximal effects in 20 minutes.	Minor and transient side effects of fear, anxiety, tenseness, restlessness, throbbing headache, tremor, weakness, dizziness, pallor, and palpitations with therapeutic doses. These effects rapidly subside with rest, quiet, recumbancy, and reassurance. Hyperthyroid and hypertensive patients are especially susceptible to the untoward pressor effects of this drug. In psychoneurotic patients, existing symptoms may be aggravated. Large IV doses may cause cerebral hemorrhage from a sharp rise in blood pressure. Can cause ventricular arrhythmias.
Levarterenol bitartrate (Norepinephrine; Levophed)	Distributed in 4-ml ampules of 1 mg levarterenol base per 1 ml. Dose is expressed in terms of base (2 mg of levarterenol bitartrate equals 1 mg of levarterenol base). Oxidizes readily and will gradually darken on exposure to light and air. Do not use if solution is brown or contains a precipitate. Destroyed in GI tract if orally ingested. Poorly absorbed from SC injection. Do not give as an IV push. Must be diluted prior to administration. Auxilliary infusions rarely used because the volume of fluid needed to correctly dilute the drug is too large. To mix an infusion drip, add 4 ml of 0.2% solution in 1000 ml D₅W or D₅S. The usual drip rate is 2–3 ml per minute initially, and should be titrated so that the systolic BP is raised to 90–120 mm Hg or CO measurements are adequate. Pressor effect is immediate and subsides minutes after infusion is discontinued. To mix a lavage, add 16 mg to 200 ml of normal saline (NS) and instill via a nasogastric tube.	Similar to those of epinephrine, but effects are usually minimal and less frequent: anxiety, insomnia, respiratory difficulty, restlessness, palpitations and transient headache. Overdoses, or regular doses in hypersensitive patients, such as those with hyperthyroidism, produce severe hypertension with violent headache, photophobia, stabbing retrosternal and pharyngeal pain, pallor, intense sweating, vomiting, cerebral hemorrhage, and convulsions. A decreased CO may be harmful to elderly patients or those with reduced cerebral or coronary flow. May cause bradycardia and potentially fatal arrhythmias, especially in patients with acute MI, hypoxemia or hypercapnea, or those receiving other drugs which increase myocardial irritability.
Isoproterenol hydrochloride (Isuprel)	Gradually darkens on exposure to air, light, and heat. Do not use if discoloration or precipitate is present. Avoid mixing with drugs that raise the *p*H above 6, such as sodium bicarbonate, because catecholamines are inactivated in alkaline solutions. Rapidly metabolized in the GI tract. Absorbed after injection or oral inhalation. Sublingual or rectal absorption is variable. Intravenous administration: IV push in extreme emergencies. Give 0.02-0.1 mg as IV or IC injection.[27] For auxilliary drips, add 1 ml of 1:5000 (0.2 mg) to 10 ml of NS or D₅W and inject over 15 minutes. For IV drip, add 1 mg to 500 ml D₅W (2 μg per ml) or 1 mg to 250 ml D₅W (4 μg per ml) and administer at a drip rate to maintain adequate ventricular rate (usually 60 beats per minute or less) or until ventricular ectopy occurs. Onset is immediate and lasts 2–3 minutes. Intracardiac administration: give 0.02–0.1 mg in extreme emergencies. SC dose is 0.2 mg every 3 hours. SL dose is 10–20 mg every 2–4 hours. For less urgent situations, 10–20 mg every 3–4 hours.[10]	Most side effects subside when drug is stopped or may abate while still in use. Nervousness, restlessness, insomnia, anxiety, tension, fear, or excitement may occur. Rarely, sweating, weakness, dizziness, mild tremor, headache, flushing, nausea, vomiting, tinnitus, light-headedness, or asthenia develop. Swelling of the parotid glands has been reported after prolonged use. Supraventricular tachycardia and ventricular arrhythmias, such as PVCs, tachycardia, and fibrillation may occur.[13] Ventricular arrhythmias are more likely to occur in patients with cardiogenic shock, acidosis, hypoxia, hypercapnea, hypokalemia, or hyperkalemia. Also more likely to occur if isoproterenol is given in conjunction with digitalis, cyclopropane, or halogenated hydrocarbon general anesthetics. Overdoses produce a slight increase in BP followed by a substantial decrease, resulting in shocklike signs and symptoms. Excess use by oral inhalation may result in decreased effectiveness. Severe paradoxic airway resistance in some patients, which does not respond until therapy withdrawn. Deaths have been reported from high doses of isoproterenol in aerosol form.
Dopamine hydrochloride (Intropin)	Do not give via IV push or auxilliary drip. Dilute before use by adding 1–2 ampules to 500 ml D₅W. Two ampules (400 mg) give a concentration of 800 μg per ml (the most frequently used). With IV administration, the onset of action occurs within 5 minutes and lasts minutes.[16,24] Begin the infusion at 2–5 μg per kg per minute and increase the rate 1–4 μg per kg per minute every 15–30 minutes up to 20–50 μg per kg per minute until the optimal effect, as measured by the BP, HR, CO, and urine flow is attained. Drug effect depends on dose and vascular bed. Aim for intermediate range. High doses result in α effects. Dose titration is extremely important and the patient response is variable. Monitor urine output and cardiac rhythm. Generally, if the pulse increases more than 15 beats per minute, the diastolic BP more than 15 mm Hg, and the systolic BP more than 30 mm Hg, decrease the infusion rate.	Most frequent side effects include ectopic beats, nausea and vomiting, tachycardia, angina, palpitations, dyspnea, headache, vasoconstriction, and dose-related hypotension and hypertension. Infrequently, widened QRS complex, aberrant conduction, bradycardia, piloerection, and azotemia develop. In case of accidental overdose, manifested by hypertension, reduce the rate of administration or temporarily discontinue the drug.

TABLE 35-2 SYMPATHOMIMETIC AMINES (Cont.)

Agent	Dosage and Administration	Side and Toxic Effects
Ephedrine sulfate, U.S.P.	Rapidly and completely absorbed after PO, IM, or SC administration. Pressor and cardiac response after IV, IM, or SC injection is 1 hour; after PO administration, response occurs in 4 hours. For direct IV administration, give 10–25 mg slowly. Parenteral adult dose should not exceed 150 mg in 24 hours. Usual adult PO dose is 25–50 mg; for SC or IM, the usual dose is 15–50 mg.	At therapeutic doses, headache, insomnia, palpitation, agitation, sweating, nausea and vomiting, and difficulty in voiding occur. Occasionally, precordial pain may occur. Higher doses can cause euphoria, confusion, delirium, and hallucinations. Acute urinary retention may be encountered in older patients with prostatic hypertrophy.
Mephentermine sulfate (Wyamine)	Store at 15–30°C. IM route: usual dose 10–80 mg; onset in 5–15 minutes; duration 1–2 hours. IV route: usual dose 20–60 mg; onset is immediate; duration is 15–30 minutes. Infusion rate is 1–5 mg per minute.	CNS-stimulating effects may cause nervousness, anxiety, weakness, and tachycardia. Arrhythmias, transient extrasystoles, AV block, and hypertension have occurred. Overdosage produces hallucinations, psychosis, and euphoria.
Metaraminol bitartrate (Aramine)	Must not be subjected to excessive heat or autoclaved. Protect from light. When diluted to 100 µg per ml, it is stable for 24 hours. It is incompatible with many other drugs. The onset of action of IV administration is 1–2 minutes, with a duration of 20 minutes. If injected IM, the onset is at 10 minutes and lasts 1 hour. When given SC, the onset is at 5–20 minutes, also lasting 1 hour. To prepare an infusion drip, dilute 15–100 mg in 500 ml NS or D_5W and administer to regulate pressures at 90–120 mm Hg systolic pressure. In emergency treatment of extreme shock, 250 µg up to 1 mg may be injected directly by IV push at 0.5 ml per minute.	Arrhythmias such as ventricular tachycardia and fibrillation may develop especially in patients with MI. Other reported reactions include hypertension, headache, flushing, sweating, tremors, dizziness, nausea, palpitations, apprehension, and when administration is stopped, hypotension. Overdosage may produce a sustained increase in BP and should be treated with 5–10 mg phentolamine IV.
Phenylephrine hydrochloride (Neo-Synephrine)	Administered for nasal congestion, 0.125, 0.25, 0.5, and 1.0% solution as a nasal spray. Since it is readily metabolized in the GI tract, it should be given parenterally when its cardiovascular effects are desired. If given IV, the onset is immediate and the duration is 15–20 minutes. The onset is 10–15 minutes when given either IM or SC, but the duration for IM is 30 minutes to 2 hours, compared with 50–60 minutes SC. For mild-to-moderate hypotension, the usual SC or IM dose is 2–5 mg, with a range of 1–10 mg. The usual IV dose is 0.2 mg, ranging from 0.1–0.5 mg. It is diluted to a 1:10 solution with sterile water for injection and given at 0.5 ml per minute. For severe hypotension and shock, an IV infusion is prepared by adding 10 mg to 500 ml NS of D_5W, giving a concentration of 1:50,000. This is infused at 100–180 drops per minute until the patient is stable, and then is maintained at 40 to 60 drops per minute. For hypotension secondary to spinal anesthesia, a 0.2 mg IV bolus should be given in emergency situations. To prevent hypotension from occurring, 2–3 mg SC or IM should be injected 3–4 minutes before the anesthetic agent is given. To prolong spinal anesthesia, 2–5 mg may be added to the anesthetic solution. To treat paroxysmal tachycardia, rapidly inject (within 20–30 seconds) 0.5 mg IV.	Overdosage may cause PVCs and short paroxysms of ventricular tachycardia, a sensation of fullness in the head and tingling of the extremities.
Methoxamine hydrochloride (Vasoxyl)	Acts in approximately 1–2 minutes after IV injection, and lasts 15–20 minutes after IM administration. It lasts approximately 1 hour after IV injection, and 1½ hours after IM administration. For severe hypotension, 3–5 mg is injected IV slowly at a rate of 1 mg per minute, followed by an IM injection for prolonged effect. To prevent hypotension secondary to spinal anesthesia, 10–15 mg IM can be given. To terminate paroxysmal supraventricular tachycardia, an average dose of 10 mg is given slowly IV at a rate of 1 mg per minute.	May cause sustained hypertension accompanied by severe headache, pilomotor erection, a desire to void, and projectile vomiting, especially with high doses.
Dobutamine hydrochloride (Dobutrex)	Requires continuous IV administration. Its plasma half-life is 2 minutes. Incompatible with alkaline solutions such as sodium bicarbonate. Reconstitute with 10 ml sterile water for injection or with D_5W. Usual rate of infusion is 2.5–10 µg per kg per minute, but rarely, 40 µg per kg per minute is required.	Precipitation of arrhythmias, although fewer than those caused by isoproterenol and dopamine.[20] May cause an increase in HR or systolic BP. A dose reduction usually reverses these effects quickly. Because it causes increased AV conduction, patients with atrial fibrillation may develop a rapid ventricular response. These patients should be on digitalis prior to therapy. Other side effects reported in 1%–3% of all patients include nausea, headache, anginal pain, palpitations, and shortness of breath.

brain. Total PVR increases, which is reflected by increases in systolic and diastolic BP and in pulse pressure.[29]

Levarterenol produces a positive inotropic effect from β_1 stimulation, resulting in increased $M\dot{V}O_2$ and cardiac work, producing less cardiac efficiency. This may increase the oxygen (O_2) deficit and extent of damages in some patients with myocardial infarction (MI). This can increase myocardial irritability and result in arrhythmias. Another β_1 action is a positive chronotropic effect. However, an increased HR is usually prevented because of the increased vagal stimulation which occurs reflexly as a result of elevated BP as sensed in the baroreceptors, and bradycardia may result. Levarterenol does not stimulate the β_2 receptors of the bronchi or peripheral blood vessels. Its main therapeutic effects are vasoconstriction and cardiac stimulation. Cardiac output will vary reflexly in response to systemic hypertension, but it is usually increased in the hypotensive patient when the BP is raised to an optimal level.

The pharmacologic actions of levarterenol are terminated by uptake and metabolism in the sympathetic nerve endings. The drug is metabolized by the liver and other tissues. Most of the drug is excreted as a metabolite in the urine.

Indications and Contraindictions. Levarterenol is a potent, rapid-acting vasopressor which restores BP in certain acute hypotensive states, such as after sympathectomy, after removal of a pheochromocytoma, with poliomyelitis, spinal anesthesia, MI, septicemia, blood transfusions, and drug reactions. Its use in hypotension associated with MI may be beneficial, but patients often have a poor prognosis. This is probably due to the increase in $M\dot{V}O_2$, cardiac work, and arrhythmias as well as to a decrease in renal blood flow, all associated with levarterenol.

Levarterenol is also used as a gastric lavage to treat hemorrhage from a variety of lesions. The solution is instilled by way of a nasogastric tube and left in the stomach for 20 minutes. After aspiration of gastric contents, the lavage may be repeated until the bleeding stops.[12]

Levarterenol should not be given to patients who are hypotensive from blood volume deficits, except as an emergency measure to maintain coronary and cerebral artery perfusion until blood volume replacement therapy can be completed. Because of the risk of increasing ischemia and of extending the area of infarction, it should not be given to patients with mesenteric or peripheral vascular thrombosis. Cyclopropane and halothane anesthetics increase cardiac irritability and may sensitize the myocardium to the action of IV epinephrine or levarterenol.

Nursing Implications. Avoid extravasation, which can cause tissue necrosis and sloughing. Check the site of infusion for free flow and observe for blanching at least at hourly intervals. The risk of tissue damage is apparently very slight if levarterenol is infused through a central line. If a peripheral vein is used, infusion should be made high in the limb, such as in an antecubital vein, through a long, pliable cannula made of teflon, polyethylene, or a similar material, which extends centrally into the patient. The addition of 5 mg to 10 mg phentolamine to each liter of levarterenol solution may be an effective antidote against sloughing should extravasation occur, without altering the pressor

effects of the drug. The site of the peripheral infusion should probably be changed every 24 to 36 hours. Impaired circulation, with or without extravasation, may be relieved by hot packs over the site and infiltration of the area with phentolamine or a local anesthetic.

Do not attempt to return BP to preshock levels, but rather aim for a BP sufficient to maintain tissue perfusion, such as 90 to 120 mm Hg. Administration which is too rapid can produce tachycardia, premature ventricular contractions (PVCs), diaphoresis, and chest pain. Propranolol blocks the positive inotropic effects of levarterenol, but may be used to treat the arrhythmias associated with it. Dangerously high BPs, which can be produced by levarterenol, should be avoided. Never leave a levarterenol infusion unattended, and always control its drip rate with an infusion pump. Record the BP every 2 minutes initially until the desired pressure is reached, and then record every 5 minuts if administration is to be continued. Headache may be a symptom of hypertension due to overdosage. Tricyclic antidepressants, some antihistamines, parenteral ergot alkaloids, guanethidine, reserpine, and methyldopa may potentiate the pressor effect of levarterenol, causing severe, prolonged hypertension.

Be aware that acidosis may inhibit the cardiac response to levarterenol. Avoid mixing the drug with sodium chloride, lactated Ringer's solution, sodium bicarbonate, aminophylline, and sodium iodide. Store in tight, light-resistant containers.

Isoproterenol Hydrochloride (Isuprel)

Isoproterenol acts on the β_1 receptors in the heart, which increases the CO and contractility, resulting in increased systolic pressure. It also stimulates the β_2 receptors in the vessels, causing vasodilation in renal and mesenteric vascular beds, and decreasing PVR. This produces a decrease in diastolic pressure. The net effect is an unchanged or decreased mean arterial pressure. Isoproterenol usually produces tachycardia through its direct action on the heart and by the baroreceptor reflexes.

CO is increased because of increased venous return to the heart and positive inotropic and chronotropic effects. This increase in CO maintains or increases systolic BP, although mean BP decreases. Isoproterenol also relaxes bronchial, gastrointestinal, and uterine smooth muscle.

Isoproterenol is metabolized by enzymes in the liver, lungs, and other tissues. In seriously ill patients, less than 15% of the dose is excreted unchanged.

Indications and Contraindications. Isoproterenol is used as a potent cardiac stimulant in heart block and septicemic shock. It is not routinely used in cardiogenic shock as it increases $M\dot{V}O_2$ and predisposes the heart to arrhythmias. It may, however, increase tissue perfusion if intense vasoconstriction is present.

Isoproterenol is used to treat hemodynamically significant bradycardia not responsive to atropine. For immediate definitive treatment of asystole or of complete heart block with a slow ventricular response, isoproterenol is the drug of choice because it is not as likely as epinephrine to precipitate ventricular fibrillation in the presence of previous cardiac damage. Like epinephrine, when given as an IV or IC injection, it slows fibrillatory activity, converting "fine" ventricular fibrillation for "coarse" ventricular fibrillation in preparation for defibrillation. (However, as described for epinephrine, hazards exist with any IC injection.) Isoproterenol is also a bronchial dilator and may be used in respiratory disorders. It is contraindicated for patients with preexisting cardiac arrhythmias, especially tachycardia and digitalis-induced arrhythmias.

Nursing Implications. The administration rate of isoproterenol, which should be controlled by an infusion pump to prevent inadvertent changes in dosage, should result in a target HR sufficient to maintain tissue perfusion. This is usually an HR of 60 beats per minute or less. However, the rate of administration should be slowed if ventricular irritability occurs. Arrhythmias may occur more readily in patients receiving potassium-depleting diuretics. A ventricular response rate above 130 beats per minute may be fatal. Cardiac, bronchodilating, and peripheral vasodilating effects are antagonized by the β-blocking agents, such as propranolol.

Store isoproterenol in tight, light-resistant containers. Do not give isoprorenol with epinephrine or other sympathomimetics because of possible additive effects and increased cardiotoxicity. However, these drugs can be given alternately. Isoproterenol is stable in lidocaine solutions, but should be administered separately, because the infusion rates may need to be regulated independently.[19] Do not mix it with barbiturates, aminophylline, phenytoin, sodium bicarbonate, calcium, or normal saline. Coadministration with cycloproprane or halogenated hydrocarbon general anesthetics may cause arrhythmias. Ergot alkaloids increase BP in patients on isoproterenol by apparently increasing isoproterenol-induced CO while causing vasoconstriction. Instruct patients receiving sublingual (SL) tablets not to swallow saliva until complete absorption has occurred.

Dopamine Hydrochloride (Intropin)

Dopamine stimulates the heart through the β_1 receptors and by releasing norepinephrine from tissue stores. In small doses (less than 10 μg per kg per minute), the CO increases from increased cardiac contractility and HR due to β_1 stimulation. However, there is no change in BP because of the balance between dopaminergic and α-receptor stimulation. In addition to the β effect of coronary artery vasodilation, the dopaminergic effect results in renal and mesenteric vasodilation, increasing the glomerular filtration rate and renal blood flow so that urine output also increases. The α effects produce vasoconstriction of skeletal muscle vascular beds. The effects of large doses are primarily vasoconstriction and blood pressure elevation.

In cardiogenic shock, dopamine may increase CO, mean arterial BP, and urine output. As CO increases, PVR falls if vasoconstriction was present prior to therapy.

Alpha-adrenergic-mediated vasoconstriction becomes the dominant effect as infusion rates increase above 10 μg per kg per minute. High doses of dopamine, 20 to 50 μg per kg per minute, may decrease urine output because the renal artery becomes constricted. A reduction in the infusion rate

may reestablish adequate urine output. Some patients require infusion rates in excess of 50 μg per kg per minute to maintain organ perfusion. The effect of high-dose dopamine on CO is variable.[15]

About 75% of a dose is metabolized in the liver, kidneys, and plasma to an inactive metabolite. It is excreted in the urine, primarily as its metabolites.

Indications and Contraindications. Dopamine is used to increase BP, CO, and urine output in patients with shock, refractory congestive heart failure (CHF), or cardiac arrest. Do not use in patients with pheochromocytoma because it may precipitate palpitations and tachycardia.

Nursing Implications. Monitor urine output and cardiac rhythm. Do not administer dopamine in the presence of uncorrected tachyarrhythmias or ventricular fibrillation. Prevent extravasation by infusing this drug into a large vein whenever possible. Administration of dopamine and furosemide will further enhance glomerular filtration rate. Avoid concurrent administration of haloperidol because it may block dopamine-produced increased perfusion. If the patient is also receiving MAO inhibitors, the initial infusion rate of dopamine should be reduced to at least one-tenth the normal rate. Dopamine in solution is stable for 24 hours, but is incompatible in alkaline solutions, such as sodium bicarbonate. Avoid mixing dopamine with any other drugs in solution.

Ephedrine Sulfate, U.S.P.

Ephedrine has both α and β effects. The α effects are primarily those of a pressor agent and nasal decongestant. Its β actions are as a cardiac stimulant and bronchodilator. Ephedrine produces a greater effect on the heart and blood vessels than does levarterenol. It stimulates adrenergic receptor sites directly and indirectly by promoting the release of norephinephrine from its storage sites in the sympathetic nerve endings.[28] It is like epinephrine, but ephedrine is effective orally, has a longer duration of action, stimulates the CNS, has some beneficial effects on the skeletal muscle weakness of myasthenia gravis and has mydriatic action.

Indications and Contraindications. The main clinical indications of ephedrine are bronchospasm, Stokes–Adams syndrome, nasal congestion, certain allergic disorders, as a pressor agent, especially during spinal anesthesia, in narcolepsy as a central stimulant, and to produce mydriasis. Ephedrine is contraindicated for patients who have shown hypersensitivity to it.

Nursing Implications. Serious cardiac arrhythmias may occur when ephedrine is given in combination with digitalis. For the same reason, ephedrine should be administered with caution to patients receiving general anesthesia, especially cyclopropane and halothane. Giving reserpine prior to ephedrine may antagonize ephedrine's actions, resulting in a diminished response. Patients receiving MAO inhibitors or tricyclic antidepressants concurrently with ephedrine may exhibit an excessive pressor response.

Mephentermine Sulfate (Wyamine)

Mephentermine has an effect similar to that of levarterenol, although it is not as potent. It is an indirect α and β receptor stimulant which releases norepinephrine, producing increased BP, CO, PVR, stroke volume (SV), and a positive inotropic effect.

Mephentermine is metabolized in the liver. Most of the drug is excreted in the urine within 24 hours. Excretion of the drug is more rapid in an acidic urine.

Indications and Contraindications. Mephentermine is used to treat hypotension secondary to ganglionic blockade and spinal anesthesia. Although it is not recommended as corrective therapy for hypotension secondary to hemorrhagic shock, it may be used as an emergency measure to maintain BP in such cases until blood or blood substitutes become available.

Mephentermine is contraindicated in the treatment of hypotension resulting from phenothiazines because it will potentiate the hypotension. Do not use it if there is a history of hypersensitivity. Do not administer it in combination with MAO inhibitors, because a hypertensive crisis can be precipitated.

Nursing Implications. Mephentermine should be used with caution in patients with known cardiovascular disease and in chronically ill patients, since the drug's action on the cardiovascular system may be profound. It should also be given with caution to patients with hyperthyroidism because they have an increased responsiveness to vasopressors. Mephentermine may be ineffective in patients receiving reserpine or guanethidine. The pressor response to this drug may be potentiated by tricyclic antidepressants. Cyclopropane and halothane can sensitize the heart to the arrhythmic action of sympathomimetic amines and cause serious ventricular arrhythmias.

Metaraminol Bitartrate (Aramine)

Metaraminol is also similar to levarterenol. It has a direct effect on the α and β adrenergic receptors, but not on β_2 sites. It has an indirect effect of releasing norepinephrine from storage sites and it may function as a false transmitter.[14]

Actions of metaraminol are an increase in total PVR with resultant increased BP, decreased blood flow to skin, skeletal muscle, and kidneys, and positive inotropic and chronotropic effects. The increased rate of impulse formation at the sinoatrial (SA) node is overcome by vagal activity as a reflex to increased arterial BP, with bradycardia usually developing.

Indications and Contraindications. Metaraminol is used in the treatment of shock and hypotension secondary to spinal anesthesia to produce vasoconstriction and cardiac stimulation. Avoid its use with cyclopropane or halothane anesthesia. Do not use it as the sole treatment of hypotension due to decreased plasma volume.

Nursing Implications. Use metaraminol with caution for patients receiving digitalis, because ectopic arrhythmias may develop. MAO inhibitors, tricyclic antidepressants,

reserpine, and guanethidine may precipitate a hypertensive crisis in patients receiving metaraminol. It may cause considerable deterioration of antibiotics mixed in an auxilliary IV unit. A precipitate may develop when metaraminol is mixed with sodium bicarbonate, narcotics, barbiturates, sodium iodide, steroids, and vitamins B and C.

Phenylephrine Hydrochloride (Neo-Synephrine)

Phenylephrine acts mainly on the α adrenergic receptors. Its effect on the heart is slight compared with that of levarterenol. It is used primarily as a nasal decongestant, but it may also be used for its vasopressor effects. Infiltrated into tissues, phenylephrine produces vasoconstriction that lasts longer than that caused by epinephrine and ephedrine. Its effects on the heart include a reduced HR and an increased SV without any change in rhythm. At therapeutic doses, little, if any stimulation of the spinal cord or cerebrum is produced.

The drug's pharmacologic effects are terminated at least partly by its uptake into tissues. Phenylephrine is metabolized in the liver and intestine. The route and rate of excretion have not been identified.

Indications and Contraindications. In addition to being a nasal decongestant, phenylephrine has several uses. It is given for maintenance of BP during spinal and inhalation anesthesia and for treatment of vascular failure in shock and shocklike states. It can be administered to treat drug-induced hypotension or hypersensitivity reactions. Phenylephrine is given to increase BP in order to reflexly terminate some attacks of paroxysmal supraventricular tachycardia. It is also used to prolong spinal anesthesia and to act as a vasoconstrictor in regional analgesia.

Parenteral administration may be contraindicated in patients with hypertension or ventricular tachycardia. It should be employed only with extreme caution in elderly patients or in patients with hyperthyroidism, bradycardia, partial heart block, myocardial disease, or severe arteriosclerosis.

Nursing Implications. The dose of phenylephrine should be adjusted according to the pressor response of the patient. If excessive elevation of BP occurs, it may be relieved immediately by administration of an α-adrenergic blocking agent, such as phentolamine. Admixture with antibiotics or any other drugs should be avoided. Concurrent use of phenylephrine with phenothiazines and reserpine can produce hypotension.

Methoxamine Hydrochloride (Vasoxyl)

Methoxamine is an adrenergic agent that increases BP by way of its potent pressor action. There is no increase in HR, and occasionally it will decrease as the BP increases.

Indications and Contraindications. Methoxamine is used for supporting, restoring, or maintaining BP during anesthesia, including cyclopropane anesthesia. It is also used to reflexly terminate some episodes of paroxysmal atrial tachycardia by raising BP. Methoxamine is contraindicated when combined with local anesthestics to prolong their action at local sites.

Nursing Implications. Avoid overdoses of methoxamine which can cause hypertension and bradycardia. Severe hypertension may develop in patients with hyperthyroidism or after injection of ergot alkaloids. Tricyclic antidepressants and MAO inhibitors may also increase the pressor effect of methoxamine. In hypotension secondary to fluid loss, methoxamine is not a substitute for replacement of blood, plasma, or saline. The increase in PVR produced by methoxamine may produce or exacerbate CHF in patients with a diseased myocardium.

Dobutamine Hydrochloride (Dobutrex)

Dobutamine is a synthetic derivative of isoproterenol. It acts directly on the myocardial β_1 receptors, increasing cardiac contractility and output. Although its primary effect is stimulation of the β_1 receptors, it also has slight β_2 and α adrenergic effects. With moderate doses, it increases cardiac contractility without major changes in arterial BP or heart rate. In high doses, it produces tachycardia and decreased PVR similar to isoproterenol. It is metabolized by the liver; metabolites are excreted in the urine and (a small percentage) in the feces.

In the treatment of CHF, dobutamine causes an increase in CO. Cardiac and renal function improve without tachycardia, PVCs, increased pulmonary or systemic vascular resistance, or tachyphylaxis.[2,6,21,22]

Indications and Contraindications. Dobutamine is indicated for short-term treatment of adults with cardiac decompensation. It is contraindicated for patients with idiopathic hypertrophic subaortic stenosis (IHSS).

Nursing Implications. Monitor the HR, BP, and electrocardiogram (ECG) of each patient. In addition, whenever possible, monitor the pulmonary artery wedge pressure (PAWP) and CO. Dobutamine may be ineffective if the patient is receiving a β-blocker, such as propranolol.

SYMPATHOLYTIC AGENTS

Alpha adrenergic blocking agents such as phenoxybenzamine hydrochloride, tolazoline hydrochloride, and phentolamine mesylate bind to α receptors, preventing excitatory responses mediated by epinephrine or norepinephrine. Vasodilation of the vascular beds results. This reduced PVR also reduces ventricular afterload. Because of increased venous capacitance, the administration of large volumes of fluids is permitted. Beta adrenergic blocking agents, such as propranolol hydrochloride and metoprolol, bind to the β receptors and, therefore, prevent the occurrence of β responses (see Table 35-3). Actions, indications, contraindications, and nursing implications are described for each sympatholytic agent. See Table 35-4 for specific information about dosage, administration and toxic effects of each.

TABLE 35-3 CLASSIFICATION OF SYMPATHOLYTIC AGENTS

Agent	Receptor Site Blocked
Phenoxybenzamine hydrochloride (Dibenzyline)	α
Tolazoline hydrochloride (Priscoline)	α
Phentolamine mesylate (Regitene)	α
Propranolol hydrochloride (Inderal)	β_1 β_2
Metoprolol tartrate (Lopressor)	β_1 β_2 (slight) α (slight)

Phenoxybenzamine Hydrochloride (Dibenzyline)

Phenoxybenzamine is a long-acting α blocking agent that increases blood flow to the skin, mucosa, and abdominal viscera. It lowers both supine and erect BPs.

Indications and Contraindications. Phenoxybenzamine is used to control episodes of hypertension and sweating that occur with pheochromocytoma, an adrenal tumor that causes an increase in the output of endogenous epinephrine and norepinephrine. Phenoxybenzamine is also used in vasospastic peripheral vascular disease associated with an increased α adrenergic activity, such as Raynaud's syndrome, acrocyanosis, and frostbite sequelae. It is contraindicated in conditions where a fall in BP is undesirable.

Nursing Implications. Phenoxybenzamine should be administered with caution in patients with renal damage or marked cerebral or coronary artery disease (CAD). Intravenous infusion of levarterenol may have to be used to combat severe hypotensive reactions. Phenoxybenzamine may aggravate symptoms of respiratory infections.

Tolazoline Hydrochloride (Priscoline)

Tolazoline is a peripheral vasodilator and α adrenergic blocking agent. It is said to promote healing and return of function by increasing blood supply to extremities. It is largely excreted unchanged by the kidneys. Little is known about the fate of tolazoline in the body.

Indications and Contraindications. Tolazoline is used in the treatment of spastic peripheral vascular disorders associated with acrocyanosis, acroparesthesia, arteriosclerosis obliterans, Buerger's disease, causalgia, diabetic arteriosclerosis, gangrene, endoarteritis, frostbite sequelae, Raynaud's disease, scleroderma, and post-thrombotic conditions such as thrombophlebitis. Tolazoline is contraindicated with known or suspected CAD and following a cerebrovascular accident (CVA).

Nursing Implications. Keeping the patients warm will often increase the effectiveness of tolazoline. Because it stimulates gastric secretions, it should be used with caution in patients with gastritis or known or suspected peptic ulcer disease (PUD). It should also be given cautiously to patients with known or suspected mitral stenosis. Parenteral administra-

TABLE 35-4 SYMPATHOLYTIC AGENTS

Agent	Dosage and Administration	Side and Toxic Effects
Phenoxybenzamine hydrochloride (Dibenzyline)	Absorption from the GI tract is variable. After PO administration, its onset is in several hours and its peak is in 3–4 days. After repeated doses, its α-adrenergic blocking effects are cumulative for about 7 days. Its half-life is approximately 24 hours. Initial dose is 10 mg PO. After at least 4 days, the daily dose is increased by 10 mg until the optimum dose is reached. Range is usually 20–60 mg daily. Usually 2 weeks or more are required to reach the optimal dosage level in most patients.	Nasal congestion, miosis, postural hypotension, tachycardia, and inhibition of ejaculation may occur. These are actually evidence of adrenergic blockade and tend to decrease as therapy is continued. Symptoms of overdosage include postural hypotension resulting in dizziness or fainting, tachycardia (particularly postural), vomiting, lethargy, and shock.
Tolazoline hydrochloride (Priscoline)	Absorbed well orally and parenterally Dosage should be individualized according to the condition being treated and the patient's response. Orally, 25 mg 4–6 times daily is given. If necessary, gradually increase to 50 mg 6 times daily. Usually 80 mg (long-acting) every 12 hours is sufficient. Parenterally, 10–50 mg 4 times daily SC, IV, or IM is administered. Start with a low dose and increase until optimal dose, as determined by appearance of flushing, is established. Intra-arterial administration should be used only when maximum benefit has been achieved orally or parenterally. This procedure should only be done by those thoroughly familiar with it. Initially, 25 mg is given slowly as a test to determine the response. Then, 50–75 mg per injection is given, depending upon the response. Only 1 or 2 injections daily are usually required to achieve maximal response. For maintenance, 2–3 injections weekly may be sufficient. Oral tolazoline may also be given to help maintain vasodilation between intra-arterial injections.	Signs and symptoms of overdosage are increased pilomotor activity, peripheral vasodilation, and skin flushing. In rare instances, hypotension to shock levels occurs. Adverse reactions are generally mild and may decrease progressively during therapy. Cardiac arrhythmias, anginal pain, marked hypertension, especially after parenteral administration, and exacerbations of PUD have occurred.
Phentolamine mesylate (Regitene)	Store in airtight containers and protect from light. The maximum effect occurs within 2 minutes of IV injection, and BP usually returns to pre-test levels within 15–30 minutes. For hypertensive episodes, give 5 mg IV. To prevent dermal necrosis, add 10 mg to each 1000 ml of levarterenol solution. To treat dermal necrosis, inject 5–10 mg diluted in 10 ml NS into the area within 12 hours following extravasation.	Overdosage results in a drop in BP to a dangerous level. Other adverse reactions include tachycardia and cardiac arrhythmias, (especially with parenteral administration), weakness, dizziness, flushing, orthostatic hypotension, nasal stuffiness, nausea, vomiting, and diarrhea.
Propranolol hydrochloride (Inderal)	Peak plasma concentrations occur 1–2 hours after a single PO dose. After IV injection they occur within 1 minute and the onset of action is immediate. The half-life is variable, usually 3–4 hours with IV administration. The half-life may decrease with decreasing renal function. Most commonly administered orally and should be taken before meals in divided doses. The dosage used in the management of hypertension must be individualized. Specific recommendations are presented in Chapter 33. For angina pectoris, the dose must also be individualized. Initially, 10–20 mg is given 3–4 times daily. This is gradually increased at 3–7 day intervals until optimum response is obtained. The average optimum dose is 160 mg per day. In the management of ventricular arrhythmias, 10–30 mg is administered 3–4 times daily. For IHSS the usual dose is 20–40 mg 3–4 times per day. For the preoperative management of pheochromocytoma, in conjunction with an α blocking agent, 60 mg in divided doses is given daily for 3 days prior to surgery. Management of an inoperable tumor requires 30 mg daily. Can be given very slowly IV in small increments of 0.1–0.2 mg at a rate not to exceed 1 mg in 5 minutes. Once dosage has been given without untoward effect, the danger is much less and increasing dosage can be given, usually up to 3–5 mg, but seldom more than 5–10 mg total.[25]	Overdosage or an exaggerated response can produce bradycardia, CHF, hypotension or bronchospasm. Other side effects include drowsiness, fatigue, fluid retention, cold extremities, rash, psychoneurotic depression, suicidal attempts, insomnia, nightmares, and toxic psychosis. Myocardial infarction and sudden death have occurred in anginal patients after abrupt withdrawal.

TABLE 35-4   SYMPATHOLYTIC AGENTS (Cont.)

Agent	Dosage and Administration	Side and Toxic Effects
	Because abrupt discontinuation of propranolol can exacerbate angina pectoris and precipitate MI and sudden death, withdraw the drug gradually over a period of several weeks.[3,23]	
Metoprolol tartrate (Lopressor)	Peak plasma concentrations are reached about 20 minutes after administration and its elimination half-life is about 4 hours.[5] The usual initial dose is 50 mg twice daily. Usual maintenance is 100 mg twice daily, with a range of 100–450 mg per day. β_1 selectively diminishes as dosage is increased	With the exception of bronchospasm, the adverse reactions and toxic effects are similar to propranolol. Adverse reactions include tiredness, dizziness, depression, CHF, bradycardia and diarrhea.

tion may produce an increase or fall in pulmonary artery pressure and total pulmonary vascular resistance.

Phentolamine Mesylate (Regitine)

Phentolamine, an α adrenergic blocking agent, produces vasodilation and cardiac stimulation. Phentolamine usually causes a drop in BP. About 10% of a parenteral dose can be recovered in the urine as active drug; the fate of the remainder is not known.

Indications and Contraindications. Phentolamine is used to prevent or control hypertensive episodes that may occur in a patient with pheochromocytoma as a result of stress or manipulation of the tumor during preoperative preparations and surgical excision. Parenterally it is used in the prevention and treatment of necrosis and sloughing following IV administration or extravasation of levarterenol. Contraindications include evidence suggestive of CAD, for example MI and angina pectoris, and hypersensitivity to phentolamine and related compounds.

Nursing Implications. Monitor the patient for marked hypotension, including symptoms of inadequate cerebral, renal, or coronary perfusion. Record the BP immediately after the phentolamine injection, then at 30-second intervals for the first 3 minutes, and at 1-minute intervals for the next 7 minutes. If using direct arterial BP monitoring, make certain that the module is correctly calibrated before administering the drug. In the event of overdosage, use levarterenol, not epinephrine, because epinephrine can produce a further drop in blood pressure. Because phentolamine and other α adrenergic blocking agents can cause tachycardia and other arrhythmias, defer administration of cardiac glycosides until cardiac rhythm returns to normal.

Propranolol Hydrochloride (Inderal)

Propranolol, a β adrenergic blocking drug, blocks the chronotropic, inotropic, vasodilator, and bronchodilator responses to β adrenergic stimulation. In doses greater than required for β blockade, propranolol exerts a quinidinelike or anestheticlike membrane action which affects cardiac action potential and depresses cardiac function. It exerts its antiarrhythmic effects by increasing electrical threshold, decreasing the height and duration of the action potential, and reducing excitability, automaticity, contractility, and the effective refractory period (Fig. 35-1). Antianginal effects are produced by the reduced $M\dot{V}O_2$ from decreased inotrop-

ism and chronotropism. Its mechanisms of antihypertensive effects are presented in Chapter 37. Propranolol is metabolized by the liver and excreted in the urine. Beta blockers may potentiate insulin-induced hypoglycemia.[1]

Indications and Contraindications. Indications for propranolol include high blood pressure, angina pectoris due to coronary atherosclerosis, pheochromocytoma, IHSS, and cardiac arrhythmias. Other interesting investigational applications are for treatment of migraine headache, anxiety, tremor, and glaucoma.

Contraindications include bronchial asthma, allergic rhinitis during the pollen season, sinus bradycardia, any heart block greater than first degree, cardiogenic shock, right ventricular failure secondary to pulmonary hypertension and CHF, unless the failure is secondary to a tachyarrhythmia treatable with propranolol. In addition, concurrent administration of propranolol with adrenergic-augmenting psychotropic drugs, including MAO inhibitors, or the administration of propranolol during the 2-week withdrawal period from such drugs, is contraindicated.

Nursing Implications. Monitor the patient for bradycardia and hypotension, and record both HR and BP prior to each administration. The patient should also be monitored for development of CHF, and at its first sign, the use of propranolol should be reassessed. Digitalis may be started at this time to improve contractility. Monitor the patient for any bronchoconstriction and, if noted, reassess the use of

Fig. 35-1. Effects of propranolol on automaticity. *Solid line* shows diagrammatic representation of transmembrane action potential from automatic Purkinje fiber. The *broken line* shows the effects of propranolol: decreased slope of phase 4 and displaced threshold potential (TP_1) toward 0 (TP_2). MDP = maximal diastolic potential; mV = millivolts; msec = milliseconds.

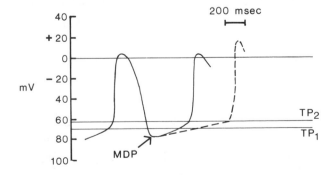

propranolol prior to the next dose. Mild wheezing may be overcome with a bronchodilating agent.

Propranolol may reduce the inotropic action of digitalis, but the effects of propranolol and digitalis are additive in depressing AV conduction and producing bradycardia.[11] It should be used with caution in patients with renal failure or impaired liver function, because the level of circulating drug will be higher, since less is metabolized and excreted. Effects of propranolol can be reversed by the administration of isoproterenol or levarterenol. Propranolol augments the hypoglycemic effects of insulin and may mask the developing hypoglycemia and tachycardia of insulin shock.[1] In addition, some clinical signs of hypertheryroidism may be masked.[8]

Propranolol impairs the ability of the heart to respond to reflex adrenergic stimuli and may increase the risk from general anesthesia and surgical procedures. Except for pheochromocytoma, therefore, withdrawal of propranolol by 48 hours prior to surgery is advised by some authorities. Propranolol must be withdrawn slowly over a period of several weeks. It is vital that patients adhere to the prescribed therapeutic regime and not discontinue taking the drug.

Metoprolol Tartrate (Lopressor)

Metoprolol is much more effective in blocking β_1 than β_2 receptors.[7] Because of its lower degree of bronchoconstriction, it may be better than propranolol for the asthmatic patient requiring β blockade.[26] Metoprolol decreases HR and force of contraction. It has antianginal activity.[18] Metoprolol is not associated with the quinidinelike effect known to result from propranolol.[9] Antiarrhythmic action is being investigated. Metoprolol has an antihypertensive effect, thought in part to be due to a decrease in plasma renin levels.[4] It is primarily metabolized by the liver and is excreted in the urine, mainly as metabolites.

Indications and Contraindications. This new cardioselective β blocker has demonstrated efficacy similar to that of propranolol in terms of antianginal and antihypertensive effects. Contraindications to propranolol apply also to metoprolol, with the exception of respiratory problems. Because of its β_1 selectivity, metoprolol may be used with caution in patients with bronchospastic disease. In patients with bronchospastic disease, because its β_1 selectivity is not absolute, a β_2 stimulating agent, such as isoproterenol, should be administered concurrently and the lowest possible dose of metoprolol used. Contraindications include bradycardia, heart block greater than first degree, cardiogenic shock, and overt CHF.

Nursing Implications. Except for bronchoconstriction, nursing implications for metoprolol are the same as those of propranolol.

REFERENCES

1. Abramson EA: Effects of propranolol on the hormonal and metabolic responses to insulin-induced hypoglycemia. Lancet ii:1386, 1966
2. Akhtar N, Mikulic E, Cohn JN et al: Hemodynamic effect of dobutamine in patients with severe heart failure. Am J Cardiol 36:202–205, 1975
3. Alderman EL, Coltart JD, Wettach GE et al: Coronary artery syndromes after sudden propranolol withdrawal. Ann Intern Med 81:625–627, 1974
4. Bengtsson C: Comparison between metoprolol and propranolol as hypertensive agents. A double-blind cross-over study. Acta Med Scand 199(1–2):71–74, 1976
5. Bengtsson C, Johnsson G, Regardh CG: Plasma levels and effects of metoprolol on blood pressure and heart rate in hypertensive patients after an acute dose and between two doses during long-term treatment. Clin Pharmacol Ther 17:400–408, 1975
6. Beregovich J, Bianchi C, D'Angelo R et al: Haemodynamic effects of a new inotropic agent (dobutamine) in chronic cardiac failure. Br Heart J 37:629–634, 1975
7. Brodgen RN, Heel RC, Speight TM et al: Metoprolol: A review of its pharmacological properties and therapeutic efficacy in hypertension. Drugs 14(5):321–348, 1977
8. Cohen GF: (Letter): Propranolol and $_{131}$I for throtoxicosis. Lancet ii:1349–1350, 1968.
9. Coltart DJ, Gibson DG, Shand DG: Plasma propranolol levels associated with suppression of ventricular ectopic beats. Br Med J 1:490–491, 1971
10. Costrini NV, Thompson WM (eds): Manual of Medical Therapeutics, 22nd ed. Boston, Little, Brown & Co 1978
11. Crawford M: Propranolol, digoxin, and combined therapy in patients with angina pectoris (abstr). Clin Pharmacol Thera 15:203, 1974
12. Douglass HO: Levarterenol irrigation. Control of massive gastrointestinal bleeding in poor-risk patients. JAMA 230:1653–1657, 1974
13. Gunnar RM, Loeb HS, Pietras RJ et al: Ineffectiveness of isoproterenol in shock due to acute myocardial infarction. JAMA 202:1124–1128, 1967
14. Harrison DC, Chidsey CA, Braunwald E: Studies on the mechanisms of action of metaraminol (Aramine). Ann Intern Med 59:297–305, 1963
15. Higgins CB, Millard RW, Braunwald E: Effects and mechanisms of action of dopamine on regional hemodynamics in the conscious dog. Am J Physiol 225:432–443, 1973
16. Holzer J, Karliner JS, O'Rourke RA: Effectiveness of dopamine in patients with cardiogenic shock. Am J Cardiol 32:79–84, 1973
17. Innes IR, Nickerson M: Norepinephrine, epinephrine, and the sympathomimetic amines. In Goodman LS, Gilman A (eds): The Pharmacological Basis of Therapeutics, 5th ed, pp 477–513. New York, Macmillan, 1975
18. Keyriläinen O, Uusitalo A: Effects of metoprolol in angina pectoris. A subacute study with exercise tests and a long-term tolerability study. Acta Med Scand 199(6):491–497, 1976
19. King JC: Guide to Parenteral Admixture, 1st ed. St. Louis, Cutter Laboratories, 1970
20. Leier CV, Heban PT, Huss P et al: Comparative systemic and regional hemodynamic effects of dopamine and dobutamine in patients with cardiomyopathic heart failure. Circulation 58:466–475, 1978
21. Leier CV, Webel J, Bush CA: The cardiovascular effects of the continuous infusion of dobutamine in patients with severe cardiac failure. Circulation 56:468–472, 1977
22. Loeb HS, Khan M, Klodnycky ML et al: Hemodynamic effects of dobutamine in man. Circulatory Shock 2:29–35, 1975
23. Miller RR, Olson HG, Amsterdam EA et al: Propranolol withdrawal rebound phenomenon. Exacerbation of coronary events after abrupt cessation of antianginal therapy. N Engl J Med 293:416, 1975
24. Rosenblum R, Frieden J: Intravenous dopamine in the treatment of myocardial dysfunction after open heart surgery. Am Heart J 83:743–748, 1972.
25. Shand DG: Drug therapy: Propranolol. N Engl J Med 293:280–286, 1975
26. Skinner C, Gaddie J, Palmer KN: Comparison of effects of metoprolol and propranolol on asthmatic airway obstruction. Br Med J 1:504, 1976

27. Smith WA: Atropine in myocardial infarction. Emergency Medicine 6:54–55, 1974
28. Sneddon JM, Turner P: Ephedrine mydriasis in hypertension and the response of treatment. Clin Pharmacol Ther 10:64, 1969
29. Vatner SF, Higgins CB, Braunwald E: Effects of norepinephrine on coronary circulation and left ventricular dynamics in the conscious dog. Circ Res 34:812–823, 1974
30. White RD: Essential drugs in emergency cardiac care. In Sladen A, Carveth SW, Goldberg AH et al (eds): Advanced Cardiac Life Support. Dallas, American Heart Association, 1975

ADDITIONAL READING

Sakamoto T, Yamada T: Hemodynamic effects of dobutamine in patients following open heart surgery. Circulation 5:525–533, 1977
Trendelburg V: Supersensitivity and subsensitivity to sympathomimetic amines. Pharmacol Rev 15:225, 1963

36

Nitrates

LORA E. BURKE, R.N., M.N.

The oldest and most important vasodilators are the nitrates. Nitroglycerin has been used sublingually for the treatment of angina pectoris since 1853. Today it still holds a dominant position among the vasodilators and is used for more than the treatment of angina.

The pharmacologic property of vasodilation is shared by the organic nitrites, nitrates, and nitrite ion; for the purpose of this discussion, the term nitrates will refer to all these agents. Actions, indications, contraindications, and nursing implications are discussed in the text. Dosage, administration, onset and duration of action, side-effects, and toxic-effects are presented in Table 36-1.

Actions

The nitrates act on both systemic and coronary vessels. Clinically, their most important effect seems to be systemic vasodilation.

Effects on Systemic Vessels. The most important and prominent action of the nitrates is on the vascular smooth muscle, with a resultant dilation of the systemic veins. This action increases the volume of these capacitance vessels and allows for a redistribution of circulating blood volume, resulting in decreased venous return, reduced filling pressures and reduced intracardiac volumes of the right and left sides of the heart (reduced preload).[15,21,24,26]

The effects of the nitrates on the arterioles and venules seems to be equal. The walls of the large arteries are relaxed, but the overall response to the nitrates is dominated by the relaxation of the relatively large veins. The predominant effect on the venous system was confirmed by one group when the intravenous (IV) administration of nitroglycerin resulted in a 45% lowering of preload with only 7% lowering of afterload.[14]

Ventricular performance, based on Starling's law of the heart, improves as the end-diastolic volume increases. It can be seen from Figure 36-1 that the patient who can benefit most from the use of these agents is one with an elevated left ventricular filling pressure (LVFP) and a low cardiac output (CO). The administration of a nitrate to this individual will reduce the LVFP and increase CO, as long as the LVFP does not fall below 15 mm Hg. Reduction of LVFP causes relief of the patient's pulmonary congestion and dyspnea.[5,10,11,19,24] The ventricular function curve can also be used to understand the consequences of administering a vasodilator (nitrate) to an individual with an already low filling pressure. The venodilation of the large capacitance vessels in the presence of low volume would result in a further reduction in filling pressure, resulting in a fall in CO, usually accompanied by a fall in blood pressure (BP) and a reflex tachycardia.

The nitrates have no direct action on the heart muscle. The changes in heart rate (HR) which may occur are secondary to changes in the vascular smooth muscle and consequently, in BP. Other changes in the heart which occur secondary to the direct action of the nitrates on the systemic capacitance vessels are a decrease in heart size, stroke volume (SV), end-systolic and end-diastolic pressures, and ejection time.[22] This results in a reduction of myocardial oxygen demand and consumption. Decreased local myocardial ischemia resulting in an improvement of local myocardial

TABLE 36-1 NITRATES

Agent	Dosage/Administration		Action		Side and Toxic Effects
			Onset	**Duration**	
Nitroglycerin (Nitrostat)	gr 1/150 (0.4 mg) to gr 1/200 (0.6 mg)	SL	2 min	15—30 min	Transient headache, vertigo, weakness, palpitation and other manifestations of postural hypotension may develop occasionally, particularly in erect, immobile patients; syncope; myocardial infarction could occur secondary to sudden, severe hypotension.
Parenteral (investigational)	Begin infusion 0.5—1.0 µg/kg/min	IV	Immediately	t½: 30 sec—2 min	Tolerance may develop with IV dose.
Ointment 2% (Nitro-Bid, Nitrol, Nitrong)	1—2 inches (15 mg nitroglycerin per inch)	Topical	20 min	3—6 hr	As above. Local skin reaction.
Amyl nitrate (Vaporole)	0.3 ml	Inhalation	30—60 sec	3 min	Mild transitory headache, dizziness, and flushing of the face are common. Nausea, vomiting, weakness, restlessness, pallor, cold sweat, incontinence, tachycardia, hypotension may occur in susceptible patients. Drug rash may occur. Transient episodes of syncope due to postural hypotension may occur, particularly in erect, immobile patients.
Erythrityl tetranitrate (Cardilate)	5—15 mg 10 mg	SL Chewable	5—10 min 5 min	2—4 hr 2—4 hr	Temporary headache may occur during first few days of therapy. Mild gastrointestinal disturbances may occur with larger oral doses.
(Tetranitol) (Erythrol tetranitrate)	5—30 mg 5—30 mg	PO PO	30 min 30 min	4 hr 2—4 hr	As above, but headache is less likely to occur with oral route.
Pentaerythritol tetranitrate (Peritrate) (Peritrate SA)	10—40 mg 80 mg	SL PO time-released	10 min 30—60 min	30 min 4—5 hr	Rash (requires discontinuation of drug), headache, gastrointestinal distress, cutaneous flushing, transient episodes of dizziness and weakness. Marked hypotension or collapse; alcohol may enhance this effect.
(Duotrate ; Metranil) (Vasitol) (Pentratol)	30—45 mg 80 mg 60 mg	PO/sustained-release PO/sustained-release PO/sustained-release	30 min 30—60 min 30 min	12 hr 12 hr 12 hr	
Isosorbide dinitrate (Isordil) (Sorbitrate)	5—10 mg 5—30 mg	SL PO	20 min 15—30 min	1½—2 hr 4 hr	Cutaneous vasodilation with flushing. Headache, transient episodes of dizziness and weakness. Drug rash and/or exfoliative dermatitis may occasionally occur. Tolerance may develop. An occasional individual exhibits marked sensitivity to the hypotensive effects of nitrate and severe responses (nausea, vomiting, weakness, pallor, perspiration and collapse) can occur even with the usual therapeutic dose. Alcohol may enhance this. Infarction could occur secondary to sudden, severe fall in blood pressure. Excessive tachycardia, increased intraocular pressure may occur.

function, is associated with this reduction. The hemodynamic effects of the nitrates are summarized in Table 36-2.

Effects on the Coronary Vessels. In most patients with angina pectoris, resistance of the coronary vessels is unaltered or decreased very transiently by the nitrates. The nitrates act on the larger coronary vessels by producing a more sustained dilation. This has also been observed in collateral vessels. It is unlikely, however, that the diseased coronary arteries dilate in response to nitrate therapy. In patients with Prinzmetal's (variant) angina, nitroglycerin reduces coronary artery spasm.

Nitrates seem to have a beneficial effect on the blood supply to the subendocardial area of the myocardium. The mechanism responsible for increased perfusion of the subendocardial regions is not clear. Vasodilation of the systemic capacitance vessels results in decreased venous return and thereby in decreased diastolic volume and pressure. The reduced pressure should allow increased blood flow to the ischemic subendocardial tissue.[22]

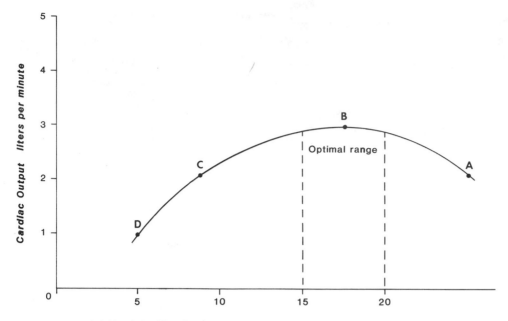

Fig. 36-1. Left ventricular function curve relating cardiac output and left ventricular filling pressure. The area between the dashed lines represents the range of optimal filling pressure. An increase in filling pressure above 22 mm Hg results in a decrease in cardiac output. Administration of a nitrate results in a nonlinear increase in CO. When the LVFP is in the optimal range there is a greater effect on CO. Administration of a nitrate (**A**) at an elevated filling pressure reduces the LVFP to the optimal range and increases CO (**B**). Administration of a nitrate at a low-filling pressure (**C**) (ascending limb of CO-LVFP curve) produces further reduction in LVFP and a proportionately greater reduction in CO (**D**).

Indications and Contraindications

The primary indications for the use of nitrates are angina pectoris and congestive heart failure (CHF). Ischemic chest pain occurs when the myocardial oxygen demand outweighs the supply, for example, an occlusion, spasm (variant angina), or narrowing of a coronary vessel, exertion, fever, anxiety, or any other reason for increased metabolism. Nitrates, regardless of the specific etiology of angina, are the treatment of choice (Chap. 22) and are frequently administered with a β-adrenergic blocking agent (Chap. 35). The urgency of the situation and the desired duration of the effect help determine which nitrate and route of administration is utilized.[7,24,26,28]

TABLE 36-2 SUMMARY OF HEMODYNAMIC EFFECTS OF NITRATES

Agent	Heart Rate	Cardiac Output*	Systemic Vascular Resistance
Nitroglycerin	slight ↑ or no change	slight ↑ or no change	slight ↓ or no change
Amyl nitrate	slight ↑ or no change	slight ↑ or no change	slight ↓ or no change
Erythrityl tetranitrate	no change	slight ↑ or no change	slight ↓ or no change
Pentarythritol tetranitrate	no change	slight ↑ or no change	slight ↓ or no change
Isosorbide dinitrate	no change	slight ↑ or no change	slight ↓ or no change

*Cardiac output response is variable and is a function of the left ventriuclar filling pressure (LVFP).

Congestive heart failure may be due to a variety of factors, functional or mechanical. The major signs and symptoms are due to elevated pressures in the systemic veins and pulmonary vascular bed, and a low CO. Figure 36-1, the left ventricular function curve, demonstrates why the nitrates are ideal agents for the treatment of pump failure.[11]

The major contraindications to the use of nitrates are low filling pressures or low diastolic arterial pressures. In patients with clinical evidence of coronary artery disease and a diastolic arterial pressure below 60 mm Hg, vasodilator therapy should be initiated with extreme caution.[11]

Sublingual Administration. Regardless of the setting or indication, the oldest and most frequently used route of administration for the nitrates is sublingual (SL). Both nitroglycerin and the longer acting SL nitrates have a rapid onset of activity with effects demonstrable as long as 30 minutes for nitroglycerin and 1–2 hours for the longer-acting forms.[19,23,25] One clear indication for the use of SL nitroglycerin is the treatment of acute attacks of angina. The long-acting nitrates are valuable adjuncts to the conventional therapy of CHF by effectively reducing LVFP, thus relieving pulmonary congestion. Nitrates are also useful in the prevention of angina.[1,28]

Cutaneous Administration. Nitroglycerin ointment contains 2% nitroglycerin in a lanolin–petrolatum base. The cutaneous administration of the ointment provides a relatively safe and effective form of vasodilator therapy with a duration of action longer than that of the other nitrate preparations. Several investigators have demonstrated beneficial hemodynamic effects of this form of nitrate therapy in the treatment of acute myocardial infarction (MI) and acute and chronic CHF.[2,5,9,22,29] Hemodynamic alterations can be seen within 15–30 minutes after application of the ointment, and a therapeutic effect may persist for 3–4 hours. The continued absorption of nitroglycerin through the skin, avoiding early passage through the portal circulation, may explain the prolonged effect of cutaneous nitroglycerin.[25] The prolonged duration of action of this form of vasodilating therapy makes it particularly useful for night-time therapy and for prolonged improvement in exercise capacity.

An advantage to the use of this route of administration is that it permits retrieval of a portion of the dose, should adverse side-effects occur. A return of hemodynamic parameters toward initial levels has been shown within 1 hour of removal of the ointment.[22] Disadvantages of cutaneous nitroglycerin include the lack of convenience in administering the drug, as compared to the sublingual and oral forms of nitrates, and the controversy and lack of knowledge regarding the proper application of this agent (site, square-inch area of application and dose/inch).[13,16,17,18,20]

Intravenous Administration (Investigational). The IV route may be chosen for nitrate therapy of an acutely ill patient in the setting of a cardiac care unit (CCU). Nitroglycerin administered IV, like the other forms of nitrates, allows a lowering of LVFP and an improvement in left ventricular function without a large reduction in mean arterial pressure. Thus, IV nitroglycerin may increase myocardial oxygen supply by maintaining coronary perfusion pressure and by its vasodilating effect on the coronary collaterals. Simultaneously, it reduces myocardial oxygen demand by reducing ventricular wall tension due to decreased preload and afterload.[12,14]

The IV administration of nitroglycerin has the advantage of prolonging the beneficial effects, and avoiding sudden falls in pressure by allowing more precise control of the dosage. Indications for IV nitroglycerin are the prevention of intra-operative hypertension, acute treatment of such valvular disease as aortic or mitral insufficiency, an attack of acute coronary spasm, systemic or pulmonary hypertension, and left ventricular failure.[7,12] At present, IV nitroglycerin is not approved by the Food and Drug Administration for routine clinical use. Another vasodilating agent, sodium nitroprusside, can be employed when intravenous therapy is required (Chap. 37). Intravenous nitroglycerin is available for investigational use.[12]

While intravenous administration has some advantages its use is necessarily restricted to an intensive care setting. Careful hemodynamic monitoring and precise control of the infusion rate is required to prevent the occurrence of dangerous systemic hypotension. If the patient requires long-term nitrate therapy, initial IV therapy should be substituted by another route while the patient is still in CCU in order that the titration of the dose can be monitored closely.

Oral Administration. It has been demonstrated that orally-administered organic nitrates are carried directly to the liver by the portal vein where they may undergo rapid degradation by a liver enzyme before entering the systemic circulation. Small doses of oral nitrates have been shown to be ineffective as anti-anginal agents. The degree of improvement observed after orally administered nitrates is frequently less than that seen after sublingual agents. However, larger doses of oral nitrates cause beneficial hemodynamic changes in the treatment of angina.

Nursing Implications

Patients in an Acute Situation. The use of nitroglycerin in patients with an acute MI may result in hypotension, causing a reduction in coronary perfusion pressure and consequently an increase in myocardial ischemia. These effects may be potentiated by saline depletion secondary to diuretic agents. The patient with an acute MI should therefore be monitored electrocardiographically and hemodynamically. If possible, assess for saline depletion by checking for postural hypotension prior to administration of nitrates. (This should have been done on admission, or as part of routine assessment.) The patient with an acute MI should be in the recumbent position, although the head of the bed may be elevated to comfort (30 degrees). However, the patient's legs should remain in the bed and not dangle over the side. The patient's HR and BP should be monitored for 5–10 minutes and the response documented. The same precautions apply to the use of other forms of nitrates, keeping in mind the onset of action and the occurrence of peak effect for the particular mode of therapy being utilized. The hemodynamic effects of SL nitroglycerin are maximal 5–10 minutes after administration, whereas peak effects of SL isosorbide dinitrate occur 15–45 minutes and the oral type 20–60 minutes after administration. Cutaneous nitroglycerin has its peak effect demonstrated 1–3 hours after application.[4,22,25]

The size of the area used in applying cutaneous nitroglycerin is an important variable affecting the hemodynamic changes which result from the use of this drug. The nurse administering this agent must be aware that the rate of absorption will also be affected by the area of application, the cutaneous blood flow of the site, and the rate of evaporation.[2,22] In one clinical investigation, nitroglycerin ointment evoked the most marked response in systolic BP when applied to the forehead and the least marked when it was applied to the ankle. The result of chest wall application corresponded closely to that of the forehead site but was of less magnitude.[16,17,18] In another clinical study, the anterior chest or flank was used. Comparable hemodynamic changes occurred when either of these sites was used with the same individual.[2,3] A study of nitroglycerin ointment application to the right anterior chest versus the upper abdomen revealed clinical differences in reduction of pressure-rate product between the two sites. The extent of the drop in pressure-rate product was greater when the abdominal site was used.[13]

One recommended method of application is to apply the ointment on the paper applicator supplied by the manufacturer and then use it to spread the ointment on a 6 × 6 inch (150 × 150 mm) area in a uniform layer. However, one should keep in mind that the size of the surface area should correspond to the dose of the ointment. A ½″ strip of nitroglycerin ointment could not be spread easily over a 36-sq. in. area without rubbing the ointment into the skin.

Whether the area should then be covered with a plastic wrap or a nonocclusive dressing has not been studied. Whatever method is used, however, must be consistent. Repeated application to the same area is likely to irritate the patient's skin. It is advisable to rotate sites within a particular anatomic area, for example the chest. The previously applied ointment must be removed with soap and water before administering a new dose.

The patient receiving IV nitrate therapy must be monitored very closely for hemodynamic changes, since IV nitroglycerin acts immediately and can cause a precipitous fall in BP. Ideally, the patient should have both an arterial and a pulmonary artery line in place so that a continuous recording of these pressures is available. The nitroglycerin infusion should be titrated in order that a certain range of arterial or pulmonary artery pressure can be reached and maintained. The IV drip must be controlled by an infusion pump. If a sudden fall in BP occurs, the infusion should be discontinued and the patient's head lowered until an adequate BP returns: This should be within a few minutes. Any patient receiving IV nitroglycerin must be kept on bed rest for the duration of the therapy. The nurse needs to explain this to the patient and to reinforce the necessity for his cooperation in this restriction. If the patient *must* get out of bed for some reason, the infusion needs to be discontinued approximately five minutes prior to the activity.

Patients in a Stable Situation. The nurse should monitor the patient's HR and BP response to SL nitroglycerin, in particular to the initial dose. If hypotension occurs, position the patient to facilitate venous return to the heart. Once the patient is ambulatory, the fact that syncope can result from relatively small doses if the patient maintains a static upright position must be kept in mind. Changes in blood volume, for example with diuresis, may have a profound effect on the patient's response to the next dose of a nitrate. Therefore, patients undergoing diuretic therapy should have their postural BP routinely assessed.

For the patient hospitalized in a nonacute setting, keeping the sublingual nitroglycerin tablets at the patient's bedside may be advisable. This permits the patient to take nitroglycerin immediately after the start of angina without waiting for his call light to be answered and the nurse to deliver the medication. Self-medication of nitroglycerin may also reduce patient anxiety. Instructions should be given on the use of nitroglycerin and the importance of reporting chest pain to the nurse.

Nursing has a vital role in patient education regarding the use of nitrates. It is important to determine whether or not the patient has taken nitroglycerin previously. The patient who has not yet required the use of this agent should be monitored by the nurse during administration of the first dose. This permits the patient to experience the response safely and to ask any questions that may arise as a result of it.

The patient must be instructed about the inactivation of nitroglycerin by exposure to light, heat, air, moisture, or prolonged periods of storage. A supply greater than two weeks should be stored in the refrigerator and the bottle should be allowed to warm to room temperature before tablets are removed. This prevents the condensation of water on the cold tablets.[6,8] Nitroglycerin ointment should be stored in a cool place, in the original container, with the tube tightly capped.

The patient should be instructed to carry only a two-week supply of tablets. These should be kept in a tightly stoppered dark glass container without much cotton filler. If the tablet crumbles easily or does not produce a slight stinging or burning sensation when placed under the tongue, the tablets should not be used, and a new supply should be obtained.[8] The patient who is taking a sustained–released preparation needs to be instructed to take it once every 12 hours and to take it on an empty stomach with an adequate amount of water.

Patients should also be informed of the possibility of postural hypotension and how to prevent its occurrence. Instructions should be given in the event of a prolonged anginal attack. Caution the patient to take two to three tablets over a 10–15 minute period; if relief is not obtained, he may be having an acute MI and should call the local paramedic system.

Since the goal of nitrate therapy is not only to shorten anginal attacks but also to prevent their occurrence and to increase exercise performance, patients need to be instructed about the prophylactic use of nitrates. Nitroglycerin or a longer-acting nitrate may be taken prior to engaging in a stressful or strenuous activity.[26] In one study, the mean time which subjects were able to exercise 2 minutes after the administration of nitroglycerin increased 51% compared to the mean time which the subjects who had received a placebo were able to exercise.[4] Exercise capacity following administration of nitroglycerin ointment has been evaluated.[27] One hour following the application of ointment, patients were able to exercise 8 minutes as compared to 5 minutes in patients who received a placebo, and most were able to perform at a higher workload. Three hours after application of the nitroglycerin ointment, the mean exercise duration was still significantly above that achieved after the placebo.

Evidence is available to suggest that tolerance can develop from chronic use of nitrates. The smallest effective dose should therefore, be administered, in order that the dosage can be increased as needed. To avoid any withdrawal effects, the gradual reduction of nitrate dosage is recommended in patients who have been receiving chronic high-dose therapy.

REFERENCES

1. AMA Department of Drugs, In cooperation with the American Society for Clinical Pharmacology and Therapeutics: AMA Drug Evaluations, 4th ed. pp 529–532. New York, John Wiley & Sons, 1980
2. Armstrong PW, Mathew MT, Boroomad K et al: Nitroglycerin ointment in acute myocardial infarction. Am J Cardiol 38:474–478, 1976
3. Armstrong PW: Standardized regimen for applying nitroglycerin ointment—Reply. Am J Cardiol 40:143, 1977
4. Aronow WS: Clinical use of nitrates: Nitrates as anti-anginal drugs (Part I). Mod Concepts Cardiovas Dis 68(6):31–35, 1979
5. Aronow WS: Clinical use of nitrates: Nitrates in congestive heart failure (Part II). Mod Concepts Cardiovasc Dis 68(7):37–42, 1979
6. Bergersen BS: Cardiovascular drugs. In Pharmacology in Nursing, 14th ed., 176–246. St. Louis, CV Mosby, 1979

7. Cain RS, Ferguson RM, Tillisch JH: Variant angina: A nursing approach. Heart Lung 8:1122–1126, 1979

8. Capilan HW: Burning sensation and potency of nitroglycerin sublingually. JAMA 219:176–179, 1972

9. Chandraratna PAN, Langevin E, O'Dell R et al: Use of nitroglycerin ointment in congestive heart failure. Cardiology 63:337–342, 1978

10. Cohn JN, Franciosa JA. Vasodilator therapy of cardiac failure (Part I). N Engl J Med 297:27–31, 1977

11. Cohn JN, Franciosa JA: Vasodilator therapy of cardiac failure (Part II). N Engl J Med 297:254–258, 1977

12. Cottrell JE, Turndorf H: Intravenous nitroglycerin. Am Heart J 96:550–553, 1978

13. Cunningham JL: Effectiveness of Nitroglycerin Ointment According to Site of Application: Hemodynamic Responses in Patients with Stable Coronary Artery Disease. Unpublished Master's thesis, University of Washington, 1980

14. Flaherty JT, Reid PR, Kelly DT et al: Intravenous nitroglycerin in acute myocardial infarction. Circulation 51:132–138, 1975

15. Fuller EO: The effect of anti-anginal drugs on myocardial oxygen consumption. Am J Nurs 80:250–254, 1980

16. Hansen MS, Woods SL, Wills RE: Relative effectiveness of nitroglycerin ointment according to site of application. Heart Lung 8:716–720, 1979

17. Hansen MS: Application site for nitroglycerin ointment. Am J Cardiol 42:1061, 1978

18. Hansen MS, Woods SL: Nitroglycerin ointment Am J Nurs 80(6):1122–1124, 1980

19. Hardarson D, Henning H, O'Rourke RA: Prolonged salutary effects of isosorbide dinitrate and nitroglycerin ointment on regional left ventricular function. Am J Cardiol 40:90–98, 1977

20. Kirby JA: Variation in Measurement of Doses of Nitroglycerin Ointment. Unpublished Master's thesis, University of Washington, 1980

21. Kovich RB, Tillisch JH, Berens SC et al: Vasodilator therapy for chronic left ventricular failure. Circulation 53:322–328, 1976

22. Meister SG, Engel TR, Gucha N et al: Sustained hemodynamic action of nitroglycerin ointment. Br Heart J 38:1031–1036, 1976

23. Needleman P, Lang S, Johnson EM: Organic nitrates: Relationship between biotransformation and rational angina pectoris therapy. J Pharmacol Exper Ther 18:489–497, 1972

24. Nickerson M: Vasodilator drugs. In Goodman LS, Gilman A (eds): The Pharmacological Basis of Therapeutics, 5th ed, pp 727–743. New York, Macmillan, 1975

25. Parker JO, Augustine RJ, Burton JR et al: Effect of nitroglycerin ointment on the clinical and hemodynamic response to exercise. Am J Cardiol 38:162–166, 1976

26. Parmley WW, Chattergee K: Vasodilator therapy. Curr Prob Cardiol 2:3–71, 1978

27. Reichek N, Goldstein RE, Redwood DR et al: Sustained effects of nitroglycerin ointment in patients with angina pectoris. Circulation 50:348–352, 1974

28. Segal BL, Kotler MN: Nitrates and propranolol for angina pectoris. Hospital Formulary 13:41–43, 1978

29. Taylor WR, Forrester JS, Magnusson P et al: Hemodynamic effects of nitroglycerin ointment in congestive heart failure. Am J Cardiol 38:469–473, 1976

37

Antihypertensives and Diuretics

JENILLE BRADLY, R.N.

and

SANDRA L. UNDERHILL, R.N., M.N.

According to the American Heart Association, 60 million Americans have elevated blood pressure (BP) (Chap. 47).[32] One way to alleviate hypertension is by drug therapy. Until the discovery of the diuretic chlorothiazide in 1956 by Sprague and Novello, there had been no truly effective way of controlling hypertension. Today, in addition to the many diuretics, there is an arsenal of drugs with different modes of action to control elevated BP, prevent the sequelae of the hypertensive state and, therefore, to extend the lives of vast numbers of patients.

Treatment of mild-to-moderate hypertension is frequently very difficult. Even though effective drugs are available, the patient may be reluctant to take them. Generally, the patient with mild-to-moderate hypertension feels well and experiences no symptoms as a consequence of his elevated BP. When started on therapy, he may feel ill because of the inherent side effects of most antihypertensive agents. Comprehensive teaching and excellent rapport must be established with the patient to achieve understanding and adherence. The nurse's role, therefore, is crucial in effective management of hypertensive patients.

Treatment regimens should be designed individually and depend upon the severity of the hypertension, the side effects of the response to the antihypertensive agent, the patient's general status, the frequency of dosage, and the cost. With complicated, multiple-dose regimens, adherence is often very poor, but can be improved considerably with daily or twice-daily medication. In order to minimize cost, untoward effects, and number of medications used, as well as to provide health practitioners involved in the management of hypertension with a rational method of treatment,

a step care approach has been suggested by the Joint National Committee on the Detection, Evaluation and Treatment of High Blood Pressure (Fig. 37-1).[30] This approach provides a systematic means of building efficacious treatment regimens without excluding individualization.

Most antihypertensive drugs are used to treat patients with essential hypertension (who are in the majority) that have a normal cardiac output (CO) and an increased total peripheral vascular resistance (PVR), rather than those with renal artery stenosis or other known cause. Antihypertensive agents affect the circulatory system in essentially three ways: reduction of the extracellular fluid (ECF) volume (diuretics); reduction of sympathetic tone, decreasing PVR (sympatholytic agents); and direct relaxation of the vascular smooth muscle, also reducing PVR (vasodilators). Some antihypertensive agents may have more than one site of action (Fig. 37-2) or may alter CO, thus contributing in more than one way. Different classes of antihypertensive agents can affect one another, either by enhancing one another's action or by countering one another's adverse effects.

The drugs discussed in this chapter are divided into two general categories: antihypertensives and diuretics. The antihypertensive agents include adrenergic neuronal, alpha (α) and beta (β) blocking agents; central acting agents; ganglionic blocking agents; and vasodilators. Although diuretics also have antihypertensive properties, they are presented separately, so as to emphasize their additional effects and uses. Actions, indications, contraindications, and nursing implications of representative drugs in each category are discussed. Specific information regarding dosage and

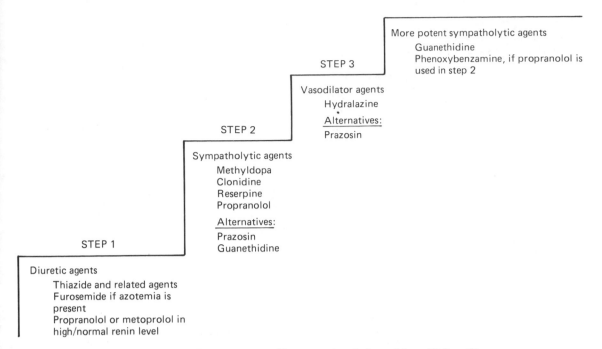

STEP 3

More potent sympatholytic agents
  Guanethidine
  Phenoxybenzamine, if propranolol is
  used in step 2

STEP 2

Vasodilator agents
  Hydralazine
  •
  Alternatives:
  Prazosin

Sympatholytic agents
  Methyldopa
  Clonidine
  Reserpine
  Propranolol

  Alternatives:
  Prazosin
  Guanethidine

STEP 1

Diuretic agents
  Thiazide and related agents
  Furosemide if azotemia is
  present
  Propranolol or metoprolol in
  high/normal renin level

Fig. 37-1.   Step care approach in the treatment of hypertension. (adapted from Wollam GL,
Vidt DG: Drug Therapy, 8:74, 1978, and Finnerty FA: Consultant, 18(2): 127, 1978)

Fig. 37-2.   Sites of action of antihypertensive agents.
(**a**) Kidney: all diuretic agents and propranolol and metoprolol;
(**b**) hypothalamus: rauwolfia alkaloids; (**c**) vasomotor center:
rauwolfia alkaloids, clonidine, methyldopa; (**d**) sympathetic
ganglion: trimethaphan, mecamylamine, pentholinum;
(**e**) postganglionic nerve fibers: rauwolfia alkaloids,
guanethidine, methyldopa; (**f**) α-adrenergic neurons (blockade):
phenoxybenzamine, phentolamine, prazosin; (**g**) β-adrenergic
neurons (blockage): propranolol, metoprolol; (**h**) arterial smooth
muscle (vasodilators): hydralazine, sodium nitroprusside,
diazoxide, prazosin (?); (**i**) blood volume: all diuretics. (Adapted
from Kochar MS, Daniels LM: Hypertension Control for
Nurses and Other Health Professionals. St Louis, CV Mosby
1978)

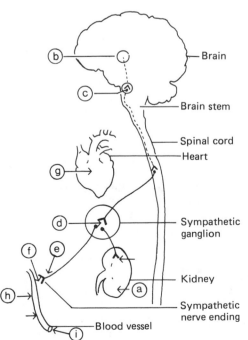

administration, drug interactions, toxic effects, and side
effects of antihypertensive agents can be found in Table
37-1. A description of general nursing care for patients
receiving antihypertensives and diuretics follows the discussions of the various categories of drugs. Drugs and
dosages used for hypertensive emergencies are listed in
Table 37-2.

ANTIHYPERTENSIVES— ADRENERGIC NEURONAL BLOCKING AGENTS

These agents deplete the stores of catecholamines in the
postganglionic nerve endings and deplete the brain amine
serotonin from the hypothalamus and vasomotor centers,
resulting in decreased PVR, CO, heart rate (HR), and renin
release. When given orally, the hypotensive response takes
7 to 14 days and lasts up to 4 weeks. As with other
antihypertensive agents, sodium (Na^+) retention occurs,
possibly because of the drop in BP. This drop in BP reduces
renal perfusion, resulting in increased tubular reabsorption
of Na^+ and enhanced secretion of aldosterone and renin.

Rauwolfia (Raudixin, Rautina)

Rauwolfia and its alkaloid reserpine (Serpasil, Sandril) are
used less now than in the past. Rauwolfia, the extract of a
shrub root native to India, was used in ancient times and
was rediscovered in 1955.

Indications and Contraindications. Rauwolfia, a step-2
drug, is indicated in the treatment of mild-to-moderate
(*Text continues on p. 488.*)

TABLE 37-1 ANTIHYPERTENSIVE AGENTS

Agent	Dosage/Administration	Drug Interaction	Toxic Effects	Side Effects
ADRENERGIC NEURONAL BLOCKING AGENTS				
Rauwolfia (Raudixin; Rautina)	50–300 mg PO q.d.	Potentiated by diuretics. Hypertensive reaction may result from use with MAO inhibitors. Arrhythmias may result from use with digitalis and quinidine.	Central depression, hypotension, ptosis, miosis, catatonia, hypothermia, depressed respirations.	Drowsiness, sedation, lassitude, bradycardia, nasal congestion, excessive salivation, nausea, vomiting, diarrhea, gastric hyperacidity, muscular rigidity, emotional alienation, depression which can be suicidal, impotence, decreased libido, nightmares, inhibition of ovarian cycle and menstruation, feminization in men
Reserpine (Serpasil; Sandril)	0.1–0.5 mg PO q.d.* May be given parenterally 0.25–5.0 mg, starting with low doses; may repeat in 4–12 hours.	As above.	As above.	As above.
Guanethidine (Ismelin)	10–300 mg PO q.d., starting with low dose and gradually increasing.	Potentiated by alcohol and diuretics. Antagonized by tricyclic antidepressants, oral contraceptives, and sympathomimetics.	Severe postural hypotension with blurred vision, dizziness, and syncope; severe diarrhea	Orthostatic hypotension, lightheadedness, lassitude, weakness, bradycardia, diarrhea, nasal stuffiness, nausea, vomiting, constipation, anorexia, depression, edema with weight gain, inhibition of ejaculation, reduced exercise tolerance, loss of scalp hair, dry mouth, rash.
ALPHA ADRENERGIC BLOCKING AGENTS				
Phentolamine hydrochloride (Regitine)	2.5 mg IV every 5 minutes, then 2.5 mg IV or IM every 2–4 hours; 100–300 mg PO q.d.*	See Chapter 35.	See Chapter 35.	See Chapter 35.
Phenoxybenzamine hydrochloride (Dibenzyline)	30–100 mg PO q.d.	See Chapter 35.	See Chapter 35.	See Chapter 35.
Prazosin (Minipres)	1–20 mg PO q.d.* starting with 1 mg b.i.d.–t.i.d. to forestall first-dose phenomenon.	Potentiated by diuretics and other antihypertensive agents.	First-dose phenomenon 30–90 minutes after ingestion. Not recommended in pregnancy.	Dizziness, headache, drowsiness, lassitude, weakness, palpitations, and nausea, which tend to disappear with continued therapy. Vomiting, diarrhea, edema, rash, nervousness occur infrequently.
BETA ADRENERGIC BLOCKING AGENTS				
Propranolol (Inderal)	Usually 30–320 mg PO q.d.* but infrequently up to 640 mg. Doses up to 3 g used in Great Britain, but not approved in United States.	See Chapter 35.	See Chapter 35.	See Chapter 35.
Metoprolol (Lopressor)	Usual initial dose 50 mg PO twice daily; maintenance dose 100 mg twice daily; dose range 100–450 mg daily.	See Chapter 35.	See Chapter 35.	See Chapter 35.
CENTRAL ACTING AGENTS				
Clonidine (Catapres)	0.1–2.4 mg PO q.d.* Usually started at 0.1 mg b.i.d. with gradual increase. Larger dose may be given at night to minimize problem of sedation. Drug should not be withdrawn abruptly.	Potentiated by diuretics and antihypertensives; potentiates depressant effects of alcohol, barbiturates, and other sedatives. Antagonized by tricyclic antidepressants.	Profound hypotension, diminished or absent reflexes, deep sedation or coma, skin pallor, decreased or irregular pulse, weakness, vomiting. Abrupt withdrawal can cause rebound hypertension (*cont. next page*)	Sedation, drowsiness, dry mouth, fatigue, weakness, and headache which usually diminishes with time. Nightmares, anxiety, nausea, vomiting, impotence, Raynaud's phenomenon, breast (*cont. next page*)

TABLE 37-1 ANTIHYPERTENSIVE AGENTS (Cont.)

Agent	Dosage/Administration	Drug Interaction	Toxic Effects	Side Effects
			that may result in hypertensive crisis and death. Rebound hypertension may be exaggerated by β blockade[3] and renovascular hypertension.[41] Not recommended during pregnancy	enlargement, edema, ECG abnormalities such as Wenkebach or ventricular trigeminy
Methyldopa (Aldomet)	0.5–2.0 g PO q.d.* For IV add to 100 ml D₅W and give slowly over 30–60 minutes. Usual dose is 250–500 mg; maximal dose is 1 g every 6 h.	Potentiated by levodopa, quinidine, diuretics, and antihypertensives. Antagonized by tricyclic antidepressants and sympathomimetics. With haloperidol, may produce a dementia syndrome. MAO inhibitors cause severe CNS stimulation and hypertensive reactions.	Liver damage, usually reversible but possibly fatal. Positive Coombs' test which may not be clinically important but may indicate hemolytic anemia. Drug fever usually in 21 days. Circumstantial evidence of fatal hypersensitivity myocarditis manifested as fatigue.[31] Not recommended during pregnancy.	Sedation, lassitude, loss of mental acuity, loss of sexual function, vertigo, nightmares, depression, parkinsonian syndrome, paresthesias, nasal congestion, dry mouth, hypotension, nausea, vomiting, breast enlargement, edema
VASODILATORS				
Hydralazine (Apresoline; Rolazine; Dralzine; LoPres)	50–300 mg PO q.d.* B.i.d. dosage may be as effective as multiple doses.[36] 10–50 mg IV produces a hypotensive response in 5–10 minutes and IM in 30 minutes. Can repeat in 4–6 hours.	Potentiated by diuretics and antihypertensives. Profound hypotension if used with diazoxide.[24] Antipyridoxine (B₆) can cause peripheral neuritis.	ECG changes of ischemia, arrhythmias, shock, acute rheumatoid state, SLE-like syndrome, other blood dyscrasias, drug fever, paresthesia, numbness, and tingling of extremities, GI hemorrhage, and depression.	Flushing, nasal congestion, headache, dizziness, palpitation, angina, anorexia, nausea, vomiting, diarrhea, edema, weakness, constipation, adynamic ileus, dyspnea, tachycardia; rarely impotence
Minoxidil	Currently under investigation in certain refractory hypertensive patients.			
Diazoxide (Hyperstat)	Usually 300 mg IV bolus in 15–30 seconds (IM or SC administration causes burning and cellulitis.) Bolus can be repeated in 10–30 minutes, then every 4–24 hours as needed. Calculated dose is 5 mg/kg.	Potentiated by diuretics and antihypertensives, especially hydralazine.[20] Potentiates warfarin.	Profound hypotension, unconsciousness, convulsions, paralysis, confusion, myocardial or cerebral ischemia, CHF, significant hyperglycemia, and abnormalities of the blood indices	Flushing, burning, itching, headache, sweating, warm sensation, weakness, nausea, vomiting, diarrhea, muscle cramps, dyspnea, chest tightness, tinnitus, anxiety, malaise, dry mouth, insomnia, dizziness, euphoria, nocturia, paresthesias, polyneuritis
Sodium nitroprusside (Nipride)	Usually 0.5–8.0 μg/kg/minute as IV drip. Mix initially with 3 ml D₅W or preservative-free sterile water, then add to D₅W 500–1000 ml. Do not use if any color except faint brown tint.	Potentiated by diuretics and antihypertensives	Severe profound hypotension; thiocynate poisoning at serum levels of 5–10 mg/100 ml, causing tinnitus, blurred vision and delirium. With renal or hepatic impairment, frank cyanide poisoning (serum levels 20 mg/100 ml) occurs, with fast, labored respirations, eventually becoming slow and shallow, widely dilated pupils, distant heart sounds, imperceptible pulse, glassy eyes, pink skin color, convulsions, absent reflexes, coma, possible death. Hypothyroidism also possible.	Nausea, vomiting, muscular twitching, agitation, diaphoresis, headache, palpitations. Retrosternal discomfort can occur with too rapid injection and diminish when infusion is slowed or stopped.

*Divided doses

TABLE 37-2 DRUGS USED FOR HYPERTENSIVE EMERGENCIES

Drug	Dosage and Administration	Onset of Action
Furosemide (Lasix)	40–60 mg every 4, 6, or 8 hours IM or IV	5 minutes
Reserpine (Serpasil; Sandril)	0.25–0.50 mg every 4 to 12 hours IM or IV	2–3 hours
Methyldopa (Aldomet)	250–500 mg in D_5W, 100–250 ml IV slowly over 30–60 minutes; repeat every 6–8 hours.	2–3 hours
Phentolamine (Regitine)	2.5–5.0 mg IV or diluted in D_5W over 5 minutes	within minutes
Diazoxide (Hyperstat)	100–150 mg IV bolus, repeat after 10–30 minutes, then every 4–24 hours. (Administer after furosemide has been given and is actively working.)	3–5 minutes
Nitroprusside (Nipride)	50 mg in D_5W 500–1000 ml; deliver 0.5–8.0 µg/kg/minute.	30–60 seconds
Hydralazine (Apresoline; Rolazine; Dralzine; LoPres)	10–50 mg IV or IM; repeat every 4–6 hours.	IM: 30 minutes IV: 5–10 minutes

hypertension and is always given in conjunction with a diuretic. It is also used for patients with tachycardia, those in need of tranquilization, or for patients who are undependable in taking medication. Reserpine can be given parenterally for accelerated hypertension. These agents are contraindicated for patients with a history of depression, peptic ulcer disease (PUD), ulcerative colitis, chronic sinusitis, and for women with a history of breast cancer. The Drug Surveillance Study and other studies suggested an increase in breast cancer with the use of reserpine[2,19,22,24] but those data were not supported by the studies of Mack[29] or O'Fallon.[35] Until the matter is settled, to be cautious seems prudent. Reserpine is contraindicated in the presence of monoamine oxidase (MAO) inhibitors, such as pargyline hydrochloride (Eutonyl).

Nursing Implications. Nurses should observe patients who have received parenteral reserpine for adverse central nervous system (CNS) effects as a result of diminished serotonin such as depression, nervousness, dulled sensorium, anxiety, nightmares and parkinsonian syndrome. If administration is parenteral, the BP should be monitored every 2 to 4 hours but less frequently with reserpine than with more powerful agents. Full antihypertensive effect does not occur for up to 3 weeks after oral administration; BP changes may not be evident until this time.

In the case of chronic hypertension, the nurse should take a careful history to ascertain whether the patient has had PUD, depression, sinus problems, or preexisting sexual dysfunction. Because ovulation may be depressed, the importance to the patient of pregnancy should be discussed. The nurse must be alert for subtle signs and symptoms of personality changes or depression. Frequently a relative or friend will call attention to such signs, which should be promptly communicated to the physician or nurse practitioner.

Guanethidine (Ismelin)

Guanethidine is a potent agent that depletes stores of norepinephrine from postganglionic nerve endings, but has little effect on the adrenal medulla or the CNS. It prevents the release of norepinephrine normally produced by nerve stimulation, thereby blunting the responsiveness of the resistance and capacitance vessels to sympathetic stimuli. This results in decreased PVR, CO, and HR, with subsequent hypotension that is more pronounced in the upright position. Renal blood flow (RBF) and glomerular filtration rate (GFR) are either unchanged or decreased. The full hypotensive effect takes 1 to 3 weeks from onset of therapy and lasts equally long after cessation of the therapy. Sodium retention also occurs.

Indications and Contraindications. Guanethidine is used as a step-4 drug in the treatment of moderate-to-severe hypertension. It is especially useful when tachycardia is present or when once-a-day drug dosage is desired. It is contraindicated for patients with pheochromocytoma, congestive heart failure (CHF) secondary to hypertension or for those taking MAO inhibitors.

Nursing Implications. Nurses should caution patients about orthostatic hypotension, which is most likely to occur upon arising in the morning, in hot weather, or after strenuous exercise, prolonged standing, or ingestion of alcoholic beverages. The patient should be taught that the symptoms of postural hypotension (faintness, dizziness, weakness, and lassitude) can be prevented by gradual assumption of an upright posture or ameliorated by sitting or lying down for a few moments.

A careful history is required prior to institution of guanethidine therapy. Because the drug may inhibit ejaculation, any preexisting sexual dysfunction in the male should be determined. The importance of athletic participation to the patient must be ascertained, because strenuous exercise may precipitate a severe hypotensive response. Prevention of the normal vasoconstriction response is augmented during hot weather or by ingestion of alcoholic beverages.

ALPHA ADRENERGIC BLOCKING AGENTS

These agents block α-adrenergic receptors and block or antagonize responses to circulating catecholamines. Although α adrenergic blocking agents are presented in more detail in Chapter 35, they are mentioned here because they are used specifically in the treatment of hypertension caused by pheochromocytoma.

Phentolamine Hydrochloride (Regitine) and Phenoxybenzamine Hydrochloride (Dibenzyline)

Indications. Phentolamine is a short-acting agent used for temporary control of severe hypertension prior to surgery for pheochromocytoma. Phenoxybenzamine is a long-acting agent used in the long-term management of hypertension due to elevated circulating catecholamines, especially in pheochromocytoma not amenable to surgery. Vlachalis's study[42] indicates that this drug may be useful in controlling moderately severe hypertension when used in conjunction with propranolol. Refer to Chapter 35 for more details.

Prazosin (Minipres)

Prazosin is a new agent frequently classified as a vasodilator. Earlier work concluded that a significant component of the action of prazosin was attributable to direct vascular smooth muscle relaxation. However, recent studies[11,34] demonstrate that this drug's primary mode of action is α adrenergic blockade. This occurs in the postjunctional (vascular) α receptors, causing vasodilation. Prazosin's action is unlike that of the other two α-blockers, which have prejunctional and postjunctional action that enhances postural drop and causes tachycardia, and increases renin activity. Prazosin is unique among existing antihypertensives. CO, HR, GFR, and RBF are unchanged. Plasma renin activity is not appreciably altered, but PVR is significantly reduced. The onset of a full hypotensive response occurs 2 hours after initiation of therapy and lasts 24 hours after cessation of therapy.

Indications and Contraindications. Prazosin can be used as either a step-2 or a step-3 drug, in the management of mild, moderate, and possibly severe hypertension. To date there are no known contraindications. However, since this is a newer agent, care should be taken to keep abreast of new data.

Nursing Implications. Nurses can be instrumental in reducing the adverse first-dose effects of prazosin (postural

hypotension, syncope, light headedness, tachycardia), which can be precipitated by exercise and Na+ depletion. Patients who are Na+-depleted may be more vulnerable to this phenomenon because they are also volume-depleted. Careful assessment of the patient's daily Na+ intake will provide useful information. First-dose effects are more likely to occur in patients taking 100 mEq (2300 mg)* or less of Na+ a day and least likely to occur in those ingesting 250 mEq (5750 mg) of Na+ per day for a week prior to therapy.[40] Thus, if a patient is on a very restricted Na+ diet, the nurse should consult with the physician concerning the possibility of adjusting the Na+ intake for several days before starting therapy. In all cases, the nurse should advise the patient of the possibility of these effects and caution him to take the first dose in a safe environment, such as the doctor's office or at home with a relative or friend in attendance. The patient should be cautioned especially against taking the initial dose prior to driving an automobile or any other potentially hazardous equipment.

BETA ADRENERGIC BLOCKING AGENTS

Propranolol (Inderal)

Although propranolol is discussed in Chapter 35, its antihypertensive uses will be presented briefly in this chapter. Propranolol is used widely as an antihypertensive agent, but its antihypertensive mechanism is poorly understood. Because of β blockade, CO is reduced, and there is a gradual loss of the reflex increase of PVR present in high CO states. Propranolol also appears to reduce sympathetic nervous system outflow through some central mechanism. In addition, propranolol lowers plasma renin activity.

Indications and Contraindications. Propranolol is recommended in the treatment of high renin hypertension[10] as a step-1 drug and, as a step-2 drug, is useful in controlling hypertension in those who have coronary artery disease (CAD), hyperkinetic states, arrhythmias, gout, or inability to tolerate postural hypotension. It is also used as adjunct therapy with hydralazine to control reflex tachycardia. Contraindications are discussed in Chapter 35.

Nursing Implications. This agent can cause fatigue and mental depression, although less commonly than reserpine. Patients and families should be warned about the possibility of these effects. They may also need assistance with adherence, since multiple and high doses of this drug are usually dispensed. Additional nursing actions are discussed in Chapter 35.

Metoprolol (Lopressor)

Metoprolol, a selective β$_1$-blocker, acts to reduce hypertension by the same action as propranolol.[5,6] Refer to Chapter 35 for additional details.

* 1 mEq Na+ = 23 mg Na+

CENTRAL ACTING AGENTS

Clonidine (Catapres)

Clonidine, a newer agent that seems to have its primary action in the CNS, directly stimulates α-adrenergic receptors, causing an inhibition of sympathetic outflow from the brain stem. It may also have a peripheral component, since total PVR is lowered, possibly by vasodilation or perhaps by reduced sympathetic tone. CO, HR, and plasma renin activity are reduced. The GFR and RBF are unchanged. Sodium is retained. The onset of the hypotensive effect occurs in 30 to 60 minutes after initiation of therapy and lasts 6 to 8 hours after cessation of therapy.

Indications and Contraindications. Clonidine is a step-2 drug indicated in the treatment of mild, moderate, and severe hypertension. It is contraindicated for unreliable patients, since abrupt withdrawal may cause hypertensive crisis. It should be used with caution for patients who may be harmed by sudden or profound hypotension, such as those with cerebral, coronary, or renal insufficiency, or those who have had a recent myocardial infarction.

Nursing Implications. In order to assess patient reliability, nurses need to determine the patient's understanding and interest in his disease and his willingness to adhere to the prescribed medical plan. The nurse should give explicit instructions about the serious consequences of abrupt cessation of this drug, which must never be allowed to happen for any reason. The patient should understand that the side effects are either self-limiting or manageable and should be brought to the attention of the physician or nurse. It is important that the patient maintain an adequate blood level of clonidine. He should be taught to anticipate occasions on which he may run out of the drug, such as during trips or because of missed doctor's appointments. In addition, the nurse should instruct the patient that alcohol potentiates this drug's effects. She should caution him against using machinery or vehicles in the presence of drowsiness or sedation.

Methyldopa (Aldomet)

In the past, methyldopa was thought to act by replacing norepinephrine at sympathetic nerve endings with methyldopa's metabolite, alpha-methylnorepinephrine, a false neurotransmitter. Nickerson,[33] Conn[12] and others cite new animal studies that demonstrate that the primary site of action is probably in the brain stem. Kersting's results[25] are compatible with this theory. The drug may act directly on the peripheral vascular system as well. CO, HR, GFR, and RBF remain essentially unchanged. The hypotensive response occurs in 4 to 6 hours after onset of therapy and persists for 24 hours after cessation.

Indications and Contraindications. Methyldopa, a step-2 drug, is indicated in the treatment of moderate-to-severe hypertension. It is especially useful in patients with CAD or CHF, or for those with impaired renal function, since it does not usually further decrease RBF and increase peripheral

vein renin activity. It can be given during all hypertensive emergencies except those caused by pheochromocytoma, because methyldopa interferes with urinary catecholamine excretion. It is contraindicated for patients with active hepatic disease, or for those who have had hepatitis as a sequelae of previous methyldopa therapy. Other contraindications include hemolytic anemia or sensitivity to the drug.

Nursing Implications. Nurses should be aware of the necessity of monitoring the hemoglobin and liver function of patients receiving methyldopa. All specimens for type and cross match should clearly state that the patient is taking methyldopa so that Coombs' test can be performed. The patient should be cautioned about operating machinery and vehicles in the presence of drowsiness and sedation. Complaints of excessive fatigue should be reported immediately to the physician or nurse practitioner.

GANGLIONIC BLOCKING AGENTS

Ganglionic blocking agents are powerful drugs that inhibit the transmission of nerve impulses through both the sympathetic and parasympathetic ganglia, resulting in vasodilation and subsequent hypotension. Severe untoward reactions, such as profound postural hypotension, paralytic ileus, circulatory collapse, and hypertensive rebound (after drug withdrawal) can occur. Mecamylamine hydrochloride (Inversine hydrochloride), pentholinum tartrate (Ansolysen), and trimethaphan camsylate (Arfonad) are rarely used in the treatment of hypertension or hypertensive emergencies today, because they have been replaced by newer drugs with more acceptable adverse effects.

VASODILATORS

Hydralazine (Apresoline; Rolazine; Dralzine; LoPres)

Hydralazine decreases BP by direct relaxation of vascular smooth muscle, with its greatest effect upon the resistance vessels. The subsequent hypotension is thought to result in baroreceptor stimulation, which in turn causes increased adrenergic discharge to the heart and peripheral vessels. This results in a sharp increase in HR and CO, which offsets much of the antihypertensive effects of the drug when used alone and results in side effects. It maintains renal and cerebral blood flow and causes Na^+ and water retention. Concomitant use with propranolol, reserpine, or guanethidine can ameliorate the reflex tachycardia. The hypotensive effect begins in 20 to 30 minutes and lasts 2 to 4 hours.

Indications and Contraindications. Hydralazine is indicated in the treatment of moderate-to-severe hypertension and for hypertensive emergencies. It is contraindicated for patients with mitral valve disease, systemic lupus erythematosus (SLE), dissecting aortic aneurysm, and CHF during hypertensive emergencies. It may be used, if needed, for patients with CAD if the patient is taking a step-2 drug. It should be used with caution, if at all, for patients with hyperdynamic circulatory states.

Nursing Implications. Nurses should monitor for an SLE-like or rheumatoid syndrome by checking the hemoglobin and soliciting symptoms of arthralgias. The electrocardiogram (ECG) should be monitored for tachycardia or changes indicating ischemia. Frequent BP monitoring is required during or after intravenous (IV) or intramuscular (IM) use.

Minoxidil

Minoxidil is a long-acting oral vasodilator currently under study. Pettinger and Mitchell[38] have shown it to be useful in the management of refractory hypertension with renal impairment. It may be superior to hydralazine.[16]

Diazoxide (Hyperstat)

Diazoxide is a powerful agent that produces rapid (3–5 minutes) hypotension by direct relaxation of the resistance vessels, consequently reducing PVR. It also exerts an effect on other smooth muscle, such as that of the uterus. CO and HR are increased, and GFR and RBF are transiently decreased. It has no direct action on the CNS. Diazoxide causes hyperglycemia and, like other antihypertensives, Na$^+$ and water retention.

Indications and Contraindications. Diazoxide is indicated in the treatment of hypertensive emergencies, especially when encephalopathy or intracranial hemorrhage are present. It is contraindicated for patients with arteriovenous shunt, coarctation of the aorta, or in pregnancy when the interruption of labor is undesirable. It should be used with extreme caution, if at all, for patients with CHF, coronary insufficiency, acute dissecting aortic aneurysm, or thiazide sensitivity.

Nursing Implications. During administration of diazoxide, nurses should ensure that the patient is recumbent and that the BP is monitored frequently. If the patient is ambulatory after therapy, the final BP measurement should be taken in the standing position. Watchfulness for signs and symptoms of cerebral and cardiac ischemia, as well as CHF and hyperglycemia, is important.

Sodium Nitroprusside (Nipride)

Sodium nitroprusside is a very powerful vasodilator which acts directly on the vascular smooth muscles of the resistance and capacitance vessels. A hypotensive response occurs in 30 to 60 seconds, but disappears as rapidly when the infusion is stopped. A slight increase in HR, a moderate reduction of PVR, and, usually, a decrease in CO ensue. In refractory heart failure or acute myocardial infarction (MI), CO and stroke volume (SV) are increased and left ventricular filling pressure is decreased. Renal blood flow and GFR are not appreciably altered.

Indications and Contraindications. Sodium nitroprusside is indicated in the treatment of essentially all hypertensive emergencies, especially those with a component of dissecting aortic aneurysm, intracranial hemorrhage, or acute left ventricular failure. It is contraindicated in the presence of arteriovenous shunt, coarctation of the aorta, or when adequate monitoring facilities are not available. It should be used with caution for patients with hypothyroidism or renal or hepatic impairment.

Nursing Implications. Nurses should be aware that this is a powerful drug with very rapid action and that profound hypotension may occur. Frequent BP monitoring is mandatory. An infusion pump should be used to administer sodium nitroprusside. Meticulous mixing and monitoring of the solution is imperative. Care must be taken so that a profound hypotensive response does not occur as a consequence of the greater potency of the fresh mix. It is imperative that the IV bag be labelled with the time that the solution was mixed and that the solution be discarded 4 hours after mixing. When a new solution is started, the infusion rate may have to be adjusted according to its effects on the BP. The IV solution must be protected from light by an aluminum foil cover. Care should be taken to explain to the patient the sudden action and value of this drug and the necessity of close monitoring. If the drug is used for an extended period, serum thiocynate levels should be monitored daily.

NURSING INTERVENTIONS IN ANTIHYPERTENSIVE DRUG THERAPY

Acute Situation

It is the nurse's responsibility to closely monitor the BP response of the patient and communicate it to the physician. Intravenous infusion of antihypertensive agents must be carefully adjusted because extreme accuracy is essential. It must be ascertained that mechanical aids, such as an infusion pump or arterial monitor, are functioning properly. Arterial lines require special observation for patency and position. The nurse should be particularly observant for signs and symptoms of severe hypotension and cardiovascular collapse, such as mental confusion, stupor, seizures, or coma. Although these can result from any antihypertensive drug, they are more commonly associated with rapid administration of the more powerful agents. The nurse should be alert for and notify the physician of any ECG changes of ischemia or arrhythmias, such as bradycardia, tachycardia, or ectopic beats. Special care should be taken to reassure the patient and to explain the use of the equipment to allay fear. It is important to understand that sudden hypotension can be as disastrous as severe hypertension, that the agents employed have powerful responses, and that elderly patients are more susceptible to the action and adverse effects of these drugs.

Chronic or Stable Situation

Baseline hemoglobin, electrolytes, blood urea nitrogen (BUN), ECG, urinalysis, and, in some cases, liver function tests should be obtained prior to the institution of and during therapy. Some antihypertensive agents will require more frequent monitoring than others because of their potency or adverse effects.

Accurate measurement of BP is crucial in the management of hypertensive patients. Proper technique and equipment are essential but often taken for granted (Chap. 14). In a stable condition, the hypertensive patient's BP should be taken in the sitting position after a 10-minute rest. However, these patients should be checked for a postural BP drop by taking the BP in the lying, sitting, and standing positions. Heart rate should also be monitored. The nurse should be aware of the antihypertensive agents most likely to cause orthostatic hypotension. The physician sets the goal of BP reduction to be achieved, usually as to as close to 140/90 as possible.[21] The nurse should discuss this with the patient in terms of making it a mutual goal, offering as much support as necessary, and emphasizing concern for and availability to the patient.

The nurse has a unique and expanding role in caring for the patient with chronic hypertension. It is frequently her responsibility to educate the patient about the rationale of lifetime drug therapy for hypertension. This requires a comprehensive understanding of the risk factors and sequelae of hypertension (Chaps. 13, 47). Because of the various side effects of each antihypertensive agent, assessment of patient reliability, preexisting symptoms, history of depression, impotence, nasal congestion, and bowel problems must be done prior to institution of drug therapy.

In order to promote patient cooperation, it is necessary to engage the patient in his own therapy while also enlisting the aid of a spouse or friend, if possible. Assessment of and response to side effects that interfere with the patient's life style is paramount, because the patient simply will not take a drug that interferes significantly with his sex life, sports life, or work life. This is especially true if he felt well prior to treatment. The nurse can provide the continuity, the access, the advocacy, and the time that these patients need and should have.

The nurse should devise a plan for teaching and monitoring each patient based on an assessment of his needs and level of comprehension. The elderly present special assessment and planning problems for the nurse. Because they live alone, have memory impairment, and have difficulties with mobility, they require careful evaluation prior to initation of drug therapy. They may forget to take medications or may take an extra dose, not remembering that it was taken before. Difficulty in getting to the bathroom may complicate diuretic therapy. An already diminished appetite may be further reduced as a side effect of some drugs. Frequently this group does not want to be a "bother" and will not volunteer problems or symptoms. Gentle probing, without judgmental questions, can establish the concerns, misconceptions, fear, hostility, passivity, or other characteristics of the patient and will provide valuable information from which to set priorities and devise a systematic approach.

The patient should be taught about his drugs on a continuing basis. Their actions, more common side effects and dangers, such as abrupt withdrawal, should be presented. Written explanations should accompany discussions with the patient and family. It should be suggested that all questions which the patient thinks of at home be written down for future discussion.

Monitoring the BP is one of the best ways to assess patient compliance to the drug regimen. This information should be shown to the patient so that he has an objective way of measuring his progress and of seeing the importance of strict adherence to this therapy. If the BP has not dropped after an appropriate interval, it can indicate inadequate drug therapy or missed medications. Questions such as "Are you having any problems with the medicine?" and "It is certainly difficult remembering to take pills, isn't it?" can help to elicit if and why the patient has not been complying. The reason may be as simple as the patient's not eating breakfast and, thus, not remembering the morning dose. However, further questioning may reveal that the patient is taking other medications that antagonize the effects of his antihypertensive drugs. (Table 37-3 lists over-the-counter drugs with sympathomimetic effects.) It is impossible to overemphasize the need to avoid such preparations if the patient has even borderline hypertension. Preparations most likely to contain sympathomimetic agents are those used to treat colds and allergies (including topical decongestants) and asthma.

The patient may not be adhering to the other components of his therapy, such as maintaining a low Na+ diet. Sodium restriction is a primary treatment for reducing increased BP.

TABLE 37-3   REPRESENTATIVE OVER-THE-COUNTER DRUGS CONTAINING SYMPATHOMIMETIC AGENTS

Cold and Allergy Products[13]

Alka-Seltzer Plus	Triaminicin
Allerest	Ursinus
Allergesic	Vasominic TD
Apcohist Allergy Tablets	Ventilade
Bayer Decongestant	
BC All Clear	**Topical Decongestants**[13]
Chlor-Trimeton Decongestant	Afrin
Codimal	Allerest
Conex DA	Contact Nasal Mist
Conex Plus	Coricidin
Contac	Dristan
Coricidin-D	Naso Mist
Coryban-D	Neo-Synephrine
D-Feda	Privine
Dristan (tablet and time	Sine-Off Once-a-Day
capsule)	Sinex L.A.
Endecon	Sinutab
Extendac	Super Anahist
Fedahist	Vicks
Fedrazil	Vicks Sinex
Ginospan	
Nazac Timed-Disintegration	**Asthma Products**[17]
Decongestant	Amodrine
Novaphed	Asma-Lief
Pyrroxate	Asthma Nefrin
Rhinidrin	Breatheasy
Sinulin	Bronitin
Sinurex	Bronkaid
Sinustat	Bronkotabs
Sinutab	Phedral
Spantac	Primatene M
Sudafed	Primatene P
Super Anahist	Tedral
Timed Cold Capsules	Thalfed
	Vaponefrin Solution
	Verequad

TABLE 37-4　SODIUM CONTENT OF SOME MEDICINALS

Type of Medicinal	Na⁺ content (mg)
LAXATIVES	
Dialose Plus capsules	38
Fleet enema	5000
Metamucil Instant Mix	250
Phospho-Soda (5 ml)	55
Sal Hepatica (1 tsp)	1000
Travad liquid (5 ml)	185
ANTACIDS	
Alka-Seltzer (1 tablet)	521
Bisodal power (10 g)	1540
Bromo Seltzer (1 capsule)	717
Calcium Carbonate and Soda	543
Creamalin	25
Eno Salts (1 tsp)	738
Fizrin (1 tablet)	673
Maalox (5 ml)	2.5
Riopan Chewables (tablet)	0.7
Riopan Liquid (5 ml)	0.7
Riopan tablets (1)	0.7
Rolaids (1 tablet)	53
COUGH FORMULAS	
Dristan (5 ml)	59
Mucomyst 1%, (10 ml)	280
Phenergan (5 ml)	51
Vicks Cough Syrup (5 ml)	54
Vicks Formula 44 (5 ml)	68
THERAPEUTICS AND DIAGNOSTICS	
Enovid (10 mg tablets)	52
Geopen (5 g)	680
Hypaque M 75% (20 ml)	200
Keflin (4 g)	249
Ovulen-28	322
Polycillin (3 g)	204
SKiodan 40% (50 ml)	1850
Surital (10 g)	1100
Viokase Powder (100 g)	2440
MISCELLANEOUS	
Carnation Slender (10 oz)	440
Kayexalate powder (15 g)	550
Nervine Effervescent (1 tablet)	544
Precision-LR (6 doses)	1500
Vivonex HN (6 doses)	2312

(Sodium in Medicinals. San Francisco, San Francisco Heart Association, 1973)

It is also important because antihypertensive drugs, except diuretics and propranolol, cause Na⁺ retention. The importance of maintaining a low Na⁺ diet must be fully understood by the patient and his family. A thorough discussion of low Na⁺ diets can be found in Chapter 47. Additionally, the patient must be apprised that there are many hidden sources of Na⁺. Over-the-counter drugs can contain large amounts of Na⁺ (Table 37-4). Patients should be cautioned that not all Na⁺-containing products taste "salty" and that they must, therefore, learn to read labels.

DIURETICS

Diuretics are the cornerstone in the management of hypertension and are the base of most regimens. A diuretic alone will satisfactorily control BP in approximately one-third of the patients with mild hypertension. Diuretics are also valuable in the management of CHF, pulmonary edema, hepatic cirrhosis, ascites, anasarca, nephrotic syndrome, corticosteroid therapy, and other expanded volume states.

There are eight distinct types of diuretics: water itself, which is not used in expanded-volume states, sulfonamide derivatives, which comprise the thiazides and related agents, loop diuretics, potassium-sparing diuretics, organomercurials, carbonic anhydrase inhibitors, osmotic diuretics, and xanthine diuretics. Natriuretics, or drugs increasing Na⁺ excretion, and saluretics, or drugs increasing sodium excretion, are terms frequently used interchangeably with the term "diuretics," which means "promoting urine." Kaliuretic is a term used to connote potassium (K⁺) excretion. Not all diuretics are equally natriuretic, saluretic, or kaliuretic.

Prior to the advent of sulfonamide diuretics, the mercurials, xanthines, and osmotic diuretics were more commonly used. Their deficiencies, restrictions, and limited mode of delivery spurred the search for better agents, such as those we use most often today. Of course the search continues for the "perfect" diuretic. The older agents, in the meantime, are still used in certain clinical situations to which they are uniquely suited. Actions, indications, contraindications, and nursing implications of representative drugs in each category are discussed in the text. General nursing care for the patient on diuretic therapy is presented at the end of this section. Table 37-5 lists specific information regarding dosage and administration, drug interactions, and toxic and side effects of diuretic agents.

SULFONAMIDE DERIVATIVES

The thiazides and related agents, which include chlorthalidone (Hygroten), quinethazone (Hydromax), and metolazone (Zaroxolyn) are the most commonly used of all diuretics, and perhaps of all therapeutic agents. The precise mechanism by which these agents act is not completely understood. They increase the excretion of Na⁺, chloride (C1⁻) and water at the distal tubule in the nephron (Fig. 37-3D). Potassium excretion is augmented because the drugs increase its secretion by the distal tubule, resulting in significant kaliuresis and potential hypokalemia. It is also thought that diuretics may reduce the vasomotor response to catecholamines, or reduce PVR, or may act by direct dilation of the arterioles. However, Bennett and co-workers[7] suggest that volume depletion is the only mechanism by which these drugs lower BP. Additionally, these drugs potentiate antihypertensive agents, since they counteract the retention of Na⁺, C1⁻, and water in common with all antihypertensive agents except propranolol. All sulfonamide derivatives except metolazone decrease GFR. Other thiazide effects include inhibition of insulin release and blockade of peripheral glucose utilization, producing hyperglycemia or aggravating preexisting diabetes mellitus.

Indications and Contraindications. The thiazides and related agents are used as step-1 drugs in hypertension. They are indicated in chronic, long-term management for most expanded-volume states, such as CHF, nephrotic syndrome, cirrhosis, and with corticosteroid therapy. They are contraindicated for patients with anuria and sensitivity to sulfonamides, and, for metolazone, should not be given to patients with severe renal impairment. Thiazides cause hyperuricemia in approximately 20% of hypertensive pa-

TABLE 37-5 DIURETIC AGENTS

Agent	Dosage/Administration	Drug Interaction	Toxic Effects	Side Effects
SULFONAMIDE DERIVATIVES				
Thiazides:				
Benthiazide (Aquatag; Exna)	50–200 mg PO q.d.*	Potentiates antihypertensives; potentiated by alcohol, barbiturates and narcotics. When administering cholestyramine, give 1 hour after thiazides. Steroids and amphotericin increase K+ loss.	Profound lethargy leading to coma; rarely rhabdomyolysis as a result of severe hypokalemia (more commonly with chlorthalidone); dilutional hyponatremia; edema in chronic CHF or liver-diseased patients; hypochloremic alkalosis; hyperglycemia, hyperuricemia	Increased serum BUN, uric acid, glucose, Ca²⁺, decreased K+ and Cl⁻; gastric irritation, nausea, vomiting, anorexia, cramping, diarrhea, constipation, dry mouth, bad taste, fever, photosensitivity, rash, blood dyscrasias, pancreatitis, respiratory distress, hypovolemia, oliguria
Chlorothiazide (Diuril)	500–1500 mg PO q.d.*			
Hydrochlorothiazide (Esidrex; Oretic; Hydrodiuril)	50–150 mg PO q.d.*			
Hydroflumethiazide (Saluron; Dicardin)	50–150 mg PO q.d.*			
Bendroflumethiazide (Naturetin)	10 mg PO q.d.			
Trichlormethiazide (Naqua; Metahydrin)	2–8 mg PO q.d.			
Methyclothiazide (Enduron; Aquatensen)	5–15 mg PO q.d.			
Polythiazide (Renese)	2–8 mg PO q.d.			
Cyclothiazide (Anhydron)	2–6 mg PO q.d.			
Thiazidelike:				
Chlorthalidone (Hygroton)	25–100 mg PO q.d.			
Quinethazone (Hydromox)	50–150 mg PO q.d.*			
Metolazone (Zaroxolyn)	2.5–5.0 mg PO q.d.			
LOOP DIURETICS				
Furosemide (Lasix)	PO: 40–160 mg q.d.*; IV: 20–40 mg in 1–2 minutes; repeat in 20 mg increments every 2 hours if needed; 100–200 mg IV in 1–2 minutes for hypertensive emergencies; IM: 20–40 mg. Do not use if solution has a yellow color. Do not mix with other drugs such as morphine, ephedrine, epinephrine, local anesthestics, because solution may precipitate. Use of more than one ampule increases chance of minute glass particles being administered.	Potentiates antihypertensive drugs; cephaloridine enhances nephrotoxicity; kanamycin enhances ototoxicity. Steroids and amphotericin increase K+ loss.	Swift and severe electrolyte and acid-base imbalance, such as hypochloremic alkalosis, hypokalemia, hypovolemia, dehydration, hypotensive prostration. Hemoconcentration can lead to circulatory collapse or possibly to fatal vascular thrombosis or embolism; rarely to sudden death from cardiac arrest with IV use; hearing loss, allergic interstitial nephritis, and blood dyscrasias can occur.	Increased serum uric acid, BUN, glucose; decreased serum K+, Cl⁻, Mg²⁺; nausea, vomiting, diarrhea, lightheadedness, photosensitivity, blurred vision, rash, tinnitus, bladder spasm, headache, sweet taste, blood dyscrasias, hypovolemia, pancreatitis.
Ethacrynic acid (Edecrin)	PO: 25–200 mg PO q.d.* after meals; preferably on alternate days; IV: 0.5–1 mg/kg, or 50 mg for average adult. IV injection should be given slowly over a period of several minutes; may be given through tubing of a running IV infusion. Observe the following precautions: Mix 50 mg per 50 ml of D₅W or normal saline; mix will precipitate in D₅W with pH of 5 or less *(cont. next page)*	As above, but in addition it potentiates warfarin.	As above, but in addition hypoglycemia with convulsions can occur in patients with uremia; liver damage; GI bleeding (more common with IV use); severe neutropenia; agranulocytosis; profuse watery diarrhea, deafness more common than with furosemide.	Blood disturbances as above. Anorexia, vomiting, nausea, diarrhea, abdominal discomfort, malaise, dysphagia, liver dysfunction, rash, chills, fever, fatigue, apprehension, mental confusion.

TABLE 37-5 DIURETIC AGENTS (Cont.)

Agent	Dosage/Administration	Drug Interaction	Toxic Effects	Side Effects
	and should be discarded. Change sites to avoid thrombophlebitis; use solution within 24 hours or discard; label with the time mixed. It is incompatible with: Normosol-M, hydralazine, procainamide, reserpine, or tolazine in saline. Do not give with blood or blood products. Do not give IM or SC.			
Ethacrynate sodium (Edecrin Sodium)	As above	As above	As above	As above
POTASSIUM-SPARING DIURETICS				
Spironolactone (Aldactone)	50–400 mg PO q.d.*	Potentiates antihypertensives and other diuretics. Effect neutralized by aspirin 600 mg.	Fatal arrhythmias from hyperkalemia. Some investigators have noted a striking increase in the incidence of breast cancer,[28] while others provide evidence against this.[23] Breast enlargement can occur.	Cramping, diarrhea, skin eruptions, drug fever, ataxia, interference with sexual function, irregular menses or amenorrhea, postmenopausal bleeding, hirsutism, deepening of the voice.
Triamterene (Dyrenium)	100–300 mg PO q.d.*	May potentiate antihypertensives.	Severe hyperkalemia; rarely severe hypotension. Other severe electrolyte imbalance	Nausea, vomiting, diarrhea, dizziness, hypotension, weakness, muscle cramps, dry mouth, anaphylaxis, photosensitivity, rash, blood dyscrasias, liver dysfunction, renal colic.
OSMOTIC DIURETICS				
Mannitol (Osmitrol)	Dosage varies with condition being treated (consult drug insert). Given only IV. Test dose may be used; (consult drug insert for criteria of proper response). Adjust infusion rate for hourly urine output of 30–50 ml. Should not be given with blood unless 20 mEq of NaCl per liter is added.	None known	Severe electrolyte imbalance; overexpansion of intravascular fluid, resulting in pulmonary edema, CHF, and water intoxication; cerebral dissection and fatal cerebral acidosis can occur.	Serum K^+, Na^+, and fluid volume can be either increased or decreased; dry mouth, thirst, headache, blurred vision, nausea, vomiting, rhinitis, arm or back pain, chills, fever, dizziness, urticaria, hypotension or hypertension, tachycardia, muscle rigidity, chest pain.
Urea (Ureaphil; Urevert)	Dosage varies with condition being treated (consult drug insert). Given as a 30% solution in $D_{5-10}W$ or in 10% invertrose in prepared mix. Rate of injection should not exceed 4 ml/minute, or 1.5 g/kg, or 120 g/24 hours.	Prolongs prothrombin time, and therefore potentiates warfarin.	As above, but in addition, hemolysis from rapid injection; convulsions and death from subdural hematoma.	Electrolyte imbalance as above; headache, nausea, vomiting, syncope, disorientation, dizziness, agitation, mental confusion, nervousness, hypotension, tachycardia, cardiotoxicity, hyperthermia, skin blebs.

* Divided doses

tients[4] and should, therefore, not be given to patients with preexisting gout. They should be administered cautiously to patients with severe hepatic impairment or pregnancy.

Nursing Implications. Monitor for signs and symptoms of hyperglycemia. In the patient with known diabetes mellitus, the need for oral hypoglycemic agents or insulin may increase. Be aware that acute attacks of gout may be precipitated by the hyperuricemia associated with thiazide therapy. This is especially true of hypertensive patients, many of whom have preexisting elevated serum uric acid levels. Hyperuricemia may be treated with colchicine, U.S.P.

LOOP DIURETICS

Furosemide (Lasix)

Furosemide is a powerful loop diuretic, so called because of its action in the medullary portion of the ascending limb of

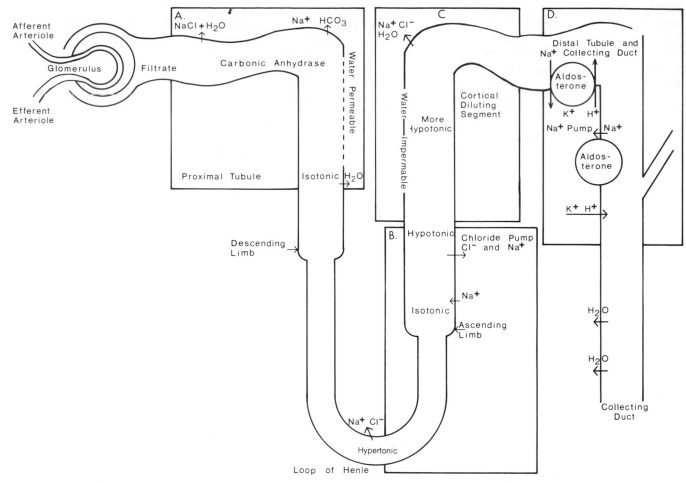

Fig. 37-3. Sites of action of diuretic agents. (**A**) The proximal tubule is the site for approximately 60% to 80% of the reabsorption of filtered Na^+. The inhibition of carbonic anhydrase at this site causes less H^+ to be generated from carbon dioxide (CO_2) and water (H_2O). Subsequently, the Na^+–H^+ exchange throughout the nephron is retarded, and more Na^+ is delivered to the distal tubule for excretion. (**B**) The ascending limb of Henle's loop, part of the medullary segment, contains the active Cl^- pump where 20% to 40% of the filtered Na^+ is delivered. Chloride is actively reabsorbed in the ascending limb, with Na^+ passively following, causing approximately 35% of NaCl to be reabsorbed. The loop diuretics inhibit this reabsorption, thus delivering more Na^+ to the distal portion of the distal tubule and collecting duct. (**C**) The proximal portion of the distal tubule, or cortical segment, normally receives 10% to 15% of the filtered Na^+. (**D**) The distal portion of the distal tubule and collecting duct contains the active Na^+ pump, which is under the control of aldosterone. Potassium and H^+ are exchanged for Na^+, so that for every molecule of Na^+ reabsorbed, one molecule of K^+ is excreted. Consequently, the more Na^+ delivered to this site, the greater is the exchange of Na^+ for K^+, producing kaliuresis and potential hypokalemia. Thiazides and related agents inhibit the reabsorption of the Na^+ in this segment. The quantity of exchange is dependent upon the aldosterone concentration. The higher the aldosterone level, the greater is the reabsorption of Na^+ and the greater the loss of K^+. The K^+-sparing diuretics antagonize the aldosterone or depress the reabsorption mechanism. (Adapted from Onesti G: Consultation in Hypertension: A Clinical Symposium. Rochester NY, Pennwalt Prescription Products, 1976)

the loop of Henle where it inhibits the reabsorption of Na^+ and Cl^- (Fig. 37-3B). Of filtered Na^+ and Cl^-, 20% to 40% is delivered to the ascending loop, where it is prevented by furosemide from being absorbed. This concentration of Na^+ and Cl^- is delivered in a large bolus to the distal tubule, where furosemide also reduces Na^+ reabsorption and increases K^+ excretion. Some data suggest that furosemide also acts on the proximal tubule, but opinions are not unanimous. Massive diuresis results, starting 30 to 60 minutes after oral administration of the drug, or 5 minutes

after IV infusion. RBF and GFR are increased. Remarkably prompt relief of symptoms of acute pulmonary edema is achieved following IV administration of furosemide. This may be related to shifting of fluid from the lung in response to the very powerful and prompt diuretic effect. In addition, PVR may be decreased prior to the diuretic effect. However, this is not well documented.

Indications and Contraindications. Furosemide is used in the treatment of CHF, pulmonary edema, refractory peripheral edema, hypertensive emergencies, nephrotic syndrome, and hepatic cirrhosis, or in moderate-to-severe hypertension in conjunction with antihypertensive agents. Its use is contraindicated for patients with increasing azotemia, metabolic alkalosis, sensitivity to sulfa drugs, pulmonary edema from cardiogenic shock, pregnancy or lactation, or those taking cephaloridine (Loridine).

Nursing Implications. Nurses must be cognizant of the potency of this agent, especially when given parenterally. Sudden, swift electrolyte imbalance can occur, especially in patients with renal or hepatic disease, who already have difficulties in maintaining homeostasis. The peripheral vasodilation which may follow IV administration can lead to postural hypotension. Patients must understand that the large quantity of urine is a desired action of the drug. The patient should be warned to call attention to new symptoms, such as hearing loss, or worsening of existing symptoms. Special mixing and administration precautions must be observed.

Ethacrynic Acid (Edecrin)

In the nephron, the actions of ethacrynic acid and furosemide are essentially the same. Renal blood flow and GFR remain essentially unchanged. Diuresis is as swift with ethacrynic acid as with furosemide.

Indications and Contraindications. Ethacrynic acid is indicated in situations requiring a powerful diuretic. It is useful in restoring effectiveness of "resistant" drug regimens in hypertensive management. Ethacrynic acid is contraindicated in the same instances as furosemide, but has a greater propensity to cause deafness.

Nursing Implications. The nurse's responsibilities are the same as those listed for furosemide. Additionally, patients also taking warfarin should be observed for an inordinately prolonged prothrombin time and its consequences. Special attention to mixing and IV administration should be observed. It should not be given as an IM or subcutaneous (SC) injection.

POTASSIUM-SPARING DIURETICS

Spironolactone (Aldactone)

Spironolactone is a direct antagonist of aldosterone, a mineralocorticoid which influences Na+ and K+ exchange at the distal tubule of the nephron (Fig. 37-3D). Normally, K+ is exchanged in the distal tubule for Na+, thus retaining Na+ in the extracellular fluid. By having this action blocked, Na+ is excreted but K+ is retained, or "spared." This action is opposite to the usual Na+ reabsorption and K+ loss, which occurs normally and with kaliuretics. Action of spironolactone is slow, taking 5 days for initiation of any effect and up to 14 days for maximal effect.

Indications and Contraindications. Spironolactone is indicated in the treatment of hyperaldosteronism and renal

vascular hypertension and when persons are resistant to other diuretics. It is most frequently used concomitantly with other diuretics to counteract the loss of K+. Spironolactone is especially useful in the management of persons who have hepatic cirrhosis with ascites, since these patients have an increased aldosterone output. It is helpful in preventing digitalis toxicity secondary to hypokalemia, and is useful for patients sensitive to sulfonamide. Spironolactone is contraindicated for patients with severe renal or hepatic disease, anuria, or hyperkalemia.

Nursing Implications. Nurses must assess the patient for hyperkalemia and Na+ depletion. Because of the serious arrhythmias that may be caused by hyperkalemia, this is a potentially fatal consequence of spironolactone therapy. Electrocardiograms should be performed periodically to assess the effects of the K+ level on the myocardium (Chaps. 9, 17). Serum Na+ and K+ should be monitored routinely. Usually patients taking diuretics are encouraged to increase K+ intake, but when taking spironolactone, they must be cautioned to avoid excessive dietary K+. Table 37-6 lists K+ contents of commonly used food products. The use of K+ supplements, such as KCl solution, Lite Salt (half NaCl, half KCl) and salt substitute (KCl), should be avoided. Since two aspirin tablets (600 mg) essentially negate the action of spironolactone,[9] the patient should be instructed to avoid the use of aspirin and over-the-counter remedies that contain aspirin.

Triamterene (Dyrenium)

Triamterene depresses reabsorption of Na+ and excretion of K+ at the distal tubule (Fig. 37-3D). However, it is not an aldosterone antagonist. Its diuretic effect is more rapid than that of spironolactone, occurring in 2 to 4 hours and lasting approximately 8 hours.

Indications and Contraindications. Triamterene is used in much the same way as spironolactone. It is used less often

TABLE 37-6 POTASSIUM CONTENT OF COMMON FOOD PRODUCTS

Food Source	Quantity	mEq K+*
Apricots, dried	¾ cup	43
Banana, medium	1	10
Carrot, raw	1 large	10
Celery, raw	1 cup	10.5
Grapefruit	½	3.5
Milk, whole or skim	1 cup	9
Molasses	5 tbsp	34
Mushrooms	10 small	14
Orange juice, canned	1 cup	11
Peanut butter	1 tbsp	2.5
Prune juice	1 cup	41
Raisins	¾ cup	20
Spinach, fresh	½ cup	20
Steak, T-bone	1 pound	24
Tomato juice	1 cup	9

* 1 mEq K+ = 39 mg K+
(Adams CF: Nutritive Value of American Foods. Agricultural Handbook No. 465, Agriculture Research Service. Washington DC, U.S. Department of Agriculture, 1975; Bowes A, Church CF: Food Values of Portions Commonly Used, 9th ed. Philadelphia, JB Lippincott, 1963; Food and Nutrition Board: Sodium Restricted Diets. Washington DC, National Academy of Sciences, 1954)

in the management of primary hyperaldosteronism. Contraindications include renal failure and hyperkalemia.

Nursing Implications. The nurse's responsibilities are the same as those listed for spironolactone. Aspirin does not alter triamterene's effectiveness.

ORGANOMERCURIALS

Mercurials are potent agents that have been used since the 16th century. They inhibit the reabsorption of Na^+ and Cl^- in the ascending limb of Henle's loop, and possibly at the proximal and distal tubules (Fig. 37-3A, B, D). To some extent they inhibit the active excretion of K^+ at the distal tubule (Fig. 37-3D). The most commonly used organomercurials used to be mercaptomerin sodium (Thiomerin), meralluride sodium (Mercuhydrin), and merethoxylline (Dicurin). However, they are used less since the development of the thiazides and loop diuretics, and will not be discussed further.

CARBONIC ANHYDRASE INHIBITORS

Acetazolamide (Diamox) and similar agents, were the first effective oral diuretics and precursors of the thiazides. By inhibiting the enzyme carbonic anhydrase, the formation of hydrogen (H^+) and bicarbonate (HCO_3^-) in the proximal and distal tubules is reduced (Fig. 37-3A, D), and Na^+ and H^+ exchange throughout the nephron is retarded. Reabsorption of water is decreased and urine volume is increased. Sodium bicarbonate and K^+ are excreted with little loss of Cl^-. Consequently, hyperchloremic acidosis may result after 24 hours of use. The loss of K^+ can be substantial, but diminishes with prolonged use. The primary use of acetazolamide is to reduce the rate of formation of aqueous humor in patients with glaucoma. It is rarely used today as a diuretic agent and therefore will not be discussed further.

OSMOTIC DIURETICS

Mannitol (Osmitrol)

Mannitol is a potent diuretic. It pulls fluid from the intracellular to the extracellular space by osmosis. This additional ECF is rapidly transferred to the intravascular compartment, increasing RBF. Mannitol is freely filtered at the glomerulus and is not reabsorbed in the renal tubules. A significant amount of this large molecule in the renal tubules serves to increase urine production through the mechanism of osmosis. Sodium, K^+, and Cl^- are removed. Mannitol is not reabsorbed or metabolized. Cellular dehydration occurs, red blood cell volume becomes concentrated, and hematocrit is decreased. Diuresis occurs in 1 to 3 hours.

Indications and Contraindications. Mannitol is sometimes used in the prevention of renal shutdown in the presence of oliguria due to shock, trauma, burns, transfusion reactions, massive hemorrhage, or any acute renal failure prior to the development of acute tubular necrosis. It is also used to reduce intraocular pressure in the treatment of acute narrow-angle glaucoma, and is useful in treating or preventing increased intracranial pressure resulting from head trauma or neurosurgery. Mannitol can be used to promote diuresis of toxic substances, such as carbon tetrachloride, barbiturates and salicylates. Contraindications include use in patients with well-established anuria due to renal failure, severe pulmonary edema, CHF, active intracranial bleeding, or severe dehydration.

Nursing Implications. Nurses must pay particular attention to the mannitol solution so that crystals are not administered. An administration set with a filter should be used. Warming the solution helps to dissolve crystals that may have formed; if it does not, discard the solution. Accurate and frequent measurement of urinary output is essential. Patients should have an indwelling urinary catheter. The patient must be closely observed for signs and symptoms of fluid overload and electrolyte imbalance. Because tissue necrosis can occur from extravasation, the site of IV infusion must be observed for inflammation and infiltration. The patient should be told to call attention to any new symptoms or the worsening of existing symptoms. Nurses should understand why this drug has been prescribed, so that the results of its effects can be closely observed. Urinary output is very accurately monitored if the purpose of mannitol administration is to increase urine production. If reduction of increased intracranial pressure is the goal, the neurologic status is particularly closely followed.

Urea (Ureaphil; Urevert)

Urea has the same mode of action as mannitol, but is used less because it has not been approved by the Food and Drug Administration (FDA) for use in the prevention of renal failure and treament of oliguiria. Compared with mannitol, it is less safe for patients with renal failure and generally carries a higher risk, such as tissue necrosis following extravasation.

Indications and Contraindications. Urea is used to reduce intracranial and intraocular pressure, to treat acute narrow-angle glaucoma and to provide urinary excretion of toxins. Urea is contraindicated in the same instances as mannitol. In addition, it should not be used for patients with frank liver failure, severely impaired renal function, sickle cell anemia with CNS involvement, and glaucoma secondary to uveitis. Urevert, which contains 10% invertose, should not be given to patients with fructose intolerance.

Nursing Implications. Nursing care is similar to that described for mannitol. In addition, the nurse should be aware that the patient's prothrombin time may be prolonged, which can result in bleeding.

XANTHINES

Theophylline (Aminophylline)

Theophylline, theobromine, and caffeine are seldom used intentionally as diuretics today, since newer agents such as thiazides are more potent. Of the xanthines, theophylline has the greatest effect upon the kidney. The rate of Na^+ and Cl^- excretion is increased by this drug through direct action on the renal tubule. Concomitant use of carbonic anhydrase inhibitors potentiates this diuresis. The cardiovascular effects of the xanthines are complex. They increase CO by enhancing myocardial contractility and causing peripheral vasodilation. This increase in CO results in increased GFR and increased RBF, augmenting the diuretic action. Xanthine's effect upon the HR and BP is variable. Coronary blood flow increases secondary to coronary artery vasodilation, but cerebral blood flow diminishes because of cerebral vasoconstriction. Theophylline causes bronchial dilation. Caffeine is a powerful CNS stimulant. In addition, it stimulates gastric secretion of acid and pepsin.

Indications and Contraindications. Theophylline is used extensively in the treatment of bronchial asthma. Xanthines may be useful in the treatment of paroxysmal nocturnal dyspnea from left ventricular failure. Caffeine may be used in counteracting the effects of CNS depression from drug overdosage, and may be taken as a stimulant when drowsiness occurs. Caffeine should be avoided by patients with gastric hyperacidity. Theophylline should be used with caution for patients with rapid HRs and for those taking caffeine. (Refer to Chap. 17 for a discussion of paroxysmal atrial tachycardia.)

Nursing Implications. Nurses should be aware that xanthines are present in many beverages and over-the-counter drugs. Caffeine, the least powerful diuretic, is present in coffee at a nearly therapeutic dose (100 mg to 200 mg per cup) and in cola drinks (35 mg to 55 mg per 12 ounces). Theobromine is present in cocoa (200 mg per cup), and theophylline is found in tea (100 mg to 150 mg per cup). Consequently, when patients use xanthines, either therapeutically or dietarily, diuresis will occur. If they are taking diuretic agents as well, they may have increased loss of electrolytes, with the net result of a more rapid disturbance in the fluid and electrolyte balance. Teaching the patient about the use and abuse of beverages and drugs containing xanthines while taking other diuretics is essential, especially if the patient is also taking digitalis.

NURSING INTERVENTIONS IN DIURETIC THERAPY

Nursing care of patients on diuretic therapy includes much of what has been stated in the section on antihypertensive drugs. In addition, there are some nursing actions specific to patients taking diuretics.

Acute Situation

It is the nurse's responsibility to ensure proper administration of the drug, with special attention to the site of injection. Frequent and accurate measurement of the patient's fluid intake, urinary output, and weight are essential. An indwelling urethral catheter may be required. If a catheter is not in place, the nurse should ensure that the patient has easy access to the bathroom, urinal, bedpan, or call bell. Special attention must be given to the confused or elderly patients who may injure themslves when attempting to get to the bathroom. BP, including assessment for postural changes, should be monitored on a periodic basis. The patient should be closely observed for signs and symptoms of electrolyte imbalance, especially when the more powerful diuretics are used.

Chronic or Stable Situation

The nurse should assess the patient's life-style, needs, and problems that may affect or be affected by these agents. Elderly patients have special problems of mobility, memory, living alone, preexisting weakness or lassitude that must be evaluated and handled. The nurse should assist the patient in devising medication schedules to meet the needs of his life-style so that the minimum amount of inconvenience is encountered and adherence is achieved. For example, a patient who routinely works on the night shift should take his diuretic when he normally wakes up rather than in the usual morning hours, so that the medication does not interfere with his sleep time. The nurse must also be conversant with the signs and symptoms of the side effects, metabolic disturbances, and toxic effects of these drugs in order to instruct the patients to call attention to them. Assessment of the drug profile of the patient is important. This includes over-the-counter preparations as well as other substances, such as caffeine, that may be ingested throughout the day but not perceived as drugs. The patient must understand that hot weather or illnesses that cause fever, vomiting or diarrhea can cause significant K^+ and Na^+ loss. In these instances, the patient should be advised to contact the nurse or physician, so that his electrolytes can be evaluated and supplemented as needed. Nurses should be especially aware that, while electrolyte imbalance usually occurs slowly, it can develop very rapidly in the elderly or in other compromised patients. The nurse should be alert for the possibility of pregnancy in younger women, since most diuretics cross the placental barrier and should be used with caution during pregnancy.

Baseline hemoglobin, serum electrolytes, creatinine, uric acid, glucose, BUN, urinalysis, weight and ECG should be obtained before therapy and monitored on a periodic basis thereafter. Care should be taken to explain to the patient the reason for these tests and for any others the physician orders to evaluate the patient's underlying disease.

In the chronic setting, the nurse has the responsibility of teaching the patient about the action of the drug and what to expect from that action. Avoid statements such as "this drug is given for fluid retention," since the patient may misinterpret this to mean that it is given to retain fluid. If the patient is told "the purpose of this drug is to help you

TABLE 37-7 DRUGS CAUSING POTASSIUM LOSS

Steroids (prescription required)[18]
Amphotericin B (Fungizone)[43]
Laxatives (over-the-counter), chronic use of any type
  Phenolphthalein or aloe
    Ex-Lax
    Agoral
    Caroid and Bile Salts
    Carter's Little Pills
    Nature's Remedy
    Feen-a-Mint
  Seena or rhubarb
    Black Draught
    Fletcher's Castoria
    Laxaid
    Swiss Kriss
Menstrual products with diuretics (over-the-counter)
  Aqua-Ban
  Pre-Mens Forte

make urine," the patient may decide that he already urinates enough and that the drug is not needed. Care should be taken to explain the value of removing the extra fluid, in the form of urine, from the body. The patient should be informed that diuretics may produce a large amount of urine, and that frequency and urgency may occur soon after taking the drug.

With few exceptions, a no-added-salt diet is instituted with diuretic therapy. Normally, an American eats 10g to 15g of salt a day, in a variety of ways. Sodium is often hidden as a preservative in medicinals or processed foods, or may be found in the water supply in many areas of the country (Chap. 47). It is frequently very difficult for a patient to stop or greatly reduce his use of salt. Consequently, the nurse should carefully explain the value of restricted Na^+, point out less obvious sources of Na^+ and stress the importance of reading labels, with special attention to the words or symbols "sodium, Na^+, sodium chloride (NaCl), soda, and salt."

The patient should also be instructed in the use of K^+ relative to the type of diuretic prescribed. Again, care should be taken to explain its importance and the reason for either increasing or decreasing its amount. Generally, 50 to 100 mEq of K^+ is ingested each day in a typical American diet. Patients taking kaliuretics need to replace the lost K^+. This can be achieved with an increase of dietary K^+ if hypokalemia has not already developed and if caloric restrictions do not preclude the use of K^+-rich foods. An additional 40 to 100 mEq of K^+ will forestall significant hypokalemia. It is also important for patients to be informed of other drugs and over-the-counter preparations that cause extensive K^+ loss (Table 37-7). The latter should be restricted and substitutions made. Licorice, which contains glycyrrhiazic acid, also can cause significant K^+ loss. Compulsive licorice eaters may manifest false aldosteronism. Licorice is also found in liquors and chewing tobacco.

REFERENCES

1. Adams CF: Nutritive Value of American Foods. Agriculture Handbook No. 465, Agriculture Research Service. Washington, DC, U.S. Department of Agriculture, 1975
2. Armstrong B, Stevens N, Doll R: Retrospective study of the association between the use of rauwolfia derivatives and breast cancer in English women. Lancet ii:672–675, 1974
3. Bailey R, Neale TJ: Rapid clonidine withdrawal with blood pressure overshoot exaggerated by beta blockade. Br Med J i:942–943, 1976
4. Beevers DC, Hamilton M, Harper JE: The long-term treatment of hypertension with thiazide diuretics. Postgrad Med J 47:639–643, 1971
5. Bengtsson C: Comparison between metoprolol and propranolol as hypertensive agents. A double-blind cross-over study. Acta Med Scand 199(1–2):71–74, 1976
6. Bengtsson C, Johnsson G, Regardh CG: Plasma levels and effects of metoprolol on blood pressure and heart rate in hypertensive patients after an acute dose and between two doses during long-term treatment. Clin Pharmacol Ther 17:400–408, 1975
7. Bennett WM, McDonald WJ, Keuhnel E et al: Do diuretics have antihypertensive properties independent of natriuresis? Clin Pharmacol Ther 22:499–504, 1977
8. Bowes A, Church CF: Food Values of Portions Commonly Used, 9th ed. Philadelphia, JB Lippincott, 1963
9. Brest NA, Onesti G, Swartz C et al: Mechanisms of antihypertensive therapy. JAMA 211:480–484, 1970
10. Buhler FR, Laragh JH, Vaughn ED et al: Antihypertensive action of propranolol: Specific anti-renin response in high and normal renin forms of essential, renal, renovascular and malignant hypertension. Am J Cardiol, 32:511–522, 1973
11. Cambridge D, Davey MJ, Massingham R: The pharmacology of antihypertensive drugs with special reference to vasodilators and alpha adrenergic blocking agents and prazosin. Med J Aust (Suppl), 2:2–6, 1977
12. Conn HF. Current Therapy. Philadelphia, WB Saunders, 1978
13. Cormier JF, Bryant BG: Cold and allergy products. Handbook of Nonprescription Drugs, 5th ed, pp 76–11. Washington, DC, American Pharmaceutical Association, 1977
14. Finnerty FA: Hypertension: Current management. Part II. Therapy. Consultant 18(2):126–139, 1978
15. Food and Nutrition Board: Sodium Restricted Diets. Washington, DC, National Academy of Sciences, 1954
16. Gottleib TB, Katz F, Chidsey CA: Combined therapy with vasodilator drugs and beta adrenergic blockade in hypertension: A comparative study of minoxidil and hydralazine. Circulation 45:571–582, 1977
17. Hak LF: Asthma products. Handbook of Nonprescription Drugs, 5th ed, pp 112–119. Washington, DC, American Pharmaceutical Association, 1977
18. Haynes RC, Larner J: Adrenocorticotropic hormone; adrenocortical steroids and their synthetic analogs; inhibitors of adrenocortical steroid biosynthesis. In Goodman LS, Gilman A (eds): The Pharmacological Basis of Therapeutics, 5th ed, pp 1472–1506. New York, Macmillan, 1975
19. Heinonen OP, Shapiro S, Tuominen L et al: Reserpine use in relation to breast cancer. Lancet ii:675–677, 1974
20. Henrick W, Cronin R, Miller PD et al: Hypotensive sequelae of diazoxide and hydralazine therapy. JAMA 237:264–265, 1977
21. Hypertension Detection and Follow-up Program Cooperative Group: Five-year findings of the Hypertension Detection and Follow-up Program. JAMA 242(23):2562–2577, 1979
22. Jick H: Reserpine and breast cancer: A perspective. JAMA 233:896–897, 1975
23. Jick H, Armstrong B: Breast cancer and spironolactone. Lancet i:368–369, 1975
24. Jick H, Slone D, Shapiro S et al: Reserpine and breast cancer. Report from the Boston Collaborative Drug Surveillance Program. Lancet i:669–671, 1974
25. Kersting F, Reid JL, Dollery LT: Clinical and cardiovascular effects of alpha methyldopa in combination with decarboxylase inhibitors. Clin Pharmacol Ther 21:547–555, 1977
26. Kochar MS, Daniels LM: Hypertension Control for Nurses and Other Health Professionals. St. Louis, CV Mosby, 1978
27. Laragh JH: Modern systems for treating high blood pressure based on renin profiling and vasoconstriction–volume analysis:

A primary role for beta-blocking drugs such as propranolol. Am J Med 61:797–810, 1976

28. Loube SH, Quirk RA: Breast cancer associated with administration of spironolactone. Lancet i:1428–1429, 1975

29. Mack T, Henderson B, Gerkins V et al: Reserpine and breast cancer in a retirement community. N Engl J Med 292:1366–1371, 1975

30. Moser M, Guyther JR, Finnerty F et al: Report of the Joint National Committee on the Detection, Evaluation and Treatment of High Blood Pressure, A Cooperative Study. JAMA 237:255–261, 1977

31. Mullick FG, McAllister HA: Myocarditis associated with methyldopa therapy. JAMA 237:1699–1701, 1978

32. National High Blood Pressure Education Program (NHBPEP). New Hypertension Prevalance Data and Recommended Public Statements, June, 1978. Presented at the American Heart Association Conference on Extending the Role of Nurses in High Blood Pressure Control, Dallas, May 2–5, 1978

33. Nickerson M, Ruedy J: Hypertensive agents and the drug therapy of hypertension. In Goodman LS, Gilman A (eds): The Pharmacological Basis of Therapeutics, 5th ed, pp 705–726. New York, Macmillan, 1975

34. Oates HF, Graham RM, Stokes GS: Mechanisms of the hypertensive action of prazosin. Arch Internat Pharmacodynamie Therapie 227:41–46, 1977

35. O'Fallon W, Abarthe DR, Kurland LT: Rauwolfia derivatives and breast cancer. Lancet ii:292–295, 1975

36. O'Malley K, Segal JL, Israili ZH et al: Duration of hydralazine action in hypertension. Clin Pharmacol Ther 18:581–586, 1975

37. Onesti G: Consultation in Hypertension: A Clinical Symposium. Rochester, Pennwalt Prescription Products, 1976

38. Pettinger W, Mitchell H: Minoxidil—An alternative to nephrectomy for refractory hypertension. N Engl J Med 289:167–171, 1973

39. Sodium in Medicinals. San Francisco, San Francisco Heart Association, 1973

40. Stokes GS, Graham RM, Gain JM et al: Influence of dosage and dietary sodium on the first dose effects of prazosin. Br Med J i:1507–1508, 1977

41. Strauss FG, Franklin SS, Lewin A et al: Withdrawal of antihypertensive therapy, hypertensive crisis in renovascular hypertension. JAMA 238:1734–1736, 1977

42. Vlachalis ND, Menlowitz M: Adrenergic blockade of diuretics in the treatment of essential hypertension. Cardiovasc Med 2(6):547–553, 1977

43. Weinstein L: Antimicrobial agents. In Goodman LS, Gilman A (eds): The Pharmacological Basis of Therapeutics, 5th ed, pp 1224–1247. New York, Macmillan, 1975

44. Wollam GL, Vidt DG: The patient with resistant hypertension. Drug Therapy 8:72–85, 1978

ADDITIONAL READING

American Hospital Formulary Service. American Society of Hospital Pharmacists, Vols I and II. Washington, DC, Revised 1-24-78

American Medical Association Drug Evaluation. AMA Department of Drugs with Society of Clinical Pharmacy and Therapeutics. Littleton, Science Group, 1977

Bagg E: Cooking Without a Grain of Salt. New York, Doubleday, 1972

Blackwell B: Drug therapy. N Engl J Med 289:249–252, 1973

Bolli P, Wood AJ, Simpson FO: Effects of prazosin in patient's with hypertension. Clin Pharmacol Ther 20:138–141, 1976

Briant RH, Reid JL, Dollery CT: Interaction between clonidine and despramine in man. Br Med J i:522–523, 1978

Cannon PJ: Physiology of the diuretics: How they work—How to pick the best one. Resident and Staff Physician 18:31–83, 1972

Cannon RT, Selding DW: Monograph: The Kidneys and Edema. Hoechst-Roussel Pharmaceuticals, in Cooperation with National Kidney Foundation and American Heart Association. Somerville, Hoechst-Roussel Pharmaceuticals, 1976

Chrysant SG, Frolich ED: Side effects of antihypertensive drugs. Am Fam Physician 9:94–101, 1974

Cooper ES, West JN: Hypertension and stroke. Cardiovasc Med 2:429–444, 1977

Dack S: Acute pulmonary edema. Hosp Med 14:112–138, 1978

deCarvalho JGR, Dunn F, Lohmoller G et al: Hemodynamic correlates of prolonged thiazide therapy: Comparison of responders and non-responders. Clin Pharmacol Ther 22:875–880, 1977

deCarvalho JGR, Frolich ED: Hypertensive emergencies. Practical Cardiology 3:50–61, 1977

Dhar SK, Freedman P: Clinical management of hypertensive emergencies. Heart Lung 5:571–575, 1976

Dollery CT, Davies DS, Draffen GH et al: Clinical pharmacology and pharmacokinetics of clonidine. Clin Pharmacol Ther 19:11–17, 1976

DuBose T, Kokko J: Renal chloride transport and control of extracellular fluid volume. Cardiovasc Med 2:967–979, 1977

Dustan HP: Evaluation and therapy of hypertension—1976. Mod Concepts Cardiovasc Dis 45(5):97–103, 1976

Dustan HP, Tarazi RI, Bravo EL et al: Diuretics and diet treatment of hypertension. Arch Intern Med 133:1007–1013, 1974

Eaton ML: Heading off adverse reactions: Methyldopa. Current Prescribing 3:58–61, 1977

Facts and Comparisons. St. Louis, Facts and Comparisons, 1980

Finnerty FA: Hypertensive crisis. Emergency Medicine 8:32–39, 1976

Finnerty FA: Hypertension: Current management. Part I. Evaluating the patient. Consultant 18(1):162–168, 1978

Finnerty FA: Hypertension: Current management. Part III. Drug and patient resistance. Consultant 18(3):53–55, 1978

Flynn JT: Hypertension: Causes and consequences. Building the right regimen for each patient. Today's Clinician 1:21–31, 1977

Foster SR, Fabre D, Cerone P: Influences on side effects of antihypertensive medications on patient behavior. Cardiovasc Nurs 14:9–14, 1978

Fournet KS: Patients discharged on diuretics: Prime candidates for individualized teaching by the nurse. Heart Lung 3:108–116, 1977

Gantt CL: Drug therapy of hypertension. Med Clin North Am 62(6):1273–1289, 1978

Gillum RF: Dietary control and prevention of essential hypertension. Practical Cardiology 4:27–31, 1978

Graham RM, Thornell JR, Gain JM et al: Prazosin: The first dose phenomenon. Br Med J ii:1293–1294, 1977

Grollman A: Adrenergic Drugs. Consultant 18:104–118, 1978

Gunnells J, Orgain E, McGuffin W: Treatment of systemic hypertension. In Hurst JW, Logue RB, Schlant RC et al (eds): The Heart, 4th ed, pp 1435–1453. New York, McGraw-Hill, 1978

Himathongkan T, Newmark SR, Greenfield M et al: Pheochromocytoma. Emergency Medicine 8:79–83, 1976

Holland OB, Kaplan NM: Propranolol in treatment of hypertension. N Engl J Med 294:930–936, 1976

Hollifield JW, Sherman K, VanderWagg RV et al: Proposed mechanism of propranolol's antihypertensive effect in essential hypertension. N Engl J Med 295:68–73, 1976

Hoobler SW, Sagastume E: Clonidine hydrochloride in the treatment of hypertension. Am J Cardiol 28:67–73, 1971

The Hypertension Handbook. Westpoint, Merck, Sharp & Dome, 1974

Johnston JM, Kem DC: Differential diagnosis of hypokalemia. Practical Cardiology 3:17–27, 1977

Kaplan NM: How to use second generation beta blockers. Current Prescribing 4:62–69, 1978

Keith T: Hypertensive crisis: Recognition and management. JAMA 237:1570–1577, 1977

Knochel J: Rhabdomyolysis and effects of potassium deficiency on muscle structure and function. Cardiovasc Med 3:247–261, 1978

Kobinger W: Pharmacological basis of the cardiovascular action of clonidine. Reprinted from Onesti G, Kim K, Moyer J (eds): Hypertension Mechanisms and Management. New York, Grune & Stratton, 1973

Koch–Weser J: The comeback of hydralazine. Am Heart J 95:1–3, 1978

Koch–Weser J: Diazoxide. N Engl J Med 294:1271–1274, 1976

Koch–Weser J: Hydralazine. N Engl J Med 295:320–323, 1976

Koch–Weser J: Hypertensive emergencies. N Engl J Med 290:211–214, 1974

Lowenstein J, Steele JM Jr: Prazosin. Am Heart J 95(2):262–265, 1978

Materson BJ: An update on diuretic agents. Consultations in Hypertension: A Clinical Symposium. Rochester, Pennwalt Prescription Products, 1976

Mazzara JT, Ayres SM: Fluid, electrolyte and acid–base disturbances in the coronary care unit. Nurs Clin North Am 7:553–554, 1972

McIntosh HD, Eknoyan G, Jackson D: Hypertension-A potent risk factor. Heart Lung 7:137–140, 1978

Moyer JH: Treatment of labile diastolic hypertension in the office setting. Practical Cardiology 3:17–25, 1977

Mroczek WJ; Consultations in Hypertension: Therapy and Long Term Management, monograph. Rochester, Pennwalt Prescription Products, 1977

Mroczek WJ, Leibel BA, Finnerty FA: Comparison of clonidine and methyldopa in patients receiving a diuretic. Am J Cardiol 29:712–717, 1972

Mudge GH: Diuretics and other agents employed in the mobilization of edema fluid. In Goodman LS, Gilman A (eds): The Pharmacological Basis of Therapeutics, 5th ed; pp 817–847. New York, Macmillan, 1975

Nies A, Shand DG: Hypertensive response to propranolol in a patient treated with methyldopa—A proposed mechanism. Clin Pharmacol Ther 14:823–826, 1973

Onesti G: Antihypertensives and their mode of action. Drug Ther 8:35–48, 1978

Onesti G, Fernandez M: Prazosin: Its usefulness in hypertension. Am Fam Physician 16:200–202, 1977

Pettinger W: Recent advances in the treatment of hypertension. Arch Intern Med 137:679–681, 1977

Physicians Desk Reference, 32nd ed. Oradell, New Jersey, Medical Economics, 1978

Putnam PP: Clonidine (Catapres): A new antihypertensive agent. Heart Lung 5:457–460, 1976

Raftos J, Bauer GE, Lewis RC et al: Clonidine in the treatment of severe hypertension. Med J Aust 1:786–793, 1973

Ram CV: Newer antihypertensive agents. Heart Lung 6:679–684, 1977

Reid JL, Dean CR, Jones DH: Central action of antihypertensive agents. Cardiovasc Med 2:1185–1194, 1977

Reisin E, Abel R, Modan M et al: Effect of weight loss without salt restriction on the reduction of blood pressure in overweight hypertensive patients. N Engl J Med 298:1–6, 1978

Report of Inter-Society Commission for Heart Disease Resources. Circulation 42:A55–95, 1970

Rodman MJ, Smith DW: Drugs acting on the heart and circulation. Clinical Pharmacology in Nursing, pp 313–342. Philadelphia, JB Lippincott, 1974

Rosenberg JM: Diuretics: Minimizing complications. Current Prescribing 3:52–59, 1977

Smith WM: Treatment of mild hypertension: Results of a ten year intervention trial. United States Public Health Service Hospital Cooperative Study Group. Circ Res 40:98–104, 1977

Stokes GS, Oates HP: Prazosin: New alpha adrenergic blocking agent in treatment of hypertension. Cardiovasc Med 3:41–47, 1978

Sung P, Samet P, Yeh, BK: Effects of clonidine and chlorthalidone on blood pressure and glucose tolerance in hypertensive patients. Curr Therapeutic Res 13:280–285, 1971

Tweeddale MG, Ogilvie RI: Antagonism of spironolactone-induced natriuresis by aspirin in man. N Engl J Med 289:198–200, 1973

Van Hoose MC, Cutler RE: Antihypertensive efficacy of metolazone alone and combined with reserpine in treatment of essential hypertension. Curr Therapeutic Res 20:266–276, 1976

Weibert RT: Heading off adverse reactions: Thiazide diuretics. Current Prescribing 3:62–69, 1977

Wilkinson P: Potassium changes during diuretic therapy. Cardiovasc Med 3:181–183, 1978

Woosley RL, Nies AS: Guanethidine. N Engl J Med 295:1053–1056, 1976

38

Anticoagulant, Antithrombotic, and Platelet Modifying Drugs

ERIKA SEIBERLER SIVARAJAN, R.N., M.A.

and

DIANNE J. CHRISTOPHERSON, R.N., M.N.

Drugs used to influence coagulation can be divided into three groups: 1. anticoagulants that inhibit clotting either by directly interfering with active coagulants (heparin sodium) or by inhibiting synthesis of clotting factors in the liver (oral anticoagulants); 2. antithrombotic agents that break down clots by activating endogenous plasminogen, which causes fibrinolysis; 3. drugs that inhibit platelet function.[77] Action, indications, contraindications, and nursing implications of some of these drugs are discussed in Table 38-1. A discussion of clotting mechanisms can'be found in Chapter 8.

ANTICOAGULANTS

An anticoagulant occurring endogenously was first discovered in 1916 by a medical student. He isolated a liver substance, later termed heparin, that interfered with animal blood clotting. The coumarin derivative dicoumarol, another substance with anticoagulant properties, was isolated in cattle that had died from hemorrhage after ingestion of large amounts of spoiled sweet clover. A substance similar in structure to dicoumarol was later synthesized by the Wisconsin Alumni Research Foundation (WARF) and named warfarin. Use of heparin and coumarin derivatives for anticoagulation in humans began in the 1930s.

Heparin

Heparin is a mucopolysaccharide that inhibits the clotting of blood by interfering with the conversion of prothrombin to thrombin. Heparin also inhibits the aggregation of platelets by thrombin. Thirty to forty times more heparin is required to inhibit the action of already formed thrombin than is required to prevent thrombin formation initially.[10,11,15,60]

Heparin is inactivated by the gastric juices of the stomach and hence must be administered intravenously or subcutaneously. The intramuscular route is associated with a high incidence of hemorrhage into the muscle tissue.[30] Heparin is metabolized by the liver and has a short half-life. It is excreted in the urine. If large doses are administered intravenously, as much as 50% of it is excreted unmetabolized through the kidney.[30] Commercial preparations of heparin are standardized according to their ability to prevent the clotting of recalcified plasma. Potency is based on units of heparin activity per milligram of the solution and has been determined by biologic assay with a United States Pharmacopeia (USP) reference standard. The USP standard is a minimum of 120 USP units per milligram of heparin.[16] Heparin does not pass through the placental barrier or into mother's milk. For this reason it is the drug of choice for pregnant women who need anticoagulant therapy.[39,60]

Indications and Contraindications. Heparin is used in the prevention and treatment of a variety of arterial and venous thromboembolic disorders. It is most effective in the treatment of venous thrombosis.[13,14] Heparin therapy has also been used in myocardial infarction (MI), cerebrovascular disease, respiratory failure, estrogen therapy, and disseminated intravascular coagulopathy (DIC).[19,23,79]

The most common use of heparin is in the treatment of patients with deep vein thrombosis (DVT), or pulmonary

(*Text continues on p. 506.*)

TABLE 38-1 ANTICOAGULANT, ANTITHROMBOTIC, AND PLATELET BEHAVIOR MODIFYING DRUGS

Agent	Dosage/Administration	Drug Interaction	Toxic Effects	Side Effects
Anticoagulant Heparin Sodium "Full-dose"	Heparin must be administered parenterally. Continuous infusion is preferred, because there is a lower incidence of bleeding with this mode of therapy.[64] An initial loading dose of 5000 USP units of heparin is given intravenously, followed by a continuous infusion at the rate of 1000 units/hour with an infusion pump (20,000–30,000 units/day). An alternative regime is 10,000 units as an intravenous bolus q. 6 h. PTT should be monitored at frequent intervals. For therapeutic benefits it is usually sufficient to administer enough heparin to prolong PTT to 1½ times the normal value. PTT 20–30 sec. Desired heparinization is 1–1½ times normal. If PTT is greater than 1½ times, further assessment is necessary.	All drugs affecting coagulation may have additive or synergistic effects with heparin.	Relatively nontoxic. Bleeding from skin and mucous membranes may result in ecchymosis, epistaxis, hemoptysis, and hematuria. Arterial hemorrhage can occur in a patient with subacute bacterial endocarditis. Anorexia, nausea, vomiting, diarrhea, urticaria, and alopecia have been reported. Acute reversible thrombocytopenia has been observed but is uncommon.[41]	Incidence of side effects is rare. Nausea, vomiting, abdominal pain, and skin rash may occur. Although heparin sensitivity and anaphylactoid reactions are rare, severe asthma, giant urticaria, rhinitis, lacrimation and fever have been encountered occasionally. Neuropathy and priapism are rare. Prolonged use may lead to mild sodium diuresis and potassium retention, and to osteoporosis and musculoskeletal pain.[15] Recommended dose regime often causes excessive or inadequate response.[59] Adjustment is often necessary.
Heparin Sodium "Low-dose"	5,000 units as subcutaneous injection 2 or 3 times/day			
Coumarin Warfarin	Dosage may vary with age and sex. Dosage is adjusted according to prothrombin time (PT). Normal PT is 12(±1) seconds. Therapeutic range is 2–2½ times the control value in the beginning. PT is done daily and dosage adjusted accordingly. Monthly checks are adequate when on long-term therapy.	See Table 38-4. Oral anticoagulants are bound to albumin in the blood (99%). Very little drug remains in the free state. Substances which displace or compete with oral anticoagulants for albumin binding sites increase serum concentrations, e.g., dilantin, imipramine. A second type of interaction is through biotransformation. Barbiturates, glutethimide, meprobamate, and phenylbutazone increase rate of metabolism of oral anticoagulants, and decrease its serum concentration. Other interactions may also occur. Absorption from gastrointestinal tract may be affected due to increased gastric pH from antacids. Interference with normal mucosal function of the bowel, due to drugs such as neomycin and colchicine, and alteration of gastrointestinal motility due to laxatives and anticholinergic drugs can alter absorption of coumarin.	Toxic effects other than bleeding in 2%–4% of patients are seldom seen. Bleeding is most common in the skin and mucous membranes of the respiratory, gastrointestinal, and genitourinary tracts resulting in ecchymosis, epistaxis, hemoptysis, melena, and hematuria. Anorexia, nausea, vomiting, diarrhea are uncommon. Rarely, urticaria and alopecia have been observed.	Hemorrhage As listed under toxic effects

TABLE 38-1   ANTICOAGULANT, ANTITHROMBOTIC, AND PLATELET BEHAVIOR MODIFYING DRUGS (Cont.)

Agent	Dosage/Administration	Drug Interaction	Toxic Effects	Side Effects
		Drugs affecting platelet function also potentiate oral anticoagulants, *e.g.,* aspirin and dipyridamole.		
Platelet-Modifying Drugs Sulfinpyrazone (Anturane)	For antiplatelet effects the dose is 400–800 mg/day by mouth, preferably taken with meals or milk.[41] In the Auturane study for prevention of recurrence of myocardial infarction, the dose was 200 mg by mouth, four times a day, started within 25–35 days after myocardial infarction.[4] For treatment of gout, the dose is 100–400 mg/day in 2–4 divided doses.	It potentiates the action of coumarin-like anticoagulants, insulin, and oral hypoglycemic agents. It also potentiates other drugs affecting coagulation. It should be used with caution when combined with sulfonamide drug therapy and also in patients with known sensitivity to phenylbutazone.	Toxic dose may result in ataxia, labored respiration, convulsion, coma.	Increased bleeding tendency results from interference with platelet function. Gastrointestinal irritation resulting in nausea, vomiting, diarrhea, epigastric pain may occur. Gastrointestinal distress may be lessened by taking the drug in divided doses with meals or milk. Hypersensitivity reactions may occur occasionally as skin rash and fever. Depression of hemopoesis has been observed experimentally in long-term administration. In the Anturane study, there was no significant increase in the incidence of side effects after 8.4 months of drug administration.[4]
Aspirin	For antiplatelet effects the dose is 325 mg, 2 or 3 times daily.[30,31] It is used alone or in conjunction with heparin and other oral anticoagulants. For antiplatelet effects it is also frequently combined with dipyridamole.	It potentiates other anticoagulant and antiplatelet drugs.	Ringing in the ears, visual disturbances, dizziness, restlessness, and confusion are evident with toxicity. Allergic hypersensitivity of skin, gastrointestinal and respiratory effects of varying severity may develop. Convulsions and cardiorespiratory arrest can be the result of salicylate poisoning. Bleeding disorders caused by thrombocytopenia may develop.[8]	Increased incidence of gout and pellagra.
Dipyridamole (Persantin)	400 mg/day taken as a single dose at night. For its vasodilator effect in the long-term treatment of angina, dose is 25–50 mg 2–3 times a day taken at least 1 hour before meals.	It is used alone or in conjunction with aspirin or oral anticoagulants. It potentiates anticoagulants, and when combined with warfarin it is more effective than warfarin alone in preventing systemic emboli in patients with prosthetic heart valves.	It is quite nontoxic.	Bleeding must be watched for. This tendency increases if drug is combined with oral anticoagulant therapy. Instances of headache, dizziness, nausea, flushing, weakness, or syncope are frequent. Gastrointestinal intolerance with nausea, vomiting, and diarrhea occurs occasionally. Because it seems selectively to dilate the large coronary arteries, a coronary steal syndrome may be precipitated with a worsening of angina pectoris. This is, however, rare.

emboli. Although heparin has been clearly demonstrated to prevent these conditions in humans, it has not had a significant impact on the mortality rate from pulmonary embolism in the past quarter century.[83] Several studies have shown that most cases of pulmonary embolism are not diagnosed during life, and therefore not treated. Two-thirds of the deaths from acute pulmonary embolism occur within 30 minutes of the embolic event.[37,38]

Low-dose heparin is becoming popular in the prophylaxis of the deep vein thrombosis. Prevention of thrombosis is accomplished with small doses of heparin sufficient to neutralize thrombin precursors but not thrombin itself.[65,83,84,85,86] In a controlled study of 4121 surgical patients, the incidence of pulmonary emboli was significantly less in patients who received low-dose heparin than in the control group of patients who were not treated.[36]

The use of heparin in the management of the patient suffering from an acute MI is controversial. Some physicians advocate a 7- to 10-day period of anticoagulation with large transmural MI to prevent DVT and the development of a mural thrombus over the infarcted myocardium. It is also advocated for patients who are in congestive heart failure (CHF), because CHF increases the incidence of DVT.[83]

Of all strokes, 20% are caused by or are accompanied by hemorrhage, and anticoagulation is contraindicated for these patients.[9] For the remaining 80% of the stroke victims, heparin therapy may be indicated.[9] Some authorities advocate heparin for the patient who is in the process of developing a stroke but not for those patients who have had a "completed" stroke. Its use to prevent a stroke in the patient with transient cerebral ischemic episodes is common, but its efficacy has not been documented.[9,30]

Heparin has also been advocated for prevention in pulmonary embolism in patients suffering from respiratory failure.[83,85] Patients receiving estrogen therapy have an increased tendency to develop venous thromboembolism, acute MI, or stroke.[86] Low-dose heparin has therefore been advocated for patients on estrogen therapy.[86]

DIC is a syndrome in which the blood is rendered incoagulable because of extensive intravascular fibrin-thrombin formation. This initial widespread clotting consumes all the available clotting factors and causes bleeding. The use of heparin in DIC is controversial since clinical results are inconsistent.[30,36,60] Those advocating heparin use do so on the premise that it arrests the intravascular coagulation and allows the restoration of normal amounts of coagulation factors.[30] Further studies are needed to establish the efficacy of heparin for this condition.

Heparin therapy is contraindicated for patients with hemorrhagic tendencies, blood dyscrasias, ulcerative gastrointestinal lesions such as colitis and diverticulitis, subacute bacterial endocarditis, threatened abortion, severe vitamin K deficiency and severe hepatic or renal disease, and for patients who have had recent surgery involving the brain or spinal cord.[16,60] It is not recommended for patients with a long history of alcohol abuse, malignant hypertension, or active tuberculosis, or for patients in need of long-range aspirin therapy. Patients in CHF appear to be more sensitive to heparin and the dosage should be adjusted accordingly.[28,30]

Nursing Implications. A trial dose of 1000 units may be advisable before a therapeutic dose is started. This is of particular importance for patients who are allergic to animal products. Heparin is prepared from pig intestine, but preparations from beef lung are available for patients who are allergic to the pig intestine.

A controlled intravenous pump system is essential for maintaining a constant rate of infusion in patients receiving full-dose intravenous heparin therapy. "Minidrip" intravenous tubing with calibrated flow of 60 drops/ml is recommended for accurate calculation of drip rates. The nurse must be aware of the number of units of heparin that the patient is receiving per hour as well as the number of drops per minute.[10,11]

The dosage of heparin is adjusted on the basis of laboratory tests of blood coagulability. There are a number of tests available; the partial thromboplastin time (PTT) is most commonly used for monitoring the effectiveness of heparin therapy. The normal control value for the PTT is 24 to 30 seconds. The heparin dose is adjusted to maintain PTT at 1½ times the control values.[83,84,85,86] A clear understanding of control and therapeutic ranges of PTT is essential (Chap. 15).

A constant watch for the symptoms and signs of bleeding should be exercised. Although routine testing of urine and stool for occult bleeding (guaiac test) is not required, observation for gross bleeding (rust-colored urine or "tarry" stools) should be made.[10,11] Common sites of bleeding such as mucous membranes should be frequently examined, and easy bruising should be looked for.

For patients receiving prophylactic "low-dose" heparin, the subcutaneous injection technique deserves attention. Usual sites of injection are the abdomen or the thigh.[10,11] Use of an ice cube to chill the abdominal site prior to injection decreases the patient's discomfort as well as causing vasoconstriction, minimizing the possibility of ecchymosis. Since use of alcohol wipes after injection increases the chances of bleeding at the site of puncture, they are best avoided. Gentle pressure applied with a sterile gauze pad aids hemostasis after the injection. The use of a template with a pattern is helpful in spacing the injections and ensuring more even absorption of the drug from the subcutaneous tissue. A small-gauge needle (25 or 27 gauge) is also recommended to minimize bleeding and discomfort.[10,11] It is recommended that the nurse keep gentle positive pressure on the piston while giving a subcutaneous injection of heparin, and that the areas not be rubbed following the injections.[10,11] Intramuscular injections are avoided because bleeding into the muscle may occur.

Since heparin is administered parenterally, it is usually given to hospitalized patients rather than to outpatients. Therefore patient education concerning heparin is not as crucial as it is concerning oral anticoagulant agents, which are frequently prescribed to outpatients.

Oral Anticoagulants

Oral anticoagulants are classified into the coumarin and the indandione derivatives (Table 38-2). The two groups of drugs differ from each other chiefly in the rate at which

TABLE 38-2 ORAL ANTICOAGULANTS

Coumarin Derivatives

Acenocoumarol (Sintrom)
Bishydroxcoumarin (Dicumarol)
Phenprocoumon (Liquamar)
Warfarin Sodium (Athrombin)
　　　　　　　(Coumadin)
　　　　　　　(Panwarfin)

Indandione Derivatives

Anisindione (Miradon)
Diphenadione (Dipaxin)
Phenindione (Danilone)
　　　　　　　(Eridione)
　　　　　　　(Hedulin)

(DiPalma JP: Drug therapy today: Precaution with anticoagulants RN 34(10):57–66, October 1971)

they are absorbed from the gastrointestinal tract.[16,87] Indandione derivatives are the most rapid-acting. The most commonly used drugs are of the former category, namely warfarin (Coumadin) and bishydoxycoumarin (Dicumarol).

Oral anticoagulants compete with vitamin K, which is essential for the manufacture of clotting factors II, VII, IX, and X in the liver. Thus the pharmacologic effect of oral anticoagulants is due to the competitive inhibition of the hepatic synthesis of vitamin K-dependent clotting factors.[30] Oral anticoagulants are highly bound to albumin in the blood (99%) with very little drug remaining in a "free" state. The small amount that is free provides the therapeutic effect of the drug. Thus any substance that will displace oral anticoagulants from albumin binding sites raises the level of the free drug in the blood and increases the therapeutic effect. Changes in the availability of vitamin K also alter the therapeutic responses to oral anticoagulants. Newborn infants and debilitated and cachectic patients are abnormally sensitive to the drugs, as are patients with decreased hepatic function and CHF. There is considerable lag time between peak plasma concentrations and therapeutic response (24–72 hours).[25,26,27] This lag time coincides with the gradual disappearance of the clotting factors.

Oral anticoagulants are metabolized by the liver, with negligible amounts being excreted in the urine. Oral anticoagulants pass through the placental barrier. For this reason these drugs are not recommended in the first trimester of pregnancy, when birth defects are likely to occur, or during the last month of pregnancy, to prevent bleeding in the newborn infant.[39] Since oral anticoagulants are not excreted in the breast milk, breast feeding of infants may be continued while the mother is on oral anticoagulant therapy.

The major side effect of oral anticoagulants is hemorrhage. When it occurs, vitamin K is usually administered intravenously. Because vitamin K antagonizes oral anticoagulants, the patients are refractory to all oral anticoagulants for several days after its administration. For this reason, judicious supplementation with vitamin K is recommended.

Indications and Contraindications. The indications for oral anticoagulant therapy are very similar to those for heparin.

Since these drugs can be given orally, they are prescribed for patients requiring long-term anticoagulation. As with heparin, the use of oral anticoagulants after myocardial infarction is variable. Some physicians advocate the use of oral anticoagulants for 2 or 3 months after the infarction to decrease the incidence of DVT and thromboembolism.[30] Oral anticoagulants are also used in the treatment of rheumatic valvular disease because they decrease the incidence of emboli, especially in severe mitral valve disease with left atrial enlargement and atrial fibrillation. After prosthetic heart valve replacement, lifelong oral anticoagulation is usually necessary to prevent the formation of clots on the prosthetic valve. For the most part use of newer heterograft valves made from animal tissue has made long-term use of anticoagulants unnecessary.[1,75] The efficacy of oral anticoagulants to prevent strokes in patients suffering from transient cerebral ischemic attacks is not proven.[9,30,77]

Patients with a history of alcohol abuse, those requiring aspirin therapy, and those with malignant hypertension or active tuberculosis should not receive the drugs, because there is an increased risk of bleeding. Oral anticoagulants can be given for a short time to patients in a moderate degree of renal failure without ill effects.

Nursing Implications. Prothrombin time (PT) or Quick Time is the laboratory test used to monitor the effectiveness of oral anticoagulant therapy. Prothrombin time is sensitive to factors II, V, VII, and X, and the normal value is approximately 12 ($\pm$ 1) seconds. The range of the PT during oral anticoagulant therapy is best expressed as a percentage of control. Optimal therapeutic range of PT is 15% to 20% of control values. At the beginning of therapy PT should be checked daily. As the patient's response is established, the test can be done less frequently. On maintenance oral anticoagulation therapy, the patient should have the prothrombin time checked at least once a month.[30] In patients receiving both heparin and oral anticoagulant drugs, PT may be checked only 5 hours after the last intravenous dose of heparin, or 24 hours after the last subcutaneous dose of heparin to exclude interaction. Since the daily dose of oral anticoagulants in the early stages of therapy is based on PT, the nurse should be familiar with the test and the normal values for the test (Chap. 15).

Nursing responsibilities include education of the patient concerning the drug and safety precautions, monitoring for symptoms and signs of hemorrhage, and the numerous interactions that oral anticoagulants have with other drugs.

An organized plan is useful to serve as a guide in teaching patients who are receiving oral anticoagulant therapy on a long-term basis (Tables 38-3 and 38-4). The teaching should focus on essentials to ensure safe self-administration of the drug, and includes 1. the importance of understanding the medication and the need for varying the dosage until stabilization has been achieved, 2. the purpose and necessity of frequent blood tests, 3. the effect of dietary intake on stabilization, 4. the prevention of accidents, 5. the risk of child bearing and, when appropriate, the need for contraception. These should include safety measures to prevent injury and bleeding (Table 38-3). It should be stressed to the patient that if injury occurs, it is essential that a medical

TABLE 38-3 SAFETY TIPS FOR PATIENTS RECEIVING ORAL ANTICOAGULANT DRUGS

1. Use electric shavers instead of razors.
2. Wear gloves while gardening.
3. Never go barefoot.
4. Do not use sharp knives to trim calluses, corns, or fingernails.
5. Use a nonslip bathmat.
6. Avoid contact sports, such as football.
7. Use sharp knives and other tools carefully; avoid power tools, such as table saws and electric scissors.
8. Use a soft bristle toothbrush; avoid use of electric toothbrushes and water-pressure devices for oral hygiene.
9. Have regular dental checkups; floss regularly to avoid gum disease and bleeding.
10. Inform dentists and all physicians that you are taking the drug.

TABLE 38-4 TEACHING OBJECTIVES FOR PATIENTS RECEIVING ANTICOAGULANT THERAPY

At the completion of the course, the patient should be able to state or demonstrate an understanding of these important matters:

1. The name and purpose of their anticoagulant medication, their dosage, and the importance of taking it every day at the same time
2. The importance of keeping laboratory appointments and stating the date when the next test is due
3. The importance of notifying the physician in the case of fever, diarrhea, minor surgery, or dental extractions
4. The importance of personal safety factors to prevent the possibility of hemorrhage. Rough contact sports are discouraged
5. The reasons for a heavier menstrual flow in the case of female patients
6. The importance of not changing their diet dramatically nor adding medications (even over-the-counter drugs, such as aspirin, antihistamines) without the physician's knowledge and approval
7. The possibility of interactions between oral anticoagulants and aspirin, antihistamines, vitamins, laxatives with mineral oil, and antibiotics
8. The importance of avoiding excess intake of alcohol and fatty foods
9. The necessity to contact a physician for nosebleeds, discolored urine, "black" stools, or an excessive menstrual flow and flank pain
10. The importance of carrying emergency identification at all times. The card should include the patient's name and address, and the name, address, and telephone number of the family physician.

TABLE 38-5 DRUG INTERACTIONS OF THE COUMARIN ANTICOAGULANTS

I. *Drugs That Diminish the Response to Oral Anticoagulants*
A. By Inhibition of Oral Anticoagulant Absorption:
Griseofulvin †
(Clofibrate)*
B. By Induction of Hepatic Microsomal Enzymes:
Barbiturates
Ethchlorvynol
Glutethimide
Griseofulvin †
(Meprobamate)
C. By Stimulation of Synthesis of Clotting Factors:
Vitamin K
(Adrenocorticosteroids)
(Estrogens)

II. *Drugs That Enhance the Response to Oral Anticoagulants*
A. By Displacement of Anticoagulant from Plasma Albumin:
Chloral hydrate
Clofibrate †
Mefenamic acid
Phenylbutazone
(Diazoxide)
(Ethacrynic acid)
(Nalidixic acid)
(Sulfinpyrazone)
(Sulfonamides, long acting)
B. By Increase in Affinity for receptor:
D-Thyroxine †
C. By Inhibition of Hepatic Microsomal Enzymes:
Chloramphenicol
Clofibrate †
(Allopurinol)
(Disulfiram †)
(Mercaptopurine †)
(Methylphenidate)
(Nortriptyline)
D. By Reduction in Availability of Vitamin K:
Anabolic steroids †
Clofibrate †
D-Thyroxine †
Broad-spectrum antibiotics
E. By Inhibition of Synthesis of Clotting Factors:
Anabolic steroids †
Glucagon †
Quinidine †
Salicylates †
(Acetaminophen †)
(Mercaptopurine †)
F. By increase in Clotting Factor Catabolism:
Anabolic steroids †
D-Thyroxine †

* If the drug name is in parenthesis, the clinical significance of the interaction is minor or has not been firmly established.
† Indicates that the mechanism is still uncertain.
(Goodman LS, Gilman A: The Pharmacological Basis of Therapeutics, 5th ed. New York, Macmillan, 1975)

checkup be sought. Women in childbearing years or women who are pregnant need to be informed about placental transfer of oral anticoagulant drugs to the fetus. Patients should be taught to observe symptoms and signs of bleeding. Urine and stool color should be checked and epistaxis, bleeding gums, and easy bruising should be looked for. Knowledge of vitamin K as the antagonist of the oral anticoagulants is very important to patients, as is drug dosage, route of administration, and side effects. Patients should also be taught about PT and its response to the dose administered. Patients who lack sufficient comprehension of safe anticoagulation therapy need to be identified, and arrangements need to be made for a public health nurse or some other resource person to assume the responsibility when these patients are discharged from the hospital on oral anticoagulant therapy. Preferably, a list of all drugs known to potentiate or inhibit the action of oral anticoagulants should be given to patients receiving oral anticoagulant therapy (Table 38-5).

ANTITHROMBOTIC AGENTS

The ideal thrombolytic agent would be one which dissolved formed clots. The major emphasis in development of thrombolytic agents has been to accelerate the body's own mechanism for dissolving a thrombus.[14,22,32,35,42,68] During clot formation a naturally occurring fibrinolytic enzyme in an inactive form, termed plasminogen or profibrinolysin, is incorporated into the interstices of the clot.[66,77,78] In the presence of an activator or kinase, a specific type of enzyme, the plasminogen, is converted to plasmin, which is a proteolytic enzyme capable of dissolving fibrin. The two drugs that are capable of activating the conversion of plasminogen to plasmin are urokinase and streptokinase.[35,45,78] Unfortunately, neither is totally satisfactory. They need to be administered intravenously 12 to 24 hours after clot formation, and they have many adverse effects. Thrombolytic therapy results in more profound alteration of the hemostatic mechanisms than does anticoagulant therapy with heparin and coumarin agents. Bleeding occurs because thrombolytic agents degrade fibrinogen as well as fibrin. They are therefore not commonly used. The indications, contraindications, and nursing implications are similar for both drugs and have therefore been combined.

Urokinase (Abbokinase)

Urokinase is a substance found in the urine of humans.[66,68,78] Its use is not accompanied by allergic reactions, but it is comparatively expensive. Urokinase has been purified and approved for use in cases of pulmonary embolism. Two forms of urokinase are available for clinical use, namely, a high-molecular-weight form and a low-molecular-weight form.

Streptokinase

Streptokinase is an activator produced by beta-hemolytic streptococci.[68,77] Since patients have a variable amount of circulating antistreptokinase (as a consequence of previous streptococcal infections), it must first be neutralized before a level of free streptokinase can be maintained in the circulation. The adverse effects of streptokinase are bleeding, pyrogenic reactions, nausea, urticaria, asthma-like attacks, and rarely, anaphylactoid reactions. A purified form of streptokinase is being used in Europe and is being considered for approval for clinical use in the United States.

Indications and Contraindications. Thrombolytic therapy is indicated for cases of pulmonary embolism and is more effective if followed by subsequent heparin therapy. Because of the high incidence of bleeding, it is reserved for cases of massive pulmonary embolism.[42] It is crucial that the drug be given within 24 hours of the embolic event. There is a potential role for thrombolytic agents in other arterial and venous thromboembolic disorders, but further studies are needed.

The use of urokinase in acute MI to dissolve the occlusive thrombus in the coronary artery and reestablish blood flow has attracted a great deal of interest, but the results are conflicting.[45] Thrombolytic therapy is expensive and should be considered experimental for uses other than the treatment of pulmonary emboli.

Because thrombolytic therapy increases the risk of bleeding it is contraindicated for patients who have had surgery within the last 10 days. Thus patients who have had a recent liver or kidney biopsy, lumbar puncture, thoracentesis or paracentesis, or extensive or multiple "cut downs" are not suitable for thrombolytic therapy. However, surgery may be performed, if indicated, soon after completion of thrombolytic therapy. It is also contraindicated in the presence of ulcerative wounds, recent trauma with possible internal injuries, visceral or internal malignancy, actively bleeding lesions of the gastrointestinal or genitourinary tract, severe hypertension, any bleeding disorders, chronic lung disease with cavitation, subacute bacterial endocarditis, rheumatic valvular disease, cerebral embolism, cerebral thrombosis, and cerebral hemorrhage, during pregnancy and during the first 10 days of the post-partum period.

Nursing Implications. Thrombolytic drugs are not commonly used and few cardiac care unit nurses will be involved in their administration. When used, strict protocols for administration and patient monitoring are established and should be closely adhered to.

The aim of the thrombolytic therapy is the production of a sufficient amount of plasmin for the lysis of intravascular deposits of fibrin. However, fibrin deposits which provide hemostasis at sites of needle punctures are also destined for lysis, and bleeding from such sites may occur. Bruising or hematoma formation, especially after intramuscular injections, is a danger during thrombolytic therapy. Hence intramuscular injections of other drugs should not be given to patients receiving thrombolytic agents. Arterial punctures should also be avoided before and during treatment with thrombolytic agents. Should arterial puncture be absolutely essential, the femoral artery must be avoided. It should be done carefully by the most experienced person on the team, using the radial or brachial artery. Pressure should be applied on the puncture site for at least 15 minutes and a pressure dressing should be applied afterwards. Also, venipuncture should be performed as infrequently as possible. Unnecessary handling of the patient should also be avoided. When bleeding is severe, whole blood transfusion, or epsilon amino caproic acid and fibrinogen, or all of these, may be needed.

AGENTS THAT MODIFY PLATELET BEHAVIOR

An occluding thrombus in the coronary artery results in MI. Hence the mechanism of thrombus formation and methods to control thrombogenesis are of interest in prevention of MI. Patients suffering from acute MI are prone to develop DVT and pulmonary emboli, and this adds further interest in finding suitable antithrombotic therapy for these patients.[31,32]

Platelet adhesion and aggregation are the initial events in the development of a thrombus in the arterial system and normally constitute the first defense against bleeding.[21,25,26,27,51,56,80,81,82] Platelet thrombus formation occurs in two phases: first, platelets adhere to the injured area; second, adenosine-diphosphate, calcium, and serotonin are released from the adhered platelets. The release of these materials leads to further aggregation of platelets and growth of the platelet plug. The evidence that platelets play a role in the development of an arterial thrombus led to the logical conclusion that inhibition of platelet function might prevent acute MI and other thromboembolic events.[31,32] Many drugs that are primarily used for other purposes seem to have an inhibitory effect on platelet aggregation. These include aspirin, sulfinpyrazone, dipyridamole, and clofibrate.[4,5,7,12,13,18,20,21,24,29,54,71,72,80,81,82] Antihistamines, pheno- thiazines, prostaglandins, dextran, and antiadrenergic agents have also been reported to exhibit antiplatelet activity. These drugs are not without side effects. This is important because their use in the prevention of thromboembolic events must be over prolonged periods to be effective, and side effects of their long-term use are largely unknown.[31,32]

General Indications for Drugs that Modify Platelet Behavior

A recent review of the role of drugs which modify platelet behavior used in the prevention of thromboembolic events listed a variety of clinical conditions for which they may be useful:[30,31] (1) transient cerebral ischemic attacks with risk of a cerebrovascular accident; (2) systemic emboli resulting from prosthetic heart valves in patients who are already receiving oral anticoagulants; (3) acute MI; (4) arteriovenous cannulas.[31,32] Other possible indications are for patients with critical lesions of the coronary artery that are not suitable for bypass surgery, documented MI with recurrence of angina, angina after coronary artery bypass surgery, new angina, coronary artery bypass grafts, and chronic angina. In the case of an acute MI or coronary artery bypass surgery, these drugs are started within 30 days of the event.

Sulfinpyrazone (Anturane)

This is a uricosuric agent used in the treatment of gout. It has been observed to lengthen platelet survival and decrease platelet turnover in gouty patients suffering from various thromboembolic disorders.[4,5,32] A similar effect has been noted in patients with prosthetic heart valves, idiopathic recurrent venous thrombosis, coronary artery disease, carotid artery stenosis, and in patients on chronic hemodialysis. Its action on prolonging platelet survival in man prompted the recent study of the effects of the drug in the prevention of sudden death in patients who had suffered MI.[4,15] The death rate during the first year after myocardial infarction was 4.9% in the group receiving sulfinpyrazone (200 mg, q.i.d.) compared with a death rate of 9.5% in the control group receiving a placebo drug. This represented a reduction of 48.5% in annual death rate in the treated group. Data on sudden cardiac death rate were even more impressive. The annual rate for sudden cardiac death was 2.7% in the treated group as opposed to 6.3% in the control group, an improve- ment of 57.2%. Rehospitalizaton for subsequent MI or cardiac arrhythmias also tended to be less frequent in the treated group.[4,5]

Indications and Contraindications. Dramatic results of the recent study have led to the use of this agent in the prevention of reinfarction and sudden death in patients who have had MIs. It is also used in maintaining patency of arteriovenous shunts in patients on chronic hemo- dialysis.[4,5,77] It is contraindicated in patients with peptic ulcer disease, impaired renal function, and bleeding disorders.

Nursing Implications. Since sulfinpyrazone produces gas- tric irritation, it should be administered with meals or milk. Patients with diabetes mellitus who are already receiving insulin or oral hypoglycemic agents should be monitored closely for hypoglycemia when sulfinpyrazone is added to their regime, since it potentiates the action of hypoglycemic agents. Sulfinpyrazone predisposes to the formation of uri- nary calculi, hence adequate fluid intake and alkalinization of the urine is recommended.

Acetyl Salicylic Acid (Aspirin)

Aspirin probably alters platelet adhesion and release, but has no effect on platelet survival.[7,9,18,25,72,77] Aspirin appears to damage platelets permanently and restoration of normal hemostatic function occurs only after the damaged platelets have been replaced by normal ones (2-7 days).[17] Prolongation of bleeding time persists for several days. Sodium salicylate and aceteminophen do not elicit this response in normal doses. It is useful in prevention of stroke and death in patients with transient cerebral ischemic attacks, but there is no evidence that aspirin prevents MI or stroke in other populations.[31,32,33,71,72,80,81] Recent evidence suggests that as- pirin is not effective in preventing reinfarctions in patients with old MI.[2]

Indications and Contraindications. Aspirin alone or with an anticoagulant drug is becoming widely used in the prevention of stroke.[9,13] It is contraindicated for patients with known sensitivity to the drug, history of gastrointestinal bleeding, and intrinsic coagulation defects. It is also not recommended for patients with severe hypertension.[17,31,32]

Nursing Implications. Aspirin should be taken with meals or milk to avoid gastric irritation. Since aspirin prescribed in these doses may cause impairment of hearing, a hearing test at the beginning of the treatment is valuable to serve as a baseline for future assessments of hearing. Bleeding tendencies should be looked for and a periodic check up of hemoglobin and hemotocrit for anemia is recommended.

Dipyridamole (Persantin)

Dipyridamole is a coronary and peripheral vasodilator. When dipyridamole is used in conjunction with oral anticoagulants for patients with prosthetic heart valves, it prevents systemic embolization.[24,74,76] The thrombus that forms around pros- thetic heart valves is a "white" thrombus, composed largely of aggregated platelets. Chronic anticoagulation with cou- marin derivatives alone appears to have little effect in preventing the formation of this type of thrombus. Dipyri- damole, when combined with warfarin, was more effective than warfarin alone in reducing incidence of systemic embolism in patients with prosthetic heart valves.[25,26,27] Combining dipyridamole with aspirin in a single dose is as effective in normalyzing platelet survival as is a larger dose of dipyridamole given alone.[34] This regimen reduces the incidence of hypotension due to dipyridamole and also reduces the cost.

Indications and Contraindications. Dipyridamole may be used in combination with oral anticoagulants and aspirin in the prevention of systemic emboli in patients with prosthetic heart valves.[31,32,34,74] Its usefulness in the prevention of acute MI has not been established.

There are no specific contraindications known. However, since it produces peripheral vasodilation, it should be used with caution by patients who are hypotensive.

Nursing Implications. When dipyridamole is prescribed in combination with oral anticoagulants or aspirin, both drugs should be taken simultaneously. They should be taken preferably at night to minimize perception of side effects. When prescribed with aspirin, dipyridamole should be taken with a glass of water or milk to prevent gastric irritation.

Dextran

Dextran is a plasma expander which interferes with the function and aggregation of platelets by coating them. It also coats erythrocytes and reduces blood viscosity, thereby preventing rouleaux formation and sludging. It also forms complexes with clotting factors, thus inhibiting coagulation.[6] Excessive doses can cause hemorrhage by virtue of the antithrombic effect of dextran.

Indications and Contraindications. Dextran is being used in the treatment of pulmonary emboli to prevent further episodes. Since it is a plasma volume expander, it may be harmful to patients in CHF.[6]

Nursing Implications. Since dextran is usually given intravenously, the infusion rate has to be carefully controlled to prevent fluid overload. Bleeding may be severe and needs to be observed for.

Other Drugs with Antiplatelet Activity

Clofibrate is a drug which is primarily used for lowering serum lipids (Chap. 39), but it is also an effective inhibitor of platelet aggregation.[29,83] There is some evidence that clofibrate is useful in the prevention of death in patients with coronary artery disease and in patients with angina, with or without prior MI. The benefit does not appear to be related to lipid lowering effects.

As mentioned earlier, beta-adrenergic blocking drugs, antihistamines, and phenothiazines exhibit antiplatelet activity but their clinical usefulness for this purpose is not being evaluated extensively.

REFERENCES

1. Altman R, Boullou F, Rouvier J et al: Aspirin and prophylaxis of thromboembolic complications in patients with substitute heart valves. J Thorac Cardiovasc Surg 72:127–129, 1976
2. Aspirin Myocardial Infarction Study (AMIS): A randomized, controlled trial of aspirin in persons recovering from myocardial infarction. JAMA 243(7):661–669, 1980
3. Andreoli KG, Fowkes VM, Zipes DP et al: Comprehensive Cardiac Care: A Text for Nurses, Physicians, and Other Health Practitioners, 4th ed. St. Louis, CV Mosby, 1979
4. Anturane Reinfarction Trial Research Group: Sulfinpyrazone in the prevention of cardiac death after myocardial infarction. N Engl J Med 298(6):289–295, 1978
5. Anturane Reinfarction Trial Research Group: Sulfinpyrazone in the prevention of sudden cardiac death after myocardial infarction. N Engl J Med 302(5):250–256, 1980
6. Bengente SE: Dextran in the prophylaxis of pulmonary embolism. World J Surg 2(1):19–25, 1978
7. Boston Collaborative Drug Surveillance Group: Regular aspirin intake and acute myocardial infarction. Br Med J i:440–443, 1974
8. Boyd EM: The safety and toxicity of aspirin. Am J Nurs 71:964–966, 1971
9. Canadian Cooperative Study Group: A randomized trial of aspirin and sulfinpyrazone in threatened stroke. N Engl J Med 299:53–59, 1978
10. Caprini JA, Zoellner JL, Weisman M: Heparin therapy—Part I. Cardiovasc Nurs 13(3):13–16, 1977
11. Caprini JA, Zoellner JL, Weisman M: Heparin Therapy—Part II. Cardiovasc Nurs 13(4):17–20, 1977
12. Coronary Drug Project Research Group: Aspirin in coronary heart disease. J Chronic Dis 29:625–642, 1976
13. Dale J, Myhre E, Storstein O et al: Prevention of arterial thromboembolism with acetyl salicylic acid. Am Heart J 94:101–111, 1977
14. Deykin D: Antithrombotic therapy: Rationale and application. Postgrad Med 65(1):135–146, 1979
15. Deykin D: Indication and techniques for the use of heparin in the treatment of thromboembolism. World J Surg 2:39–43, 1978
16. Di Palma JP: Drug therapy today: Precaution with anticoagulants. RN 34(10):57–66, 1971
17. Donosco E: Aspirin, platelets and cardiovascular disease. Council on Clinical Cardiology, American Heart Association, Dallas, Texas 1(4):1–4, 1974
18. Elwood PC, Cochrane AL, Burr ML et al: A randomized controlled trial of acetylsalicylic acid in the secondary prevention of mortality from myocardial infarction. Br Med J i:436–440, 1974
19. Ewy GA: Anticoagulant in patients with acute myocardial infarction. Practical Cardiology 4:25–33, 1978
20. Folts JD, Crowell EB, Rowe LL: Platelet aggregation in partially obstructed vessels and its elimination with aspirin. Circulation 54:365–370, 1976
21. Folts JD, Rowe LL: Platelet aggregation in stenosed coronaries: Mechanism of sudden death? (abstr). Am J Cardiol 41:425, 1978
22. Fratantoni JC, Ness P, Simon TL: Thrombolytic therapy: Current status. N Engl J Med 293:1073–1078, 1975
23. Frishman WH, Ribner HS: Anticoagulation in myocardial infarction: Modern approach to an old problem. Am J Cardiol 43:1207–1213, 1979
24. Gent AE, Brook CGD, Foley TH et al: Dipyridamole: A controlled trial of its effect in acute myocardial infarction. Br Med J 4:366–368, 1968
25. Genton E, Gent M, Hirsh J et al: Platelet inhibiting drugs in the prevention of clinical thrombotic disease—Part I. N Engl J Med 293(23):1174–1178, 1975
26. Genton E, Gent M, Hirsh J et al: Platelet inhibiting drugs in the prevention of clinical thrombotic disease—Part II. N Engl J Med 293(24):1236–1240, 1975
27. Genton E, Gent M, Hirsh J et al: Platelet inhibiting drugs in the prevention of clinical thrombotic disease—Part III. N Engl J Med 293(25):1296–1300, 1975
28. Glazier RL, de Takatz G, Wessler S et al: Forum: Small dose prophylactic heparin: Does it prevent venous thrombosis? Mod Med 45:37–42, 1977
29. Glynn MF, Murphy EA, Mustard JF: Effect of clofibrate on platelet economy in man. Lancet ii(7513):447–448, 1967

30. Goodman LS, Gilman A: The Pharmacological Basis of Therapeutics, 5th ed. New York, Macmillan, 1975
31. Haft JI: Role of blood platelets in coronary artery disease. Am J Cardiol 43:1197–1206, 1979
32. Haft JI: Seminar on thrombosis: Introduction. Am J Cardiol 43:1195, 1979
33. Hansten PI: Drug Interactions, 3rd ed. Philadelphia: Lea & Febiger, 1976
34. Harker LA, Sichter SJ: Studies of platelet and fibrinogen kinetics in patients with prosthetic heart valves. N Engl J Med 283:1302–1305, 1970
35. Hirsh J, Hale GS, McDonald TG et al: Streptokinase therapy in acute major pulmonary embolism: Effectiveness and problems. Br Med J 4:729–734, 1968
36. International Multicenter Trial. Prevention of fatal postoperative pulmonary embolism by low doses of heparin. Lancet ii:45–51, 1975
37. Kakkar VV: The current status of low dose heparin in the prophylaxis of thrombophlebitis PE. World J Surg 2:3–18, 1978
38. Kakkar VV: The current status of low dose heparin prophylaxis against venous thromboembolism. Scottish Med J 23(4):327–329, 1978
39. Kelly JG, O'Mally K: Clinical pharmokinetics of oral anticoagulants. Clin Pharmacokinet 4:1–15, 1979
40. Koch–Weser J, Sellers EM: Drug interactions with coumarin anticoagulants—Part I. N Engl J Med 285(9):487–497, 1971
41. Koch–Weser J, Sellers EM: Drug interactions with coumarin anticoagulants—Part II. N Engl J Med 285(10):547–558, 1971
42. Levine WG: Anticoagulant, antithrombotic, and thrombolytic drugs. In Goodman LS, Gilman A (eds): The Pharmacological Basis of Therapeutics, 5th ed. New York, Macmillan 1975
43. Martin EW et al: Hazards of Medication, 2nd ed. Philadelphia, JB Lippincott, 1978
44. Marx JL: Blood clotting: The role of prostaglandins. Science 196:1072–1075, 1977
45. Maurice P: Urokinase use held not justified in myocardial infarction (abstr). Medical News 2(2):1, 1978
46. McCarthy ST, Robertson D, Turner JJ et al: Low dose heparin as a prophylaxis against deep venous thrombosis after acute stroke. Lancet ii(8042):800–801, 1977
47. McNicol GP: The fibrinolytic enzyme system. Postgrad Med (suppl) 49:10–12, 1973
48. Meltzer LE, Dunning AJ: Textbook of Coronary Care. Philadelphia, Charles Press, 1972
49. Meyers FH, Jawetz E, Goldfien A: Anticoagulants and vitamin K. In Review of Medical Pharmacology, 3rd ed, p 161–172. Los Altos, Lange Medical Publications, 1972
50. Meyers FH, Jawetz E, Goldfien A: Vitamins and other therapeutic nutritional agents. In Review of Medical Pharmacology, 3rd ed, pp 417–420. Los Altos, Lange Medical Publications, 1972
51. Moncada S, Vane JR: Arachidonic acid metabolites and the interactions between platelets and blood-vessel walls. N Engl J Med 300(20):1142–1147, 1979
52. Moore K, Maschak BJ: How the patient can reduce his risks of anticoagulation. Nursing 7:24–29, 1977
53. Morris GK: Oral anticoagulant prophylaxis against venous thromboembolism. Scottish Med J 23(4):325–327, 1978
54. Moschos CB, Lahiri K, Lyons M et al: Relation of microcirculatory thrombosis to thrombus in the proximal coronary artery: Effect of aspirin, dipyridamole, and thrombolysis. Am Heart J 86:61–68, 1973
55. Mustard JF, Kinlough-Rathbone RL, Jenkins CSP et al: Modification of platelet function. Ann NY Acad Sci 201:343–359, 1972
56. Mustard JF, Packham MA: Factors influencing platelet function: Adhesion, release, and aggregation. Pharmacol Rev 22:97–187, 1970
57. O'Brien JR: The mechanisms of venous thrombosis: Anticoagulants, aspirin, and heparin. Mod Concepts Cardiovasc Dis 42(3):11–15, 1973
58. Oliva PB, Breckenridge JC: Arteriographic evidence of coronary arterial spasm in acute myocardial infarction. Circulation 56:366–374, 1977

59. Packham MA, Warrior ES, Glenn MF et al: Alteration of response of platelets to surface stimuli by pyrazole compounds. J Exper Med 126:171–188, 1967
60. Poller L: Anticoagulant treatment. Practitioner 221(1322):211–216, 1978
61. Roberts WC: Relationship between coronary thrombosis and myocardial infarction. Mod Concepts Cardiovasc Dis 41(2):7–10, 1972
62. Rodman MJ, Smith DW: Clinical Pharmacology in Nursing. Philadelphia, JB Lippincott, 1974
63. Rodvien R, Mielke CH: Platelet and antiplatelet agents in strokes. Current Concepts of Cerebrovascular Disease 13(2):5–8, 1978
64. Sackett D: Patients and therapies: Getting the two together. N Engl J Med 298:276–279, 1978
65. Salzman EW, Deykin D, Shapiro RM et al: Management of heparin therapy. N Engl J Med 292:1046–1050, 1975
66. Sasahara AA, Myers TM, Cole C et al: The urokinase pulmonary embolism trial: A national cooperative study. Circulation (suppl II) 47:1–108, 1973
67. Sasahara AA, Sharma GVRK, Parisi AF: New developments in the detection and prevention of venous thromboembolism. Am J Cardiol 43:1214–1224, 1979
68. Sherry S: Streptokinase, urokinase: Do they really work? Mod Med, November 1, 72–76, 1976
69. Simon L, Likes K: Hypoprothrombinemic response to ice cream. Drug Intelligence and Clinical Pharmacy 12:121–122, 1978
70. Simon TL, Ware JM, Stengle JM: Clinical trials of thrombolytic agents in myocardial infarction. Ann Internat Med 79(5):712–719, 1973
71. Smith G: Dipyridamole-Aspirin. Drug-Therapy Information Newsletter 3(6):1–2. Seattle, University of Washington, 1975
72. Smith JB, Willis AL: Aspirin selectively inhibits protoglandin production in human platelets. Nature 231:235–237, 1971
73. Strandness DE: Invited commentary in response to Kakkar. World J Surg 2(1):17–18, 1978
74. Sullivan JM: Effect of dipyridamole on the incidence of arterial emboli after cardiac valve placement. Circulation (Suppl 39–40):1–19, 1969
75. Sullivan JM: Pharmacologic control of thromboembolic complications of cardiac-valve replacement. N Engl J Med 279:576–580, 1968
76. Sullivan JM, Harken DE, Gorlin R: Pharmacologic control of thromboembolic complications of cardiac valve replacement. N Engl J Med 284:1391–1394, 1971
77. Tsu EC: Antiplatelet drugs in arterial thrombosis: A review. American Hospital Pharmacy 35:1507–1515, 1978
78. Urokinase Pulmonary Embolism Trial Study Group: Urokinase/streptokinase embolism trial phase 2 results. JAMA 229:1066–1316, 1974
79. Veterans Administration Cooperative Clinical Trial. Anticoagulants in acute myocardial infarction. JAMA 225:724–729, 1973
80. Weiss HJ: Platelet physiology and abnormalities of platelet function, Part I. N Engl J Med 293(11):531–541, 1975
81. Weiss HJ: Platelet physiology and abnormalities of platelet function, Part II. N Engl J Med 293(12):580–588, 1975
82. Weiss HJ, Aledorf LM, Kochwa S: The effect of salicylates on the hemostatic properties of platelet in man. J Clin Invest 47:2169–2180, 1968
83. Wessler S: Control of heparin therapy. Prog Hemost Thromb 3:311–329, 1976
84. Wessler S: Prevention of venous thromboembolism by low dose heparin: A 1976 status report. Mod Concepts Cardiovasc Dis 44(6):105–109, 1976
85. Wessler S, Gitel SN: Low dose heparin: Is the risk worth the benefit? Am Heart J 98(1):94–101, 1979
86. Wilson JR, Lampman J: Heparin therapy: A randomized prospective study. Am Heart J 97(2):155–158, 1979
87. Wood JE: The cardiovascular effects of oral contraceptives. Mod Concepts of Cardiovasc Dis 41(8):37–40, 1972

39

Antilipid Drugs

ERIKA SEIBERLER SIVARAJAN, R.N., M.A.

Atherosclerotic lesions develop in regions of intimal and subintimal deposition of lipid materials.[7] Hyperlipidemic disorders are discussed and a classification is outlined in Chapters 11 and 22.

Treatment of hypertension, discontinuation of smoking, and dietary therapy usually precede the use of hypocholesterolemic drugs. The effects of drug-induced lowering of serum cholesterol and other lipids on morbidity and mortality due to atherosclerosis or coronary artery disease (CAD) have not been determined but many physicians believe that use of antilipid drugs is justified pending further evaluation.

A raised level of serum cholesterol is related to CAD. Whether the use of antilipid drugs can prevent CAD from developing, prevent future myocardial infarctions or prolong the life of patients who have CAD are questions which remain unsatisfactorily answered.

The largest study undertaken in an attempt to answer the last two questions confirmed that the blood cholesterol levels can be lowered, but showed that they have little effect on heart disease morbidity and no effect on prolongation of life.[1,2] It was found that nicotinic acid reduces the incidence of nonfatal myocardial infarctions but has other side-effects (for example, more atrial fibrillation, thromboembolic events, and gall stones). Clofibrate does not alter outcome, and estrogens and dextrothyroxins may have potentially harmful effects.[1,2,6,10] These drugs are used only after very careful consideration of other therapeutic alternatives, such as diet and exercise.[9] Treatment of hyperlipoproteinemia, effectiveness of selected drugs, and partial ileal bypass surgery are discussed in Chapter 22. Actions, indications, contraindications, and nursing implications are discussed in this chapter. Dosage, administration, drug interaction, side-effects, and toxic-effects are presented in Table 39-1.

Clofibrate (Atromid-S)

Clofibrate reduces triglyceride and to a lesser extent cholesterol concentration in plasma. Among its many actions, it restricts very low-density lipoprotein (VLDL) release from the liver and its removal from plasma by increasing the activity of lipoprotein lipase. As a result, elevated plasma levels of prebeta lipoproteins (VLDL) which are rich in triglyceride, are reduced by 30%–40%. To a lesser extent clofibrate also reduces the cholesterol-rich low-density lipoprotein (LDL) by 15%–20%.[5,7] The higher the initial blood levels, the greater are the observed decreases. In certain disorders, particularly hypertriglyceridemia, high-density lipoprotein (HDL) cholesterol is increased by clofibrate. Clofibrate also corrects abnormal platelet adhesiveness, reduces fibrinogen levels and increases fibrinolysis.

Indications and Contraindications. Clofibrate is used as an adjunct for patients who do not respond adequately to diet and other measures for reduction of elevated serum cholesterol, especially beta lipoproteins, and triglyceride. Clofibrate has a greater depressant effect on VLDL, which are rich in triglyceride, than on the LDL, which are rich in cholesterol. Broad beta disease, or Type III hyperlipidemia, is particularly responsive to clofibrate and is now considered the best evidence that antilipid drugs are effective. Clofibrate is the drug of choice in the treatment of a symptomatic hyperlipidemia, such as for xanthomas which cannot be treated with diet alone. The skin lesions frequently regress with clofibrate therapy as in Type III hyperlipidemia. Clofibrate may also be used in secondary hyperlipidemia such as for diabetes mellitus and lipemic retinopathy. Although its effect is still unestablished, it is used for asymptomatic

TABLE 39-1 ANTILIPID DRUGS

Agent	Dosage/ Administration	Drug Interaction	Toxic Effects	Side-Effects
Clofibrate (Atromid-S)	500 mg four times a day or 1 g three times a day orally.	It potentiates oral anticoagulant drugs. Dosage of oral anticoagulant should be reduced by one-half to maintain the prothrombin time at the desired level.	Gallstone formation and pancreatitis, possible increased incidence of cancer, arrhythmias, thromboembolic events, impotence, and gastrointestinal complaints. Myositis and myopathy are seen in azotemic patients who accumulate very high levels of drug because of diminished renal excretion.	Nausea and "flu-like" symptoms may occur, but they usually disappear on continuing treatment. Other gastrointestinal symptoms such as vomiting, loose stool, dyspepsia, flatulency, and abnormal distress have been reported but they are uncommon. Headache, dizziness, fatigue, muscle cramping, weakness, skin rash, urticaria, and pruritus have also been reported. Dry brittle hair has been noted by some women and alopecia has also occurred in isolated cases. Side-effects are surprisingly infrequent in view of the requirement to take the drug continuously for years. Liver function tests (SGOT) may be depressed during the early part of the treatment, but they return to normal on continuation of therapy.
Choles-tyramine (Questran)	Dose is initially 8–16 g/day, slowly increased every 2–4 weeks to a maximum dose of 24 g/day. It may be taken in two, three, or four divided doses.	Cholestyramine may interfere with absorption of fat-soluble vitamins and acidic compounds such as digitalis, thiazides, warfarin, thyroid preparations, tetracycline, and phenylbutazone. These medications should be taken at least 1 hour before cholestyramine.	None known in adults. Hyperchloremia is reported in small children.	Major side effects are gastrointestinal. Constipation is common, especially in older patients. Heartburn, nausea, vomiting, abnormal cramps, and abdominal distention may occur. Adjustment in dosage usually alleviates these side effects.
Nicotinic Acid (Niacin)	Initial dose is 100 mg orally three times a day. The daily dose is increased by 200 to 300 mg every 4–7 days until maintenance dose of 3 to 9 g/day is reached.[8] It is administered with or shortly after meals to reduce gastrointestinal irritation. It may be taken with cold but not hot beverages.	Niacin may potentiate vasodilation or postural hypotensive effects of anti-hypertensive and ganglionic blocking drugs.		The most common side effect is flushing with itching and a feeling of vasodilator effects which occurs within 1–2 hours and may last up to several hours. A tolerance to this effect often develops so it becomes less bothersome within a few weeks. Heartburn and nausea, vomiting and diarrhea may occur. Skin may become dry and brown pigmentation may appear.[7] Liver function may be depressed and jaundice may manifest itself. Hypotension and anaphylaxis have been reported following intravenous administration.
Dextrothy-roxin (Choloxin)	Dosage range is 4–8 mg/day.	Potentiates the effects of anticoagulant drugs. Need for insulin may be increased in diabetic patients.	Dosage in excess of 8 mg/day may cause signs of hyperthyroidism and may precipitate angina in patients with coronary artery disease.	
Beta Sitosterol	Dose is available in suspension 3 g/15 ml.	Decreases or prevents absorption of dietary cholesterol.		Increase in the bulk and looseness of stools.[5]

patients with common endogenous hyperlipidemia to prevent coronary occlusion and other atherosclerotic diseases, but probably less frequently since the publication of the World Health Organization study in which the prevention was not conclusively demonstrated.[10]

Clofibrate is contraindicated for patients with impaired renal and hepatic function, primary biliary cirrhosis, pregnancy, and nursing mothers. It is used with caution for patients with a history of jaundice or hepatic disease, renal dysfunction, peptic ulcer, gout, and for those who are taking hypoglycemic agents or anticoagulants.

If clofibrate is prescribed in conjunction with anticoagulants, the dosage of the anticoagulant needs to be reduced (usually cut in half) to maintain prothrombin time at the desired level and prevent bleeding complications. The mechanism for this interaction is not understood, but it is probably related to displacement of oral anticoagulant bound to the albumin fraction in the plasma.

Nursing Implications. Since hyperlipidemia is frequently genetically determined, members of the patient's family, especially children and young brothers and sisters, should be screened for abnormal lipid levels. Dietary counseling can be directed to several members of the household.

Serum cholesterol and triglyceride levels should be determined at the start of treatment and periodically thereafter (every 2 weeks for the first few months). Refer to Chap. 15 for laboratory standards. These can be graphed and used to reinforce both dietary and medication regimes and to enhance compliance with instructions. There are seasonal variations in serum cholesterol (peak increases) during winter and later summer and decreases in fall and spring). These factors need to be considered when discussing changes in lipid values with patients. Clofibrate is generally withdrawn after three months if the response is not adequate. Frequent liver function tests, periodic complete blood counts, and renal function tests are advocated. Patients also taking oral hypoglycemic agents should be observed for episodes of hypoglycemia.

Nicotinic Acid (Niacin)

Nicotinic acid partially blocks the release of free fatty acids from adipose tissue, which are not transported to the liver and resecreted as triglyceride. The dosage given to correct hypercholesterolemia is much in excess of its requirement as a vitamin and causes side-effects of cutaneous flushing. The side effects can be subdued by starting with a small dose and gradually increasing it to the desired level. Nicotinic acid produces vasodilation by direct action on vascular smooth muscle, primarily in cutaneous vessels. It can also cause histamine release. Nicobid, a timed-release form of nicotinic acid, helps to minimize these vascular side-effects.

Indications and Contraindications. Nicotinic acid in large doses causes reduction in VLDL and LDL levels and is prescribed in hyperlipidemia types II, IV, and V.

It is contraindicated in patients with known hypersensitivity to niacin or niacinamide, hepatic dysfunction, active peptic ulcers, gastric hemorrhage, or severe hypotension. It should be used with caution for patients with glaucoma, gout, diabetes, angina, and gall bladder disease.[4]

Nursing Implications. The patient must be told that the vasodilatory effect occurs within minutes of oral ingestion and may last for a few minutes to an hour. Follow up and close monitoring of symptoms and individualized adjustment of dosage are essential. Patients should be cautioned against exposure to direct sunlight if their skin is sensitive. Symptoms can be minimized if the medication is taken with meals.

Fluorometric tests to determine urinary catecholamines may result in falsely high readings.

Cholestyramine (Questran)

Cholestyramine is a resin that is insoluble in water and is not absorbed in the gastrointestinal tract. In the small intestine the chloride ion is exchanged for bile acids. The binding of bile acids interrupts the enterohepatic circulation and thus the conversion of cholesterol to bile acids is increased, as well as the synthesis of cholesterol.[8] Cholestyramine binds bile salts in the intestine; they are excreted in stool instead of being reabsorbed. Liver cholesterol is then broken down to replace the missing bile salts. This process can lead to a 20%–25% reduction in blood cholesterol.[3] The plasma level of LDL decreases because the rate of its removal from the circulating plasma increases. In patients with type IIa hyperlipoproteinemia, plasma cholesterol is usually lowered by 20%–25% below the level achieved by diet.

Indications and Contraindications. Cholestyramine is given only for type II hyperlipoproteinemia, specifically type IIa, in which only LDL levels are elevated. At times, cholestyramine causes plasma triglyceride to rise in patients with hypercholesterolemia because of an increase in VLDL.

Cholestyramine is contraindicated for patients who have complete biliary obstruction. It has not been established whether it is safe to use the drug during pregnancy and lactation. Cautious use is recommended for patients with steatorrhea and impaired renal function.

Nursing Implications. Cholestyramine may bind drugs given concurrently; other medications should therefore be administered at least 1 hour before or 4–6 hours after the cholestyramine dose.

The drug is unpalatable, and has initial side-effects. For these reasons, it may be discouraging to patients to continue taking this drug. The nurse should encourage the patients that side-effects diminish and offer suggestions as to how the drug may be taken.

It is usually easiest to ingest this powder when mixed with orange juice, grapefruit juice, lemonade, applesauce, puddings, gelatins, yogurt, or oatmeal. Constipation can be alleviated if the patient takes bran supplements or stool softeners. At very high doses, cholestyramine may interfere with absorption of fat-soluble vitamins. Supplementary vitamins should probably be given to all patients on cholestyramine therapy.

Dextrothyroxine (Choloxin)

A hyperthyroid state, due either to an overactive gland or to thyroid hormone ingestion, decreases cholesterol levels by increasing the rate of excretion and metabolism of cholesterol beyond the rate of synthesis. This is accomplished by an increase in the catabolism and excretion of cholesterol by the liver. Dextrothyroxine is a less active isomer of the naturally occurring l-thyroxine. While it is less active as a thyroid hormone, large doses are required to produce a cholesterol-lowering effect and most attribute its cholesterol-lowering effect to induced hyperthyroidism. Caution must be exercised in its use, because there is a very narrow range (4–8 mg/day) between the dosage which increases metabolism and that which may precipitate angina. Dextrothyroxine sodium was one drug discontinued early in the Coronary Drug Project Trial because of an unexpectedly high number of deaths in the treatment group; particularly among those with certain risk factors at entry.[2]

Indications and Contraindications. Dextrothyroxine reduces cholesterol and triglyceride levels in hyperlipidemia by lowering both beta and pre-beta lipoproteins. Its use is contraindicated for patients with angina pectoris or myocardial infarction because it may increase metabolic demands.

Nursing Implications. New symptoms, signs of cardiac disease or an increase in angina, especially if associated with exercise, should be elicited from the patient.

Beta Sitosterol

Beta sitosterol is a naturally occurring plant oil which interferes with cholesterol absorption. It is used when there is an increase in endogenous cholesterol synthesis. Its only side-effects are an increase in the bulk and looseness of stools. There are no known toxic-effects. Beta sitosterol seldom returns cholesterol levels to normal but is nevertheless useful in lowering elevated cholesterol levels in endogenous hypercholesterolemia.

REFERENCES

1. Coronary Drug Project Research Group. Findings leading to further modification of its protocol with respect to dextrothyroxine. JAMA 220:996–1008, 1968
2. Coronary Drug Project Research Group. The Coronary Drug Project. Clofibrate and niacin in coronary heart disease. JAMA 231:368–386, 1975
3. Eder MA: Drugs used in the prevention and treatment of atherosclerosis. In Goodman LS, Gilman A (eds): The Pharmacological Basis of Therapeutics, 5th ed, pp 744–752. New York, Macmillan, 1975
4. Govoni LE, Hayes JE: Drugs and Nursing Implications, 3rd ed, pp 141–142. New York, Appleton-Century-Crofts, 1978
5. Hazzard WR: A pathophysiologic approach to managing hyperlipedemia. Am Fam Physician 14(2):78–87, 1976
6. Krasno LR, Kidera GJ: Clofibrate in coronary artery disease: Effect on morbidity and mortality. JAMA 219:845–851, 1972
7. Meyers, FH, Jawetz E, Golfein A: Review of Medical Pharmacology, 3rd ed. Los Altos, Lange Medical Publishers, 1972
8. Schlant RC, Digirolamo M: Modification of risk factors in the prevention and management of coronary atherosclerotic heart disease. In Hurst JW, Logue RB, Schlant RC, et al (eds). The Heart, Arteries and Veins, 4th ed, pp 1311–1344. New York, McGraw-Hill 1978
9. Turpeinen O: Effect of cholesterol-lowering diet on mortality for coronary heart disease and other causes. Circulation 59(1):1–13, 1979
10. World Health Organization Committee of Principal Investigators. A cooperative trial in the primary prevention of ischemic heart disease using clofibrate. Br Heart J 40:1069–1118, 1978

SECTION F
PACEMAKERS AND ELECTRICAL HAZARDS

40

Pacemakers

JANET B. HASKIN, B.S.N., R.N.

The nurse's role in pacemaker therapy is becoming increasingly more important and complex, and the nurse is becoming more responsible than ever before. She must know the signs and symptoms that denote the need for a pacemaker and the modes of pacing; she must also be versed in the related patient care. Today, with techniques advancing and equipment becoming more sophisticated, it is equally important that the nurse be skilled in recognizing, diagnosing, evaluating, and solving pacemaker problems. Her role in patient and family teaching as well as in follow-up care in this area is a prime responsibility.

HISTORY AND ORIGIN OF PACING

As early as the 1700s Volta developed the concept that electrical energy is produced during cardiac and other muscular contraction. Galvani's experiments with frogs' legs in 1791 demonstrated that muscle would also respond to external electrical stimulation. Clinical application of these phenomena was limited and sporadic until the early part of the 20th century. Transvenous cardiac pacing with an increase in heart rate (HR) was demonstrated in dogs in 1927, but this technique was not applied to humans until 1959. Closed-chest cardiac stimulation was first used in 1952 by Zoll, but long-term use did not prove feasible.[7]

Open-heart surgery initiated secondary complications of heart block. A technique was developed to pace the myocardium by use of an external pulse generator attached to two wires leading from the heart muscle through the closed chest. In 1960, an entire pacemaker unit (electrode wires and pulse generator) was implanted into a patient with a power source adequate to last for several years.[7]

Since then, research and development has produced a wide variety of types of reliable pacemakers. From a survey completed through 1975 it was reported that 156,000 patients in the United States were living with pacemakers; 57,000 new pacemakers were implanted in 1975 and approximately 60,000 batteries were replaced.[21]

BASIC PRINCIPLES OF PACEMAKER THERAPY

The purpose of a cardiac pacemaker is to provide an artificial electrical stimulus to the heart muscle when either the impulse initiation or the intrinsic conduction system is defective. Both temporary and permanent pacemaker units are used, the type being determined by the patient's physiological need.

Components of a Pacemaker

Basically, both temporary and permanent pacemakers are the same and consist of two to three elements.

Pulse Generator (Pacer Box). The electrical supply source to provide the stimulus consists of batteries and electrical circuitry. Some units also have a sensing mechanism designed to interpret particular information about the patient's own rhythm.

Catheter with Electrodes (Lead Wire). A conductive material (wire), which delivers the electrical stimulus to the myocardium by way of negative (cathode) and positive (anode) electrodes (also called stimulating electrodes), is enclosed in an insulated catheter. In order for the stimulus to be delivered, the electrode must have very close or direct contact with the heart muscle. Some catheters also have a sensing electrode. These electrodes transmit information that is received about the patient's own heart rhythm through the sensing electrode to the sensing circuitry in the pulse generator. Two types of pacer catheters are used, unipolar and bipolar, which will be described later.

Bridging Cable (Optional—Used in Temporary Pacemakers). An extension wire can be used between the pulse generator and the electrode catheter if the pulse generator is secured someplace other than at the site of insertion. This can be for patient comfort (the pacer box is relatively heavy and can be placed, for instance, on an intravenous pole rather than on the arm) or patient safety (if the patient is confused and is likely to change the pacer settings or disconnect the pulse generator from the pacer catheter).

Electrical Current Flow

To have a better understanding of how the pacemaker unit functions, it is necessary to have the basic concept of electrical current flow. Electricity flows from a negative pole to a positive pole, or vice versa. To complete the circuitry over which the current can pass, there must be a path of conductive material between the negative and positive terminals of a battery. This path can be a wire, a muscle, or any conductive solution, such as saline. The current flow may be stopped by disconnecting or removing from contact any of the items used to complete the electrical circuit. If one applies the above principles to a pacemaker unit, one can understand how it operates.

TYPES OF PACEMAKER CATHETERS

Bipolar Pacer Catheter

A bipolar pacing catheter consists of a pacing catheter with two closely spaced electrodes at the end; the distal electrode is negative, the proximal, positive. This type is used for both temporary and permanent pacing (Fig. 40-1).

Unipolar Pacer Catheter

The distal electrode (cathode) is in contact with the myocardium, whereas the indifferent (positive or anode) electrode is outside the heart. This type of catheter senses natural heart signals better because it has a larger surface area and also shows a more prominent pacer spike (the narrow vertical line or "blip" seen on the electrocardiogram which is produced when the electrode elicits a stimulus). Unipolar catheters are generally used for permanent pacemakers, but can also be used for temporary pacemakers. Some literature advances the theory that a unipolar catheter

is less likely to induce ventricular tachycardia or ventricular fibrillation. These arrhythmias are more likely to be initiated at the anode. This is because of the shorter refractory period and lower excitation threshold at the anode than at the cathode (Fig. 40-2).[24]

CLASSIFICATION OF PACEMAKERS

The classification of pacemakers can be very confusing to the reader; each resource may use a slightly different outline and terminology. Although an international classification exists, it is not yet widely used.[20] (See Tables 40-1, 40-2). Pacemakers are generally identified according to location and mode of action.[30,33]

Location refers to the area of the heart where the stimulating or pacing electrode is placed, for example, the atrium or ventricle. Thus, if the stimulating electrode is in the ventricle, the pacemaker is classified as ventricular. If it lies in the atrium, the pacemaker is classified as atrial.[29,30,33]

Mode of action is described as a preprogrammed delivery from the circuitry in the pulse generator. Classification is based on the presence or lack of a sensing mechanism. When the sensing electrode is located in the atrium, the pacing circuitry senses the patient's natural atrial depolar-

Fig. 40-1. Bipolar Pacer Catheter. (*1*) The pulse generator delivers an electrical stimulus at a predetermined rate. (*2*) The stimulus travels down the negative electrode wire. (For learning purposes the positive and negative wires are exposed; normally they are insulated from each other and are within a catheter.) (*3*) The electrical stimulus is delivered to the myocardium. (Catheter is positioned at the apex of the right ventricle.) (*4*) Current spreads through cardiac muscle and then to the positive electrode wire. (*5*) Current returns to the battery, completing the circuit. (Courtesy of Dr. Thomas A. Preston)

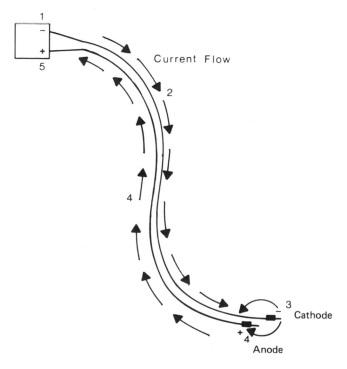

Current Flow

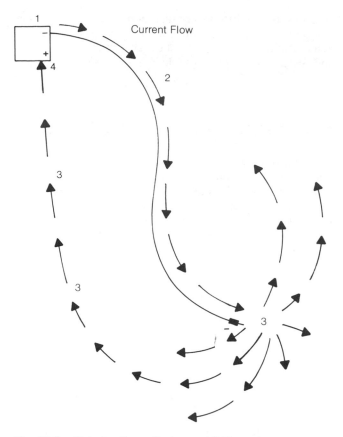

Current Flow

Fig. 40-2. Unipolar Pacer Catheter. (*1*) The pulse generator delivers an electrical impulse. (*2*) The stimulus travels down the negative electrode. (*3*) Current comes out at the end of the electrode, stimulates the myocardium, and completes the circuit by coming out through the body tissues to the indifferent (positive) electrode. (*4*) The positive electrode consists of a large metal plate attached to the outside of the pulse generator, or is often the external capsule of the pulse generator. (Courtesy of Dr. Thomas A. Preston)

ization. The patient's natural ventricular depolarization is sensed when the sensing electrode is in the ventricle.

All pacemakers that have a sensing mechanism have a preset escape interval, which is the time between the patient's own depolarization (ectopic or sinus beat) and the initial pacemaker impulse. When a natural beat fails to appear before a preset escape interval, the pacemaker will automatically fire and initiate a paced beat. The escape interval in most pacing units is comparable to the automatic interval, or the time between two consecutive paced beats or pacer spikes.[29] In a few selected types of pacemakers, however, the escape interval may be shorter or longer than the automatic interval.[19]

Modes of Pacing

There are four modes of pacing:
1. Fixed-Rate (*Asynchronous, competitive, continuous)
   a. Ventricular
   b. Atrial
2. Demand (*Standby, noncompetitive, QRS-complex inhibited)

*Other synonymous terms used in the literature.

TABLE 40-1 INTERNATIONAL PACEMAKER CLASSIFICATION: THREE LETTER IDENTIFICATION CODE

1st Letter	2nd Letter	3rd Letter
CHAMBER PACED	CHAMBER SENSED	MODE OF RESPONSE
V—VENTRICLE	I—INHIBITED	
A—ATRIUM	T—TRIGGERED	
D—DOUBLE CHAMBER	O—NOT APPLICABLE	

First letter. The paced chamber is identified by V for ventricle, A for atrium or D for double—both atrium and ventricle.

Second letter. The sensed chamber of either, is again V for ventricle, A for atrium.

Third letter. The mode of response if any, is either
  I   for inhibited, a pacemaker whose output is blocked by a sensed signal, or
  T   for triggered, a unit whose output is discharged by a sensed signal.
  O   indicates a specific comment is not applicable.

Examples of application of the terminology to existing conventional pacemakers would be
  1. Medtronic demand, VVI
  2. Biotronik IRP-44, VVT
  3. Cordis Atricor, VAT
  4. A-O bifocal, DVI
  5. General Electric fixed rate, VOO

(Parsonnet V, Furman S, Smyth NPD: Implantable cardiac pacemakers status report and resource guideline. Circulation 50(4):A21–35, 1974. By permission of the American Heart Association, Inc.)

a. Ventricular
   b. Atrial
3. Synchronous
   a. Ventricular
   b. Atrial
4. Bifocal (*Sequential, atrioventricular sequential)

Fixed-Rate. This type of pacemaker delivers an electrical impulse at a preset fixed rate to the heart and functions quite independently of cardiac activity. It does not have a sensing mechanism (capacity of the circuitry in the pulse generator to determine the heart's own electrical activity and inhibit the release of pacing impulses) and, therefore, is not sensitive to the patient's own rhythm. Some permanent units are manufactured to allow the rate to be changed by means of an external magnet or programmer, or by manipulation of a variable-rate control with a triangular needle inserted percutaneously into the unit.[7]

There are several major disadvantages of the ventricular fixed-rate mode. Atrial and ventricular activity are not synchronized and, therefore, the efficiency of the atria as a pump is lost. Cardiac output (CO) is increased 15% to 20% by synchronized atrioventricular (AV) contraction.[11] For some patients whose CO is already compromised, this factor can be of considerable importance.

The possibility also exists that competitive rhythms between the pacemaker and the patient's own natural rhythm may develop. If the pacing stimulus happens to occur during the vulnerable period—the peak and early downslope of the T wave—ventricular tachycardia or fibrillation may occur.[6]

An advantage of the fixed-rate unit is the simplicity of the circuitry, which reduces the chance of pacemaker

TABLE 40-2 INTERNATIONAL PACEMAKER CLASSIFICATION OF SUGGESTED NOMENCLATURE CODE FOR IMPLANTABLE CARDIAC PACEMAKERS

Chamber Paced	Chamber Sensed	Mode of Response	Generic Description	Previously Used Designation
V	O	O	Ventricular pacing, no sensing function	Asynchronous, fixed rate, set rate
A	O	O	Atrial pacing, no sensing function	Atrial fixed rate, atrial asynchronous
D	O	O	AV pacing, no sensing function	AV sequential fixed rate (asynchronous)
V	V	I	Ventricular pacing and sensing, inhibited mode	Ventricular inhibited, R inhibited, R blocking, R suppressed, noncompetitive inhibited, demand, standby
V	V	T	Ventricular pacing and sensing, triggered mode	Ventricular triggered, R triggered, R wave stimulated, noncompetitive triggered, following: R synchronous, demand: standby
A	A	I	Atrial pacing and sensing, inhibited mode	Atrial inhibited, P inhibited, P blocking, P suppressed
A	A	T	Atrial pacing and sensing, triggered mode	Atrial triggered, P triggered, P stimulated, P synchronous
V	A	T	Ventricular pacing, atrial sensing, triggered mode	Atrial synchronous, atrial synchronized, AV synchronous
D	V	I	AV pacing, ventricular sensing, inhibited mode	Bifocal sequential demand, AV sequential

(Parsonnet V, Furman S, Smyth NPD: Implantable cardiac pacemakers status report and resource guideline. Circulation 50(4):A21–35, 1974. By permission of the American Heart Association, Inc.)

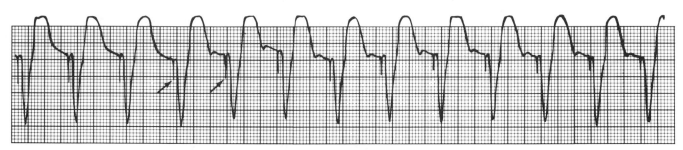

Fig. 40-3. ECG, Fixed Rate Pacemaker: ventricular, lead MCL$_1$. The pacemaker delivers stimuli continuously at a constant rate to the ventricles regardless of the intrinsic rhythm. A pacemaker spike (*arrows*) precedes each ventricular depolarization. A wide QRS complex follows (left bundle branch block pattern) due to late depolarization of the left ventricle.

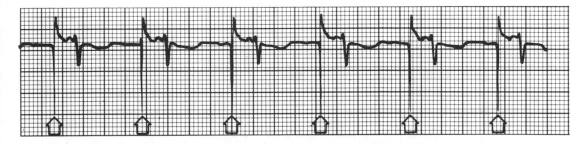

Fig. 40-4. ECG, Fixed Rate Pacemaker: atrial, lead MCL$_1$. The pacemaker initiates each atrial depolarization. A pacing stimulus artifact (*arrows*) precedes each P wave.

failure. Fixed-rate pacemakers are used infrequently today and would most likely be used for second- and third-degree AV block. (Figs. 40-3, 40-4, 40-5).

Demand. Pacemakers of this type are used for both atrial and ventricular pacing. Each has a sensing mechanism built into the pulse-generator circuitry. There may also be a separate sensing electrode(s) located in either the atrium or the ventricle. If the patient's natural rhythm fails to appear before a predetermined escape interval (programmed into the pulse-generator circuitry), the pacing unit will activate and deliver an electrical stimulus. The pacemaker fires only when needed or on demand, and, therefore, does not compete with the patient's own rhythm. For example, if the pacemaker rate has been preset at a rate of 60 beats per minute (bpm) and the patient's heart rate falls below 60 bpm, the demand pacemaker will activate. It will fire at a fixed rate of 60 bpm until the sensing mechanism again senses a natural beat.

a. Types used for pacing the ventricle

    1. R wave-inhibited (ventricular inhibited, QRS complex-inhibited).

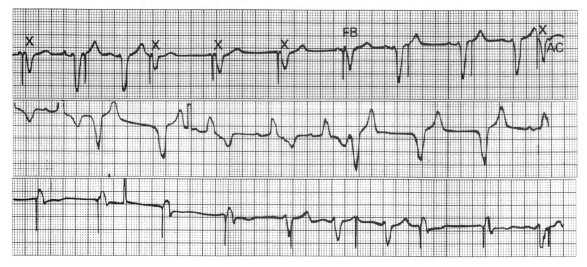

Fig. 40-5. ECG, Fixed Rate Pacemaker: competitive pacing. The patient's own sinus rhythm competes with a fixed-rate ventricular pacemaker rhythm (*X*). Note frequent ventricular fusion beats (*FB*), a combination of a pacemaker-induced beat and an intrinsic beat, and occasional areas showing the "R-on-T phenomenon." There is an atrial captured beat (*AC*). The underlying ECG abnormality is incomplete trifasicular block consisting of bifasicular block (RBBB with left anterior hemiblock) and advanced AV block. (Chung EK: Reprinted by permission of PW Communications from Primary Cardiology 4:50, 1978)

The stimulating and the sensing electrodes are both located in the ventricle. The sensing mechanism senses the ventricular depolarization and does not activate and fire a stimulus until the preset escape interval has been exceeded. As in any demand pacemaker, the unit functions as a fixed-rate pacemaker if it does not receive any inhibiting impulses. This type is commonly used for both temporary and permanent pacing. Conditions requiring R wave-inhibited pacemakers are AV block, sinoatrial (SA) arrest, and electrical overdrive (Fig. 40-6).

2. R wave-triggered (QRS-triggered, ventricular stimulated, ventricular synchronized)

Both sensing and pacing electrodes are in the ventri-

cle. This type is programmed to deliver an electrical stimulus during the patient's own QRS complex (during the absolute refractory period); on the ECG the pacing spike will be seen in the middle of the QRS complex. The patient's own ventricular depolarization triggers the pacemaker to fire and indicates that the sensing mechanism is working properly. The pacer spike somewhat distorts the configuration of the QRS complex and can, therefore, cause problems in evaluating acute injury and interpreting certain arrhythmias, such as atrial fibrillation with a rapid ventricular response. (Fig. 40-7).[29]

3. Hysteresis pacemaker

The hysteresis pacemaker is a demand pacemaker

Fig. 40-6. ECG, Demand Pacemaker: ventricular R-wave inhibited. (**A**) Several examples of the pacer sensing right-side PVCs (beats 5 and 7); the PVCs may have been induced from the tip of the pacer wire itself. (**B**) Paced beats (*PB*), intrinsic beats (*IB*), and a fusion beat (*FB*).

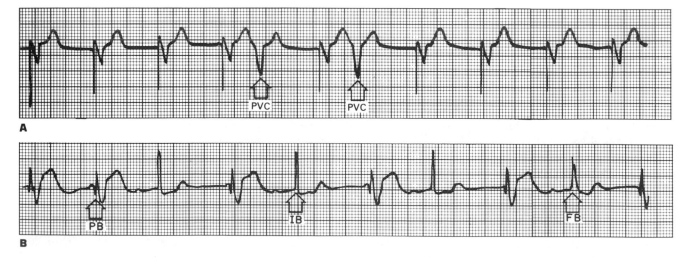

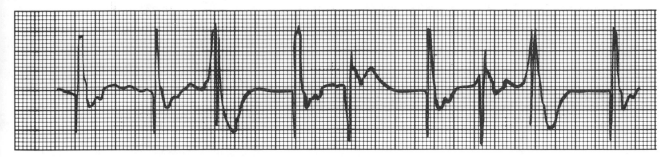

Fig. 40-7. ECG, Demand Pacemaker: ventricular R-wave triggered. Pacemaker stimuli artifacts are seen during the patient's own QRS complexes (beats 3, 5, 7, 8). Other beats are pacemaker escape beats. (Spence MI, Lemberg L: Heart Lung 3(5):823, 1974)

with the sensing and pacing electrodes located in the ventricle. The feature that makes this type unique is that the escape interval is longer than the pacing interval. For example, when the pacemaker paces at a rate of 70 impulses per minute but does not turn on until the patient's intrinsic rate drops to 60 bpm or below, there is a 10-beat hysteresis. This type is advantageous in that it can preserve sinus rhythm because it allows for the normal physiological responses in the body, such as slowing of the HR during rest or sleep. Pacemakers such as this can be used for patients with bradyarrhythmia, for example, intermittent AV block, or incomplete bilateral bundle branch block. It has a decided disadvantage for the

patient with frequent premature ventricular contractions (PVCs). The longer pause can lead to a long ineffective ventricular cycle, thus reducing CO. Most important, the nurse needs to be aware that such pacemakers exist lest she misinterpret the longer escape interval for a malfunctioning pacemaker (Fig. 40-8).[19]

b. Types used for pacing the atrium

1. P wave-inhibited atrial
   Both sensing and pacing electrodes are in the atrium. This type acts as a demand pacemaker; it activates and fires a stimulus when a natural atrial depolarization fails to appear after a predetermined time

Fig. 40-8. ECG, Demand Pacemaker: ventricular hysteresis. Leads V₁, II, and V₅ were taken simultaneously by using a three-channel ECG recorder. The tracing shows a ventricular demand pacemaker-induced ventricular rhythm (rate: 67 beats per minute) with intermittent sinus beats (*S*). Note that the pacemaker escape interval (1.08 second) is much longer than the consecutively occurring pacing intervals (0.86 second) because of hysteresis. There are occasional ventricular fusion beats (*FB*). (The numbers in this figure represent hundredths of a second.) (Papa, LA, Abkar KB, Chung EK: Heart Lung 3(6):983, 1974)

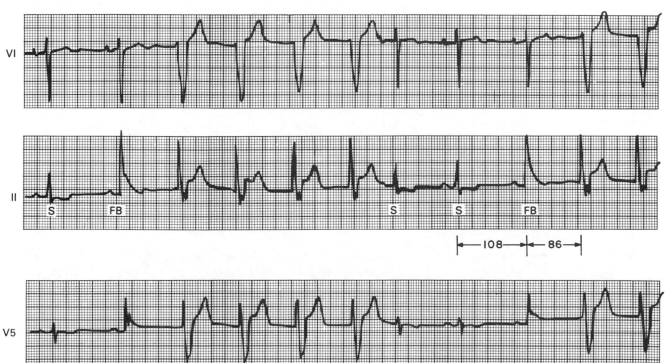

interval. The patient's intrinsic AV conduction system must be intact in order for this pacemaker to be beneficial (Fig. 40-9).[29]

2. P wave-triggered atrial

Both pacing and sensing electrodes are located in the atrium. The pacer stimulus artifact can be seen within the P-wave morphology and, like the R wave-triggered pacer, acts in a demand mode until the sinus node

fails to fire and the escape interval is exceeded. Conditions requiring a P wave-triggered atrial pacemaker are SA block, sinus arrest, and sinus bradycardia (Fig. 40-10).[29]

Synchronous. This type is also a demand form of pacing but of a particular type.

a. For stimulation of the ventricle

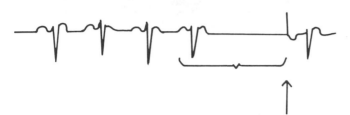

Fig. 40-9. ECG, Demand Pacemaker: P-wave inhibited atrial, lead MCL₁. When a P-wave fails to appear before a preset interval, the atrial pacemaker stimulus fires (*arrow*). (Adapted from Spence MI, Lemberg L.: Heart Lung 3(5):824, 1974

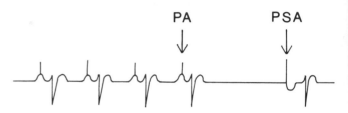

Fig. 40-10. ECG, Demand Pacemaker: P-wave triggered atrial, lead MCL₁. The pacer artifact (*PA*) can be seen during the P-wave. When block occurs, the pacer stimulus artifact (*PSA*) appears at the end of the escape interval and precedes the P wave. (Adapted from Spence MI, Lemberg L: Heart Lung 3(5):824, 1974)

Fig. 40-11. ECG, Synchronous Pacemaker: P-Wave triggered ventricular. Effect of exercise on atrial synchronous cardiac rate. (**A**) and (**B**). Electrocardiograms made with the patient at rest; the atrial rate is below 60 bpm and the automatic pacer rate is 60 impulses per minute. (**A**) Two P waves appear preceding QRS complex, but as they occur too late after the preceding QRS complex, they do not stimulate the succeeding QRS complex. (**B**) Two complexes (*arrows*) occur at an appropriate interval and stimulate a pacer impulse. The P-wave at S is a PAC and produces an appropriate but early pacer response. (**C**) Electrocardiogram made during mild exercise. Atrial synchrony is at an interval of 0.84 second (72 impulses per minute). (**D**) After moderate exercise, synchrony is at an interval of 0.66 second (91 impulses per minute). (Furman S, Escher DJW: Principles and Techniques of Cardiac Pacing, p 156. New York, Harper & Row, 1970)

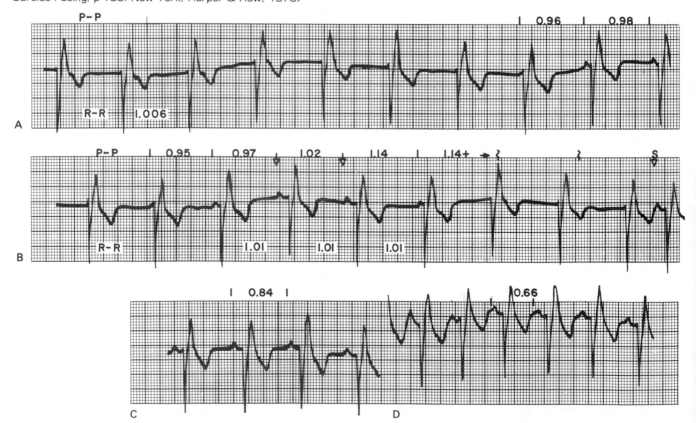

P wave-triggered ventricular pacing (atrial synchronized ventricular, atrial-triggered) uses two electrodes: a sensing device in the atrium and a stimulating electrode in the ventricle. The atrial sensing electrode perceives the patient's own atrial depolarization, waits for a preset interval (simulates the PR interval) and then triggers the ventricular pacemaker to fire. Normal cardiac sequence is best simulated when atrial and ventricular activity are synchronized. As a safety feature, should a rapid atrial rhythm occur that exceeds a certain rate limit, the ventricular pacemaker fires independently at a fixed rate. Like other demand pacemakers, it has a preset escape interval, and if atrial depolarization does not appear after a certain interval, the ventricular pacemaker fires. This type is most often used in children who have AV block. A major benefit is an increasing HR to accompany the body's physiological demand (Fig. 40-11).

b. For stimulation of the atrium

The QRS-inhibited atrial pacing electrode is located in the atrium, but the sensing electrode is in the ventricle. Ventricular rates faster than the programmed escape interval suppress firing of the atrial pacemaker. When a ventricular depolarization fails to appear within the preset interval, the atrial pacemaker will fire.(Fig. 40-12).[29]

Bifocal. This type is used for stimulation of both the atrium and the ventricle. They function as either a continuous sequential atrial and ventricular pacemaker or as a QRS-inhibited sequential atrial and ventricular pacemaker (bifocal demand).

a. Continuous sequential atrial and ventricular pacing

Stimulating electrodes are located in both the atrium and ventricle. This type acts as a fixed-rate pacemaker delivering continuous stimuli to the atrium and ventricle in sequence. A problem with competitive rhythms can exist because there is no sensing mechanism. Conditions indicating this type are symptomatic sinus bradycardia, AV block, and the need to increase CO by AV synchrony (Fig. 40-13).

b. QRS-inhibited sequential atrial and ventricular pacing (bifocal demand)

This type is classified as a combined atrial and ventricular pacemaker, because both areas have stimulation electrodes. However, sensing electrodes are located only in the ventricle. Both atrial and ventricular pacemakers are QRS-inhibited. The bifocal pacemaker can simulate normal cardiac sequence by sequentially stimulating the atrium and ventricle at a preset fixed interval. It can also stimulate the atrium alone or remain totally dormant. This pacemaker is sensitive to the patient's ventricular depolarization and is programmed to shut off or inhibit both atrial and ventricular pacing stimuli. The escape interval of the atrial pacemaker is designed to be shorter than that of the ventricular pacemaker. Thus, the time difference between these two escape intervals defines the AV sequential delay, or PR interval, which affects ventricular filling time. Conditions that indicate this type of pacemaker are sick sinus syndrome, acute or chronic AV block, overdrive, reciprocating tachycardia, and the need to improve CO by AV synchrony. (Fig. 40-14).[3,29]

INDICATIONS FOR PACING

Impulse conduction of the heart normally originates in the SA node and proceeds throughout the electrical conduction system in an orderly, predictable manner. In the young as well as in the aged, a considerable number of pathologic and physiological conditions can develop that alter or interrupt this normal pattern. These conditions determine the need for either a temporary or a permanent pacemaker.

Clinically, the patient may be totally asymptomatic or may manifest several symptoms. Among the more common are lightheadedness, dizziness, syncope (Stokes–Adams at-

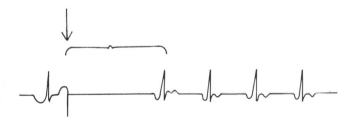

Fig. 40-12. ECG, Synchronous Pacemaker: QRS-inhibited atrial, lead MCL₁. An atrial pacemaker stimulus fires (*arrow*) when a QRS complex fails to appear before a preset escape interval. (Adapted from Spence MI, Lemberg L: Heart Lung 3(5):824, 1974)

Fig. 40-13. ECG, Bifocal Pacemaker: Continuous sequential atrial and ventricular pacing. Stimulus artifacts capture the atria and then the ventricles with a delay equal to the normal PR interval. (Spence MI, Lemberg L: Heart Lung 3(5):824, 1974)

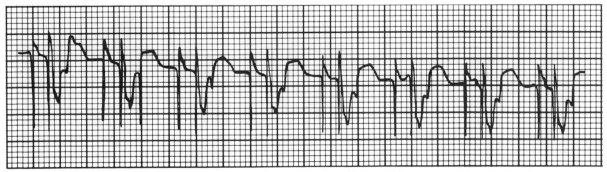

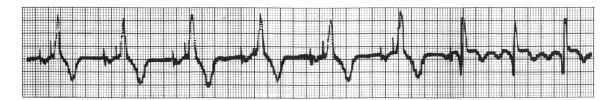

Fig. 40-14. ECG, Bifocal Pacemaker: QRS-inhibited sequential atrial and ventricular pacing (demand). At the right end of the trace, the ventricular stimulus artifact is inhibited initially. Both atrial and ventricular pacemaker stimuli are inhibited when NSR returns. (Spence MI, Lemberg L: Heart Lung 3(5):825, 1974)

tacks*), easy fatigability, forgetfulness, confusion, poor exercise tolerance, and congestive heart failure (CHF). Prerenal azotemia, loss of consciousness, seizures, circulatory arrest or even death can occur as well. The common denominator in these instances is a marked decrease or temporary absence of CO, regardless of the arrhythmia.

Cardiac pacing was initially used for the treatment of complete heart block (CHB). Since then, the use of pacing has increased considerably. The main reason for pacing, however, remains the presence of an inappropriately slow HR (Tables 40-3, 40-4).

TEMPORARY PACEMAKERS

Temporary pacing is used for emergency as well as electively. Methods of pacing temporarily are external, epicardial, transthoracic, and, most commonly, transvenous or endocardial.

External Pacing

Although external pacing is a very easy and rapid method, it is rarely used today. Metal electrode plates (covered with electrolyte jelly) fastened to the chest, or metal needles placed subcutaneously deliver electrical current to the external chest wall from a pulse generator. Electrodes are placed at the cardiac apex (V_4 or V_5 position) and along the left sternal border, ensuring that the ventricles lie between them. Threshold for ventricular capture will vary from 15 to 100 volts (V) or 50 to 200 milliamperes (mA).[23] It is very painful for the patient because this type of pacing necessitates using large amounts of current in order to deliver adequate impulses through the chest wall (skin is a poor conductor.) Other problems encountered are skin burns, skeletal muscle twitching, and a high incidence of failure to stimulate the heart.[6,8,23,36]

Epicardial Pacing

Temporary epicardial pacing is used after cardiac surgery if the patient develops arrhythmias or if CO needs to be temporarily augmented. While the heart is exposed, wire

electrodes are loosely sutured either on the atrial or the ventricular surface, or both. Sometimes a third electrode (indifferent) is placed subcutaneously. The terminals of the catheter(s) are then brought through the chest wall and attached to an external pulse generator, as needed. The origin of wires can be identified by using different lengths, or by labels. If the patient does not need to be paced, it is a nurse's responsibility to see that the exposed wires are

TABLE 40-3	ETIOLOGIES OF CONDUCTION ABNORMALITIES	
Conditions causing conduction abnormalities	**Cause or mechanism**
1. After-effects of cardiac surgery	Surgical trauma or edema; anatomic location of surgery; poppets of prosthetic valves may injure the conduction system.
2. Myocardial infarction (MI)	Transient ischemia to SA or AV node with increase in vagal stimulation to other areas of conduction system.
3. Drug toxicity or drug overdose (cardiac drugs or any medication)	Impulses are slowed or not formed in SA node; entire conduction system may be suppressed.
4. Electrolyte imbalance (hyperkalemia, hypocalcemia, hyponatremia)	Suppression or absence of impulse formation; interatrial and AV conduction slowed.
5. Sclerodegenerative disease (Lev's or Lenegre's)	Fibrosis, sclerosis, or both, of the conduction system.
6. Calcific valve disease (aortic or mitral)	Interruption of the conduction system.
7. Infectious disease (syphilis, Chagas' disease, myocarditis)[35]	Produces myocarditis; syphilitic involvement of the His bundle
8. Congenital	Usually associated with other congenital anomalies affecting the conduction system.
9. Coronary artery disease	Progressive atherosclerosis with ischemia to the SA and AV nodes

(Adapted from Furman S, Escher DJW: Principles and Techniques of Cardiac Pacing. New York, Harper and Row, 1970; TA Preston, personal communication.)

---

* Stokes–Adams attacks is a term commonly used to describe intermittent transient episodes of dizziness, syncope, unconsciousness or convulsions resulting from sudden disturbances of ventricular rhythm caused by partial or complete AV block. The heart block reduces blood flow to the brain and thus causes cerebral ischemia.[8,9]

TABLE 40-4 INDICATIONS FOR PACING

I. Heart Block
  a. Second-degree heart block
    1. Mobitz I
    2. Mobitz II
  b. Third-degree heart block
II. Arrhythmias in the absence of heart block
  a. Sinoatrial disease (sick sinus syndrome)
    1. Sinus bradycardia
    2. Sinus arrest
    3. SA block
    4. Atrial fibrillation with high-grade AV block, resulting in a slow ventricular rate
  b. Tachyarrhythmias
    1. Supraventricular
      a. Paroxysmal atrial tachycardia
      b. Atrial flutter
      c. Tachybrady syndrome
    2. Ventricular
      a. PVCs
      b. Ventricular tachycardia
III. Prophylaxis (pacemaker may be inserted as a preventive measure)
  a. Before surgery
    (Anesthesia can increase preexisting block.)
  b. Before diagnostic studies
    (Preexisting block or disease)
    Examples: cardiac catheterization or stress test for which pacing rather than exercise is used to increase the heart rate
  c. Prior to inserting permanent pacemaker
    Examples: emergency control for patients with Stokes–Adams syndrome or for patients with pacemaker failure.

(Adapted from Furman S, Escher DJW: Principles and Techniques of Cardiac Pacing. New York, Harper & Row, 1970; TA Preston, personal communication)

adequately insulated and the surrounding site is kept clean and dry (Chap. 41). Usually within a week, when the patient's condition is considered stable, the wires will be pulled out through the chest wall.[6,36] Because of the possibility of cardiac tamponade, the nurse should check for paradoxical blood pressure (BP) while the wires are in place as well as after their removal (Chap. 14).

Transthoracic Pacing

Transthoracic pacing is used in emergencies and involves either threading a myocardial pacing wire through a percutaneous cardiac needle or inserting a catheter by means of an introducer through the chest wall into the myocardium. The cardiac needle or introducer is then withdrawn, leaving the electrode in place. The electrodes are subsequently attached to a pulse generator. If time permits during insertion, the terminal ends of the pacing catheter should be attached with alligator clamps to the V lead on the electrocardiograph (ECG) machine. Myocardial contact with the pacer wire is manifested by elevation of ST segments and 10 to 20 millivolt (mV) signals. This procedure runs a high risk of coronary artery injury or bleeding, or both, resulting in pericardial tamponade.[8]

Transvenous or Endocardial Pacing

Transvenous or endocardial pacing involves threading an electrode catheter through a vein into the heart (either right atrium or right ventricle) and attaching the terminal positive and negative poles to an external pulse generator. The physician has a choice of five veins to use and his selections may be dictated by personal preference or by preexisting conditions, or both. Any approach has its advantages and drawbacks. Consideration must also be given to the probability of permanent pacing, because the vein cannot be reused once a cutdown has been performed. Veins used are the antecubital basilic, femoral, subclavian, and external or internal jugulars.

Antecubital Approach. For this approach, the catheter is inserted into the heart by way of the superior vena cava. Arm motion can cause a high incidence of electrode movement and displacement, which can stop the pacing or perforate the ventricle. Incidence of phlebitis is greater in the antecubital vein than in the others. A disadvantage for the patient is not being able to flex his arm and being therefore unable to feed and wash himself without assistance.

Femoral Approach. This approach ensures a rapid and relatively easy route. A cutdown is not necessary and the catheter can be inserted with a percutaneous guide. The catheter is easily passed through the inferior vena cava to the right ventricle. This avoids the superior vena cava in which the wire must make a J loop in order to pass through the tricuspid valve. The latter maneuver often requires lengthy manipulations to position the electrode from the right ventricular outflow tract to a more stable site in the apex. With the femoral approach, after traversing the tricuspid valve, the catheter tip is initially very often directed toward the apex of the heart. In a study of 100 patients, the incidence of catheter dislodgment, phlebitis, and formation of thrombi was low using this route.[34] If phlebitis does occur, it is of a more serious nature in the femoral area because of involvement with this major vein. Some institutions allow the patients with femoral catheters to ambulate. If walking is limited, the incidence of complications is low. There are also many psychological benefits to the patient who is permitted out of bed. When assisting the patient to get up and sit in the chair, care should be taken that hip flexion is minimal. Similarly, a bed patient in a high Fowler's position may be subject to catheter dislodgment.

Jugular and Subclavian Approach. Because the jugular and subclavian veins are used for permanent pacing, they are usually excluded as sites for temporary catheters. Ease of insertion is certainly a plus for using these routes. Anatomic location allows the patient to ambulate freely without risk of catheter dislodgment. Pneumothorax, air embolism, and puncture of the subclavian artery have all been reported as complications.

Methods of Temporary Pacemaker Catheter Insertion

The pacemaker catheter can be placed by "blind insertion" at the patient's bedside or using fluoroscopy, which may also be available for bedside use at some hospitals. Although in the literature opinions on the use of the "blind method" are divided,[8,36] this method has been successful (TA Preston, personal communication).

Either a "hard wire" or a "semi-floater" unipolar or bipolar catheter is used. One type of catheter has a balloon between the two stimulating electrodes and can be floated into place in a manner similar to that of a Swan–Ganz pulmonary artery catheter (See box below).[28]

Catheter	Advantages	Disadvantages
Hard wire	Easier to manipulate and position under fluoroscopy Reusable	Larger diameter Because it is stiffer it can more easily perforate the right ventricular wall. Restricts movement of patient, if in femoral vein, due to its being larger and stiffer.
Semi-floater	Smaller diameter More flexible Better for "blind" insertion because it will not perforate so easily Can be used in femoral vein, and patient is able to ambulate	Should only be used once

(From T. A. Preston, personal communication)

While the nurse need not be overly concerned with learning detailed information about equipment, she should be familiar with the types and uses of equipment in her own setting.

Positioning. When "blind" insertion is used, the electrode catheter is advanced under ECG monitoring. The precordial or V lead of the ECG machine is attached to the end of the pacer catheter by means of alligator clamps. The electrode serves as an exploring intracavitary lead and determines the position of the electrode tip. Specific ECG tracings will be seen during insertion (Fig. 40-15). If ventricular pacing is desired, the catheter is advanced until it is securely lodged in the apex beneath the trabeculae. This is a very stable position and has the lowest pacing thresholds. Generally, the lower the pacing threshold, the better the contact between the electrode and the endocardium. Limited success has been achieved with the electrodes positioned in the outflow tract of the right ventricle.[25,34]

In atrial pacing, the difficulty lies in securely positioning the catheter so that the electrodes can maintain contact with the endocardium. It is not possible to wedge the catheter, and only partial success has been obtained with special catheters designed to hook into stable positions. The areas of the coronary sinus and right atrial appendage seem to offer the best pacing.[25]

Stimulation Threshold. Once the catheter is in position, it is connected to the pulse generator and tested for stimulation threshold. The stimulation threshold is the least amount of electrical energy or current required to elicit ventricular contraction. If positioning is adequate, the threshold should be less than 1.5 mA. The mA setting on the pulse generator should then be set at two to three times the stimulation threshold.[36]

Because of a number of factors, the threshold can either increase or decrease within hours. Fibrosis around the tip of the catheter and the administration of certain drugs can cause an increase in the threshold. In the presence of myocardial ischemia, electrolyte imbalance (for example, hypokalemia), drug toxicity (for example digoxin) or hypoxia, the threshold will be lower. Ventricular fibrillation threshold is thought to be 10 to 30 times the stimulation threshold[36] and markedly lower in the presence of an acute myocardial infarction (MI).[23]

Sensitivity Threshold. If demand pacing is to be used, the sensitivity threshold is determined. This is the level at which the sensing electrode is able to sense accurately the patient's own QRS complexes. There is a sensitivity dial on most pulse-generator pacemakers; as the dial is turned clockwise, the sensitivity increases. Some older models do not have a separate sensing dial but do have a dial labeled "fixed pacing" and "demand pacing." The sensitivity increases as the dial is turned toward the demand mode.

Site Care. The catheter is then either sutured or well taped at the site of insertion, covered with povidone iodine (Betadine) ointment and then a sterile dressing. The site of insertion will determine the accessories used for the patient's comfort and safety.

External Pulse Generator

Several companies produce pulse generators, and although the cover designs may differ, their function is similar (Fig. 40-16). Most models have clear plastic shields to protect the dials from being tampered with. If not, clear tape can be used to prevent the settings from accidentally being changed, or else the whole generator can be encased in a rubber glove and taped on the end. Not all pacemaker models have insulated terminals and, therefore, the catheter tips remain partly exposed. The danger of ventricular fibrillation resulting from even minute amounts of current leakage is magnified by the presence of a low-resistance pathway (the catheter) in direct contact with the myocardium. For insulation, the ends must be covered with a rubber glove, and rubber gloves must be worn by everyone working with them.

It should be mentioned that most manufacturers state that pulse generators are made to withstand a current of up to 400 watt-seconds during defibrillation. However, if time permits, the pulse generator should be turned off and the wires disconnected from the pacemaker terminals. This will prevent diversion of the current from its cardiac pathway and the possibility of damaging the generator.[36]

External pulse generators are powered by mercury transistor batteries with a service life of around 500 hours. The procedure for changing batteries varies with the model; some models continue pacing for a short time even while the battery is being changed. Cleaning the box can be accomplished by wiping it with alcohol or water, or gas-

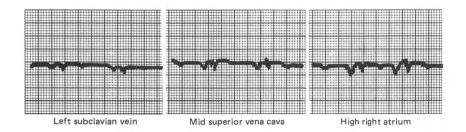

Left subclavian vein   Mid superior vena cava   High right atrium

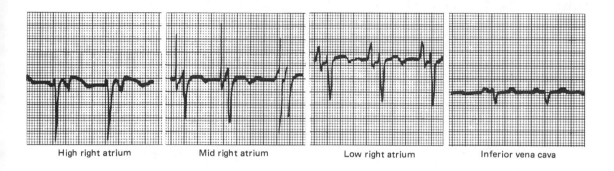

High right atrium   Mid right atrium   Low right atrium   Inferior vena cava

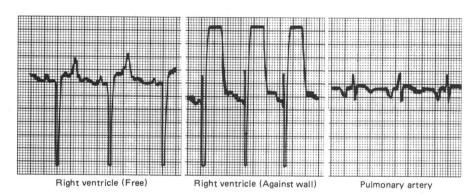

Right ventricle (Free)   Right ventricle (Against wall)   Pulmonary artery

Fig. 40-15. Sequence of ECG tracings during temporary pacemaker placement. As the pacing catheter approaches the right atrium, the amplitude of the P waves increases progressively. Since atrial depolarization is inferiorly directed in this patient, P waves recorded above the atria have a negative deflection, whereas those low in the atria and in the inferior vena cava are positive. As the catheter enters the ventricle, the QRS amplitude increases markedly, and a QS complex is inscribed. When the catheter tip touches the endocardial surface, marked ST-segment elevation is seen. As the electrode passes into the pulmonary artery (for demonstration purposes only) the QRS amplitude diminishes, and a negative P wave is inscribed since the catheter tip is again above the level of the atria. (Bing OHL, McDowell JW, Hantman JN, et al: Reprinted by permission from N Engl J Med 287(13):651, 1972)

sterilizing it with ethylene oxide after use on an infected patient.

Electrocardiographic Patterns

When the electrical stimulus is delivered from the pulse generator, a vertical line is seen on the ECG tracing. The spike, which may be positive, negative, or isoelectric in relation to the baseline, may be difficult or impossible to see. If a pacemaker is functioning properly, it is a misconception that a stimulus artifact will be identifiable in any lead that one happens to be recording. If P waves or pacemaker spikes are not easily visible in a particular lead, try monitoring lead aVR which has the smallest QRS-complex and T-wave excursions. Sometimes lead aVR may be the only lead in which pacer artifacts can be seen.[16] The pacer spike will be larger in unipolar pacing than in bipolar and may distort the ECG pattern. The shape of the pacer-induced P wave or QRS complex will differ from that of the intrinsic beat.

Transvenous endocardial pacing of the right ventricle will result in a left bundle branch block pattern (LBBB pattern), negative in leads V_1, II and aVR and positive in lead I. The limb leads will show left axis deviation (Fig. 40-

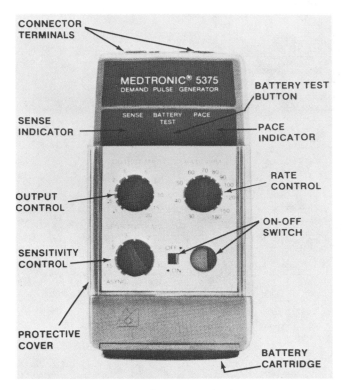

Fig. 40-16. An example of an external pulse generator (Medtronic, Model 5375). (Medtronic Technical Manual p 8, 1977)

17).[30] Epicardial transthoracic left ventricular pacing displays a right bundle branch block (RBBB) pattern (Chap. 17).

It is important to be aware that fusion beats will commonly occur with a properly functioning pacemaker, because the ventricles are being partly activated by a natural impulse and partly by the pacemaker. The natural QRS complex begins slightly before the time when pacemaker inhibition would have occurred; the combination produces a wide QRS complex with a pacemaker spike. The escape interval will be equal to that programmed for the pacemaker.[30]

Heart Sounds

With a right ventricular pacemaker, one can hear a paradoxically split second heart sound that is due to the delay in left ventricular depolarization. A change in intensity of the patient's heart sounds may indicate that perforation of the myocardium by the pacemaker has caused cardiac tamponade.

Nursing Responsibilities and Interventions

Before Catheter Insertion

1. If time permits, explain the procedure to patient and family, using audiovisual aids available. The teaching must be geared to the patient's level of understanding. Often, although the doctor has talked with the patient, the procedure may need to be explained in simpler terms.
2. Obtain the patient's or a family member's signature to a statement of informed consent.
3. Shave the area surrounding the insertion site, as needed, to prevent infection and discomfort from the tape.
4. Check the patency of the intravenous (IV) line or heparin lock.
5. Collect equipment:
   a. skin preparation solutions such as those with iodine base
   b. local anesthetic (lidocaine, 1% or 2%)
   c. pacer catheter which has been selected by the physician
   d. alligator clamps
   e. bridging cable
   f. percutaneous introducer or 14-gauge needle
   g. sterile dressings and tape
   h. sterile towels
   i. masks and sterile gowns and gloves
   j. cutdown tray, if needed
   k. suture with needle
6. Test the pulse generator and change batteries if nec-

Fig. 40-17. Typical ECG obtained by stimulating the apex of the right ventricle. Note the LBBB and left axis deviation. (Vera Z, Awan NA, Amsterdam EA et al: Heart Lung 4(3):448, 1975)

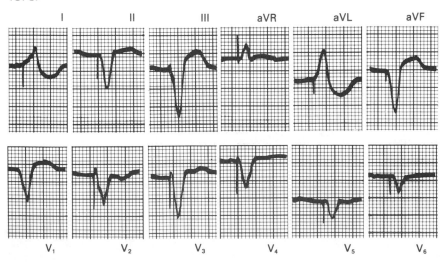

essary (date of battery change should be noted on the pacemaker box).

7. Have emergency equipment available.
8. Have emergency drugs ready for use; lidocaine (mechanical irritation with pacer wire often induces PVCs during insertion), atropine, and isoproterenol.
9. Check all equipment in room and all equipment to be used, to see that it is properly grounded and electrically safe.
10. Sedate patient, if necessary.
11. Attach the electrocardiograph machine to the patient.

During Catheter Insertion

1. Assist the physician as needed.
2. Monitor cardiac rhythm closely.
3. Check level of local anesthesia with patient. Is he feeling any pain?
4. Give emotional support to patient. This can be a very frightening experience for the patient, and often the doctor is so busy with the procedure itself he cannot take time to explain to the patient what is happening. Simple explanations will prove invaluable, allaying fears and fostering cooperation.

After Catheter Insertion

1. Obtain ECG for baseline determination of catheter position.
2. Obtain chest film, lateral if possible (to ensure that the catheter tip is anterior in the right ventricle) to determine catheter position.
3. Selectively restrict the patient's motion to prevent pacer wire dislodgment:
   a. Antecubital approach—An armboard should be used to immobolize the arm. The pulse generator can be secured on the arm with either gauze or an Ace bandage. Newer models come with specially made Velcro straps for this purpose. Padding around the elbow as well as underneath the pacer box can usually prevent pressure areas from developing (Fig. 40-18). Abduction of the patient's arm can be prevented by positioning him with pillows in bed, or securing his arm to his body with an Ace wrap or gauze bandage if he is sitting up or ambulating. If the patient is oriented and cooperative, these last measures may not be necessary. If the generator is one of the older models, the area of connection between the terminal pacer wires and the pacer box should be covered with a nonconductive material such as a rubber glove for added precaution. The extremity should be elevated slightly with a pillow to facilitate venous return, and pulses should be checked distally to determine adequacy of circulation.
   b. Femoral approach—Usually a bridging cable (extension) is used between the terminal ends of the catheter and the pulse generator. The pulse generator can be fastened to the thigh area, but for the patient's comfort (because of its weight), it may be better carried around the waist by using an Ace bandage, gauze, or specially designed Velcro belt. If this is not satisfactory for the patient, the pacer box can be placed in a cloth bag and suspended on an IV pole on or adjacent to the bed.
   c. Jugular or subclavian approach—An extension cable is used and the pulse generator can be attached at the patient's waist or on an IV pole adjacent to or on the bed.
4. Enforce bed rest initially; the unit policy and physicians orders vary regarding increased activity.
5. Record, on nursing care plan and in nursing notes:
   a. Date and time of insertion
   b. Type of wire inserted and location of insertion
   c. Mode of action, that is, demand or fixed
   d. Note if the pacer is on or off
   e. Rate setting of pacer
   f. The threshold and mA setting; record with date and time of test.
6. Check and record stimulation threshold and, if appropriate, sensitivity threshold at least once every eight hours (Table 40-5).
7. Attach a monitor rhythm strip to the chart at least every 4 hours. Measure rate and automatic interval to confirm that pacer is functioning properly.
8. Change dressing daily, using sterile technique:
   a. Cleanse surrounding area, using an antiseptic solution such as a povidone iodine swab (an antiseptic germicidal iodine preparation).
   b. Apply povidone iodine (Betadine) ointment at catheter insertion (recent studies have noted resistance of some organisms, including *Candida albicans*, to

Fig. 40-18. One method of securing the pulse generator and immobilizing the patient's arm when the anticubital vein is used for pacemaker insertion. (Winslow EH, Marino LB: Am J Nurs 75(4):586, 1975)

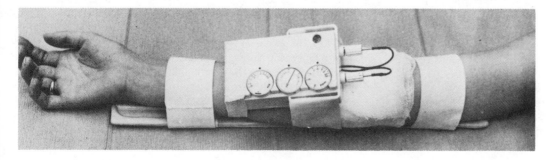

TABLE 40-5 PROCEDURE FOR TESTING STIMULATION THRESHOLD OF A TEMPORARY PACEMAKER

PURPOSE:

To determine the lowest voltage (mA) of electrical current necessary to elicit atrial or ventricular contraction

EQUIPMENT:

Pulse generator and pacemaker catheter
Cardiac monitor and write-out

PROCEDURE:

1. Give brief explanation to the patient.
2. At nurses' station, turn the monitor write-out to "direct."
3. If the patient is not pacing at the time of threshold testing, temporarily increase the rate per minute on the pulse generator until the paced rhythm overrides the patient's intrinsic rhythm.
4. While observing the continuous or intermittent paced rhythm on the monitor, gradually decrease the mA setting on the control dial (counterclockwise) until a pacemaker spike is elicited but does not capture a beat. Next, very slowly increase the mA setting on the control dial (clockwise) until a QRS complex follows each pacing impulse. The amount of current used when 1:1 capture first occurs is the stimulation threshold. The mA threshold, then, is the number on which the dial is set at that time.
5. The mA setting on the pulse generator should then be increased to two to three times the stimulation threshold.
6. If rate has been temporarily increased for testing purposes, decrease it to the ordered rate.
7. Record mA stimulation threshold and mA setting on the nursing notes as well as on the patient's nursing care plan.

antibiotic ointment.) The fungicidal properties of the Betadine ointment make it superior in efficacy to antibiotic ointment.[12]
  c. Apply dry sterile dressing and tape (make sure entire exposed catheter is covered).
  d. Record date of dressing change on outer dressing and in nursing notes.
9. During dressing change, watch for any signs of infection or cellulitis (not uncommon with pacemaker insertions). Check area for any redness, swelling, drainage, unusual tenderness, warmth, and pain. Chart your observations.
10. Check body temperature every 4 hours.
11. Be aware of other potential complications:
  a. Phlebitis
  b. Thrombosis
  c. Perforation of the myocardium by the wire as indicated by:
    1. Pericardial friction rub
    2. BP with a paradox greater than 10 mm Hg
    3. Muffled heart sounds
    4. Change in polarity of pacer spike
  d. Hiccoughing (pacing the phrenic nerve) or intercostal muscle twitching may indicate perforation by

catheter, pacer-wire dislodgment, or excessively high mA setting.
12. Be aware of the patient's electrolyte status, especially the serum potassium level, throughout the pacing period.
13. Be aware of safety precautions:
  a. Anyone handling exposed wires should wear rubber gloves.
  b. Be sure that all equipment in the room is properly grounded.
  c. Be sure that no electrical equipment such as a shaver is used.
  d. Remember that properly grounded radios and televisions may be used in patient's room but should not be touched by the patient or come in contact with the bed.

Trouble-Shooting Temporary Pacemaker Malfunction

The nurse can identify and resolve most pacemaker malfunction problems by using a logical approach. She must, however, have a thorough knowledge of the components of a pacemaker and understand its unique characterisitcs. Most of the problems that will be encountered fall into three areas:

1. Failure to stimulate appropriately.
2. Failure to capture appropriately. Capture refers to an electrical stimulus which produces effective depolarization.
3. Failure to sense appropriately.

The guidelines in Tables 40-6, 40-7, 40-8 are directed mainly toward the demand QRS-inhibited pacemaker as it is most frequently used in a cardiac care unit (CCU).

Conversion of a Temporary Transvenous Bipolar Electrode Pacing System to a Unipolar Electrode Pacing System

A temporary bipolar pacing catheter that does not sense appropriately may be converted to a unipolar pacemaker (Table 40-8). In order to accomplish this conversion, the catheter wire which is attached to the positive terminal is disconnected. An ordinary ECG limb electrode is attached to the patient's arm or leg. Try the right arm for the indifferent electrode first, and if this does not give adequate sensing, try the left arm or leg. An alternative method is to suture a small electrode beneath the skin, but this method is not as desirable because it often results in muscle-twitching around the indifferent electrode. Connect the positive terminal of the catheter to the limb electrode. This should improve the sensing function of the pacemaker (Fig. 40-23)[25]

Once the conversion to a unipolar system is made, the nurse has several responsibilities. The conducting paste or jelly under the limb electrode is changed every 8 hours in order to avoid drying and loss of electrical contact. The electrode is firmly fixed in place with either the strap or tape. Exposed wires are adequately insulated with dry dressings and a rubber glove, as needed. Remember to

TABLE 40-6   FAILURE OF THE TEMPORARY PACEMAKER TO STIMULATE APPROPRIATELY*

Problem	Possible source of problem	Nursing action

Marked variations in the automatic interval
  a. see Figure 40-19.
  b. "runaway" pacemaker (rapid, inappropriate release of electrical impulses)†
  See Fig. 40-20.
Intermittent or complete absence of the pacing artifact (Fig. 40-21)
	Battery failure
	Disconnections between catheter, bridging cable, or pulse generator
	Pacer may be oversensing or undersensing.
	Pulse generator failure
		Measure automatic interval.
		Check connections between catheter and pulse generator.
		Rule out failure of pacemaker to sense properly. Pacer sensitivity may need adjusting. See Table 40-8.
		Change batteries.
		If the pulse generator is not discharging after batteries are changed, change the box.
		If the patient is symptomatic because of the intrinsic arrhythmia, have atropine ready or isoproterenol drip on hand.
		Perform cardiopulmonary resuscitation, if necessary, until problem is solved.

* Refers to the inappropriate release or absence of electrical current from the pulse generator.
† Appropriate intervention is simply to disconnect pacer box from pacer wires.
(Spence MI, Lemberg L: Cardiac pacemakers IV. Complications of pacing. Heart Lung 4(2):286–295, 1975)

TABLE 40-7   FAILURE OF THE TEMPORARY PACEMAKER TO CAPTURE APPROPRIATELY*

Problem	Possible source of problem	Nursing action

Pacing artifact present but not followed by QRS complex (or if pacing is atrial, not followed by P wave; Fig. 40-22).	Pacing threshold inadequate
	Catheter out of position
		Check the pulse generator to determine
		  1. Threshold
		    (Increase voltage on generator, initially by only 1-2 mA)
		  2. That all connections between catheter and pulse generator are intact.
		Reposition the patient.
		  1. Move his arm if the catheter is in the antecubital area;
		  2. Turn the patient on either side for possible establishment of better catheter contact with the endocardium.
		Take 12-lead ECG and determine catheter position (check leads, I, II, aVF, and V.)
		Obtain chest film
		  1. If patient is stable, take anterior–posterior and lateral views.
		  2. If unstable, use a portable anterior–posterior x-ray.
		If patient is symptomatic, have atropine or isoproterenol drip ready. Initiate cardiopulmonary resuscitation, if necessary, and call the doctor.

* Refers to stimulus that is released from the pulse generator but fails to elicit a response; *i.e.*, depolarization of the atria or ventricles. To ensure proper capture, each component of the pacemaker unit must be functioning correctly: 1. voltage delivery adequate 2. stimulating circuits functioning properly 3. catheter properly positioned and intact.
(Spence MI, Lemberg L: Cardiac pacemakers IV. Complications of pacing. Heart Lung 4(2):286–295, 1975)

explain what you are doing to ensure the patient's cooperation.

PERMANENT PACEMAKERS

Direct myocardial stimulation for permanent cardiac pacing can be either epicardial by thoracotomy (transthoracic or mediastinal), or endocardial by the transvenous approach.

Epicardial Approach

The transthoracic approach ensures greater reliability because the electrodes are stable; also, it can offer a much greater selection of modes of pacing. The anterior chest is opened on the left between the fifth and sixth ribs. The sensing or the pacing electrodes, or both, are sutured to the exterior surface of the right or the left ventricle or the atria and threaded through a connecting subcutaneous tunnel to

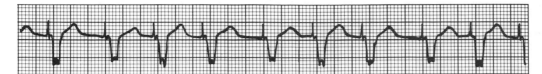

Fig. 40-19. An ECG trace showing variation in the rate of stimulus discharge. (Spence MI, Lemberg L: Heart Lung 4(2):288, 1975)

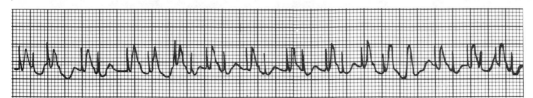

Fig. 40-20. An ECG trace of a "runaway" pacemaker. The pacemaker is firing at approximately 270 impulses per minute and capturing the ventricles when the stimuli fall outside of the refractory period of the previous beats. (Spence MI, Lemberg L: Heart Lung 4(2):287, 1975)

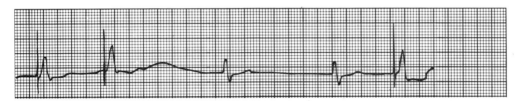

Fig. 40-21. An ECG trace showing intermittent absence of the pacing stimulus. (Spence MI, Lemberg L: Heart Lung 4(2):288, 1975)

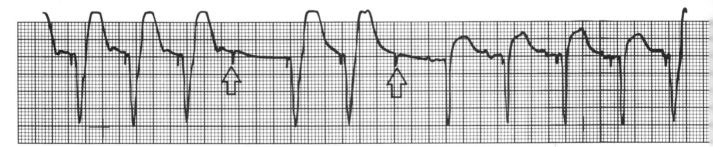

Fig. 40-22. Failure of a temporary pacemaker to capture appropriately (*arrows*). Note pacemaker spikes occurring at regular intervals (Lead MCL₁).

the abdominal wall, either above or below the waist, and attached to the pulse generator (Fig. 40-24).

The epicardial method is used for children because the fixed length of the transvenous type of catheter will not allow for vertical growth of the chest. The mediastinal approach involves opening the chest in the midline, thus avoiding entering the pleural cavity. The electrodes are attached to the epicardium (sometimes electrodes are screwed into the myocardium) and threaded through a subcutaneous tunnel to a newly created pocket that houses the power source.[1,8]

Transvenous Approach

By far the majority of permanent pacemakers are implanted transvenously. There are several advantages to this method. The procedure is a relatively minor one, can be performed under local anesthesia, and has a lower morbidity and mortality rate. A thoracotomy, which can be contraindicated in aged or debilitated patients, is not necessary. The cephalic, and external and internal jugular veins are the most commonly used. A small incision is made just above the clavicle, usually on the right, but sometimes on the left, side of the neck, and the electrode is threaded into the vein. The catheter is advanced to the right ventricle and lodged beneath the trabeculae in the apex area. (Refer to Fig. 16-19 for chest film of correct placement.) A separate incision is made below the clavicle and a tunnel is burrowed beneath the subcutaneous fat up to the neck-vein incision. The electrode catheter is passed down through the tunnel to the battery-powered pulse generator. A subcutaneous pocket is formed in which to place the pulse generator, sometimes encased in a Dacron pouch (Fig. 40-25). Connective tissue eventually grows into the Dacron fibers of the pouch and firmly anchors it to the chest wall.[31] The generator is tested, its threshold determined, and the incision closed. The skin layer over the pulse generator protrudes about one-half inch above the normal skin surface.

TABLE 40-8 FAILURE OF THE TEMPORARY PACEMAKER TO SENSE APPROPRIATELY*

Problem	Possible Source of Problem	Nursing Action
ELECTROMAGNETIC INTERFERENCE— can cause pacemaker inhibition or cause it to revert to a fixed mode of pacing.	An electrical source such as an electric razor. Faulty sensing mechanism in circuitry. Failing battery pack Pacemaker's refractory period—all demand pacemakers, by design, have an absolute refractory period after a beat is sensed, as well as after the emission of an impulse and capture. Therefore, very early beats such as premature atrial contractions (PACs) and PVCs may not be sensed and may not recycle the pacemaker.	Remove all potential sources of interference from room. Reduce sensitivity on pulse generator (making it less sensitive to external electrical signals). Change pulse generator. If patient is symptomatic, immediately changing to a fixed-rate mode should relieve symptoms (watch for competitive rhythm). Change batteries.
OVERSENSING— sensing electrical activity other than QRS (such as T waves) can cause a prolonged automatic interval.	Sensitivity set too high	Reduce sensitivity on pulse generator.
UNDERSENSING— not sensing appropriately	Sensitivity set too low	Increase sensitivity on pulse generator.
PARTIAL SENSING— a short escape interval caused by incomplete recycling of the sensing mechanisms.	Poor positioning of catheter electrodes or low voltage of intracavitary signals.	Reposition patient. Record ECG to determine catheter position. Inform physician that the catheter may have to be repositioned.
IMPROPER SENSING— a competitive rhythm can develop and cause the pacer spike to fall during a vulnerable period of the T wave.	Faulty sensing mechanism. Sensitivity set too low. Malpositioned catheter.	Check to see that pacer is on demand mode, not fixed rate. Reposition the patient. Increase the sensitivity. If patient's own rhythm is adequate, turn pacer box off. Increase the rate to overdrive the underlying rhythm. Try repositioning the patient appropriately for site of catheter insertion. Record ECG to determine catheter position. Order chest film.
UNDERSENSING— Failure to sense a spontaneous beat (such as PVC) because of the vector of the beat in relation to the electrodes.	Intracavitary signals or voltage less than 2 mV at the catheter tip may fail to trigger the sensing mechanism. Adequate sensing of spontaneous beats is sometimes unattainable with a bipolar electrode system because low signals are seen by the sensing electrodes. By changing to a unipolar system, a larger interelectrode distance is created, which picks up a greater voltage for a given signal.	Call the physician to 1. Determine intracavitary voltage. The sensed signal can be measured by an intracardiac ECG tracing taken from the pacemaker wires. Hook right arm and left arm leads to the two pacer wires and turn ECG to lead I. 2. See if catheter needs to be repositioned. 3. Change the bipolar catheter into a unipolar system. (See p. 532 and Fig. 40-23 for directions.)

*Refers to inappropriate release or absence of a stimulus release at the proper time. (Preston TA, Yates JD: Heart Lung 2(4): 533–538, 1973; Spence MI, Lemberg L: Heart Lung 4(2): 286–295, 1975; Vinsant MD, Spence MI, Hagen DC: A Commonsense Approach to Coronary Care: A Program, pp. 203–219. St. Louis, CV Mosby, 1975)

Permanent Pulse Generators

Power sources for permanent pacemakers are numerous: mercury-zinc batteries (lifespan from 2-5 years), lithium-salt batteries (lifespan from 7-10 years), and nuclear-powered (radioactive plutonium) batteries, first used in the early 1970s (projected lifespan 20 or more years).[15] Since 1979, however, lithium-salt batteries have almost exclusively replaced mercury-zinc batteries. The primary reasons for this are improved reliability (because mercury-zinc batteries cannot be hermetically sealed, the chances for current leakage increase), increased longevity, and a slower failure

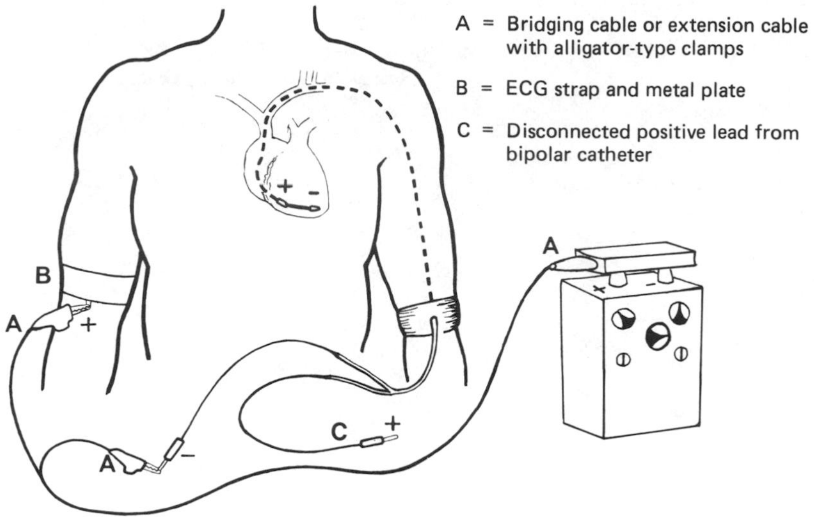

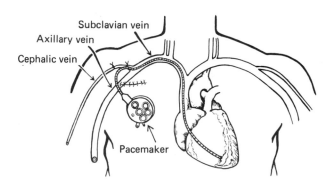

A = Bridging cable or extension cable with alligator-type clamps

B = ECG strap and metal plate

C = Disconnected positive lead from bipolar catheter

Fig. 40-23. Conversion of a temporary transvenous bipolar electrode to a unipolar electrode pacing system. Connecting the positive terminal of the external pulse generator via a bridging cable or extension with alligator clips (**A**) to a body surface electrode (**B**) instead of to the positive catheter electrode (**C**). *All* exposed connections must be insulated with a rubber glove or similar material. (Adapted from Preston TA, Yates JD: Heart Lung, 2(4):535, 1973)

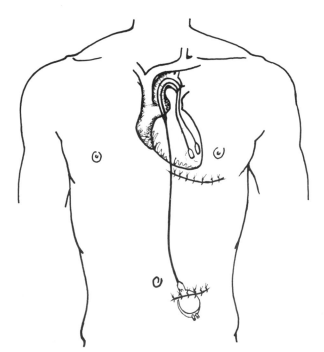

Fig. 40-24. Transthoracic installation of a permanent pacemaker.

Subclavian vein

Axillary vein

Cephalic vein

Pacemaker

Fig. 40-25. Transvenous installation of a permanent pacemaker.

mechanism once the batteries begin deteriorating (months for lithium-salt vs. 1-2 weeks for mercury-zinc batteries) (TA Preston, personal communication). Batteries in some units can be recharged transcutaneously by induction coils and an external charging console. This can be done weekly or monthly at home.[1,15]

Nursing Responsibilities and Interventions

The intensity of nursing care provided preoperatively and postoperatively depends on the approach used for permanent implantation. The following objectives should be kept in mind:

1. Prevention of postoperative complications
2. Prevention of pacemaker complications
3. Prevention of infection
4. Patient teaching

Preoperative Nursing Care.

1. Avoid placing ECG monitoring electrodes over potential incision site (above the right or left clavicles) to prevent skin breakdown. When using the MCL_1 or MCL_6 monitoring system, the negative electrode can be moved from the left anterior shoulder to left posterior shoulder without interfering with the electrocardiographic pattern. The ground electrode can be placed anywhere on the body. For convenience, it may be moved to the right posterior shoulder.

2. Hold informal discussion(s) with patient and family to assess their level of knowledge and understanding regarding the reason for a pacemaker and what it does (refer to the following patient teaching section). Show model catheter and pulse generator. Use heart model and drawing. Mention skin protrusion.

3. Teach patient range of motion exercises to arm and shoulder on operated side (to prevent loss of shoulder function postoperatively). Have patient redemonstrate and practice.

4. Review importance of coughing and deep breathing postoperatively. Demonstrate and redemonstrate.

5. Do routine preoperative preparation for pacemaker patients (this varies with hospitals):
   a. Obtain signed forms of consent for operation.
   b. Scrub surgical area for 10 minutes with solution such as Prepodyne (1% iodine) the night before and on the morning of procedure.
   c. Give nothing by mouth after midnight.
   d. Begin sedation, as ordered.
6. Insert patent IV line.

Postoperative nursing care.

1. Take frequent vital signs until they are stable (for example, every 15 minutes times four, every 30 minutes times four, and every hour times four).
2. Take temperature every 4 hours.
3. Order bed rest, up to 24 hours, mainly to reduce the risk of the catheter being dislodged (transvenous approach only).
4. Encourage coughing, deep breathing, and turning to prevent atelectasis and accumulation of bronchial secretions (every 1–2 hours).
5. Check operative site for any bleeding, swelling, or discharge. Usually the dressing will be removed on the first postoperative day by the surgeon; sutures will be removed in approximately one week, usually after the patient's discharge.
6. Administer prescribed pain medication as needed.
7. Record baseline 12-lead ECG after return to the unit, and periodically obtain monitor strips to determine proper functioning. To test a demand or synchronous ventricular pacemaker, a magnet can be placed on the skin over the location of the pulse generator. The magnet will activate a switch that reverts the pacer to a fixed rate. There will be an initial pause before the generator begins firing.
8. Watch for cardiac arrhythmias. The potential for ventricular irritability is high shortly after surgery, for several reasons. The stiff catheter causes some myocardial injury. Catheter movement is not uncommon until adequate fibrosis has developed, usually 48 to 72 hours after implantation. The amount of energy (in mA) delivered is higher than the desired level but will dissipate somewhat as fibrosis develops. If arrhythmias persist they will need to be suppressed with medication. (See Chap. 26 for differentiation of right-side versus left-side PVCs.)
9. Note on patient's care plan and nursing notes:
   a. Date and time of insertion
   b. The type of pacemaker
   c. The selected rate.
10. Be aware of other potential complications:[1,18]
    a. A break in a wire (look for absence of pacing stimulus on monitor even though pulse generator is discharging.)
    b. Perforation of the right ventricle by the catheter tip into the left ventricle or pericardium
    c. Rejection of pacemaker unit (can occur at any time from 1 week to one year).
    d. Pressure necrosis of the skin overlying the pulse generator.

PATIENT TEACHING AND PSYCHOLOGIC ASPECTS

Acceptance of a Pacemaker

The first introduction to a pacemaker for many patients is under less than ideal learning conditions, such as during an emergency when the patient is symptomatic. Fear of the unknown and of dying are real feelings for patients during such an event. The patient's anxiety level is undoubtedly high, and therefore learning and retention are minimal. It is a prime opportunity and an obligation for the nurse to be the intervening factor toward helping a patient to understand the principles behind pacemakers. Initial pacemaker teaching, help in the recognition of fears, and emotional support given by the nurse undoubtedly influence the patient's present and long-term acceptance of his pacemaker.

Most persons requiring a pacemaker are 50 to 80 years old. Chronic disease and degenerative alterations that accompany aging are prevalent in this age bracket. Factors such as reduced hearing, vision, perception, memory, judgment, and motor skills influence the learning process.

A patient's reaction toward and acceptance of a pacemaker will be influenced by many factors: past experiences, usual reactions to stress and anxiety, self-concept before illness, level of education, severity of the present illness, and required change in living patterns that it may necessitate. Despite physical ailments such as decreased hearing, decreased retention, and/or impaired vision, elderly people can learn. The nurse needs to be aware of the person's handicap(s) and individualize the teaching plan accordingly.[13]

Many patients have expressed fears associated with the need for a pacemaker: fear of dying from pacemaker failure and dependency on a life-support system. Verbal and nonverbal cues can alert the nurse that such fears exist. However, some patients may never reveal their inward thoughts unless specifically questioned, for example, about describing feelings of living with a pacemaker.[27] Helping a patient to identify and discuss his fears, to learn about his pacemaker, and how to live with it should alleviate some of these fears. Although dependence upon the pacemaker is inevitable, the nurse can help the patient to distinguish areas of his life in which he is not dependent on others, and encourage him to accept help with the activities that he cannot manage alone.[27]

A study involving 30 patients showed many of the patient's problems in adjusting to a permanent pacemaker and in taking an active part in its maintenance were related to a lack of accurate information about what to expect or how to ensure normal functioning of the pacemaker.[27] Motivation must be present before learning can take place. That is, learning is most effective when a person feels he needs to know something. The nurse's role is to encourage a readiness to learn. If the desired behavior change is urgent, the nurse may need to use direct supervision to ensure that this change occurs.[26]

Regardless of dependency on an outside support system, some hospitalized patients may never be in the acceptance stage and ready to learn, while others may not possess the capabilties to learn or to care for themselves. In these instances, the nurse should involve the family, public health nurse, or another responsible person.

With any patient, there is a definite need to involve family members. Their interest, acceptance, and support affect the patient and may well influence the patient's reliability in follow-up care. Since sharing common problems is reassuring, pacemaker group sessions at the hospital or in the community may be of benefit.

Patient Teaching

A teaching plan must be realistic and geared to the individual's needs. The more the patient can actively participate, the more meaningful his learning is. To evaluate teaching effectiveness and retention of material, the nurse should ask the patient to describe in his own words the concepts discussed and to redemonstrate the skills presented. The following areas should be covered with either the patient or someone who will be responsible for his care.

Anatomy and Physiology of the Heart. An introductory part of the teaching plan should be a simple, concise discussion of the structure of the heart and its basic function as a pump which delivers oxygen and nourishment to the cells in the body. The normal conduction system should also be briefly described, as well as the alteration in the patient's conduction mechanism. What the patient has been told by his physician and how much he understood and retained should be determined by the nurse.

Pictures or models are helpful. If the patient can actually visualize with the help of these tools what is being discussed, the information is more meaningful to him. An excellent booklet to give every patient is the American Heart Association's *Living With Your Pacemaker*.[14] Most pacemaker manufacturing companies furnish a similar booklet for patient teaching. Having written material to refer to after discharge is invaluable for many patients.

Introduction to a Pacemaker. The basic function of the patient's artificial pacemaker should be discussed next. He needs to be aware of its type: for example, if the pacemaker wire will be in the atrium or ventricle and if it will work at a fixed rate or on demand. An actual pulse generator and catheter that can be handled by the patient will prove helpful. Again, pictures and drawings will help the patient to visualize implantation. An important fact to emphasize is that the pacemaker is an entirely closed and sealed system.[13] Patients who initially have a temporary pacemaker may think the pulse generator and paraphernalia must be worn externally forever.

Pacemaker Failure. The patient must be aware of why he is learning to take his own pulse. He should understand that the pulse reflects heart action and pacemaker function.[13] If he does not grasp this concept, any amount of teaching may fail. A former patient who recently returned for a battery replacement was questioned about pulse taking, to which he replied: "Oh, I stopped taking that a long time ago; it was always regular." Some important points to discuss with the patient and family are

1. The meaning of battery failure

2. The approximate length of time the pulse generator is expected to last

3. Knowing ways in which the patient himself can detect battery failure, the most common being HR change (usually a slowing of 5–10 bpm). A patient with a fixed-rate pacemaker should call his doctor if his pulse ranges 5 bpm above or below the set rate.[15] Rather than slowing at battery exhaustion, a few pulse generators will increase their rate. Such information should accompany the battery pack. Rarely, a "runaway" pacemaker is encountered. If the patient discovers a rapid pulse rate not associated with physical activity or emotional stress, he should call his doctor.

4. Taking the pulse. The teacher should first demonstrate the procedure and then the patient should perform a return demonstration.

5. Practicing pulse taking repeatedly. Pulse-taking can be taught in a series of steps. The patient will learn to find his pulse, identify and understand its rhythmic pattern, and count the pulse accurately for a full minute.[13]

6. Having a clock or watch at home with a second hand. Some kitchen timers will work as well.

7. Counting the pulse daily for one full minute *at rest* and recording the rate

8. Knowing his normal pulse range. The patient can determine this by evaluating daily recorded pulses for 1 month after he has returned to his normal living pattern.[15]

9. Knowing the rate at which the pacemaker is set

10. Knowing when to call the doctor. The patient should be aware that his pulse will not necessarily be regular (unless he has a fixed-rate pacemaker). For example, he may be having premature atrial contractions (PACs) or premature ventricular contractions (PVCs) that do not perfuse peripherally. Consequently, at times the pulse rate may be irregular and slower than the set pacemaker rate. It does not necessarily mean a generator problem. It is important that the person understand that he should call the doctor to determine the cause, if the condition persists.[15]

11. Emphasizing the need for his participation in detecting battery failure (daily pulse taking) as well as the importance of keeping clinic appointments.

12. The possibility of arranging for a public health nurse to visit the patient or family periodically

Symptoms of Pacemaker Failure. It is imperative that the patient understand that his pulse must be counted when he is symptomatic as well as asymptomatic. PVCs can result in a low pulse, causing the patient to be symptomatic. These symptoms then, may or may not be associated with battery failure. A multitude of symptoms can mimic battery failure. The patient may experience dizziness, lightheadedness, syncope, chest pain, shortness of breath, peripheral edema, palpitations, loss of consciousness, and confusion. With the majority of patients in an older age group, any of these can be common. If any prolonged hiccoughing or chest wall muscular twitching occurs, the nurse should advise the patient to call the doctor.

Each patient should be given a pacemaker identification card. Figure 40-26 is an example. Most manufacturers provide a similar card. Some doctors may also suggest that their patients wear an emergency identification wrist bracelet or necklace.

Electromagnetic Interference. Information from manufacturers varies regarding electrical and mechanical interferences with the functioning of pacemakers. Many of the newer models have metallic shielding that will keep out most interfering signals. Therefore, unless specific instructions are included from the pacemaker's manufacturer, it is best to give general directions to the patient.

1. The interference will not break or destroy the pacemaker. However, it may switch it over to a fixed rate, or temporarily shut it off so that the pacer will not sense the patient's heart beat.

2. Most electrical and mechanical devices can be used safely; however, the patient should have the following information:

    A. Electric hair clippers and shavers are unlikely to interfere with pacemakers but patients should not operate them directly over the pulse generator area.

    B. Keep at least 3 feet away from microwave ovens. Many airlines heat their food in microwave ovens; so, if the patient is flying, he should arrange to be seated as far away as possible from these appliances.

    C. Avoid arc welding equipment completely.

    D. Gasoline engines (cars, lawn mowers, snowmobiles, boat motors), electric motors (large shop tools and high-frequency signals from cautery and diathermy machines) are sources of danger. Be sure electric motors are properly grounded, avoid leaning directly over any running engines or motors.

    E. The metal in the pacemaker unit triggers the metal detectors in airport screening devices. Screening personnel need to be notified that you have a pacemaker. Your identification card may be necessary for clearance.

    F. Use caution near antitheft devices: some clothing, jewelry, and department stores have such equipment, which can temporarily affect pacemaker function. If the patient becomes symptomatic when entering a store or waiting in the checkout line, he should move away from the detection area and inform the clerk about the pacemaker.

    G. Stay away from the power transmitters and towers of radio, television, and radar. This does not include antennas found in the home.[5,10,17,31]

3. The general rule of thumb is that if the patient becomes dizzy or feels "unusual" in the presence of one of these devices he should move 5 to 10 feet away from it and count his pulse. If interference has caused the symptom, the pulse will return to normal when the person moves away from the source.[15] Be sure that the patient tells any of his other medical doctors or his dentist that he has a pacemaker so that certain equipment can be avoided.

Care of Pacemaker Site. The nurse should provide information about skin care in the area where the pulse generator is located:

PACEMAKER IDENTIFICATION CARD
🛡 **American Heart Association**

Name _____
Address _____
Phone _____ Blood type _____

I am wearing a pacemaker In an emergency, contact:

Doctor _____
Phone _____
Address _____
Type of Pacemaker _____

Type of leads _____
Manufacturer _____
Date of Implant _____
Hospital _____
Phone _____
Address _____
Paced rate _____
Model _____
Serial number _____

Please! Carry this card at all times
It will help others assist you in an emergency

Fig. 40-26. Pacemaker identification card. (Living with Your Pacemaker, p 13. Dallas, American Heart Association, 1979. By permission of the American Heart Association, Inc.)

1. Advise the patient to keep the incision clean and dry until it is completely healed and the sutures have been removed. No showering is initially permitted but a tub bath is appropriate, providing the surrounding area is kept dry.

2. Mention initial temporary discoloration (bruising) in the site after surgery. Instruct the patient to report any redness, discoloration, drainage, pain, heat, or swelling around the pacemaker or lead sites. Patients who are thin or have pulse generators in the upper chest are more prone to develop skin problems.[15]

3. Advise selection of loose-fitting underwear and clothing to avoid skin breakdown due to pressure.

Pacemaker Replacement. The patient should be aware of the procedure for an anticipated battery change. With prior information, some misconceptions or anxiety can be alleviated.

1. Briefly explain pacemaker replacement: use of local anesthetic, removal of old generator, and connection of new one to the same catheter (leads generally not replaced unless a problem exists).

2. Explain need for a short hospital stay to monitor pacemaker's function, generally 24 to 48 hours.

Medications. Many patients will be on cardiac drugs as well as diuretics and electrolyte supplements. To avoid any misunderstanding, the patient needs to know that he should continue to take these medications as ordered. He needs to be aware that the pacemaker and the medicines are to aid the heart, but are used for different reasons.

Physical Activity. The patient should have a clear understanding of his activity or physical limitations, if any. This will depend somewhat on his cardiac status prior to the pacemaker insertion. Most patients will be able to resume their previous activity level. In one study involving 30 patients, over 75% of them described their life styles as improved. Some patients who had lived with a slow pulse for a number of years described an increase in energy after pacemaker implantation.[27]

FOLLOW-UP CLINIC

Follow-up of pacemaker function is important. Periodic checks ensure that pacemaker failure can be predicted before clinical failure occurs. Battery failure generally does not occur suddenly; voltage weakens over a period of days or weeks. The most common sign of battery failure is rate variation, usually a decrease in rate of 5 to 10 bpm. A few models will increase in rate or revert to a fixed rate.

By keeping accurate records at periodically scheduled intervals, the doctor will be able to determine when these changes take place. Premature replacement, and hence unnecessary expense for the patient, can be avoided.

The frequency of pacemaker function checks will be determined by various factors: the type of pulse generator, the patient's age and reliability, his compliance with pulse taking, and travel distance from the clinic. Methods of surveillance range from a check-up in a doctor's office to an elaborate, computerized hospital pacemaker clinic.

Periodic Appointments

Follow-up appointments at a hospital clinic or doctor's office should be made periodically where HR and an ECG can be taken.

Trans-Telephone Method

Electrodes and a small transmitting unit are used in conjunction with a home telephone. The patient attaches his ECG electrodes on each wrist, places his phone receiver in his transmitting unit and transmits data over the phone to the receiving unit. Electrical impulses are changed into signals that are transmitted over the phone. At the receiving unit, the signals are changed into their original form as electrical impulses and recorded as the ECG. During recordings, patients with demand pacemakers use magnets which convert the mode to a fixed rate. While this method does not provide direct contact with the patient, it does allow conversation. For patients living a considerable distance from a doctor or clinic, this method provides some means for checking on the patient. Pacemaker rate and function can be easily determined.

Phone Monitoring

A pacemaker emits a small radio frequency with each electrical impulse. If the patient holds a portable transistor radio tuned to a low frequency over the pulse generator, the signal can be heard as a click. The patient's rate can then be counted over the phone. This method is usually restricted to fixed-rate pacemakers and has the distinct disadvantage of relaying very limited information.

Pacemaker Clinics

At regular intervals ECG strips are taken and brief patient exams are performed. Additionally, a waveform analysis is done. Waveform analysis consists of analyzing a visual display of the electrical impulse, generally rectangular or trapezoidal, that is emitted from the pacemaker. The duration or width of this impulse, which reflects the length of time (in milliseconds) necessary for the emission of the electrical stimulus, usually increases with battery failure. By proper analysis, very subtle changes in battery condition can be detected earlier than by any other method available.[4,8,22]

REFERENCES

1. Andreoli KG, Fowkes VH, Zipes DP et al: Artificial cardiac pacemakers. Comprehensive Cardiac Care, 3rd ed, pp 244–265. St. Louis, C. V. Mosby, 1975.
2. Bing OHL, McDowell JW, Hantman J et al: Pacemaker placement by electrocardiographic monitoring. N Engl J Med 287(13):651, 1972
3. Chung EK: Pacing by different modes. Primary Cardiology 4:50–52, 1978
4. Czerwinski B: Trans-telephonic surveillance for pacemaker patients. Am J Nurs 77(5):828–829, 1977
5. The Effects of Other Devices, Pacing Your Heart, Minneapolis, Medtronic, 1977
6. Escher DJW: Medical aspects of artificial pacing of the heart. Cardiovasc Nurs 8(1):1–4, 1972
7. Furman S: Fundamentals of cardiac pacing. Am Heart J 73(2):261–277, 1967
8. Furman S: Management of heart block. In The Twenty-Eighth Hahemann Symposium, Critical Care Medicine, pp 133–143. New York, Grune & Stratton, 1974
9. Furman S, Escher DJW: Principles and Techniques of Cardiac Pacing. New York, Harper & Row, 1970
10. Germain CP: Helping your patient with an implanted pacemaker. RN 37(8):30–35, 1974
11. Harthorne J: Selections of various types of cardiac pacemakers. In Norman J, Rickards A (eds): Proceedings of the Pacemaker Colloquium, pp 24–29. Arnhem the Netherlands, Tamminga, bv, 1976
12. Kaminski MV Jr, Harris DF: Prolonged uncomplicated intravascular catheterization. Am J I.V. Therapy 3:19–23, 1976
13. Kos BA, Culbert PA: Teaching the patient with a pacemaker. Cardiovasc Nurs 6(6):57–60, 1970
14. Living With Your Pacemaker. Dallas, American Heart Association, 1979
15. Manwaring M: What patients need to know about pacemakers. Am J Nurs 77(5):825–830, 1977
16. Marriott HJL, Gozensky C: Electrocardiogram problems created by pacemakers. Cardiovasc Nurs 12(1):1–6, 1976.
17. Medtronic Technical Manual, Model 5375. Minneapolis, Medtronic, 1977
18. Nursing Care of Patients with Internal or External Pacemakers. DHEW Publication No. (NIH) 75-226. Washington, D.C., U.S. Government Printing Office, 1974
19. Papa LA, Abkar KB, Chung EK: Pacemaker hysteresis. Heart Lung 3(6):982–984, 1974
20. Parsonnet V, Furman S, Smyth NPD: Implantable cardiac pacemakers status report and resource guideline. Circulation 50(4):A21–35, 1974
21. Parsonnet V, Manhardt M: World survey on long-term follow-

up of cardiac pacing. In Watanabe Y (ed) Cardiac Pacing, pp 569–571. Amsterdam, Excepta Medica, 1977

22. Parsonnet V, Myers GH, Gilbert L et al. Follow-up of implanted pacemakers. Am Heart J 87(5):642–653, 1974
23. Post MR, Killip T: Application of cardiac pacing to acute myocardial infarction. In Meltzer LE, Dunning AJ (eds) Textbook of Coronary Care, pp 341–356. Philadelphia, Charles Press, 1972
24. Preston TA: A comparison of bipolar and unipolar permanent stimulation electrodes. In Norman J, Richards A (eds): Proceedings of the Pacemaker Colloquium, pp 55–60. Arnhem, Netherlands: Tamminga bv, 1976
25. Preston TA, Yates JD: Management of stimulation and sensing problems ed. St. Louis, C. V. Mosby, 1972
26. Redman BK: The Process of Patient Teaching in Nursing, 2nd ed. St. Louis, C. V. Mosby, 1972
27. Rossel CL, Alyn IB: Living with a permanent cardiac pacemaker. Heart Lung 6(2):273–279, 1977
28. Schnitzler RN, Caracta AR, Damato AN: Floating catheter for temporary transvenous ventricular pacing. Am J Cardiol 31:351–354, 1973
29. Spence MI, Lemberg L: Cardiac pacemakers I. Modalities of pacing. Heart Lung 3(5):820–827, 1974
30. Spence MI, Lemberg L: Cardiac pacemakers IV. Complications of pacing. Heart Lung 4(2):286–295, 1975
31. Sweetwood H: Patients with pacemakers. Nursing '77 7(3):44–51, 1977
32. Vera Z, Awan NA, Amsterdam EA et al: Cardiac pacemakers: Indications and complications. Heart Lung 4(3):444–451, 1975
33. Vinsant MD, Spence MI, Hagen DC: Electrical intervention in acute MI. A Commonsense Approach to Coronary Care: A Program, pp. 203–219. St. Louis, C. V. Mosby, 1975
34. Weinstein J, Groj J, Mazzara JT et al: Temporary transvenous pacing via the percutaneous femoral vein approach. Fundamentals of clinical cardiology. Am Heart J 5:695–705, 1973
35. Wenger NK: Myocarditis. In Hurst JW, Logue RB, Schlant RC et al (eds): The Heart, 3rd ed, p 1326. New York, McGraw-Hill, 1974
36. Winslow EH, Marino LB: Temporary cardiac pacemakers. Am J Nurs 75(4):586–591, 1975

ADDITIONAL READING

Furman S: Recent developments in cardiac pacing. Heart Lung 7(5):813–826, 1978

Haddad M, Weisberger C, Chung E: Reciprocal beats initiated by artificial pacemaker. Heart Lung 5(1):124–126, 1976

Kallenbach J, Miller RN, Obel IWP: Runaway temporary pacemaker. Heart Lung 6(3):517–518, 1977

Kitchen JG, Goldreyer GN: Demand pacemaker for refractory paroxysmal supraventricular tachycardia. N Engl J Med 287(12):596–599, 1972

Spence M, Lemberg L: Cardiac pacemakers: III. Pacemakers in the management of reciprocating tachycardias. Heart Lung 4(1):128–133, 1975

41

Electrical Hazards in the Cardiac Care Unit

SUSAN L. WOODS, R.N., M.N.

Despite the advantages of a CCU, its environment subjects the patient to potential electrical hazards. The following topics are discussed in this chapter: the vulnerability of the CCU patient; the principles of electricity; electrical shock; sources of current; isolated power systems; equipotential grounding; electrical safety.

The Vulnerability of the CCU Patient

The patient in the CCU is vulnerable to electrical hazards because he is connected to a cardiac monitor and thus can become part of an electrical circuit. The CCU patient may be connected to more than one electrical device, such as a portable suction machine, a hypothermia blanket, an electrocardiograph, a vaporizer, or an electrical bed, and any of these electrical devices can leak current. Leakage current is current conveyed from accessible parts of an appliance to ground or to other accessible parts of an appliance.[4] If the current leakage in any one of these devices exceeds the threshold of resistance of the patient's skin, then the leakage current runs off to ground through a circuit that includes the patient's body (Fig. 41-1).[1,7] Resistance is a measure of the difficulty of electrons to flow through a material.[5] If the equipment is properly grounded, leakage current is channeled through a ground wire away from the patient to a distant point. If the equipment is not grounded, current leakage can be conducted through anything with a low enough resistance. The patient with a temporary pacemaker electrode in place is particularly vulnerable, because that device provides a low-resistance pathway directly to the heart. If a piece of electronic equipment leaks current, and a connection is made between the indwelling electrode and the leakage current, current may flow through the heart, resulting in ventricular fibrillation.

Principles of Electricity

For current to flow, the following criteria must be met: (1) there must be a complete, closed circuit; (2) there must be a difference in potential (voltage) between two points in a circuit. Ohm's law describes the relationship between voltage (in watts/second), resistance (in ohms), and current (in amperes) (current = voltage/resistance). Thus, a low-resistance pathway allows more current to flow than a high resistance pathway does. If the voltage is reduced the current flow is reduced.[8] Electricity flows from higher levels of voltage to lower levels of voltage. Earth (ground) is the lowest level of voltage.[3] A conducting pathway between an electrical circuit or equipment and the earth or some other conductive body is the ground.[4]

In the United States, alternating current (a series of sine waves with maximum excursion above and below an isoelectric point) is delivered at a rate of 60 cycles per second. Standard wall receptacles provide 110–120 milliamperes if the person in contact with the circuit offers a resistance of 1000 ohms. The polarity of the wall receptacle, if the opening for the ground prong slot is on top, is as follows: the left slot of the receptacle has a potential of approximately 115 volts alternating current, whereas the right slot is neutral and close to zero potential.[4]

The tissue surrounding the heart acts as a resistor, and opposes current flow. The skin has a resistance of 50,000 to 100,000 ohms. This resistance is reduced if the skin is moist and abraded (skin oil is removed).[3] Conducting cath-

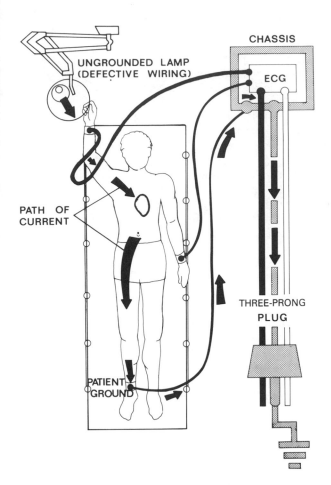

Fig. 41-1. Electrical hazard caused by providing an alternative pathway for grounding the current. As the defectively wired lamp is touched, the electricity accumulated in the metal frame takes the alternative low-resistance pathway and a potentially lethal current passes through patient's heart to the ground lead. (After Directions in Cardiovascular Medicine. 7. The Heart and Electrical Hazards, p 22. Sommerville NJ, Hoechst Pharmaceutical, 1973)

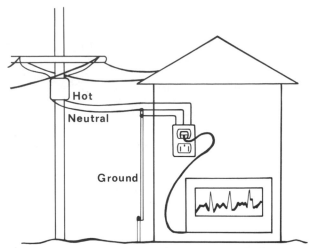

Fig. 41-2. Simplified schema of power entering a building. Note that one of the current-carrying conductors (neutral wire) is connected to the ground at the point at which power enters the building. (From Mylrea KC. Reprinted with permission from the January issue of Nursing 76, copyright © 1976, by Intermed Communications, Inc., Horsham, PA)

Fig. 41-3. Simplified drawing of the wiring of incoming power line and connection to a medical device in a modern hospital. Note that the hot wire is at the same potential relative to both cold and ground wires, both of which are essentially at the same (zero) potential. (After Directions in Cardiovascular Medicine. 7. The Heart and Electrical Hazards, p 11. Sommerville NJ, Hoechst Pharmaceutical, 1973)

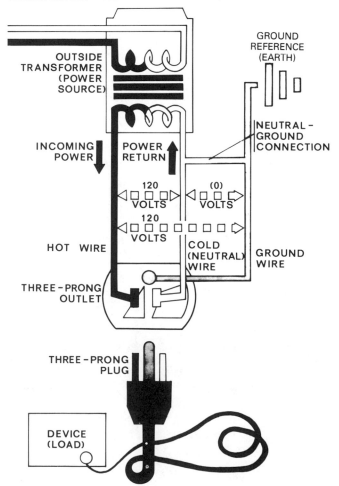

eters inserted into the heart offer a low-resistant pathway by which current can flow. Such catheters are: pacing electrode catheters (resistance 70 ohms); Dacron cardiac catheter filled with saline (resistance 300,000 ohms). But when a metal guide is used, it offers only 20 ohms resistance.[8]

Electrical Power to the Hospital

Figure 41-2 illustrates how electrical power enters the hospital.[5] Two wires (hot and neutral lines) carry current to the two slotted holes in the electrical outlet. A third wire is connected to the circular hole in the electrical outlet and is attached to a copper pipe (ground) which is driven into the earth at a point at which the power enters the building. At this point the neutral line is also connected to the ground. Current flows from the hot line (high voltage) to the neutral line (near zero voltage) or to the ground wire or through any conductive surface in the hospital that is connected to ground (Fig. 41-3).[2] Thus, current will flow from the hot line to any grounded object if a conductive path is provided.

Electrical Shock

One milliampere applied to the body can be felt (macroshock); 5 to 10 milliamperes applied to the body will result in sustained muscular contraction; 50 to 100 milliamperes applied to the body can cause ventricular fibrillation; and 1000 to 5000 milliamperes applied to the body results in sustained myocardial contraction and severe burns at the point of electrical contact. One hundred microamperes, imperceptible to human touch, applied directly to the heart (for example, via a pacing catheter) results in ventricular fibrillation (microshock).[5] Current applied by direct contact to the heart is very concentrated (high-current density). Current applied to the chest is more diffuse (low-current density).

Sources of Currents

Leakage Current. In electronic equipment, voltage difference exists between the "hot" wiring inside and the metal housing. This can result in current flow to the metal housing. Also, if the "hot" wire within the equipment is not properly

Fig. 41-4. An electrical hazard in the CCU. The nurse can complete the circuit by simultaneously touching the metal portion of the electrical bed (which is leaking current) and the external ends of the patient's pacemaker catheter. Current flows from the electrical bed to the ECG ground through the low-resistance pathway (pacemaker electrode) through the patient's heart. (After Directions in Cardiovascular Medicine. 7. The Heart and Electrical Hazards, p 22. Sommerville NJ, Hoechst Pharmaceutical, 1973)

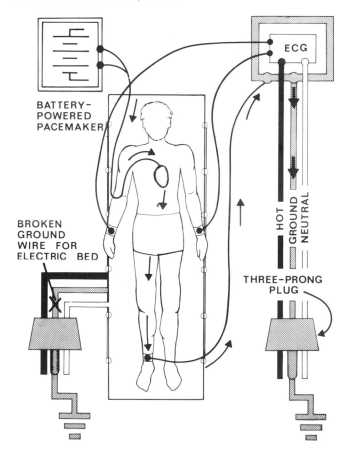

insulated, leakage current can flow to the equipment housing.

Ten microamperes, measured between patient connector terminals on the equipment and ground, is the maximum amount of leakage current that a patient with a low-resistance intracardiac catheter can tolerate from any device with which he is in contact. Battery operated devices provide maximum protection to the patient from electrical shock because the device is not part of the electrical circuit.[8]

Equipment Fault. Electronic equipment that is not grounded or has a defective ground can cause current to flow through the patient to another piece of grounded equipment with which the patient is in contact (Fig. 41-4).

Isolated Power System

Some hospitals use an isolated power system in which current flows only from one isolated line to the other rather than to the ground. An isolation transformer can break the neutral connection to ground. Thus, the conventional system can be converted to an isolated power system (Fig. 41-5). This system appears to offer many advantages over the conventional power system, but in actuality it is impossible to maintain perfect isolation of the lines from ground.[5] Also, isolation transformers are costly, require maintenance, and do not eliminate all types of hazards. Additional hazards are introduced by the ground fault detectors of this system.[6]

Equipotential Grounding

This system maintains equal voltage of all conductive surfaces eliminating current flow, because no voltage exists between the surfaces. Equipotential grounding is achieved by connecting all conductive surfaces (metal bed frame, electrical equipment) to one ground reference point. This point is then attached by a copper conductor to a ground tie point at the electrical distribution panel.[5] Thus, if all ground conductors in the environment are at the same electrical potential, no current will flow through an object or person in contact with two conductors.[6]

The ground wire, contained within the plug and the cord, connects the metal housing of patient equipment to the ground contact within the electrical outlet. This provides for the safe flow of leakage current from the equipment housing to ground. If the equipment is not properly grounded, however, then leakage current will seek the path of least resistance to ground.[5]

Electrical Safety

Equipment in the room of a patient with a heart catheter should meet the following standards:[5]

1. The exposed end of the electrically conductive portion of the catheter (wires or fluid) should not be handled unless plastic or rubber gloves are worn. The external end of the catheter should not come in contact with any instrument or conductive surface other than the point at which it is intended to be connected.

2. All electrical equipment must be properly grounded and inspected regularly to detect leakage current.

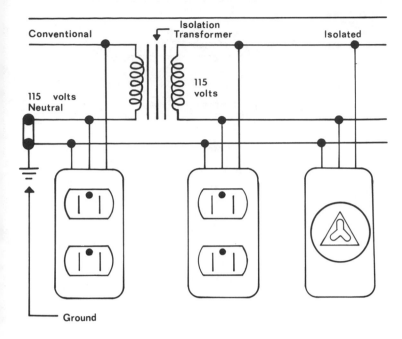

Fig. 41-5. An isolation transformer. An isolation transformer changes a conventional power system (neutral side connected to ground) to an isolated power system (neither side connected to ground.) (From Mylrea KC. Reprinted with permission from the January issue of Nursing 76, Copyright © 1976, by Intermed Communications, Inc., Horsham, PA)

3. If the metal terminals holding the pacing catheter are exposed, they should be covered securely with a nonconductive material which prevents or decreases current flow, for example, a plastic or rubber glove.

Any electrical device brought into the CCU should be checked to determine the amount of leakage current in accordance with the Biomedical Electrical safety guidelines of the state or city. The equipment should be assigned to one or possibly two of the electrical risk-leakage-current classes described below:

1. Risk I: Applies to all equipment that does not normally contact a patient.

2. Risk II: Applies to all equipment that is attached to a patient, but not directly to his heart. This risk class also applies to equipment without patient attachments that the patient is likely to touch.

3. Risk III: Applies to all equipment with isolated inputs that are attached directly to the patient's heart.

Table 41-1 summarizes the maximum leakage current (measured under worst conditions) allowable within each of the three classifications.

The patient should be prevented from contacting the conductive parts of electrical equipment. Also, a nurse or anyone attending the patient in his room may serve as the current path between an improperly grounded machine and the patient. Many electrical beds are not safe enough for use in the CCU. They may leak large amounts of current and surround the patient with a low-resistance path to ground. Hydraulic and mechanical beds are safer to use in electrically-sensitive areas.[6]

All alternating current (AC) receptacles and grounded surfaces should be inspected and tested. Tests should include:[6]

1. Determination of resistance between ground points

2. Determination of the current that will flow through a resistor (equivalent to a myocardial impedance—500 ohms) when it is connected to two separate points

3. Determination of polarity, since the receptacle may have been improperly repaired between checks

4. Determination of broken or dead outlets

Since static electricity is also potentially harmful, carpeting is not recommended in the CCU. Methods of abolishing static electricity are not perfect; grounding the carpet creates an additional grounded surface, and further exposes the patient to electrical hazard.[6]

Preventive maintenance is essential if electrical hazards are to be avoided. Table 41-2 lists an example of a mainte-

(*Text continues on p. 548.*)

TABLE 41-1   MAXIMUM-RISK LEAKAGE-CURRENT DATA

Class	Where Measured	Maximum Allowable Leakage-Current
RISK III	Between patient connector terminals on the equipment and ground	10 microamperes
RISK III	Between an appropriate current-limiting resistor connected to a 120-volt alternating current and to each patient attachment point. Equipment is properly connected to the supply.	20 microamperes
RISK III	In the ground wire (green) of the equipment power cord or between equipment case and ground	100 microamperes
RISK II	Between patient attachment point or points and ground	50 microamperes
RISK II	In the ground wire of the equipment power cord or between equipment case and ground	100 microamperes
RISK I	In the ground wire of the equipment power cord or between equipment case and ground	500 microamperes

(Biomedical Electrical Safety Guidelines. State of Washington Department of Social and Health Services, Health Service Division, March, 1979)

TABLE 41-2 PREVENTIVE MAINTENANCE SCHEDULE

	Hospital Maintenance	Biomedical Engineer or Technician	Nurse	Frequency of Maintenance
Cardiac Monitors—ECG Machine				
1. Cable continuity (repair)	x			3 months
2. Strain relief (repair)	x			3 months
3. Leakage current and condition of power cord	x			1 month
4. Ground wire continuity:				
permanently installed	x			3 months
portable units	x			1 month
5. Workability of knobs			x	weekly
6. Cathode-ray tube image			x	weekly
7. Alarm limits			x	weekly
8. Common mode rejection ratio, input impedance, noise level, frequency response, maximum gain, sensitivity, linearity		x		6 months
9. Calibration marker	x	x		3 months
10. Sweep/paper speed	x	x		3 months
11. Rate meter	x	x		3 months
12. Interaction between controls		x		3 months
13. Transient leakage spikes		x		3 months
14. Internal component check		x		6 months
Defibrillators				
1. Strain relief	x			3 months
2. Continuity of cables	x			3 months
3. Ground integrity and power cord condition	x			3 months
4. Meter movement (needle should move smoothly)			x	after use
5. Paddle surface condition			x	after use
6. Charge and/or discharge relay operation			x	after use
7. Proper sterilization of internal paddles			x	after use
8. Proper accessories on portable cart			x	daily and after use
9. Proper storage of defibrillator			x	daily and after use
10. Leakage current	x			1 month
11. Workability of control knobs			x	after use
12. Automatic discharge		x		3 months
13. Wave shape and energy		x		6 months
14. Storage capacitor leakage (for DC defbrillators)		x		3 months
15. Condition of internal discharge resistor		x		3 months
16. Deterioration of internal components due to age or otherwise		x		6 months
17. Capability of rapid, successive discharges		x		6 months
18. Synchronizing (or cardioverting)		x		6 months
19. Actual isolation of "isolated" paddles		x		6 months
20. Review of "emergency call" system performance		x		6 months
21. Condition of rechargeable batteries		x		6 months
22. Electrical condition of paddles and paddle cables		x		6 months
Pacemakers				
1. Pulse amplitude and rate		x		6 months
2. Amplitude control linearity		x		6 months
3. If line operated-leakage current, power cord and strain relief	x			monthly
4. Use of battery log			x	during use
5. Cable continuity	x			monthly
6. Demand/automatic modes of pacing		x		6 months
7. Internal component check		x		6 months
8. Refractory period		x		6 months
Pressure or temperature transducers				
1. Leakage current, condition of power cord and strain relief	x			3 months
2. Impedance pathway to ground		x		6 months
3. Calibrating resistor		x		6 months
4. Sensitivity		x		6 months
5. Drift		x		6 months
6. Linearity		x		6 months
7. Frequency response		x		6 months
8. Calibrate against a known external reference		x		6 months

TABLE 41-2 PREVENTIVE MAINTENANCE SCHEDULE (Cont.)

	Hospital Maintenance	Biomedical Engineer or Technician	Nurse	Frequency of Maintenance
Portable x-ray machine				
1. Leakage current	x			3 months
2. Condition of power cord, strain relief	x			3 months.
Power distribution system				
1. Wall outlet check	x			6 months
2. Common grounds	x			6 months
3. Isolation transformers including ground fault monitors		x		6 months
Electrical beds				
1. Check function	x			on delivery and every month if bed is moved from one location to another; otherwise every 6 months.
2. Continuity of ground wire	x			
3. Inspect power cord and strain relief	x			
4. Leakage current	x			
Lamps				
1. Check function	x			on delivery
2. Continuity of ground wire	x			annual
3. Leakage current	x			annual
Ancillary				
1. Hypothermia unit (leakage current, power cords)	x			3 months
2. Suction units (leakage current, power cords)	x			3 months
3. Nurse's call button	x			3 months
4. Hydrotherapy unit (leakage current, grounding, power cord)	x			3 months

For detailed test methods, see:
(1) National Fire Protection Association (NFPA) Standards
    a. NFPA 56A: Use of Inhalation Anesthetics (Flammable and Nonflammable)
    b. NFPA 76A: Essential Electrical Systems for Health Care Facilities
    c. NFPA 70: National Electrical Code
    d. NFPA 101: Life Safety Code
(2) Association for the Advancement of Medical Instrumentation (AAMI)
    a. AAMI SCL-P: Safe Current Limits
    (Report of Inter-Society Commission for Heart Disease Resources. Electronic equipment in critical care areas. Part II: The electrical environment. Part III. Selection and maintenance program. Circulation 44:A249–A250, 1971. By permission of the American Heart Association, Inc.)

TABLE 41-3 ELECTRICAL SAFETY GUIDELINES IN THE CARDIAC CARE UNIT

General Precautions for all Devices

1. Do not use "cheater" adaptors, multiple-outlet adaptors, or extension cords in the CCU. Do not disconnect the plug from the wall by grasping the power cord.
2. Report any device and remove it from service if:
    a. It has been dropped or otherwise physically abused, or if liquid has been spilled into it
    b. Anyone has received a shock in connection with its use
    c. There is evidence of overheating, by smell or touch.
3. Also immediately report any of the following:
    a. Any wire, especially a power cord, that has frayed, worn, burned, or cut insulation
    b. Any plug that is broken, bent, or loose
    c. Cable connectors that are loosely connected to the cable, or to the instrument panel, or that do not hold securely
    d. Switches that are loose, or do not snap definitely from one position to another
    e. Control knobs that are loose or do not turn smoothly
    f. Switches, knobs, or other controls that do not consistently produce the expected result when they are operated
    g. Any event suggests to the user that a device is not operating normally.

4. Report any wall receptacles that are loose, damaged, or do not supply power. All receptacles should be of the three-wire type.
5. There is a potential decrease in patient safety when two or more line-operated devices are connected to a patient, therefore:
    a. Presently available electrical beds are not recommended for use in patient-monitoring areas.
    b. Disconnect patient cable from oscilloscope monitor when taking standard 12-lead ECG (merely turning off the power switch does not protect the patient)
    c. If two separate line-powered machines must be connected to the same patient, they should be plugged into adjacent receptacles. Devices plugged into different remote receptacles (such as a wall plug in the corridor outside the operating suite) should not be brought near the patient.
6. Battery operated equipment should be encouraged

Precautions for Monitors and Electrocardiographs

1. Do not use a monitor or electrocardiograph to check the position of a pacing catheter or a pericardiocentesis needle unless it is battery operated or known to have a leakage current of less than 10 microamperes (as measured through the ground wire or between the leads to ground) in the situation in which it is being used.

547

TABLE 41-3 ELECTRICAL SAFETY GUIDELINES IN THE CARDIAC CARE UNIT (Cont.)

2. Report any of the following:
   a. Poor quality tracing on the oscilloscope screen (slanted, bowed, out-of-focus, dim, off-center, partly off-screen) or if there is excessive blanking, interference, or difficulty in identifying ECG complexes
   b. Automatic direct writers that fail to trigger on time or are not self-centering
   c. Rate-meter malfunction (incorrect rate, alarm failure)
   d. Any alarm malfunction
   e. ECG tracings of poor quality

Precautions for Defibrillators

1. Report any of the following:
   a. Bent paddles
   b. Meter that does not operate smoothly (for example, if needle movement is "jerky" or stepwise.)
   c. Circuit breaker that opens or failure of defibrillator to operate even temporarily
   d. Inability to defibrillate or cardiovert even for a brief period
   e. Unusually long charging time

f. Defibrillator which does not hold its set charge.
2. Be sure synchronization is *off* for defibrillation, *on* for cardioversion
3. No one should touch the patient, bed, defibrillator, or its cart during discharge
4. Keep paddles and handles clean, because jelly on the handles provides a conductive pathway at the time of discharge

Precautions for Pacemakers

1. Use only battery-operated pacemakers
2. Keep an accurate log of battery use, including date of manufacture of battery (or at least date of purchase) and hours of use, and whether pacemaker is in "demand" or "continuous" mode of operation.
3. Use a fresh battery every time pacemaker is used, and test the battery before it is installed
4. Keep the terminals of the pacemaker and the tips of the pacing catheter covered with nonconductive material at all times during use
5. Unless easily explained, report immediately any apparent deviation from the expected, for example, inability to pace, unusual changes in apparent threshold, inability to sense R waves, inaccurate rate

(Report of Inter-Society Commission for Heart Disease Resources. Electronic equipment in critical care areas. Part II: The electrical environment. Part III: Selection and maintenance program. Circulation 44:A237–261, 1971. By permission of the American Heart Association, Inc.)

nance schedule and persons or departments responsible. Each hospital must design a schedule that meets the needs of that institution.[6] Safety guidelines for electrical equipment are listed in Table 41-3.

There should be a good working relationship between the CCU nurses and the hospital electrical engineers, each helping to teach the other, and cooperating for the benefit of the patient.

REFERENCES

1. Biomedical Electrical Safety Guidelines. State of Washington Department of Social and Health Services, Health Service Division, March, 1979
2. The Heart and Electrical Hazards. Directions in Cardiovascular Medicine, No. 7. Sommerville, New Jersey, Hoechst Pharmaceuticals, 1973
3. Hochberg HM: Effects of electrical current on heart rhythm. Am J Nurs 71(7):1390–1394,1971
4. Mhyre N: Testing for Hospital Safety in Hospitals, 2nd ed. Seattle, Medical Computer Service Association, 1975
5. Mylrea KC, O'Neal LB: Electricity and electrical safety in the hospital. Nursing 76, 6(1):52–59, 1976
6. Report of Inter-Society Commission for Heart Disease Resources. Electronic equipment in critical care areas. Part II: The electrical environment. Part III: Selection and maintenance program. Circulation 44:A237–261, 1971
7. Sharp L, Rabin B: Nursing in the Coronary Care Unit, pp 168–170. Philadelphia, JB Lippincott, 1970
8. Starmer CF, McIntosh HD, Whalen RE: Electrical hazards and cardiovascular function. N Engl J Med 284(4):181–186, 1971.

ADDITIONAL READING

Aronow S, Bruner JM, Siegal EF et al: Ventricular fibrillation associated with an electrically operated bed. N Engl J Med 281(7):31–32, 1969

Bronzino JD: Technology for Patient Care. St. Louis, C. V. Mosby, 1977

Bruner JM: Hazards of electrical apparatus. Anesthesiology 28(2):396–425, 1967

Burchell HB: Hidden hazards of cardiac pacemakers. Circulation 24:161–163, 1961

Chisholm LA, Telden R, Dolan AM: Proceedings: A patient safety program for small hospitals. Biomed Sci Instrum 10:125–128, 1974

Cromwell L, Weibell FJ, Pfieffer EA et al: Biomedical Instrumentation and Measurement. Inglewood Cliffs NJ, Prentice-Hall, 1973

Dornette WH: Safety standards and the standard of care. J Leg Med: 2(6):49, 1974

Essential Electrical Systems for Hospitals, (NFPA 76A). Boston, National Fire Protection Association, 1973

Feldtman RW, Derrick JR: Hospital electrical safety. Am Fam Physician 13(3):127–137, 1976

Hoenig SA, Scott DH: Medical Instrumentation and Electrical Safety. New York, John Wiley & Sons, 1977

Life Safety Code (NFPA 101). Boston, National Fire Protection Association, 1976

Lubin D: Electrical safety. Hospitals 43:57–60, 1969

Merkel R, Sovie M: Electrocution hazards with transvenous pacemaker electrodes. Am J Nurs 68:2560–2564, 1968

National Electrical Code (NFPA 70). Boston, National Fire Protection Association, 1975

Parker B and Ritterman SA: An inspection procedure for hospital room electrical systems. Med Instrum 9(2):108–111, 1975

Pfeiffer EA: A simulator for teaching electrical safety procedures in the hospital. Med Instrum 9(2): 103–105, 1975

Report on Inter-Society Commission for Heart Disease Resources: Electronic equipment in critical care areas. Part I: Status of devices currently in use. Circulation 43:A–101, 1971

Ross AS: Electrical hazards for cardiac patients. N Engl J Med 281(7):390, 1969

Sovie MD, Fruehan CF: Protecting the patient from electrical hazards. Nurs Clin North Am 7(3):469–480, 1972

Standards for Use of Inhalation Anesthetics (NFPA 56A). Boston, National Fire Protection Association, 1973

Stanley PE: Electrical shock hazards, I and II. Hospitals 45:58–73, 1971

Starmer CF, Whalen RE, McIntosh HD: Hazards of electric shock in cardiology. Am J Cardiol 14:537–546, 1964

Thierer J, Perhus S, McCracken ML et al: Standards for Nursing Care of the Critically Ill. Reston VA, Reston Publishing Co, 1981

von der Mosel HA: Is your CCU electrically safe? Med Surg Rev 6(5):28–32, 1970

Walter CW: Electrical hazards in hospitals. Hosp Pract 5(12):53–56, 1970

Whalen RE, Starmer CF, McIntosh HD: Electrical hazards associated with cardiac pacemaking. Ann NY Acad Sci 111:922–931, 1964

Whalen RE, Starmer CF: Electrical shock hazards in clinical cardiology. Mod Concepts Cardiovas Dis 36(2):7–12, 1967

Winslow EH, Marino LB: Temporary cardiac pacemakers. Am J Nurs 75:586–591, 1975

Using Electrically-Operated Equipment Safely with the Monitored Cardiac Patient. Hewlett-Packard, Medical Electronics Division, 1971

Zalis EG, Conover MH: Electrical hazards of ECG monitoring. Understanding Electrocardiography, pp. 168–180. St Louis, C. V. Mosby, 1972

SECTION G
CARDIAC REHABILITATION

42

Cardiac Rehabilitation: Activity and Exercise Program

ERIKA SEIBERLER SIVARAJAN, R.N., M.A.

Rehabilitation programs for patients recovering from myocardial infarction (MI) vary in intent, scope, type, and delivery. This is due, in part, to an insufficient number of appropriately trained personnel, limited monetary resources, and a lack of research data regarding effectiveness of existing methods and programs. This chapter emphasizes one approach to cardiac rehabilitation. Key concepts, principles, and guidelines are stressed. Specific models of programs serve as examples only.

Rehabilitation programs are usually directed toward the four phases of illness:

Phase I: Cardiac Care Unit (acute illness)

Phase II: Recovery during the remainder of hospitalization

Phase III: Convalescence at home

Phase IV: Long-term conditioning

In instituting specific rehabilitation programs during these four phases, it is necessary to keep the following factors in mind:

1. Assessment of activity and exercise tolerance
2. Reponse to activity and exercise
3. Activity prescription
4. Exercise prescription

In this chapter, general principles of patient assessment used to prescribe activity and exercise, and aspects of assessment pertinent to specific phases of rehabilitation will be discussed.

Activity refers to movements which are accomplished in the course of meeting human physiologic needs, including activities of daily living such as shaving, bathing, dressing, eating, walking, and driving a car.[13] *Exercise* refers to physical exertion such as calisthenics, walking, jogging, swimming at prescribed rates to prevent deconditioning, improve health, correct physical deformity or disability, and provide for cardiovascular conditioning.[13]

ASSESSMENT OF ACTIVITY AND EXERCISE TOLERANCE

A thorough assessment is necessary in order to individualize the activity and exercise prescribed and to start the patient at an appropriate level of activity or exercise. This assessment is essential, at any phase of illness for the individual patient. The first part of the assessment serves as a one time history to be documented in the nurse's notes. The second part of the assessment provides an evaluation before, during, and after each change of activity or exercise level.

Initial activity levels or exercise prescriptions are based on the patient's tolerance as may be predicted from: (1) the patient's history, and (2) the patient's cardiovascular and respiratory response to activity and exercise.

History

Age. Physical fitness declines with age, hence older persons can tolerate less activity.

Sex. There are physiologic differences in the working capacity of men and women. Women generally have more endurance but they are capable of a lesser intensity of workload than men because of a smaller muscle mass in proportion to total body weight.[3]

Weight. Assessment of weight in relation to height is made to establish whether the person has a normal weight or is over-, or underweight. Generally, the intensity and type of exercise prescribed has to be modified for the very obese or the very small patient. Obesity, based on the body-mass index, is defined as at least 20% above ideal weight.[19] Very obese patients may not be able to perform calisthenics or other vigorous exercises, since musculoskeletal injuries may result from the excess weight. Swimming or walking may be the only recommended exercise for these patients.

Physique. Posture, flexibility, equilibrium, and agility should be directly observed, and assessed, since these factors are related to the ease of exercise performance and workload.

Physical Impairments. Patients with problems affecting locomotion, such as hemiplegia, amputations, joint or bone disorders, and other orthopedic or neurologic problems, expend more energy on the same type of activity or exercise than do other patients, because of their mechanical inefficiencies. Most of the usual exercises prescribed for cardiac patients cannot be performed as easily by these patients and the pacing may have to be modified.

Motivation. It is also important to assess the person's attitude toward exercise. Patients who have not exercised in the past and who lack motivation may need special encouragement in order to develop the habit of regular exercises.

Previous Activity Level. The exercise prescription and the response to exercise would be different for a 42-year-old man who was an athlete before the heart attack than for an 84-year-old woman who has been sedentary all her life and needs help with managing her apartment. Assessment of the patient's level of activities before this illness should take into consideration three areas; activities at home, work, and recreation. It is useful to assess the average level of energy expenditure as well as peak energy expenditures. This can be done by asking, "What are some of the most strenuous activities or sports you engage in?" While it is difficult to quantify this type of information, the use of metabolic equivalents (METS) may help.

The concept of METS in assessing activity and exercise is helpful to nurses as well as to patients. One MET is defined as the approximate energy expended per minute while sitting quietly in a chair.[2] Thus, other activities can be quantitated as multiples of this baseline measurement. MET level estimates are available for self-care activities in the hospital, for housework, recreational activities, and a variety of occupational activities. One limitation of METS is that it is an average estimate of energy expended for a given activity, and if that activity is performed at a faster or slower rate, or by a person of less than average skill, then the MET estimate becomes inaccurate. However, the overall concept of quantifying a variety of activities in METS and prescribing activity or exercise according to the patient's current level of function is a useful one.

Cardiovascular History. A detailed knowledge of the duration of cardiovascular impairment in the past is essential.

Specifically, information about previous myocardial infarction, valvular diseases, exercise-induced arrhythmias, or other cardiac problems, should be obtained. Presence of angina or claudication in response to activity or exercise in the past tends to influence the attitude of the patient to the activity and exercise prescribed. Detailed information about the intensity of activity that precipitated the angina, location and radiation of the pain, and measures that eased or relieved the pain are important, since these factors form the basis for comparing the patient's performance of future activity and exercise.

Detailed assessment of the patient as outlined above provides guidelines for an initial activity and exercise prescription appropriate for the patient and the phase of rehabilitation. Continued assessment of the patient's response to the activity or exercise prescribed is not only essential to monitor progress, but to detect any untoward responses that might require modification of the prescription.

The patient's reactions to or acceptance of the prescription should be determined first and the prescription modified to suit the individual's needs and requirements. Circumstances may impose difficulties in complying with the program and these have to be acknowledged when a prescription is made. For example, if regular jogging is difficult in winter, an indoor activity such as stationary bicycling may substitute. Detailed assessment of respiratory and cardiovascular responses to exercise is also essential.

Other Health Problems. Other health problems that would influence, limit, or contraindicate exercise should be assessed in each patient. Patients with chronic renal failure who are on dialysis are usually anemic and may not be able to perform exercises. Tolerance to activity and exercise may also be diminished in patients with chronic respiratory disease due to hypoxia. In a diabetic patient, activity may change the insulin requirements. Patients with severe psychologic disturbances may have difficulty adhering to an exercise program. Such factors must be taken into account when prescribing activity or exercise.

Cardiovascular and Respiratory Responses to Activity and Exercise

Normal cardiorespiratory responses to exercise are described in Chapter 7. Cardiovascular and respiratory responses to activity and exercise in patients after MI will be discussed here, because they pertain to the overall assessment of the patient.

Subjective Responses. Some of the adverse subjective responses either due to limited tolerance or to over exertion include fatigue, shortness of breath, chest pain, dizziness, and palpitations.

All complaints of symptoms by the patient should be assessed carefully. Fatigue, a symptom often reported by patients, is usually overlooked as being too vague. However, fatigue is a reliable symptom that correlates well with objective measurements of the patient's exercise capacity.[4] The location, radiation, intensity, and duration of chest pain, if present, needs to be noted. The circumstances that precipitated the chest pain should be examined so that preventive steps can be taken in the future.

Dizziness is indicative of reduced cerebral perfusion, as a result of a decrease in cardiac output with or without hyperventilation from anxiety. Palpitations may be due either to rapid heart rates or to premature contractions, indicating myocardial irritability. The patient's description of irregularities or changes in pulse should be assessed through such objective measurements as systolic blood pressure (SBP), heart rate (HR), and electrocardiogram (ECG), and a simple test of hyperventilation.

Objective Responses. Skin color, temperature, and perspiration provide information about the relative stress of a given activity. Flushing accompanied by warm sweating means that the effort put forth by the patient is sufficient to increase heat production. The body's compensatory mechanism of vasodilation in the skin in order to dissipate heat is a normal response to exercise. In contrast, pale or cyanotic skin that is cool and clammy indicates that the exercise represents either an excessive strain, resulting in a fall in cardiac output with compensatory vasoconstriction, or patient anxiety, which also results in vasoconstriction to the skin.

Respiratory rate is noted and recorded. Any shortness of breath which does not subside with cessation of exercise should be further evaluated to determine presence of heart failure.

HR should be measured in the following manner: (1) at rest; (2) in response to activity and exercise; (3) during the recovery period after activity or exercise. Since increases in HR increase myocardial oxygen requirements, a resting tachycardia (more than 100 beats/minute) indicates that exercise should be postponed. The common reasons for resting tachycardia in patients with acute myocardial infarction are anxiety, fever produced by myocardial injury, and heart failure. HR increases during activity and exercise in direct proportion to the workload until it reaches a peak that coincides with exercise capacity. Maximal attainable HR decreases with age, just as exercise capacity declines with age. The increase in HR tolerated by a patient depends on the phase of rehabilitation as well as on the patient's condition.

SBP rises with an increase in activity level. An SBP that fails to rise, or falls below the usual resting levels, should be cause for concern, since it implies that the left ventricle is not capable of generating enough force to increase or maintain stroke volume during exercise. The activity or exercise should then be stopped and the level of effort be reduced at future exercise sessions.

Pressure-rate product is an indirect indication of myocardial oxygen consumption and is easily calculated by multiplying SBP and HR.[11] Pressure-rate product increases with exercise, indicating increasing myocardial oxygen consumption. In patients with coronary artery disease (CAD), when the increased myocardial oxygen demand cannot be met, the signs of ischemia, such as angina and electrocardiographic changes, will appear. If the pressure-rate product at which ischemic signs occur is known, measures can be taken to reduce either HR or SBP by modifying the activity and exercise intensity, or by using drugs such as propranolol.

Biofeedback techniques and relaxation exercises can also be taught to the patient to help keep the pressure-rate product below the critical level.

Electrocardiographic (ECG) Responses. Both heart rhythm and changes in the ST segment should be assessed. When arrhythmias are present, the time of their occurrence and whether they increase or decrease in response to activity should be recorded.

A rehabilitation program should have preestablished criteria in regard to activity and exercise to be prescribed in the presence of arrhythmias. Indications for stopping or postponing exercises until further therapy is initiated or until the arrhythmia spontaneously subsides are:

1. An increase in frequency and severity of premature contractions.
2. Any tachyarrhythmia which results in a HR greater than an upper limit of HR set for that patient, for example, paroxysmal tachycardia, atrial fibrillation with ventricular response greater than the patient's upper limit.
3. Arrhythmias that are a new manifestation or those that are preexisting and increase in severity with exercise are reason to postpone exercise until further assessments are made. If the patient is started on medication, its efficacy should be evaluated before exercise is resumed.
4. Serious arrhythmias such as ventricular tachycardia, defined as three or more consecutive ventricular premature beats, demand immediate cessation of activity or exercise. However, activity may be continued in the presence of known preexisting arrhythmias such as premature contractions which do not produce any hemodynamic changes.

PHASES OF REHABILITATION

Phase I—Cardiac Care Unit (Acute Illness)

Objectives. The purpose of instituting rehabilitation efforts during the patient's stay in the cardiac care unit (CCU) is to prevent anxiety, depression, and deconditioning due to prolonged bedrest and inactivity.

Bedrest has always been regarded as an essential aspect of the treatment of MI. The objective of this form of therapy is to reduce myocardial oxygen requirements and permit the damaged myocardium to heal. The criteria for determining the duration of bedrest and the initiation of ambulation have been based on subjective impressions rather than on objective evidence.

The reason given by those advocating prolonged bedrest is that in the acute stage of tissue damage, exercise may increase the risks of arrhythmia, reinfarction, ventricular rupture, and ventricular aneurysm. The tradition of prolonged bedrest and restricted activity during convalescence was based on inferences about possible adverse effects of even mild activity on myocardial healing.[12] In view of the deleterious effects of prolonged bedrest, this practice is being increasingly questioned. The potentially harmful effects of bedrest for patients with uncomplicated myocardial infarction have been amply documented.[1,20]

Evidence of deconditioning can be found as early as the second or third day of bedrest.[21] There is a decrease in physical work capacity, an increase in HR response to effort, a decreased adaptability to change posture, resulting in orthostatic hypotension, and a tendency to thrombus formation in the veins (Chap. 30).[15] These changes are especially critical in the cardiac patient who has compromised cardiovascular function due to recent MI with venous stasis or congestive heart failure and possible hypotension. Prolonged bedrest may also evoke feelings of helplessness and dependency and may contribute to a loss of confidence and the promotion of invalidism. Those arguing for a more "liberal regime" of earlier ambulation indicate that there is a reduced risk of the aforementioned side-effects of bedrest as well as a lesser likelihood of cardiac failure due to reduced pulmonary congestion during ambulation.

Early ambulation has few complications as shown by Abraham and co-workers.[1] It should be emphasized that there is no scientific evidence to date that early ambulation of MI patients has definite physiologic benefits. Until such evidence is forthcoming, early ambulation can be justified only on the theoretic grounds of preventing the known complications of prolonged bedrest.

There is wide variation in the opinions of practicing physicians as to the duration of bedrest, but there has been a trend toward earlier mobilization and discharge of patients after MI.[1,6,20] Whether patients run a high or low risk of subsequent complications can be identified early in their hospitalization.[14,18] It has been recommended that patients who are free of complications (representing up to 40% of some groups) can be mobilized quickly.[18] Thus, in-hospital efforts to support the patients without complications in the physical and psychologic rehabilitation should begin relatively early, given assurance that the process of infarction is completed and that there is no continuing evidence of ischemia, heart failure, or electrical instability.[22]

There still remain, however, over 50% of the patients who have transient complications during the initial phase of hospitalization and who progress much more slowly through their convalescence. While patients in this group may benefit greatly from earlier rehabilitation, they are often excluded from such programs. Appropriate guidelines are necessary to ensure that the infarction process is complete and that subsequent cardiovascular stability has been established before patients with transient complications can be safely entered into programs of early low-level graded exercise. Rehabilitation in patients with complications is important and should be approached cautiously.

Activities and Exercises. While patients are still on bedrest they can be given a MET chart (Table 42-1) outlining activities in the sequence in which they may be resumed. The chart helps them to understand the need for reducing energy expenditure immediately after a heart attack and resuming activities gradually.

Patients with no complications after their infarction and those who have become free from transient complications after myocardial infarction and who have no evidence of shock, failure, intractable angina, or uncontrolled arrhyth-

mias, and are free of resting tachycardia for at least 24 hours after MI, can be started on self-care activities and in passive and active dynamic exercises in the CCU.[22]

During the acute phase of illness, energy expenditure should be limited to 1.5–2.0 METS, which permits the patient to feed himself, wash his hands and face, shave, and use a bedside commode with assistance. Passive and active exercises include flexion and extension of arms and legs as well as planned changes in posture, such as sitting upright on the edge of the bed, legs dangling unsupported for short periods of time. In addition to self-care activities and exercises, many programs also attempt to meet psychologic needs by providing educational opportunities, such as reading or watching television. Now that duration of stay in the CCU tends to be shorter, there is less of a need for an organized recreational program. An example of a program recommended by the American Heart Association is available in booklet form. A condensed version is found in the textbook *The Heart*[22] and is outlined in Table 42-2. These activities should be carried out under direct supervision of an experienced CCU nurse or physical therapist along with continuous ECG monitoring and, more importantly, with frequent measurement of SBP and HR and evaluation of symptoms and signs.

Indications that there is an inappropriate increase in exertion during the acute CCU phase are:

1. Unexpected fatigue, weakness or dyspnea
2. Development of or increase in angina pectoris
3. The occurrence of important disturbances in rhythm or conduction
4. Increase in ischemic changes seen in electrocardiogram, such as a greater than 1-mm ST segment depression, or a greater than 1-mm ST segment elevation during the activity or exercise
5. Increase in HR by more than 20 beats over the resting rate or a HR exceeding 110 beats/minute.
6. Fall in SBP of 20 mm Hg below the usual resting level, or a failure of SBP to increase over the resting level

The occurrence of any of these signs is an indication that additional rest should be instituted and the activity or exercise plan reevaluated and revised. Many cardiac centers have developed guidelines and programs that offer the patient gradually progressive physical activity under careful supervision. Information and education provided to patients and families will offer reassurance and reduce the anxiety commonly encountered during the first few days of hospitalization, when enforced bedrest and restricted physical activity evoke feelings of helplessness and vulnerability.

Phase II—Recovery During the Remainder of Hospitalization

Along with the trend toward early ambulation, there is also a trend toward early discharge from the hospital after an acute MI. The average day of discharge in hospitals in the Seattle area is day 10 after MI, ranging from four to more than twenty days. Since the duration of hospitalization has been considerably shortened, there is less time available to prepare the patient for self-care activities at home. Hence, the rehabilitation program for the remainder of hospitali-

TABLE 42-1   ENERGY COST (IN METS) OF ACTIVITY AND EXERCISE

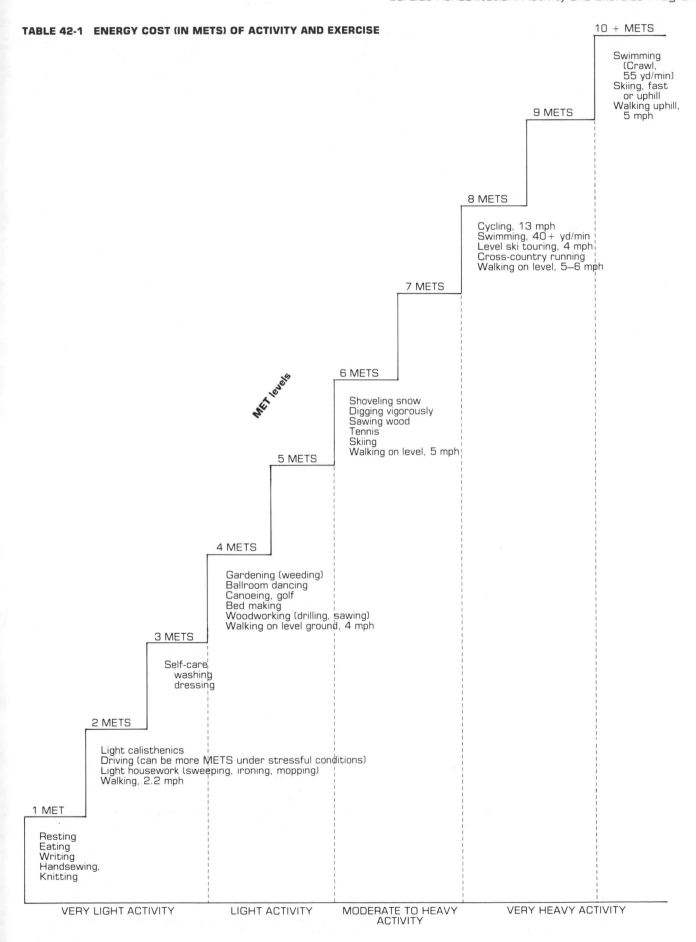

10 + METS

Swimming
(Crawl,
55 yd/min)
Skiing, fast
or uphill
Walking uphill,
5 mph

9 METS

8 METS

Cycling, 13 mph
Swimming, 40 + yd/min
Level ski touring, 4 mph
Cross-country running
Walking on level, 5–6 mph

7 METS

6 METS

Shoveling snow
Digging vigorously
Sawing wood
Tennis
Skiing
Walking on level, 5 mph

MET levels

5 METS

4 METS

Gardening (weeding)
Ballroom dancing
Canoeing, golf
Bed making
Woodworking (drilling, sawing)
Walking on level ground, 4 mph

3 METS

Self-care
washing
dressing

2 METS

Light calisthenics
Driving (can be more METS under stressful conditions)
Light housework (sweeping, ironing, mopping)
Walking, 2.2 mph

1 MET

Resting
Eating
Writing
Handsewing,
Knitting

VERY LIGHT ACTIVITY   LIGHT ACTIVITY   MODERATE TO HEAVY
ACTIVITY   VERY HEAVY ACTIVITY

TABLE 42-2   FOURTEEN-STEP MYOCARDIAL INFARCTION REHABILITATION PROGRAM

Step	Exercise	Ward activity	Educational and craft activity
1	Passive ROM to all extremites (5 times ea); patient to do *active* plantar and dorsiflexion of ankles several times/day	Feeding self, sitting with bed rolled up to 45°, trunk and arms supported by over-bed table	Initial interview and brief orientation to program
2	Repeat exercises of Step 1	1. Feed self 2. Partial a.m. care (wash hands, face, brush teeth) in bed 3. Dangle legs on side of bed (1 time)	Light recreational activity, such as reading
3	Active assistive exercise in shoulder flexion; elbow flexion and extension; hip flexion, extension, and rotation; knee flexion and extension; rotation of feet (4 times ea)	1. Begin sitting in chair for short periods as tolerated, 2 times a day 2. Bathing whole body 3. Use of bedside commode	More detailed explanation of program. Continue light recreation
4	Minimal resistance, lying in bed in above ROM, 5 times ea. Stiffen all muscles to the count of 2 (3 times)	1. Increase sitting 3 times a day 2. Change gown	Begin explanation of what is an MI. Give patient pamphlets to read. Begin craft activity: 1. Leather lacing 2. Link belt 3. Hand sewing, embroidery 4. Copper tooling
5	Moderate resistance in bed at 45° above ROM exercises; hands on shoulder, elbow circling (5 times ea. arm)	1. Sitting ad lib 2. Sitting in chair at bedside for meals 3. Dressing, shaving, combing hair—*sitting down* 4. Walking in room, 2 times a day	Continue education about healing of heart, reasons for early restrictions in activity
6	1. Further resistive exercises sitting on side of bed, manual resistance of knee extension and flexion (7 times ea). 2. Walk to bathroom and back (note if patient needs help)	1. Walk to bathroom, ad lib if patient can tolerate 2. Stand at sink to shave	Continue craft activity or supply patient with another one. Patient may attend group meetings in a wheelchair for no more than 1 hr
7	1. Standing warm-up exercises: a. Arms in extension and shoulder abduction, rotate arms together in circles (circumduction), 5 times ea arm. b. Stand on toes, 10 times. c. May substitute abduction, 5 times ea leg. 2. Walk length of hall (50 ft) and back at average pace	1. Bathe in tub 2. Walk to telephone or sit in waiting room (1 time day)	May walk to group meetings on the same floor
8	1. Warm-up exercises: a. Lateral side bending 5 times ea side. b. Trunk twisting, 5 times ea side. 2. Walk 1½ lengths of hall, down 1 fl stairs, elevator up	1. Walk to waiting room, 2 times a day 2. Stay sitting up most of the day	Continue all previous craft and educational activities
9	1. Warm-up exercises: a. Lateral side bending, 10 times ea side. b. slight knee bends, 10 times with hands on hips. 2. Increase walking distance, walk down one flight of stairs	Continue above activities	Discussion of work simplification techniques and pacing of activities
10	1. Warm-up exercises: a. Lateral side bending with 1-lb weight (10 times) b. Standing—leg raising leaning against wall, 5 times ea 2. Walk two lengths of hall and downstairs, take elevator up	Continue all previous ward activities	1. Patient may walk to OT clinic and work on craft proj. for ½ h. a. Copper tooling; b. woodworking; c. ceramics; s. small weaving project; e. metal hammering; f. mosaic tile 2. Discussion of patient's home exercises
11	1. Warm-up exercises: a. Lateral side bending with 1-lb weight, leaning against wall, 10 times ea side. b. Standing, leg raising, 5 times ea. c. Trunk twisting with 1-lb weight, 5 times ea. side. 2. Repeat part 2 of Step 10	Continue all previous ward activities	Increase time in OT clinic to 1 hr.
12	1. Warm-up exercises: a. Lateral side bending with 2-lb weight, 10 times b. Standing—leg raising, leaning against wall, 10 times ea. c. Trunk twisting with 2-lb weight, 10 times 2. Walk down two flights of stairs	Continue all previous ward activities	Continue craft activity with increased resistance
13	Repeat all exercises of Step 12	Continue all previous ward activities	Complete all projects
14	1. Warm-up exercises: a. Lateral side bending with 2-lb weight, 10 times ea. side. b. Trunk twisting with 2-lb weight, 10 times ea. side. c. Touch toes from sitting position, 10 times 2. Walk up flight of 10 stairs and down	Continue all previous ward activities	Final instructions about home procedures and activities

ROM = range of motion
OT = occupational therapy
Source: Wenger, NK, Gilbert, CA: Rehabilitation of the myocardial infarction patient. In Hurst WJ, Logue RB, Schlant RC, Wenger NK (eds): The Heart, Arteries and Veins, 4th ed., pp 1303–1311. New York, McGraw Hill, 1978

zation should be progressive, yet cautious. Both the physical status and the expected activity level after discharge differ widely; thus, objectives should be clearly defined and individualized for each patient.

Objectives. Rehabilitation during the remainder of hospitalization is aimed at helping patients to reach the activity level required for self-care by the time they are ready to return home. To accomplish this, the aims are to:

1. Demonstrate to patients their physical capabilities in a safe, controlled setting with close monitoring of the ECG and SBP
2. Enable patients to recognize their symptoms in response to activity, and to use these symptoms and signs to guide their activity
3. Reduce the duration of the patient's hospitalization
4. Increase the patient's cardiovascular functional capacity
5. Increase the patient's confidence, reduce anxiety and depression, and improve psychologic state through an improved self-image.

It is believed that depression is the most formidable problem in cardiac convalescence and rehabilitation. The "homecoming depression," very common in infarction patients, is often the result of a feeling of weakness and fatigue upon return home. This weakness, interpreted by the patient as a loss of capacity, may initiate depression or further compound an already existing state of depression.[7] Hackett suggests that physical conditioning is the most important means of preventing or reducing depression, by raising the patient's self esteem and feeling of independence.[8] The physical activity program has the advantage of focusing on what the patient can do in the midst of all the "don'ts", and it stands out as "affirmation of life." There are no adverse clinical effects from early mobilization after MI; indeed, there are benefits from this approach.[1]

Activities and Exercises. During this phase of recovery, patients are encouraged to sit up in a chair for gradually increasing periods of time. All self-care activities such as walking to the bathroom, showering, and bathing are gradually resumed with the help of MET tables to guide patients in their progress.

Calisthenic exercises for the upper extremities and trunk may be started together with a gradually progressive walking program (Tables 42-3 and 42-4). Patients progress from walking in the room to walking in the hospital corridor, and then to climbing the stairs. At this time physical activities are interspersed with rest periods. Physical activity is avoided for 1 hour after meals when the patient is not in a basal state. Isometric exercises are also avoided because of the excessive pressure workload which they impose on the heart.

Criteria similar to those specified for Phase I are used to identify an excessive, disproportionate, or adverse response to a particular level of activity and to indicate a need to decrease or stop the exercises. Using predetermined guidelines to evaluate responses, exercise under supervised conditions has been safe this early after MI.[21]

An important aspect of rehabilitation during this phase is to teach the patient to recognize the onset of adverse symptoms such as shortness of breath, chest pain, palpita-

TABLE 42-3 CALISTHENICS

University of Washington Cardiac Rehabilitation Study Calisthenics	Repetitions/ 30 sec.	Metronome beats/min.
1	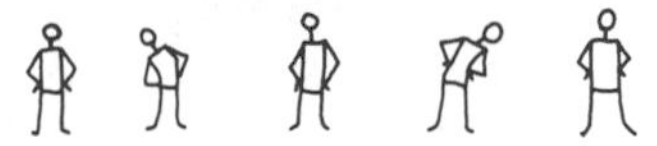 X8	(66)
2	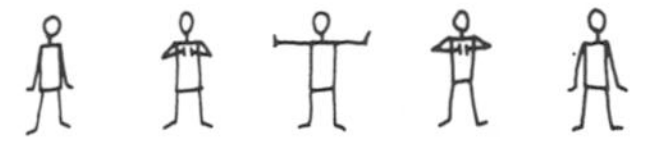 X14	(112)
3	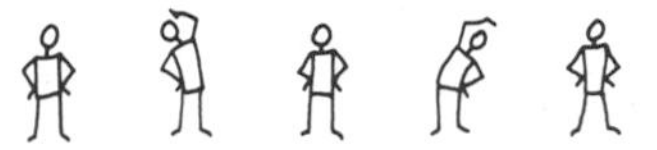 X8	(66)
4	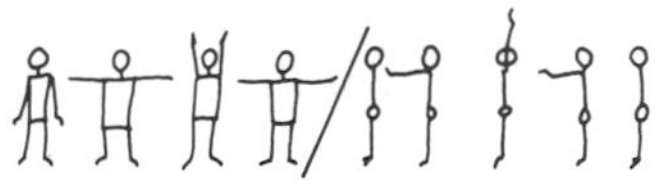 X7/7	(112)
5	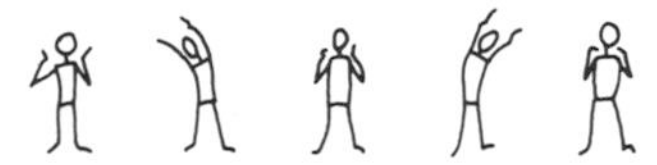 X8	(66)
6	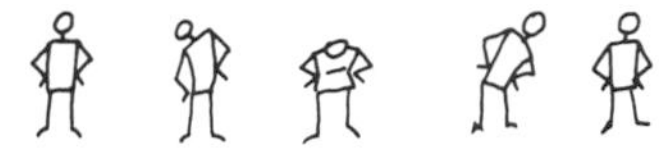 X7	(80)
7	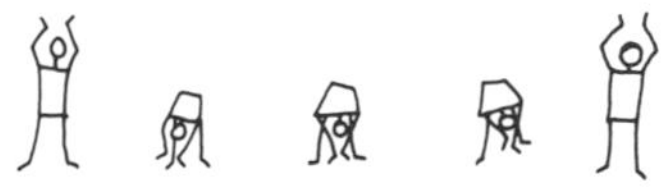 X8	(66)
8	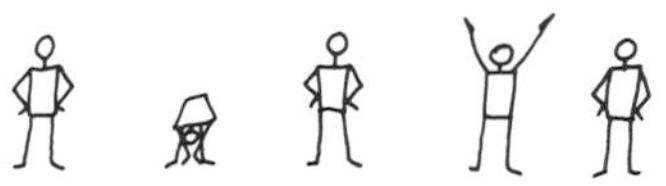 X8	(66)

Adapted from St. Mary's Hospital Cardiac Rehabilitation Center, Minnesota

TABLE 42-4 HOME WALKING PROGRAM

Rate (mph)	Distance	Time Range (min.)	Approximate METS
	440 ft.	5.0	1.5
	660 ft.	7.5	
	880 ft.	10.0	
	1100 ft.	12.5	
	1320 ft.	15.0	
	1320 ft. (¼ mile)	10–15	
1½	¼ mile	5–10	1.8
1½	½ mile	15–20	
2	½ mile	10–14	2.2
2+	¾ mile	20–25	
2¼	¾ mile	14–20	2.8
2	1 mile	25–30	
2½	1 mile	20–25	3.0
3	1 mile	15–20	3.1
2½	1½ miles	30–35	
3	1½ miles	25–30	
2½	2 miles	40–45	
3	2 miles	35–40	
3½	2 miles	30–35	3.6
3¼	2½ miles	40–45	
3¾	2½ miles	35–40	
3+	3 miles	50–55	
3½	3 miles	45–50	
4	3 miles	40–45	4.0
4½	3 miles	40	4.8

Instructions to Patients: Aim at walking the distance prescribed within the range of minutes for that step. If you have any difficulty with the distance or time, return to a previous step. If you experience discomfort, follow the guidelines for "Slow Down Precautions," and "Contact Your Physician Precautions," pp. 20–42.

tions, and dizziness. These symptoms and excessive increase in HR serve as warning signals of undue cardiovascular exertion. Patients should be taught to take their own pulse in the hospital under the nurse's supervision. Repeated practice will help build confidence in patients. Using their own pulse as an indicator of undue exertion, they can perform and monitor activities of daily living and exercise. This will help patients keep their activities or exercises to a level that does not induce adverse symptoms or signs. The relatives and friends of the patient should be included in this teaching and must be made aware of the activities and exercises prescribed for the patient. This may help avoid tension and discord between the patient and family members who are well-meaning but often overprotective.

Assessment of Responses to Activity and Exercise. At the time of discharge home, most patients should be able to perform activities at peak levels of about 3.5–4.0 METS for short duration, which corresponds to many common activities at home (Table 42-5). The actual level of activity at which a patient can perform may be assessed by a low-level treadmill test, which requires an energy expenditure of about 3.5 METS for completion. In many centers, low-level treadmill testing or some form of submaximal exercise testing is done the day before discharge from the hospital.[13,17] (Some physicians prefer to do this test on the first or second office visit after discharge from the hospital.) The purpose of such testing is to establish the level of walking that a patient can tolerate without adverse effects. One such testing protocol is described in Chapter 18, page 252. The test is 12 minutes in duration, starting at a very slow speed of 1.2 mph at 0% incline.[16,17] For some patients this is a symptom-limited test. The patient is stopped at the onset of any adverse responses or complaint of fatigue. The highest HR achieved by the patient without onset of adverse symptoms is noted. The patient is advised not to exceed this HR during activities at home.

Phase III—Convalescence at Home

This phase begins at the time of the patient's discharge home and extends to return to work or prior level of involvement. Although most hospitals provide adequate activity, exercise, and teaching opportunities during hospitalization for MI patients, conditioning and maintenance programs are not available at every facility. In many instances, these programs are postponed for three or four months after MI. During the transition period from discharge home to enrollment in a conditioning program, patients are often left to fend for themselves, with very little assistance other than infrequent visits to their physicians. Clearly, the nurse can play an important role in filling this gap in professional guidance during these crucial months.

Objectives. The objectives during this phase of rehabilitation are:

1. To increase activities and exercises to a level required for return to work or previous activities
2. To provide psychologic support to patients and their families during the recovery process

Patients are usually concerned with their physical abilities in relation to job and leisure activities, including sexual

TABLE 42-5 MET LEVEL FOR RECREATIONAL, SELF-CARE, HOME MAINTENANCE, AND OCCUPATIONAL ACTIVITIES

MET Level	Recreational, Self-Care, Home Maintenance	Occupational
1.5 or less	Watching TV Painting Sewing Conversation	
1.8– 2.2	Walking 1.2 mph Driving Playing the piano Self-care activities Playing cards	typing desk work operating electrical office machinery
2–3	Walking 2 mph Level cycling 5 mph Golf with power cart	manual typing light janitorial shoesmith, tailor, locksmith auto, radio, TV repair bartending hand dusting, dusting floor, vacuum cleaning scrubbing floors
3–4	Walking 3 mph Cycling 6 mph Golf, pulling bag cart Gardening[3] (raking, hoeing, weeding) Pushing power mower[2]	cleaning windows making beds machine assembly trailer-truck in traffic
4–5	Walking 3.5 mph Cycling 8 mph Swimming 20 yards/ min. Light carpentry Golf, carrying clubs Table tennis	painting, paperhanging, masonry light carpentry carrying (carpets, food, bags) washing floors[5] stripping beds[3]
5–6	Walking 4 mph Cycling 10 mph Stream fishing Digging garden Ice or roller skating 9 mph	stair climbing, slowly walking fast (4 mph) scrubbing[3]
6–7	Walking 5 mph Cycling 11 mph Ski touring 2½ mph Downhill skiing Splitting wood Singles tennis Snow shoveling Folk and square dancing Mowing lawn with push mower	shoveling 10/min, of 10 pounds digging ditches
7–8	Jogging 5 mph Cycling 12 mph Vigorous downhill skiing	pushing wheelbarrow[5] carrying heavy load >80 pounds planing wood[3]
8–9	Running 5½ mph Cycling 13 mph Ski touring 4 mph Squash and handball	shoveling 10/min. of 14 pounds
>9 METS		shoveling 10/min. of 16 pounds

activity. (Sexual counseling is discussed in Chapter 46.) They need specific information about how to perform activities safely and which activities to avoid, or postpone until later. The exercise prescription needs to be concise, precise, and individualized to each patient's functional capacity, personal preferences, interests, and needs. The rationale for this prescription must be well understood by the patient in order to assure adherence to the plan and to strengthen motivation. Recommendations about exercise should be made with the same care and precision that is used for other therapies such as drugs. As Haskell points out, "an overdose of exercise can produce new clinical manifestations of coronary artery disease, including cardiac arrest and sudden death, while inappropriate restrictions can result in cardiovascular deconditioning, psychologic trauma and economic disability."[9]

Activities and Exercises. Most light housework and hobbies can be resumed at this time. Patients can perform activities of daily living requiring 3–4 METs of energy expenditure if they were able to finish the low-level treadmill test without adverse symptoms. Activities requiring prolonged, vigorous effort of arms and shoulders, such as scrubbing floors, wringing clothes, making beds, and carrying such heavy objects as a suitcase should be postponed. This type of activity involves isometric muscle contractions and creates a disproportionate workload on the heart in relation to total energy expended.[10]

Patients are very apprehensive about the safety of resuming activities that were part of their lifestyle before their illness. The more common questions that patients have are about visiting with friends and relatives, driving, going to the movies, gardening, and doing other chores around the house. Resumption of activities is of particular importance to patients because boredom quickly sets in, especially during the recuperation period prior to return to work. These specific anxieties and questions need to be talked out with a health professional. Useful approaches in helping patients evaluate the components of a given task are these:

1. Description of activity: The degree of effort, the rate of work, and the emotional component involved in performing the activity, all need to be ascertained
2. Type of muscle: Does the activity require isometric or isotonic muscle contractions, or both? Which are the muscle groups used predominantly?
3. Duration: Is the activity continuous or can it be interrupted with rest periods?
4. Frequency: How many times each day a task may be done.
5. Environmental conditions: The temperature, humidity, wind-chill factor, and altitude need to be ascertained.
6. Terrain: Is the activity to be performed in water, on land, on level surface, or on hilly terrain?

By analyzing the components of a task as outlined above, the nurse, therapist, and patient can better understand the appropriate energy expenditure required to perform the task. Patients can then be advised on a more individual basis. Patients who tolerate the activities well, without undue fatigue or symptoms, can progress to an exercise program. An appropriate unsupervised exercise would be a prescribed walking program which gradually increases the intensity and duration of exercise from week to week. The information in Table 42-4 is useful in prescribing a walking program. The walk should be of a specified speed and distance and should be repeated 2–3 times a day until the patient returns to work. Initially, patients are asked to increase the distance rather than the speed, in order to build up endurance. When the patient returns to work the duration of exercise should be lengthened. Keep in mind that it is easier to maintain the exercise program if the frequency is reduced to once a day and a minimum of three times a week.

These walking programs build up strength and endurance in the lower extremity muscles. Pre-exercise warm-ups and calisthenics for conditioning upper extremity and trunk muscles, which were taught during the hospital phase (Phase I and II) of recovery, are continued and gradually increased in number (Table 42-3). New calisthenics of higher MET levels are gradually added to the program.

The decision to return to work depends on many factors: the severity of the infarction; the presence of any residual complications; the rate of progress in the rehabilitation program; the functional level of activity; the strenuousness of the job to be returned to; the financial needs; and family support and obligations. The decision should be a mutual one between the patient and family, the employer, and rehabilitation team.

Assessment of Responses to Activity and Exercise. Assessment of response to activity and exercise increasingly becomes the responsibility of the patient. The patient is taught to monitor his pulse and is advised not to exceed the upper limit of a designated HR during the walking program for the first few weeks after discharge. Other responses, such as presence of premature contractions, are explained to the patient and he is taught to monitor their frequency as well as their relationship to exercise. Any symptoms, for example, shortness of breath, can be taken as symptoms of overexertion. If angina occurs, the patient is asked to grade it on a numerical scale from zero to ten. The patient is asked specifically: "If zero is no discomfort, and ten is the worst discomfort you have ever experienced, what number would you give the discomfort you now feel?" Recording this number helps to determine if angina is increasing, remaining stable, or decreasing. For patients who complain of symptoms such as dizziness, fainting, or palpitation, or who report frequent "skipped beats" while taking their pulse, ambulatory ECG monitoring may provide information about the cause of such symptoms.

Patients are also taught to recognize the symptoms and signs of overexertion so that they may reduce the speed at which the activity or exercise is performed. The list of symptoms for which "slow-down precautions" need to be initiated may include:

1. Elevated HR persisting for 10 minutes after exercise
2. Extreme shortness of breath lasting more than 10 minutes after exercise.
3. Prolonged fatigue lasting 24 hours or more
4. Side-stitch, a sharp stabbing pain in the upper abdomen, under the ribs, when exercising
5. Pain in joints, shins, heels, and calf muscles
6. Flare-up of arthritic conditions
7. Insomnia that was not present prior to exercise program
8. Nausea or vomiting after exercise

A list of "contact your physician precautions" before continuing exercise may include:

1. Abnormal heart action, such as irregular pulse, palpitations, sudden very slow pulse, or a sudden burst of rapid pulse
2. New or prolonged pain, pressure, or discomfort in chest, arms, or throat
3. Dizziness, lightheadedness, cold sweat, fainting

Phase IV—Long-term Conditioning or Maintenance Program

Depending on the specific program of rehabilitation that the patient has been advised to participate in, and also depending on available community resources, this phase of rehabilitation may be accomplished by the continuation of an ongoing program or the beginning of a more formal group rehabilitation program.

Objectives. The goals of phase IV of rehabilitation are:
1. To retain a physical working capacity commensurate with the occupational needs and leisure time interests of the patient.
2. To obtain and maintain optimal cardiovascular functional capacity.

The specific aim is to increase aerobic capacity and aid in conditioning, thereby restoring optimal health, and preventing or slowing progression of the underlying disease process. The benefits of such a program are a functional bradycardia with concomitant increase in stroke volume. The increase in aerobic capacity is primarily due to improved peripheral oxygen extraction. Beneficial side-effects often emphasized are less fatigue and improved sleeping patterns.

Assessment of Responses to Exercise

The important consideration in recommending a maintenance program is whether the patient can exercise on his own or whether the exercise should be performed only in a group program under medical supervision. Exercise testing is used to determine exercise capacity prior to beginning an exercise program and also to identify high-risk individuals. Since some patients with CAD are more susceptible to sudden cardiac death or reinfarction, it is reasonable to subject patients to exercise testing in order to identify those who exhibit life-threatening exertional arrhythmias, or exertional hypotension. There is controversy about prescribing an exercise program for these individuals. Even those who do advocate exercise for these high-risk individuals agree that they should exercise only in a group program under medical supervision if they wish to exercise at high intensity, for example, to jog. The starting exercise prescription can be based on the results of this exercise test. (See Chap. 18 for exercise testing protocols.) Exercise testing can also be used to monitor progress.

In prescribing exercises, the following general principles must be kept in mind:
1. The exercises should involve major muscle groups to provide cardiovascular conditioning.
2. The exercises selected should preferably be dynamic (isotonic) rather than isometric. Dynamic exercises provide cardiovascular conditioning, whereas isometric exercises can be more stressful, without producing a cardiovascular conditioning effect. However, if a patient's job requires isometric effort, isometric exercises may be phased in gradually.
3. The exercise should start at a low level and progress gradually to the desired intensity. To derive cardiovascular benefit, exercises should be performed 3–5 times a week for about 30 minutes each time. The intensity of exercise is individually determined from the patient's performance on the exercise test. If the patient exercises without supervision, he is advised to exercise at an

TABLE 42-6 REHABILITATION EXERCISE LEVELS IN PHASE IV

LEVELS	1	2	3	4	5	6	7	8	9	10
WARM-UP	WALK 3	WALK 3	WALK 3	WALK 3	WALK 3	WALK 3	WALK 3	WALK 3	WALK 3	WALK 3
WALK & JOG	Walk fast 1	Jog ¼	Jog ½	Jog 1	Jog 1¼	Jog 2	Jog 3	Jog 4	Jog 8	
	Walk slow 1	Walk 1	Walk 2	Walk 2	Walk 2	Walk 1½	Walk 1	Walk 1	Walk 1	
	Walk fast 1	Jog ¼	Jog ½	Jog 1	Jog 2	Jog 2	Jog 3	Jog 4	Jog 8	Jog 20
	Walk slow 1	Walk 2	Walk 2	Walk 2	Walk 2	Walk 2	Walk 2	Walk 1	Walk 1	
	Walk Fast 1	Jog ¼	Jog ½	Jog 1	Jog 2	Jog 3	Jog 4	Jog 4		
	Walk slow 1	Walk 2	Walk 2	Walk 2	Walk 2	Walk 2	Walk 2	Walk 1½		
CALISTHENICS	6	8	10	12	15	15	15	15	15	15
WALK & JOG	Walk slow 1	Walk 1	Walk 2	Walk 2	Walk 2	Walk 2	Walk 1	Walk 1	Walk 1	
	Walk fast 1	Jog ¼	Jog ½	Jog 1	Jog 1	Jog 2	Jog 3	Jog 4	Jog 8	Jog 20
	Walk slow 1	Walk 2	Walk 2	Walk 2	Walk 2	Walk 2	Walk 2	Walk 1	Walk 1	
	Walk fast 1	Jog ¼	Jog ½	Jog 1½	Jog 2	Jog 3	Jog 3	Jog 4½	Jog 8	
	Walk slow 1	Walk 2	Walk 2	Walk 2½	Walk 2½	Walk 2	Walk 2	Walk 2		
	Walk fast 1	Jog ¼	Jog 1	Jog 1	Jog 2	Jug 3	Jog 4	Jog 5		
COOL-DOWN	2	2	2	2	2	2	2	2	2	2
TOTAL LAPS WALKED	17	15	17	17½	17½	16½	15	12½	9	5
TOTAL LAPS JOGGED	—	1½	3½	6½	10¼	15	20	25½	32	40
TOTAL DISTANCE (MILES)	1.00	1.00	1.25	1.50	1.75	2.00	2.25	2.50	2.75	3.00

16.6 Walk Laps = 1 Mile (1.6 km)
14.5 Jog Laps
Source: CAPRI (Cardiopulmonary Research Institute, 914 E. Jefferson, Seattle, WA 98122)

intensity sufficient to raise HR to 60% but not to exceed 80% of the maximal HR achieved during exercise testing.[9] Patients in supervised programs may perform exercises at higher intensities corresponding to 70%–85% of maximal HR. This range of HR is called the training range. Alternatively, some programs prescribe exercises using age-predicted HR ranges from tables. The exercise intensity induced by this method is based on average numbers and is not based on the person's observed maximal capacity. The limitation of using this approach has to be recognized.

4. Each exercise session should be preceded by stretching and warm-up exercises. This avoids sudden cardiovascular exertion and also helps prevent muscle injury. Exercises should be followed by a gradual cool-down.

Group programs may be preferable to individual exercise because they provide camaraderie and structure and may improve adherence to long-term habit of exercise. Many community group exercise programs are available. An example of a gradually progressing exercise program incorporating the above principles is shown in Table 42-6.

Physical rehabilitation programs do not change the nature of CAD but may enhance compensatory adaptation to the disease process and minimize or delay further disability.[5] Furthermore, they improve cardiovascular fitness and help the patients achieve an improved level of function. Most patients report that they feel better, have greater stamina and improved confidence, and feel an enhancement in quality of life. A positive attitude that develops in patients helps greatly in returning them to productive life and in generating a sense of usefulness. Such individual responses make it more than worthwhile to pursue rehabilitation efforts that at best can have the added benefits of reducing mortality and morbidity from the epidemic of coronary artery disease.

REFERENCES

1. Abraham AS, Sever Y, Weinstein M et al: Value of early ambulation in patients with and without complications after acute myocardial infarction. N Engl J Med 292:719–722, 1975
2. Acker J: Early ambulation of post-myocardial infarction patients. A. Early activity after myocardial infarction. In Naughton JP, Hellerstein HK (eds): Exercise Testing and Exercise Training in Coronary Artery Disease, pp. 311–314. New York, Academic Press, 1973
3. Åstrand PO, Rodahl K: Textbook of Work Physiology, 2nd ed. New York, McGraw-Hill, 1977
4. Borg G: Perceived exertion as an indicator of somatic stress. Scand J Rehabil Med 2–3:92–98, 1970
5. Bruce RA: The benefits of physical training for patients with coronary heart disease. In Ingelfinger FG, Ebert RV, Finland M, et al (eds): Controversy in Internal Medicine. Philadelphia, WB Saunders, 1974
6. Duke M: Bedrest in acute myocardial infarction. Am Heart J 83:486–491, 1971
7. Hackett TP, Cassem NH: Psychological adaptation to convalescence in myocardial infarction patients. In Naughton JP, Hellerstein HK (eds): Exercise Testing and Exercise Training in Coronary Heart Disease, pp. 253–262. New York, Academic Press, 1973
8. Hackett TP, Cassem NH: Patient Psychology: Coronary Care. Dallas, AHA Publication, 1975
9. Haskell W: Physical activity following myocardial infarction. In Amsterdam EA, Wilmore JH, DeMaria AN (eds): Exercise in Cardiovascular Health and Disease, pp. 344–363. New York, Yorke Medical Books, 1977
10. Jackson DH, Reeves TJ, Sheffield LT et al: Isometric effects on treadmill exercise response in healthy young men. Am J Cardiol 31:344–350, 1973
11. Kitamura K, Jorgensen CR, Gobel FL et al: Hemodynamic correlates of myocardial oxygen consumption during upright exercise. J Appl Physiol 32:516–522, 1972
12. Mallory GK, White PD, Salcedo-Salgar J: The speed of healing of myocardial infarction. Am Heart J 18:647–671, 1939
13. Mansfield LW, Sivarajan ES, Bruce RA: Exercise testing of myocardial infarction patients prior to hospital discharge: A quantitative basis for exercise prescription. Cardiac Rehabilitation 8:17–20, 1978
14. McNeer JF, Wallace AG, Wagner GS et al: The course of acute myocardial infarction: Feasibility of early discharge of the uncomplicated patient. Circulation 51:410–413, 1975
15. Saltin B, Blomqvist G, Mitchell JH et al: Response to exercise after bedrest and after training. Circulation 38:1–78, 1968
16. Sivarajan ES, Lerman J, Mansfield LW et al: Progressive ambulation and treadmill testing of patients with acute myocardial infarction during hospitalization: A feasibility study. Arch Phys Med Rehabil 58:241–247, 1977
17. Sivarajan ES, Snydsman A, Smith B et al: Low-level treadmill testing of 41 patients with acute myocardial infarction prior to discharge from hospital. Heart Lung 6:975–980, 1977
18. Swan HJC, Blackburn HW, Sanctis RD et al: Duration of hospitalization in the uncomplicated completed acute myocardial infarction. Am J Cardiol 37:413–419, 1976
19. Thomas AE, McKay DA, Cutlip MB: A nomograph method for assessing body weight. Am J Clin Nutr 29:302–304, 1976
20. Tucker HH, Carson PH, Bass NM et al: Results of early mobilization and discharge after myocardial infarction. Br Med J 1:10–13, 1973
21. Wenger NK: Coronary Care: Rehabilitation After Myocardial Infarction. New York, AHA Publication, 1975
22. Wenger NK, Gilbert CA: Rehabilitation of the myocardial infarction patient. In Hurst WJ, Logue RB, Schlant RC, Wenger NK (eds): The Heart, Arteries and Veins, 4th ed, pp 1303–1311. New York, McGraw-Hill, 1978

ADDITIONAL READING

Comoss PM, Burke EA, Swails SH: Cardiac Rehabilitation: A Comprehensive Nursing Approach. Philadelphia, JB Lippincott, 1979

Ellestad MH, Blomquist GC, Naughton JP: Standards for Adult Exercise Testing Laboratories. American Heart Association Subcommittee on Rehabilitation Target Activity Group, Circulation 59:412A–430A, 1979

Erb BD, Fletcher GF, Sheffield TL: Standards for Cardiovascular Exercise Treatment Programs. American Heart Association Subcommittee on Rehabilitation Target Activity Group, Circulation 59:1084A–1090A, 1979

Fardy PS, Bennett JI, Reitz NL et al: Cardiac Rehabilitation. St. Louis, CV Mosby, 1980

Hellerstein HK: Specifications for Exercise Testing Equipment. American Heart Association Subcommittee on Rehabilitation Target Activity Group, Circulation 59:849A–853A, 1979

Sivarajan ES, Bruce RA: Early exercise testing after myocardial infarction. Cardiovasc Nurs 17:1–5, 1981

Wilson PK, Fardy PS, Froelicher VF. Cardiac Rehabilitation, Adult Fitness, and Exercise Testing. Philadelphia, Lea & Febiger, 1981

43

Cardiac Rehabilitation: Lifestyle Adjustments

KATHERINE M. NEWTON, R.N., M.A.

and

ERIKA SEIBERLER SIVARAJAN, R.N., M.A.

What happens to patients when they return home after a myocardial infarction (MI)? How do they adjust to the many changes they face? How do they make decisions regarding life-style changes such as smoking, dietary restrictions, and medication routines? Health care personnel as well as patients are confronted with questions such as these during recovery from MI. The purpose of this chapter is to discuss the various life-style adjustments implied in these questions. Specifically discussed are 1. the adjustment of MI patients and their families to the practical, everyday problems they face in adapting to life-style changes, and 2. the issues and approaches that nurses should consider in preparing programs to assist patients during this time. Exercise, psychologic aspects of recovery, education, and sexual activity during recovery are presented in chapters 42, 44, 45, and 46 respectively.

CONVALESCENCE—WHAT PATIENTS WANT TO KNOW

Homecoming can be a stressful event for the patient, the spouse, and the family. The successful adjustment of patients during hospitalization and the recovery period increases chances of successful recovery and return to work.[9,12,14,28,45] Depression, anxiety, weakness, disturbed sleep patterns, and concern regarding sexual performance are common during the recovery phase.[10,14,26,27,45,46] Spouses of these patients may experience guilt, fear, depression, anger, anxiety, and a sense of loss.[2,4,17,35]

The causes of these reactions are undoubtedly multiple,

but it has become clear that one of the greatest needs of patients during this time is information.[6,18,31] Many hospitals now incorporate inpatient teaching as a part of their cardiac rehabilitation program.[8,21,29,44] These programs are vital in helping reduce patients' anxiety, and reassure them that fellow patients have similar anxieties. However, the hospitalization period is not an ideal time for learning because the psychologic reactions commonly experienced by patients (fear, anxiety, depression, denial) and such medications as tranquilizers interfere with perception and retention. Thus, although in-hospital teaching fulfills an important function, much of the information is quickly forgotten after discharge.[29,30] Patients often feel very well in the hospital after the first few days of acute illness; during this time their activities are restricted to those requiring very minimal levels of oxygen consumption. Therefore, it is difficult for them to appreciate the fatigue they may experience when they return home, as a result of the psychologic stress and physical demands imposed by their daily routine. Diets and other instruction often make perfect sense in the hospital but become frustrating and confusing when attempted at home in the context of a family routine. Patients are often told that they need to "relax!" without specific guidelines as to how this goal may be accomplished. (Some patients actually end up worrying about relaxing.)

It has become increasingly clear that in-hospital teaching and routine posthospital visits to the physician do not adequately meet the needs of patients recovering from MI. Nurses are well prepared both educationally and experientially to help these patients meet their needs. Through counseling and interviewing of groups and individuals the major concerns to patients and their spouses have been identified.[1,2,6,30,31] Some are discussed in depth here, with suggestions for nursing intervention. A comprehensive list can be found in Chapter 45.

Cause of Myocardial Infarction

"Why me?" is perhaps the single most commonly expressed sentiment of the patient after an MI. If it is the first MI and there were no prior symptoms, the patient may have difficulty comprehending the event and its implications. As patients discuss and relive their attack, they may realize retrospectively that the "shortness of breath," "feeling in their chest," or "indigestion" they experienced for a time before the MI was in fact angina. This recognition may generate anger or frustration as they wonder if recognizing these symptoms might have enabled them to prevent their MI. Sometimes patients experience guilt or remorse at not having taken steps against such risk factors as obesity, inactivity, or smoking. They may view their MI as a warning, and believe that their survival is a second chance, to "do things right from now on."

Discussing risk factors and the causes of coronary artery disease may help relieve the guilt which patients and spouses feel, and can serve to put the event in perspective. The following points may be helpful in this respect:

1. Risk factors are not absolutes. Some people have every risk factor and never experience an MI. Other patients suffer an MI yet have none of the risk factors.
2. Many of the most important risk factors (age, sex, diabetes, and heredity) cannot be controlled.
3. Coronary artery disease is a long-term process. In the majority of cases, therefore, it is unlikely that MI is precipitated by any one event. It is not known exactly why MI occurs when it does. This is very important for those who associate their MI with an activity such as walking, intercourse, arguing, or travel. (See also Chap. 13.)

Dietary Changes and Alcoholic Beverages

Altering eating habits may be extremely frustrating and unpalatable for an entire family.[30,31] Even without physician recommendations, patients often plunge wholeheartedly into changing their entire way of eating, cutting down on calories, salt, cholesterol, and saturated fats. It is something they can "do" at a time when there are many "don'ts." Many of the cookbooks in print today promise a life without heart disease if one were just to stop eating salt, or fats and cholesterol, or sugar. This information is not inherently bad or harmful. However, these overly simplified promises need to be put into perspective. We have no conclusive evidence that people with coronary artery disease can arrest or reverse the process, or prolong their life, by changing the fats and cholesterol in their diet.[37] We do know that reducing the intake of sodium is important for the person with hypertension or congestive heart failure.

For patients who have been advised to modify their diets, specific lists of items to choose and to avoid, and discussions of shopping ideas are extremely valuable (see Tables 43-1 and 43-2). Those who are trying to reduce their intake of

saturated fats should be taught to read labels and to compare the ratio of polyunsaturated to saturated fats (P/S ratio). (See Table 43-3.) It provides a tool for choosing among brands rather than relying on particular brand names, since product ingredients change frequently. The American Heart Association has many publications that help with dietary changes. Given these basic guidelines and principles, many patients become quite ingenious at developing their own dietary creations. It is also important that the diet be reviewed

TABLE 43-1 SAMPLE SUGGESTIONS FOR LOW CHOLESTEROL AND FAT-MODIFIED DIETS

Avoid	Use
Eggs (limit to 3/week)	Egg substitutes
Butter, lard, meat fat, coconut and palm oils, hydrogenated oils	Margarines (first ingredient, liquid oil), liquid oils (corn, safflower, sesame, sunflower)
Whole milk and whole milk products, cream, half and half, sour cream	Lowfat, nonfat, or buttermilk cottage cheese
Cheeses from cream or whole milk	Farmer's, Sapso, Baker's low-fat mozarella cheeses
Nondairy creamers	Powdered nonfat or lowfat milk
Duck, goose, shrimp	Chicken, shellfish, turkey, fish
Fatty meats: spareribs, sausages, bacon, liver, organ meats, lunchmeats	Lean meats: beef, veal, pork, ham, lamb (trim *all* fat)
Butter rolls, eggbread, cheese bread, commercial rolls	Whole wheat and enriched white bread, French bread, English muffins, oatmeal, rye bread, pumpernickel, biscuits, muffins, pasta, cereals
	Fruits and vegetables

TABLE 43-2 SAMPLE SUGGESTIONS FOR SODIUM-RESTRICTED DIETS

Avoid	Substitute with (or use instead)
Table salt	Salt subsitutes, other seasonings
Salted, smoked, or canned fish	Fresh meats and fish
Processed cheeses or cheese spreads	Nonprocessed cheeses
Sauerkraut, pickles, canned vegetables	Fresh or frozen vegetables
Bacon, bacon fat	Vegetable oil, margarine
Canned soups, dried soup mixes, instant soup, bouillion cubes	Homemade soups
Breads or crackers with visible salt, salted snack foods	Products without visible salt
Salt seasonings, seasoning mixes, soy sauce	Onion and garlic powder, pepper

TABLE 43-3 SAMPLE FOOD LABELS INGREDIENTS, CHOLESTEROL CONTENT, AND RATIO OF POLYUNSATURATED TO SATURATED FATS

A. Ingredients: liquid safflower oil, liquid soybean oil, partly hydrogenated soybean and cottonseed oils, water and milk products, salt . . .

Nutrition information:

Serving size:	1 Tbsp.	Fat:	11 grams
Calories:	100	poly-unsaturated:	5 grams
Protein:	0 grams	saturated:	2 grams
Carbo-hydrate:	0 grams	Cholesterol:	0 mg

B. Ingredients: partly hydrogenated soybean oil, water, salt, whey . . .

Nutrition information:

Serving size:	1 Tbsp.	Fat:	11 grams
Calories:	100	poly-unsaturated:	1 gram
Protein:	0 grams	saturated:	2 grams
		Cholesterol:	0 mg

By reading the above labels of comparably priced products, the buyer learns that product A is made with liquid corn oil as its largest ingredient, whereas product B has partly hydrogenated oil as its greatest ingredient. This is reflected in the ratios of polyunsaturated to saturated fats in the two products. The products have approximately the same caloric content and no cholesterol.

may have very little consequence, whereas drinking with friends in a smoke-filled room, after a big meal, may impose a stress on the myocardium.[36]

Recurrence of Chest Pain

The recurrence of chest pain, especially if the patient did not experience angina either prior to the infarction or during hospitalization, may be terrifying, not only for the patient but for the spouse as well. When patients first return home, they are often acutely aware of every ache and pain, wondering "Is this it? Is it going to continue?". Anxiety and fear, through increased sympathetic stimulation, may raise the HR and blood pressure (BP), thus increasing myocardial oxygen consumption, resulting in prolonged episodes of angina. Talking about the various sensations assists the patient to differentiate minor aches and pains from angina (for example, "I have one over here on the right that just lasts a second, that's just muscle. Then there's the feeling in my arm if I walk up a hill; I think that's angina"). Helping patients recognize the pattern of their angina, what brings it on, and how to anticipate events that might cause it, is one way to enable the patient to gain a sense of control in a situation that seems at first very much out of control. Myths and fears must also be dispelled. Reassuring explanations that angina does not mean "a little heart attack every time," and that nitroglycerin is not a "crutch," addictive, or dangerous, and that a headache does not mean something is wrong but that the nitroglycerin is working, may help reduce the anxiety that surrounds chest pain.

Medications

Specific, written instructions for medications are essential. Teaching about medications is too often done as the patient is on the way out of the hospital. Teaching about medications should be an early part of discharge planning and should preferably include the spouse as well as the patient. On return visits, patients should be asked if they take their medicines, at what times they take them, how they react to them, and if their medication schedule is causing difficulties for them.

Individualization can make medication schedules much more acceptable. Many patients will disturb their sleep because they have been told to take their pills every 6 hours. Prior to discharge, medication plans can be drawn up, taking into consideration the medication, activity schedules, sleep patterns, work patterns, and the reason for giving the drug.

Return to Work

Numerous factors influence the decision to return to work, including the patient's physical capacity relative to the job, the availability of other financial resources, and the patient's age, but above all, emotional factors.[45,46] Those who plan to return to work, express anxieties by such questions as: When should I return to work? Can I work full time or part time? Can I return to the same duties or different ones?

Patients should be cautioned that returning even to a desk job can be stressful or tiring at first. (It may be tiring even for a healthy person after a vacation.) It is also important

with whoever does the cooking and food shopping. There is no need to throw out everything in the cupboard and start over. Such a requirement is not only discouraging but is an expense that some households cannot afford if financial stress has resulted from the illness, medical expenses, and loss of work. Many helpful cookbooks are now available on low-fat and low-cholesterol, or low-sodium diets and a few include both restrictions (see suggested references). The nurse can also help the patient set priorities for these restrictions. Multiple restrictions are often difficult and expensive. For the person on a mild sodium restriction, for example, specially prepared low-sodium foods are an unnecessary expense.

The use of community resources is beneficial in some cases. Community classes in nutrition may be available from the local Heart Association. For patients who need to lose weight, programs that make use of techniques of behavior modification are meeting with success. Third-party payment may cover part of the cost of these programs.

Patients frequently inquire about the effects of alcohol. The following are some of the points about alcohol that should be explained: 1. "One drink" equals one 12-oz can of beer, 4 ounces of wine, or one single (1-½ oz) drink of hard alcohol—the amount of alcohol in these drinks is equal; 2. alcohol is not a risk factor of coronary artery disease, although in excessive amounts it can create other problems; 3. alcohol tends to raise the heart rate (HR) and thus make the heart work harder; 4. the setting in which alcohol is consumed is important—a quiet, relaxing drink at home

to prepare patients for the reactions and questions from friends and acquaintances. Some patients, after their MI, find that they are suddenly expected to be the expert on everyone else's aches and pains. A comment often heard is: "They all want me to tell them it's not their heart." Or, they may be the unwilling recipient of everyone else's horror stories about an aunt, brother, or father who had a heart attack. Well-meaning friends or relatives can cause anxiety with comments such as: "My father was kept in bed for 6 weeks. Should you really be walking like that?" Rehearsing possible responses to these remarks ["It troubles me to hear you say that," or, "My doctor (or nurse or therapist) is giving me specific instructions and told me times have changed since then"] helps prepare the patient for such comments and offsets any possible anxiety. The patient can also be told ahead of time to report these situations to the nurse, especially if they cause anxiety. Explaining the rationale for earlier ambulation, hospital discharge, and return to work can reassure the patient and spouse that these recommendations are safe and beneficial.

Current and Future State of Health

It is understandable that patients are concerned with how to improve their health and prevent a recurrence of an MI. To this end, some will "shop" for or make bargains: "I know if I just quit smoking and exercise I can live until I'm 80." Providing reassurance without arousing or supporting false promises is often difficult at this stage, but such efforts are necessary. Often, just allowing patients an opportunity to explore and voice their hopes and expectations enables them to work through these feelings. This is one benefit of a group meeting in which patients can help one another face reality. When one voices unrealistic expectations, another often adds a note of reality with comments such as: "Well, I guess no matter what you do, when your time comes it comes," or, "Well, none of us can live forever."

Physical Effects of Smoking

Smoking is the risk factor about which we can offer patients the most encouragement. It is well documented that, for persons who quit smoking, the risk of MI decreases markedly.[22] It is also common knowledge that patients who stop smoking breathe easier and taste food better. The stern advice of the physician to quit smoking still has the greatest influence in encouraging patients to give up cigarettes.[25,32] Individual counseling sessions and smoking withdrawal clinics have also proved helpful.[39] Both the American Heart Association and American Lung Association provide self-help pamphlets on request.

Diagnostic Tests and the Healing Process

Patients are often curious about how their MI was diagnosed. Questions such as: "They told me my enzymes were up. What does that mean?" or, "Will my heart attack always show on the electrocardiogram, or will it go back to normal when it heals?" are frequently raised. Many patients seek more specific information concerning the extent and location of their infarct and the healing process. Frequently they use this information to reassure themselves. "My doctor said it was just a little one on the bottom—I hear that's not as bad as one in the front." Their concern focuses on their future, the restrictions on activity, when they can return to work, and the effects on their physical capacity. Questions also arise about the risks, benefits, and purposes of treadmill testing, scanning procedures, and cardiac catheterization.

Because few patients have actually seen a heart, or even pictures of an MI, misconceptions about what has happened are the rule. Asking them what they think happened to their heart is a helpful starting point. Some think it is a hole, or tear, and this creates concern that it may leak or rupture. Specific information about what an infarct looks like (a bruise) and how it heals: "With time it forms a scar that replaces the damaged muscle but does not contract" helps patients better understand the need for rest during recovery.

Stress and Relaxation

There is evidence that a person's behavior pattern may be predictive of the development of coronary artery disease.[7,33] This has been described in Chapter 11. Because this idea has been popularized by books and articles written for the general public, patients often have questions about this topic.[11]

Patients face many potentially stressful situations as they recover from their MI (e.g., being at home all day, changes in their bodily responses to activities, adaptation to illness, financial adjustments, retirement, returning to work, family adjustments). Patients may or may not react to these situations with a stress response, but even those who appear to be visibly stressed (rapid speech, clenched teeth or fists, anger) may not recognize this stress in themselves. Others who appear calm may admit to "holding things in" and feeling stressed in some situations.

There are several recognized methods of relaxation; most of them are relatively easy to learn and can provide a means of helping people deal with stressful situations (Table 43-4).

TABLE 43-4   RELAXATION TECHNIQUES

Progressive Relaxation (Jacobson): Directed toward relaxation of major muscle groups by contraction and relaxation of various muscles. May not be advisable in early recovery after MI because of isometric component.[19,20]

Autogenic Training (Luthe): Repetition of autosuggestive phrases to oneself to induce physiologic and mental relaxation.[24]

Relaxation Response (Benson): Promotes relaxation using approach of
1. quiet environment; 2. mental device such as word or phrase to be repeated; 3. passive attitude; 4. comfortable position to induce a response of relaxation. Twice a day for 20 minutes.[5]

Biofeedback (Schwartz and Shapiro): Provides feedback about autonomic responses (blood pressure, heart rate, galvanic skin response, muscle tension) through instrumentation which may assist patients in recognizing and controlling these responses to promote relaxation.[34]

Transcendental Meditation (Maharishi Mahesh Yogi): Promotes relaxation by having patient sit comfortably with eyes closed and repeat a "mantra" silently. Suggested practice is 20 minutes twice a day.[42,43]

However, patients should realize that although twenty minutes of relaxation twice a day may be helpful, reduction of the overall stress level is the main objective. It helps also to emphasize that while it may not be possible to change the situations which produce stress, patients can change the way that they react to it. This is a matter of 1. recognizing events which are stressful; 2. recognizing one's own physical and emotional responses to these stresses; 3. consciously choosing to react to these situations in a new way; 4. practicing these new responses. It takes thought and practice to learn new responses to stressful situations, especially those related to the family.

Women with Myocardial Infarction: Special Considerations

Very little information is available about the special needs of women following MI. While women face many of the same concerns as men, they also encounter unique problems. Yet most of the literature apparently is written specifically for the man with an MI, which creates confusion about whether the same instructions also apply to women. It may very well be that women need different information. A distressing finding in one study of life adjustment after MI was that women had a more difficult postinfarction rehabilitation course than did men.[38] Fewer returned to work, fewer returned to sexual activity (40% of women vs. 93% of men), and more were anxious or depressed. Of 13 women, six died within 1 year, and all six women were unmarried. A high incidence of type A behavior was demonstrated in these women. It is clear that women may need special consideration during rehabilitation. Many of the women MI patients are housewives and are thus working in their own homes. Unlike their male counterparts who are removed from their jobs temporarily, women convalescing from MI may find it difficult to limit household activities to self-care only. The disruption in family life may make recovery in the home more stressful for the woman. Guilt about neglecting the husband and children when she is not able to perform the usual chores is often a major stress.

Career and working women face more stress than do their male counterparts, partly because of the lingering traditional belief that women should stay at home and raise a family. Career women who suffer an MI may tend to place undue blame for the MI on their choice of life-style. Some even contemplate giving up their careers. These factors should be taken into consideration in rehabilitation efforts directed toward working women.

Women who suffer an MI during the childbearing years need to be cautioned about using the pill as a method of birth control, since the incidence of thromboembolic events is increased with use of oral contraceptives, especially among smokers. When anticoagulants are prescribed for a woman during her menstrual years, she should be advised to contact her physician if excessive bleeding occurs.

Return to sexual activity has been delayed for some women after MI because their spouses are overprotective and fear that sex may hurt their wives' heart conditions. Although similar apprehensions are voiced by women when the man is recovering from the MI, they do not seem to withhold involvement in resuming sexual activity.[38] Women patients should be encouraged to discuss sexual matters openly with their partners. When the woman has suffered the MI, the spouse is less inclined to participate in the wife's rehabilitation than are wives to participate in that of their husbands. The delay in sexual rehabilitation may be prevented by encouraging women patients to bring their spouses or sexual partners to counseling sessions, which may help to dispel misunderstandings.

THE USE OF GROUPS IN REHABILITATION

The use of groups in the rehabilitation process is receiving increasing attention as cardiac rehabilitation programs develop. One of the essentials for the formation of a group is the presence of a common purpose or goal. In the case of the patient who has had an MI, the common need for information, reassurance, and emotional support lends itself readily to group intervention. There is no strong research evidence that documents the benefits and advantages of group intervention; however, patients and health professionals who have participated in such groups report that they serve a useful function.[2,6,13,15,16,17,18,31,40,41] Early work with groups of cardiac patients showed that patients were reluctant to explore their feelings. Rather than discuss their feelings, they focused on their physical condition and the practical realities of day-to-day problems.[1,2] With time, however, patients demonstrate an ability to support and assist one another in problem solving in an atmosphere of friendliness and sharing.

Philosophy and Purpose

The philosophy behind the use of group discussion and the purpose of the particular group must be clear to the group leaders and to the participants. This helps to set the stage and gives the participants some idea of what is expected of them. Table 43-5 lists some factors to be considered in developing a program of group teaching and counseling. These factors are discussed below.

TABLE 43-5 FACTORS TO BE CONSIDERED IN DEVELOPING A GROUP TEACHING AND COUNSELING PROGRAM

LEADERSHIP

PHILOSOPHY AND PURPOSE

PUBLIC RELATIONS AND COMMUNITY INVOLVEMENT

MEMBERSHIP CRITERIA

SETTING, LENGTH, NUMBER

CONTENT, FORMAT, STYLE

ADDITIONAL RESOURCES

SIZE

COST

REFRESHMENTS

Leadership

Groups have been led by nurses, psychologists, psychiatrists, social workers, physicians, and chaplains. Whoever assumes leadership of the group should be familiar with group dynamics and the essentials of group leadership. Since group meetings may uncover serious problems (physical, emotional, and family), leaders must know their own limits and recognize when it is appropriate to turn problems to other resource persons (counselor, psychologist, physician, or social worker). The leader(s) must have at least some knowledge of cardiovascular disease, MI, and recovery in order to answer questions and clarify misconceptions. Co-leadership at times may be a good way of meeting these various needs.

When group discussions were first used for patients with MI, there was concern that the emotional effects of the group interactions could lead to angina or more severe cardiac emergencies. It has therefore been suggested that the leader have experience in dealing with these emergencies or that medical backup be available.[15] The need for this service has not appeared in any published reports on cardiac groups but it should be considered, especially for patients that join early after MI.

Public Relations and Community Involvement

The issue of how to deal with the referring physician and the community concerns depends largely on how the group is established. The patients may come from one hospital or several and may be referred by few or many physicians. It is important to reassure the physicians that the patients will not be given advice contrary to their practices. This issue can be sensitive and troublesome for all persons involved, depending on the degree of autonomy allowed the rehabilitation group by the physicians. The situation is different for an agency or group which assumes total responsbility for rehabilitation as compared to one in which rehabilitation is managed by the physician, with classes or groups being offered by the hospital nurses. When persons other than the primary physician assume responsibility for rehabilitation, conflicting recommendations may arise. One approach is to share information with the patients and their spouses so that they can make their own choices. Another is to explain the reasons why the physician has made certain recommendations.

Community involvement will vary with the size of the community and the services available, as well as with the special interests of its citizenry. Hospital-employed nurses who wish to establish an outpatient teaching and counseling program will have to use their skills to recruit administrative and physician support. Clear proposals which include philosophy, content, expected costs, and documentation of expected benefits are essential in proposing a group program.

Membership Criteria

While groups can be conducted for patients and spouses together, or for patients alone, there is general agreement that spouses as well as patients benefit from the exchange. At least two investigators have found that the group benefited when patients and spouses met together, and others have also suggested this approach.[3,12,13,18,40] Unmarried patients may wish to bring partners, close friends, or relatives to the group. Patients' children may also benefit from attending some or all of the sessions. Separate group meetings may be held for children who share serious concerns about how their life-style may be affected by their parents' condition. Another consideration is whether patients who have had an MI and those who have undergone cardiac surgery should meet together or separately, or meet together for some sessions and separately for others. Membership in these groups may be rotated or fixed, depending upon the size of the group or community, how soon after the MI the patient is to enter the group, and the structure of the group. Rotating membership allows patients who are further along in the recovery process to give encouragement to newcomers, while fixed membership may be more beneficial if group process is heavily emphasized.

Physical Setting, Length, and Number of Sessions

The philosophy and purpose of the group are important considerations in determining the setting and the length and number of sessions. The setting may vary from a formal classroom to an informal discussion over refreshments. The length of the sessions should be geared to how sick the patients have been, as well as to how soon after their MI they begin. Most groups generally meet for 60 to 90 minutes. The number of sessions is determined by their structure, that is, whether they are open-ended or outlined for specific content.

Content, Format, Style

Considerations of content, format, and style are in large part determined by the objectives. It has become possible to predict many of the common concerns of MI patients and their spouses from the findings of early research in this area.[2,6,15,18,30] Thus specific content must be presented in the group. However, unstructured meetings are also necessary to allow free discussion. In such instances, an open-ended approach can be used to encourage discussion about specific problems, concerns, or suggestions from members of the group.

The use of such audiovisual aids as films, cassette tapes, flip charts, a loan library of helpful references, and printed material is beneficial. These resources not only provide valuable information but stimulate discussion. A sample of a series of structured classes, intended to give content and also allow time for discussion, is presented in Table 43-5.

Additional Resources

In groups where discussion and expression of feelings are encouraged, individual concerns related to emotional, sexual, vocational, dietary, or medical matters may arise and may be beyond the purpose of the group or the skill of the leader. In such instances it is important that the leader feel comfortable in saying "I do not know." At times it may be

TABLE 43-6 SUGGESTED OUTLINE: ORGANIZING CONTENT FOR OUTPATIENT TEACHING AND COUNSELING SESSIONS

CLASS 1—Anatomy and Physiology

I. The Circulatory System
   a. The blood vessels
   b. The heart
   c. The coronary circulation

II. Coronary Artery Disease

III. Angina
   a. Definition
   b. Causes
   c. Symptoms
   d. Things that differentiate it from MI
   e. Things that differentiate it from other "aches and pains"
   f. Treatment
   g. When to call for help

IV. Heart Attack
   a. Definition
   b. Symptoms and signs
   c. Causes
   d. Diagnosis: ECG, enzymes, history
   e. Healing

V. Care After an MI
   a. The Cardiac Care Unit
   b. The medical unit
   c. Returning home

CLASS 2—Risk Factors

I. Smoking
   a. Physiologic effects
   b. Benefits of stopping
   c. Ways of stopping

II. Hypertension
   a. Definition
   b. Causes
   c. Physiologic effects
   d. Symptoms
   e. Treatment

III. Obesity

IV. Sedentary Lifestyle
   a. Effects of inactivity
   b. Benefits of regular exercise

V. Nonmodifiable Risk Factors
   a. Diabetes
   b. Sex
   c. Age
   d. Family history

CLASS 3—Diet Changes

I. Weight Control
   a. Rationale
   b. Methods

II. Cholesterol Reducing Diets
   a. Rationale
   b. Definitions—Cholesterol, saturated fats, monosaturated fats, polyunsaturated fats
   c. Methods for change, substitutions

III. Low-Sodium Diets
   a. Rationale: congestive heart failure, hypertension
   b. Methods for change, substitutions

IV. Coffee

V. Alcohol

CLASS 4—Activity and Exercise

I. Definitions of activity and exercise

II. Benefits
   a. Physiologic
   b. Psychologic

III. Energy expenditure
   a. METS: applications to daily activities
   b. Considerations for exercise: graded, interval principle
   c. Energy-saving techniques

IV. General principles for exercise
   a. Dynamic versus isometric
   b. Warm-up and cool-down
   c. Exercise period: clothing, when, where
   d. General precautions

V. Community exercise programs

CLASS 5—Emotional Reactions to MI

I. Common reactions to MI

II. Use of support systems

III. Stress and the heart

IV. Relaxation techniques

CLASS 6—Returning to a Meaningful Life

I. Retirement versus return to work

II. Returning to sexual activity.

---

appropriate to bring an outsider into the group to deal with these concerns. Other situations may call for individual referral and require that resource persons be available to deal with problems that are beyond the leader's skill.

Another resource that cannot be overemphasized is the telephone. Patients and family members are usually encouraged to ask questions and voice concerns before they are discharged from the hospital. The problem is that they often do not know what to ask until they are confronted with a new problem or situation. If questions must be saved for the visit to the physician or the next group meeting, there may be a period of anxiety, sleeplessness, or discord among family members. Often these concerns go unvoiced unless the group leader or the physician specifically asks about them.

Weekly or biweekly telephone calls by a nurse to the patient or to the spouse, or both, can serve as a time to answer questions and give reassurance about diet, somatic and emotional difficulties, and activity.[6,15,29,45] Others have encouraged patients to call the nurse in the cardiac care unit if they have questions. Patients will often use this resource as a means of reassuring themselves of the legitimacy of a question before "bothering" the physician. It must be clearly explained that this is not a medical emergency number. The community medical emergency number should also be distributed at discharge, with instructions to patients that it be placed on the telephone with the patient's address. During a stressful situation, people often forget their own address, or a visitor making the call may not know it.

The structure of a rehabilitation program intended to help modify life-style and risk factors is dependent on the expertise of the personnel, and the resources and finances available. It is most important that the objectives of the program be clear, that the program be well planned and structured, and that patients be offered specific information and skills. The use of contracts puts patients in charge of their own health care. The program must be flexible to accommodate individual needs. Diet, weight loss, and stress management can be offered in individual modules and referred to patients, depending on need and choice. It must be recognized that patients vary both in their readiness for such commitment and in acceptance of the time required to effect change.

REFERENCES

1. Abramson EE: Behavioral approaches to weight control: An updated review. Behav Res Ther 15:355–363, 1977
2. Adsett CA, Bruhn JG: Short-term group psychotherapy for postmyocardial infarction patients and their wives. Can Med Assoc J 99:577–584, 1968
3. Anderson DE: Cardiac rehabilitation: The crucial month. Med J Aust 64:124–127, 1977
4. Baile WF, Engle BT: A behavioral strategy for promoting treatment compliance following myocardial infarction. Psychosom Med 40:413–419, 1978
5. Benson H: The Relaxation Response. New York, Avon, 1975
6. Bilodeau CB, Hackett TP: Issues raised in a group setting by patients recovering from myocardial infarction. Am J Psychiatry 128:105–110, 1971
7. Blumenthal JA, Williams RB, Kong Y et al: Type A behavior patterns and coronary atherosclerosis. Circulation 58:634–639, 1978
8. Boggs B, Malone D, McCullock C: A coronary teaching program in a community hospital. Nurs Clin North Am 13:457–472, 1978
9. Bruhn JG, Wolf S, Philips BV: A psycho-social study of surviving male coronary patients and controls over nine years. J Psychosom Res 15:305–313, 1971
10. Crawshaw JE: Community rehabilitation after acute myocardial infarction. Heart Lung 3:258–262, 1974
11. Friedman M, Rosenman RH: Type A Behavior and Your Heart. Greenwich, Fawcett Publications, 1974
12. Garrity TF, Klein RF: Emotional responses and clinical severity as early determinants of six-month mortality after myocardial infarction. Heart Lung 4:730–737, 1975
13. Golden LH, Golden NP, Dibiase J: Crisis intervention for cardiac outpatients. Medical Insight 4:18–23, 1972
14. Gulledge AD: The psychological aftermath of a myocardial infarction. In Gentry WD, Williams RB (eds): Psychological Aspects of Myocardial Infarction and Coronary Care, pp 107–123. St. Louis, C. V. Mosby, 1975
15. Hackett TP: The use of groups in the rehabilitation of the postcoronary patient. In Konig K, Denolin H (eds): Advances in Cardiology, pp 127–135. Basel, S Karger, AG, 1978
16. Halhuber MJ: Health education in cardiac rehabilitation. In Konig K, Denolin H (eds): Advances in Cardiology, pp 146–152. Basel, S Karger, AG, 1978
17. Harding AL, Morefield M: Group intervention for wives of myocardial infarction patients. Nurs Clin North Am 11:339–347, 1976
18. Ibrahim MA, Feldman JG, Sultz HA et al: Management after myocardial infarction: A controlled trial of the effect of group psychotherapy. Int J Psychiatry Intern Med 5:253–268, 1974
19. Jacobsen E: Anxiety and Tension Control. Philadelphia, JB Lippincott, 1964
20. Jacobson E: Progressive Relaxation. Chicago, University of Chicago Press, 1938
21. Johnson BL, Cantwell JD, Fletcher GF: Eight steps to inpatient cardiac rehabilitation: The team effort—Methodology and preliminary results. Heart Lung 5:97–111, 1976
22. Kannel WB, Doyle JT, Fredrickson DT et al: American heart association ad hoc committee on cigarette smoking and cardiovascular diseases, revision of 1971 statement, pp 161–167. Dallas, American Heart Association, 1975
23. Kelty MF: Ethical concerns in behavior change. In Weiss E (ed): Proceedings of National Heart and Lung Institute Working Conference on Health Behavior, pp 161–167. Maryland, National Institute of Health, 1975
24. Luthe W: Autogenic Therapy, Vols I–VI. New York, Grune & Stratton, 1969
25. Mallaghan M, Pemberton J: Some behavioral changes in 493 patients after an acute myocardial infarction. British Journal of Preventive and Social Medicine 31:86–90, 1977
26. McGill AA: Review of literature and cardiovascular rehabilitation. In Weiss E (ed): Proceedings of National Heart and Lung Institute Working Conference on Health and Behavior, pp 242–280. Maryland, National Institute of Health, 1975
27. Mulcahy R: The rehabilitation of patients with coronary heart disease, a clinician's view. In Stocksmeier V (ed): Psychological Approach to the Rehabilitation of Coronary Patients, pp 52–61. Berlin, Springer-Verlag, 1976
28. Mullen PD: Health education for heart patients in crisis. Health Services Reports 88:669–675, 1973
29. Pozen MW, Stockmiller JA, Harris W et al: A nurse rehabilitator's impact on patients with myocardial infarction. Medical Care 15:830–837, 1977
30. Rahe RH, Scalzi C, Shine K: A teaching evaluation questionnaire for post-myocardial infarction patients. Heart Lung 5:759–766, 1975
31. Rahe RH, Tuffli CF, Suchor RJ et al: Group therapy in the outpatient management of post-myocardial infarction patients. Int J Psychiatry in Medicine 4:77–88, 1973
32. Raw M: Persuading people to stop smoking. Behav Res Ther 14:97–101, 1976
33. Rosenman RH, Brand RJ, Scholtz RI et al: Multivariate prediction of coronary heart disease during 8.5 year follow-up in the western collaborative group study. Am J Cardiol 37:903–909, 1976
34. Schwartz GE, Shapiro DC, Ferguson E et al: Behavioral methods in the treatment of hypertension. Ann Intern Med 86:626–636, 1972
35. Skelton M, Dominion J: Psychological stress in wives of patients with myocardial infarction. Br Med J II:101–103, 1973
36. Smith JW: Alcohol and disorders of the heart and skeletal muscles. In Estes RJ, Heinemann ME (eds): Alcoholism, Development, Consequences and Interventions, St. Louis, C. V. Mosby, 1977
37. Stamler J: Lifestyles, major risk factors, proof and public policy. Circulation 58:3–19, 1978
38. Stern MJ, Pascale L, Ackermann A: Life adjustment postmyocardial infarction. Arch Intern Med 137:1680–1685, 1977
39. Thompson EL: Smoking education programs 1960–1976. Am J Public Health 3:250–257, 1978
40. Toth A, Toth S: Post-coronary patients receive group therapy. Hosp Prog 58:72–75, 1977
41. Wallace N: Group education after myocardial infarction, is it effective? Med J Aust 2:245–247, 1977
42. Wallace RK: Physiological effects of transcendental meditation. Science 167:1751–1754, 1970
43. Wallace RK, Benson H: The Physiology of meditation. Sci Am 226:85–90, 1972
44. Wenger NK, Mount F: An educational algorithm for nursing. Cardiovasc Nurs 9:11–15, 1974
45. Wishnie HA, Hackett TP, Cassem NH: Psychological hazards of convalescence following myocardial infarction. JAMA 215:1295–1296, 1971
46. Wynn A: Unwarranted emotional distress in men with ischemic heart disease (IHD). Med J Aust 2:847–851, 1967

ADDITIONAL READING

An Active Partnership for the Health of Your Heart: 1. Your Heart Attack and Your Future, 2. Signals for Action, 3. You are What You Eat, 4. Prescription for Health, 5. Move into Action, 6. Quit for Life, 7. Your Heart Surgery, 8. Stress and Relaxation. Dallas, American Heart Association, 1979

Cambre S: The Sensuous Heart. Atlanta, Pritchett & Hull Associates, 1978

Eshleman R, Winston M: The American Heart Association Cookbook. New York, Ballantine Books, 1973

Guidelines for Cardiac Patient and Family Teaching After Hospitalization, Ad Hoc Committee to Develop Guidelines for Cardiac Patient and Family Teaching. Seattle, American Heart Association of Washington, 1976

Jacobson E: Self Operations Control, A Manual of Tension Control. Chicago, National Foundation for Progressive Relaxation, 1964

MacRae NM: How to Have Your Cake and Eat It Too. Anchorage, Alaska Northwest Publishing Company, 1975

Miller RA: How to Live with a Heart Attack and How to Avoid One. Radnor, Chilton Book, 1977

Scalzi CC, Burke LE, Greenland S: Evaluation of an inpatient education program for coronary patients. Heart Lung 9:846–853, 1980

Scheingold LD, Wagner NN: Sound Sex and the Aging Heart. New York, Human Sciences Press, 1974

Schoenberg J, Stichman J: How to Survive Your Husband's Heart Attack. New York, David McKay Co, 1974

Selye H: Stress Without Distress. New York, JB Lippincott, 1974

Waldo M: The Low Salt, Low Cholesterol Cookbook. New York, GP Putnam's Sons, 1961

Walker T, Winston P, Purcell JA et al: Heart Attack! What Now? Atlanta, Georgia Heart Association, 1972

Waltz J: Food Habit Management. Mercer Island, Northwest Learning Associates, 1978

White J, Fadiman J (eds): Relax. USA: The Confucion Press, 1976

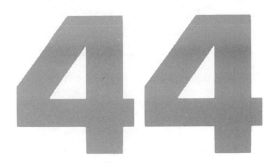

Myocardial Infarction: Behavioral Responses of Patient and Spouse

CYNTHIA C. SCALZI, R.N., M.N.

and

LORA E. BURKE, R.N., M.N.

In the past decade there has been an increased emphasis on the behavioral or psychologic aspects of the care of the patient who has had a myocardial infarction (MI). Medical and nursing emphasis has been placed on the value and importance of understanding human behavior and the responses of anxiety, denial, depression, and anger commonly observed in patients with heart disease. However, there has been a lack of emphasis, both in the literature and in practice, on identifying specific behavioral response patterns and interventions for assisting the patient and the patient's family in the adaptation process.

This chapter presents a framework for viewing the process by which the patient and spouse adapt psychologically to an MI. Five stages in the process are identified and the behavioral responses that characterize each stage are described. Tables have been used to parallel the responses of the patient and the spouse. Each behavioral response (anxiety, denial, depression, anger, guilt, and sexual aggressiveness) is described in terms of the common manifestations, primary causes, and specific nursing interventions for both patient and spouse. By viewing a behavioral response as part of a normal pattern, the nurse will be able to identify where the person is in the process of adaptation and intervene more effectively.

PROCESS OF ADAPTATION

Since an MI may present the patient and spouse with a sense of loss, such as loss of health and loss of income, the concepts of loss and grief provide the fundamental basis for the process of adaptation presented in this chapter.[2,3,5] Loss has been defined as the actual or threatened withdrawal of a valued object, or person, or a part of self. The loss of a valued object is considered to be the event preceding the emotional responses of grieving.[2,3,5] The behavioral adaptation responses that characterize each of the phases of loss as they relate to the patient after MI are given in Figure 44-1.

Shock and Disbelief

The first phase occurs immediately after the heart attack. The patient experiences a stunned numbness from the suddenness of the attack and responds with anxiety and denial in a manner characteristic of this phase. The spouse, too, reacts with highly anxious behavior and expressions of guilt and self-accusations. This phase persists for the first 24 to 48 hours.

Developing Awareness

The second phase usually begins after the first 48 hours. Once the patient has regained some hemodynamic stability, the intense fear of death decreases. As the shock of the initial event wears off, it becomes more difficult for the patient to maintain a state of denial. The reality of the heart attack begins to penetrate the consciousness during this time. "Why me?" or "Why my husband?" is a question frequently asked. The possible consequences of the event, and the feelings of emptiness and frustration that result lead to anger and depression in both patient and spouse during the second phase.

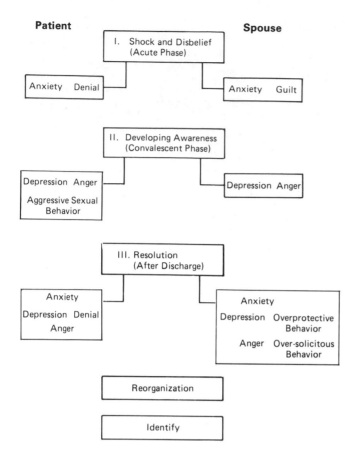

Fig. 44-1. Phases of adaptation.

Resolution

The third phase begins after discharge from the hospital and may last for 3 months. The patient begins to deal with the consequences of the infarction and faces the reality of the limitations imposed, even if they are only temporary. The convalescing patient starts to relinquish some of the dependence that accompanied the acute state and begins to see that he has choices to make, such as which risk factors to reduce. During this third phase the patient begins to deal with the feelings of being vulnerable and of being less than whole. In moving through this phase of the adaptation process, the patient assumes responsibility for setting realistic goals and the means to achieve them. The behavioral responses of this phase may include all those previously experienced. For the spouse, the anxiety created by discharge is frequently exhibited as overprotective and oversolicitous behavior.

Reorganization

The fourth phase usually occurs 2 to 6 months after discharge. The individual is recovering from the emotional trauma and begins to reorganize his life-style as related to diet, exercise, and so on, in order to accommodate the restrictions imposed by the MI.

Identity

This is the final phase, which begins when the person has successfully completed the process of adaptation. He has accepted his loss and is now able to identify himself with others who have had an MI.

It is difficult to identify one or two specific behavioral characteristics of the final two phases. Organized rehabilitation programs are available now more than in the past for individuals who have had a heart attack. It is anticipated that these programs will provide an environment to obtain information about behavioral characteristics of these later phases. There is evidence to suggest that the attitudes of the spouses influence the degree to which a patient participates in rehabilitation programs and complies with the medical regimen.

Two points need to be made before discussing the specific behavioral responses. First, the intensity of the response will vary according to the person's perception of the event and its consequences. Second, the phases are not distinct but overlap one another. The patient, in the phase of developing awareness, may find the loss too painful and may resort to denial, and so revert to an earlier phase. The nurse, who spends the most time with the patient, is in a key position to observe changes in behavior, to recognize deviations from the usual pattern, and to provide guidance through the process of adaptation (Table 44-1).

ANXIETY

Anxiety is an uncomfortable feeling or apprehension that can be either vague or very intense and occurs as a reaction to threats to one's self-esteem or personal security.[15]

A person's perception of a situation directly determines the responses to that situation. If the situation is perceived as threatening, anxiety results.

Anxiety is significant because it forms the basis for the other behavioral responses. For example, a patient may perceive a heart attack as a threat to life, job, and self-image, all of which produce anxiety. The responses used to cope with that anxiety may vary; a person may deny it exists, may retaliate with anger, or may withdraw into a state of depression. The spouse and children adopt emotional concerns similar to those of the patient. All families interviewed in one study demonstrated significant anxiety for the patient's recovery and for their own role in promoting or hindering it.[19] Individual family members can also differ in the manner in which they cope with anxiety. Their responses may vary from severe panic to total withdrawal from the acute situation.

Nursing Intervention

For the patient who has had an MI, there are at least three predictable periods when the anxiety level is high: 1. on admission; 2. upon transfer from the cardiac care unit (CCU); 3. prior to discharge. One implication for nursing care is the need for consistent nursing personnel to antici-

(*Text continues on page 575*)

TABLE 44-1   NURSING MEASURES IN RELATION TO BEHAVIORAL RESPONSE PATTERNS COMMONLY OBSERVED IN MI PATIENTS AND SPOUSES

For Patient	For Spouse
I. ANXIETY	**I. ANXIETY**
A. Manifestations	**A. Manifestations**
1. Increased verbalization	1. Increased verbalization
2. Inability to concentrate, understand, or retain information	2. Inability to concentrate, understand, or retain information
3. Restlessness or insomnia	3. Change in sleep patterns
4. Apprehension and tenseness	4. Apprehension and tenseness
5. Tremulousness	5. Tremulousness
6. Arrhythmia, angina, and elevated blood pressure	6. Frequent phone calls of inquiry
7. Hypervigilance	7. Hypervigilance
	8. Change in appetite
	9. Weeping or tearfulness
B. Primary causes	**B. Primary causes**
1. Fear of death or chronic disability	1. Fear of patient's death or chronic disability
2. Uncertainty of etiology of illness and prognosis	2. Uncertainty about own role in the patient's recovery
3. Being subjected to the strange complex environment and frightening procedures of a CCU	3. Fear that in a strange complex environment patient may have no support system
4. Development of complications (arrhythmias and cardiac arrest) in self or others	4. Lack of information or misconceptions about patient's condition, treatment, and prognosis
5. Threat to self-image	5. Threat to the family structure
6. Misinterpretation of information and misconception of experience (*i.e.*, perceiving the general physical weakness as proof of irreversible heart damage)	6. Feelings of helplessness
C. Nursing intervention	**C. Nursing intervention**
1. During periods of severe anxiety, maintain consistent, continuous nurse–patient contact; consistency of personnel assists development of patient's trust and facilitates an accurate assessment.	1. Severe anxiety may result in panic-like disorganized behavior. Nurse must take an active, sometimes directive role in assisting the spouse to set priorities and plan initial activities.
2. Give initial and repeated orientation to CCU routines, equipment, and procedures.	2. Give initial and repeated explanations of treatment program and of patient's progress.
3. Assess the patient's experience with earlier illnesses, hospitalization, and severe stress and its relationship to current condition.	3. Assess spouse's experiences with illness, hospitalization, and severe stress.
4. Assess coping mechanisms previously adopted under severe stress.	4. Assess coping mechanisms previously adopted under severe stress.
5. Solicit expressions of concern and invite questions.	5. Provide time for spouse to express concern and to ask questions.
6. Prepare for each change or move in the patient's physical environment (transfers from the CCU to a convalescent unit or to home).	6. Prepare spouse and family for patient's transfer, and involve them in discharge planning.
	7. Make daily phone calls or periodic daily reports to spouse about patient's condition.
II. DENIAL	**II. GUILT**
A. Manifestations	**A. Manifestations**
1. History of ignoring symptoms prior to admission	1. Outward expression ranging from questioning her role in causing the heart attack to lambasting herself for being totally at fault.
2. Avoidance of discussing the heart attack or its significance	2. Over solicitous or over protective behavior.
3. Minimization of severity of his condition and its consequences	3. Constant vigil at hospital a possibility
4. Secondhand description of his/her condition ("The doctor says I. . . .")	
5. Verbal acknowledgment of having had a heart attack but disregard for activity and diet restrictions	
6. Attempt to keep interactions on a social, humorous level; appearance of being overly cheerful	
7. Repetition of same questions to different staff members, as if "shopping around" for desired answers.	
B. Primary cause	**B. Primary cause**
1. Patient, unable to control the medical events, focuses on parts of existence that he can control; copes with anxiety or threatening situations by ignoring, rejecting, or refusing to believe that they exist.	1. Spouse perceives own past behavior as contributing to the patient's MI, *e.g.*, being too demanding.

(Table continues on page 574)

TABLE 44-1   NURSING MEASURES IN RELATION TO BEHAVIORAL RESPONSE PATTERNS COMMONLY OBSERVED IN MI PATIENTS AND SPOUSES (Cont.)

For Patient

C. Nursing intervention

1. Assess whether denial is inhibiting the treatment plan; is it verbal or active denial?
2. If verbal, listen but do not reinforce the denial or force acceptance of a fact that he is not ready to cope with.
3. If active (*i.e.*, if he disregards activity restrictions) assess the consequences of his actions. Are they detrimental? Conveying concern and allowing more control of environment are more successful than "threats."
4. Assess the threat producing the need for denial. What does this illness mean to the patient?

III. DEPRESSION

A. Manifestations

1. Sad look, listlessness, and disinterest

2. Expressions of pessimism or hopelessness
3. Short verbal responses
4. Slowness in movement and speech
5. Patient withdrawn (appears to sleep more, wants curtains to remain drawn).
6. Loss of appetite
7. Crying

B. Primary cause

1. Patient becomes less able to maintain denial, becomes more aware of what has happened to him, and begins to think about how it will affect his future.
2. May feel powerless, hopeless, or helpless
3. Thought content is centered on injury to self-esteem, particularly loss of job, independence, fears of sexual impotence, invalidism, and premature old age.

C. Nursing intervention

1. Voice your observations (*i.e.*, "You look really down."; "You seem to be depressed").
2. Let patient know that it is normal to feel this way and that depression is a common experience after a coronary.
3. Solicit and listen to the patient's feelings, assess how he perceives his illness.
4. Allow and encourage tearfulness or crying; can be done either verbally or nonverbally, through your presence or use of touch, or both.
5. Manipulate environment, *e.g.*, radio, television, reading material; increase or decrease the number of visitors.
6. Encourage participation in hospital rehabilitation programs that emphasize early mobilization.

IV. ANGER

A. Manifestations

1. Open opposition to treatment regimen, *e.g.*, removing monitor leads, refusing oxygen or IV line

2. Expressions of disappointment or frustration, *e.g.*, "I'll never get that promotion."
3. Passive-aggressive behavior, *e.g.*, forgetful of restrictions, getting out of bed
4. Sarcasm

5. Withdrawal, depression
6. Voices anger or resentment which may be directed at staff, spouse, or aspects of the treatment program *e.g.*, diet, activity restrictions.

For Spouse

C. Nursing intervention

1. Allow spouse to express feelings of guilt.

2. Help interpret facts for spouse, (*i.e.*, multiple causes of a MI).

3. If spouse's behavior is interfering with patient's care, place restrictions on her behavior, *i.e.*, limit visiting time.

III. DEPRESSION

A. Manifestations

1. Sad look, listlessness, and disinterest in anything except spouse and effects of this event on self and family.
2. Expressions of pessimism or hopelessness
3. Change in sleep patterns
4. Change in appetite
5. Tearfulness, crying

B. Primary cause

1. Spouse begins to think about the impact of this event on their future relationship (may be concerned about a temporary role reversal).

2. Spouse may feel powerless to help the patient.
3. Spouse's depression may result from patient's depression or emotional state.

C. Nursing intervention

1. Voice your observations of spouse's behavior.

2. Prepare spouse for possible occurrence of these feelings (in self as well as the patient).

3. Provide opportunity for spouse to express concerns.

4. Allow tearfulness and crying and be supportive through your presence or use of touch, or both.

IV. ANGER

A. Manifestations

1. Expressions of disappointment or frustration, *e.g.*, "We'll never be able to take that vacation we had planned."
2. Passive-aggressive behavior, *e.g.*, not honoring visiting regulations
3. Withdrawal or depression when away from patient

4. Spouse may speak angrily to people or about situations that she perceives as being responsible or contributing to the patient's coronary, *e.g.*, boss, children, marital problems, or the patient's life-style.

TABLE 44-1   NURSING MEASURES IN RELATION TO BEHAVIORAL RESPONSE PATTERNS COMMONLY OBSERVED IN MI PATIENTS AND SPOUSES (Cont.)

For Patient

B. Primary causes
1. Feelings of frustration and loss of self-esteem
2. Feelings of disappointment (in self, spouse, etc.), a sense of unfairness or a feeling of unmet needs
3. An assertive protection against feelings of helplessness or loss of control
4. Guilt feelings for having temporarily abandoned his responsibilities

C. Nursing intervention
1. Acknowledge the angry or hostile feelings, *i.e.*, listen to patient without reproach.
2. Explore the cause of the anger (it may be appropriate).
3. Let the patient know that these feelings are normal.
4. Be matter-of-fact about the patient's expressions of anger to prevent him from feeling guilty about being angry.
5. If the patient becomes extremely hostile or angry, do not try to clarify or reason with him at the time.

For Spouse

B. Primary causes
1. Feelings of frustration caused by mate's illness
2. Feelings of disappointment (in mate, self, etc.), a sense of unfairness or a feeling of unmet needs.
3. An assertive protection against feelings of helplessness or loss of control

C. Nursing intervention
1. Acknowledge the angry or hostile feelings, *i.e.*, listen to the spouse without reproach.
2. Explore the cause of the anger (it may be appropriate).
3. Let the spouse know that these feelings are normal.
4. Be matter-of-fact about the spouse's expressions of anger to prevent feeling guilty about being angry.
5. If the spouse becomes extremely hostile or angry, take her away from the patient area. Do not try to clarify or reason with her at the time.
6. Explain the patient's behavior to the spouse, *i.e.*, that he may not really be angry at her but that she is a safe target on which he can vent these feelings.

V. AGGRESSIVE SEXUAL BEHAVIOR

A. Manifestations
1. Frequent seductive comments (*i.e.*, overt bids for dates after discharge)
2. Flirtatious compliments, frequently accompanied by attempts to hold, fondle, or kiss parts of the nurse's body
3. Deliberate exposure of genitals while being assisted with bath, use of urinal, linen change, and so forth
4. Frequent boasts about past sexual interests and prowess

B. Primary Cause
1. Fear of sexual inadequacy or impotence compounded by forced position of dependency, loss of self-sufficiency, and loss of physical strength; the perceived threat produces anxiety; the aggressive sexual behavior attempts to counteract the anxiety

C. Nursing Intervention
1. Assess what the patient is seeking by this behavior.
2. If the patient's sexual behavior makes you uncomfortable and is unacceptable by your standards, be very honest and simply tell him that.
3. Ask the patient if there was something that you might have done to stimulate his behavior.
4. Accept the patient's flirtatious compliments, since they are frequently an attempt to bolster his ego.
5. Assess previous patterns of sexual activity (refer to Chap. 46).
6. Arrange sexual counseling for patient and spouse prior to discharge (refer to Chap. 46).
7. Identify patient or family, or both, who may have physical or psychologic problems and make appropriate community referral (rehabilitation programs, risk-factor reduction clinics, psychologic counseling, etc.).

---

pate, plan, and prepare the patient and family during these periods.

The need for a consistent nurse on each shift cannot be overemphasized. The patient and family need to relate to the same nurse in order to develop trust and an understanding of the scope of assistance available. The nurse, in turn, has the advantage of being able to assess, coordinate, and institute a plan of nursing care based on a knowledge of the patient as an individual. This consistent contact provides an opportunity to observe more accurately any changes in the patient's physical and behavioral responses. At the same time, the nurse will know what information has been given the patient and family, and can better evaluate what they understand and what must be clarified or reexplained.

The nurse has a primary role in assessing the patient and planning patient care. Since the patient's expectations are based on previous experience, the nurse needs to assess or gather information about the patient's earlier experiences with illness, hospitalization, and with relatives or friends who have had heart attacks. Because the patient's past experiences may influence or color his expectations of the current situation, the nurse is in a position to alter the plan of care as need be. For example, a patient may tell the nurse that a previous hospitalization was very upsetting because the physicians and nurses never explained anything. On the basis of this information, the nurse may make an additional effort to explain daily routines and what the patient can anticipate during the remainder of hospitalization. The patient's need for information should be written on the nursing care plan and communicated to the staff on the other shifts. Learning the manner in which the patient has reacted to stress in the past will provide the nurse with a basis for comparing his response to the current situation. If the patient is asked how he has handled stress in the past, at work or at home, he may explain that he tends to get very angry but holds his feelings in. This gives the nurse a clue that it may be more difficult for this patient to express his feelings, and that depression may be anticipated.

How successful the specific nursing interventions will be in reducing and alleviating anxiety depends on the nurse's ability to listen, observe, and solicit information with which to identify the patient's perception of his condition as it changes from day to day. Initially, the patient's anxiety may be "free-floating"; he knows he is anxious but he cannot identify the cause or causes. As time progresses, he will be able to identify and admit the cause of his anxiety. For example, the patient may state that his primary concern is fear that he will not be able to return to his former job as a fireman. Once the cause of the anxiety has been identified, the nurse and patient can look at it realistically. Is there something that the nurse, the patient, or someone else can do to change the situation? If not, the nurse can acknowledge an understanding of the patient's concern, indicating at the same time that there is nothing that can be done about it right now. Attempts should be made to bring the patient back to the reality of the current situation. This approach may not alleviate the patient's concern, but it may redirect his focus to something he can do immediately.

In the same vein, information concerning the spouse's anxiety should be collected to identify appropriate interventions. The nurse should assess the degree or level of the spouse's anxiety, previous methods of coping with stress, and available support system. What is the spouse's perception of the problem? Is it realistic? For many spouses, the patient's heart attack may precipitate a crisis. Feelings of helplessness and isolation may exaggerate the panic and disorganized behavior that is frequently observed. For example, a nursing assessment may reveal that a spouse has never before experienced such stress and, as a result, feels very helpless, with no idea of whom to call or what to do. This brief assessment suggests that the spouse is facing a new experience or problem that cannot be readily solved by using coping mechanisms that have worked in the past. Under these circumstances the nurse should take an active role in temporarily assisting the spouse to make decisions and plan short-term activities.

Periodic interviews with the spouse or family members can provide necessary information to validate the nursing assessment of the patient's responses. Soliciting expressions of concern and questions from the patient and family demonstrates that the nurse is prepared to assist the patient and identify what is expected of him in his new role as patient.

Too frequently, patients learn informally and haphazardly how to be a "good patient."[9] ". . . I did learn what kind of information to report and to whom; what kind of information I could expect to elicit and from whom; what mood or feeling expression would be acceptable and to whom; what kinds of request for assistance would be responded to positively, and the like. I also learned what not to do or say."[9] This was written by a nurse about her own experiences on learning to be a patient. The situation described indicates that a patient can be inhibited from revealing his feelings and reactions, thereby causing significant information to be withheld. The patient may not know what information is significant and unintentionally neglect to report it. To avoid such a situation, the nurse should take the initial responsibility of explaining to the patient and family what is expected of them, what they can expect in turn, why certain questions are being asked, and what kind of information they should report. The nurse should tell the patient and the family that they are expected to ask questions and seek clarification. This is not just their right but their responsibility as well.

PREPARATION OF THE PATIENT AND FAMILY FOR TRANSFER FROM THE CCU

1. Begin preparation shortly after admission.
2. Explain that stay in the unit is only temporary.
3. If possible, arrange a meeting between the nurse from the convalescent unit and the patient and family before the transfer takes place.
4. Explain how environment and routines will differ on the convalescent unit (*i.e.*, methods of monitoring and ratio of staff to patients).
5. Emphasize transfer as a positive step toward recovery.
6. Try to avoid making sudden transfers, especially at night, since they increase anxiety and disorientation.
7. If possible, have a relative of the patient with the patient at time of transfer.
8. Begin nursing assessment and care plan in the CCU and discuss these with the nurse or nursing team that will care for the patient after transfer from the CCU.
9. If possible, maintain some contact between CCU nurses and patient after transfer to the convalescent unit.

PREPARATION OF THE PATIENT AND FAMILY FOR DISCHARGE FROM HOSPITAL

1. Begin preparation as soon as acuteness of the situation subsides.
2. Establish a multidiscipline approach (*i.e.*, cooperation between nurse, physician, dietitian, social worker), with the nurse responsible for coordination.
3. Go over some of the essential areas to be covered with the patient and family, including progression of physical activity, medications, and dietary modifications (see also Chaps. 42 and 43).
4. Prepare the patient and family for the emotional responses commonly experienced after discharge, which should include
   a. A warning that the patient may experience a "homecoming" depression. (It should be emphasized that this is a common temporary response usually associated with fatigue.)
   b. A caution to the spouse about the tendency to become overprotective and oversolicitious (*i.e.*, fear of leaving the house, monitoring of all phone calls, etc.).
   c. A statement to the spouse and the children that the patient is likely to be more irritable and quick-tempered during the convalescence at home.
   d. A caution to the spouse and children not to alter their normal responses or activities, in an attempt to maintain an unusually calm, placid environment in the home.
5. Provide the patient and family with information regarding their local medical resources (*i.e.*, phone numbers of paramedics, physician, and CCU) to allay anxiety and provide reassurance.
6. Provide information regarding local post-MI rehabilitation programs.
7. Identify the patient or family, or both, who may have problems (physical or psychologic), and make appropriate community referral (rehabilitation programs, risk-factor reduction clinics, psychologic counseling, etc.).

A final point in the discussion of anxiety is the nurse's role in anticipatory planning and preparation of the patient and family for changes or moves in his physical environment. Preparation for anticipated changes greatly reduces the stress and anxiety when the change occurs.[10] Before these changes take place, the nurse should become familiar with such guidelines as those in the charts on page 576 in preparing the patient for transfer from the CCU and discharge from the hospital.

DENIAL

Denial is a normal defense mechanism used to alleviate anxiety by reducing the perception of the threat. Here denial is defined as behavior that indicates a failure to accept either an obvious fact or its meaning to the individual in the situation.[11]

A person who is suddenly confronted with an acute MI has not had time to prepare for the experience of being a patient. He experiences a period of shock and disbelief, during which time the use of denial is common for the first 24 to 48 hours but may extend well into convalescence. The use of denial seems to be more prolonged in younger patients between the ages of 30 and 40.[16]

During the first few days of hospitalization, the patient must slowly work through a sense of "I can't believe this has happened" to an acceptance of the reality of the heart attack and its impact. At the same time, his perception and senses are numbed by sedatives and overwhelmed with new and frightening experiences. According to Levine,[13] "the patient may not be deliberately refusing to believe what has happened to him. He simply can't believe it." For many patients, the use of denial at this time serves a beneficial purpose.

Nursing Intervention

The nurse must first assess whether the patient's denial is interfering with the medical plan of care. Is the denial verbal or active? In other words, is the denial only stated, or is it manifested in the patient's behavior or activities. Temporary denial is a normal, functional, necessary, adaptive maneuver for many patients. It becomes subject to intervention when it is prolonged (1–2 weeks), or disruptive to the plan of care, or detrimental to the patient's welfare. This is considered active denial.

A common approach used by physicians and nurses to counteract this behavior is to threaten the patient with the possible consequences of his action. For example, "If you get out of bed and walk to the doorway, you may have another heart attack." The patient has more than likely already walked to that doorway several times before being seen. Nothing happened to him then, so why should he pay attention to the warning now? As many of us have learned from similar experiences, threats do not work.

Levine feels that denial has become a label of convenience which has decreased our perception of the patient's need.[13] This indicates that a patient's use of denial has come to mean he is viewed as not considering his condition to be as severe as the nurse or physician perceives it to be.

An alternative approach requires some adaptation on the part of the nurse and the physician. The first step is to assess accurately the likely consequences of the patient's not following the prescribed activity regimen. Observation and measurement of physiologic parameters (for example, vital signs, fatigue, shortness of breath) provide clues to the actual rather than the threatened consequences. By conveying concern and allowing the patient more control over his environment, the nurse will be more successful in altering or modifying his behavior. This may call for a compromise on the part of the physician to liberalize or alter instructions about activity, while the patient on his part agrees to function within prescribed limits over which he now has some control.

GUILT

The predominant feeling expressed by spouses of coronary patients is guilt. If the spouse is a woman, she feels greatly responsible. Women are likely to feel responsible for their husbands' attacks because they frequently see themselves as protectors of their husbands' health.[1,2] The expression of guilt and the continuous search for the cause of the MI seems most evident during the first few days of the hospitalization, particularly when the prognosis is still questionable.

Nursing Intervention

Allowing the spouse to express feelings of guilt may reduce the anxiety felt. The fears and self-accusations of many spouses are based on unrealistic perceptions that can be clarified by the nurse. Once the nurse interprets the facts about the causes of a heart attack, and the spouse is able to understand and accept these explanations, anxiety may lessen. Some spouses will hold on to their guilt until the feelings become too painful to suppress. If this occurs, the feelings may be transferred through anger onto other individuals. Oversolicitous behavior on the part of a spouse helps compensate for any feelings of neglect in the past. As long as this behavior does not interfere with the care of the patient or exhaust the spouse, it should be allowed. If the behavior becomes inappropriate, or interferes with the patient's care, then the nurse should intervene and place some restrictions on visiting time. A spouse is frequently helped when medical or nursing personnel give permission to go home for the night. The spouse who experiences much guilt may need this extra assurance.

DEPRESSION

After the first 2 or 3 days in CCU, the patient's shock of what has happened begins to wear off and reality sets in. Denial recedes as the patient's thoughts turn to how this heart attack will alter his way of life. At this point, the patient's concern may be centered on one specific anticipated change, or several life-style adjustments that must be made.

Such thoughts can lead to anger or depression, especially in patients between 50 and 60 years of age ("Why did this have to happen to me?").[16] On the other hand, the patient may feel guilty for having caused the heart attack ("If only I had quit that job or stopped smoking. . . ."). Feelings of helplessness are often present and reinforced by the forced dependency in the CCU. Depression may continue well into the convalescent period, at which time the patient may become more withdrawn and unwilling to participate in the plan of care.

Depression on the part of the spouse may not be as overtly manifested, but it is nevertheless a common emotional response to the situation, especially when future family relationships appear to be in jeopardy. Frequently the family's uncertainties are compounded by many misconceptions about heart attacks, their causes and effects. The family may experience further complicated feelings of guilt (aimed at themselves for having caused the attack) and anger (directed unconsciously toward the patient for becoming sick and upsetting future plans).[18] Since such feelings of anger and guilt are rarely put into words, they fester internally, giving rise to more extensive depression. Thus the goal of nursing intervention is to assist the patient and family to express these feelings in order to avoid the build-up of suppressed emotions and to clarify any possible misconceptions.

Nursing Intervention

It is not difficult to recognize depression and to reflect these observations verbally, for example, "You look really down." Such statements inform the patient or spouse that the nurse is concerned and willing to provide an opportunity to discuss the situation. Patients may become very concerned about their depression, particularly if they have cried. For many men, instability can be very upsetting and may prompt them to try even harder to hold their feelings in for fear of crying in front of someone. For this reason, it is important that the nurse tell the patient and spouse that depression is common and to be expected. By soliciting information and listening to the patient's feelings, the nurse can assess how this patient perceives his illness.

Caring for the patient who is severely depressed is an extremely difficult undertaking and can drain the nurse emotionally, especially when efforts to find a solution for the patient's dilemma prove ineffectual. Often the nurse, in turn, becomes mildly depressed. To avoid this cycle of depression, the nurse should not be overly solicitous in working with a depressed patient. It does not help a patient when the nurse takes command; rather it underscores his helplessness and increases his dependency and feelings of inadequacy. The best approach is to acknowledge that the patient is depressed, but expect him to do whatever he is capable of doing. The patient may become angry because the nurse does not seem sympathetic or helpful. While such a response may make the nurse feel uncomfortable, it is better not to take anger personally or become defensive, but rather to maintain a matter-of-fact approach and listen without showing approval or disapproval. This method of handling the situation will prevent the patient from feeling guilty for expressing his anger.

As with other kinds of emotional responses, the spouse often reflects the patient's depression. Since the spouse and the nurse are frequently faced with a similar situation, it is important for both to work closely together. To this end, the nurse should explain to the spouse that feelings of helplessness, frustration, and depression are normal responses. At the same time, the spouse should be instructed not to be overly supportive or protective because that will only increase the patient's dependency.

One final intervention that effectively reduces depression in postinfarction patients is participation in a cardiac rehabilitation program. Hospital programs that emphasize early mobilization with systematic progression of physical activity have demonstrated beneficial physical and emotional effects.[4] An active mobilization program has one strong advantage for nurses caring for depressed patients—it is something the patient can do! In a long list of don'ts—don't smoke, don't eat so much, and so forth—a program of progressive activity reaffirms to the patient and family that the patient is not an invalid.

ANGER

Anger is a response to the anxiety an individual experiences when faced with a threat that leaves him feeling powerless to deal with it. The patient who suddenly finds himself ill in a CCU may very well perceive his illness as a threat to his self-esteem, to his goals, to his role in family and society, and to his life. The behavioral response will be influenced by the perception of the threat. While anger and hostility are terms used interchangeably by some authors, anger need not be linked to hostility, but can be viewed as a normal response to illness. The feelings of anger that the patient experiences may be dealt with in one of three ways: 1. they may be expressed in an indirect manner; 2. they may be turned inward; 3. they may be openly expressed.

Since societal and cultural standards frequently do not allow overt expressions of anger, many patients find indirect ways of expressing this emotion. For example, expressing disappointment may be an expression of repressed anger, as indicated in the following statement: "We had planned to take a trip across the country when my retirement began next month, but now we will never be able to make it." On the other hand, feelings of resentment may be sublimated through humor and sarcasm, or through forgetfulness. The individual who constantly forgets activity restrictions or the visiting regulations may be expressing anger in a passive-aggressive manner. At the same time, feelings of anger can stir feelings of guilt which in turn further inhibit the patient from expressing his feelings openly. In such instances, the patient may withdraw to avoid showing his feelings. While the deeper feelings of anger may be internalized, the more superficial feelings generated by the forced dependency of hospitalization may be the only ones expressed openly. Thus it is not uncommon for the patient to transfer feelings onto those individuals who are in the immediate environment, including the nurse, spouse, or other close family members, especially if they are perceived as being less threatening and less vital to survival. The physician upon whom the patient feels more dependent is less likely to receive the brunt of the patient's anger.

The spouse may also experience feelings of anger and resentment based on disappointment in self and mate, a sense of unfairness, anxiety in the face of stress, and concern about the eventual outcome.[14] Since these feelings are rarely directed openly toward the sick patient, it is the nurse, social worker, or physician who may be the recipient of such feelings. Like the patient, the spouse may find outward expression of anger unacceptable, and therefore internalize it, or express it in less overt ways, for example, by passive-aggressive behavior.

Nursing Intervention

The basic intervention technique for a nurse facing an angry patient or spouse is assessment of the behavioral response. To carry out this function effectively, it is important to recognize that passive-aggressive behavior or frequent expressions of frustration about the medical regimen are often covert displays of anger. Conveying a sense of awareness that the patient or spouse is troubled, and a willingness to explore the cause, will provide an atmosphere in which feelings can be expressed. At the same time, the nurse must be prepared for two possible negative reactions: the support and understanding extended to the patient and family may be met by silence, or by an angry outburst. In this last instance, the nurse should endeavor not to take it personally or become defensive. Trying to defend, clarify, or reason with the individual at this point may only increase the anger. It is beneficial to listen and then explain to the patient that you will return to discuss this after you both have had an opportunity to give it some thought. It is important that you return, allowing enough time to lapse for the built-up emotion to subside and to enable discussion to proceed in a more objective perspective. Since patients frequently vent their anger at their spouses because they are the safest targets, it is helpful if the nurse prepares the spouse for this possibility. If the patient or spouse, or both, are able to share their concerns and vent their anger, they will be able to deal with the loss they are experiencing and move onward in the process of psychologic adaptation.

AGGRESSIVE SEXUAL BEHAVIOR

Very little has been written about aggressive sexual behavior in the cardiac patient. Even less has been written on how to deal with it. However, this type of exaggerated sexual behavior is quite common and can be observed in various stages of hospitalization and in patients of various ages.

A study by Rosen and Bibring[16] reports that this behavior was most common in 30-year-old male patients who had heart attacks, though at the University of California, Los Angeles, the nursing personnel reported that it was the 50- to 60-year-old male patients who displayed this behavior most readily.[17] The findings in this second instance may be related to the crisis encountered by men in their fifties as they shift from the active orientation of youth (with its emphasis on autonomy, virility, and external achievement) to a more passive outlook of later years. A heart attack can accentuate this conflict and intensify the patient's need to prove that he is still virile.

Psychiatric literature has proposed that inappropriate sexual behavior results from anxiety, which in turn causes the patient to regress to an earlier, sexually immature developmental level. In the male patient who has had an MI, sexually aggressive behavior attempts to counteract anxiety—anxiety that results from a threat to his self-image and fears of sexual inadequacy or impotence.[17]

Nursing Intervention

The nurse should try to assess what the patient is seeking through this behavior. What are the consequences of his behavior? What happens when the patient deliberately exposes his genital organs or makes frequent seductive comments? In many instances the nurse tries to ignore the behavior, then becomes uncomfortable, embarrassed, anxious, frightened, and, finally, withdraws from the situation.

To assess what the patient is seeking, the nurse must be aware of how she feels and reacts toward his behavior. Does she become embarrassed and flustered? In most cases the patient is trying to achieve some reaction to his sexuality or response to his overtures. If the nurse is aware of her reaction, then she may try to alter her response the next time the behavior occurs. How will the patient respond if she does not become embarrassed or flustered? He will probably change his behavior.

If aggressive sexual behavior continues or becomes more exaggerated, then the nurse may need to be more direct. For example, she may simply tell him that his behavior makes her uncomfortable, or she may ask if there was anything that she said or did to cause his behavior. In most cases this question will shift the uncomfortable feeling back to the patient. He may then say, "No," and apologize, or proceed to explain why he acted as he did.

The patient perceives his heart attack as a threat to his sexuality and attempts to counteract his fears of inadequacy or impotence through aggressive sexual behavior. Rather than focus on the patient's fear of sexual inadequacy, the nurse can assist him to feel adequate as a human being. Feeling more competent as a person may reduce his need to prove his masculinity.

Finally, sexual intercourse should be discussed with the patient and spouse prior to discharge. Aggressive sexual behavior gives the nurse an overt sign of the patient's fear and anxiety about sex. Not all patients exhibit this behavior, but all coronary patients, either in the hospital or after discharge, experience some anxiety about resuming sexual relations. Much of the anxiety is due to misconceptions and unrealistic fears that can be reduced through adequate sexual counseling. (Refer to Chap. 46 for detail.)

This chapter has presented a framework for viewing the process of psychologic adaptation following an MI. We have introduced the concept that reactions to an MI have a pattern, and that behavioral responses of the patient or spouse occur in a sequence. The pattern will be relatively consistent from one patient to another and from one spouse to another, but the duration of the phases and the intensity of the responses will vary.

The importance of assessing behavior from the perspective of the individual patient or spouse needs to be emphasized. The nurse is in a key position to observe changes in behavior, to recognize deviations from the usual pattern, and to help the patient or spouse move forward in the process of adaptation. To assist in the process, the nurse must be able to assess accurately the manifestations, identify the behavior, assess the cause, intervene, and evaluate the results of the intervention.

We conclude with the words of a respected colleague:

There seems to be an undue reliance on previously established facts—or a tendency to consider the textbook or journal presentation of a clinical condition or situation as representing the truth, the whole truth, and nothing but the truth. The facts are, of course, that individuals are unique and textbooks present generalizations, and that proof of truth in an absolute sense is nearly impossible. While we need to call upon our generalizations, we also need to be free enough and flexible enough to recognize the novel and incorporate this into our analysis of patient conditions and situations.[9]

REFERENCES

1. Adsett CA, Bruhn JC: Short-term group psychotherapy for post-myocardial infarction patients and their wives. Can Med Assoc J 99(12):577–584, 1968
2. Burke LE: Anticipatory Grief in Spouses of the Critically Ill. Unpublished Master's Thesis, UCLA School of Nursing, 1978
3. Carlson CE: Grief and mourning. In Carlson GE (ed): Behavioral Concepts and Nursing Interventions, pp 95–116. Philadelphia, JB Lippincott, 1970
4. Cassem NH, Hackett TP: Psychological rehabilitation of myocardial infarction patients in the acute phase. Heart Lung 2(3):382–388, 1973
5. Engel GL: Psychological responses to major environmental stress. In Engel GL (ed): Psychological Development in Health and Disease, pp 273–282. Philadelphia, WB Saunders, 1962
6. Hackett TP, Cassem NH, Wishnie HA: The coronary care unit: An appraisal of its psychological hazards. N Engl J Med 279(25):1365–1370, 1968
7. Harding GL, Merifield MA: Group intervention for wives of myocardial infarction patients. Nurs Clin North Am 11(2):339–347, 1976
8. Hellerstein HK: Rehabilitation of the post-myocardial infarction patient. Hospital Practice, 7:45, 1972.
9. Johnson DE: Cardiac care in the first person. In American Nurses' Association Clinical Sessions. New York, Appleton-Century-Crofts, 1973
10. Kiening MM: Denial of illness. In Carlson CE (ed): Behavioral Concepts and Nursing Intervention, pp 9–28. Philadelphia, JB Lippincott, 1970
11. Kiening MM: Denial of illness. In Carlson CE (ed): Behavioral Concepts and Nursing Intervention, pp 187–206. Philadelphia, JB Lippincott, 1970
12. Klein RF, Kliner VA, Zipes DP et al: Transfer from a coronary care unit. Arch Intern Med 122:104–108, 1968
13. Levine ME: The intransigent patient. Am J Nurs 70:2106–2111, 1970
14. Roberts SL: Hostility and Anger. In Roberts SL (ed): Behavioral Concepts and the Critically Ill Patient, pp 199–223. New Jersey, Prentice-Hall, 1976
15. Rollo M: The Meaning of Anxiety. New York, Ronald Press, 1950
16. Rosen I, Bebring GL: Psychological reaction of hospitalized male patients to a heart attack. Psychosomat Med 28:808–821, 1966
17. Scalzi CC: Nursing management of behavioral responses following an acute myocardial infarction. Heart Lung 2(1):62–69, 1973
18. Twerski AJ: Psychological consideration on the coronary care unit. Cardiovasc Nurs 7:65–68, 1971
19. Wishnie HA, Hackett TP, Cassem NH: Psychological hazards of convalescence following a myocardial infarction. JAMA 215:1292–1296, 1971

ADDITIONAL READING

Aquilera DA, Messick JM: Crisis Intervention: Theory and Methodology. St. Louis, C. V. Mosby, 1974
Crate MA: Nursing functions in adaptation to chronic illness. Am J Nurs 65(10):72–76, 1965
Gentry WD, Williams RB (eds): Psychological Aspects of Myocardial Infarction and Coronary Care, 2nd ed. St. Louis, C. V. Mobsy, 1979

APPENDIX **A**

A Message for Families

Our visiting hours are designed to provide the patient with the essential rest and care needed during his stay in the coronary care unit (CCU). Just as we plan each patient's medical and nursing care to meet his individual needs, we attempt to do the same with visiting hours. Visitors can be like medicine—in the correct amounts and at properly spaced intervals they can be very therapeutic for the patient. We will attempt to learn each patient's needs and incorporate this into his care.

Some General Guidelines

The CCU is open for visiting 24 hours/day except from 8 A.M. to 11 A.M. We discourage visitors during this period because the doctors and nurses are making rounds, x-rays and blood tests are being done, and the nurses are giving baths.

In order to provide time for rest and treatments between visits, we encourage you to plan visits about every two hours, and have them last 15–20 minutes.

Visitors are limited to two at a time.

Mealtimes are often more enjoyable for patients when they have company, so we encourage you to visit during these times: lunch, 12–1; dinner, 5–6.

In order to prevent any embarrassment on the part of the patient who may not be ready for a visitor, and to prevent other interruptions, we request that you always stop and use the gray phone outside the double fire doors. Identify yourself and the patient you wish to visit, and the nurse will tell you if it is appropriate for the patient to have a visitor at that time.

If you wish to speak with your relative's doctor, a good time for this is between noon and 3 P.M.

Phone Communication

In order to ensure that our patients get undisturbed rest, the hospital operator is not permitted to connect calls directly to patient's rooms while they are in the CCU. There is, however, a portable phone available for patients who need to place an outside call. It is advised to keep them to a minimum, and business calls must be approved by the doctor.

While your family member is in the CCU you can receive condition reports by calling this number: _____. Designate one member of the family to make calls inquiring about the patient's condition. This person can then give the information to other family members and friends. Your cooperation in this will enable nurses to devote more time at our patient's bedside.

We encourage you to remember yourself and also get adequate rest. If there are any changes in the patient's condition, we will notify you regardless of the hour.

There is a waiting room (visitor's lounge) on 4-West, down the hall from the K elevators. There is a phone in this lounge through which your relatives and friends may contact you. The nurses in the CCU can also contact you when the patient is available for visitors. A blackboard is in the lounge so that messages may be left for you when you are not there. The number for this phone is: _____.

Services in the Hospital

Across the hall from the waiting room on 4-West there are rest rooms and pay phones.

There is a cafeteria, canteen (a room with several food machines) and a gift shop on the first floor.

The cafeteria serves at the following hours:

	Weekdays	Weekends
Breakfast:	6:30–10:00	7:30–10:00
Lunch:	11:00– 3:00	11:00– 3:00
Dinner:	4:30–11:00	3:30– 6:45

The canteen is open 24 hours a day and is located at the north end of the cafeteria.

The gift ship is open 9:00 A.M. till 7:30 P.M. on weekdays and 9:00 A.M. till 5:00 P.M. on weekends. (Depending on the availability of volunteers, hours for the gift shop may vary on weekends.)

Hospital admissions office is located on the first floor across from the gift shop.

The chapel is located near the admissions office.

Additional Professional Services

In addition to the team of doctors and nurses, we also have a social worker, financial aide, psychiatrist, and clergymen who are happy to assist you or answer any questions. The CCU nurses can help you make appointments with any of these people.

In addition, we have a dietitian who makes rounds daily to discuss dietary preferences and assist the patient with menu planning.

Parking

Instructions on hospital parking are available in English and Spanish at the information and service center on the first floor. If the hospitalization will be more than a week, please see a CCU nurse for special parking permit information.

For a complete listing of hotels, check with the information desk in the main lobby.

We encourage you and your family to ask questions and to inform us of any special concerns you have.

45

Education of the Patient and Family

CYNTHIA C. SCALZI, R.N., M.N.

and

LORA E. BURKE, R.N., M.N.

A heart attack places special stresses on the patient and family, which affects their motivation and ability to learn. Experience with persons adapting psychologically to a myocardial infarction (MI), discussed in Chapter 44, shows that variations in readiness to learn are to be anticipated. The degree of adaptation varies with the severity of the infarct, the change in lifestyle it necessitates, the meaning that change in lifestyle has for the patient and those close to him, and the usual response patterns. Familiarity with the patient's common concerns and responses can enable the nurse to provide the information needed to facilitate movement through the stages of adaptation.

This chapter presents the authors' philosophy regarding the patient's education and the nurse's responsibility in this activity. Selected principles of learning and assessment of readiness to learn are discussed. The importance of communication between members of the health team about the progress and evaluation of teaching is emphasized. Tables are used to illustrate the objectives, content, and suggested methods of teaching for each of the stages of adaptation to an MI. The scope of content, instructional aids, and educational resources for teaching the patient with coronary artery disease and family are outlined and discussed.

STATEMENT OF PHILOSOPHY

A philosophy for educating patients and their families is based on beliefs and values regarding the teaching–learning process that determine and reflect what is presented. For purposes of this discussion, learning is defined as a change in human behavior that persists over a period of time.[4] Teaching is defined as an activity that involves the intention to produce learning but not necessarily success in doing so.[6] More specifically, teaching–learning can be viewed as an interaction between the patient who has a need to learn, and the nurse who identifies that need and provides appropriate information or responses. Often we are unable to know exactly how and to what extent providing information (teaching) contributes to or causes lasting behavioral change (learning). For this reason, it can be said that all nursing interactions with patients and families potentially contribute, in a broad sense, to teaching–learning. For example, each time nurses are with patients, they are assessing the needs of the patients, some of which can be met by providing information. Therefore teaching need not be viewed as a separate activity but rather as an integral part of nursing practice.

Inherent in this philosophy is the belief that patients and families have the right to receive information about diagnosis, treatment, and prognosis in terms that they can understand (see Appendix A). Where the patient is viewed as a member of a family unit to which he will return, it is essential that other members of the family be included in the educational process. Within this context it is a responsibility of the professional nurse to provide information that will allow the patient to make informed decisions or choices.[2] It is also a nursing responsibility to identify appropriate resources and to coordinate the participation of other members of the health team in the educational process. Finally, the individual's right to determine his own course must be respected, in which case he may accept, adopt, or reject the information that is provided.

It is important to note that this philosophy of the teaching–learning process has determined the principles of learning advocated here and the importance placed on nursing assessment. The principles selected reflect specific values regarding optimal conditions for learning. The factors to be assessed reflect the value placed on an individualized approach to the education of the patient.

PRINCIPLES OF LEARNING

Because of the complexity of factors involved in patient teaching (for example, intellectual ability, psychologic status, effects of illness) the following principles are recommended to guide the health team in their teaching activities.

1. *Learning is more effective when the patient is ready to learn.*[6] Experiential readiness and motivation together constitute readiness to learn. Experiential readiness means that the individual has had previous experiences which prepare or enable him to learn what is to be taught. Motivation, an incentive to learn, may not be present initially but may be developed through teaching. Redman points out that it is not unusual for a person to become motivated after he gains some knowledge and no longer feels at a loss.[8] An example is the patient with an MI who may be so overwhelmed by the numerous changes that need to be made that he may exhibit little interest in learning about his illness. Once he gains some knowledge and has some misconceptions clarified, he may become more motivated to learn.

2. *People vary in their readiness to learn about health because of the differences in their general educational background, intellectual ability, and attitudes toward acceptance of responsibility.*[6] These factors will influence the integration and the speed with which learning takes place. It should be noted that a person's educational level should not be equated with his ability to learn.

3. *Learning is more effective when the content is relevant to the patient and his problem.* Therefore, the sequence varies according to the problem.

4. *Learning is more effective when the patient participates in setting the goals.* If the learner assists in defining the goal, there is an increased chance he will understand the goal and will want to achieve it. The nurse can assess the capabilities of the patient and should determine whether the goal is realistic for the patient to meet, for example, the nurse will assist the patient to incorporate a program of regular exercise into his lifestyle.

5. *Learning is enhanced when associations between ideas are strengthened.*[6] Comparing the healing process of a skin laceration to that of the myocardium after an infarct provides such an association.

6. *Learning is more effective if extended over a period of time.* Because of the amount of material to be learned and the brief period of hospitalization, the patient's retention of information is increased when the teaching is carried out over the postdischarge phase. Repetition of material at that time will also increase retention.

7. *Retention of material learned is proportional to the number of senses involved in the learning.*[6] Thus the combination of printed material with verbal instruction is preferable to the use of either one separately.

The simultaneous employment of several of these seven principles make the nurse's teaching most effective.

ASSESSMENT

There are four objectives for assessing a patient and family for teaching:

1. To obtain data appropriate to them as individuals;
2. To identify the sequence of topics and the teaching methods to be used;
3. To evaluate the presentation and acquisition of the information;
4. To coordinate the teaching with the readiness of the patient and family to receive it.

When such guidelines are used, an individualized teaching plan will be the result. It will include what will be taught, in what sequence, when the teaching will be done, and the methods that will be utilized. The teaching plan will be based on information derived from the assessment of the following factors:

1. Demographic variables such as age, level of education, socioeconomic and marital status are easily obtained from the medical records and by interviewing the patient. This information can provide insight into the patient's home life, for example, his emotional support system and the financial resources available. Religious or cultural beliefs which might influence the patient's attitude toward the illness are also assessed in this category. The age and educational level of the patient are crucial in the nurse's selection of appropriate instructional aids, for example, evaluating the value of using sophisticated printed material as against simple audiovisual tapes (Fig. 45-1).

2. The patient and family's preexisting knowledge and misconceptions about heart attacks and the subsequent treatment and prognosis. Asking the patient about his experience or those of the family or friends often elicits this information.

3. The presence of risk factors for coronary heart disease: family history of heart disease, male sex, hypertension, cigarette smoking, high levels of blood fats (cholesterol and triglycerides), diabetes mellitus, physical inactivity, psychologic stress.

4. The patient's readiness to learn. Such readiness may be indicated when the patient asks questions regarding the disease process, treatment, prognosis, and such matters. To accelerate this readiness it is essential for nurses to encourage the patient and family to ask questions.

5. The stage of the patient's adaptation to the illness. Knowing this aids in planning teaching objectives. (Refer to chart on p. 589.)

6. On-going assessment of individual's major concerns or problems will determine the sequence of content that is presented.

```
┌─────────────────────────────────────────────────────────────────────────┐
│                                                                           │
│   Date of Admission: _____  Dx: _____   │
│   Date of MI:  _____  Cardiac Hx: _____    │
│   Date of Trans. CCU → COU: _____  Estimated Date of D/C: _____   │
│   Major Health Problems: _____    │
│   _____     │
│                                                                           │
│   Risk Factors: (Check, if positive)                                      │
│   _____ Family Hx.       _____ Hypertension      _____ Ambitious Personality │
│   _____ Smoking          _____ High Cholesterol  _____ Many Stresses in Life │
│   _____ Overweight       _____ Diabetes                               │
│   Activity Style of Patient: _____    │
│   Social Background: _____    │
│   M  S  W  D  Occupation: _____    │
│   Lives with: _____  Type of Dwelling: _____    │
│   Level of Education: _____                                 │
│   Hobbies:_____                                                 │
│   Patient's Primary Learning Interest: _____    │
│   Family's Primary Learning Interest: _____    │
│   Additional Comments and/or Significant Information: _____    │
│   _____     │
│   _____     │
│   _____     │
│                                                                           │
└─────────────────────────────────────────────────────────────────────────┘
```

Fig. 45-1. Cardiac patient and family education inventory. (Developed by L. E. Burke, 1976)

Content	Teaching Done: (Date & Initial)	Reinforcement Given—Date	Need for Further Teaching? Comments: (List any pamphlets or Teaching Aids Used)
Acute Phase			
—Purpose of CCU			
—Monitor alarms			
—Reason for restrictions in unit (Visiting)			
—IVs, oxygen			
—ECGs, x-ray, blood tests			
—Support hose—purpose			
—Moving legs in bed			
—Expectation of patient to ask questions			
—Reporting chest pain, SOB			
—Gradual progression of activity			
Preparation for Transfer From CCU			
—No longer need constant nursing care and observation (sign of progress)			
On Intermediate Care Unit			
—Progression from monitored to unmonitored bed			
—Continue to report any symptoms to nurse			
Preparation for Discharge			
—Relation of activity to healing process			
—Guidelines for evaluating activity tolerance			
—Continue progression of activity (such as driving, sexual activity, walking program)			
—Chest pain and treatment			
Teaching Re:			
—Medications			
—Need for follow-up with physician			
—Alteration of risk factors			

Fig. 45-2. Teaching record. (Adapted by L. E. Burke from patient education forms used at Grady Memorial Hospital, Atlanta)

7. Assessment of the patient's and family's anxiety and the effect of this anxiety on learning and retention.
8. A continuous assessment of the patient's and family's progress in the learning process, for example, how much retention and integration of information has occurred (Fig. 45-2).

SCOPE OF CONTENT

For various reasons, many patients do not receive instruction on each item listed in the chart on this page. Of those who do receive instruction on each topic, many will not remember being told about it and will need to be instructed more than once. Because the patient may initially not be interested in, or be able to deal with learning about the MI, and because the hospitalization phase is continuing to shorten, a few topics should receive priority. Topics which should be explained, clarified, and reinforced during the first month after an MI are the healing process and its relationship to the gradual progression of activity, guidelines for activity at home, warning signs expected, psychologic reactions to an MI, medications, and such community resources as the paramedics. The patient should be questioned regarding these topics on a return visit to a clinic, physician's office, or rehabilitation program.

When possible, all material listed in the chart should be presented to the patient and spouse at least once during the hospital course. Because of the stress caused by the sudden illness, and medications given to patients, retention of information during the acute phase is limited. This seems to indicate a need for printed material that the patient can take home and refer to after discharge.

TEACHING METHODS

Teaching is the provision of information to another person or group of persons. The three basic methods of teaching are lecturing, discussion, and demonstration. All three approaches will be discussed in this section. The choice of a teaching method is determined primarily by the content of the material to be presented, and the content is determined by assessment of the patient's major problems or concerns. It should be emphasized that the actual content and sequence of its presentation are determined by the patient and the family rather than by the nurse. In practice, most teachers use a combination of the three methods and interchange them as the situation warrants.

Lecturing

This is the presentation of information to a group using a highly structured format. Its strongest point is that it is an efficient method of providing a great deal of material to a few or many people. Depending on the lecturer's skills, it can also be an interesting way of learning. The weaknesses of this method are that it often does not provide an opportunity for student–teacher exchange and also does not

---

SCOPE OF TEACHING CONTENT FOR MI PATIENT

Risk factors
The normal heart and circulation
The coronary arteries
The disease process
Diagnosis of a heart attack
The healing process
Progression of activity
Suggested progression of activity during the acute stage
Suggested progression of activity during the subacute stage
Suggested progression of activity during the convalescent stage
The first 1 to 2 weeks after discharge from the hospital
A walking program at home
Activity guidelines
Sexual intercourse after a heart attack
Psychologic factors
Dietary suggestions
Smoking
Alcohol
Medication
Nitroglycerin
Community resources

---

guarantee that the student is actively thinking about the material being presented. Learning through the lecture method can be enhanced by adding elements of the other methods, for example, by providing a time period after the lecture for discussion of the material, or by encouraging questions from the participants during the lecture, or by adding some demonstration to the lecture.

The lecture method can be best used with MI patients in the postdischarge phase, in the context of a rehabilitation program. The patients are then in much the same stage of adaptation. Teaching hospitalized MI patients by means of classroom lecture is less successful for a few reasons: the patient with an acute MI has a short attention span, and is preoccupied with himself and his condition and therefore may not do well in a group setting. Patients find excuses for not attending classes when they have to leave their bedside. A successful variation on the lecture method, that of presenting the lecture on videotape, was introduced by Bracken and associates.[3] After the individual or group videotape sessions, a nurse visits each patient so that anything unclear in the material can be clarified and questions answered. The use of such an approach needs to be seriously considered for several reasons: the method ensures a uniform presentation of content, the teaching can be done by those who are most skilled, and more patients can be reached in a lesser amount of time.

Discussion

The second teaching method involves an exchange of ideas between persons. This technique is less structured than the lecture method and thus is more suitable for a small group. Discussion provides greater assurance that each individual comprehends the material. It also allows the teacher to adapt the material to the level of the group and to individuals in the group, for example, adjusting the vocabulary for people of lower socioeconomic groups, and providing a less structured learning environment. Redman[8] cautions one to look at the cultural values of the members of the group when implementing the discussion approach because this method is readily accepted by middle-class Americans, but not always by other ethnic groups. The discussion approach is probably best when a change in or a development of an attitude is desired. This approach may be used at any time with the MI patient but is particularly appropriate and advantageous for teaching on a one-to-one basis during the acute phase. At this time, the patient may be anxious or depressed and does best with individual discussions which allow him to express his apprehensions, interpretations, and so on, to someone, with some degree of privacy. The individual discussion approach is the ideal way to teach about more sensitive topics, such as resumption of sexual activity after an MI.

The major weakness of the discussion method is that it is time-consuming and therefore may be costly and inefficient, especially if a large number of people have to be reached. Bilodeau demonstrated successful use of this method with a group of patients convalescing after MI.[3]

Demonstration

The third teaching method, demonstration, can be defined as an acting out of a procedure accompanied by an explanation. This can be a demonstration of a motor skill, such as taking one's pulse; or of an intellectual skill, such as knowing under what circumstances to call the paramedics. The demonstration method is selected in order to provide the learner with a clear idea of how to perform a particular task. It is thus essential that the demonstration be accurate and clearly visible to the learner. It is beneficial at this point to allow the individual to practice the skill under supervision and in a setting that closely resembles the circumstances under which the activity will be performed. It is also helpful to provide feedback to the person on his performance. An example would be to have the patient check his pulse before and after an ambulation period, just as he would do after activity at home. The nurse would also check the patient's pulse rate in order to provide verification of his accuracy.

Instructional Approach

There are two instructional approaches: individual and group. When choosing which to use, one needs to consider several factors. First, whether the patient is ready to learn. If one were to consider teaching a group of five patients who have had an acute MI and are in different phases of adjustment and interested in learning different content, the group approach may prove less than successful. If one were to consider teaching this same group of five individuals a few months after their MI, the group approach may be quite successful and present great potential for the members to learn from each other. At this later stage, each patient has been experimenting with what he has been taught and has learned from trial and error what efforts have helped reduce his risk factors. These individuals are usually eager to share their experiences and knowledge, and therefore do well in a group setting.

Second, the amount of staff time available for teaching the patients and families is another factor that will influence the approach chosen. If the situation is such that only one nurse is available to teach, the group approach may be the only choice. Under such circumstances, printed take-home material should be available to compensate for using this approach, since the group approach is not the optimal way to teach patients in the acute phase.

The individual approach is appropriate and beneficial at any time when teaching the MI patient and family. It is almost essential if learning is to occur in the acute phase, and is highly recommended as the approach in teaching about sensitive topics. The patient who has a limited education and is not fluent in English, or who is emotionally unstable, seems to do best with the individual approach.

INSTRUCTIONAL AIDS

There is a wealth of printed material and teaching aids to assist the nurse in presenting information to the patient. Again, when choosing instructional aids, it is important to consider many factors. Information can be presented through printed material, audiovisual aids, and physical objects.

Printed Material. Printed material can take the form of diagrams or illustrations, pamphlets, booklets, or flip charts. When choosing printed material as a teaching aid, one should look at the type of print size, the complexity or simplicity of the diagrams, and the general format, as well as the vocabulary and sentence length. Important factors to examine are the accuracy of the information and whether or not the views presented are in agreement with the teaching procedure and standards of the institution.[6]

The use of printed material with the MI patient, especially when supplemented with individual instruction is much more successful than either approach used alone. There are several advantages to using printed material: it is always available, the patient is able to set his own pace of learning, and it is economical in the use of the instructor's time.

The amount of information to be taught to a patient with coronary heart disease continues to increase at the same time that the length of hospitalization decreases. When the patient is taught only by verbal instruction, retention is markedly reduced. It is estimated that the average patient remembers only 50% of the information given by the physician in a single encounter. Studies have shown varying amounts of recall, depending on the specific type of information provided.[5,9] A general finding is that as the proportion of information provided increases, the amount of information forgotten also increases. Another study showed that after discharge the MI patient has barely any recall of what was presented during the hospital phase.[7] This finding does not negate the need for teaching the MI patient during the acute phase of illness, since the provision of information frequently reduces the patient's anxiety. Limited retention emphasizes the need to use printed take-home material to reinforce what has been presented verbally during the patient's hospitalization. Refer to Figures 45-3 and 45-4 for samples of printed information.

About Your Medication .... NITROGLYCERIN

PURPOSE:

Nitroglycerin (NTG) used in the treatment of angina—a discomfort which results from an inadequate supply of oxygen to the heart muscle because of narrowing of the coronary arteries.

Nitroglycerin works within 3 to 5 minutes, to relieve this discomfort in 2 ways: (1) it dilates the coronary arteries, thus delivering more blood to the heart muscle; (2) it reduces the work load of the heart, thus decreasing the heart's demand of oxygen.

DOSE:

Your doctor has prescribed _____mg. (_____ gr.) tablets for you. Take 1 tablet every 3–5 minutes to relieve angina discomfort.

SPECIAL INSTRUCTIONS:

Place the nitroglycerin tablet under your tongue and let it dissolve. If you accidentally swallow the tablet, take another one immediately. **Nitroglycerin is ineffective if swallowed.** Do not drink liquid while the tablet is in your mouth.

A fresh nitroglycerin tablet will be bitter tasting and may cause stinging when placed under the tongue. If the tablet you take is not bitter or does not cause stinging, it is probably no longer good. Take another tablet immediately.

If possible, sit down when taking nitroglycerin.

Take one tablet every 3–5 minutes for any of the following symptoms:

—pain in the chest, neck, shoulders, arms, elbows, or between the shoulder blades
—pain in the jaw, teeth, or earlobe
—a tightness, squeezing, or pressure sensation in the chest
—a choking feeling in the throat
—a heaviness, numbness, tingling or ache in either arm, elbow, or hand
—a feeling of indigestion

If the discomfort has not been relieved after taking 3 nitroglycerin tablets over 15 minutes, call the paramedics or fire department to bring you to the nearest Emergency Room.

Fig. 45-3. Sample medication card. (Medication information sheet utilized on cardiac units, UCLA Hospital, Los Angeles)

Audiovisual Aids. One principle of learning stresses that retention is increased when more than one sense is involved in the learning. The use of audiovisual aids builds on this principle, since it involves sight and hearing. A mass of material is available in the form of audio cassette teaching tapes, film strips, and closed-circuit television films. Instructional aids of this type can be made by the nurses or purchased as part of a commercially prepared educational package. Use of audiovisual materials ensures a uniform presentation of content to patients and families, and this can be supplemented with individual follow-up sessions by the nurse.

Many of the same factors that need to be assessed during the selection of printed materials also need to be considered when choosing audiovisual aids. It is important to present material at the intellectual level of the patient. This is a factor that needs to be assessed prior to the purchase of teaching aids. If a broad diversity exists among the intellectual and educational levels of the patient population, a variety of materials may be needed to ensure an individualized approach.

Physical Objects. This category could include heart models, pills, pacemakers, or prosthetic heart valves that can be used in teaching the cardiac patient. Whenever possible, it is best to use the actual object rather than a model of it. This approach involves more than the senses of sight and hearing, because it allows the individual to touch the actual objects and become familiar with their size and texture.

Depending on the situation, the availability and sophistication of instructional devices will vary. It is important to remember that research has shown that the message presented to the patient is more important in terms of teaching effectiveness than is the actual channel of communication used to present it. Therefore, the importance of the content should not get lost in the attractiveness of the communication medium.

Resources. When setting up an education program for patients or when just looking for resources for teaching a particular patient, it is well to remember that several agencies within the community can often provide assistance. For the patient with coronary heart disease, one of the most valuable sources is the American Heart Association. Many of the local affiliates have a catalog or a list of aids that are available for patient teaching. This includes many pamphlets on coronary heart disease, diet, risk factors, angina, pacemakers, and so on. Booklets developed by nurses for teaching the patient with coronary heart disease are also available for purchase as a single item or in bulk from some local affiliates. Private publishers often send flyers to hospitals to advertise patient education materials. Some institutions develop their own instructional aids in printed form and have them mimeographed. The crucial element is the provision of take-home instructions which are appropriate and accurate.

RISK FACTORS

A short time ago you were told by your doctors that you have had a heart attack. Probably one of the first questions to cross your mind at that time was "WHY ME?". If you asked your doctors or nurses "WHY ME?", they probably told you that medical science has not yet discovered the answer to your question. Right now we cannot predict who will have a heart attack nor do we know exactly why certain individuals have heart attacks and others do not. But even though we don't have these answers, research has provided some clues about the occurrence of heart disease. For example, research has shown us that people with certain habits, attributes, and styles of living have an increased risk of having a heart attack. These specific habits, attributes, and styles of living are called *"coronary risk factors."*

You may be asking yourself "HOW DOES THIS AFFECT ME NOW THAT I'VE ALREADY HAD A HEART ATTACK?". (Basically, you are now aware that you have a tendency toward heart disease.) Now is the time for you and your health team to look at your risk factors and assist you in taking steps to either modify or eliminate them. *The goal now is to minimize your risk of future heart trouble.*

Below is a list of the physical and psychological coronary risk factors. As you read each one, think about whether it applies to you. You may wish to comment or use the checklist in the space provided.

RISK FACTORS	Yes, this applies to me
1. **FAMILY HISTORY OF HEART DISEASE:** The tendency for heart disease can be inherited. Do you have close relatives (particularly parents, grandparents, sisters or brothers) who have had heart attacks, high blood pressure or strokes in the middle age years?	
2. **MALE SEX:** Males between the ages of 35 and 55 have a six times greater risk than do women of the same age. After the age of 55, however, women quickly rise to the same risk level as men.	
3. **HYPERTENSION** (HIGH BLOOD PRESSURE): High blood pressure increases the work the heart must do to assist you through normal daily activities.	
4. **CIGARETTE SMOKING:** Research currently indicates that smokers increase their risk of premature heart disease by three to six times over non-smokers.	
5. **OVERWEIGHT:** If you are overweight the heart must work harder to pump blood to the extra area of your body. Your health team is available to discuss the weight range that would be best for you.	
6. **HIGH LEVELS OF BLOOD FATS** (CHOLESTEROL AND TRIGLYCERIDES): People with an increased amount of saturated fats such as cholesterol and triglycerides in their blood have a much greater chance of developing coronary artery disease. Because your heart attack temporarily causes the blood fats to increase, we cannot test cholesterol and triglyceride levels while you are in the hospital. Your doctor will be able to run this test two to three months after discharge.	
7. **DIABETES MELLITUS:** Persons with diabetes (high levels of sugar in the blood) have an increased risk of developing atherosclerosis. This means that fats are deposited in the arteries of the body, including the arteries which supply the heart with oxygen. If you are diabetic, it is important to control your weight and your blood sugar level to reduce this risk.	
8. **PHYSICAL INACTIVITY:** Some studies indicate that people who lead an inactive life or who exercise sporadically, run a higher risk of heart disease than do people who exercise on a regular basis.	
9. **PSYCHOLOGICAL STRESS:** Tension and psychological stress are considered by some to be one of the most important risk factors. Recent changes in one's life can also lead to increased worry, tension and stress.	

Fig. 45-4. Teaching tool for risk factor modification
Sample of printed educational material. (Burke LE, Cain R, Scalzi CC: As the Beat Goes On, Los Angeles, American Heart Association; 1976)

TEACHING—LEARNING PROCESS FOLLOWING MI
ACUTE PHASE
(SHOCK AND DISBELIEF)
Time: Approximately 24—48 hours after MI

1. *ASSESSMENT OF BEHAVIORAL RESPONSES*
   Patient: Anxiety, denial
   Spouse: Anxiety, guilt

2. *TEACHING OBJECTIVES*
   To reduce anxiety
   To assess major concerns of patient and spouse
   To begin to develop a trusting relationship, *e.g.,* clarify
   role expectations of patient, family, and nurse.

3. *TEACHING CONTENT*
   Initial and repeated orientation to all routines, equipment, and procedures
   On the basis of the nursing assessment of major
   concerns, provide necessary information, *e.g.,*
   causes of a heart attack/risk factors.
   Inform the patient of what he can expect from you
   regarding teaching, including the scope of content.
   Inform the patient that the nurses expect him and his
   spouse to ask questions.

4. *TEACHING METHOD*
   Individual instruction with patient and spouse
   Instructional aids:
      Teaching booklet to introduce scope of content
      Family guide (Chap. 44, Appendix A)

5. *EVALUATION OF TEACHING/EVIDENCE OF LEARNING*
   Reduction of anxiety, *e.g.,* reduced restlessness and
   hypervigilance of the cardiac monitor
   Ability to identify and express major concerns

SUBACUTE—CONVALESCENT PHASE
(DEVELOPING AWARENESS)
Time: After first 48 hours through discharge

1. *ASSESSMENT OF BEHAVIORAL RESPONSES*
   Patient: Depression, anger, aggressive sexual behavior
   Spouse: Depression, anger

2. *TEACHING OBJECTIVES*
   To prepare for transfer from CCU (Chap. 44, p. 576)
   To continue to reassess the major concerns of patient
   and spouse; to determine readiness and sequence
   of content to be taught
   To explain and discuss expectations during the convalescent phase, *e.g.,* daily progression of activity
   and reporting of any symptoms
   To assess understanding of information received, current level of knowledge, and misconceptions
   To prepare for discharge (Chap. 44, p. 576)

3. *TEACHING CONTENT*
   Changes in environment, routines, staffing ratio, and
   level of activity
   On the basis of assessment of major concerns, provide
   the appropriate information. Major concerns and
   degree of readiness to learn will vary, *e.g.,* primary
   concern of spouse on day 10 may be related to
   resumption of sexual activity, while the primary
   concern of the patient on day 10 may be related to
   return to work.

Daily progression of activity, diet, medication, tests,
and procedures
Reinforcement of invitation to patient and spouse to
ask questions and express their concerns. Emphasis
by the nurse of her role in providing and clarifying
information
Essential content prior to discharge: progression of
activity, diet, medications, medical follow-up, and
reporting of symptoms

4. *TEACHING METHOD*
   Individual instruction
   Instructional aids
      Printed materials
      Audiovisual tapes
      Physical objects

5. *TEACHING EVALUATION/EVIDENCE OF LEARNING*
   Reduced anxiety about the transfer process
   Cooperation by the patient in the progression of activity
   and in reporting any symptoms
   Increase in both patient and spouse initiating questions
   relevant to their concerns or problems
   Ability to direct questions to the appropriate member
   of the health team, *e.g.,* physician, dietician, nurse
   Participation in planning for discharge by asking questions relevant to changes in their life-style, *e.g.,*
   stair climbing, dining out

AFTER DISCHARGE
(RESOLUTION; REORGANIZATION; IDENTITY)
Time: Discharge to 1 year after MI

1. *ASSESSMENT OF BEHAVIORAL RESPONSES*
   Any or all of the previous responses

2. *TEACHING OBJECTIVES*
   To assess understanding of information received, current level of knowledge, and misconceptions
   To clarify existing misconceptions
   To provide the patient and spouse with additional
   instruction in content needed for setting realistic
   goals and for making informed choices
   To evaluate the acquisition of knowledge by the patient
   and spouse

3. *TEACHING CONTENT*
   Varies with the nursing assessment (refer to Scope
   of Content, p. 585)

4. *TEACHING METHOD*
   Individual or group instruction
   Instructional aids:
      Printed material
      Audiovisual aids
      Physical objects

5. *EVALUATION OF TEACHING/EVIDENCE OF
   LEARNING*
   Patient and spouse are able to demonstrate verbally
   the acquisition of knowledge, *e.g.,* are able to explain
   the proper use of NTG.
   Patient and spouse demonstrate behaviorally their
   understanding of information, *e.g.,* by reporting to
   M.D. sudden weight gain or a change in the patient's
   pattern of angina.

TEACHING—LEARNING PROCESS

The teaching—learning process has been defined as an
interaction in which the patient has a need to learn and the
nurse identifies that need and provides the appropriate
information or response. The charts shown here were
developed to outline the steps in this process for the patient
and spouse.

The first step is nursing assessment, or the collection of
information with which to individualize a teaching plan.
The factors to be assessed have been previously discussed;
they include demographic variables, the patient's or spouse's
preexisting knowledge, misconceptions and apprehensions,
and the stage of adaptation. This information will enable
the nurse to proceed to the second step of setting realistic
teaching objectives. Identification of the teaching content,

step 3, then becomes relatively easy, because it is based on the previous steps. For example, a nursing assessment may reveal that the patient is in the subacute phase of illness and is beginning to develop awareness (see chart on acute phase). The patient is exhibiting some depression and is at present concerned with what caused the heart attack. The nurse's teaching objectives are to assess the patient's previous knowledge and understanding of coronary risk factors and to provide needed clarification and information.

The fourth step is the selection of the teaching method and use of instructional aids. This is determined primarily by the content being presented. For the depressed patient, the nurse would probably make use of individual instruction, for example, the informal lecture–discussion method, with supplementary printed material (see Figs. 45-3 and 45-4).

The final step, evaluation, is an on-going process that has several important purposes: 1. to provide a measurement of the patient's knowledge and understanding; 2. to provide a basis of direction for future instruction; 3. to provide the nurse with feedback on the effectiveness of the teaching plan and process.

In conclusion, it is important to be aware that the patient with coronary heart disease, as well as his family members, experience numerous stresses during the acute phase of the illness. The stresses limit their ability to learn and retain information, and this fact has several implications that warrant emphasis. First, nurses have the responsibility for an on-going assessment of what has been learned and what needs to be learned, particularly during the outpatient phase of illness. The nurse must be aware of educational resources available, regardless of the practice setting, and be able to coordinate teaching–learning with other members of the health team. The use of printed take-home material provides the patient and family with an accurate source of information to which they can refer. It also serves to reinforce the content previously presented, while enabling them to learn at their own pace. Finally, assessment of the major concerns or problems of the patient and family determines the actual content and the sequence of its presentation. Guidelines for planning patient and family teaching are based on the adaptation model of Chapter 44, thus facilitating teaching as a part of the nursing process.

REFERENCES

1. American Hospital Association: A Patient's Bill of Rights. Chicago, American Hospital Association, 1975
2. American Nurses' Association: The Professional Nurse and Health Education. Kansas City, American Nurses' Association, 1975
3. Bilodeau CB, Hackett TP: Issues raised in a group setting by patients recovering from myocardial infarction. Am J Psychiatry 128:73–78, 1971
4. Bracken MB, Bracken MA, Landry GB Jr: Patient education by videotape after myocardial infarction: An empirical evaluation. Arch Phys Med Rehabil 58:213–219, 1977
5. Gagne RM: The Conditions of Learning, 3rd ed. New York, Holt, Rinehart & Winston, 1977
6. Joyce CRB, Caple G, Mason M et al: Quantitative study of doctor-patient communication. Q J Med 38:183–194, 1969
7. Redman BK: Client education therapy in treatment and prevention of cardiovascular diseases. Cardiovasc Nurs 10:1–5, 1974
8. Redman BK: The Process of Patient Teaching in Nursing, 3rd ed. St. Louis, CV Mosby, 1976
9. Waitzkin H, Stoeckle JD: The communication of information about illness. Adv Psychosom Med 8:180–215, 1972

APPENDIX **A**

A PATIENT'S BILL OF RIGHTS

The American Hospital Association presents a Patient's Bill of Rights with the expectation that observance of these rights will contribute to more effective patient care and greater satisfaction for the patient, his physician, and the hospital organization. Further, the Association presents these rights in the expectation that they will be supported by the hospital on behalf of its patients, as an integral part of the healing process. It is recognized that a personal relationship between the physician and the patient is essential for the provision of proper medical care. The traditional physician-patient relationship takes on a new dimension when care is rendered within an organizational structure. Legal precedent has established that the institution itself also has a responsibility to the patient. It is in recognition of these factors that these rights are affirmed.

1. The patient has the right to considerate and respectful care.

2. The patient has the right to obtain from his physician complete current information concerning his diagnosis, treatment, and prognosis in terms the patient can be reasonably expected to understand. When it is not medically advisable to give such information to the patient, the information should be made available to an appropriate person in his behalf. He has the right to know, by name, the physician responsible for coordinating his care.

3. The patient has the right to receive from his physician information necessary to give informed consent prior to the start of any procedure and/or treatment. Except in emergencies, such information for informed consent should include but not necessarily be limited to the specific procedure and/or treatment, the medically significant risks involved, and the probable duration of incapacitation. Where medically significant alternatives for care or treatment exist, or when the patient requests information concerning medical alternatives, the patient has the right to such information. The patient also has the right to know the name of the person responsible for the procedures and/or treatment.

4. The patient has the right to refuse treatment to the extent permitted by law and to be informed of the medical consequences of his action.

5. The patient has the right to every consideration of his privacy concerning his own medical care program. Case discussion, consultation, examination, and treatment are confidential and should be conducted discreetly. Those not directly involved in his care must have the permission of the patient to be present.

6. The patient has the right to expect that all communications and records pertaining to his care should be treated as confidential.

7. The patient has the right to expect that within its capacity a hospital must make reasonable response to the request of a patient for services. The hospital must provide evaluation, service, and/or referral as indicated by the urgency of the case. When medically permissible, a patient may be transferred to another facility only after he has received complete information and explanation concerning the needs for and alternatives to such a transfer. The institution to which the patient is to be transferred must first have accepted the patient for transfer.

8. The patient has the right to obtain information as to any relationship of his hospital to other health care and educational institutions insofar as his care is concerned. The patient has the right to obtain information as to the existence of any professional relationships among individuals, by name, who are treating him.

9. The patient has the right to be advised if the hospital proposes to engage in or perform human experimentation affecting his care or treatment. The patient has the right to refuse to participate in such research projects.

10. The patient has the right to expect reasonable continuity of care. He has the right to know in advance what appointment times and physicians are available and where. The patient has the right to expect that the hospital will provide a mechanism whereby he is informed by his physician or a delegate of the physician of the patient's continuing health care requirements following discharge.

11. The patient has the right to examine and receive an explanation of his bill regardless of source of payment.

12. The patient has the right to know what hospital rules and regulations apply to his conduct as a patient.

No catalog of rights can guarantee for the patient the kind of treatment he has a right to expect. A hospital has many functions to perform, including the prevention and treatment of disease, the education of both health professionals and patients, and the conduct of clinical research. All these activities must be conducted with an overriding concern for the patient, and, above all, the recognition of his dignity as a human being. Success in achieving this recognition assures success in the defense of the rights of the patient.

46

Sexual Counseling
CYNTHIA C. SCALZI, R.N., M.N.

The expressions of human sexuality—touching, holding, intercourse, fantasy—protect men and women against feelings of isolation, while offering an opportunity to be free of tension and stress. For patients with heart disease, however, the exact opposite is often the case. Sexual intimacy, particularly coitus, is frequently seen as stressful and even life-threatening.

The impact of a myocardial infarction (MI) for many patients engenders fears of sexual inadequacy. The two major fears experienced by MI patients are the fears of imminent death and the loss of physical capacity.[4] The loss of physical capacity is frequently perceived by patients as a severe threat to self-esteem and to their concept of masculinity or femininity. During the course of hospital convalescence the patient begins to question his or her ability to return to work, to undergo emotional stress, and to perform physical activities (work related, sexual, and recreational). "The patient experiences a general fear of being impotent to face the continuing challenges of life, and this anxiety is symbolized in the inability to perform sexually."[24] Without adequate sexual counseling, the patient and spouse must rely on their own knowledge, myths, and misconceptions to cope with their fears of sexual inadequacy, impotence, and coital death.

This chapter presents the need for counseling and the physiologic and psychologic factors that must be considered in sexual counseling. Counseling techniques are suggested. A framework for a nursing assessment of sexual patterns and guidelines for patient instruction are provided. The common sexual dysfunctions experienced by cardiac pa-

tients and the implications for sexual therapy as a method of treatment are discussed.

NEED FOR SEXUAL COUNSELING

Lack of effective sexual counseling and its consequences have been described in a study of male post-MI patients.[23] Of the population studied, two–thirds received no advice regarding sexual activity, while the remaining one–third received vague and nonspecific advice. Among these men, 65% reported a marked and lasting reduction in the frequency of intercourse. Permanent impotence was reported by 10%. The behavior patterns reported in this study, moreover, showed no consistent association with age or severity of disease.[23]

A second study, done by H. K. Hellerstein and E. H. Friedman, reported similar findings. Of 48 post-MI patients interviewed, 24 men reported a significant decrease in the frequency of sexual activity. When they were questioned about the cause of this decrease, the following factors were mentioned: changes in the patient's sexual desire, fear of having another heart attack, feelings of depression, spouse's fear, and symptoms of coronary disease.[7]

In a later study, R. Koller and others[10] pointed out that reduced sexual activity after a myocardial infarction may lead to frustration and marital problems, which in turn can impede recovery. It is imperative, then, that medical and nursing staff take responsibility for giving specific advice on sexual activity to MI patients and their partners. Nurses may be particularly appropriate for this role because of the close interpersonal relationship that develops between a patient and a nurse in a critical care setting.

FACTORS TO BE CONSIDERED

Physical Status of the Patient

The assessment of the patient's physical status will indicate when sexual activity can be comfortably resumed. The following considerations should be noted: the patient's general health and tolerance for physical activity prior to the MI; the extent of the myocardial damage; the frequency and severity of angina or arrhythmias; and the patient's ability to tolerate progression of activity.

Prior to discharge from the hospital the patient's physical status should be evaluated with either a low-level treadmill test, a Holter-type portable electrocardiographic electromagnetic tape recording made during moderate exercise, or by a two-flight stair climbing test, followed by a resting electrocardiogram (ECG).[21] The stair climbing test reported by Siewicki has been shown to provide a hemodynamic challenge similar to that of sexual activity. Before sexual activity is resumed, the patient's physical status should be further evaluated during a post-discharge visit to the physician's office or in the outpatient clinic by means of exercise testing (Chap. 18). Such testing provides specific information which the physician and nurse can use in counseling and which may also reduce the patient's fear about resuming sexual activity.

A more accurate physiological measure may be obtained by ECG electromagnetic tape recording monitoring of the patient's sexual activity in the privacy of the home. This test has been called a "sexercise" tolerance test[7] and provides the physician and nurse with definite physiological information on an individual, with which they can modify their future counseling and instruction.

Physiological Effects of Sexual Activity

Regarding the physiological cost of sexual intercourse, H. K. Hellerstein and E. H. Friedman provided the first important findings. They studied 48 post-MI patients and 43 normal patients prone to coronary heart disease to determine the differential effects of sexual activity and other daily activities. It was concluded that in both groups the physiologic cost of sexual activity is modest for middle-aged, middle-class, long-married men.[7] In the 14 patients monitored by Holter-recording at home during coitus, heart rate response was minimal, with the peak rate averaging 117.4 beats/minute (range 90–144). The average heart rate for the period 2 minutes before orgasm and two minutes after orgasm was 97.5 (range 85.0–102.2).

Blood pressure was measured during bicycle ergometry exercise tests at a point at which the heart rate was equal to that recorded during intercourse. The average blood pressure was 127/85 mm Hg at rest and 162/89 mm Hg at the peak heart rate which had occurred during coitus (see Table 46-1). However, physical exercise, such as riding a bicycle, elevates the cuff blood pressure in the arms, but not the central aortic pressure.[16] Since this latter pressure can be elevated in sexual activity, the blood pressure recordings reported here may not accurately describe the blood pressure levels during intercourse.

It was previously thought that coital positions which do not involve isometric exercises (for example, patient on bottom, or side to side) cause less of an increase in both cuff and central aortic blood pressure. However, a recent study by E. Nemec et al on normal males showed no significant differences when positions using sustained isometric arm and shoulder muscle contraction (for example patient on top) were compared with positions that do not use isometric exercise (Table 46-1).[13]

In some studies metabolic energy expenditures (METs) have been used in comparing the cardiovascular cost of sexual activity with that of other daily living activities (where the MET equals the energy expenditure/kilogram of body weight/minute of an average individual sitting quietly in a chair). The average man who has completely recovered from

TABLE 46-1 CARDIOVASCULAR RESPONSES DURING SEXUAL ACTIVITY AND STAIR CLIMBING

Researchers	Subjects	Activity	Mean Maximal Heart Rate (beats/min.)	Mean Maximal Blood Pressure	Pressure Rate Product (Heart Rate × Systolic Blood Pressure) 100
Hellerstein and Friedman	Males with ASHD;* average age 47.5 years	Sexual inter-course	117.4	162/89[1]	190
Nemec	Normal males; average age 29.3 years	Sexual inter-course	On top: 114 On bottom: 117	On top: 163/81[2] On bottom: 161/77	On top: 189 On bottom: 183
Siewicki and Mansfield	Normal males; average age 29.7 years	Stair climbing test	127	145/72[3]	185

1. Recorded during ergometric exercise on bicycles at heart rate noted during sexual activity
2. Recorded during sexual activity by use of an automatic ultrasonic device
3. Recorded by arm cuff method at specified intervals.

(Adapted from Siewicki B: All about Sex—After a Coronary. Copyright © 1977, American Journal of Nursing Company. Reprinted from the American Journal of Nursing, April, Vol 77, Nr. 4)
* ASHD = atherosclerotic heart disease

an uncomplicated myocardial infarction has a maximum capacity of eight to nine METs. Activity at maximum heart rate during coitus is approximately five METs for less than 30 seconds. During pre- and post-orgasm periods, the energy cost is about 3.7 METs. Thus the energy cost of sex for the average cardiac patient is relatively small. If the cardiac patient can walk on a treadmill at 3–4 miles/hour, climb stairs, or pass a Master's test without increase in blood pressure, heart rate, or electrocardiographic changes, his exercise capacity is 5–6 METs. This level of ability is well above the work requirements for sexual activity.[6]

Another common method for assessing a patient's readiness to resume sexual activity after an MI is the two-flight stair climbing test. B. J. Siewicki and L. W. Mansfield[21] evaluated the cardiovascular effects of stair climbing, using standardized measurements. Heart rates were obtained with a Holter monitor, and blood pressures were taken by the arm-cuff method at specified intervals. The mean pressure rate product (an indicator of myocardial oxygen uptake) fell well within the normal range of values reported by others evaluating sexual activity (Table 46-1).[7,13] Thus the myocardial oxygen requirement of this two-flight test is probably similar to that required for sexual activity. This requires that the health professionals counseling patients define a flight of stairs and explain the specified rate of climb. The recommended "two flights of stairs at a brisk rate" should be at least 20 steps in 10 seconds or 2 steps per second.[21]

An individual's fatigue and experience of cardiovascular symptoms during sexual activity must be evaluated in the light of previous research findings.[6,7,16,21] The physician may want to prescribe the use of nitroglycerin or propranolol to reduce the workload on the heart during sexual intercourse, rather than counsel abstinence. Exercise training in a cardiac rehabilitation program may be recommended. Research has shown that the physically conditioned MI patient can perform a given level of effort (such as sexual intercourse) at a significantly lower heart rate and lower systolic blood pressure than can the untrained cardiac patient.[22]

Psychological Effects of an MI

There are a number of psychosocial variables which may influence when and with what degree of comfort the MI patient resumes sexual intercourse. Two primary psychological responses have been documented: (1) anxiety that interferes with sexual functioning; and (2) depression or a grief response that alters libido.[5,7,17] Anxiety may result from a fear of possible cardiac symptoms or fear of coital death. The sexual partner frequently shares this anxiety and may communicate this feeling covertly, thereby reinforcing the patient's anxiety. Another factor that may contribute to this anxiety is the patient's perceived change in body image. The strong emotional symbolism of the heart may result in a severe body image disturbance, in which the patient describes himself or herself as being "less of a man" or "less of a woman." These feelings frequently disrupt communication between the couple and may lead to sexual dysfunction.

A study by I. Rosen and G. L. Bibring[15] describes the "middle age crisis" of men between the ages of 50–60, who are experiencing the conflict over the shift from the active orientation of youth to the passive attitude of later years. When a heart attack occurs, it accentuates the impact of aging and may increase fears of sexual inadequacy.

Many MI patients experience a moderate-to-severe depression secondary to losses incurred with the disease.[5,15] This depression, which is part of a normal grief response, may last for days, weeks, or months after the patient has been discharged. A decrease in libido, as well as occasional impotence, may be experienced during this period. In group therapy sessions, convalescent male cardiac patients have expressed feelings of diminished libido and fear of death during intercourse. They also expressed feelings of anxiety that exist at a preconscious level for many years following an MI; a feeling shared by spouses.[1,3]

Almost all coronary patients experience depression during and immediately after hospitalization. This emotional state involves an inability to invest emotionally in another person, and feelings of guilt. Moreover, these feelings are further compounded by the forced dependency of the hospital setting. The result is an erosion of feelings of self worth and sexual attractiveness. During this time the spouse can provide much needed support. Many husbands and wives of cardiac patients find themselves in a state of psychological trauma, wanting to reassure their spouses of their love and concern, and yet fearing the consequences of sexual activity. Their fears may be displaced into avoidance of sex, over-protection, or resentment of their responsibility for the health status of their partners. All these factors combine to create a climate which may be more detrimental to the patient than the underlying pathologic condition.

SEXUAL COUNSELING

The goal of sexual counseling is to provide the patient and spouse with information they need in order to make their own choices about sexual activity. The nurse's role is not to lay down rules, but to help the patient and spouse combat their fears, guilt, and lack of knowledge in this area.

Counseling Techniques

Information should be provided early in the patient's hospitalization. The topic can be introduced soon after admission to the cardiac care unit (CCU) by telling the patient that most individuals who have suffered a myocardial infarction are able to return to usual or modified activities after a period of convalescence. Sexual activity is included in the list of activities. During instruction of the post-MI patient and spouse, the topic of sexual intercourse should be included in discussions of physical activity. If printed material, tapes, or other audiovisual aids are used in conjunction with staff teaching, it is helpful to have a physical activity section devoted to this topic. Early inclusion of this subject may assist patients to voice their questions, fears, and fantasies regarding future sexual functioning. It also identifies sexual activity as an area that will be discussed by medical and nursing staff prior to discharge.[18]

Separate counseling sessions for the patient and the spouse are advantageous. Interviewing each one individually allows each the opportunity to express personal concerns which may cause discomfort if discussed before the other party. Patients may be concerned about future extramarital or casual sexual experiences, but may be hesitant to discuss these in the presence of their spouse. Spouses, on the other hand, may be fearful of coital death on resumption of intercourse, but reluctant to share their anxiety with their mates. A joint session prior to discharge ensures the couple of hearing the same information and gives the nurse the opportunity to reinforce information given in the individual sessions.[18]

For the purpose of sexual assessment and counseling, three sessions are ideal. Some couples may not need all three, and nurses must be sensitive to the cues the patient

and his sexual partner give in this regard. There is no standard. Obviously, privacy is an essential component of these counseling sessions. Unfortunately, this is often difficult to achieve in the usual hospital setting.

Assessment and Instructions. Table 46-2 outlines the assessments necessary for sexual counseling. The rationale for the assessment questions is presented and guidelines for patient instruction are discussed.

Sexual counseling is an important adjunct to the rehabilitation of all MI patients, although to date there are no published data substantiating its effectiveness. A current research project, however, has shown that patients who received appropriate sexual counseling returned to a pre-MI

TABLE 46-2 SEXUAL COUNSELING OF CARDIAC PATIENTS

Assessment	Rationale	Instructions

1. Previous patterns of sexual activity:
  a. availability of sexual partner
  b. frequency (e.g., times/wk or mo)
  c. average duration of coitus (8 min vs 30 min)
  d. usual time of day (a.m., p.m.)
  e. favored position(s) (male on top, male on bottom, side by side)
	1. Goal of counseling—a return to pre-MI level of sexual activity. Specific assessment of patterns (a-c) gives baseline information which:
	  a. indicates the need for sexual counseling
	  b. identifies *previous* stressful (physiologically and emotionally) sexual patterns
	  c. provides information needed to individualize instructions
		1. General principle: intercourse like any other physical activity places a demand on cardiovascular system. Recommendations:
		  a. adopt more familiar positions which impose less strain
		  b. patterns: avoid intercourse:
		   —after a heavy meal
		   —after excessive intake of alcohol
		   —when extremely *fatigued*
		   —under time pressure
		   —with unfamiliar partner*

2. Past experience with chest pain during sexual stimulation or intercourse	2. Not an uncommon experience. If the patient has had chest pain during sexual activity, increased fear and anxiety may be anticipated in the patient and the partner.	2. Instructions regarding the prophylactic use of nitroglycerin:
		  —take prior to sexual intercourse or any activity that the patient knows might precipitate chest pain
		  —apply information regarding the *purpose, side effects,* and *how to take* nitroglycerin

3. History of sexual difficulty 1–3 mos prior to the heart attack
  a. kind: women inorgasmia
   men erectile difficulty, premature ejaculation
  b. frequency: *how many times* in past 3 months
  c. surrounding circumstances (stressful patterns)
  d. medications before and after MI
  e. preexisting disease states which may cause sexual dysfunction (e.g., diabetes mellitus)
	3. Previous sexual difficulty, particularly impotence in men, appears to be a common experience. Periodic sporadic episodes of sexual difficulty are normal and commonly associated with fatigue and emotional stress. However, sexual difficulty prior to the MI tends to increase fears of sexual inadequacy and permanent impotence.
	Some drugs which affect sexual response are:
	—Reserpine: decrease libido, impotence, or both
	—Aldomet: impotence, lack of sexual desire, and disorders of ejaculation
	—Inderal: increased fatigue with decreased sexual desire
		3. Information should emphasize that this is a common experience that is frequently associated with stressful life patterns (fatigue, working long hrs, emotional stress, etc.)
		Under similar circumstances this may occur periodically after a heart attack, particularly if there is anxiety.

4. Patient and partner's understanding of when they can resume sexual activity	4. Expectations, information acquired, and misconceptions can be identified and, if necessary, clarified in the instructions	4. Resumption of sexual activity† (6–8 weeks after MI)
		  a. Physical conditioning programs enhance exercise tolerance and ability to participate in intercourse
		  b. There are certain warning signals patient should know and report to physician:
		   —rapid heart rate, rapid breathing or both, that persist (4–5 min. after orgasm)
		   —feeling of extreme fatigue the day after intercourse
		   —chest pain during or after intercourse

*There is a greater physical and emotional stress due to performance anxiety associated with new sexual experiences.
†Also determined by the physician's assessment of the extent of recovery and the patient's ability to tolerate progression of physical activity
(Scalzi C and Dracup K: Sexual Counseling of Cardiac Patients, Heart Lung 7(5):840–845, 1978)

level of sexual activity more quickly than did patients who did not receive such counseling.[20] Further research needs to be done in this area.

Instruction regarding sexual activity, as in other areas involving rehabilitation following an MI, requires coordination among the members of the health team and follow-up of the patient and spouse. Discharge often activates issues and concerns not felt during the period of hospitalization, which can be effectively dispelled by sexual counseling in the outpatient setting. This means that nurses working in community settings must be as knowledgeable as their colleagues in acute care settings with regard to sexual counseling of cardiac patients and their spouses.

During the hospital or outpatient counseling sessions, the nurse can assess the presence of longstanding sexual dysfunction (for example, inorgasmia, erectile failure) about which he or she feels unprepared to counsel. A referral for appropriate sexual therapy can be made if the patient or couple desires. For this reason, it is important to discuss some of the common sexual dysfunctions experienced by cardiac patients, and to differentiate between sexual counseling and sexual therapy as a mode of treatment.

Sexual Dysfunctions

The following discussion is not intended to cover all sexual dysfunctions, but only those commonly experienced by patients who have had an MI.[1,7,19,23]

Male Dysfunction. The two major manifestations of sexual dysfunction in post-MI men are erectile failure and premature ejaculation. Erectile difficulty may be experienced in varying degrees, such as failure of the penis to harden sufficiently, loss of firmness after hardening, or complete flaccidity.[8,19] This discussion is limited to the cardiac patients with secondary impotence, that is, patients who functioned well for some time prior to the development of their erectile difficulty. Premature ejaculation is cited in the literature as the most common of the male sexual dysfunctions.[8] Kaplan defines premature ejaculation as a condition wherein a man is unable to exert voluntary control over his ejaculatory reflex, with the result that once he is sexually aroused, he reaches orgasm very quickly.[8] W. H. Masters and V. Johnson define a premature ejaculator as one who cannot control his ejaculatory process for a sufficient length of time to satisfy his partner in at least 50% of their coital experiences.[11] Although reliable data supporting this phenomenon in a population of cardiac patients is not available, clinical experience suggests that secondary premature ejaculation is indeed quite prevalent in post-MI patients. Secondary again connotes that function had been normal before this sexual problem developed.

Female Dysfunction. Secondary inorgasmia is defined as an inability to achieve orgasm in situations where similar arousal in the past would have produced orgasm. Despite the lack of documentation, clinical experience suggests that temporary secondary inorgasmia is commonly experienced by women after MI.

Decreased Sexual Desire. This problem is characterized by an inhibition of the general arousal aspect of the sexual response and appears to be a commonly reported experience in both men and women after MI.[1,7,19,23] Both men and women experience impairment of the vasocongestive component of the sexual response. The woman has difficulty lubricating, while the man experiences erectile difficulty.

GOAL OF SEXUAL COUNSELING

The causes of sexual dysfunction in individuals with cardiac diseases is not precisely understood. Nevertheless, there are data that suggest a strong relationship between the lack of adequate information (inadequate sexual counseling) and the presence of fears and misconceptions with the development of these secondary sexual dysfunctions in both men and women who have had MI.[7,19,23] Sexual therapy is considered an accepted mode of treatment for existing primary or secondary sexual dysfunction.

Sexual Therapy

Until recently, sexually dysfunctional patients who were physically ill and disabled have been virtually ignored. However, increasing attention and clinical application of sexual therapy to patients with physical illness suggest a good prognosis.[19]

Sexual therapy has flourished in the past decade, stimulated by basic research[11,12] and a social climate in which public attention has focused on human sexuality. In brief, behaviorally-oriented approaches to the treatment of sexual dysfunction[2,3,8] are based on the concept that such problems are caused by sexual ignorance, performance anxiety and culturally-influenced inhibition. It is widely accepted that sexual dysfunctions are more frequently caused by psychogenic problems than by physical illnesses. This knowledge has resulted in a justifiable enthusiasm for treating psychogenic sexual dysfunctions.

One of the limitations of sex therapy is that in most of the university-based therapy clinics, treatment entails the participation of two cooperating individuals. The prescribed exercises which are crucial components of sex therapy are structured interactions between sexual partners. They simply cannot be conducted alone. This poses a problem for the single person with a sexual dysfunction.

Since the educational and clinical requirements for training sexual therapists is from one to two years in most university programs, this is not something that most nurses and physicians are qualified to do.[9] Nevertheless, it is realistic to expect nurses and physicians to assess and identify sexual dysfunctions and refer patients requesting treatment to the appropriate centers. There are sexual dysfunction clinics in most of the large university medical centers across the country, and at present these provide the most reliable treatment for patients with primary sexual dysfunction, or for persistent problems following an MI.

REFERENCES

1. Adsett CA, Bruhn JG: Short-term group psychotherapy for myocardial infarction patients and their wives. Can Med Assoc J 199:577, 1968
2. Annon JS: The Behavioral Treatment of Sexual Problems. Volume 1—Brief Therapy. Honolulu, Enabling Systems, 1975
3. Bilodeau CJ, Hackett TP: Issues raised in a group setting by patients recovering from initial myocardial infarction. Am J Psychiatry 128:73, 1971
4. Cassem NH: The nurse in the coronary care unit. In Gentry WD, Williams RB (eds): Psychological Aspects of Myocardial Infarction, p. 88. St. Louis, C. V. Mosby, 1975
5. Cassem N, Hackett T: Psychological rehabilitation of myocardial infarction patients in the acute phase. Heart Lung 2:383, 1973
6. Green AW: Sexual activity and postmyocardial infarction patient. Am Heart J 89:246, 1975
7. Hellerstein HK, Friedman EH: Sexual activity and the post-coronary patient. Arch Intern Med 125:992, 1970
8. Kaplan HS: The New Sex Therapy. New York, Brunner-Mazel, 1974.
9. Klein RF, Dean A, Wilson M et al: The physician and post-myocardial infarction invalidism. JAMA 194:123, 1965
10. Koller R, Kennedy JW, Butler JC et al: Counseling the coronary patient on sexual activity. Postgrad Med 51:134, 1972
11. Masters WH, Johnson V: Human Sexual Inadequacy. Boston, Little, Brown & Company, 1970.
12. Masters WH Johnson V: Human Sexual Response. Boston, Little, Brown & Co 1966
13. Nemec E, Mansfield L, Kennedy JW: Heart rate and blood pressure responses during sexual activity in normal males. Am Heart J 92:276, 1976
14. Puksta N S: All about sex . . . after a coronary. Am J Nurs 77:602, 1977
15. Rosen I, Bibring GL: Psychological reactions of hospitalized male patients to a heart attack. Psychosom Med 28:808, 1966
16. Rowell LB, Brengelmann GL, Blackmon JR et al: Disparities between aortic and peripheral pulse pressures induced by upright exercise and vasomotor changes in man. Circulation 37:954, 1968
17. Scalzi CC: Nursing management of behavioral responses following an acute myocardial infarction. Heart Lung 2:62, 1973
18. Scalzi C, Dracup K: Sexual counseling of cardiac patients. Heart Lung 7:5, 1978
19. Scalzi C, Loya F, Golden J: Sexual therapy of patients with cardiovascular disease. West J Med 126:243, 1977
20. Scalzi, CC, Burke LE, Greenland S: Evaluation of an inpatient educational program for coronary patients. Heart Lung 9:846, 1980
21. Siewicki BJ, Mansfield LW: Determining readiness to resume sexual activity. In All about sex . . . after a coronary, Am J Nurs 77:604, 1977
22. Stein RA: The effect of exercise training on heart rate during coitus in the post-myocardial infarction patient. Circulation 55:738, 1977
23. Tuttle WB, Cook WL, Fitch E: Sexual behavior in post-myocardial infarction patients. Am J Cardiol 13:140, 1964
24. Wagner NN: Some sexual aspects of the rehabilitation of cardiac patients. In Stockmeier U (ed): Psychological Approach to the Rehabilitation of Coronary Patients, p 119. New York, Springer-Verlag, 1976

SELECTED CARDIOVASCULAR PROBLEMS

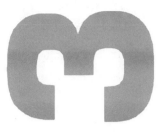

PART 3

47

High Blood Pressure
KATHRYN A. LEE, R.N., M.N.

High blood pressure is the most common risk factor of cardiovascular disease in developed and developing countries today. In Europe and in the United States, the past 30 years have seen a slow decline in the mortality rate from hypertensive heart disease, primarily because of the development of successful therapy with antihypertensive drugs.

This chapter will include definitions and classifications of high blood pressure, the pathophysiologic processes involved, and the management strategies relative to the field of nursing. For a discussion of antihypertensive medications, see Chapter 37. For a review of physiologic mechanisms controlling normal blood pressure, refer to Chapters 5 and 6.

DEFINITIONS

High blood pressure, or systemic arterial hypertension, is not a single disease state but a disorder with many causes, a variety of symptoms, and a range of responses to therapy. Hypertension is best thought of as a pressure somewhere on the high end of a continually rising scale. The greater the blood pressure, systolic or diastolic, the higher are the morbidity and mortality, regardless of age, sex, and ethnicity. The difficulty of distinguishing normal from abnormal blood pressure makes any definition of hypertension an arbitrary one.

The World Health Organization[154] reviewed the standard deviations from the normal population curve for blood pressures and arbitrarily defined "normal" blood pressure as that at or below the 95th percentile of the population, or as below either 140 mm Hg systolic or 90 mm Hg diastolic (using disappearance of the fifth Korotkoff sound) in the adult. "Borderline" hypertension encompasses values between 140/90 mm Hg and 160/95 mm Hg, and "definite" hypertension is 160/95 mm Hg and higher. For children, hypertension is defined by pressures above the 95th percentile (Table 47-1).

For therapists to deal effectively with hypertension, researchers have additionally defined a range of diastolic blood pressure levels for mild, moderately severe, and severe hypertension. Mild hypertension ranges from 90 to 104 mm Hg diastolic and applies to about 75% of the population with high blood pressure.[37] Moderately severe hypertension ranges from 105 mm Hg to 114 mm Hg diastolic and applies to about 15% of the population with high blood pressure. About 10% of the hypertensive population is severely hypertensive, with diastolic pressures of 115 mm Hg and greater.[69]

Many researchers prefer to adjust their definitions to fit age groups rather than standard deviations from the mean for an entire population. These definitions allow a higher range of normal for the older adult. However, blood pressure does not appear to increase with age in isolated societies where atherosclerosis is not a significant problem and where the prevalence of hypertension and obesity in the elderly is low. An operational definition of hypertension in adults, such as Kapan's[74] appears to be clinically useful. He bases his definition of hypertension on blood pressure levels associated with a 50% increase in mortality rates: males under age 45 with a blood pressure greater than 130/90 mm Hg; males over 45 with a pressure greater than 145/95 mm Hg; and all adult females with pressures greater than 160/95 mm Hg.

TABLE 47-1   BLOOD PRESSURE LEVELS AT THE 95TH PERCENTILE IN CHILDREN, BY AGE GROUP

Age	Systolic Pressure	Diastolic Pressure	Mean Arterial Pressure
0–6 months	110	60	77
6 months–3 years	112	80	91
4–5 years	115	84	94
6–10 years	130	90	103
11–15 years	138	90	106
16–21 years	140	90	107

In children, high blood pressure is defined as a pressure, diastolic or systolic, above the 95th percentile. Diastolic pressure stabilizes from age 6, whereas systolic pressure continues to rise slowly throughout adolescence.

(Richard GA et al: Adv Pediatr 24:339–398, 1977. Copyright © 1977 by Year Book Medical Publishers, Inc, Chicago. Reproduced with permission)

CLASSIFICATIONS OF HIGH BLOOD PRESSURE

High blood pressure can be graded as mild, moderate, or severe, according to the levels of pressure (see above) or it can be referred to by the degree of its severity: labile, benign, or malignant (accelerated). These terms, however, give no clue as to etiology, and are often misleading.[83] "Labile" (sometimes called borderline or prehypertension) hypertension is a meaningless term, since everyone exhibits fluctuations in blood pressure. About 10% of all hypertensive individuals are classified as labile, and only 25% of these people progress to sustained hypertension; the term "benign" has a false association with lower morbidity; and "malignant" hypertension, often reversible with proper treatment, is not always fatal. High blood pressure is most often classified by etiology as idiopathic (primary, essential) if the cause is unknown, or secondary if the causative factor is evident.

Idiopathic (Primary, Essential) Hypertension

It was originally thought among the medical professionals that, if no cause for a person's hypertension could be determined, a higher blood pressure must be necessary ("essential") for getting blood through narrowed arterioles. It was felt that any attempt to lower that pressure would result in inadequate perfusion to the tissues. At least 90% of all hypertensive adults have no medically discernible disorder responsible for their high blood pressure, at least with the current level of diagnostic knowledge available. But it has been demonstrated repeatedly that the original hypothesis was in error; lowering blood pressure will reduce morbidity and mortality rates.

Prevalence of Idiopathic Hypertension. The results of epidemiologic studies conclude that approximately 20% to 30% of American adults (25 million people) have idiopathic hypertension at a value of 160/95 mm Hg and higher. Less than 1% of children and 3% to 4% of adolescents are affected, but hypertension affects 70% of persons over age 40.[37,52]

There are marked geographic differences in blood pressures between and within ethnic groups. A survey conducted in 1973 found that the prevalence of hypertension among persons with low annual incomes (less than $5,000) was three times that of persons with incomes higher than $15,000.[54] In the United States, the prevalence is twice as high for urban blacks as for urban whites of all ages and incomes. The likelihood of developing hypertension appears to be highest among black women, with black men a close second.

Subcategories of Idiopathic Hypertension. According to some researchers, subcategories of idiopathic hypertension can be based on plasma renin activity.[85] Plasma renin activity indicates how much renin-induced vasoconstriction is maintaining the blood pressure at any given point in time and varies with the state of sodium balance. In the presence of water deficit or excess body sodium, for example, fluid volume increases and maintains the blood pressure, thereby reducing the need for renin (see Chap. 6 for mechanisms maintaining normal blood pressure).

About 30% of the cases of idiopathic hypertension are characterized by low plasma renin activity.[84] Low plasma renin activity levels are evident in conditions of expanded fluid volume, catecholamine deficiency, and hyperkalemia (Table 47-2). Response to diuretic therapy is highly successful in this group. High plasma renin activity, occurring under conditions of depleted fluid volume, diminished renal

TABLE 47-2   FACTORS INFLUENCING PLASMA RENIN ACTIVITY

	Factors Inhibiting Renin Release	Factors Stimulating Renin Release
FLUID VOLUME	EXPANSION Excess sodium Increased fluids Excess mineralocorticoids Supine posture	DEFICIT Sodium restriction Fluid loss due to diuretics, hemorrhage, or gastrointestinal losses Upright posture
CATECHOLAMINE	DEFICIT resulting primarily from adrenergic blocker agents	EXCESS resulting primarily from 1. stress 2. hypoglycemia 3. trauma 4. exercise 5. hyperthyroidism 6. pheochromocytoma
ANTIHYPERTENSIVE DRUG THERAPY	Propranolol Methyldopa Reserpine Clonidine Guanethidine Prazosin	Thiazides Spiroaldactone Diazoxide Nitroprusside Hydralazine Furosemide
RENAL CONDITIONS	Decreased renal tissue	Decreased renal perfusion pressure
SERUM POTASSIUM	Hyperkalemia	Hypokalemia

The status of fluid volume, catecholamine level, potassium level, and drugs are some factors known to influence the amount of renin released.

(After Kaplan NM: Clinical Hypertension, 2nd ed. Baltimore, Williams & Wilkins, 1978; Laragh JH: Hosp Pract 9(1):61–73, 1974; Moser M: Hypertension: A Practical Approach. Boston, Little, Brown & Co, 1975)

perfusion, and catecholamine excess, accounts for about 15% of the cases of idiopathic hypertension.[84] Individuals with high plasma renin respond well to beta-adrenergic blocking agents such as propranolol (Inderal).

The majority of hypertensive persons have a normal level of plasma renin activity. It may be that a normal renin level is the only true indicator of idiopathic hypertension and that further research into low and high renin levels will reveal distinct pathologic causes.

Secondary Hypertension

Although secondary hypertension affects less than 10% of all hypertensive adults, more than 80% of the hypertension that occurs during childhood is secondary to a specific physiological condition.[52] Table 47-3 summarizes the types of health problems that occur with, or lead to, hypertension in children as well as adults. In addition to fluid overload, hypertension can be induced by drugs and foods, organ dysfunction, tumors, and pregnancy.

Exogenous Compounds. Hypertension can result from a wide variety of exogenous agents. Vasoconstriction can result from chronic use of sympathomimetic drugs. (See Table 37-3 for a list of over-the-counter medications containing sympathomimetic agents.) Nicotine and caffeine can increase blood pressure by stimulating release of catecholamines and stimulating the myocardium. Amphetamines and tricyclic antidepressants (imipramine derivatives) can induce hypertension by preventing the reuptake of catecholamines. Patients taking tricyclic antidepressants and the antihypertensive agent guanethidine may experience severe hypertension if the antidepressant is suddenly discontinued.

Hypertension can result from stimulation of mineralocorticoid activity following administration of adrenocorticotropin hormone (ACTH) or corticosteroids. Exogenous steroid therapy causes the adrenals to release ACTH-sensitive mineralocorticoids which act to retain sodium and thus expand fluid volume. Ingestion of large amounts of glycyrrhizin (an aldosterone-like compound found in licorice, some liquors, and chewing tobacco) can also stimulate mineralocorticoid activity.

Persons taking monoamine oxidase inhibitors and ingesting sympathomimetics, caffeine, chocolate, or large amounts of tryptophan, tyramine, or dopamine-containing foods can develop hypertension. Tyramine releases stored catecholamines from postganglionic nerve endings and monamine oxidase inhibitors increase the amount of norepinephrine and serotonin in the central nervous system to potentiate the effect of the tyramine, tryptophan or dopamine. Within an hour the blood pressure increases briefly and the patient may complain of headache, nausea, and palpitations. In some instances the hypertension from this combination of compounds has been known to result in cerebrovascular accidents.

The first reports of hypertension following the use of oral contraceptives, published in 1962 and 1967,[17,86,153] revealed that as many as one of every five women taking oral contraceptives containing more than 0.05 mg (50 µg) of estrogen will develop mild, moderate, or severe hypertension.

This risk depends on age, medical history, ethnicity, prior history of toxemia of pregnancy, smoking habits, and the duration of contraceptive use.[88]

The mechanism involved in hypertension secondary to

TABLE 47-3 SECONDARY CAUSES OF HIGH BLOOD PRESSURE

Exogenous

Sympathomimetic agents	Amphetamine Caffeine Adrenalin Dopamine Nicotine Methyldopa Tyramine
Tricyclic antidepressants Phenacetin-containing analgesics Licorice Chewing tobacco Steroid therapy Monoamine oxidase inhibitors	Isocarboxazid (Marplan) Isoniazid Nialamide (Niamid) Pargyline (Eutonyl) Phenelzine (Nardil) Procarbazine Tranylcypromine (Parnate)
Tryptophan- and tyramine-containing foods	Chicken liver Pickled herring Yeast extract Broad beans Matured cheeses (especially cheddar) Beer Wines (especially Chianti)
Oral contraceptives Trace metals, minerals, and electrolytes	Cadium Zinc Lead Selenium Mercury Calcium Magnesium Potassium Sodium

Cardiovascular Disorders

Coarctation of the aorta
Patent ductus arteriosus
Polycythemia hypertonica

Endocrine Disorders

Adrenal cortex	Primary aldosteronism Secondary aldosteronism Cushing's syndrome Excess deoxycortisol Congenital adrenal hyperplasia Adenoma
Adrenal medulla Hypothyroidism Hyperparathyroidism Acromegaly	Pheochromocytoma

Neurologic disorders

Autonomic hyperreflexia
Excessive rapid-eye-movement sleep
Increased intracranial pressure
Ganglioneuromas, neuroblastomas, and tumors of the posterior fossa
Sleep apnea syndrome

(Table continues on page 604)

TABLE 47-3 SECONDARY CAUSES OF HIGH BLOOD PRESSURE (Cont.)

Kidney Disorders

Renal artery stenosis Unilateral	Tumor Hypoplasia Renal tuberculosis Pyelonephritis Hydronephrosis Single cysts

Bilateral	Acute/chronic renal failure
	Polycystic disease
	Pyelonephritis
	Glomerulonephritis
	Nephropathy from gout,
	  diabetes, and phenacetin
	  abuse
	Lupus erythematosus
	Progressive systemic
	  sclerosis
	Periarteritis nodosa
	Amyloidosis
	Radiation nephritis

Renin-secreting tumors	Wilms' tumor
	  (nephroblastoma)
	  (paraganglioma)
	Hemangiopericytoma
	Renin-producing pulmonary
	  carcinoma

Surgical Procedures Involving the Cardiovascular System

Pregnancy

	Preeclampsia Eclampsia

oral contraceptives is unknown. It is known, however, that estrogens increase the hepatic synthesis of angiotensinogen, the substrate necessary for renin synthesis. However, progesterone has also been implicated in causing hypertension.[95] Regardless of the possible causes, studies indicate that the risk of developing hypertension more than doubles after the first five years of oral contraceptive use,[124] and the death rate from hypertension and heart disease compared with that among women not using oral contraceptives is 10:1.[10,148] When the drug is discontinued, 80% of these hypertensive women will return to normotensive states within 3 to 18 months.

Although research findings do not agree, excessive amounts of trace metals, particularly cadmium, may be responsible for hypertension. Contact with cadmium comes primarily from working with rechargeable batteries and appears to influence cardiac output, renin secretion, and sodium and water excretion.[8] An excess amount of cadmium has been found at autopsy in hypertensive individuals and in cigarette smokers. Furthermore, victims of myocardial infarction exposed to soft water supplies have less evidence of atherosclerosis but twice the amount of cadmium deposits at autopsy.[130] The exact mechanism for cadmium's ability to increase blood pressure remains unknown at this time.

Low serum magnesium and serum potassium levels have also been associated with hypertension.[105] Findings that hard water, containing calcium and magnesium, may have some protective value from coronary artery disease and cardiovascular mortality have prompted studies of calcium ingestion.[131]

Cardiovascular Disorders. Increased viscosity, such as in the case of a particular form of polycythemia (Gaisbock's disease) can result in hypertension. Coarctation of the aorta is a rare cause of hypertension in the adult. At rest, cardiac output, heart rate, and oxygen uptake are increased in cases of coarctation of the aorta, but stroke volume remains normal. With exercise, cardiac output increases while the heart rate and oxygen uptake remain normal and an abnormally high systolic blood pressure results in an extremely wide pulse pressure.

Adrenal Gland Disorders. Adrenal gland dysfunction is responsible for no more than 3% of all cases of hypertension, and primary aldosteronism accounts for most of that 3%.[99] Despite high fluid volume, excess production of aldosterone continues in cases of primary aldosteronism, and is responsible for the inappropriate retention of more sodium and water from the distal renal tubule and collecting duct.

Secondary aldosteronism, excessive aldosterone secretion resulting from stimulation of the renin–angiotensin–aldosterone system, can occur when renal blood flow diminishes. Renal artery stenosis, malignant hypertension, and congestive heart failure are some causes of reduced renal blood flow.

Hypertension occurs in about 85% of persons with idiopathic Cushing's Syndrome[111] and in 20% of persons undergoing steroid drug therapy.[73] Hypertension results because of cortisol's ability to cause sodium retention and thus volume expansion.

Congenital adrenal hyperplasia is an inherited enlargement of the adrenal glands, accompanied by enzyme defects which result in excessive mineralocorticoid secretion. Two forms of congenital adrenal hyperplasia have hypertension as part of their clinical presentation: 11-beta-hydroxylase deficiency and 17-alpha-hydroxylase deficiency.

Tumors of the adrenal medulla can also cause dramatically elevated blood pressures above 300/160 mm Hg. Pheochromocytomas are catecholamine-secreting tumors of chromafin tissue, 90% of which are found within the adrenal medulla. If these same tumor cells are located outside the adrenal medulla or anywhere along the sympathetic chain, they are called paragangliomas. Pheochromocytomas account for only 0.5% of all hypertension[99] but if these tumors go unrecognized, death is likely to occur because the patient may develop an accelerated type of hypertension. Death can also result from surgery if the pheochromocytoma has not been diagnosed before or at the time of surgery.

Other Endocrine Disorders. Hypertension commonly occurs with untreated hypothyroidism. In persons with hypothyroidism, cardiac output diminishes and peripheral vascular resistance increases. The systolic blood pressure tends to drop while the diastolic pressure rises, creating a narrow pulse pressure.[3,44] Hyperparathyroidism accounts for only 1% of all patients with hypertension but as many as 50% of these individuals present with hypertension.[13,16,123] Although the actual cause is unknown, hypertension develops in 30% to 40% of individuals with acromegaly (excessive growth hormone)[94] and excess aldosterone levels are always documented in these patients.[27]

Neurologic Disorders. Many different neurologic disorders can induce hypertension. Quadriplegics whose spinal cord is transsected at or above the sixth thoracic vertebra may respond to stimuli, such as a full bladder, by developing sudden severe hypertension as a result of autonomic hyperreflexia. Hypertension can result from increased intracranial pressure secondary to such problems as subarachnoid hemorrhage and subdural hematoma. Up to 70% of patients with ruptured intracranial aneurysms or intracerebral hemorrhage are hypertensive,[126] and about 50% of all patients diagnosed with sleep apnea syndrome are hypertensive.[151]

Tumors in the cerebellum or in other parts of the posterior fossa can cause excessive catecholamine secretion. Any tumor putting pressure on nearby sympathoadrenal pathways or irritating the posterior hypothalamus and brain stem medulla will cause blood pressure to increase because of excessive catecholamine stimulation.

Ganglioneuromas are benign tumors of sympathetic nervous system origin that increase blood pressure. Neuroblastomas, on the other hand, are highly malignant tumors of ganglionic cells in the sympathetic nervous system that can be responsible for hypertension. Ganglioneuromas and neuroblastomas may be related to pheochromocytomas found in the adrenal medulla.

Although rapid-eye-movement (REM) sleep is not a neurologic disorder, the bursts of sympathetic activity that occur during REM sleep cause peripheral vasoconstriction and are responsible for variable increases in mean arterial blood pressure of as much as 13 mm Hg in hypertensive persons.[78] When REM-suppressing medications are suddenly discontinued, or when patients who have been deprived of sleep are allowed to sleep, a REM-rebound effect occurs and the amount of REM sleep can actually double.[70] This rebound has relevant implications for patients with a history of angina or other cardiac disorders who may become symptomatic during REM sleep (Chap. 31).

Kidney Disorders. Congenital or acquired renal dysfunction can cause hypertension as a direct result of renal artery disease or of unilateral or bilateral renal disease. Any renal disorder that retards the excretion of sodium, and therefore water, or increases the secretion of renin is apt to cause hypertension. Table 47-3 lists the specific renal disorders known to be responsible for hypertension. Although it is often difficult to pinpoint whether renal failure causes hypertension or results from hypertension, patients with chronic renal failure are the largest group of patients with kidney dysfunction to present with hypertension. Renal vascular disease accounts for only 10% of the hypertension originating from renal dysfunction.

Systemic diseases, such as progressive systemic sclerosis (scleroderma), lupus erythematosus, and periarteritis nodosa, can lead to hypertension. Hypertension occurs initially in 50% to 75% of the persons with a diagnosis of polycystic disease, but 90% have hypertension by the time the disease progresses to renal failure.[103] Renal nephropathy can result from gout (hyperuricemia), diabetes, and chronic abuse of phenacetin-containing drugs. Renin-secreting tumors, such as Wilms' tumor (nephroblastoma, embryonal carcinosarcoma), hemangiopericytoma, and renin-producing pulmonary carcinoma, can also be responsible for severe hypertension.

Surgical Procedures. Hypertension can develop after such procedures as coronary artery bypass graft surgery, closure of atrial–septal defects, and aortic valve replacements. The resulting hypertension is thought to be due to activation of sympathetic reflexes. As many as one in every three patients will develop short-term hypertension within 2 hours after bypass surgery.[31] One-half of the patients having surgery to close an atrial–septal defect will experience hypertension[21] and patients undergoing aortic valve replacements have a 50% chance of developing hypertension.[87]

Pregnancy-Induced Hypertension. Hypertension during pregnancy constitutes a significant cause of maternal and infant morbidity and mortality. It is usually present before delivery, but can also occur during or after delivery and is of variable duration. It is responsible for as many as 33% of all deaths of mothers giving birth, and for a high percentage of prematurity and growth retardation in the infant.[154]

Blood pressure normally decreases during the first two trimesters of pregnancy and slowly rises to normal during the third trimester. The normal cardiovascular changes that occur during pregnancy include increases in plasma volume, the number of red blood cells, and cardiac output, whereas blood viscosity decreases. A 15-degree left-axis deviation on electrocardiogram is also normally seen during pregnancy.[150]

Because of the normal changes in cardiovascular status during pregnancy, the definition of adult hypertension previously discussed cannot apply. Hypertension in pregnancy is defined as a 30 mm Hg elevation in systolic pressure or a 15 mm Hg elevation in diastolic pressure above the woman's normal pressure. If her normal blood pressure is unknown, hypertension in pregnancy is diagnosed at a pressure of 140/90 mm Hg or higher on two separate occasions at least 6 hours apart.[147,150]

Preeclampsia is defined as hypertension developing after 20 weeks of gestation and includes the appearance of edema and proteinuria. A woman with a history of hypertension has as much as a 30% chance of developing preeclampsia, compared with the normotensive woman's 12% chance. Women with mean arterial pressures greater than 90 mm Hg (130/70, 120/75, 110/80 mm Hg) during the second trimester carry a higher risk of developing preeclampsia and eclampsia and of stillbirth. Eclampsia includes signs and symptoms of preeclampsia and is extended to include seizures and coma. Eclampsia occurs in one of every 2,000 deliveries in the United States.[74]

PATHOGENESIS OF HYPERTENSION

In order to understand the pathology of hypertension, one must have a good understanding of the normal mechanisms controlling blood pressure. This was discussed in detail in Chapter 6 and will be briefly summarized.

Blood pressure is a product of cardiac output and total peripheral vascular resistance. There are three main mechanisms regulating these two interacting variables to keep blood pressure within normal limits:

1. Nervous system control (the immediate response of vasoconstriction)
2. Renal control of blood volume (excretion of sodium and water to reduce fluid volume, or retention of sodium and water to increase fluid volume)
3. Humoral changes (causing vasoconstriction and vasodilation)
   a. renin–angiotensin–aldosterone system
   b. E_2 prostaglandins
   c. kinins
   d. corticosteroids
   e. vasopressin (antidiuretic hormone)

These mechanisms are all closely interrelated and operate to maintain blood pressure in hypertensive as well as normotensive individuals. In hypertension, however, the renal control mechanism is altered by many factors, including the humoral agents listed above, and the pressure becomes maintained at a higher set point.

Altered Hemodynamics

Autonomic Nervous System Control. Nervous system control of blood presure is a short-term mechanism involving the autonomic nervous system and baroreceptor stimulation. Because hypertensive individuals are very sensitive to intravenous noreinephrine, it is thought that there must be a circulating factor in the plasma, perhaps cholesterol, that sensitizes vascular smooth muscle to the vasoconstrictive effects of norepinephrine. Steroids have also been implicated in this hypersensitivity because of their ability to inhibit the uptake of norepinephrine into vascular smooth muscle. Rosendorff and his colleagues[121] hypothesize a biochemical defect preventing normal activation of the enzymes involve in norepinephrine synthesis. This is supported by evidence of a high angiotensin/norepinephrine ratio in the cerebrospinal fluid of hypertensive persons.

Renal Control. The kidney has both prohypertensive and antihypertensive action. Any condition that results in water and sodium retention will lead to hypertension in susceptible persons by affecting the renal control of blood volume. When fluid is retained, a series of compensatory mechanisms come into play, as depicted in Figure 47-1. Autoregulation, as discussed in Chapter 5, attempts to return the flow to normal by increasing resistance by way of vasoconstriction. This vasoconstriction results in diminished cardiac output and the increased pressure across the glomeruli results in increased urinary output. In fact, the normal kidney would double its output of urine if it were to operate at 15% higher pressure.

If this compensatory mechanism is in operation over a long time, it is possible that autoregulation would continue increasing the peripheral vascular resistance in order to normalize the blood flow through the tissues. The ultimate effect is hypothesized to be an elevated pressure because of the highly increased resistance compared with the slightly reduced cardiac output. Eventually the blood pressure may become high enough to return cardiac output to normal, but then the person would be very hypertensive.[53]

The hypertensive state can now serve to prevent further retention of sodium and water because the kidneys have reached a higher set point and need the hypertension to maintain normal fluid balance. Anesthesiologists are well

Fig. 47-1. Renal control mechanism in sustained fluid volume excess. When fluid is retained, blood pressure and cardiac output increase. Autoregulation attempts to normalize the blood flow by vasoconstriction. Over time, the increased peripheral vascular resistance from constant vasoconstriction returns the cardiac output to normal, but blood pressure remains very high in order to do so.

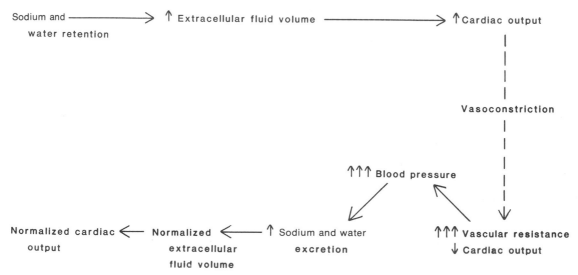

aware that hypertensive persons can become severely oliguric if blood pressure is lowered to a normal mean of 100 mm Hg during surgery.

Humoral Control. In addition to changes in fluid volume, conditions that stimulate the renin–angiotensin–aldosterone mechanism may lead to hypertension in certain persons. Renin is released from the granular cells of the afferent glomerular arteriole (juxtaglomerular apparatus) in response to three mechanisms: reduced pressure in the afferent renal arterioles, depleted sodium in the distal tubule, and sympathetic stimulation of beta-adrenergic receptors in the juxtaglomerular apparatus (see Fig. 47-2, Table 47-2).

As depicted in Figure 47-2, renin, a peptidase-class enzyme, is released into the circulation and acts upon the glycoprotein precursor angiotensinogen which is secreted from the liver to produce angiotensin I, an inactive decapeptide. With the help of a converting enzyme, angiotensin I is converted to the active octapeptide, angiotensin II.[127] Although it has a short half-life (from 1–2 minutes), angiotensin II is an extremely potent vasoconstrictor. It restores renal perfusion by increasing blood pressure quickly and

stimulating release of aldosterone. Aldosterone promotes reabsorption of sodium, and thus water, from the distal tubule, thereby expanding the extracellular fluid volume and causing blood pressure to increase.

In summary, the interaction between renal and humoral control of blood pressure, even high blood pressure, can be thought of as a product of fluid volume and the extent of vasoconstriction. On the basis of renin and sodium values, one researcher has classified causes of hypertension on a spectrum from excessive vasoconstriction to excessive fluid volume (Table 47-4).[84]

There is increasing evidence of a connection between prostaglandin deficiency and hypertension. Prostaglandins are found throughout the body and are rapidly synthesized and released in response to adrenergic stimulation. E_2 prostaglandin, normally found in the inner zone of the renal medulla, acts as a potent antihypertensive agent by inhibiting norepinephrine.[143] Almost all the E_2 prostaglandin is degraded as it passes through the lungs but some of the E_2 prostaglandin may form A_2 prostaglandin which is not so readily degraded by lung enzymes. Muirhead and his associates[102] implanted fragments of the renal medulla, con-

Fig. 47-2. Humoral interactions resulting in increased blood pressure. Renin released into the circulation acts on angiotensinogen to eventually produce angiotensin II, an extremely potent, short-acting vasoconstrictor, which thereby increases blood pressure and also stimulates aldosterone secretion. Aldosterone helps as well to increase blood pressure by causing sodium and water retention. If there is a deficiency in prostaglandins, potent antihypertensive agents stimulated by kinins, hypertension can also result.

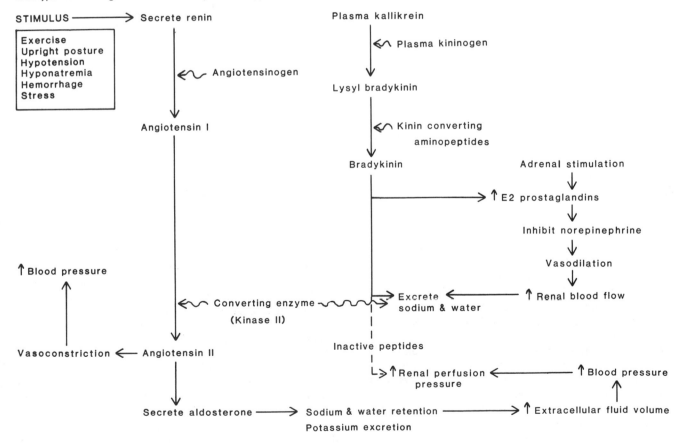

TABLE 47-4   SPECTRUM OF EXCESSIVE VASOCONSTRICTION TO EXCESSIVE FLUID VOLUME

Excessive Fluid
Volume

Primary aldosteronism
Bilateral polycystic kidney disease
Cushing's syndrome
Pregnancy-induced hypertension
Low-renin hypertension (responsive to diuretics)
Bilateral renovascular hypertension

Normal-renin hypertension

Low-renin hypertension (unresponsive to diuretics)
High-renin hypertension
Toxemia of pregnancy
Unilateral renovascular hypertension
Oral contraceptive-induced hypertension
Scleroderma
Accelerated hypertension
Malignant hypertension

Excessive
Vasoconstriction

Causes of high blood pressure can be arranged on a spectrum from excessive vasoconstriction and high levels of renin to excessive fluid volume and sodium and water retention.
(After Laragh JH: Hosp Pract 9(1):61–73, 1974)

taining prostaglandins, under the skin of hypertensive rats and the blood pressure dropped. Thus, it was hypothesized that an E_2 prostaglandin deficiency can result in hypertension (see Fig. 47-2).

Kinins, formed from kininogen by kallikreins, stimulate the secretion of E_2 prostaglandins and also increase blood flow to cause diuresis and natriuresis (see Fig. 47-2). When the body is tilted to an upright position, kinin concentration drops, renal blood flow diminishes, and sodium and water are retained.[63] Persons with idiopathic hypertension appear to have low levels of urinary kallikrein and persons who are on low salt diets appear to have high urinary kallikrein levels.

Vascular Changes Associated with Hypertension

In a normal artery, the intima is a smooth-surfaced inner lining and the media is the middle layer consisting of smooth muscle fibers which expand and contract, thus dilating and constricting the vessel. The adventitia is the outer layer of connective tissue that serves to anchor the vessel to surrounding structures (Chap. 5). Under conditions of sustained hypertension, with increased peripheral resistance of more than 3 months' duration, the layers of the normal artery change.

Arteries may undergo any of three major pathologic changes associated with hypertension: atherosclerosis if the artery is large, arteriosclerosis if the artery is smaller, and fibrinoid arteriolar necrosis, which occurs as a result of accelerated hypertension. The morphology of these three types of lesions is different, but focal endothelial damage occurs with all of them (Chap. 10).

Atherosclerosis. Hypertension appears to accelerate the process of atherosclerosis by disrupting the endothelium and forcing plasma and lipoproteins into the intimal and subintimal layers of the vessel. Plaques then develop which set the stage for atherosclerosis.[48] Constantinides[24] has discovered that the endothelium overlying these atherosclerotic plaques is much more permeable than is the endothelium overlying normal vessel walls. Whether the injury causes the increased permeability or whether the increased permeability results in the injury remains to be studied. Nevertheless, the abnormal gaps between the endothelial cells of the large arteries allow water and salt (calcium, sodium, chloride) content to increase and the wall becomes edematous.

Atherosclerosis affects primarily the aorta and large- to medium-sized arteries in which there is more elastin content than smooth muscle fiber content. It develops in areas where pressure is high, such as the bronchial arteries, and not in areas where pressure is low, as in the pulmonary arteries. It is the most common vascular pathology associated with cerebral infarction and systolic hypertension in the elderly.

Arteriosclerosis. Arteriosclerosis is responsible for most cases of cerebrovascular disease, peripheral vascular disease, and their sequelae. Arteriosclerotic lesions occur in smaller arteries and arterioles and are classified as hyperplastic or hyalinotic.

Hyperplastic arteriosclerosis occurs when the increased pressure either causes smooth muscle cells to proliferate and migrate or stimulates actin microfilaments in the endothelium to act as pseudomuscle cells. Whatever the mechanism for the hyperplasia, the endothelium eventually becomes separated from the internal elastic membrane of the intima by layers of smooth or pseudosmooth muscle, and the result is thickened vessels with narrowed lumens.

In addition to hyperplastic arteriosclerosis, hyaline arteriosclerosis (also called hyalinosis, fibrinoid arteritis, or lipohyalinosis) may occur. Hyaline arteriosclerosis is a condition of patchy subintimal lesions consisting of fibrin and other plasma elements. The patchy fibrotic lesions also result in thickening and narrowing of the arterioles and cause peripheral vascular resistance to become fixed.

Fibrinoid Arteriolar Necrosis. Fibrinoid necrosis occurs in the small arterioles and indicates accelerated (malignant) hypertension. The medial layer has patchy areas of hyaline arteriosclerosis, which extend into the intima, and inflammation is apparent in the adventitia. These lesions are found primarily in the kidneys, but also occur in all other organ tissues excluding skin and skeletal muscle. The pathogenesis of fibrinoid arteriolar necrosis will be covered in more detail in the discussion of accelerated hypertension.

Systolic Hypertension and the Elderly Patient

With aging, arterial changes associated with systolic hypertension take place in the heart, brain, and kidney. During normal exercise, systolic blood pressure increases because of a pressor reaction reflecting sympathetic stimulation of the heart, but the superimposed atherosclerosis increases the systolic pressure even more because of the loss of elasticity.

The slowly evolving process of atherosclerosis begins in childhood and reaches clinical expression during middle and old age. The aorta and large arteries become less distensible to pulsatile flow because of the atherosclerotic process and are less able to accommodate the ejected stroke volume. As a result, cardiac output diminishes while peripheral resistance increases. After age fifty, peripheral resistance increases at the rate of 1% every year.[14] Cardiac output decreases 50% over a 50-year period.[14,19]

The increased peripheral resistance, resulting from the lack of distensibility, leads to increased intraventricular pressure, which is necessary for ejection of blood through the rigid aorta. This increased resistance accounts for the increased systolic pressure. A wide pulse pressure may be present because the indistensible aorta causes the diastolic pressure to fall rapidly.

Although research findings regarding advantages of treating high blood pressure in elderly patients are inconclusive at this time, a blood pressure that has been increasing gradually over the years should probably be reduced *slowly* with the stepped care method described in Chapter 37. If long-standing hypertension is reduced too rapidly in the elderly, the diminished responsiveness of their baroreceptors can cause weakness and syncope from postural hypotension.

COMPLICATIONS OF HIGH BLOOD PRESSURE

Target organs subjected to vascular damage as a result of hypertension include the heart, aorta, peripheral vessels, kidney, retina, brain, pancreas, adrenals, intestines, and liver. Hypertension has been categorized into three stages by the extent of organ damage, and these stages are summarized in Table 47-5. The degree of organ involvement correlates well with the level of the blood pressure and has an important predictive value in terms of a patient's prognosis, the type of antihypertensive therapy most likely to be successful, and the urgency with which treatment should be initiated.

Heart and Vasculature

The cardiac complications of hypertension are left ventricular hypertrophy, ischemic heart disease, and acute heart failure. Hypertension forces the left ventricle to increase its force of contraction in order to open the aortic valve against elevated aortic diastolic pressure. If the increased pressure is sustained, the muscle fibers thicken and the ventricular wall enlarges. Thus, one result of systemic hypertension on the heart is hypertrophy of the left ventricle.

The elevated systolic pressure and the left ventricular hypertrophy serve to compensate for the increases in peripheral resistance. However, myocardial work and oxygen consumption increase because of the compensatory left ventricular hypertrophy. When the heart can no longer meet the demands for increased oxygen, symptoms of failure occur. Early signs and symptoms of heart failure include dyspnea, orthopnea, nocturia, and diminished exercise tolerance. The signs and symptoms can progress to peripheral edema, positive hepatojugular reflux, and hepatic tenderness.

Electrocardiographic changes indicating left ventricular hypertrophy include a progression from increased QRS voltage to depressed ST segment and inversion of the T wave. Left ventricular changes seen on x-ray films include rounding and increased convexity of the lateral cardiac shadow in the posterior–anterior view. The posterior border of the heart overlaps the spine and obliterates the posterior–inferior cardiophrenic recess in the lateral or oblique view. A fourth heart sound reflects the decreased compliance of the left ventricular wall, and a third heart sound confirms heart failure.[22]

With hypertension, there is a threefold risk of developing coronary artery disease. Coronary artery disease remains the most common sequela and the leading cause of death in hypertensive individuals (see Chap. 13). Hypertrophy of the medial layer of the coronary vessels, the vessel wall edema, and the accelerated arteriosclerosis resulting from the sustained hypertensive state lead to diminished perfusion through sclerotic coronary vessels. The elevated diastolic pressure helps facilitate increased perfusion because most of the coronary blood flow occurs during diastole.[143] The hypertrophy of the heart and the increased distance between

---

TABLE 47-5   STAGES OF HIGH BLOOD PRESSURE CLASSIFIED BY EXTENT OF ORGAN DAMAGE

Stage I	No objective signs or symptoms of organ dysfunction are evident by examination
Stage II	At least one sign of organ involvement is present: 1. Left ventricular hypertrophy on physical examination, chest x-ray, electrocardiograph, echocardiograph, etc. 2. Generalized and focal narrowing of arterioles in the retina 3. Proteinuria or a slightly elevated plasma creatinine concentration

Stage III	The appearance of signs and symptoms as a result of various target organ damage
	1. Cardiovascular: Left ventricular failure
	                       Dissecting aneurysm
	                       Arterial occlusive disease
	                       Angina pectoris or myocardial infarction
	2. Brain: Cerebral, cerebellar, or brain stem hemorrhages
	                       Hypertensive encephalopathy
	                       Intracranial thrombosis
	3. Optic fundi: Retinal hemorrhages and exudates with or without papilledema
	4. Kidney: Renal failure

(After World Health Organization Technical Report Series #628, Geneva, 1978)

the capillary bed and the cells make the heart highly sensitive to any impairment of coronary blood flow. Because atherogenesis is accelerated by hypertension, maintenance of blood pressure by the hypertrophied ventricle becomes self-defeating (see Chap. 2). The result is angina pectoris, or if the vessel is severely impaired, myocardial infarction. With treatment, the blood pressure decreases and, because the oxygen requirement is decreased more than the coronary flow, the likelihood of angina is reduced.

The aorta is not exempt from changes in vessel wall structure. Hypertension can lead to dilatation of the aorta and may precipitate formation of an aneurysm in the thorax or abdomen which may rupture (Chap. 53). Patients will commonly complain of dyspnea, nausea and vomiting, and sudden onset of lacerating ("tearing"), unremitting interscapular pain which can radiate anteriorly, superiorly, and inferiorly. Aneurysms are associated with degenerative changes in the medial layer of the aorta, especially in elderly individuals with hypertension.[75] Peripheral artery disease, evidenced by intermittent claudication and ischemia of the feet, is also accentuated by hypertension.

Congestive heart failure and pulmonary edema can result from left ventricular hypertrophy because the incompetent left ventricle is unable to expel the necessary blood volume.[113] Without treatment, congestive heart failure has a poor 5-year survival rate of 60% for men and 40% for women.[72] But congestive heart failure is very responsive to therapy; with long-term treatment, the ventricular hypertrophy can be reversed and death rarely occurs (see Chap. 27).

Kidney

All persons dying from the sequelae of hypertension show a greater incidence of pathologic changes in small renal arteries at autopsy than do normotensives. Increased permeability of the vessels, hypertrophy, and edema of the arterioles progressively result in diminished renal perfusion, obstructed renal arteries, hyalinosis of capillaries in the nephron (glomerulus), and tubular atrophy.[144]

With the increased permeability, proteins leak out into the tubules and patients develop proteinuria. Patients may complain of nocturia because of the kidney's limited ability to concentrate urine. Azotemia, as indicted by elevated blood urea nitrogen and creatinine levels, will also be present if nephrons have been damaged and renal perfusion has been diminished.[144]

The 5-year survival rate for persons treated for accelerated hypertension in the absence of azotemia is 60%, but only 25% if azotemia is present.[110]

Optic Fundi

The condition of the retina is a reliable index of the severity and prognosis of hypertension because it is the only place where arterioles can be seen by noninvasive examination techniques. Evidence of vessel damage in the retina indicates blood vessel damage elsewhere.

Hypertensive retinopathy is classified according to changes in the optic fundus using a grading scale originally developed by Keith, Wagener, and Barker and modified by many practitioners, including Kohli and Elwood.[81] One form

of the grading scale is outlined in Figure 47-3 together with characteristic funduscopic findings. Grade I indicates recent onset, or a labile course, of hypertension. Grade II confirms the occurrence of sclerosis and is diagnostic of diastolic hypertension of at least 110 mm Hg for more than a 2-year period. Grade III findings include soft, cotton-wool exudates and striate hemorrhage in addition to the arteriolar narrowing. The venules can also appear sclerotic and spastic. Grade III hypertensive retinopathy indicates an accelerating phase of severe hypertension. The grade IV finding of papilledema signals the onset of severe retinopathy as a result of malignant hypertension.

Brain

Like renal, retinal, and coronary vessels, the cerebral vessels undergo similar changes in hypertensive persons and the effects are just as detrimental. Even in mildly hypertensive persons the risk of cerebrovascular disease is four times higher than in normotensive persons.

Hypertension is a clearly identifiable risk factor in the stroke-prone person. In all industrially developed countries, stroke is a major complication of hypertension, especially in Asia (Japan, Korea, and China). Fortunately, the incidence of stroke has been gradually decreasing since the 1950s when effective drug treatment for high blood pressure was initiated, and is now 30% less than it was 25 years ago.[93]

One effect of sustained hypertension is the shifting of autoregulation upward into a higher range of pressures so that the brain remains protected, but the person is less able to compensate for drastically reduced blood pressure. The other effect of hypertension involves the following four different pathologic changes in the cerebral vasculature.[48]

Cerebral Infarct. Cerebral infarcts are responsible for 80% of the strokes and transient ischemic attacks (TIAs) occurring in hypertensive individuals. They occur in hypertensive persons because of the accelerated atherosclerosis in the large carotid and cerebral vessels nourishing the brain. Cerebral infarcts occur primarily in the elderly population with less severe hypertension because of large vessel thromboembolic disease. As many as 20% of patients with TIAs (episodes of focal, reversible neurologic deficits of sudden onset and of less than 24 hours' duration) will have a stroke within 5 years. Studies have demonstrated that a reduction in blood pressure will decrease the frequency of TIAs.

Hyalinosis. In small vessels, hyalinosis causes the formation of microaneurysms, which weaken and rupture during the early stages of the process and usually result in massive intracerebral hemorrhage into the ventricular system. Intracerebral hemorrhage accounts for 10% of strokes in hypertensive persons[93] and is most likely to occur as a result of a severe, acute hypertensive crisis.

Lacunar Infarct. If the hyalinotic lesions fail to rupture, chronic hyalinosis results in occlusion of the cerebral artery lumen and a lacunar infarct occurs. Lacunar infarcts (lacunae) are small cystic infarctions of up to 1.5 cm in diameter that occur in deep small vessels located in the basal ganglia, internal capsule, thalamus, forebrain, base of

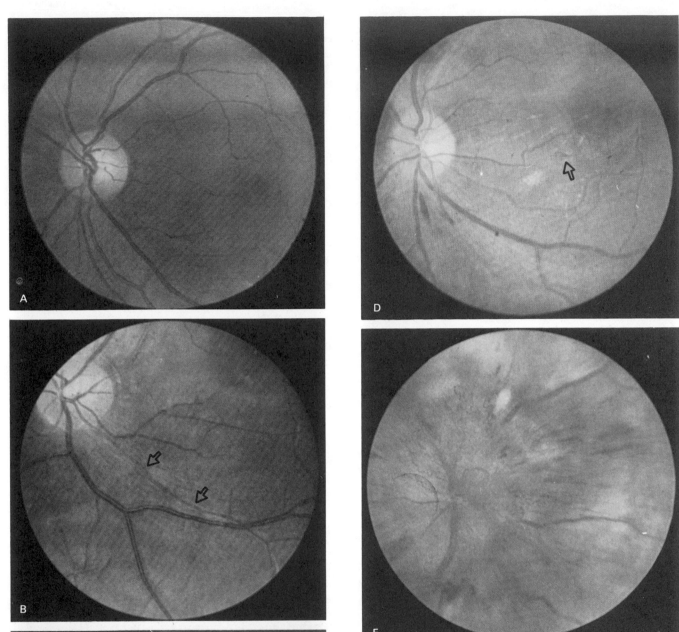

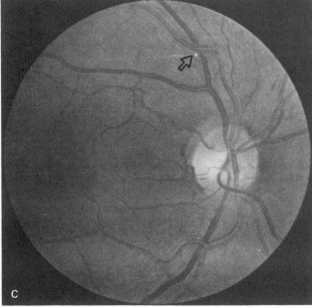

Fig. 47-3. Funduscopic Changes by Grade of Retinopathy. (**A**) Normal fundus: optic disk is healthy and pink, and retinal arterioles are wide. (**B**) Grade I (benign): a minimal amount of narrowing of the arterioles in relation to venules characterizes vasoconstriction. (**C**) Grade II (semibenign): narrowing and arteriole—venule crossing phenomenon is evidenced by the underlying venule tapering (nicking) with the tip toward the arteriole at both sides. (**D**) Grade III (semimalignant): at this point, the arterioles appear pale and tortuous and are diffusely narrowed. Striated hemorrhage occurs in the nerve fiber layer and appears as flame-shaped whitish flecks. Punctiform hemorrhage can also be present. (**E**) Grade IV (malignant): in addition to hemorrhage, tortuosity, and narrowing, papilledema (edema of the optic disk) is also seen. The disk appears elevated, and the disk margins are often indistinct or blurred. In the early stages of papilledema (as this picture indicates), the optic disk remains transparent but, in advanced situations, it appears greyish—white and atrophic. (Irinoda K [ed]: Colour Atlas and Criteria of Fundus Changes in Hypertension. Philadelphia, JB Lippincott, 1970)

the pons, and in the cerebellum. Lacunar infarction can be manifested as two different syndromes: a motor syndrome resembling Parkinson's disease but without the characteristic pill-rolling tremors or cogwheel rigidity and unrelieved by L-dopa therapy; and a syndrome resembling a multi-infarct dementia, with symptoms of inappropriate behavior, forgetfulness, and loss of intellect.

Hemorrhage. Hemorrhage from cerebral aneurysms constitutes about 6% of the strokes in hypertensive individuals.[93] An aneurysm forming in a major intracerebral vessel (berry aneurysm) may cause a subarachnoid hemorrhage when it ruptures. Charcot–Bouchard aneurysms, which form on smaller arterioles, can also rupture.

Occipital morning headache is the earliest symptom of brain tissue damage from hypertension. Symptoms progress from complaints of fatigue, irritability, and forgetfulness, to confusion, focal neurologic signs, seizures, and coma, as hypertension enters the accelerated phase. If treatment is initiated promptly, recovery is possible unless irreversible brain damage has occurred. Without treatment, hypertensive encephalopathy or intracerebral hemorrhage results from malignant hypertension and there is an 80% fatality rate.[43]

Accelerated (Malignant) Hypertension

An accelerated form of hypertension can develop suddenly in a normotensive individual, or in persons with idiopathic or secondary hypertension. Roughly 1% of all hypertensive persons, particularly blacks, males, and the middle-aged, can enter into an accelerated phase.[128] A sudden acceleration in blood pressure can be triggered by such things as severe emotional stress, increased salt intake, or abrupt discontinuation of antihypertensive medication, but any disease process that produces hypertension can result in an accelerated form. There is a 90% mortality rate at the end of 1 year if a hypertensive crisis goes untreated. The majority die as a result of renal failure, cerebral sequelae, or heart failure.[36,43,46]

Accelerated hypertension presents an immediate threat to all organs except skeletal muscle and skin. It is important to recognize that the signs and symptoms of accelerated hypertension are target-organ responses to the *rate* of acceleration in blood pressure, and not to the absolute level of blood pressure. Although lesions can be found in the pancreas, intestines, spleen, and adrenal glands, the most common site for damage is the kidney.

The signs and symptoms of renal damage are due primarily to lesions affecting the afferent arterioles, which cause them to become stiff, thickened, and less responsive to changes in renal perfusion. Signs of renal damage include azotemia, proteinuria, oliguria or anuria, hematuria, and renal failure with or without uremia.

Neither are the brain, heart, and vasculature exempt from the effects of accelerated hypertension. Acute damage to small vessels in the brain can produce an encephalopathy, the symptoms of which include headache, nausea and vomiting, decreasing level of consciousness, seizures, increased intracranial pressure, and coma. Cardiac failure or a dissecting aortic aneurysm can also result. Because red blood cells are lysed in the small arterioles undergoing

fibrinoid necrosis, patients may be anemic, with low platelet counts and high reticulocyte counts. This type of anemia is known as microangiopathic hemolytic anemia.

Accelerated hypertension is defined as a sudden onset of markedly increased diastolic pressure greater than 120 mm Hg and development of signs and symptoms indicating acute target-organ damage. Most clinicians make no clear distinction between the two terms, but because of the connotation of "malignant" hypertension, accelerated hypertension is the preferred term.

Malignant hypertension should probably be distinguished from accelerated hypertension by the added presence of papilledema (grade IV retinopathy) when the optic fundi are examined (see Fig. 47-3e). Papilledema is associated with increased intracranial pressure and indicates that the acceleration has advanced to involve retinal vessels that are at the nerve head. The patient may complain of blurred vision or other visual impairment. The presence of papilledema signifies a very poor prognosis and the term "malignant" hypertension is probably more appropriate if this sign is documented.

Pathology and Consequences of Malignant Hypertension. As mentioned earlier, the underlying pathology of malignant hypertension is fibrinoid arteriolar necrosis of the medial smooth muscle layer, which can extend into the intima. The vessel wall is suddenly invaded by fibrinoid material and proliferative inflammation of the intima occurs, especially in the afferent arterioles and the small interlobular arteries of the kidney. The lumen size diminishes because the intima becomes thickened with layers of collagen.[28,48] There is no relationship between the absolute level of the pressure and the incidence or severity of the necrosis.

The fibrinotic necrosis occurs in an irregular fashion along the vessel and causes areas of dilatation and constriction. The fulminating, necrotic lesions in the arterioles can rupture and cause small hemorrhages in the target organs. In the areas surrounding the necrosis, plasma exudate is visible and thought to be a result of the vessel's high filling tension, causing overstretching of the smooth muscle fibers in the media. This overstretching creates gaps in the endothelium which increase the permeability and allow plasma, with its fibrin contents, to exude into the vessel wall and severely narrow the lumen. Whether the necrosis is secondary to the overstretching or a toxic factor in the plasma exudate remains to be ellucidated.

This pathologic process and the consequences of malignant hypertension are readily apparent when the retina is examined (see Fig. 47-3e). These retinal changes indicate the effects of accelerated pressure on vessels elsewhere, especially in the kidney, where malignant hypertension is particularly devastating. Renal failure can result rapidly from the fibrinoid necrosis occluding afferent glomerular arterioles and causing ischemia. Because of the ischemia, the glomeruli atrophy and the kidney shrinks.

Hypertensive Encephalopathy (Vascular Crisis, Bright's Disease). In addition to renal failure, heart failure, and dissecting aortic aneurysms, malignant hypertension can also cause encephalopathy. Rarely encountered clinically because of modern antihypertensive therapy, the most prominent signs of this type of hypertensive crisis are sudden, severely elevated blood pressure and neurologic symptoms that derive from vascular lesions primarily in the brain stem and basal ganglia.[23] A diagnosis of hypertensive crisis is confirmed only when administration of antihypertensive medication resolves the symptoms of neurologic dysfunction.

There are two hypotheses to explain the cause of hypertensive encephalopathy. One is that ischemia initiates vasospasm: excessive intra-arterial pressure results in vasospasm, diminished cerebral blood flow, and increased capillary permeability, and hence ischemia. The outcome of the vasospasm is focal or diffuse hemorrhage of cerebral capillaries. The other is that hypertensive encephalopathy results from a defect in cerebral autoregulation: the blood pressure increases above an upper limit and breaks through the autoregulatory threshold (Chap. 5). The "breakthrough" increases the permeability of the cerebral arterioles, veins, and venules, and results in cerebral edema.[90,106]

PROGNOSIS

Hypertension is directly responsible for 60,000 deaths every year in the United States. Of all deaths in the United States, 20% result directly or indirectly from hypertension.[42] The impact of hypertension on the black American is even more astounding. Hypertension is responsible for four times as many deaths in black males (66 per 100,000) and black females (58 per 100,000) than in white males (16 per 100,000).[42]

During the 1940s a downward trend in deaths secondary to stroke, congestive heart failure, accelerated hypertension, and renal failure began with the introduction of antihypertensive drug therapy. However, since the incidence of severe hypertension has been reduced, the incidence of myocardial infarctions at mild levels of hypertension has increased fourfold.[15] One-half of all myocardial infarctions in middle-aged men occur with hypertension classified as mild, or diastolic pressures under 100 mm Hg.

Stroke remains the leading sequela of severe hypertension at diastolic pressures greater than 110 mm Hg. At diastolic pressures under 110 mm Hg there are ten cases of myocardial infarction for every case of stroke. At pressures greater than 110 mm Hg, there are only two cases of myocardial infarction for every case of stroke. One-fourth of the fatal strokes due to hypertension occur at pressures greater than 110 mm Hg.[42]

Hypertension and other risk factors of coronary artery disease appear additive. Three primary risk factors were examined in men between the ages of 30 and 59 over a 10-year period.[89] The three risk factors are: 1. diastolic pressure greater than 90 mm Hg; 2. serum cholesterol greater than 250 mg/dl; 3. smoking. Of the men in the study, 2% had myocardial infarctions if no risk factors were present. If one factor was present, the incidence was almost 5%. Each additional factor was responsible for doubling the occurrence of myocardial infarctions: if two factors were present, the risk was 9%, and if all three factors were present, the risk was 17%.

With higher levels of blood pressure, the prognosis

TABLE 47-6　A COMPARISON OF TEN-YEAR MORTALITY RATES FOR TREATED AND UNTREATED HYPERTENSIVE PATIENTS BY DEGREE OF SEVERITY

Type of Hypertension	Untreated (%)	Treated (%)
Benign, uncomplicated hypertension	72	24
Benign, complicated by stroke or myocardial infarction	95	61
Accelerated hypertension without azotemia	100	52
Accelerated hypertension with azotemia	100	94

(After Perry HM Jr, Wessler S, Avioli LV: JAMA 210(5):890–895, 1969)

worsens. The Veteran's Administration study documented a morbidity rate of 55% in individuals with an untreated diastolic pressure of 90 to 114 mm Hg. With untreated diastolic pressures above 115 mm Hg, there was an 80% morbidity rate. This and other studies documented that treatment can prevent a morbid event in 90% of those with diastolic pressures above 115 mm Hg and 67% of those with pressures of 90 to 114 mm Hg.[69]

Without treatment, a patient with accelerated hypertension has a negligible rate of survival (Table 47-6). Patients treated with a grade III retinopathy still have a 5-year mortality rate of 30%, but grade IV retinopathy can increase the death rate to as high as 75%.[110]

DIAGNOSTIC ASSESSMENT OF THE HYPERTENSIVE PATIENT

Hypertension is an easily diagnosed health care problem. Diagnosing hypertension does not require the use of expensive equipment or laboratory analysis, and causes no real inconvenience or pain to the patient. However, the diagnosis itself carries the connotation of disability, diminished activity, lack of job opportunities or advancement, and a change in life-style that most people have difficulty accepting.

The quiet, asymptomatic nature of hypertension presents the greatest problem in establishing its diagnosis. In our society, people usually visit health care providers only for symptomatic relief and this behavior is reinforced by focusing only on the complaint and not on preventive practice. Persons with mild or moderately severe hypertension usually have no symptoms. Because of the lack of symptoms, about half of the hypertensive population in the United States are unaware of their condition.[54]

The normal circadian fluctuations in blood pressure do not allow an accurate diagnosis of hypertension from a single office visit; in fact, the highest daytime diastolic pressure can be higher than the nighttime systolic pressure.[98] Furthermore, a patient's blood pressure can be elevated during an office visit because of apprehension, pain, or preexisting illness. Authorities generally agree that one blood pressure reading is fairly reliable from visit to visit and does have some predictive value, but they generally recommend at least three readings, on two different occa-

TABLE 47-7 RECOMMENDED ACTION AFTER PATIENT'S INITIAL BLOOD PRESSURE IS MEASURED

Blood Pressure	Population	Initial Action
Diastolic 120 mm Hg or higher	All adults	Prompt evaluation and treatment
160/95 mm Hg or higher	All adults	Confirm hypertension within one month
140/90 to 160/95 mm Hg	Under age 50	Reevaluate within 2–3 months
140/90 to 160/95 mm Hg	Over age 50	Reevaluate within 6–9 months

(Joint National Committee on Detection, Evaluation, and Treatment of High Blood Pressure. Washington DC, DHEW Publication No. 79–1088, 1977)

TABLE 47-8 RECOMMENDATIONS AFTER INITIAL BLOOD PRESSURE MEASUREMENT IS REEVALUATED

Diastolic Blood Pressure	Follow-up Action
120 mm Hg and higher	Immediate evaluation and treatment
105–119 mm Hg	Treatment is indicated
90–104 mm Hg	Individualized treatment program based on presence of other risk factors
Less than 90 mm Hg	Reevaluate once every year

(Joint National Committee on Detection, Evaluation, and Treatment of High Blood Pressure. Washington DC, DHEW Publication No. 79–1088, 1977)

sions, before the diagnosis is established and any form of antihypertensive drug therapy is initiated (Table 47-7, Table 47-8).

The objective of a medical assessment for hypertension is to determine whether the cause is curable and to assess the damage, if any, to target organs. The assessment should include a careful history and analysis of other risk factors, a urinalysis to rule out renal disease, and serum laboratory tests to determine the impact of hypertension on target organs, assess for secondary causes, and establish baseline data for follow-up evaluation should drug therapy prove necessary. A cardiac examination, funduscopic examination, chest x-ray, and electrocardiogram may also be indicated. The completeness of the examination will depend on the person's age, health history, severity and duration of the hypertension, and the probability of a secondary cause.

The diagnosis of idiopathic hypertension is reached by excluding secondary causes. However, most practitioners feel that an exhaustive search for a cause is unwarranted for every patient, because less than 10% of all hypertension is related to a secondary cause. An extensive assessment would be warranted if the patient is under age thirty or over age fifty, has had no response to antihypertensive drug therapy previously instituted, cannot tolerate the therapeutic dosage of antihypertensive medication prescribed, or has an accelerated phase of previously well-controlled hypertension.[37]

MEDICAL MANAGEMENT OF THE HYPERTENSIVE PATIENT

Management of hypertension is not a straightforward process. The Chicago Heart Association Study of 1967–1972 revealed that less than 20% of all hypertensive persons were getting effective treatment.[101] For adherence to therapy, a program tailored to the individual hypertensive patient is essential. Before the introduction of antihypertensive medications 30 years ago, thereapy was limited to sedation with barbiturates, surgery, drastic diets, and even phlebotomy. Today most therapy is directed toward reducing the blood pressure to the lowest possible level without introducing adverse effects, maximizing adherence to therapy, and ensuring that the complications and expense of therapy do not outweigh the benefits.

It appears to be more cost-effective, in terms of the practitioner's time and the direct cost of medication and management of adverse drug effects, to begin with a conservative approach in the case of the 70% who are mildly hypertensive. Conservative management would reduce the risk of hypertensive heart disease by helping individuals change poor health habits. Weight reduction, diets to reduce intake of salt and cholesterol, an exercise program, and efforts to reduce smoking and stress are some topics to discuss when counseling the hypertensive patient.

A careful assessment of all risk factors is essential before reaching a decision on the type of management strategy to adopt. If the person is young, has no evidence of organ damage, and has no family history of hypertension, the long-term effects of drug therapy (hypokalemia, gout, carbohydrate intolerance, and so on) may not warrant a more aggressive therapy for mild hypertension than the conservative approach mentioned above. However, a black, overweight, diabetic woman with a positive family history, who smokes heavily and has hypercholesteremia, would require more drastic medical intervention.

If conservative therapy is ineffective, or if one or more risk factors is present, the patient should probably be treated with drug therapy because the benefits of drug management, even with the possibility of side effects, will far outweigh their expense and inconvenience.

If the patient has a diastolic pressure above 105 mm Hg, drug therapy is definitely necessary and the cost of therapy, with its possibility of side effects, is far outweighed by the improved quality of life and the number of productive life-years gained. In determining the cost of hypertension to the American work force, one survey found that hypertensive persons missed an average of 51 days from work during a 1-year period. This was double the number of days for normotensive persons.[54] However, when considering the need for more health care providers to treat the many cases of mild hypertension, it is estimated that health care costs would increase $2.8 billion, but the incidence of myocardial infarction and stroke would decrease 15%.[149]

Even if the hypertension has persisted for many years,

the asymptomatic older person is still at increased risk. Although some physicians fear that reducing the pressure may harm the older person by decreasing the perfusion through their sclerosed vessels, the Veteran's Administration study negated that fear, and demonstrated that even elderly patients who have had their blood pressure lowered live longer. Because of decreased baroreceptor responsiveness, the elderly may have a problem with postural hypotension if the pressure is reduced too fast during antihypertensive therapy. An elderly patient with cerebrovascular, coronary, or renal insufficiency would also be particularly vulnerable to suddenly lowered blood pressure. Unless side effects occur, a slow, controlled reduction in blood pressure is recommended for the elderly patient.

There are basically two approaches to the treatment of hypertension: interference with renal control mechanisms and inducement of hypovolemia to lower total body sodium and interference with neural control mechanisms by giving large doses of adrenergic blockers. Because as many as 85% of all hypertensive persons have low or normal plasma renin activity levels, Klahr[79] suggests starting treatment with drugs that interfere with renal control and also stimulate renin (diuretics such as the thiazides). If there is no response to the diuretic therapy within 2 months, or if there are significant side effects, Klahr suggests adding or substituting drugs (such as the beta blocker propranolol) that will alter the sympathetic nervous system activity or deal with the hyperreninemia. (Refer to Table 47-2 for drugs which potentiate or inhibit renin secretion.)

The "Stepped Care" approach, as illustrated in Figure 37-1, is a simplified practical scheme for the medical management of hypertensive individuals and is often used by physicians.[37,132,138] This approach involves introducing low doses of drugs with the highest likelihood of effectiveness and adherence and the lowest risk of adverse effects. For a complete discussion of drug therapy in hypertension, refer to Chapter 37.

NURSING MANAGEMENT DURING ACUTE HYPERTENSIVE CRISIS

Before there were any effective drugs with which to treat severe hypertension, the incidence of hypertensive crisis was nearly 8%. Today, with a successful antihypertensive program, the incidence is less than 1%. Even though it is rare, considering the large number of people with chronic hypertension, hypertensive crisis presents an immediate threat to life and prompt action to reduce the blood pressure is essential. The rapidity with which blood pressure is reduced depends on the patient's age, level of the diastolic pressure, and the evidence for impending organ failure (pulmonary edema, papilledema, encephalopathy, or severe azotemia). If lowered blood pressure can be maintained while the vascular lesions heal, malignant hypertension can be reversed.[36,75,90]

Individuals most likely to become critically hypertensive include primarily poorly controlled hypertensives, and those who suddenly discontinue their medication.[5,61] The severity of withdrawal symptoms depends on the dose taken, but a

TABLE 47-9 CLINICAL SITUATIONS IN WHICH PATIENTS REQUIRE IMMEDIATE REDUCTION IN BLOOD PRESSURE

1. Sustained diastolic pressure of more than 100 mm Hg, and
   a. sudden onset of cerebral dysfunction
   b. acute left-ventricular failure
   c. myocardial infarction
2. Leaking or dissecting aortic aneurysm
3. Accelerated hypertension from any cause
4. Toxemia of pregnancy when life of fetus or mother is immediately threatened by convulsions, left-ventricular failure, or fetal distress
5. Uncontrolled hypertension in patients requiring immediate surgery
6. Refractory hypertension greater than 120 mm Hg in kidney transplant patients

(After Keith TA: JAMA 237(15):1570–1577, 1977)

sudden surge in secretion of norepinephrine can occur with any of the centrally acting agents, such as clonidine, methyldopa and propranolol. Situations requiring immediate intervention to reduce blood pressure to normotensive levels are listed in Table 47-9.

The goal of aggressive therapy is to decrease the blood pressure to within normal limits within 24 to 48 hours, depending on the presence or absence of coexisting complications. Action must be taken within minutes if left ventricular failure, encephalopathy, or intracerebral hemorrhage occurs. Reduction of blood pressure can be more gradual and not necessarily to normal limits if acute cerebral or myocardial infarction or severe renal failure is present.[47]

Sodium nitroprusside (Nitrostat) has been used since 1951 and is still considered the drug of choice in hypertensive emergencies by most physicians because of its immediate vasodilating effect and its short duration. For a complete discussion of nitroprusside and other drugs used in hypertensive crisis, see Chapter 37.

With the hazards inherent in nitroprusside and other current drug therapy (Chap. 37), the vasodilatory and natriuretic effects of the prostaglandins look rather promising. When commercially available for general use, prostaglandins can be given intravenously to lower blood pressure within 15 to 30 seconds, with a minimum of side effects.[128]

NURSING MANAGEMENT OF PATIENTS WITH CHRONIC HYPERTENSION

Patients with chronic hypertension can have problems centering on inability to control their pressure or on poor adherence to antihypertensive therapy. The factors responsible for poor control or nonadherence are many but can be eliminated or reduced by quality patient assessment, supervision, and teaching. Table 47-10 outlines possible nursing diagnoses for initiating a plan of care for the patient with chronic hypertension. Since these problems are amenable to nursing intervention primarily in the form of patient education,[51] a teaching plan for the patient with newly diagnosed hypertension is presented in Table 47-11. The nurse–patient activities and outcome criteria found in the teaching plan can be used concurrently as plans and goals for the nursing diagnoses established from Table 47-10.

TABLE 47-10 PATIENT PROBLEM LIST FOR CHRONIC HIGH BLOOD PRESSURE

I. *Lack of Blood Pressure Control Secondary to*
1. Overweight condition
2. Excessive sodium intake
3. Lack of exercise
4. Extreme stress
5. Excessive smoking
6. Inappropriate medication administration, due to
   a. misunderstanding dose schedule
   b. over-the-counter drug interactions
   c. misunderstanding of necessity for control, not cure

II. *Poor Adherence to Prescribed Therapy Secondary to*
1. Inappropriate understanding of high blood pressure, due to
   a. past experiences
   b. apprehension
   c. conflicting advice from friends
2. Lack of family's understanding and support
3. Denial of health problem
4. Distrust of health-care system or provider
5. Drug side effects, such as
   a. orthostatic hypotension
   b. hypokalemia
   c. hyperuricemia
   d. sexual dysfunction
6. Not following prescribed drug therapy for various reasons:
   a. unpleasant taste of potassium supplement
   b. gastrointestinal side effects
   c. not feeling symptomatic
   d. forgetting to take medication
   e. belief that medications are a waste of time
   f. belief that treatment is worse than the problem
   g. fear of side effects
   h. too expensive
   i. fear of addiction
   j. embarrassment around friends and family

This list of probable problems together with their cause(s) constitutes nursing diagnostic statements that may be applicable in any hypertensive patient's situation. Refer to Table 47-11 for possible goals and actions to use in conjunction with the patient's diagnosed problem.

As nurses dealing primarily with long-term hypertensive patients, our role has been defined by the National Task Force on the Role of Nursing in High Blood Pressure Control; it involves six specific client outcomes or goals within three general areas of nursing practice:[45,46,118]

1. To assist the patient and family in recognizing behaviors that promote health
   Goals
   a. Stable blood pressure at the desired level
   b. Minimal target organ damage
2. To assist the patient and family to cope with, and adhere to, the demands of the therapy program
   Goals
   a. Successful adjustments to diagnosis and therapy
   b. Minimal side effects from drug therapy
3. To instruct, guide, and support patients in achieving and maintaining self care
   Goals
   a. Understanding of hypertension and prescribed therapy
   b. Responsibility for self care
   c. Stable blood pressure at desired level

Promoting Health

To carry out nursing's first role of helping patients and their families to enhance the quality of their lives, an understanding of the factors influencing the development of hypertension and heart disease is essential (see also Chap. 13 on risk factors for coronary artery disease).

Hypertension is the major risk factor contributing to the high incidence of cardiovascular death, and it is one of the few controllable ones. Because the evidence for controllable environmental factors is as strong as the evidence for uncontrollable genetic inheritance of hypertension, importance should also be placed on efforts to help hypertensive persons maintain good health care practices. Individuals not genetically inclined toward hypertension can tolerate many environmental factors without developing hypertension, but persons who are genetically predisposed to developing hypertension may not manifest high blood pressure until an environmental factor, such as high salt or cholesterol intake, stress, smoking, or increased weight, is superimposed.

Countries in which individuals are physically active throughout their lives do not have evidence of hypertension in the older age groups. With acculturation more sugar, fat, meat, and salt are consumed, activity decreases, and weight and blood pressure increase with age.

Weight Control. The results of many studies indicate a direct relationship between obesity, defined as a weight 20% above the body-mass index (weight/height^2), and hypertension.[30,66,140] The finding that increased weight can increase blood pressure has been explained physiologically as a disproportion between the capacity of the aorta and an increased cardiac output. As body mass increases, the cardiac output increases but the capacity of the aorta cannot increase and the result is hypertension.

Studies of populations in Framingham, Massachusetts, and Evans County, Georgia, both reveal that overweight individuals have from four to eight times the risk of developing hypertension.[71,146] To rule out inheritable tendencies, blood pressure levels in twins were studied: differences in blood pressure correlated highly with differences in weight.[34]

Weight reduction lowers blood pressure in both sexes and at all ages and levels of blood pressure[116] and can reduce the prevalence of hypertension in the United States by 50%.[146] Follow-up of a group of patients who lost about 5 kg over a 6 month period revealed that their systolic blood pressure dropped an average of 28 mm Hg and their diastolic pressure, an average of 20 mm Hg.[116] Hypertensive people in Evans County, Georgia, between 1960 and 1962 lost an average of 18 pounds and lowered their blood pressure an average of 18 mm Hg systolic and 13 mm Hg diastolic.[146] Thus it appears that counseling patients toward a weight-reduction program is a good way of controlling the blood pressure as an initial step in hypertensive persons who are overweight. Furthermore, it is relatively inexpensive and virtually free of side effects.

Sodium Consumption. Eating is an important part of every culture, but a person's appetite for salt appears to have no relationship to physiologic requirement. Since 1 g of salt (¼ tsp) is required for each liter of water ingested, only about 3 g of salt is required for the average adult's daily water intake of less than 3 liters from food and liquid.[96] A child requires no more than 700 mg of salt per kilogram of body weight,[115] but Americans' diets average a total daily intake of 10 g to 15 g of salt.

TABLE 47-11 TEACHING PLAN FOR THE PATIENT WITH HIGH BLOOD PRESSURE

Content Area	Nurse—Patient Activity	Outcome Criteria
A. *Pathology of high blood pressure*		A. *The patient/family are able to*
1. Definition of blood pressure, including concepts of arterial circulation systolic pressure diastolic pressure peripheral resistance	1a. Establish rapport with patient and family. b. Assess readiness to learn and level of understanding regarding blood pressure. c. Explain that blood pressure is determined by sounds that result from the vibration of blood against the arterial wall. d. Explain systolic pressure as the pressure which occurs when the heart actually beats; it is the first number recorded; the first sound heard through the stethoscope; it measures how hard the heart works to pump blood. e. Explain diastolic pressure as the pressure between heart beats; the second number recorded; the last sound heard through the stethoscope; the pressure arteries exert on the blood as it flows through. f. With visual aids, explain how vasoconstriction and vasodilatation influence pressure through the blood vessels.	1. Define and state the limits of normal blood pressure. Distinguish the systolic from diastolic pressure as recorded. State what happens when there is a state of increased or decreased peripheral resistance.
2. Definition of high blood pressure	2a. Assess understanding of high blood pressure. b. Include in explanation that "hypertension" is not synonomous with high anxiety or tension and that "high blood pressure" is not the same as "high blood" or the opposite of "low blood" (anemia).	2. Define high blood pressure accurately. Differentiate between normal and abnormal blood pressure.
3. Causes and contributing factors in the onset of high blood pressure	3a. Assess cause/contributing factors for patient's high blood pressure. b. Discuss the cause, or lack of apparent causes, as appropriate. c. Discuss relevant contributing factors.	3. Explain the most likely reason for development of high blood pressure.
4. Effects of high blood pressure on the body Lack of symptoms ("silent killer")	4a. Explain that the higher the blood pressure, the greater the likelihood of organ damage. b. Explain that there are usually no symptoms until hypertension has progressed too far and reinforce that hypertension is symptomless. c. Outline the consequences of high blood pressure on blood vessels and organs in the body: heart failure kidney failure stroke	4. State that high blood pressure can exist without symptoms. State effects of high blood pressure on the heart and blood vessels, kidneys, and brain.
5. Control versus cure	5a. Explain that high blood pressure is a life-long problem and patient should not stop treatment regardless of side effects or feeling better. Also explain that drug or dose can be altered. b. Inform patient of what desired blood pressure (goal) is for him. c. Encourage patient and family to express feelings. d. Encourage family's participation in the patient's treatment program. e. Reassure that concerns are normal, common, and expected. f. Avoid saying "normal" blood pressure and use the term "well-controlled" when patient reaches desired goal.	5. Distinguish control from cure. State personal goal for blood pressure level. State when and how family members can help and is able to ask family for that assistance. Request information for friends and relatives about blood pressure control and management.
B. *General Well-being*		B. *The patient is able to*
1. Dietary habits and weight control	1a. Assess patient's weight compared with ideal and consult with dietitian. b. Explain effects of excess weight on workload of the heart, hypertension, and general health. c. Emphasize that losing 5 pounds will make a difference in blood pressure. d. Explain effects of excess cholesterol and sugar on vasculature and show pictures, if available. e. Give diet instructions in writing to patient and family.	1. State what desired weight should be Recognize need for weight loss to improve health. Verbalize need to lose weight if necessary. Accept diet instructions. Be within 5 pounds of desired weight by 6 months.
2. Smoking	2a. Explain importance of eliminating or decreasing smoking. b. Discuss with patient a plan to quit smoking. c. Inform of counseling and support through local clinics of the American Cancer Society.	2. Reduce number of cigarettes smoked by one half (or eliminate smoking entirely) by 3 months.

(Table continues on page 618)

TABLE 47-11 (Cont.)

Content Area	Nurse—Patient Activity	Outcome Criteria
3. Alcohol	3a. Explain alcohol's high caloric content and its effect as a vasodilator and a depressant. b. Check alcohol's synergistic effects with patient's medication. c. Inform patient verbally and in writing about alcohol's interaction with prescribed medication.	3. Explain effects of alcohol on the body. Explain how alcohol would affect the prescribed medication patient is taking.
4. Exercise	4a. Explain importance of regular, moderate, frequent exercise program, unless contraindicated. b. Determine what patient enjoys and encourage that activity, if practical. c. Instruct patient to increase daily exercise until walking briskly 30 minutes/day.	4. Verbalize importance of activity and exercise program. Ambulate 30 minutes/day briskly, without fatigue or complaints of intermittent claudication. Verbalize positive enjoyment of exercise program.
5. Caffeine	5a. Explain caffeine's stimulating effect on the heart. b. Encourage patient to decrease the amount of coffee, tea, cola, etc. in diet or eliminate caffeine entirely from diet. c. Offer other suggestions for fluid intake: caffeine-free coffee, juices, water, etc.	5. State effect of caffeine on heart. Reduce amount of caffeine intake by one half in a 3-month period.
6. Stress management	6a. Encourage patient to verbalize feelings. b. Assist patient to identify stressors in his environment. c. Explore ways to help cope with stress: avoiding hurrying leisurely meals well-space appointment calendar d. Help patients distinguish stressors which can be avoided and those which are unavoidable. e. Instruct patient in relaxation techniques if desired and appropriate for patient as a tool in self-management of hypertension. e. Recommend counseling to change life-style.	6. Identify two stressors in environment. Eliminate one of those two stressors within 6 months. Verbalize willingness to learn a relaxation technique. Accept counseling if necessary.
C. *Low Sodium Diet*[59]		C. *The patient/family are able to*
1. Effects of sodium on the body and sodium's relationship to high blood pressure	1a. Establish rapport with patient and family. b. Assess patient and family understanding of sodium and its relation to fluid retention and high blood pressure. c. Explain relationship of sodium to blood pressure and explain reason for low sodium diet. d. Gather data on patient's diet history and cultural patterns to establish diet plan. e. Determine effects of altering food preparation on family members. f. Formulate a diet plan in accordance with patient's cultural preferences, financial means, and seasonal variations. g. A 5 g sodium diet requires no added table salt, slight salting during cooking, avoidance of obviously salty foods, and reduced amount of canned, frozen, and "fast" foods. h. Clarify any confusion.	1. Explain rationale for low sodium diet.
2. Foods containing sodium	2a. Give patient and family a list of foods and nonprescription medications containing sodium (see Chap. 37, Table 37-4). b. Teach patient to avoid foods high in sodium: milk products, processed foods, prepared foods, canned or frozen foods, and "fast" foods. c. Instruct patient in reading labels and recognizing sodium-containing products. d. Inform patient where to obtain specific product information (see section on Teaching Aids).	2. Identify favorite foods from list of high, moderate, and low sodium content foods. List common food groups to avoid or minimize.
3. The components of salt a. Salt vs sodium b. mg vs mEq	3a. Explain that salt consists of sodium and chloride. b. Discuss conversion of mEq to gm or mg. c. Teach patient to convert mEq to mg: 1 teaspoon salt = 2.4 g salt = 2,400 mg salt = 960 mg sodium (Na+) = 42 mEq	3. Name components of normal table salt. Easily convert mEq to mg and teaspoons of salt and pure sodium.
4. Other alternatives Exchange lists[59] Other sources of seasoning Salt substitute	4a. Explain the flexibility of an "exchange list" for commonly used items; *i.e.,* One glass milk = ½ cup peanuts. 4 ounces cottage cheese = ½ cup jello instant pudding. 2 slices bacon = 14 potato chips.	4. Recognize that occasional substitution of a favorite food for items in the prescribed diet can be done if the amount of sodium is equivalent State what type of diuretic he is taking and if a salt substitute can be

TABLE 47-11 (Cont.)

Content Area	Nurse—Patient Activity	Outcome Criteria
	b. Have patient consider alternatives to use of salt for flavoring foods: lemon juice, fresh garlic or onion instead of garlic salt, catsup, or steak sauces. c. Caution patient to avoid soy sauce, monosodium glutamate, etc. in flavoring foods.	used safely. State the components of salt substitute.

D. Medications
  1. Schedule for medication administration
	1a. Clarify with patient that antihypertensive medication is not like an antibiotic that can be taken only for a short period and then discontinued; that the dose should not be reduced to save money nor increased to obtain an even better effect.
	b. Stress that the medication is only effective (in dilating vessels, or whatever mechanism is pertinent) if taken and that the effect wears off over a specified amount of time.
	c. Reinforce that patient should assume he will take the medication for the rest of his life.
	d. Help patient construct a simple, convenient schedule for taking the medication.
	Let the patient offer suggestions to space out b.i.d. or t.i.d. doses.
	Help patient to discover ways to cue his medication-taking with an associated daily activity like eating, brushing teeth, etc.
	e. Tailor the medication schedule to fit the patient's personal habits/needs/schedule.
	f. Write down the name of the medication(s), dosage, appearance, and times to be taken.
	g. Instruct patient to store medication in a prominent location and mark a calendar to signify that the dose was taken.
	h. If the patient has been noncompliant with medication therapy
	  1. Explore reasons why medication was not taken
	  2. Work with patient and family to change the circumstances or the medication
		D. The patient and family are able to
		  1. Verbalize importance of following treatment regime as prescribed
		State:
		a. which pill to take
		b. what the pill looks like
		c. when to take the pill
		d. what to do if a dose is missed
		Mark doses taken on a calendar.
		Renew prior to exhausting current supply.
		Request advice on financial resources available to assist with cost.

2. Sudden withdrawal of medication	2a. Warn patient of effects of suddenly discontinuing their medication: rebound hypertensive effects (crisis) b. Instruction patient that medication should not only be stopped under physician's supervision and should be tapered off slowly.	2. State the consequences of sudden discontinuation of antihypertensive medication. Explain appropriate situation for discontinuing medication.
3. General knowledge of possible side effects (see Chap. 37, Table 37-1).	3a. Explain that some side effects are possible because the medication affects nerves and nerves control other functions of the body in addition to blood pressure. b. Emphasize that the patient will not necessarily have any side effects, but should be aware of possible effects beforehand and what to do about them should they occur. c. Make a list for the patient of a few of the more common side effects and action to take should they occur. d. Consider using the American Heart Association pamphlet entitled "What You Need to Know to Help Your Doctor Control Your High Blood Pressure," which contains pertinent side effects of common antihypertensives and action to take if they occur. e. Sympathize with patient—some effects can be very annoying. f. Recognize that the patient who feels fine and asymptomatic prior to starting therapy will be annoyed by taking medication and by side effects which may occur. g. Emphasize that taking the medication requires far less effort than treating complications of high blood pressure if and when they should occur. h. Encourage patient not to be too discouraged if treatment continues indefinitely.	3. State important side effects of his medication and what action to take if side effects occur. Seek advice prior to taking nonprescription medications. Verbalize feelings and annoyances.
4. Hypokalemia	4a. Assess if diuretic can be taken as a single dose to minimize potassium loss. b. Teach patient symptoms of potassium deficit: weakness, fatigue, leg cramps. Provide a list if necessary.	4. State symptoms of potassium deficit. Select favorite foods which are high in potassium.

(Table continues on page 620)

TABLE 47-11 (Cont.)

Content Area	Nurse—Patient Activity	Outcome Criteria
	c. Teach patient about foods high in potassium: dried fruits, nuts, etc. Provide list if necessary (see Chap. 37, Table 37-6).	
	d. Inform patient that potassium deficit will be treated when level drops below 3.0 or there are complaints of symptoms.	
	e. If using potassium supplements, instruct patient to mix medication in chilled fruit juice, preferably orange juice, and to take it after meals to minimize the distaste and gastric irritation.	
	f. Inform patient that it is very difficult to obtain adequate amounts of potassium from dietary sources alone: normal dietary intake of potassium should be 50—100 mEq/day (4 glasses of orange juice, or 7 bananas, contain 60 mEq potassium).	
	g. Teach patient that 1 mEq potassium = 39 mg.	
	h. Consider use of potassium-sparing diuretic.	
5. Postural hypotension	5a. Explain why patient will feel dizzy/faint when he stands suddenly from a lying position if volume is depleted or there is excessive vasodilatation.	5. Explain why dizziness occurs. State what to do if feels dizzy when arising from a lying position.
	b. Caution patient to dangle before getting up.	
	c. If dizziness persists more than 1—2 minutes, instruct patient to sit down, lie down, and either decrease or omit the next dose of medication; if dizziness continues, instruct patient to notify physician.	
	d. If necessary, teach patient to sleep with head elevated; not to stand still for more than a few minutes; avoid standing in sun or drinking alcohol because of vasodilatory effects.	
	e. Assess whether the medication can be taken at bedtime to minimize postural effects.	
6. Sexual dysfunction	6a. Be aware that sexual dysfunction can occur with all drugs except Apresoline, Lasix, Minipress, and Capoten.	6. Discuss sexuality status with practitioner.
	b. Also be aware that dysfunction can result from many other causes: alcohol, diabetes, stress, marital difficulties, etc.	
	c. Do not suggest that patient will have dysfunction during initial teaching of medication side effects. Discuss side effect at a later date if patient indicates a problem.	
E. *Taking the blood pressure*		E. *The patient/family are able to*
1. Ability to take blood pressure	1a. Assess patient for hearing, visual acuity, manual dexterity, and coordination.	1. Verbalize willingness to learn to take blood pressure
	b. Assess patient's or family member's willingness to learn and readiness to participate in self care.	
2. Appropriate environment	2a. Instruct patient in importance of limiting noisy environment; avoiding chills that vasoconstrict; avoiding other discomforts.	2. Describe appropriate environment for taking blood pressure
	b. Instruct to rest for 5 minutes prior to taking the blood pressure.	
3. Suitable position	3. Instruct patient to assume a position of comfort with arm resting at heart level and avoiding isometrics (tensing arm muscles).	3. Assume proper position for taking blood pressure
4. Well-functioning equipment	4. Instruct patient to make sure needle on manometer is at zero prior to inflation of the cuff, and that glass cover is intact.	4. Identify properly functioning equipment
5. Reading the gauge and adjusting the pressure-control valve	5. Help the patient to become familiar with reading the gauge and adjusting the flow valve.	5. Accurately read a mercury gauge or needle gauge at various points on the scale. Open and close the pressure control valve without difficulty
6. Brachial pulse and cuff placement	6a. Assist patient to find the brachial pulse.	6. Find brachial pulse. Apply cuff snuggly
	b. Assist patient to find the center of the cuff bladder which is then placed 1—2 inches above the spot where the elbow bends (antecubital fossa).	
	c. Assist patient to apply cuff snuggly.	

TABLE 47-11 (Cont.)

Content Area	Nurse—Patient Activity	Outcome Criteria
	d. Assist patient to place the bell of the stethoscope firmly, but not too hard, over the artery. The bell can be sewn into the cuff or held in place by 2 wide elastic bands.	
7. The actual procedure	7a. Explain the procedure to the patient prior to starting: Inflating the cuff compresses the artery and obstructs the flow of blood temporarily; deflating the cuff decreases the pressure and reestablishes the blood flow. b. Instruct patient in cleansing the earpieces prior to initiating the procedure. c. Show patient how the stethoscope earpieces should be placed in the ears (directed forward for better acuity). d. Stress the importance of keeping the tubing from rubbing and creating excess noise. e. Have patient inflate the cuff to 20—30 mm Hg above last known blood pressure reading* and deflate at a slow, steady rate of 2 lines per second (2—4 mm Hg per second). f. Caution patient to never stop or reinflate cuff during procedure because of increased inaccuracy. g. Inform patient that pressure can be rechecked again after waiting 1—2 minutes. h. If patient has difficulty hearing blood pressure sounds, instruct him to raise arm over head and inflate the cuff. Then lower the arm and take the reading. i. Reinforce the fact that a single reading is not significant in and of itself. The trend is what is significant.	7. Correctly take 3 accurate blood pressures as the practitioner listens with a double stethoscope

* If a professional is taking the blood pressure, it is still recommended that the cuff be inflated to 20—30 mm Hg above cessation of the palpated brachial pulse or radial pulse.

Five content areas are outlined with appropriate teaching activities and outcome criteria for evaluating the success of the educational program. It can be used in conjunction with Table 47-10 to formulate a plan of care for the patient with high blood pressure.

Consuming more salt than the body needs leads to hypertension only in susceptible persons. If about ¼ tsp of salt is retained per day in the body, an adult can potentially accumulate a liter of fluid during a week's time.[29] Experiments with sodium-sensitive rat strains suggest that if they are never allowed salt in their diet, they will remain normotensive and live a normal life span. If sodium is introduced into their diet, hypertension develops and they die prematurely.

Polynesians who migrated to New Zealand experienced a reduction in the amount of exercise and a change in diet from fish and coconut to increased proteins, refined carbohydrates and calories. They also doubled their intake of salt. In a survey of the migrating population, children 5 to 9 years old had a significantly higher blood pressure than those who did not migrate.[4]

Japanese farmers, who consume an average of 20 g to 25 g of salt per day, have a high incidence (84%) of systolic pressures above 140 mm Hg, whereas people in areas with low salt intake (less than 4 g/day) have a low incidence of hypertension.[131] Korean men, whose salt intake averages 25 g per day, have higher blood pressures than Belgians of larger weights who ingest about 11 g of salt per day.

People consume salt from a variety of sources: water, natural foods, processed foods, and table salt. Fortunately, the purchase of table salt by consumers has decreased over the past few years. Unfortunately, the consumption of processed and prepared foods has increased, and with it, the salt content. Salt is added to prepared foods because of the toxic effect it has on microorganisms. Prior to 1970, partially in an attempt to satisfy the parents' taste, commercially prepared baby food had 5 to 100 times as much salt as the natural product.[26,35] Today, no salt is added to manufactured baby foods, but a comparison of baby food prepared at home showed some startling results: salt content is significantly higher than that of the manufactured product of the 1960s because the parent appears to be using processed and prepared foods to make the baby food.[77]

Potassium content is depleted during the food processing. The reduced potassium has clinical implications because potassium appears to counteract the blood pressure-raising effects of sodium.[96,145] If sodium is held at a constant level in experiments with rats, the blood pressure will increase as the potassium in their diet is lowered. In patients with hypertension, it may be that sodium intake is sufficiently high to cause an elevated blood pressure and the potassium intake is not adequate enough to mask the elevation. When thiazide diuretics were introduced in the treatment of hypertension, the necessity for sodium-restricted diets became overlooked. Potassium loss from eating high-sodium diets is augmented when a diuretic is taken. When persons taking 50 mg of hydrochlorothiazide increased their salt intake from 3 g to 6 g, the amount of medication had to be increased to 100 mg in order to prevent hypokalemia and to obtain a satisfactory blood pressure level.[32] Because high salt intake reduces the effectiveness of antihypertensive medications, people should lower their sodium intake, even when taking a diuretic.

Food products that contribute to high salt intake are sometimes easily recognized (potato chips, peanuts, etc.) but sometimes not so easily recognized (baked goods, bottled water, cheese, processed meats, V₈ Vegetable juice, white processed breads, water, and medications). The salt content of various water supplies can be quite significant (Table 47-12). Refer to Chapter 37 and Table 37-4 for a list of the medications containing sodium. Another problem is inherent in prescribing food products that have been developed to reduce the intake of animal fats (egg substitutes and imitation animal products made from vegetables) because of their high sodium content.

Rigid low-salt diets (less than 1 g of salt, or about 500 mg of sodium) will reduce blood pressure in a high percentage of patients, even those with severe hypertension, but compliance becomes so poor that it is better to ask people to comply with a moderately low salt diet. One example of a rigid diet is the Kempner Rice Diet of the 1950s in which dieters were not even allowed to lick gummed labels or stamps or to wash their dishes with soap![129]

Moderately low-salt diets (salt intake reduced from 10 g to 5 g, or from 4 g of sodium to 2 g) can drop blood pressure about 10/7 mm Hg.[100,107] Two years on a moderately low salt diet can accomplish the same effect as antihypertensive drug treatment or reduce the amount of medication used. A moderate sodium restriction can be accomplished by limiting processed foods, table salt, and obviously heavily salted foods.

In counseling patients and their families about sodium and dietary restrictions, the results are less than encouraging. A survey in 1973 found that of the 60% who were even counseled to eat less salt, a third said that they often added salt, and another third said that they almost never added salt to their food. It was of further interest to note that more than 60% of the college-educated hypertensive population said that they often added salt to their foods.[54] For better adherence to sodium-restricted diets, an intense teaching program is necessary for all hypertensive patients.

Smoking. Patients should be counseled to quit smoking or reduce the number of cigarettes they smoke. But the evidence that smoking causes hypertension is not as strong as the evidence that obesity does. In fact, the Framingham Study data revealed that blood pressure was lower in those who smoked than in those who had quit smoking. The difference may have been due to subsequent weight gain,[50,72] but confirmation is needed.

Nicotine increases catecholamine discharge and causes an increase in heart rate and blood pressure. Smoking two cigarettes will increase mean arterial blood pressure by as much as 12 mm Hg.[25] Chain smokers, because of the continual release of catecholamines, exhibit a higher than normal blood pressure.[109] Smoking also has some effect on vascular tissue. Researchers have found severe damage to the umbilical vasculature and placental villi in mothers who smoke during pregnancy.[2] Whether this has any detrimental effects on the fetus is still under investigation.

There are indications that women who smoke heavily shorten their lives by an average of 19 years and increase the likelihood of dying suddenly from acute heart disease. If they use oral contraceptives, the risk is even greater. In a retrospective study of women dying from sudden heart

TABLE 47-12 SODIUM AND POTASSIUM CONTENT IN WATER SUPPLIES OF CITIES IN THE UNITED STATES*

Location	Na^+ (mg) per 100 ml	K^+ (mg) per 100 ml
Aberdeen, SD	20	2
Albany, NY	0.2	0.2
Albuquerque, NM	5	0.7
Annapolis, MD	0.2	0.2
Ann Arbor, MI	2	0.5
Atlanta, GA	0.2	0.2
Augusta, ME	0.2	0.2
Austin, TX	3	0.5
Baltimore, MD	0.3	0.2
Bangor, ME	0.2	0.1
Baton Rouge, LA	9	0.2
Beloit, WI	0.5	0.2
Biloxi, MS	23	0.6
Birmingham, AL	2	0.3
Bismarck, ND	6	0.6
Boise, ID	2	0.3
Boston, MA	0.3	0.2
Brownsville, TX	6	0.3
Buffalo, NY	0.7	0.3
Burlington, VT	0.2	0.1
Carson City, NV	0.4	0.3
Charleston, SC	1	0.3
Charleston, WV	0.3	0.2
Charlotte, NC	0.3	0.1
Charlottesville, VA	0.2	0.1
Cheyenne, WY	0.3	0.2
Chicago, IL	0.3	0.1
Cincinnati, OH	0.7	0.3
Cleveland, OH	1	0.3
Columbia, SC	0.4	0.2
Columbus, OH	5	0.6
Concord, NH	0.2	0.1
Crandall, TX	170†	0.5
Dallas, TX	3	0.5
Denver, CO	3	0.2
Des Moines, IA	1	0.4
Detroit, MI	0.3	0.1
Dover, DE	2	0.5
Durham, SC	0.4	0.2
El Paso, TX	7	0.6
Ephrata, PA	0.3	0.2
Evansville, IN	2	0.5
Fargo, ND	5	0.7
Frankfort, KY	0.3	0.1
Galesburg, IL	30	2
Galveston, TX	34	0.7
Harrisburg, PA	0.2	0.1
Hartford, CT	0.2	0.1
Helena, MT	0.3	0.2
Houston, TX	16	0.6
Huntington, WV	3	0.2
Indianapolis, IN	1	0.3
Iowa City, IA	0.5	0.3
Jackson, MS	0.4	0.2
Jacksonville, FL	1	0.2
Jefferson City, MO	3	0.4
Jersey City, NJ	0.3	0.2
Kansas City, KS	4	0.4
Kansas City, MO	10	3
Lansing, MI	1	0.5
Lincoln, NE	3	0.7
Little Rock, AR	0.1	0.1
Los Angeles, CA		
Aqueduct source	6	0.6
Metropolitan source	17	0.6
River source	5	0.5
Louisville, KY	2	0.3
Madison, WI	0.4	0.2
Manchester, NH	0.2	0.1
Marison, OH	17	0.7
Memphis, TN	2	0.3
Miami, FL	2	0.3
Milwaukee, WI	0.3	0.1
Minneapolis, MN	0.5	0.3
Minot, ND	25	0.6
Montgomery, AL	0.8	0.1
Montpelier, VT	0.1	0.1
Nashville, TN	0.3	0.2

TABLE 47-12 (Cont.)

Location	Na⁺ (mg) per 100 ml	K⁺ (mg) per 100 ml
Nevada, MO	33	0.7
Newark, NJ	0.2	0.1
New Haven, CT	0.3	0.1
New Orleans, LA	1	0.4
New York, NY	0.3	0.2
Oakland, CA	0.3	0.1
Oklahoma City, OK	10	0.8
Olympia, WA	0.5	0.3
Omaha, NE	8	1
Philadelphia, PA	2	0.4
Phoenix, AZ	11	0.7
Pierre, SD	9	0.5
Pittsburgh, PA	6	0.5
Portland, ME	0.2	0.1
Portland, OR	0.1	0.1
Providence, RI	0.2	0.1
Raleigh, NC	0.4	0.1
Reno, NV	0.5	0.1
Richmond, VA	0.7	0.2
Rochester, MN	0.7	0.2
Rochester, NY	0.3	0.2
Sacramento, CA	0.3	0.2
Santa Fe, NM	0.4	0.1
St. Louis, MO	5	0.5
St. Paul, MN	0.5	0.3
Salem, OR	0.2	0.1
Salt Lake City, UT	0.8	0.2
San Diego, CA	5	0.5
San Francisco, CA	1	0.3
Seattle, WA	0.2	0.1
Sioux Falls, SD	1	0.4
Springfield, IL	0.8	0.3
Syracuse, NY	0.2	0.1
Tallahassee, FL	0.3	0.1
Topeka, KS	1	0.5
Trenton, NJ	0.1	0.1
Tucson, AZ	3	0.3
Washington, D.C.	0.3	0.3
Wichita, KS	5	0.5
Wilmington, DE	0.8	0.1

* City or state water departments should be consulted for current information regarding constituents of specific water supplies.

† An extreme example. This water is rarely ingested, but is used for cooking.

(Billf CE et al: J Am Diatet Assoc 25:312–313, 1949. Copyright by American Dietetic Association. Reprinted with permission)

disease, 62% smoked more than 20 cigarettes per day and their mean age at death was only 48 years. Among women who died of other causes, only 28% were heavy smokers and their average age of death was 67 years.[137]

Alcohol Intake. Studies indicate that 80-proof alcohol (in amounts of 30 to 75 ml) increases heart rate and cardiac output. There is little change in peripheral vascular resistance because of the vasodilation induced by the alcohol. However, vessels in the viscera constrict to compensate for the peripheral vasodilation, with the result that systolic pressure can climb very high and be accompanied by a rise in the diastolic pressure.[80]

Consumption of more than 60 ml of alcohol per day appears to double the number of people with hypertension above 160/95 mm Hg that consumption of half that amount would cause.[72] Patients can be reassured that there probably is a safe amount of alcohol that can be consumed without developing hypertension. Less than 30 ml of alcohol (24 oz of beer or 7 oz of wine) per day is probably not harmful and may in fact be beneficial, if it reduces anxiety.

Psychologic Stress and Personality. Stress should be considered a factor in the development of hypertension or in the maintenance of a hypertensive state, but it is unlikely to actually cause hypertension.[134] If certain individuals perceive events that occur in their environment as threatening, they initiate defense mechanisms that cause blood pressure to increase. Stress, conflicts, frustration, uncertainties, and even overwork can potentially increase blood pressure. To date, no relationship between hypertension and personality or way of perceiving the environment has ever been proved.[49,135]

In a breed of hypertension-sensitive rats, researchers kept salt ingestion just below the level required to induce hypertension and found that the rats became hypertensive when exposed to approach–avoidance stress.[40] To stimulate psychologic stress in humans, individuals with borderline hypertension were asked to carry out mental arithmetic. An increased amount of catecholamine was excreted as a result of this experimentally imposed stress, and this indicates a possible link to hypertension.[69]

If a person lives in an urban area for more than twenty years, there is a significant increase in blood pressure. Some of the increase in pressure may be a result of the increase in psychologic stress, as well as a result of a different diet and increased weight associated with an urban life-style. People working in stressful occupations, for example, air traffic controllers, are four times as likely to have blood pressures greater than 140/90 mm Hg as are persons with less stressful occupations.[20]

In addition to the stresses of a particular occupation or of urban living, there is also a positive correlation between hypertension and persons of high intellectual achievement. Studies report that developing high blood pressure is three times more likely if a person is concerned with academic grades and is in the top 10% of the class.[135]

Age, Sex, and Familial Tendency. Mean arterial blood pressure progressively increases with age. Blood pressure averages 103/57 mm Hg in the 5-year-old child and 111/67 mm Hg in the 12-year-old.[112] Females tend to have a steady increase in systolic pressure, but males have a rapid increase during childhood and a more gradual increase after age 20, so that by middle age, women surpass men in systolic pressure. The diastolic pressure increases gradually in both sexes.[54]

More and more evidence has been gathered to indicate that hypertension is initiated during early childhood. Children as young as 2 years from high-risk families have been reported to be hypertensive. Children have a 41% risk of developing idiopathic hypertension if both parents are hypertensive, but a 28% risk if only one parent is hypertensive. The risk of developing hypertension (greater than 160/100 mm Hg) is four times higher in siblings of hypertensive adults than in the general population.[33]

In looking at the total population, up to 60% of the variance in blood pressure can be accounted for by genetic factors. In studies of adult twins, the variance was as high as 80% even if the twins had lived apart for many years.[98] Adopted children, no matter the age at which they are adopted, have a higher correlation with biologic relatives than with their adoptive parents.[11]

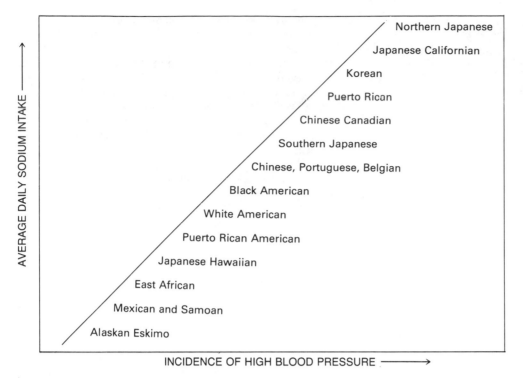

↑ AVERAGE DAILY SODIUM INTAKE

Northern Japanese
Japanese Californian
Korean
Puerto Rican
Chinese Canadian
Southern Japanese
Chinese, Portuguese, Belgian
Black American
White American
Puerto Rican American
Japanese Hawaiian
East African
Mexican and Samoan
Alaskan Eskimo

INCIDENCE OF HIGH BLOOD PRESSURE ⟶

Fig. 47-4. Incidence of high blood pressure in different populations, by amount of sodium intake. (Meneely GR, Battarbee HD: Am J Cardiol 38(6):768–785, 1976; Meneely GR, Dahl LK: Med Clin North Am 45(2):271–283, 1961)

Ethnic Differences. No ethnic group is considered immune to the development of hypertension. Studies generally conclude that after 10 years in the United States, foreign-born men have the same incidence of hypertension as those born in the United States.[74] Japanese men have a higher blood pressure than Japanese migrants of equivalent weights living in California and a lower blood pressure than Japanese migrants living in Hawaii.[152] Chinese people exhibit an increase in blood pressure after emigrating to Canada.[82] Mexicans and Samoans have a low incidence of hypertension, but the Japanese and the Portuguese are intermediate between the Chinese on the one hand and the residents of the United States and Western Europe on the other (Fig. 47-4).

Black persons living in the United States have more severely elevated blood pressures, ranging from 5 to 10 mm Hg higher than that of their white contemporaries.[119] Hypertension is twice as prevalent among blacks as among whites, and death from hypertension is four times higher,[41,66] yet black children in East Africa have lower systolic pressures at all ages than does the black population in the United States.[112]

The First National Conference on Hypertension among Puerto Ricans[104] announced that Puerto Ricans living in New York have a lower rate of hypertension than both the total United States population and the population living in Puerto Rico. The incidence of hypertension appears to increase with the length of stay in New York, but this may be reflecting a trend toward increased weight. The mortality from hypertension is higher in Puerto Rico than in the United States.

Maximizing Patient Adherence to Therapy

Results of many studies indicate that about 75% of all hypertensive patients are not obtaining effective antihypertensive therapy.[141] For some patients, it is a matter of not being aware of their hypertensive state. For others it is a matter of inadequate control despite medical follow-up; and for still others, nonadherence with the therapy program outlined for them can occur as a result of many influencing factors.[125]

Before undertaking efforts to maximize a patient's adherence to anti-hypertensive therapy, health care providers should feel certain that hypertension is a severe health problem, that a treatment program can be an effective control measure, and that the benefits of reducing blood pressure are not outweighed by the expense to the health care system and to the patient, or by side effects from the therapy.[68]

In developing a framework for managing a patient with hypertension, a distinction between adherence and compliance is useful to the practitioner. Compliance merely means that the patient does what he or she is told to do, and the outcome can be all but encouraging. Adherence implies a basis for long-term cooperation between patient and practitoner such that the patient willingly and actively participates in his therapy program.[142] Adherence is essential for the patient with a chronic problem such as hypertension.

There are many factors to consider when assessing the patient's motivation for adherence to the prescribed treatment. The greater the impact on the person's life style, the less likely one is to comply. Practitioners should consider

TABLE 47-13 COST OF ANTIHYPERTENSIVE MEDICATIONS BY EXPENSE PER 100 TABLETS OR CAPSULES*

Common Antihypertensive Medications	Amount
Hydrochlorothiazide 50 mg	$ 3.99
Propranolol 10 mg	5.99
Propranolol 40 mg	9.99
Methyldopa	10.99
Lasix 40 mg	12.49
Dyazide	12.99
Spiroaldactone	19.35

* As of June 1981.

convenient appointment times, minimal waiting time and transportation and parking problems when scheduling outpatient visits. The duration of therapy, expense of medication, complexity of the therapy, and side effects from the drug therapy are also factors that can reduce the likelihood of complete adherence.[55]

For people on long-term therapy for a chronic problem such as hypertension, there is an increased chance of progressive deterioration in motivation to continue treatment indefinitely. A survey of hypertensive steelworkers revealed that slightly more than half complied with at least 80% of their therapy program after 6 months.[57]

The expense of medication should also be considered as a factor. Thiazides cost as little as $4.00 for 100 capsules, whereas spiroaldactone can cost $20.00 for the same number. Table 47-13 lists some of the more common antihypertensive medications and their cost per 100 tablets. The more complex the therapy program, for instance adding potassium supplements and a diuretic to digoxin therapy or taking vitamins three times a day instead of just once, the less likely it is that the patient will comply with the therapy.[12]

Side effects from antihypertensive drugs have not been found to be a major factor for noncompliance. About 15% complain of adverse effects, but less than 3% stop taking their medication because of a side effect.[54] Side effects include lethargy (37%), gastrointestinal disturbances (21%), sleep disturbances (20%), and sexual dysfunction (20%). It is interesting to note that persons taking placebos complain of the same side effects: lethargy (16%), sleep disturbances (14%), sexual dysfunction (10%), and nasal stuffiness (20%).[141]

Hypertension has been called the "silent killer" because of its lack of symptoms. The lack of symptoms in hypertensive patients can also contribute to nonadherence. Compared with persons who have complaints of specific symptoms, asymptomatic patients are only 60% as cooperative in following treatment.[57] Interestingly, when individuals with hypertension were surveyed, as many as 72% said that they could tell when their blood pressure was elevated. They complained of dizziness, headache, feeling nervous, getting flushed, or feeling tired. Fortunately, however, three out of four of these people still took their medication even if they did not feel that their blood pressure was elevated.[54]

The lack of symptoms can contribute to what Podell and his colleagues[113] describe as a "disease denial–rationalization syndrome." One reason for poor patient adherence, they argue, is the patient's attempt to deny the seriousness of his condition. Patients can gain support for their denial by badgering the physician into relaxing standards and goals of treatment. For instance, if the physician says the patient should have a return visit in 1 month, the patient is likely to test the seriousness of his condition and ask if returning for a visit in two months would be acceptable.

The Health Belief Model. The major factor determining adherence is inherent in the patient's health values and beliefs. The health belief model, proposed in various forms by Hochbaum,[60] Rosenstock,[122] and Becker,[6,7] balances the amount of perceived threat of loss of health with the perceived benefits of therapy. The model incorporates a strong motivation for health that can compete with other life goals and attractions, a realistic understanding of one's susceptibility to complications, and a perception of how severely disrupted one's life-style will be if complications occur. It is interesting to note that as many as 94% agree with the seriousness of hypertension although only 33% believe that they are susceptible to hypertension.[54,78]

Assessment of components of these personal health beliefs can be used to predict the patient's readiness for cooperating with any prescribed treatment program and can be manipulated during nurse–patient interaction to enhance adherence to prescribed therapy. From the patient's initial perspective, there can be few benefits in treating his lack of symptoms considering the difficulties and negative experiences encountered in the health care system.[62] An example of a hypertension assessment form which incorporates the patient's health beliefs can be found in Figure 47-5.

Educating the Patient for Self-Care. In order to help motivate the patient to achieve and maintain self-care, personal responsibility for control of hypertension should be emphasized. Even mildly hypertensive persons need to understand the concept of hypertension and its association with a shorter life span and a higher rate of morbidity and mortality (Table 47-6). It should be made clear to the patient that he must make the choice of either following the prescribed medical treatment program or becoming incapacitated by a stroke, heart failure, or kidney failure.

In keeping with the health belief model, patient adherence to prescribed treatment is enhanced by a realistic understanding of the disease process and its potential complications. To help the patient understand the problem of hypertension, nursing's primary role is in developing a plan for educating the patient so that the negative aspects of therapy are minimized and adherence is enhanced. The more information the patient has about the health problem, the fewer are his readmissions to the hospital, the shorter is the length of stay if he is admitted, and the more responsibility he takes for self-care.[120]

Although the demands of a lengthy, complex therapy program can reduce adherence, establishing a satisfactory relationship with the practitioner[62] and fostering family support can improve the patient's cooperation. These two principles should be incorporated into any teaching plan for a patient, since positive interactions with others help patients to cope with the demands of the therapy program. A teaching plan should also incorporate skills in problem solving, as outlined in the teaching plan in Table 47-11 under the content area "scheduling for medication administration," so

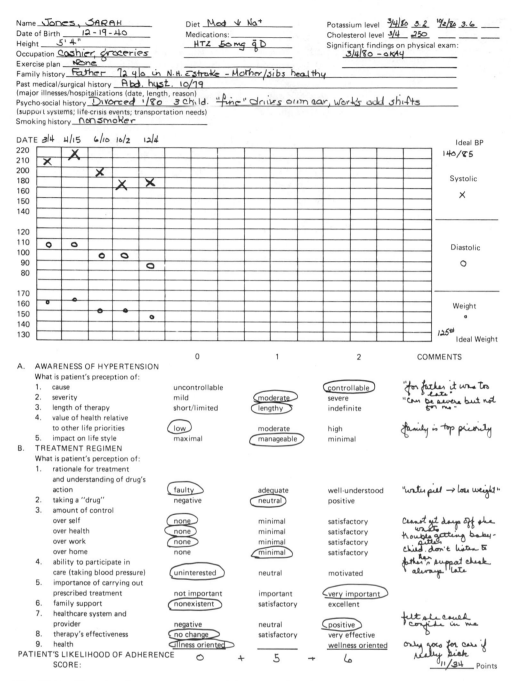

Name _Jones, SARAH_   Diet _Mod ↓ Na⁺_   Potassium level _3/4/80_ _3.2_ _½/80_ _3.6_
Date of Birth _12-19-40_   Medications: _____   Cholesterol level _3/4_ _250_ ___ ___
Height _5' 4"_   _HTZ 50 mg q̄ D_   Significant findings on physical exam:
Occupation _Cashier, groceries_   _3/4/80 - OKAY_
Exercise plan _none_
Family history _Father 72 y/o in N.H. stroke - Mother/sibs healthy_
Past medical/surgical history _Abd. hyst. 10/79_
(major illnesses/hospitalizations (date, length, reason)
Psycho-social history _Divorced 1/80 3 child. "fine" drives own car, works odd shifts_
(support systems; life-crisis events; transportation needs)
Smoking history _nonsmoker_

DATE 3/4 4/15 6/10 10/2 12/4   Ideal BP
                                                                    140/85
220
210
200   Systolic
180
160
150
140

120
110   Diastolic
100
90
80

170
160   Weight
150
140
130   125# Ideal Weight

                        0   1   2   COMMENTS

A. AWARENESS OF HYPERTENSION
    What is patient's preception of:
    1. cause   uncontrollable   (controllable)   "for father it was too late"
    2. severity   mild   (moderate)   severe   "can be severe but not
    3. length of therapy   short/limited (lengthy) indefinite   for me."
    4. value of health relative
        to other life priorities (low)   moderate   high   family is top priority
    5. impact on life style   maximal   (manageable) minimal
B. TREATMENT REGIMEN
    What is patient's perception of:
    1. rationale for treatment
        and understanding of drug's
        action   (faulty)   adequate   well-understood "water pill → lose weight"
    2. taking a "drug"   negative   (neutral)   positive
    3. amount of control
        over self   (none)   minimal   satisfactory   Cannot get days off she
        over health   (none)   minimal   satisfactory   works
        over work   (none)   minimal   satisfactory   trouble getting baby-
        over home   none   (minimal)   satisfactory   sitter
    4. ability to participate in   child. don't listen to
        care (taking blood pressure) (uninterested) neutral motivated   father's support check
    5. importance of carrying out   her always late
        prescribed treatment   not important important (very important)
    6. family support   (nonexistent) satisfactory excellent
    7. healthcare system and   felt she could
        provider   negative   neutral   (positive)   confide in me
    8. therapy's effectiveness (no change) satisfactory very effective only goes for care if
    9. health   (illness oriented)   wellness oriented really sick
PATIENT'S LIKELIHOOD OF ADHERENCE
    SCORE: 0   +   5   +   6   11/34 Points

Fig. 47-5. Hypertension assessment tool for assessing the patient with high blood pressure using the health belief model. An example of how this tool was used for one patient is presented. After assessing Mrs. Jones and her awareness of what high blood pressure is and her perception of the prescribed therapy, the items circled can be totaled at the end and can give an indication of her likelihood to adhere to the therapy. Mrs. Jones has a score of 11 points out of a possible 34. A score below 17 indicates increased difficulty with adherence and a score above 17 indicates a greater likelihood of adherence. From the assessment, a plan of care can then be outlined for patients like Mrs. Jones. (Foster S, Kousch DC: Am J Nurs 78(5):829–832, 1978)

that adherence does not diminish as the supervision of the patient is reduced.

A survey of patients reveals some of the more common reasons for discontinuing therapy. In order of frequency these include:

1. No longer feeling that the medication is needed
2. Feeling well

3. Receiving poor instructions
4. Becoming dissatisfied and discouraged
5. Lacking financial means
6. Lacking family support
7. Experiencing drug side effects[18]

All these reasons can be influenced by educating the patient.

Snow[136] suggests that many low-income Americans of Puerto Rican, Mexican, and Southern heritage may have tried home remedies such as vinegar and honey or epsom salts to "open the pores and let excess blood be sweated out," before they enter the health care system. When dealing with any individual, a primary step in beginning to teach that person about his health care problem is to determine what has already been tried and, if harmless, one may consider allowing irrational remedies to continue, while at the same time adding behaviors based on scientific principles as the patient becomes more open to suggestions.[136]

Patient teaching for control of hypertension consists of as many as five different content areas. (See Table 47-11 for an example of areas to include for the patient with chronic hypertension.) Concepts of normal circulation and blood pressure as well as a description of the pathogenesis of hypertension and its effect on the patient should be carefully explained in order to provide the patient with a basic understanding of the underlying process.

When assessing the patient's level of understanding, one may be surprised to discover misconceptions about high blood pressure and its causes. Some individuals may think it is due to spicy foods or old age. Because some individuals may misinterpret the word "hypertension" and rationalize its cause as being due to too much stress or tension, or having a "hyper" personality, the American Heart Association has advocated use of the term "high blood pressure" instead of hypertension. Even then, some individuals may mistakenly assume that high blood pressure means the opposite of low blood, or anemia, and that it is the result of the heart pumping too fast, or having too much thick blood.[54,136] Factors contributing to hypertension should therefore be explained, and general measures to promote health emphasized. The vasoconstrictive effects of caffeine (coffee, tea, cola, medications, etc.) should also be explained to the patient as appropriate.

In addition, patients will need counseling on such things as weight control, exercise, and stress management. It is more appropriate, cost-effective, and professionally responsible to modify these factors than to treat all patients with drugs. See Chapter 22 for a complete discussion of various stress management options available to patients. Yoga and biofeedback have been shown to lower mean arterial blood pressure in hypertensive patients[108,114] as much as 12 mm Hg. The effects of medication are still inconsistent[114] and further study in this area is necessary before the results can be summarized.[39,58] Altering one's way of interacting with the environment, such as with relaxation techniques, will decrease sympathetic tone and can lower blood pressure and reduce the amount of medication required in some instances.[9,108,134]

A discussion of the effects of sodium on the body and a list of the sodium content in common foods, beverages, and condiments should be part of any hypertensive patient's teaching plan (Tables 47-14, 47-15, 47-16). With inadequate teaching, patients have been known to use garlic salt, soy sauce, or other condiments to flavor foods as substitutes for salt. One relevant conclusion reached by the Harris Survey[54] is that, the higher the level of awareness about the effects of salt, the less salt will be added to food.

If drug treatment is used, a patient-education program should also include formulation of a simple schedule for taking antihypertensive medications and a brief discussion of side effects. Knowing what to expect will reduce the patient's anxiety, but a careful assessment should be made before going into detail on the possible side effects of the medications. Patients should be very clearly informed of the hazard of suddenly stopping their medication treatment and developing rebound hypertension that can lead to a hypertensive crisis.[61] Patients should also be given lists of food groups high in potassium, if it is relevant to their medication therapy. It is very difficult to correct a potassium deficiency with dietary measures, and the caloric intake can be greatly increased if dietary measures are resorted to (see Tables 37-6 and 37-7 for lists of the potassium content in foods and for drugs which cause hypokalemia). Salt substitute can be used unless the patient has renal failure or is using a potassium-sparing diuretic.

One last aspect of patient/family education concerns self-blood pressure measurements. With few exceptions, teaching the patient or a family member to monitor the blood pressure is reassuring to the patient and helps in guiding therapy,[1,57] although adherence is probably not directly enhanced.[56] Some practitioners feel that it contributes to anxiety and makes the patient too conscious of his blood pressure,[101] but for the appropriate patient, self-monitoring and charting pressures to visualize the effects of therapy will probably enhance adherence to therapy. The noncompliant steelworkers mentioned earlier were taught to take their own blood pressures and to graph the results. At the end of a 6-month period, compliance had increased 21%.[57]

The teaching plan presented in Table 47-11 can be used in part or in its entirety for patients with newly diagnosed hypertension. Other items that may help nurses to educate their hypertensive patients are readily available.

Available Teaching Aids. The National High Blood Pressure Information Center of the National Heart, Lung, and Blood Institute has teaching materials and posters available for the consumer, practitioner, and program planner. Their material is directed toward Spanish-speaking as well as English-speaking people. They also have a list of addresses to write for free or low-cost booklets listing sodium content of foods, recipes, and tips on seasoning, shopping, and eating out. A catalog of audiovisual aids available for preview, rent, or sale can be obtained by writing to High Blood Pressure Information Center, 120/80 National Institutes of Health, Bethesda, Maryland 20205, or by calling (301) 652-7700. The information center has also rated a wide variety of educational publications according to content and reading level. Explicit low-sodium diets are available but may be obtained only with a physician's written consent.

The American Heart Association has many pamphlets, among them a booklet entitled, "How You Can Help Your Doctor Treat Your High Blood Pressure," which is available through local chapters of the American Heart Association. It includes lengthy explanations of normal blood pressure, causes of high blood pressure, treatment for hypertension, and some side effects of antihypertensive drugs, as well as information on what action can be taken should side effects occur.

TABLE 47-14 SODIUM CONTENT OF COMMON FOODS

Food	Amount	Sodium (mg)	Calories (kcal)
Bacon	1 strip	51	30
Biscuits, baking powder	1 2-inch biscuit	219	130
Cake, commercial			
angel food	1 piece	66	115
chocolate frosted	1 piece	131	170
white frosted	1 piece	113	175
Cake, homemade			
angel food	1 piece	127	120
chocolate frosted	1 piece	117	185
white frosted	1 piece	115	185
Cheese:			
American	1 oz	210	119
Brick	1 oz	210	111
Camembert, domestic	1 oz	210	89
Cream cheese, natural	1 oz	75	112
Low-sodium (Cheezola)	1 oz	165	90
Parmesan	1 oz	220	118
Pasturized processed:			
American cheese	1 oz	341	111
Cheese spread	1 oz	488	86
Roquefort	1 oz	210	110
Swiss	1 oz	213	111
Chocolate candy bar,			
plain	1 bar	33	182
Chow mein, homemade	½ cup	287	102
Chow mein, canned	½ cup	290	38
Cocoa, mixes	1 tbsp	38	39
Coconut	2 tbsp	3	99
Cold cuts	1 oz	390	91
Cookie, commercial, misc.	1 cookie	60	71
Homemade, chocolate chip	1 cookie	70	103
Homemade, sugar	1 cookie	32	44
Crab, canned regular	¼ cup	400	40
Crackers			
Graham	5	94	54
Saltine	5	165	65
Doughnut	1	175	137
Dried beef	1 oz	1290	60
Fish sticks	1 oz	53	52
Frankfurters	1	550	155
French fries, salted	½ cup	276	233
Ham	1 oz	330	60
Jello	½ cup	61	71
Lobster, regular, canned	1 oz	63	28
Meat, canned	1 oz	370	88
Olives	3	493	50
Pancakes	1 4-inch pancake	191	104
Peanut butter	2 tbsp.	182	175
Pickle			
Dill, large	1	714	5
Sweet, chip	1	71	1
Pie, fruit	⅛ of pie	452	385
Pizza			
Commercial	1 piece	647	245
Homemade	1 piece	729	234
Potato chips	1 oz	102	170
Pot pie			
Beef	1	1024	448
Turkey	1	876	423
Chicken	1	876	510
Pretzels, small	5	252	58
Pudding, homemade			
Chocolate	½ cup	67	178
Vanilla	½ cup	78	133
Pudding, commercial			
Chocolate	½ cup	155	150
Vanilla	½ cup	119	160
Salmon, regular, canned	1 oz	157	51
Sardines, canned	1 oz	247	61
Sauerkraut	½ cup	560	14
Sausage	1 oz	287	104
Soup, canned			
Chicken noodle	1 cup	979	62
Split pea	1 cup	922	142
Vegetable beef	1 cup	1025	77
Spaghetti, canned	1 cup	955	190
Sweet roll	1	195	158
Tomato paste	½ cup	50	106
Tuna, regular, canned in oil	1 oz	240	60

TABLE 47-14 (Cont.)

Food	Amount	Sodium (mg)	Calories (kcal)
TV dinner			
Beef	1	820	347
Ham	1	1177	307
Pork	1	712	416
Meat loaf	1	1221	366
Swiss steak	1	1075	250
Chicken	1	1083	548
Fish	1	1319	326
Waffle, homemade	1 4-inch section	309	181

(Margie JD, Hunt JC: Living with High Blood Pressure: The Hypertensive Diet Cookbook, pp. 244–246. Bloomfield, NJ, HLS Press, 1978)

TABLE 47-15 SODIUM CONTENT OF COMMON BEVERAGES

Beverage	Sodium (mg)/ 6 ounces	Potassium (mg)/ 6 ounces
Coffee		
Brewed	0.6 mg	101.4 mg
Instant	1.4	66.3
Sanka		
Instant	0.2	85.8
Freeze-dried	0.3	89.7
Ground roast	2.0	156.0
Tea	0	97.5
Cola	15–30	0
Perrier water	2.3	
Milk	97.0	
Buttermilk	234.0	
Tomato Juice	292.0	
V8 vegetable juice	654.0	
V8 juice (low sodium)	45.0	
Motts apple juice	2.1	
Beer	12.5	
Beef broth (1 pkg.)	812.0	
Bouillon	586.5	

(From Iannaccone ST, Potter JD, Robertson SP: JAMA 244(5):436–437, 1980; Medical Letter 19(16):485, 1977)

TABLE 47-16 SODIUM CONTENT OF FOOD ADDITIVES AND CONDIMENTS

Food	Amount	Sodium (mg)
Baking powder	1 teaspoon	239
Baking soda	1 teaspoon	1360
Catsup	1 tablespoon	156
Heinz 57 sauce	1 tablespoon	284
Mustard	1 tablespoon	188
Pickle relish	2 teaspoons	135
Salad dressings		
French	1 tablespoon	205
Roquefort	1 tablespoon	164
Thousand Island	1 tablespoon	105
Italian	1 tablespoon	314
Soy sauce	1 tablespoon	1099
Worcestershire sauce	1 tablespoon	250

(Margie JD, Hunt JC: Living with High Blood Pressure: The Hypertensive Diet Cookbook, pp. 244–246, Bloomfield, NJ, HLS Press, 1978)

The Nutrition Department of General Mills has lists of the sodium content in various food products. Drug manufacturers have patient-education materials available also: Pfizer Laboratories, makers of Minizide, has a patient education kit which contains a 6-minute record on helpful hints for the hypertensive patient; Squibb & Sons publishes a pamphlet entitled: "Too Many Blacks Die from the Effects of High Blood Pressure."

Nursing journals have a variety of teaching aids which can be copied for distribution to hypertensive patients.[91] "How to Measure Your Blood Pressure at Home" and "Teaching Guidelines for Sodium Restricted Diets"[59] are two examples.

In order to meet our goals in working with hypertensive patients, nurses need to be involved not only in the detection of hypertension in the general population, but also in patient education. Nurses need to invest the majority of their time in educating the public, and especially individuals with hypertension, in all aspects of hypertension. Appropriate teaching will maximize patient self-care and adherence to therapy, and will reduce the amount of time spent in hospital beds from complications of hypertension.

REFERENCES

1. Aagaard GN: Treatment of hypertension. Am J Nurs 73(4):620–623, 1973
2. Asmussen I: Effects of maternal smoking on the fetal cardiovascular system. In Lauer RM, Shekelle RB (eds): Childhood Prevention of Atherosclerosis and Hypertension, pp 235–250. New York, Raven Press, 1980
3. Attarian E: Myxedema and hypertension. N Y State J Med 63(19):2801–2804, 1963
4. Beaglehole R: Social factors and blood pressure in children. In Lauer RM and Shekelle RB (eds): Childhood Prevention of Atherosclerosis and Hypertension, pp 313–321. New York, Raven Press, 1980
5. Becker CE, Benowitz NL: Hypertensive emergencies. Med Clin North Am 63(1):127–140, 1979
6. Becker MN, Drachman RH, Kirscht JP: A new approach to explaining sick-role behavior in low-income populations. Am J of Public Health 64(3):205–216, 1974
7. Becker MH, Maiman LA, Kirscht JP et al: Patient perceptions and compliance: Recent studies of the health belief model. In Haynes RB, Taylor DW, Sackett DL (eds): Compliance in Health Care, pp 78–109. Baltimore, Johns Hopkins University Press, 1979
8. Beevers DG, Campbell BC, Goldberg A et al: Blood–cadmium in hypertensives and normotensives. Lancet 2:1222–1224, 1976
9. Benson H: Systemic hypertension and the relaxation response. N Engl J Med 296(20):1152–1156, 1977
10. Beral V: Mortality among oral contraceptive users. Lancet 2:727–731, 1977
11. Biron P, Mongeau J, Bertrand D: Familial aggregation of blood pressure in adopted and natural children. In Paul O (ed): Epidemiology and Control of Hypertension, pp 397–405. New York, Stratton Intercontinental Medical Books, 1975
12. Blackwell B: The drug regimen and treatment compliance. In Haynes RB, Taylor DW, Sackett DL (eds): Compliance in

Health Care, pp 144–156. Baltimore, Johns Hopkins University Press, 1979

13. Blum M, Kirsten M, Worth MH Jr: Reversible hypertension—caused by the hypercalcemia of hyperparathyroidism, vitamin D toxicity, and calcium infusion. JAMA 237(3):262–263, 1977

14. Brandfonbrener M, Landowne M, Shock NW: Changes in cardiac output with age. Circulation 12(4):557–566, 1955

15. Breckinridge A, Dollery CT, Parry EHO: Prognosis of treated hypertension. Q J Med 39(155):411–429, 1970

16. Brinton GS, Jubiz W, Lagerquist LD: Hypertension in primary hyperthyroidism: The role of the renin–angiotensin system. J Clin Endocrinol Metabol 41(6):1025–1029, 1975

17. Brownrigg GM: Toxemia in hormone-induced pseudopregnancy. Can Med Assoc J 87(8):408–409, 1962

18. Caldwell JR, Cobb S, Dowling MD et al: The dropout problem in antihypertensive treatment. J Chronic Dis 22(8/9):579–592, 1970

19. Chrysant SG, Frohlich ED, Papper S: Why hypertension is so prevalent in the elderly—and how to treat it. Geriatrics 31(10):101–108, 1976

20. Cobb S, Rose RM: Hypertension, peptic ulcer, and diabetes in air traffic controllers. JAMA 224(4):489–492, 1973

21. Cockburn JS, Benjamin IS, Thomson RM et al: Early systemic hypertension after surgical closure of atrial septal defect. J Cardiovasc Surg 16(1):1–7, 1975

22. Cohn JN, Limas CJ, Guiha NH: Hypertension and the heart. Arch Intern Med 133(6):969–979, 1974

23. Conomy JP: Impact of arterial hypertension on the brain. Postgrad Med 68(2):86–97, 1980

24. Constantinides P: The morphological basis for altered endothelial permeability in atherosclerosis. Adv Experi Med Biol 82:969–974, 1977

25. Cryer PE, Haymond MH, Santiago JV et al: Norepinephrine and epinephrine release and adrenergic mediation of smoking-associated hemodynamic and metabolic events. N Engl J Med 295(11):573–577, 1976

26. Dahl LK: Salt in processed baby foods. Am J Clin Nutr 21(8):787–792, 1968

27. Dluhy RG, Williams GH: Primary aldosteronism in a hypertensive acromegalic patient. J Clin Endocrinol Metabol 29(10):1319–1324, 1969

28. Dranov J, Skyler JS, Gunnells JC: Malignant hypertension: Current modes of therapy. Arch Intern Med 133(5):791–801, 1974

29. Dustan HP: Obesity and hypertension. In Lauer RM, Shekelle RB (eds): Childhood Prevention of Atherosclerosis and Hypertension, pp 305–312. New York, Raven Press, 1980

30. Dustan HP, Tarazi RC, Bravo EL: Diuretic and diet treatment of hypertension. Arch Intern Med 133(6):1007–1013, 1974

31. Estafanous FG, Tarazi RC, Viljoen JF et al: Systemic hypertension following myocardial revascularization. Am Heart J 85(6):732–738, 1973

32. Fallis N, Ford RV: Electrolyte excretion and hypertensive response. JAMA 176(7):581–584, 1961

33. Feinleib M, Garrison R, Borhani N et al: Studies of hypertension in twins. In Paul O (ed): Epidemiology and Control of Hypertension, pp 3–20. New York, Stratton Intercontinental Medical Books, 1975

34. Feinleib M, Garrison RJ, Havlik RJ: Environmental and genetic factors affecting the distribution of blood pressure in children. In Lauer RM, Shekelle RB (eds): Childhood Prevention of Atherosclerosis and Hypertension, pp 271–279. New York, Raven Press, 1980

35. Filer LJ Jr: Availability of suitable foods in the marketplace. A. Are suitable low-salt foods available in the market? In Lauer RM, Shekelle RB (eds): Childhood Prevention of Atherosclerosis and Hypertension, pp 411–417. New York, Raven Press, 1980

36. Finnerty FA Jr: Aggressive drug therapy in accelerated hypertension. Am J Nurs 74(12):2176–2180, 1974

37. Finnerty FA Jr: Workup and treatment of the average hypertensive patient. Compr Ther 4(12):40–45, 1978

38. Foster S, Kousch DC: Promoting patient adherence. Am J Nurs 78(5):829–832, 1978

39. Frankel BL, Patel DJ, Horowitz D et al: Treatment of hypertension with biofeedback and relaxation techniques. Psychosom Med 40(4):276–293, 1978

40. Friedman R, Iwai J: Genetic predisposition and stress-induced hypertension. Science 193(4248):161–162, 1976

41. Freis ED: Age, race, sex and other indices of risk in hypertension. In Laragh JH (ed): Hypertension Manual, pp 31–41. New York, Dun-Donnelly Publishing Co, 1974

42. Freis ED: The clinical spectrum of essential hypertension. Arch Intern Med 133(6):982–987, 1974

43. Frohlich ED: Hypertensive crisis. Hospital Medicine 13(1):32–51, 1977

44. Fuller H Jr, Spittell JA, McConahey WM et al: Myxedema and hypertension. Postgrad Med 40(4):425–428, 1966

45. Giblin E: Controlling high blood pressure. Am J Nurs 78(5):824, 1978

46. Giblin EC, Ackerman AM, Anderson MA et al: Guidelines for educating nurses in high blood pressure control. Report of the Task Force on the Role of Nursing in High Blood Pressure Control. Washington DC, DHEW, PHS (NIH) Publication No. 80–1241, March, 1980

47. Gifford RW Jr: Management and prognosis in complicated hypertension. In Moser M (ed): Hypertension: A Practical Approach, pp 151–176. Boston, Little, Brown & Company, 1975

48. Goldby FS: The pathology of hypertension. In Marshall AJ, Barritt DW (eds): The Hypertensive Patient, pp 266–292. Great Britain, Pitman Medical, 1980

49. Gomez OL: Psychological factors of arterial hypertension. In Velasco M (ed): Arterial Hypertension, p 3–5. Oxford, Excerpta Medica, 1977

50. Gordon T, Kannel WB, Dawber TR et al: Changes associated with quitting cigarette smoking: The Framingham study. Am Heart J 90(3):322–328, 1975

51. Green LW: Educational strategies to improve compliance with therapeutic and preventive regimens: The recent evidence. In Haynes RB, Taylor DW, Sackett DL (eds): Compliance in Health Care, pp 157–173. Baltimore, Johns Hopkins University Press, 1979

52. Greenfield D, Grant R, Lieberman E: Children can have high blood pressure, too. Am J Nurs 76(5):770–772, 1976

53. Guyton AC, Hall JE, Norman RA Jr et al: Physiology of blood pressure regulation. In Lauer RM, Shekelle RB (eds): Childhood Prevention of Atherosclerosis and Hypertension, pp 251–262. New York, Raven Press, 1980

54. Harris L, and Associates: The public and high blood pressure. A Survey Conducted for the National Heart and Lung Institute, June, 1973

55. Haynes RB: Determinants of compliance: The disease and the mechanics of treatment. In Haynes RB, Taylor DW, Sackett DL (eds): Compliance in Health Care, pp 49–62. Baltimore, Johns Hopkins University Press, 1979

56. Haynes RB: Strategies to improve compliance with referrals, appointments, and prescribed medical regimens. In Haynes RB, Taylor DW, Sackett DL (eds): Compliance in Health Care, pp 121–143. Baltimore, Johns Hopkins University Press, 1979

57. Haynes RB et al: Improvement of medication compliance in uncontrolled hypertension. Lancet 1:1265–1268, 1976

58. Henry JP: Relaxation methods and the control of blood pressure. Psychosom Med 40(4):273–275, 1978

59. Hill M: Helping the hypertensive patient control sodium intake. Am J Nurs 79(5):906–909, 1979

60. Hochbaum G: Public participation in medical screening programs. Washington, DC, PHS Publication No. 572, U.S. Government Printing Office, 1958

61. Hubbell FA, Weber MA: Adverse effects of sudden withdrawal of antihypertensive medication. Postgrad Med 68(2):129–138, 1980

62. Hulka BS: Patient–clinician interactions and compliance. In Haynes RB, Taylor DW, Sackett DL (eds): Compliance in Health Care, pp 63–77. Baltimore, Johns Hopkins University Press, 1979

63. Hulthén UL, Lecerof H, Hokfelt B: Effect of upright tilting

on kinins as compared to renin activity in the renal venous blood from patients with essential hypertension. Acta Med Scand 203(5):411–414, 1978

64. Iannaconne ST, Potter JD, Robertson SP: Sodium content of bottled sparkling water. JAMA 244(5):436–437, 1980

65. Irinoda K (ed): Colour Atlas and Criteria of Fundus Changes in Hypertension. Philadelphia, JB Lippincott, 1970

66. Johnson AL, Cornoni JC, Cassel JC et al: Influence of race, sex, and weight on blood pressure behavior in young adults. Am J Cardiol 35(4):523–530, 1975

67. Joint National Committee on Detection, Evaluation, and Treatment of High Blood Pressure. Washington DC, DHEW Publication No. 79–1088, 1977

68. Jonsen AR: Ethical issues in compliance. In Haynes RB, Taylor DW, Sackett DL (eds): Compliance in Health Care, pp 113–120. Baltimore, Johns Hopkins University Press, 1979

69. Julius S, Schork MA: Predictors of hypertension. Ann N Y Acad Sci 304:38–52, 1978

70. Kales A et al: Effectiveness of secobarbital with intermediate term use: Sleep laboratory studies. Sleep Research 5:69, 1976

71. Kannel WB, Brand N, Skinner JJ et al: The relation of adiposity to blood pressure and development of hypertension: The Framingham study. Ann Intern Med 67(1):48–59, 1967

72. Kannel WB, Sorlie P: Hypertension in Framingham. In Paul O (eds): Epidemiology and Control of Hypertension, pp 553–592. New York, Stratton Intercontinental Medical Books, 1975

73. Kaplan NM: Adrenal causes of hypertension. Arch Intern Med 133(6):1001–1006, 1974

74. Kaplan NM: Clinical Hypertension, 2nd ed. Baltimore, Williams & Wilkins, 1978

75. Keith TA: Complications and treatment of acute hypertension. Compr Ther 4(12):18–31, 1978

76. Keith TA: Hypertension crisis—Recognition and management. JAMA 237(15):1570–1577, 1977

77. Kerr CM Jr, Reisinger KS, Plankey FW: Sodium concentration of homemade baby foods. Pediatrics 62(3):331–335, 1978

78. Khatri IM, Freis ED: Hemodynamic changes during sleep. J Appl Physiol 22(5):867–873, 1967

79. Klahr L: Modern treatment of essential arterial hypertension. In Velasco M (ed): Arterial Hypertension, pp 59–64. Oxford, Excerpta Medica, 1977

80. Klatsky AL, Friedman GD, Siegelaub AB: Alcohol and hypertension. Compr Ther 4(12):60–68, 1978

81. Kohli RK, Elwood CM: Treating acute hypertensive crisis with sodium nitroprusside. Am Family Phys 15(1):141–145, 1977

82. Krakower A: The blood pressure of Chinese living in eastern Canada. Am Heart J 9(3):396–404, 1934

83. LaBarthe DR: Problems in definition of mild hypertension. Ann N Y Acad Sci 304:3–14, 1978

84. Laragh JH: An approach to the classification of hypertensive states. Hosp Pract 9(1):61–73, 1974

85. Laragh JH: Essential hypertension: New concepts in diagnosis and treatment. Compr Ther 4(12):10–17, 1978

86. Laragh JH, Sealey JE, Ledingham JGG et al: Oral contraceptives—Renin, aldosterone, and high blood pressure. JAMA 201(12):918–922, 1967

87. Layton C, Monroe J, Brigden W et al: Systemic hypertension after homo-graft aortic valvar replacement—A cause of late homograph failure. Lancet 2:1343–1347, 1973

88. Ledingham JGG: Secondary hypertension. In Marshall AJ, Barritt DW (eds): The Hypertensive Patient, pp 230–233. Great Britain, Pitman Medical, 1980

89. Lew EA: High blood pressure, other risk factors and longevity: The insurance viewpoint. In Laragh JH (ed): Hypertension Manual, pp 43–70. New York, Dun-Donnelley Publishing Co, 1974

90. Lowenthal DT: Hypertensive crisis and postcrisis management. Compr Ther 4(12):32–39, 1978

91. Maloney R: Helping your hypertensive patients live longer. Nursing 78(10):26–35, 1978

92. Margie JD, Hunt JC: Living with High Blood Pressure: The Hypertensive Diet Cookbook. Bloomfield, NJ, HLS Press, 1978

93. Matsumoto N, Whisnant JP, Kurland LT et al: Natural history of stroke in Rochester, Minnesota, 1955 through 1969: An extension of a previous study, 1945 through 1954. Stroke 4(1):20–29, 1973

94. McGuffin WL Jr, Sherman BM, Roth J et al: Acromegaly and cardiovascular disorders. Ann Intern Med 81(1):11–18, 1974

95. Meade TW, Chakrabarti R, Haines AP et al: Haemostatic, lipid, and blood-pressure profiles of women on oral contraceptives containing 50 μg or 30 μg oestrogen. Lancet, 2:948, 1977

96. Meneely GR, Battarbee HD. High sodium-low potassium environment and hypertension. Am J Cardiol 38(6):768–785, 1976

97. Meneely GR, Dahl LK: Electrolytes in hypertension: The effects of sodium chloride. Med Clin North Am 45(2):271–283, 1961

98. Miall WE: Genetic considerations concerning hypertension. Ann N Y Acad Sci 304:18–25, 1978

99. Moore TJ, Williams GH: Adrenal causes of hypertension. Compr Ther 4(12):46–52, 1978

100. Morgan T, Gillies A, Morgan G et al: Hypertension treated by salt restriction. Lancet 1:227–230, 1978

101. Moser M: Hypertension: A Practical Approach. Boston, Little, Brown & Co, 1975

102. Muirhead EE, Brown GB, Germain GS et al: The renal medulla as an antihypertensive organ. J Lab Clin Med 76(4):641–651, 1970

103. Nash DA Jr: Hypertension in polycystic kidney disease without renal failure. Arch Intern Med 137(11):1571–1575, 1977

104. National High Blood Pressure Education Program. First Conference on Hypertension Among Puerto Ricans, Summary Report. National Heart, Lung, and Blood Institute, National Institutes of Health Summary Report. New York, United States Department of Health, Education and Welfare, NIH Publication No. 80–1962, April, 1980.

105. Neri L, Johansen HL: Water hardness and cardiovascular mortality. Ann N Y Acad Sci 304:203–219, 1978

106. Olsen F: Increased permeability for plasma components of the cerebral vessels during acute angiotensin hypertension in rats. Acta Pathol Microbiol Scand Section A, 85A(5):572–576, 1977

107. Parijs J, Joossens JV, VenderLinden L et al: Moderate sodium restriction and diuretics in the treatment of hypertension. Am Heart J 85(1):22–34, 1973

108. Patel C: 12-month follow-up of yoga and bio-feedback in the management of hypertension. Lancet 1:62–64, 1975

109. Paul O: Complications of mild hypertension. Ann N Y Acad Sci 304:59–63, 1978

110. Perry HM Jr, Wessler S, Avioli LV: Survival of treated hypertensive patients. JAMA 210(5):890:895, 1969

111. Plotz CM, Knowlton AI, Ragan C: The natural history of Cushing's syndrome. Am J Med 13(5):597–614, 1952

112. Pobee JO: The status of cardiovascular diseases in the setting of diseases of environmental sanitation and hygiene and malnutrition: The West African (Ghana) experience. In Lauer RM, Shekelle RB (eds): Childhood Prevention of Atherosclerosis and Hypertension, pp 465–472. New York, Raven Press, 1980

113. Podell RN, Kent D, Keller K: Patient psychological defenses and physician response in the long-term treatment of hypertension. J Fam Pract 3(2):145–149, 1976

114. Pollack AA, Weber MA, Case DB et al: Limitations of transcendental meditation in the treatment of essential hypertension. Lancet 1:71–73, 1977

115. Prineaus RJ, Gillum RF, Blackburn H: Possibilities for primary prevention of hypertension. In Lauer RM, Shekelle RB (eds): Childhood Prevention of Atherosclerosis and Hypertension, pp 357–366. New York, Raven Press, 1980

116. Reisin E, Abel R, Modan M et al: Effect of weight loss without salt restriction on the reduction of blood pressure in overweight hypertensive patients. N Engl J Med 298(1):1–6, 1978

117. Richard GA, Garin EH, Fennell RS et al: A pathophysiologic basis for the diagnosis and treatment of the renal hypertensions. Ad Pediatr 24:339–398, 1977

118. Robinson AM: Detection and control of hypertension: Challenge to all nurses. Am J Nurs 76(5):778–780, 1976
119. Rose G: Epidemiology. In Marshall AJ, Barritt DW (eds): The Hypertensive Patient, pp 1–21. Great Britain, Pitman Medical, 1980
120. Rosenberg SG: A case for patient education. Hospital Formulary Management 6(6):14–17, 1971
121. Rosendorff C, Bloom DS, Stein MG: Vascular hypersensitivity to norepinephrine in hypertension. In Velasco M (ed): Arterial Hypertension, pp 32–34. Oxford, Excerpta Medica, 1977
122. Rosenstock IM: Why people use health services. Milbank Memorial Fund Quarterly 44(3):94–127, 1966
123. Rosenthal FD, Roy S: Hypertension and hyperparathyroidism. Br Med J 4(5837):396–397, 1972
124. Royal College of General Practitioners. Oral Contraceptives and Health, p 37. London, Pitman Publishing Corporation, 1974
125. Sackett DL, Snow JC: The magnitude of compliance and noncompliance. In Haynes RB, Taylor DW, Sackett DL (eds): Compliance in Health Care, pp 11–22. Baltimore, Johns Hopkins University Press, 1979
126. Sandok BA, Whisnant JP: Hypertension and the brain. Arch Intern Med 133(6):947–954, 1974
127. Schmid PG, Abboud FM: Neurohumoral control of vascular resistance. Arch Intern Med 133(6):935–945, 1974
128. Segal JL: Hypertensive emergencies: Practical approach to treatment. Postgrad Med 68(2):107–125, 1980
129. Seymour FI: Rice, Dietary Controls and Blood Pressure. New York, Froben Press, 1951
131. Shaper AG, Clayton DG, Stanley F: Water hardness and hypertension. In Paul O (ed): Epidemiology and Control of Hypertension, pp 163–176. New York, Stratton Intercontinental Medical Book Corporation, 1975
130. Shaper AG: Soft water, heart attacks, and stroke. JAMA 230(1):130–131, 1974
132. Shapiro AP, Bartsch GE, Berge KG et al: Five-year findings of the hypertension detection and follow-up program I. Reduction in mortality of persons with high blood pressure, including mild hypertension. II. Mortality by race, sex and age. JAMA 242(23):2562–2577, 1979
133. Shapiro AP, Schwartz GE, Ferguson DCE et al: Behavior methods in the treatment of hypertension—A review of their clinical status. Ann Intern Med 86(5):626–636, 1977
134. Shapiro AP, Schwartz GE, Redmond DP et al: Non-pharmacologic treatment of hypertension. Ann N Y Acad Sci 304:222–235, 1978
135. Shekelle RB, Harburg E, O'Malley P et al: Psychological factors and high blood pressure in adolescents. In Lauer RM, Shekelle RB (eds): Childhood Prevention of Atherosclerosis and Hypertension, pp 323–330. New York, Raven Press, 1980
136. Snow LF: Folk medical beliefs and their implications for care of patients—A review based on studies among black Americans. Ann Intern Med 81(1):82–96, 1974
137. Spain DM, Siegel H, Bradess VA: Women smokers and sudden death: The relationship of cigarette smoking to coronary disease. JAMA 244(7):1005–1007, 1973
138. Stamler J: The mass treatment of hypertensive disease: Defining the Problem. Ann N Y Acad Sci 304:333–358, 1978
139. Stone RA, DeLeo J: Psychotherapeutic control of hypertension. N Engl J Med 294(2):80–84, 1976
140. Strasser T: Primary prevention: The role of the World Health Organization. In Lauer RM, Shekelle RB (eds): Childhood Prevention of Atherosclerosis and Hypertension, pp 473–476. New York, Raven Press, 1980
141. Syme SL: Drug treatment of mild hypertension: Social and psychological considerations. Ann N Y Acad Sci 304:99–106, 1978
142. Taylor DW, Sackett DL, Haynes RB et al: Compliance with antihypertensive drug therapy. Ann NY Acad Sci 304:390–403, 1978
143. Taylor SH: Pathogenesis: The circulation in hypertension and cardiovascular reflexes. In Marshall AJ, Barritt DW (eds): The Hypertensive Patient, pp 39–112. Great Britain, Pitman Medical, 1980
144. Tobian L Jr: Hypertension and the kidney. Arch Intern Med 133(6):959–967, 1974
145. Tobian L: Salt and hypertension. Ann N Y Acad Sci 304:178–197, 1978
146. Tyroler HA, Heyden S, Hames CG: Weight and hypertension: Evans County studies of blacks and whites. In Paul O (ed): Epidemiology and Control of Hypertension, pp 177–204. New York: Stratton Intercontinental Medical Book Corporation, 1975
147. Valenzuela GG, Bodkhe RR: Effect of pregnancy-induced hypertension upon placental prostaglandin metabolism: Decreased prostaglandin $F_2\alpha$ catabolism with normal prostaglandin E_2 catabolism. Am J Obstet Gynecol 136(2):255–256, 1980
148. Vessey MP, McPherson K, Johnson B: Mortality among women participating in the Oxford/family planning association contraceptive study. Lancet 2:731–733, 1977
149. Weinstein MC, Stason WB: Economic considerations in the management of mild hypertension. Ann N Y Acad Sci 304:424–436, 1978
150. Welt SI, Crenshaw MC: Concurrent hypertension and pregnancy. Clin Obstet Gynecol 21(3):619–648, 1978
151. Williams RL, Karacan I: Sleep disorders: Diagnosis and treatment, p 16. New York, John Wiley & Sons, 1978
152. Winkelstein W Jr: Cooperative studies of blood pressure in Japanese in Japan, Hawaii and the United States. In Paul O (ed): Epidemiology and Control of Hypertension, pp 101–115. New York, Stratton Intercontinental Medical Book Corporation, 1975
153. Woods JW: Oral contraceptives and hypertension. Lancet 2:653–654, 1967
154. World Health Organization. Arterial hypertension. WHO Technical Report Series, #628, Geneva, 1978

ADDITIONAL READING

Secondary Hypertension

Adrián-Garbi O: Endocrine aspects of arterial hypertension. In Velasco M (ed): Arterial Hypertension, pp 37–39. Oxford, Excerpta Medica, 1977
Barajas L, Bennett CM, Conner G et al: Structure of a juxtaglomerular cell tumor: The presence of a neural component. Lab Invest 37(4):357–368, 1977
Bonnin JM et al: Hypertension due to a renin-secreting tumour localised by segmental renal vein sampling. Aust N Z J Med 7(6):630–635, 1977
Charro AL, Hofeldt FD, Becker N et al: Adrenocortical function in acromegaly. Am J Med Sci 266(3):211–218, 1973
Dluhy RG: Adrenal function testing. Compr Ther 4(12):53–59, 1978
Ferriss JB et al: Clinical, biochemical and pathological features of low-renin ('primary') hyperaldosteronism. Am Heart J 95(3):375–388, 1978
Gavras H, Gavras I, Cannon PJ et al: Is elevated plasma renin activity of prognostic importance in progressive systemic sclerosis? Arch Intern Med 137(11):1554–1558, 1977
Label M, Talbot J, Grose J et al: Adenocarcinoma of the kidney and hypertension: Report of 2 cases with special emphasis on renin. J Urol 118(6):923–927, 1977
Mang HYL, Markovic PR, Chow S et al: Solitary intrarenal cyst causing hypertension. NY State J Med 78(4):654–656, 1978
Mathias CJ, Christensen NJ, Corbett JL et al: Plasma catecholamines during paroxysmal neurogenic hypertension in quadriplegic man. Circ Res 39(2):204–208, 1976
Messerli FH, DeCarvalho JGR, Mills NL et al: Renal artery stenosis and polycystic kidney disease. Arch Intern Med 138(8):1282–1283, 1978
Ohmori H et al: Extrarenal renin-secreting tumor associated with hypertension. Acta Pathol J 27(4):567–586, 1977
Robertson PW, Klidjian A, Harding LK et al: Hypertension due to a renin-secreting renal tumour. Am J Med 43(6):963–976, 1967

Roe DA: Interactions between drugs and nutrient. Med Clin North Am 63(5):985–1007, 1979

Snow MH, Piercy DA, Robson V et al: An investigation into the pathogenesis of hypertension in acromegaly. Clin Sci Mol Med 53(1):87–91, 1977

Souadjian JV, Schirger A: Hypertension in acromegaly. Am J Med Sci 254(5):629–633, 1967

Weidmann P et al: Curable hypertension with unilateral hydronephrosis. Ann Intern Med 87(4):437–440, 1977

Pathogenesis

Berry CL: Hypertension and arterial development: Long-term considerations. Br Heart J 40(7):709–717, 1978

Brown JJ et al: Renal hypertension: Role for renin. Postgrad Med J (Suppl 3) 53:31–34, 1977

Brunner HR, Laragh JH, Baer L et al: Essential hypertension: Renin and aldosterone, heart attack and stroke. N Engl J Med 286(9):441–449, 1972

Byrom FB: The Hypertensive Vascular Crisis—An Experimental Study. New York, Grune & Stratton, 1969

Correa–Suárez R: The effect of vasodilators on the renin–angiotensin–aldosterone system. In Velasco M (ed): Arterial Hypertension, pp 96–103. Oxford, Excerpta Medica, 1977

Cubeddu LX, Talmaciu R, Klahr L et al: Dopamine–β–hydroxylase in essential hypertensive patients. In Velasco M (ed): Arterial Hypertension, pp 9–12. Oxford, Excerpta Medica, 1977

Ferrario CM, Barnes KL, Brosnihan KB et al: Cardiovascular effects of angiotensin II mediated by the central nervous system. In Velasco M (ed): Arterial Hypertension, pp 50–55. Oxford Excerpta Medica, 1977

Fujishima M, Onoyama K, Oniki H et al: Effect of acute hypertension on brain metabolism in normotensive, renovascular hypertensive and spontaneously hypertensive rats. Stroke 9(4):349–353, 1978

Goldstein DJ, Fingielman S, Nahmod VE: The brain renin angiotensin system: Facts and hypothesis. In Velasco M (ed): Arterial Hypertension, pp 13–18. Oxford, Excerpta Medica, 1977

Guyton AC, Young DB, Hall JE et al: The renal–blood volume mechanism for regulation of arterial pressure. In Velasco M (ed): Arterial Hypertension, pp 27–31. Oxford, Excerpta Medica, 1977

Harnish A, Pearce ML: Evolution of hypertensive retinal vascular disease: Correlation between clinical and postmortem observations. Medicine 52(6):483–533, 1973

Hollander W: Hypertension, antihypertensive drugs and atherosclerosis. Circulation 48(5):1112–1127, 1973

Kirkendall WM, Hammond JJ, Overtuff ML: Renin as a predictor of hypertensive complications. Ann NY Acad Sci 304:147–160, 1978

Lawton WJ, Fitz AE: Urinary kallikrein in normal renin essential hypertension. Circulation 56(5):856–859, 1977

Liard JF: Cardiogenic hypertension. Int Rev Physiol 18:317–355, 1979

Reis DJ, Dampney RAL, Doba N et al: Central control of blood pressure: A proposed localization of the 'tonic vasomotor center' of the medulla. In Velasco M (ed): Arterial Hypertension, pp 6–8, 19–23. Oxford, Excerpta Medica, 1977

Safar ME, Weiss YA, London GM et al: Differences in the mechanisms of borderline and permanent hypertension. Postgrad Med J (Suppl) 53:35–39, 1977

Velasco M, O'Malley K, McNay JL et al: Mechanisms of minoxidil-induced increase in plasma renin activity in hypertensive patients. In Velasco M (ed): Arterial Hypertension, pp 45–59. Oxford, Excerpta Medica, 1977

Ethnicity and Hypertension

Bays RP, Scrimshaw NS: Facts and fallacies regarding the blood pressure of different regional and racial groups. Circulation 8(5):655–663, 1953

Cassel J: Studies of hypertension in migrants. In Paul O (ed): Epidemiology and Control of Hypertension, pp 41–61. New York, Stratton Intercontinental Medical Book Corporation, 1975

Chávez I: The incidence of heart disease in Mexico. Am Heart J 24(1):88–98, 1942

Edwards KEC: Prevalence of early age onset of hypertension in a selected group of blacks. University of Washington thesis, 1976

Hatano S: Hypertension in Japan: A review. In Paul O (ed): Epidemiology and Control of Hypertension, pp 63–99. New York, Stratton Intercontinental Medical Book Corporation, 1975

Ito PK: Comparative biometrical study of physique of Japanese women born and reared under different environments. Human Biology 14(3):279–351, 1942

Kilcoyne MM, Thomson GE, Branche G et al: Characteristics of hypertension in the black population. Circulation 50(5):1006–1013, 1974

Moser M: Epidemiology of hypertension with particular reference to racial susceptibility. Ann NY Acad Sci 84(17):989–999, 1960

Page LB: Dietary sodium and blood pressure: Evidence from human studies. In Lauer RM, Shekelle RB (eds): Childhood Prevention of Atherosclerosis and Hypertension, pp 291–303. New York, Raven Press, 1980

Page LB, Vandervert D, Nader K et al: Blood pressure, diet, and body form in traditional nomads of the Qash'gai tribe, Southern Iran. Acta Cardiol 33(2):102–103, 1978

Swartz H: Differences in mean adolescent blood pressure by sex, age, ethnic origin, obesity and familial tendency of hypertension. University of Washington Master's thesis, 1974

Switzer S: Hypertension and ischemic heart disease in Hiroshima, Japan. Circulation 28(3):368–380, 1963

Yano K, Rhoads GG, Kagan A: Coffee, alcohol and risk of coronary heart disease among Japanese men living in Hawaii. N Engl J Med 297(8):405–409, 1977

Aging

Babu TN, Nazir F, Rao DB et al: What is 'normal' blood pressure in the aged? Geriatrics 32(1):73–76, 1977

Caird FI, Judge TG: Assessment of the Elderly Patient. London, Pitman Medical, 1974

Landowne M, Brandfonbrener M, Shock NW: The relation of age to certain measures of performance of the heart and the circulation. Circulation 12(4):567–576, 1955

Papper S: The effects of age in reducing renal function. Geriatrics 28(5):83–87, 1973

Wilkie FL, Eisdorfer C, Nowling JB: Memory and blood pressure in the aged. Exper Aging Res 2(1):3–16, 1976

Risk Factors and Hypertension

Aronow WS, Goldsmith JR, Kern JC et al: Effect of smoking cigarettes on cardiovascular hemodynamics. Arch Environ Health 28(6):330–332, 1974

Ashley FW, Kannel WB: Relation of weight change to changes in atherogenic traits: The Framingham Study. J Chronic Dis 27(3):103–114, 1974

Blumenthal S: Precursors in childhood of primary hypertension in the adult. Ann NY Acad Sci 304:28–32, 1978

Crane MG, Harris JJ, Winsor W III: Hypertension, oral contraceptive agents, and conjugated estrogens. Ann Intern Med 74(1):13–21, 1971

Evans RI: Deterring smoking in adolescents: A social–psychological perspective. In Lauer RM, Shekelle RB (eds): Childhood Prevention of Atherosclerosis and Hypertension, pp 459–464. New York, Raven Press, 1980

Farquhar JW: Changing cardiovascular risk factors in entire communities; The Stanford Three-Community Project. In Lauer RM, Shekelle RB (eds): Childhood Prevention of Atherosclerosis and Hypertension, pp 435–440. New York, Raven Press, 1980

Holland WW, Chinn S, Wainwright A: Weight and blood pressure in children. In Lauer RM, Shekelle RB (eds): Childhood Prevention of Atherosclerosis and Hypertension, pp 331–341. New York, Raven Press, 1980

Kannel WB: Hypertension, blood lipids, and cigarette smoking as co-risk factors for coronary heart disease. Ann NY Acad Sci 304:128–139, 1978

Kannel WB, Castelli WP, Gordon T: Serum cholesterol, lipoproteins, and the risk of coronary heart disease. The Framingham Study. Ann Intern Med 74(1):1–12, 1971

Kannel WB, Hjortland MC, McNamara PM et al: Menopause and risk of cardiovascular disease. Ann Intern Med 85(4):447–452, 1976

Kannel WB, McGee D, Gordon T: A general cardiovascular risk profile: The Framingham Study. Am J Cardiol 38(1):46–51, 1976

Keys A, Taylor HL, Blackburn H et al: Coronary heart disease among Minnesota business and professional men followed fifteen years. Circulation 28(3):381–395, 1963

Lauer RM, Clarke WR: Immediate and long-term prognostic significance of childhood blood pressure levels. In Lauer RM and Shekelle RB (eds): Childhood Prevention of Atherosclerosis and Hypertension, pp 281–290. New York, Raven Press, 1980

McMahon FG, Cole PA, Ryan JR: A study of hypertension in the inner city. Am Heart J 85(1):65–71, 1973

Medical Letter: Coffee and cardiovascular disease. 19(16):65–66, 1977

Miller CL, Stein RF, Grim C: Personality factors of the hypertensive patient. Int J Nurs Studies 16(3):235–251, 1979

Perry HM, Perry EF: Metals and human hypertension. In Paul O (ed): Epidemiology and Control of Hypertension, pp 147–162. New York, Stratton Intercontinental Medical Book Corporation, 1975

Platt R: Heredity in hypertension. Lancet, 1:899–904, 1963

Puska P, Tuomilehto J, Nissinen A et al: Changing the cardiovascular risk in an entire community: The North Karelia Project. In Lauer RM, Shekelle RB (eds): Childhood Prevention of Atherosclerosis and Hypertension, pp 441–451. New York, Raven Press, 1980

Rosenman RH, Brand RJ, Sholtz RI et al: Multivariate prediction of coronary heart disease during 8.5 year follow-up in the western collaborative group study. Am J Cardiol 37(6):903–909, 1976

Sackett DL: Studies of blood pressure in spouses. In Paul O (ed): Epidemiology and Control of Hypertension, pp 21–39. New York, Stratton Intercontinental Medical Book Corporation, 1975

Seltzer CC: Effect of smoking on blood pressure. Am Heart J 87(5):558–564, 1974

Shapiro AP: An experimental study of comparative responses of blood pressure to different noxious stimuli. J Chronic Dis 13(4):293–311, 1961

Stamler J, Berkson DM, Dyer A et al: Relationship of multiple variables to blood pressure—Findings from four Chicago epidemiologic studies. In Paul O (ed): Epidemiology and Control of Hypertension, pp 307–356. New York, Stratton Intercontinental Medical Book Corporation, 1975

Stamler J, Lindberg HA, Berkson DM et al: Prevalence and incidence of coronary heart disease in strata of the labor force of a Chicago industrial corporation. J Chronic Dis 11(4):405–420, 1960

Tibblin G: Raising a smoke-free generation in Sweden. In Lauer RM, Shekelle RB (eds): Childhood Prevention of Atherosclerosis and Hypertension, pp 453–458. New York, Raven Press, 1980

Truett J, Cornfield J, Kannel W: A multivariate analysis of the risk of coronary heart disease in Framingham. J Chronic Dis 20(7):511–524, 1967

Yamori Y: Gene-environment interaction in the pathogenesis of hypertensive diseases. In Lauer RM and Shekelle RB (eds): Childhood Prevention of Atherosclerosis and Hypertension, pp 263–269, New York, Raven Press, 1980

Zinner SH, Levy PS, Kass EH: Familial aggregation of blood pressure in childhood. N Engl J Med 284(8):401–404, 1971

Sodium and Hypertension

Langford HG, Watson RL: Electrolytes and hypertension. In Paul O (ed): Epidemiology and Control of Hypertension, pp 119–130. New York, Stratton Intercontinental Medical Book Corporation, 1975

Langford HG, Watson RL, Thomas JG: Salt intake and the treatment of hypertension. Am Heart J 93(4):531–532, 1977

Schechter PJ, Horwitz D, Henkin RI: Sodium chloride preference in essential hypertension. JAMA 225(11):1311–1315, 1973

Tobian L: Current status of salt in hypertension. In Paul O (ed): Epidemiology and Control of Hypertension, pp 131–146. New York, Stratton Intercontinental Medical Book Corporation, 1975

Watt BK, Merrill AL: Composition of foods. United States Department of Agriculture, in Agriculture Handbook # 8. Washington, DC, U.S. Department of Agriculture, 1963

Wotman S, Mandel ID, Thompson RH Jr et al: Salivary electrolytes and salt taste thresholds in hypertension. J Chronic Dis 20(11/12):833–840, 1967

Intervention in Hypertension

Balossi EC, Hauger-Klevene JH: Down with high blood pressure; A theme with a warning for physicians. Bull Pan American Health Organization 13(3):249–252, 1979

Deeds SG, Bernheimer E, McCombs NJ et al: Patient behavior for blood pressure control—Guidelines for professionals. JAMA 241(23):2534–2537, 1979

Friedman H, Taub HA: A six-month follow-up of the use of hypnosis and biofeedback procedures in essential hypertension. A J Clin Hypnosis 20(3):184–188, 1978

Frohlich ED: Mild essential hypertension: Benefit of treatment. Ann NY Acad Sci 304:68–73, 1978

Gantt CL: Drug therapy of hypertension. Med Clin North Am 62(6):1273–1289, 1978

Hartshorn JC: What to do when your patient's in hypertensive crisis. Nursing 80(7):37–45, 1980

Moser M: How you can help your doctor treat your high blood pressure. Dallas, Am Heart Assoc, 1974

Moses C: Drug treatment of mild hypertension: Adverse consequences. Ann NY Acad Sci 304:84–95, 1978

Perry HM Jr, Goldman AI, Laving MA, Schnaper HW et al: Evaluation of drug treatment in mild hypertension: VA-NHLBI feasibility trial. Ann NY Acad Sci 304:267–288, 1978

Schnaper HW: Use of paramedical personnel in routine antihypertensive treatment. Ann NY Acad Sci 304:381–385, 1978

Sheiner LB, Melmon KL: The utility function of antihypertensive therapy. Ann NY Acad Sci 304:112–122, 1978

Ward GW, Bandy P, Fink JW: Treating and counseling the hypertensive patient. Am J Nurs 78(5):824–828, 1978

Ziesche S, Franciosa JA: Clinical application of sodium nitroprusside. Heart Lung 6(1):99–103, 1977

Patient Education and Compliance

Binn MA: Beliefs about hypertension: The benign essential hypertensive adult. Master's Thesis, University of Washington, 1979.

Griffith EW, Madero B: Primary hypertension—Patients' learning needs. Am J Nurs 73(4):624–627, 1973

Long ML, Winslow EH, Scheuhing MA et al: Hypertension—What patients need to know. Am J Nurs 76(5):765–770, 1976

Loustau A: Using the health belief model to predict patient compliance. Health Values: Achieving High Level Wellness 3(5):241–245, 1979

McKenney JM, Slining JM, Henderson HR et al: The effect of clinical pharmacy services on patients with essential hypertension. Circulation 48(5):1104–1111, 1973.

Schoof CS: Common questions patients ask. Am J Nurs 80(5):926–927, 1980

Stein FR, Miller CL, Grim CE: Factors contributing to a nursing protocol on hypertensive patients with essential and secondary hypertension. Int J Nurs Studies 16(4): 329–336, 1979

48

Valvular Disorders

SANDRA L. UNDERHILL, R.N., M.N.

Valvular heart disease is a common form of heart disease.[14] Most disorders of the heart valves are a consequence of chronic rheumatic disease. The incidence of rheumatic fever is still common in other countries but has declined in the United States. Consequently, rheumatic valvular disease has also decreased in the U.S. Rheumatic heart disease primarily involves the left heart valves, especially the mitral valve. However, isolated involvement of one valve is rare. Rheumatic valvular lesions in rank of order of occurrence are mitral stenosis, mitral insufficiency, aortic stenosis, and aortic insufficiency. The order of frequency of involvement correlates with the hemodynamic stress placed upon each of the valves. The closed mitral valve is subjected to a higher stress by systemic arterial systolic pressure than the closed aortic valve, which is subjected to systemic diastolic pressure.

Each of these four valvular disorders, including mitral valve prolapse, is described in this chapter. In rheumatic heart disease, the tricuspid valve is infrequently involved, and the pulmonic valve is only rarely affected; disorders of these valves are therefore not discussed. Because of their complex nature, combined valvular disorders are beyond the scope of this text. Nonrheumatic causes of valvular disease are briefly discussed under pathology. Surgical intervention and the nursing care of the patient with valvular disease are presented at the end of the chapter.

MITRAL STENOSIS

Pathology

In response to recurrent rheumatic endocarditis, the valvular leaflets and chordae tendineae become fibrous. The two commissures fuse and the chordae tendineae shorten (Fig. 48-1). Normally blood flows into the left ventricle through the principal orifice, which leads to the ventricular chamber, as well as through multiple secondary orifices, which are spaces formed where the chordae attach to the leaflets (Fig. 48-2). The principal orifice is reduced and the secondary orifices may be obliterated in rheumatic mitral stenosis.

Fig. 48-1. Rheumatic mitral stenosis. View is from left atrium looking down to the valve. (Eliot and Edwards: In Hurst JW, Logue RB, Schlant RC et al (eds): The Heart, 4th ed, p 955. New York, McGraw-Hill, 1978)

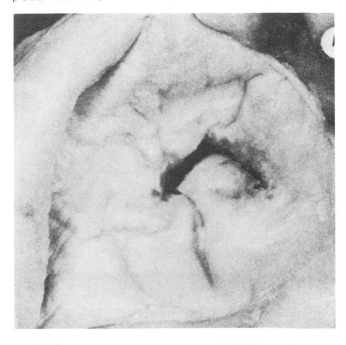

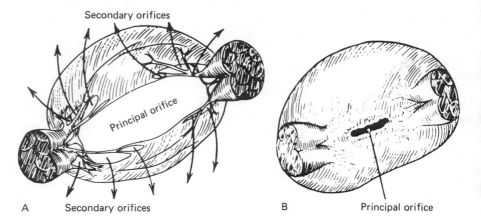

Fig. 48-2. (**A**) The normal mitral valve with principal and secondary orifices. (**B**) The stenotic mitral valve with narrowed principal orifice and obliterated secondary orifices. (Bonnabeau RC Jr, Stevenson JE, Edwards JE: J Thorac Cardiovasc Surg, 49:265, 1965)

Rarely, nonrheumatic mitral stenosis occurs as a result of a congenital lack of one of the papillary muscles, causing a parachute deformity of the mitral valve.[15]

Pathophysiology

Before hemodynamic consequences develop from mitral stenosis, the cross section of the mitral valve area must be reduced from 4–6 cm² to 2.5 cm² or less. This does not occur suddenly, but takes place gradually over many years. Normally, there are no pressure gradients. A pressure gradient is defined as a difference in the pressure between two chambers when the valve which separates them is open. In mitral stenosis a pressure gradient exists between the left atrium and left ventricle in diastole. Because the velocity of blood flow through the stenotic mitral valve cannot be increased, left atrial pressure (LAP) rises, the left atrium dilates, pulmonary artery pressure (PAP) increases, and the right ventricle hypertrophies. Mitral stenosis spares rather than stresses the left ventricle, a situation which is unique among acquired valvular disease (Fig. 48-3).

Pulmonary vascular changes may occur in patients with severe mitral stenosis as a result of structural changes in the arterioles and arteries, and of vasoconstriction of the small arteries. This increase in vascular resistance protects the pulmonary arteries from large increases in right ventricular output and protects the patient from resultant symptoms of pulmonary congestion. If pulmonary hypertension is not present and the mitral stenosis is moderate to severe, the normal distribution of pulmonary blood flow may be reversed. That is, the upper lobes of the lungs will be perfused better than the lower lobes, a condition that is also common in left heart failure from other causes. The exact cause of pulmonary hypertension in mitral stenosis is not known, although several theories have been suggested. The vasoconstriction may be a reflex initiated by elevated pressures in the left atrium, pulmonary veins and pulmonary capillaries. More likely it occurs because of alveolar hypoventilation from excess transudation of fluid from the pulmonary capillaries. Pulmonary vasoconstriction is usually reversible following surgical correction of the stenosis.

Clinical Findings

Patients with mitral stenosis who have a valve area greater than 2.5 cm² are generally asymptomatic. As the valvular orifice narrows, symptoms appear insidiously and are initially precipitated by exercise. The increased venous return that occurs during exercise causes LAP to rise, as the enlarged blood volume is unable to move through the stenotic valve. Patients can be divided into two groups: younger patients with elevated LAP, a normal cardiac output (CO), and pulmonary congestion; and older patients with high pulmonary vascular resistance, variable degrees of right heart failure and low CO. Patients in the younger group usually manifest respiratory symptoms such as paroxysmal dyspnea, hemoptysis, or pulmonary edema. The older patients most likely demonstrate findings consistent with low CO, for instance dyspnea, fatigue, and weakness.[32] Dyspnea, which is well correlated with increased PAP and pulmonary artery wedge pressure (PAWP), is the most important symptom associated with mitral stenosis; it occurs in both patient groups. Chronic right heart failure produces peripheral edema and hepatic engorgement. Atrial fibrillation, from

Fig. 48-3. Simultaneous left atrial and left ventricular pressure tracing in mitral stenosis. The diastolic pressure gradient is indicated by the cross-hatched area. (Schlant: In Hurst JW, Logue RB, Schlant RC et al (eds): The Heart, 4th ed, p 974. New York, McGraw-Hill, 1978)

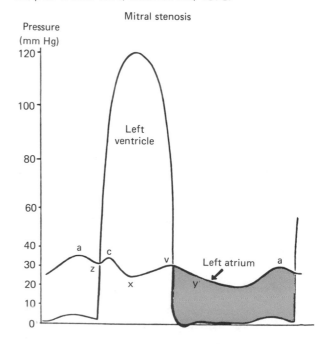

dilatation of the left atrium, occurs in 40% of patients with mitral stenosis, usually older patients with long-standing valvular disease. Once atrial fibrillation occurs, left ventricular filling is reduced, the heart rate (HR) increases, and blood tends to stagnate in the atria. Because of this circus movement of blood, mural thrombi are likely to form on the walls of the atria and in the appendages, resulting in pulmonary or systemic embolization.

Physical Assessment

Blood pressure (BP) is generally not affected by mitral stenosis unless the disease has progressed to the point of causing low CO. The pulse is usually normal to palpation, although the amplitude may be diminished in long-standing disease. The rhythm may be regular or irregularly irregular, as in atrial fibrillation. The point of maximal impulse (PMI) is normal. A sternal lift may be present, indicating right ventricular hypertrophy (RVH). On auscultation there are four principal findings: a loud apical first sound (closure of the stenotic mitral valve); an opening snap (OS) (the snapping of the stenotic valve into the ventricle during early diastole in response to the rapidly changing pressure gradients); a rumbling apical diastolic murmur with presystolic accentuation during sinus rhythm (blood flowing with difficulty and under increased pressure through the stenotic valve, and moving with increased force during atrial kick); and an increased pulmonic second sound associated with pulmonary hypertension. The intensity of the murmur changes with blood flow and may disappear altogether in endstage disease. Exercise and placing the patient in the left lateral position increase the intensity of the murmur. An apical S_3 gallop is rare, because the left ventricle is protected from failure and the boundary between rapid and reduced filling times is obscured by the stenosis; however, an S_3 gallop may be heard along the left sternal border as an indicator of right ventricular failure (Fig. 48-4).

Diagnostic Tests

Electrocardiogram. The electrocardiogram (ECG) is not specific for mitral stenosis and is often not a good indicator of the severity of the disease. In normal sinus rhythm (NSR), if left atrial enlargement has occurred, characteristic P mitrale is seen.

If atrial fibrillation is present, a large fibrillatory wave in V_1 is thought to be indicative of rheumatic heart disease, although large fibrillatory waves may also be seen with hypertension or with idiopathic paroxysmal atrial fibrillation. About 10% of patients with tight mitral stenosis have a flat fibrillatory baseline, indicating the irreversibility of the atrial fibrillation.

There may be no QRS abnormalities associated with mitral stenosis. The right ventricle usually does not hypertrophy, except with concurrent pulmonary hypertension. In mitral stenosis classic RVH almost always means a PAP greater than 35 mm Hg (see Chap. 17).

Echocardiogram. Mitral stenosis can be diagnosed by echocardiogram (see Chap. 20).

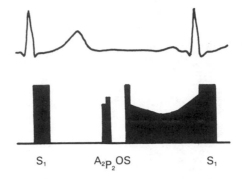

S_1 A_2P_2OS S_1

Fig. 48-4. Heart sounds in mitral stenosis: loud S_1, OS, diastolic murmur, and increased P_2. (Adapted from Frank MJ, Alvarez-Mena SV: Cardiovascular Physical Diagnosis, p 157. Copyright © 1973 by Year Book Medical Publishers, Inc., Chicago)

Chest X-Ray Chest x-ray findings correlate well with the severity of the lesion and the stage of the disease. The heart shape becomes "mitralized," or boxy in appearance, although the overall heart size remains normal. The left atrium may become very large (giant left atrium) and there may be increased vascular markings in the upper lobes of the lungs (see Chap. 16).

Cardiac Catheterization. Cardiac catheterization is an important diagnostic test of mitral stenosis. The most important finding in mitral stenosis is a pressure gradient across the mitral valve, with elevated LAP or PAWP. Left atrial pressure no longer mirrors left ventricular pressure during diastole, but rather, falls gradually. The gradient across the valve depends on the severity of the stenosis, the duration of diastole and the stroke volume (SV). Therefore, with a small SV, slow HR, and mild stenosis there may be little, if any gradient (see Chap. 19).

Medical Plan

Mitral stenosis, if untreated, has a gradual downhill course that may be accelerated by conversion to atrial fibrillation, or by pregnancy, bacterial endocarditis, or embolization.[5] Definitive therapy for mitral stenosis is surgical, but management by medical therapy is often required to control some aspects of the disease process. Several characteristics of the best candidate for surgical correction of mitral stenosis have been identified: Class II cardiac patient (New York Heart Association) (see Chap. 14), 30 to 50 years of age, no appreciable cardiac enlargement or valve calcification, and progressive symptoms of at least 2 years' duration.[8]

The medical care of rheumatic mitral valvular disease focuses on treating acute pulmonary edema or congestive heart failure (CHF), controlling atrial fibrillation, and treating or preventing embolization, bronchopulmonary infection, bacterial endocarditis, and recurrences of rheumatic fever.[32]

Acute pulmonary edema is managed by diuretics and opiates. In patients with mitral stenosis, digitalis is used to treat CHF by controlling the rapid ventricular response during atrial fibrillation. Propranolol may also be useful in controlling the ventricular rate in patients who are unable to tolerate the dose of digitalis required. Quinidine is prescribed in hopes of maintaining NSR, although atrial systole may or may not return with NSR. Anticoagulants are necessary for the treatment of peripheral or pulmonary emboli. Penicillin is specifically used as prophylaxis against bacterial endocarditis and recurrent rheumatic fever, and antibiotics and pulmonary toilet are used when respiratory infections occur.

MITRAL INSUFFICIENCY

Pathology

The pathologic picture is the same in rheumatic mitral insufficiency (mitral regurgitation) as in mitral stenosis, but the fibrotic and calcific changes occur in such a way that the valve leaflets are prevented from closing rather than opening (Fig. 48-5). Common causes of nonrheumatic mitral insufficiency seen in an acute cardiac care setting are mitral valve prolapse, which will be discussed separately, coronary artery disease (CAD), and bacterial endocarditis. Coronary artery disease results in ischemia or infarction of the papillary muscles, preventing their adequate contraction, which is necessary for mitral valve closure. Bacterial endocarditis may cause valvular perforation or rupture of the chordae tendineae.[8] Less common causes of nonrheumatic mitral insufficiency are genetic and congenital abnormalities. Left heart failure from any cause may result in left ventricular enlargement to such a degree that the atrial annulus becomes dilated and the valve is no longer large enough to cover the enlarged orifice. However, this occurs rarely, because the mitral valve leaflets are so large that they are prevented from closure only with extreme ventricular enlargement.

Fig. 48-5. Mitral insufficiency. Unopened mitral valve from above. (Eliot and Edwards: In Hurst JW, Logue RB, Schlant RC et al (eds): The Heart, 4th ed, p 956. New York, McGraw-Hill, 1978)

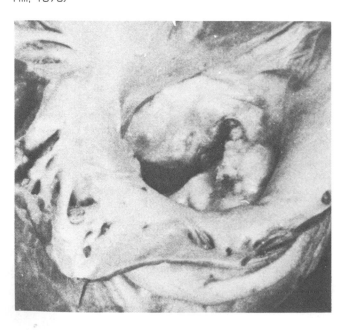

Pathophysiology

Mitral insufficiency is the result of inadequate valve closure and regurgitant flow from the ventricle back into the atrium during ventricular systole. In mitral insufficiency, the output of the left ventricle is divided into systemic and regurgitant flow. The amount of forward versus backward flow depends on the severity of the insufficiency and the degree of resistance to the outflow through the aortic valve. Regurgitant flow increases in proportion to the cross-sectional area of the insufficient mitral valve. Any factor causing increased resistance at the aortic valve, for example increased peripheral vascular resistance (PVR) or aortic stenosis, causes more regurgitant flow. In addition, as forward output decreases, a reflex vasoconstriction occurs in order to maintain BP and perfuse vital organs.[21] This causes more regurgitant flow and consequently more vasoconstriction. If this resistance decreases, for example with afterload reduction, regurgitant volume lessens and systemic output improves (see Chap. 27).

Mitral insufficiency results in increased preload of both the left ventricle and the left atrium. Regurgitant output is returned from the left atrium to the left ventricle during diastole, so that both the normal amount of blood plus the additional regurgitant volume is presented for ejection during systole. Left atrial volume is also increased because of the additional regurgitant flow. This "high volume" work causes dilatation and hypertrophy of both left-side chambers. Usually only a slight rise in left ventricular diastolic pressure accompanies the increase in diastolic volume, because the left ventricle is able to increase its compliance.

When mitral insufficiency is a result of rheumatic heart disease it usually coexists with some degree of mitral stenosis.[30] A calcified mitral valve that is immobile or "fixed" may produce an insignificant degree of stenosis but a considerable regurgitant flow. Because of the amount of blood returned to the left atrium during ventricular systole, a hemodynamic "block" may occur during diastole, which prevents adequate ventricular filling. This effect is enhanced by atrial fibrillation and by rapid ventricular rate.[32]

Clinical Findings

Mitral insufficiency usually progresses slowly, and in the absence of bacterial endocarditis, patients may remain symptom-free for decades or their entire lives. Early symptoms of mitral insufficiency are exertional dyspnea, palpitation, and easy fatigability, which are characteristically relieved by rest. These symptoms are usually insidious but may be precipitated abruptly by acute illness: systemic embolization, atrial fibrillation, pulmonary edema from other causes,[32] pulmonary infection,[11,32] pulmonary emboli,[11] bacterial endocarditis, spontaneously ruptured chordae, and systemic hypertension.[14] Pulmonary edema and hemoptysis are not as common as in mitral stenosis. Right heart failure is a late development and is usually progressive and intractable.

Physical Assessment

Examination of the apex reveals a PMI that is hyperdynamic, is displaced downward and to the left, and is abnormally wide,

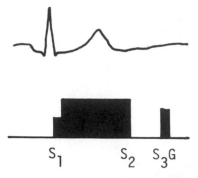

Fig. 48-6. The holosystolic murmur of mitral insufficiency with an S_3 gallop. (Frank MJ, Alvarez-Mena SV: Cardiovascular Physical Diagnosis, p 136. Copyright © 1973 by Year Book Medical Publishers, Inc., Chicago)

extending over two intercostal spaces. With marked left dilatation there may be a parasternal impulse easily confused with RVH. On auscultation a loud holosystolic murmur can be heard at the apex, radiating to the axilla and the back. It is high-pitched, blowing, and superficial in quality, and it may be accompanied by a systolic thrill. In severe mitral insufficiency, an S_3 gallop and a short diastolic rumbling murmur may be heard. An opening snap occurs in approximately 10% of patients, indicating leaflet mobility. Leaflet rigidity accounts for the absence of an opening snap in severe mitral insufficiency (Fig. 48-6).[14,32]

Diagnostic Tests

Electrocardiogram. The ECG in patients with even hemodynamically significant mitral insufficiency may be normal or at least non-specific. In longstanding disease either atrial fibrillation or P mitrale in NSR will be present. Evidence of left ventricular hypertrophy (LVH) is not always present. Right or biventricular hypertrophy may be documented in patients with severe pulmonary hypertension (see Chap. 17).

Echocardiogram. Echocardiograms provide no diagnostic information in rheumatic mitral insufficiency (see Chap. 20).

Chest X-Ray. Left atrial and ventricular enlargement in patients with mitral insufficiency can be demonstrated by chest x-ray. The use of fluoroscopy can sometimes demonstrate abnormal systolic expansion of the left atrium even though the size appears normal on routine chest x-ray. With pulmonary hypertension, right ventricular enlargement may be seen. If CHF is not present, the lung fields appear normal in spite of cardiomegaly (see Chap. 16).

Cardiac Catheterization. Depending on atrial compliance, the LAP and the PAWP tracings may be normal or elevated in the presence of even severe mitral insufficiency. If the degree of incompetence is very severe, or the insufficiency is so acute that there is little left atrial enlargement, the LAP curve increases in early systole as regurgitant blood enters the left atrium (Fig. 48-7). This is diagnostic of mitral insufficiency and is termed "ventricularization" of the left

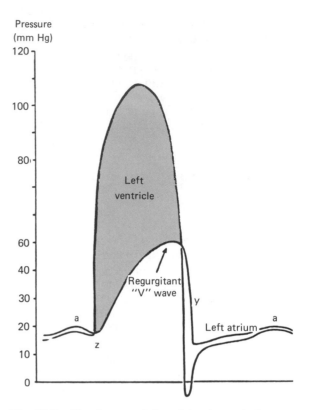

Fig. 48-7. Simultaneous left atrial and ventricular pressure tracings in severe mitral insufficiency. (Schlant RC: In Hurst JW, Logue RB, Schlant RC et al (eds): The Heart, 4th ed, p 975. New York, McGraw-Hill, 1978)

atrium if the pressure curve resembles that of the left ventricle. Assessment of the percentage of insufficiency and calculation of the mitral valve area can be done using ventriculography (see Chap. 19).

Medical Plan

Medical therapy for rheumatic mitral valve disease is discussed earlier with mitral stenosis. In mitral insufficiency, digitalis improves CHF by increasing the contractile state of the left ventricle. If mitral insufficiency is acute, as in papillary muscle rupture, or if symptoms of low forward output associated with elevated PAWP appear in the patient with chronic disease, afterload reduction should be used. In patients with mitral insufficiency nitroprusside has been shown to improve forward flow and reduce regurgitant volume by reducing aortic impedance.[21,27] For chronic cases, oral or percutaneous nitrates are sometimes utilized.

Selection of patients who will benefit from surgical treatment of mitral regurgitation is difficult, because postoperative left ventricular function is variable and cannot be easily predicted. Evaluation of myocardial performance by preoperative ventriculography may demonstrate what appears to be an efficiently contracting ventricle. However, once the incompetent valve is replaced, rather than pumping against a reduced afterload (secondary to regurgitant flow), the ventricle must eject blood against full systemic resistance. If the left ventricle is already compromised, valvular replacement can result in left ventricular failure. For this reason, and because of postoperative complications, replacement of the mitral valve is usually postponed until the patient is in functional class III category (New York Heart Association) (Chap. 14).[5,8] Most often these patients have a long history of fatigue, edema, and cardiomegaly. However, if the mitral insufficiency is acute, as in rupture of the papillary muscle, emergency surgery has been done with some success.

MITRAL VALVE PROLAPSE*

Pathology

Cells in the middle tissue layer of the mitral valve, the spongiosa, proliferate, causing intermittent encroachment upon the outermost collagen layer of the leaflet, the fibrosa. This increase in cells causes the leaflet to become voluminous in size. The fibrosa is consequently weakened, permitting abnormal degrees of prolapse of the valve toward the left atrium. The posterior leaflet is the most frequently involved (Fig. 48-8).

Secondary lesions are found in the valve leaflets and on the left ventricular endocardium. Fibroelastic thickening occurs on the atrialis, the closing aspect of the leaflets, in the area of prolapse in response to hemodynamic stresses and injury. In addition, collagenlike material pads the ventricular aspect in the concavity of the leaflet. During systole, as the posterior papillary muscle contracts, the chordae are stretched and rub the endocardial wall, creating a friction lesion. There is a surprisingly high incidence of mitral valve prolapse in apparently healthy subjects. The question has been raised whether this is indeed a pathologic state or simply a normal variation.[33]

Pathophysiology

Leaflet enlargement (redundancy) causes systolic prolapse of the mitral valve into the left atrium. With continuing ballooning, the supporting structures of the valve, the chordae tendineae and papillary muscles, are stressed, contraction of the papillary muscle is reduced, and mitral insufficiency, although usually hemodynamically insignificant, occurs.[2] Theoretically, if the papillary muscle is pulled very hard its blood supply might be blanched, causing systolic ischemia.[14] It is also thought that as the mitral valve prolapses, myocardial wall tension in the area of the papillary muscles may increase, causing a localized discrepency between O_2 supply and demand within the mitral valve apparatus.[1,14] Local coronary artery spasm from mild focal trauma is also thought to be a factor.[10]

Clinical Findings

Prolapse of the mitral valve occurs in both sexes, although it is more common in females, with a peak incidence in the fourth decade.[33] Familial occurrence has been well established.[3]

* Synonyms include Barlow's syndrome, click-murmur syndrome, and floppy, myxomatous, mucinous, hooded, billowing, or balloon mitral valve.

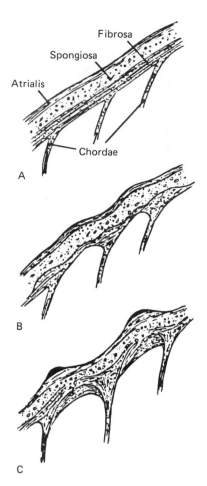

Fig. 48-8. (**A**) Normal composition of the mitral leaflet. (**B**) Increase in the spongiosa layer with encroachment upon the fibrosa. (**C**) Multiple interruptions in the fibrosa, fibroelastic thickening of the atrialis, and collagen-like padding on the ventricular aspect of the leaflet. (Shrivastava S, Guthrie RB, Edwards JE: Modern Concepts of Cardiovascular Disease, 46(12):58, 1977. By permission of the American Heart Association, Inc.).

Some patients are asymptomatic. However, atypical chest pain is common and is usually the presenting symptom. It is sharp, is localized to the left chest, and may resemble ischemic pain. Its duration is usually short, although it may last for hours. This pain is not necessarily associated with electrocardiographic abnormalities or related to exertion but is frequently precipitated by fatigue. Chest pain may be secondary to papillary muscle ischemia or spasm of a coronary artery.[10,20] Both atrial and ventricular ectopic beats occur, but the mechanism is not known. Focal ischemia has been suggested as a reason for ventricular arrhythmias. Another postulated cause is mechanical stimulation of the myocardium from chordal tension on the papillary muscle or friction of the chordae against the endocardial wall.[33]

Mild, progressive dyspnea may be related to hyperventilation. Fatigue, palpitations, presyncope, and syncope may be associated with arrhythmias.[10] Chest pain, fatigue, and effort intolerance may be cyclic in nature, improving for long periods without apparent reason.[11] In extremely advanced cases, symptoms of CHF may be evident (Chap. 27).

Some patients are reported to be emotionally unstable

and very anxious. The cause of these symptoms is unknown. Because their hearts seem normal but their chest pain persists, these patients may have been accused of being neurotic.[3] It has also been suggested that cerebral embolism from microemboli off the prolapsed valve may be the cause of the neuropsychiatric symptoms.[33]

There are several complications associated with mitral valve prolapse. Rupture of chordae tendineae can occur; these patients demonstrate symptoms of mitral insufficiency. Another potential complication is bacterial endocarditis occurring at the area of faulty valve contact, or more rarely at the friction lesions. (see Chap. 50). Sudden cardiac death has been widely associated with mitral valve prolapse in the past but is actually quite uncommon in patients with this condition. Sudden cardiac death occurs most often in patients with a history of electrocardiographic abnormalities of repolarization, such as T-wave inversion and prolonged Q-Tc interval, and ventricular ectopic beats.[11,35] Sudden death is probably secondary to ventricular fibrillation.[11]

Physical Assessment

The BP and pulse are normal in mitral valve prolapse. The rhythm may be regular, or irregular from ectopic beats. Inspection and palpation of the precordium most often are unremarkable, except in extreme cases of mitral insufficiency. Auscultatory findings are usually sufficient to diagnose prolapsed mitral valve. The first heart sound is followed by a nonejection or a mitral click and a crescendo-decrescendo murmur which continues to and sometimes through the second sound. The click is thought to result from tensing of the prolapsed leaflet with gradual "give" in the supporting structures.[11] The late systolic murmur is indicative of regurgitant flow through the prolapsed incompetent valve.

The murmur is heard best at the apex and is high-pitched and musical. Certain vasoactive maneuvers can be done to elicit a change in the murmur. Any decrease in heart size slackens chordopapillary support, promoting earlier prolapse. This causes both the click and the murmur to move closer to S_1 (Fig. 48-9). The easiest method of reducing left

Fig. 48-9. (**A**) Click-murmur (SC = systolic click) heard in mitral valve prolapse when the patient is supine. (**B**) Both click and murmur move closer to S_1 when the patient stands. (Frank MJ, Alvarez-Mena SV: Cardiovascular Physical Diagnosis, p 148. Copyright © 1973 by Year Book Medical Publishers, Inc., Chicago)

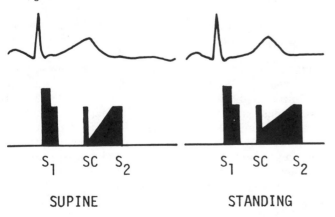

SUPINE   STANDING

ventricular size is by having the patient stand, although a Valsalva maneuver, isoproterenol, and amyl nitrate have the same effect.[20] However, because standing also increases BP, the murmur becomes louder in the erect position,[2] which makes it the maneuver of choice.

A precordial honk may also be present. It is diamond-shaped, sometimes very brief, and may be superimposed on the murmur. This sound is intermittent and may alternate with the click. It is thought to result from leaflet resonance.[11]

Diagnostic Tests

Electrocardiogram. With prolapse of the mitral valve, the ECG may be normal or show a variety of nonspecific changes. ST-segment elevation or depression and T-wave inversion in the inferior (II, III, AVF) and left lateral (V_5 and V_6) leads are most frequent.[3,14,20] Prolonged Q-Tc interval and prominent U waves have also been noted. Premature ventricular contractions (PVCs) are the most commonly noted arrhythmias, although premature atrial contractions (PACs) paroxysmal atrial tachycardia (PAT), atrial fibrillation and flutter, and ventricular tachycardia and fibrillation are seen. Mobitz II and complete atrioventricular (AV) block can occur. It is thought that myocardial fibrosis or degeneration of the sinoatrial and AV nodal arteries may contribute to these blocks (see Chap. 17).[3]

Echocardiogram. Prolapsed mitral valve can be accurately diagnosed by echocardiography. (see Chap. 20).[16]

Chest X-Ray. The chest x-ray is usually normal in patients with mitral valve prolapse. In advanced cases, evidence of LVH and CHF may be seen.

Cardiac Catheterization. Ventriculography provides information about which mitral leaflet or leaflets are involved, although no definite criteria have yet been established that delineate normal from variant systolic posterior movement. This same information can usually be determined noninvasively by echocardiography. The matter of the superiority of the echocardiogram versus catheterization for diagnosis of mitral valve prolapse has not been resolved.[20] Coronary angiography may be necessary to rule out CAD as the cause of persistent chest pain.

Medical Plan

Medical management is directed toward relief of symptoms. Chest pain does not always respond to drug therapy. Nitroglycerin provides relief for some patients. Some physicians feel that propranolol has little effect,[11] while others report a good effect.[3] It is suggested that, when explaining this atypical chest pain to the patient, one compare it to a headache, which is bothersome and usually of little consequence, and point out that remission is spontaneous.[11] Chest pain may be induced by nervous hyperventilation precipitated by palpitations. These arrhythmias should be treated. Quinidine is usually not effective, although propranolol has been shown to be of some benefit. Propranolol reduces focal ischemia by decreasing myocardial O_2 demand. By reducing the force of the contraction, it is thought, it also reduces the tug on the papillary muscles and friction against the endo-cardium. If severe mitral insufficiency develops, the mitral valve may need to be replaced. All patients with prolapsed mitral valve should have prophylaxis against bacterial endocarditis (see Chap. 50). The prognosis is generally good. Extreme care must be taken to avoid making the patient into a cardiac cripple.[3]

Nursing Care

Nursing care should be concerned with the physiologic as well as the psychologic well-being of the patient. Special care should be given to patients who are emotionally unstable or extremely anxious. The asymptomatic patient should understand that prolapsed mitral valve may be a normal variation rather than a disease.

Because response to drug therapy is so unpredictable, the symptomatic patient with chest pain may need to learn to live with the pain. Since fatigue frequently precedes pain, the patient should get adequate rest and avoid overly tiring situations as much as possible. Concern over the significance of chest pain should be played down, although its discomfort cannot be ignored. The use of chest-pain medication should be explained to the patient (see Chaps. 35, 36). If arrhythmias are being treated, the antiarrhythmic drug prescribed must be understood by the patient (see Chap. 34). The patient should also be aware of the importance of keeping follow-up appointments. All patients with prolapse of the mitral valve must have the concept of prevention of bacterial endocarditis thoroughly explained (see Chap. 50).

AORTIC STENOSIS

Pathology

Rheumatic involvement of the aortic valve causes fusion of the commissures with thickening and fibrosis of the cusps, eventually resulting in valve calcification. If all three commissures are affected, the valve becomes immobile and aortic insufficiency also results (Fig. 48-10).

Nonrheumatic aortic stenosis almost always results from a congential bicuspid valve. Calcification is usual in long-standing aortic stenosis from any cause. Benign calcification of the valve often occurs in persons 70 or more years of age.

Pathophysiology

Aortic stenosis results in increased afterload, forcing the left ventricle to hypertrophy with little or no dilation. This tremendous concentric hypertrophy may allow left ventricular output to remain essentially normal for many years. Ventricular systolic pressures are elevated and may reach 260 to 300 mm Hg. These high pressures can only be sustained for short periods, for instance during mild exertion. Left ventricular end-diastolic pressures (LVEDP) may be elevated even at rest because of reduced ventricular compliance, which is associated with hypertrophied muscle rather than with heart failure. Atrial contraction contributes significantly to final diastolic filling and a more forceful

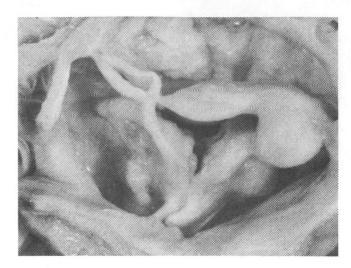

Fig. 48-10. Stenotic aortic valve viewed from above. (Eliot RS, Edwards JE: In Hurst JW, Logue RB, Schlant RC et al (eds): The Heart, 4th ed, p 963. New York, McGraw-Hill, 1978)

ventricular ejection (Starling's law.) A marked reduction in CO with development of pulmonary edema can result from the loss of this atrial kick. Left atrial pressure, which may rise to 30 to 35 mm Hg during atrial systole, does not produce pulmonary edema unless the mean LAP is also elevated. During the later stages of aortic stenosis, as left ventricular failure develops, CO decreases, LVEDP increases, the left atrium fails, and pulmonary edema and right heart failure result.[30]

Clinical Findings

Symptoms of aortic stenosis occur because of reduced CO, increased cardiac workload and increased end-diastolic pressures. The normal adult cross-sectional aortic valve area ranges from 2.5 to 3.5 cm², but with pure aortic stenosis typical symptoms do not develop until the orifice is reduced to a critical point of 0.5 to 0.7 cm². The classic symptoms are effort syncope, angina pectoris, and dyspnea. Syncope may result from activation of the stretch receptors of the left ventricle as the LVEDP increases with exertion. These receptors relay inhibitory afferent impulses to the vasomotor center, preventing the normal vasoconstriction reflex that occurs during exercise.[7] Significantly reduced CO resulting in reduced cerebral and cardiac perfusion also contributes to effort syncope. The reduced cardiac perfusion can cause either tachyarrhythmias or bradyarrhythmias, which further diminish both cerebral and coronary blood flow. Rarely, syncope may be secondary to advanced AV block from conduction system disease. Angina pectoris may occur even in the absence of significant CAD, precipitated by the very high myocardial oxygen consumption of the hypertrophied left ventricle and reduced coronary blood flow. However, angina in the older male patient may be the result of coexisting CAD. Survival time is approximately 2 years following the appearance of syncope and non-CAD-related angina pectoris. Dyspnea is related to left heart failure, which occurs when LVEDP increases after systolic pressure is no longer able to maintain forward flow. CHF in the patient with aortic stenosis is an ominous sign. Sudden death remains an everpresent threat; it occurs in 14% to 18% of all patients with aortic stenosis, including those who are asymptomatic, usually during periods of strenuous activity. It is probably due to ventricular fibrillation.[31]

Physical Assessment

BP is usually normal in patients with aortic stenosis. An indication of the severity of the stenosis may be reflected by the pulse pressure, which decreases to 30 mm Hg or less in severe disease. However, moderate systolic hypertension, which is not uncommon in the elderly patient, invalidates pulse pressure as a reliable measure of SV (see Chap. 14). Atrial fibrillation usually does not occur unless there is coexisting mitral stenosis. In advanced disease the carotid pulse characteristically is small, slow-rising, and sometimes prolonged. The pulse may be normalized if aortic insufficiency is also present.

The apex impulse is relatively quiet in aortic stenosis. The PMI is not necessarily displaced unless there is left heart failure, but the impulse is quite prolonged. A presystolic heave may be present. Four findings are characteristically noted on auscultation (Fig. 48-11). A diamond-shaped ejection murmur is usually heard best in the aortic area and may be accompanied by a thrill. The murmur and thrill may radiate to the carotid arteries. Occasionally this murmur is loudest at the apex and may be mistaken for the murmur of mitral insufficiency. This occurs most frequently in the elderly patient. The second finding is a loud click which is heard best at the apex and may be mistaken for a split S_1. Clicks result from the upward movement of a mobile valve and are, therefore, not usually heard in rheumatic or calcified stenosis. Another finding is an absent aortic second sound resulting from the inability of the aortic valve to close. Finally, an S_4 gallop is frequently heard, but is very nonspecific. An S_3 gallop appears only in the presence of marked left ventricular failure.[31]

Diagnostic Tests

Electrocardiogram. The ECG is not a good index of the severity of aortic stenosis. It is almost always normal if the pressure gradient is less than 50 mm Hg, and it may remain normal even with severe disease. However, LVH is present in the majority of patients. P mitrale is occasionally seen in NSR.[14,31] Commonly noted are left anterior hemiblock and left bundle branch block, and complete AV block may be seen with calcific aortic stenosis.[22]

Echocardiogram. The use of echocardiography in the diagnosis and quantification of aortic stenosis is disappointing (see Chap. 20).[16]

Chest X-Ray. As with electrocardiography, chest x-rays can be deceptively normal even with severe disease. Heart size may be within normal limits or only slightly enlarged, although cardiomegaly is often evident in advanced disease. A barium swallow may demonstrate left atrial enlargement. A calcified aortic ring may be visualized most commonly in patients over 35 years old with severe stenosis. Poststenotic aortic dilatation, which occurs only in patients with severe obstruction, is due to the stream of blood passing through the stenotic lesion. A "jet" lesion, or intimal fibrosis, develops, resulting in wall change and dilatation of the aorta.[19,31]

Cardiac Catheterization. A systolic pressure gradient between the left ventricle and the aorta is diagnostic of aortic stenosis. This pressure gradient can be increased during exercise. Significant stenosis is reflected by a gradient greater than 50 mm Hg. CO may be normal or low. An accentuated atrial kick can be observed on the pressure tracing. Left ventriculography is used to estimate ventricular contractility, rule out mitral insufficiency, and differentiate valvular from subvalvular or supravalvular stenosis (Fig. 48-12).

Medical Plan

Surgical therapy is the only definitive treatment for significant aortic stenosis; it is recommended when left ventricular heart failure, syncope, or angina develop. Because of the risk of sudden death, some physicians recommend surgery even in asymptomatic patients who have gradients greater than 50 mm Hg,[32] while others prefer to wait until symptoms

Fig. 48-12. Simultaneous aortic and left ventricular pressure tracings in aortic stenosis. The pressure gradient is demonstrated by the shaded area. (Adapted from Schlant RC: In Hurst JW, Logue RB, Schlant RC et al (eds): The Heart, 4th ed, p 821. New York, McGraw-Hill, 1978)

Fig. 48-11. The systolic ejection murmur of aortic stenosis with an ejection click (EC), S_4 gallop and absent A_2. (Adapted from Frank MJ, Alvarez-Mena SV: Cardiovascular Physical Diagnosis, p 141. Copyright © 1973 by Year Book Medical Publishers, Inc., Chicago)

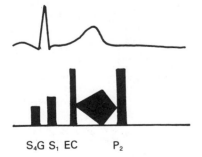

S_4G S_1 EC P_2

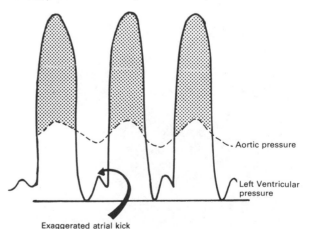

Aortic pressure

Left Ventricular pressure

Exaggerated atrial kick

appear. In order to reduce the possibility of sudden death, strenuous physical activity must be stopped in all patients with significant disease until the stenosis can be surgically corrected.

Medical treatment is used to manage the symptoms of the stenosis until surgery can be performed. CHF (Chap. 27) and angina pectoris (Chap. 22) are treated as they occur. Asymptomatic patients do not require medical therapy.

AORTIC INSUFFICIENCY

Pathology

Rheumatic aortic insufficiency has the same underlying pathogenesis as rheumatic stenosis, many times causing these lesions to coexist. Scarring, rolling, retraction, stiffening, and eventual calcification of the leaflets prevent closure of the cusps and allow regurgitation of blood to occur (Fig. 48-13). Nonrheumatic causes of aortic insufficiency include bacterial endocarditis, syphilitic aortitis, cystic medial necrosis, dissecting aortic aneurysms, traumatic tears of the aorta, and congenital bicuspid valves.[15,32]

Pathophysiology

Volume overload of the left ventricle occurs during aortic insufficiency from the combination of blood entering normally from the left atrium and regurgitant blood reentering through the incompetent aortic valve. Retrograde flow occurs during diastole when pressures are lowest in the ventricle and highest in the aorta. The left ventricle dilates and hypertrophies as a result of this volume overload. In free aortic insufficiency, hearts become so enlarged (500 g to 1000 g) that they are termed "ox heart" or "cor bovinum."

Several compensatory mechanisms exist to maintain normal cardiac function despite valvular incompetence. In

Fig. 48-13. Insufficient aortic valve viewed from above. (Eliot RS, Edwards JE: In Hurst JW, Logue RB, Schlant RC et al (eds): The Heart, 4th ed, p 960. New York, McGraw-Hill, 1978)

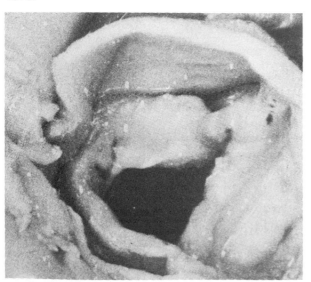

long-standing aortic insufficiency, the left ventricle remains compliant, allowing a large increase in volume with normal end-diastolic pressure. A more forceful contraction (Starling's law) and a prolonged systolic ejection time result in an increased SV, which commonly may be twice normal and occasionally as much as 200 to 300 ml/m². This allows a normal CO and response to exercise to be maintained. Interestingly, exercise produces beneficial results in these patients by decreasing reflux: the tachycardia of exercise shortens diastolic time, while the reflex vasodilation decreases afterload. In order to maintain myocardial perfusion, which can be compromised by the increased cardiac workload and the decreased diastolic perfusion pressure, coronary blood flow shifts from diastole to systole. Early in the course of the disease, forward flow is maximized by a lowered PVR. In more advanced stages, unfortunately the PVR increases, causing retrograde flow to increase as well.

In acute aortic insufficiency with sudden increases in left ventricular volume there is not sufficient time for compensatory mechanisms to develop. Large refluxes into a relatively indistensible left ventricle cause the LVEDP to rise, forward flow to decrease, and heart failure to ensue rapidly. Death results unless the pressure gradient can be quickly reduced.[17,22,32]

Clinical Findings

Significant aortic insufficiency may be present for many years or even a lifetime without the development of symptoms. The first symptom likely to be noted is an awareness of the hyperdynamic heart and pulse; for instance, visible throbbing in the neck and palpitations, especially while lying on the left side. Dizziness, accentuated by rapid postural change, occurs often and is thought to be from pronounced pressure changes in the cerebral vessels. Dyspnea from moderate exertion occurs commonly but is not necessarily progressive. However, when the patient reaches the point that dyspnea is precipitated by normal activity, a rapid downhill course follows.

More than 50% of patients with aortic insufficiency eventually develop angina pectoris. As an isolated symptom it does not necessarily represent a poor prognostic sign, but when angina becomes atypical, prolonged, or worse at night and is accompanied by CHF, the situation becomes serious. The cause of angina pectoris with aortic insufficiency is not fully understood. In the later stages of aortic insufficiency the compensatory vasodilation diminishes and vasoconstriction occurs, increasing left ventricular work, volume, and pressure. CAD may be totally or partially responsible for chest pain in the older age group. Once CHF clearly develops, the chances of sudden death are increased. A distinctive syndrome has been noted in advanced cases when death appears imminent: tachycardia, sweating, flushing, paroxysmal hypertension, and severe chest pain. It is thought that CHF develops at night because of mobilization of edema fluid. This may result in sympathetic storm because of the additional stress placed on the system. Myocardial oxygen consumption increases, as does PVR. Consequently, as the reflux worsens, angina develops and pulmonary congestion becomes more severe.

Physical Assessment

There are many peripheral signs apparent with moderate-to-severe aortic insufficiency. A rapidly rising and collapsing ("water-hammer" or Corrigan's) pulse is characteristic with significant aortic insufficiency (Fig. 48-14). The forceful ventricular contraction causes a rapid upstroke, while the retrograde flow and peripheral vasodilation result in diastolic collapse. Systolic hypertension, decreased diastolic pressure (sometimes as low as 40 mm Hg), and a widened pulse pressure are numerical indicators of the bounding pulse. Visible pulsations may be seen in the carotid, subclavian, and brachial arteries. Occasionally, a double systolic peak (pulsus bisferiens) can be felt if firmer than usual pressure is exerted over the carotid pulse during its descent (Fig. 14-9A). However, this sign can also be felt in persons without aortic disease who have increased CO or extremely compliant vessels. In severe aortic insufficiency, systolic BP may be from 20 to 60 mm Hg higher in the legs than in the arms (Hill's sign). This is probably an accentuation of the normal BP response in the lower extremities. Capillary pulsation (Quinke's sign), representing peripheral vasodilation, can be observed as alternating flushing and paling of the nail beds. When listening to overly large arteries "pistol shot" sounds can be heard and a to-and-fro murmur (systolic and diastolic) can then be elicited with slight compression by the stethoscope (Durozier's sign). Head bobbing with each aortic pulsation (DeMusset's sign) is also characteristic of hemodynamically significant aortic insufficiency.

The apex impulse may be the most reliable physical indicator of the severity of aortic insufficiency. Typically, the heart is hyperdynamic with a prolonged systolic thrust and palpable diastolic filling wave. Because of LVH and dilatation, the PMI is displaced downward and to the left, and becomes holosystolic. A diffuse precordial heave may be present in advanced cardiac failure.

On auscultation there is a diastolic murmur that starts with the second sound and is decrescendo, high-pitched, and blowing. The intensity of the murmur varies with the pressure gradient and decreases through diastole (Fig. 48-15). In mild aortic insufficiency a soft (grade I–II/VI) murmur heard best in the left third intercostal space next to the sternum (Erb's point) may be the only physical finding. As the severity of the lesion increases, the murmur becomes louder and longer, and can be easily heard along the left sternal border. However, hemodynamic significance of the regurgitation does not always correlate with the

Fig. 48-14. Comparison of (**A**) normal pulse contour with (**B**) water-hammer pulse (Bates B: A Guide to Physical Examination, 2nd ed., p 144. Philadelphia, JB Lippincott, 1974)

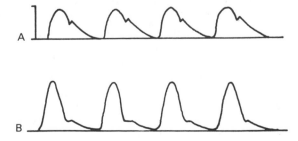

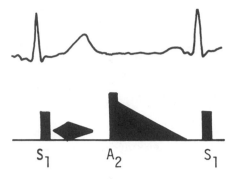

Fig. 48-15. Diastolic murmur of aortic insufficiency with early systolic murmur. (Frank MJ, Alvarez-Mena SV: Cardiovascular Physical Diagnosis, p 153. Copyright © 1973 by Year Book Medical Publishers, Inc., Chicago)

intensity of the murmur. For instance, during severe heart failure, LVEDP rises, the pressure gradient between the left ventricle and aorta decreases, less reflux occurs, and the intensity of the murmur decreases. If the murmur has a musical or "seagull" quality and is heard to the right of the sternum, the etiology is thought to be nonrheumatic. Changing the position of the patient may increase the intensity of the murmur: leaning forward on all fours, or recumbent. Raising the BP, for instance by administering phenylephrine or by having the patient perform an isometric handgrip, may also increase the murmur's intensity. Whatever the maneuver, the patient must be instructed to stop breathing or the murmur may be masked by breath sounds.

An early systolic murmur is commonly heard with significant aortic insuffiency. The augmented systolic flow causes a functional aortic stenosis (high flow through a nonstenotic valve), which is not significant. An apical diastolic rumble (Austin Flint murmur) may be heard, especially when heart failure develops. It must be carefully differentiated from the murmur of mitral stenosis. An early systolic click that sounds somewhat like the second half of a split S_1 may represent a "pistol shot" sound in the central arteries. In free aortic insufficiency an S_3 gallop is commonly heard.

Diagnostic Tests

Electrocardiogram. The ECG in mild to moderate aortic insufficiency may be normal. In significant regurgitation LVH may be noted, and with advanced disease, left atrial enlargement can be seen. Atrial fibrillation, which is rare without concomitant mitral valve disorders, is usually associated with progression of the disease. The ECG can also be normal with severe, acute aortic insufficiency.

Echocardiogram. Although it has limited usefulness in the diagnosis of aortic insufficiency, the echocardiogram is helpful in the evaluation of left ventricular function and in the establishment of coexisting mitral disease[16,22] (see Chap. 20).

Chest X-Ray. Chest x-rays are usually normal in mild to moderate aortic insufficiency. As the left ventricle dilates from more significant regurgitation, the heart takes on a boot-shaped appearance. With further progression of the disease, CHF occurs, the left atrium enlarges, and pulmonary congestion becomes apparent. Cardiac size can be normal with severe acute aortic insufficiency.

Cardiac Catheterization. Physical findings and noninvasive tests are sufficient to establish the diagnosis of aortic insufficiency, although cardiac catheterization may be performed prior to surgery. The extent of regurgitation can be visualized by aortography and quantified by left ventricular angiography.

Medical Plan

Once symptoms of aortic insufficiency have developed, the aortic valve should be surgically replaced. It is recommended that surgery be performed on patients regardless of symptoms if LVH can be documented on chest x-ray and the ECG, and if the systolic BP is 140 mm Hg or more with a diastolic BP of 30 mm Hg or less.[34] Until that time no treatment may be needed, although the patient should be followed up at regular intervals. CHF and angina pectoris should be managed medically until surgery can be performed.

Sudden, acute aortic insufficiency requires immediate medical intervention. Afterload reduction therapy, such as nitroprusside infusion, improves forward flow by reducing two major factors contributing to ejection impedence: arteriolar resistance and aortic stiffness. Left ventricular preload is reduced by several mechanisms: venodilatation, causing venous pooling and a decreased venous return; improvement in ventricular emptying because of less impedence; and reduction of regurgitant volume because of a greater forward flow. This therapy may maintain a sufficient forward output to allow time for the aortic valve to be surgically replaced.[25]

SURGICAL TREATMENT OF VALVULAR DISEASE

Mitral Commissurotomy

Instead of valvular replacement, closed mitral commissurotomy may be selected in pure mitral stenosis if the cusps are still pliable. Indications of valve mobility are: a loud, delayed S_1, an opening snap and absence of radiographic evidence of valve calcification. After a right anterolateral thoracotomy is performed, the surgeon's finger is inserted through an incision in the atrial appendage into the left atrium and gently into the stenotic valve. If this simple finger fracturing does not adequately increase the size of the mitral orifice, an expandable metal dilator is inserted transventricularly into the orifice.[26] The operative risk in closed mitral commissurotomy is small, with a mortality rate of about 2%. Postoperative complications include the postcommissurotomy syndrome (30%), which consists of fever, chest pain, and numerous other signs and symptoms, atrial fibrillation (24%–44%), arterial embolization (2%) and, rarely, significant mitral insufficiency.[23] Of patients surviving surgery initially, 80% to 85% have good results, but stenosis recurs in approximately 20% of these patients after

5 to 10 years.[8] Many surgeons prefer using open mitral commissurotomy because atrial thrombi can be seen and the valve can be dissected under direct observation. If valve replacement is indicated, the open technique provides a direct approach to the valve. After mitral commissurotomy the postoperative course is usually uncomplicated. Postoperative care is similar to that for patients who have had open heart surgery[24] (see Chap. 24).

Mitral Annuloplasty

Mitral annuloplasty is a reconstruction of the insufficient mitral valve. If patients are selected carefully, good results can be obtained. This procedure is no longer widely used, having been replaced by the use of prosthetic valves.

Mitral Valve Replacement

Surgical candidates with mitral insufficiency or stenosis who cannot undergo commissurotomy have mitral valve replacement instead. Open heart surgery (see Chap. 24) is required for insertion of all prosthetic valves. For mitral replacement a median sternotomy is performed, the mitral valve, chordae tendineae, and papillary muscles are excised, and the appropriate prosthetic valve is sutured into place (Fig. 48-16). After mitral valve replacement many patients experience a transient period of low CO. This may last from 3 to 12 hours after surgery, but output gradually increases, often returning to normal.

Aortic Valve Replacement

Complete aortic valve excision and replacement is the treatment of choice for patients with aortic insufficiency or stenosis. A median sternotomy is performed, and after total cardiopulmonary bypass has begun, the aortic valve is exposed by a transverse aortotomy. The diseased valve is then removed and replaced by a prosthesis.

Prosthetic Valves

Recent advances in the surgical therapy and prognosis of valvular disease are due in part to the development of improved artificial valves. More than 50 different prosthetic and bioprosthetic valves have been used since 1960. Before a decision is made to use a particular artificial valve, factors in valve design, specifically durability, thrombogenic potential, and hemodynamic properties, are weighed against annulus size and certain clinical considerations, such as the desirability of long-term anticoagulation.[12] A complete description of all models of artificial valves is beyond the scope of this book, but the most important types will be discussed.

Central flow valves more nearly simulate normal blood flow. At present only biologic valves achieve this flow pattern. The Hancock stabilized glutaraldehyde valve (Fig. 48-17A) is the most widely used valve of this type. These are porcine aortic valves and can be used to replace any heart valve. These valves are nonviable tissues that are essentially nonthrombogenic. Some physicians feel that this may be the prosthesis of choice for mitral valve replacement.[9] Morbidity and failure rate with the Hancock valve is low. Anticoagulants are not necessary for patients in NSR.[12] These valves which have been in clinical use since 1970

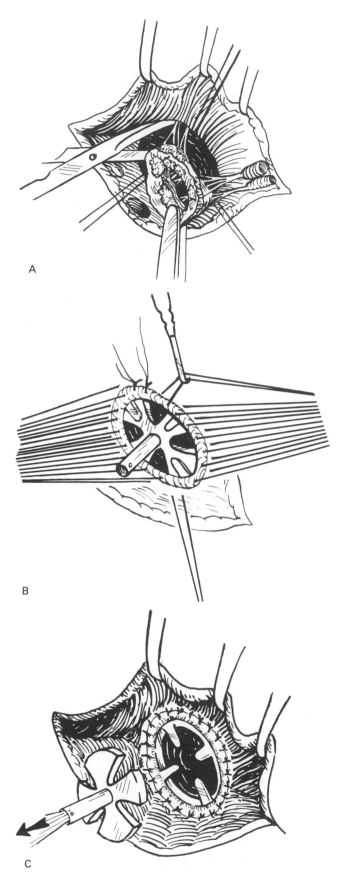

Fig. 48-16. Mitral valve replacement. (**A**) The diseased valve is excised, and (**B**), (**C**) replaced by a prosthesis sutured into the annulus. (Cooley DA, Norman JC: Techniques in Cardiac Surgery, p 144. Houston, Texas Medical Press, 1975).

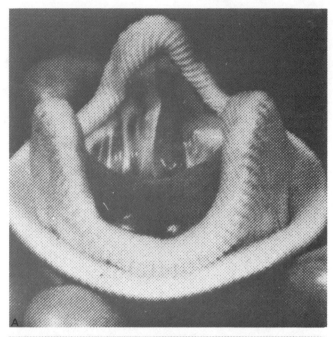

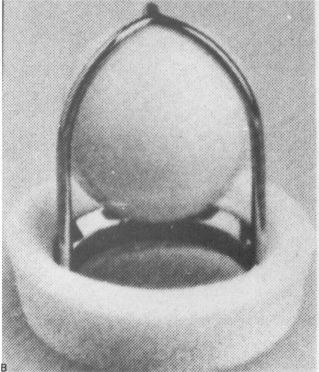

Fig. 48-17. Commonly used prosthetic and bioprosthetic valves. (**A**) Hancock stabilized gluteraldehyde valve (central flow). (**B**) Starr-Edwards ball valve (lateral flow). (*Cont. on page 648*)

may require replacement more often than synthetic valves. The Carpentier–Edwards and the Angell–Shiley valves are two new models of gluteraldehyde-stabilized porcine heterografts. Other biologic valves include pulmonic autografts, viable and nonviable homografts, and tissue valves, such as the Ionescu–Shiley pericardial or the dura-mater valve.[9,12,28,36]

Lateral flow valves are synthetic prostheses which direct blood away from the normal central flow. The Starr–Edwards ball valve (Fig. 48-17B) presently consists of a metal cage

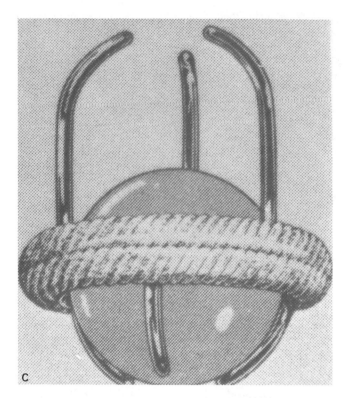

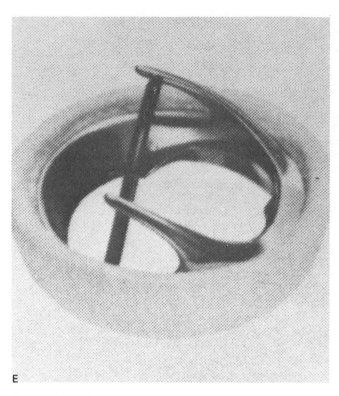

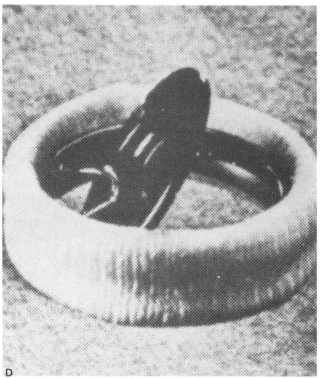

Fig. 48-17. (*Cont.*) Commonly used prosthetic and bioprosthetic valves. (**C**) Smeloff-Cutter ball valve (lateral flow). (**D**) Björk-Shiley disc valve (lateral flow). (**E**) Lillehei-Kaster disc valve (lateral flow). (Cohn LH, Collins JJ: Primary Cardiology, 4(4):15, 1978)

boembolism; hemolytic anemia from the destruction of red blood cells by the valve; ball variance from lipid adsorption into the silastic ball (manufactured prior to 1965), changing its diameter and causing it to either stick in the cage or escape from it; intimal thickening around the coronary ostia after aortic valve replacement because of high velocity of centrifugal flow around the valve;[5] strut cloth wear and cloth embolization; and obstruction of the orifice.[12] Hemolytic anemia can be detected by periodically checking the hematocrit. Other signs that may help in the definitive diagnosis of hemolytic anemia are a fall in serum haptoglobin and increases in serum lactic dehydrogenase, carbon monoxide production, and urinary iron excretion.[5] Smeloff–Cutter (Fig. 48-17C) and Braunwald–Cutter are other types of ball valves in use. Disc valves have a flat lens suspended in an abbreviated cage. Because of a high incidence of strut and lens wear, clinical trials of the disc valve have been disappointing. The Björk–Shiley (Fig. 48-17D) and Lillehei–Kaster (Fig. 48-17E) valves are tilting disc valves that allow some amount of central flow. Although the incidence of thromboembolism is lower with disc valves, anticoagulants are recommended with these as well as with all synthetic valves.

NURSING INTERVENTION

Nursing functions in the care of the patient with valvular disease can be divided into three areas: primary prevention of valvular disease; acute and chronic care of patients with

with three struts and an enclosed hollow stellite ball. Changes in chamber pressure cause the ball to move back and forth in its cage, opening and closing the valve. Important declines in long-term morbidity and mortality from thromboembolism in this valve have occurred with the advent of cloth-covered ring and struts in 1967. The Starr–Edwards valve has an excellent durability record. Complications involving the use of this valve include throm-

valvular disease, including secondary prevention; and post-surgical management. As in all nursing care, the nursing process must be followed and outcome criteria used to evaluate the care given.

Primary Prevention

Rheumatic heart disease, the most common cause of valvular disease, can be prevented. Nurses functioning in community health-care centers should be responsible for detection of β-hemolytic streptococcal infections. Once streptococcal infection is diagnosed, nurses should teach the adult patient and the young patient and parents the importance of complying with the medical therapy. For patients already rheumatic but without valve involvement, teaching should focus on the prevention of future streptococcal infections which would cause recurrent endocarditis (see Chap. 50). Nurses skilled in the area of physical assessment should screen for previously undetected heart murmurs and refer these patients to specialists for proper follow-up.

Nursing Care of the Patient with Acute or Chronic Valvular Disease

When the patient is admitted to the cardiac care unit, a nursing assessment, including a history and physical examination (Chap. 14), should be done as soon as feasible in order to plan appropriate care. On-going patient assessment, repeated as often as necessary, will provide important information concerning patient progress.

In acute cases, patient care does not focus upon valvular disease and its implications *per se* but rather on providing for patient understanding of the situation and assisting the patient to obtain symptomatic relief. These symptoms include those of CHF and shortness of breath, syncope, and fatigue (Chap. 27) and anginal pain (Chap. 22). Specific nursing actions for the patient with acute endocarditis are described in Chapter 50.

Before discharge, the patient and family must understand diet restriction, if any; medications, usually one or more of the following: digoxin (Chap. 34), quinidine (Chap. 34), diuretics (Chap. 37), potassium chloride supplement, anticoagulants (Chap. 38), and the prophylactic use of antibiotics (Chap. 50); activity restrictions, which for those with aortic stenosis require a specific exercise prescription but for others is self-limiting; the need for compliance and follow-up; and when to notify the physician of symptoms. This teaching must be documented for future reference.

Nursing care for the chronically ill or stable patient with valvular disease may center on different problems. The difficulties of coping physically or psychologically with valvular disease may not have become apparent until after discharge, and appropriate counseling interventions are usually needed. Referrals may be helpful. Teaching begun during the acute phase should be continued and reemphasized for the chronically ill patient and the family.

Presurgical and Postsurgical Nursing Management

In addition to routine preoperative teaching for cardiac catheterization (Chap. 19) and open-heart surgery (Chap.

24), specific information about valve prostheses should be given. The physician may have already discussed the particular artificial valve to be used, including some of its implications. The nurse should reinforce this teaching by further discussion and encouragement of questions.

For general postoperative nursing care of the patient after open-heart surgery, refer to Chapter 24. In addition, the nurse should be alert for early signs of valvular failure, for instance perivalvular leaks manifested by murmurs of either mitral reguritation or aortic insufficiency, and subsequent CHF.

Prior to discharge, the patient and family must be aware of any changes in the therapeutic regime. The importance of follow-up care should again be stressed.

REFERENCES

1. Aranda JM, Befeler B, El-Sherif N et al: Mitral valve prolapse. Recent concepts and observations. Am J Med 60(7):977–1004, 1976
2. Barlow JB, Bosman CK, Pocock WA et al: Late systolic murmurs and non-ejection ("mid-late") systolic clicks. Br Heart J 30:203–218, 1968
3. Barlow JB, Pocock WA: The problem of nonejection systolic clicks and associated mitral systolic murmurs: Emphasis on the billowing mitral leaflet syndrome. Am Heart J 90(5):636–655, 1975
4. Bates B: A Guide to Physical Examination, 2nd ed, p 185. Philadelphia, JB Lippincott, 1979
5. Behrendt DM, Austen WG: Current status of prosthetics for heart valve replacement. Prog Cardiovasc Dis 15(4):369–401, 1973
6. Bonnabeau RC Jr, Stevensen JE, Edwards JE: Obliteration of the principal orifice of the mitral valve: A rare form of 'Restenosis.' J Thorac Cardiovasc Surg 49(2):264–268, 1965
7. Brody MJ, Abboud FM: Tissue perfusion. Frohlich ED (ed): Pathophysiology, 2nd ed, pp 29–48. Philadelphia, JB Lippincott, 1976
8. Brockman SK: Surgery of the cardiac patient. Silber EN, Katz LN (eds): Heart Disease, pp 1301–1390. New York: Macmillan, 1975
9. Buch WS, Pipkin RD, Hancock WD et al: Mitral valve replacement with the Hancock stabilized gluteraldehyde valve. Clinical laboratory evaluation. Arch Surg 110(11):1408–1415, 1975
10. Buda AJ, Levene DL, Myers MG et al: Coronary artery spasm and mitral value prolapse. Am Heart J 95(4):457–462, 1978
11. Cobbs BW Jr: Clinical recognition and medical management of rheumatic heart disease and other acquired valvular disease. Hurst JW, Logue RB, Schlant RC et al (eds): The Heart, 3rd ed, pp 826–971. New York, McGraw-Hill, 1974
12. Cohn LH, Collins JJ: Cardiac valve replacement: Tissue or prosthetic? Primary Cardiol 4(4):14–19, 1978
13. Cooley DA, Norman JC: Techniques in Cardiac Surgery. Houston, Texas Medical Press, 1975
14. Crawley IS, Morris DC, Silverman BD: Clinical recognition and medical management of rheumatic heart disease and other acquired valvular disease. Valvular heart disease. In Hurst JW, Logue RB, Schlant RC et al (eds): The Heart, 4th ed, pp 992–1067. New York, McGraw-Hill, 1978
15. Eliot RS, Edwards JE: Pathology of rheumatic fever and chronic valvular disease. In Hurst JW, Logue RB, Schlant RC, et al (eds): The Heart, 4th ed, pp 952–965. New York, McGraw-Hill, 1978
16. Feigenbaum H: Echocardiography, 2nd ed, pp 107–118, 146–155, 161–164. Philadelphia, Lea & Febiger, 1976
17. Ford PJ: Valvular heart disease. Price SA, Wilson LM (eds): Pathophysiology, pp 357–371. New York, McGraw-Hill, 1978
18. Frank MJ, Alvarez-Mena SV: Cardiovascular Physical Diagnosis. Chicago, Year Book Medical Publishers, 1973

19. Friedberg CK: Diseases of the Heart, Vol III, 3rd ed, p 1133. Philadelphia, WB Saunders, 1966
20. Gottlieb R, Chung EK: Mitral valve prolapse-click syndrome. Chung EK (ed): Quick Reference to Cardiovascular Disease, pp 87–94. Philadelphia, JB Lippincott, 1977
21. Harshaw CW, Grossman W, Munro AB et al: Reduced systemic vascular resistance as therapy for severe mitral regurgitation of valvular origin. Ann Intern Med 88(3):312–316, 1975
22. Humphries JO: Valvular heart disease. Chung EK (ed): Quick Reference to Cardiovascular Disease, pp 69–86. Philadelphia, JB Lippincott, 1977
23. Kirklin JW, Karp RB: Surgical treatment of acquired valvular disease. Hurst JW, Logue RB, Schlant RC et al (eds): The Heart, 3rd ed, pp 971–984. New York, McGraw-Hill, 1974
24. Kirklin JW, Karp RB: Surgical treatment of acquired valvular heart disease. Hurst, JW, Logue, RB, Schlant, RC et al (eds): The Heart, 4th ed, pp 1081–1093. New York, McGraw-Hill, 1978
25. Miller RR, Vismara LA, DeMaria AN et al: Afterload reduction therapy with nitroprusside in severe aortic regurgitation: Improved cardiac performance and reduced regurgitant volume. Am J Cardiol 38(5):564–567, 1976
26. Netter FH: The Ciba Collection of Medical Illustrations, Vol 5. In Yonkman FF (ed): Heart, p 192. Summit, NJ, CIBA, 1969
27. Palank EA: Vasodilation therapy: Its role in treatment of acute left ventricular failure and mitral regurgitation. Military Medicine 142(6):472–474, 1977
28. Pluth JR, McGoon DC: Current status of heart valve replacement. Mod Concepts Cardiovasc Dis 43(1):65–70, 1974
29. Schlant RC: Altered cardiovascular function of congenital heart disease. Hurst JW, Logue RB, Schlant RC et al (eds): The Heart, 4th ed, pp 813–830. New York, McGraw-Hill, 1978
30. Schlant RC: Altered cardiovascular function of rheumatic heart disease and other acquired valvular disease. Hurst JW, Logue RB, Schlant RC et al (eds): The Heart, 4th ed, pp 965–981. New York, McGraw-Hill, 1978
31. Shaffer AB: Congenital heart disease. In Silber EN, Katz LN (eds): Heart Disease, pp 565–696. New York, Macmillan, 1975
32. Shaffer AB, Silber EN: Rheumatic fever and rheumatic heart disease. Silber EN, Katz LN (eds): Heart Disease, pp 697–758. New York, Macmillan, 1975
33. Shrivastava S, Guthrie RB, Edwards JE: Prolapse of the mitral valve. Mod Concepts Cardiovasc Dis 46(12):57–71, 1977
34. Spagnulo M, Kloth H, Taranta A et al: Natural history of aortic regurgitation. Circulation 44(3):368–380, 1971
35. Winkle RA, Lopes MG, Popp RL et al: Life threatening arrhythmias in the mitral valve prolapse syndrome. Am J Med 60(7):961–967, 1976
36. Zuhdi N: The porcine aortic valve prosthesis: A significant alternative. Ann Thorac Surg 21(6):573–575, 1976

ADDITIONAL READING

Ahmand R, Manohitharajah SM, Deverall PB: Chronic hemolysis following mitral valve replacement. A comparative study of the Björk–Shiley, composite-seat Starr–Edwards, and frame-mounted aortic homograft valves. J Thorac Cardiovasc Surgery 71(2):212–217, 1976
Allard JR, Fraser G, Dobell ARC: Sudden hemolysis indicating prosthetic valve dysfunction. Can J Surg 19(3):272–273, 1976
Austen WG, Hutter A: Acquired mitral and tricuspid valvular disease. In Sabiston DC (ed): Davis-Christopher Textbook of Surgery, 10th ed, pp 2050–2074. Philadelphia, WB Saunders, 1972
Barrett-Boyes BG, Roche AHG, Whitlock RML: Six year review of freehand aortic valve replacement using antibiotic sterilized homograft valves. Circulation 55(2):353–361, 1977
Harris FA, DeMaria AN, Amsterdam EA: Exercise testing in patients with valvular heart disease. Amsterdam EA, Wilmore JH, DeMaria AN (eds): Exercise in Cardiovascular Health and Disease, pp 234–244. New York, Yorke Medical Books, 1977
Hohn AR, VanPraagh S, Moore AAD et al: Aortic stenosis. Circulation (Suppl 3) 31–32:III 4–12, 1965
Hurst JW, Logue RB, Schlant RC, et al (eds): The Heart, 4th ed. New York, McGraw-Hill, 1978
Katholi RE, Nolan SP, McQuire LB: Living with prosthetic heart valves. Am Heart J 92(2): 162–167, 1976
Kirklin JW, Pacifico AD: Surgery for acquired valvular disease, Part 1. N Engl J Med 288(3):133–140, 1973
Kirklin JW, Pacifico AD: Surgery for acquired valvular disease, Part 2. N Engl J Med 288(4):194–198, 1973
Muller WH Jr, Nolan SP: Acquired disorders of the aortic valve. Sabiston DC (ed): Davis-Christopher Textbook of Surgery, 10th ed, pp 2042–2049. Philadelphia, WB Saunders, 1972
Nitter-Hauge S: Haemolysis after mitral valve replacement with Björk–Shiley and Lillehei–Kaster disc valve prosthesis. Br Heart J 38(9):977–980, 1976
Peterson KL, Tsuji IJ: Myocardial adaptations in aortic valve disease. West J Med 126(6):461–463, 1977
Pine M: Homograft and prosthetic aortic valve replacement: A comparative study. Circulation (Suppl 3) 54:84–89, 1976
Pipkin RD, Buch WS, Fogarty TJ: Evaluation of aortic valve replacement with a porcine xenograft with long-term anticoagulation. J Thorac Cardiovasc Surg 71(2):179–186, 1976
Pluth JR, Broadbent JC, Barnhorst DA et al: Aortic and mitral valve replacement with cloth-covered Braunwald-Cutter prosthesis. A 3 year follow-up. Ann Thorac Surg 20(3):239–248, 1975
Rasmassen K, Anderson A, Myhre E et al: Hemolysis during acute exercise in patients with aortic ball valve prosthesis. Acta Med Scand 188(4):281–286, 1970
Rhodes GR, McIntosh CL: Evaluation of hemolysis after replacement of A–V valves with porcine xenograft (Hancock) valves. J Thorac Cardiovasc Surg 73(2):312–315, 1977
Roberts DL, DeWeese JA, Mahoney EB et al: Long-term survival following aortic valve replacement. Am Heart J 91(3):311–317, 1976
Santinga JT, Batsakis JT, Flora JD et al: Hemolysis in the aortic prosthetic valve. Chest 69(1):56–61, 1976
Schlant RC, Nutter DO: Heart failure in valvular disease. Medicine 50(5):421–451, 1971
Shappell SD, Marshall CE, Brown RE et al: Sudden death and the familial occurrence of mid-systolic click, late systolic murmur syndrome. Circulation 48(5):1128–1134, 1973
Smith HJ: The natural history of rheumatic aortic regurgitation and indications for surgery. Br Heart J 38(2):147–154, 1976
Starr A, Herr RH, Wood JA: Mitral replacement. Review of six years' experience. J Thorac Cardiovasc Surg 54(3):333–358, 1967
Trenouth RS, Phelps NC, Neill WA: Determinants of left ventricular hypertrophy and oxygen supply in chronic aortic valve disease. Circulation 53(4):644–650, 1976
Wanderman KL, Dvilansky A, Yoran C et al: Hemolysis in Starr–Edwards cloth-covered mitral valve prosthesis. Am Heart J 90(3):405–406, 1975
Which Prosthetic Valve? Lancet i:619–620, 1976

49

Cardiomyopathies
GENE TROBAUGH, M.D.

A cardiomyopathy is a heart muscle abnormality characterized by (a.) ventricular dilatation; (b.) wall thickening out of proportion to physical conditioning; (c.) focal or global reduction in contractility; or (d.) electrocardiographic conduction disturbances.

The cardiomyopathies are difficult to classify because both the etiology and pathophysiology are unknown or poorly understood. About 20% of individuals with abnormal ventricular function have a clinical setting that suggests a cardiomyopathy. Table 49-1 outlines the major cardiomyopathies. About half of these patients have dilated ventricles associated with alcohol, the peripartum period, viral myocarditis, or conditions of unknown etiologies. The other half have a hypertrophic myocardiopathy characterized by a thick-walled left ventricle which has a small-to-normal cavity with increased contractility.

In addition, other uncommon conditions cause cardiomyopathies (Table 49-2). Cardiomyopathies associated with these diseases can be present with a combination of dilatation, electrocardiographic conduction disturbances, or evidence for constriction-simulating constrictive pericarditis. Ischemic heart disease or rheumatic heart disease can mimic many of these conditions; therefore, evidence for these etiologies must be sought. They account for approximately 60% and 20% of patients with abnormal ventricular function, respectively.

In addition, a classical description of angina or infarction (for example, substernal chest pain radiating to the arm or jaw) may not necessarily be caused by coronary artery disease (CAD). Viral infections have been documented to produce a similar clinical pattern, and there may be other etiologies as well. The thickened mitral leaflets associated with rheumatic heart disease can also be produced by viral infections. These common diagnoses need, therefore, to be made thoughtfully.

CARDIOMYOPATHIES CAUSING DILATATION OF THE VENTRICLES

Alcoholic Cardiomyopathy

Alcohol appears to have a direct toxic effect on the heart, reducing its ability to contract. The individual with a cardiomyopathy associated with alcohol intake may be difficult to recognize, particularly in the early stages, because the clinical manifestations of congestive heart failure may not be present. In a group of nine patients with a history of significant alcohol consumption, normal electrocardiograms, and normal cardiothoracic ratios on chest x-rays, Asokan and colleagues found that the percentage of blood ejected with each beat (ejection fraction) was typically reduced, ranging from 36%–53% (mean value of 46%, lower limit of normal = 50%).[3] One patient also had an abnormally high end-diastolic volume index (140 ml/M^2, upper limit of normal = 100 ml/M^2) associated with an ejection fraction of 34% in spite of a normal chest x-ray (cardiothoracic ratio of 0.46). The cardiothoracic ratio, however, gives a poor estimate of end-diastolic volume (r = .36 from a consecutive series of 42 patients from our hospital). Asokan et al also noted that the contractility index of their patients was approximately half the normal value. One of the important messages that can be derived from their study is the significance of careful

TABLE 49-1 A CLASSIFICATION OF THE COMMON CARDIOMYOPATHIES

A.	**Cardiomyopathies causing dilatation**
	Associated with alcohol (not necessarily "alcoholic")
	Peripartum
	Viral (also mimics "rheumatic" disease)
	Unknown etiologies
B.	**Hypertrophic cardiomyopathies**
	Obstructive
	Nonobstructive

TABLE 49-2 OUTLINE OF THE LESS COMMON CARDIOMYOPATHIES

Endocrine: Thyrotoxicosis, carcinoid, diabetes (?), pheochromocytoma

Neuromuscular: Duchenne's pseudohypertrophic dystrophy, limb-girdle dystrophy, facioscapulohumeral dystrophy, Friedreich's ataxia, dystrophia myotonica

Unknown etiology: Sarcoid

Nutritional: Beri-beri (thiamine deficiency)

Toxic: Cobalt, anthracyclines

Obliterative: Endomyocardial fibrosis, Loeffler's eosinophilic disorder

Infective: Chagas' disease (trypanosomiasis), schistosomiasis

Infiltrative (restrictive): Amyloid

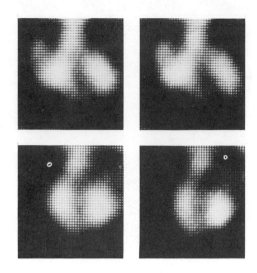

Fig. 49-1. Radionuclide ventriculogram showing enlargement and poor contractility of both ventricles.

review of the patient's clinical status by a physician or nurse who has taken the time to differentiate features of minimal heart failure (slight decrease in exercise tolerance, or slight increase in frequency of premature ventricular contraction, or duration in a rapid or an irregular cardiac rate associated with drinking. Patients who have been drinking heavily frequently may have increased atrial or ventricular ectopy, including ventricular tachycardia.

Arrhythmias may be noted at any stage. Even social drinkers can experience an increase in premature ventricular contractions or the onset of atrial fibrillation. Patients with a history of paroxysmal atrial tachycardia may notice an increase in frequency of premature ventricular contraction, or duration in a rapid or an irregular cardiac rate associated with drinking. Patients who have been drinking heavily frequently may have increased atrial or ventricular ectopy, including ventricular tachycardia.

In the later stages, the heart dilates and myocardial contractility is reduced. There is no satisfactory substitute for abstinence from further intake of alcohol. In those individuals whose disease has progressed to overt heart failure, treatment with conventional measures (digitalis, diuretics) has not been satisfactory without total abstinence from alcohol. Patients in overt heart failure should be anticoagulated because of a risk of emboli (both pulmonary and systemic). Overt heart failure is biventricular; both ventricles are enlarged and contract poorly. Figure 49-1 demonstrates the minimal change in size from diastole to systole for both the left and right ventricles. The dilatation and poor contractility demonstrated on this radionuclide ventriculogram are nonspecific and would also have been found for any of the dilated cardiomyopathies. Some investigators have evaluated the role of prolonged bedrest (up to a year or more) in a hospital and have generally noted a reduction in heart size.[19] In this setting, the consumption of alcohol is also minimized or eliminated. After resumption of their usual activities outside of the supervised setting,

their hearts typically enlarge again, associated with a progressive downhill course.

At autopsy, the heart is found to be dilated. The nonspecific pathologic findings in the myocardial wall include areas of patchy fibrosis and all degrees of muscle fiber degeneration mixed with other muscle fibers that are hypertrophied.[6] The structural changes noted by electron microscopy, although still nonspecific, are widespread throughout the myocardium. Extensive mitochondrial degeneration is noted. Since these structures are the site of the biochemical oxidative (energy producing) pathways, this disruption of energy utilization probably contributes to the clinical findings.

A direct myocardial toxicity of alcohol appears likely; but because of the cardiomyopathy which was caused by the addition of cobalt to beer in the mid-1960s to produce a better "head," it is possible that additional constituents also play a role.[2] The amount of alcohol required to reduce contractility or to produce left ventricular dilitation is uncertain, and some individuals may be much more sensitive than others. Individuals showing a predilection for cardiac damage may be a separate group from those who develop liver damage.[6]

Peripartum Cardiomyopathy

Peripartum cardiomyopathy is a complication of pregnancy, manifesting itself in approximately 1.2 patients per 10,000 women.[9] Women over 30, those who are delivering twins, and those who are manifesting toxemia are at increased risk. Patients are at risk during the last month of pregnancy (7%) and during the first five months post-partum (93% of cases).

All patients initially have signs of left heart failure, typically with moderate respiratory distress and a gallop rhythm.[9] Since both ventricular chambers are typically dilated, both mitral and tricuspid regurgitation may be present. Right heart failure is also present in about 50% of the women, as indicated by peripheral edema and right upper abdominal discomfort from an enlarged, congested liver. As with other dilated cardiomyopathies, emboli (both pulmonary and systemic) frequently occur and may lead to chest pain that may suggest ischemic heart disease.

The chest x-ray can be used to evaluate the course of recovery and the risk of having a subsequent pregnancy.[9] The heart size returns to normal in approximately 50% of the patients within 6 months. Further, functional status generally returns to New York Heart Association functional class I (in approximately two-thirds of patients) or to functional class II (see Table 14-1 for an explanation of the functional classes). Of eight patients who had 21 pregnancies, only two patients in this group manifested a temporary deterioration during three pregnancies. There was no permanent deterioration and there were no deaths due to peripartum cardiomyopathy in this group. In those patients whose cardiomegaly lasted longer than 6 months, however, a subsequent pregnancy was associated with a 50% probability of death because of heart failure. In these remaining 10 patients, 8 died with manifestations of chronic congestive heart failure. The average duration of survival in these patients was 4.7 years.

In addition to treatment for congestive heart failure, all patients with cardiomegaly should be anticoagulated because of the risk of emboli. Patients with cardiomegaly should be aware of the risk of subsequent pregnancies.

The etiology of peripartum cardiomyopathy is unknown.[9] Pathologically, the deterioration of the heart cannot be distinguished from other dilated cardiomyopathies, showing variable degeneration of some muscle fibers along with hypertrophy of other fibers.

Viral Myocardiopathy

A myopericarditis of viral etiology is frequently regarded as a transient and benign infection. However, the viral etiology of a myocardiopathy may be more prevalent than is generally recognized and may account for many of the "unknowns" in Table 49-1. It is difficult to prove that an increase in viral antibody titers is related to acute myocardial injury, because of the frequency of "colds." The impression that viral-caused injury to the heart may be common comes from (1) animal studies involving mice and monkeys,[16] (2) pathologic studies using immunofluorescence,[5] and (3) case reports documenting the possibility of this type of involvement in man.[8,23]

In addition to causing temporary inflammation, it is now clear that viral infection, particularly from Coxsackie B5, may simulate either ischemic heart disease (dilatation of the left ventricle with focal contraction abnormalities) or the clinical spectrum of rheumatic heart disease. Desa'neto and co-workers recently documented a case of Coxsackie B5 viral myopericarditis that presented with chest pain characteristic of a myocardial infarction, subsequent typical enzyme changes and a pyrophosphate myocardial scan documenting a focal uptake in the infero-lateral wall.[10] The patient, whose coronary arteries were normal by cardiac catheterization, was subsequently documented as having a rise in Coxsackie serotype B5 antibody titers. Other patients with myocardial infarction following a viral type of upper respiratory infection have been reported.[8] Woods et al found that approximately 10% of 233 patients felt to have acute myocardial infarction by ECG Q waves and typical serum enzyme criteria also had significant increases in Coxsakie

B neutralizing antibody titers.[23] Other investigations have shown that valvular thickening and fusion of chordae tendinae, usually associated with rheumatic heart disease, can have a viral etiology.[5,7]

HYPERTROPHIC CARDIOMYOPATHY

In the patient with hypertrophic cardiomyopathy, the walls of the ventricle are thickened and myocardial contractility is increased. The overall heart size is normal or nearly normal. The hypercontractile state is manifested by an increase in the percentage of blood ejected with each beat (increased ejection fraction) as well as a greater percentage of the blood volume ejected earlier in systole.[12]

Patients are usually asymptomatic until the second decade of life or of the disease, although occasionally hypertrophic cardiomyopathy may be present in both infants and the elderly. In patients with ideopathic hypertrophic subaortic stenosis, approximately two-thirds have a left ventricular outflow tract obstruction, either at rest or one that can be provoked by certain drugs such as isoproterenol (hypertrophic obstructive cardiomyopathy). Other individuals do not have an outflow obstruction, either at rest or caused by provocation. This condition is called hypertrophic non-obstructive cardiomyopathy. The significance of a new or increased obstruction upon provocation is unknown.

From a clinical point of view, many features of the obstructive or nonobstructive hypertrophic cardiomyopathies are similar. The initial symptoms of both can be dyspnea, presyncope (dizziness), syncope, or even sudden cardiac death. Dyspnea is probably related to an elevated end-diastolic pressure, an adaptation which permits increased flow into a non-compliant, thick-walled left ventricle.[22] When the elevated end-diastolic pressure approaches the osmotic pressure of the blood, fluids are not as readily absorbed in capillary alveoli, leading to the sensation of dyspnea. Physical findings associated with the elevated left ventricular end-diastolic pressure and the strong atrial contraction needed to force blood into the noncompliant ventricle are a palpable presystolic tap and an audible fourth heart sound. If a left ventricular outflow tract obstruction is present, a murmur may be heard, and tends to be maximal near the apex. This location can make differentiation from the murmur of mitral regurgitation a clinical challenge. The murmur frequently increases during the Valsalva maneuver.

Patients with an outflow tract obstruction may also have mitral regurgitation, but it is generally mild, although occasionally moderate in severity. About 90% of the patients will have chest discomfort. In about half of these patients, the chest pain would be considered typical of angina, although only about 10%–15% have coincidental CAD. The basis for this chest pain is uncertain. Their peripheral arterial pulse may feel bounding because of the initial rapid ejection of blood from the heart. This feature should help separate these patients from those with fixed aortic stenosis. The peripheral pulse in patients with obstruction may also feel as though it has two components (bisferiens), which is related to a mid-systolic decrease in flow. This is generally felt to be related to an obstruction of the left ventricular outflow tract by the focal hypertrophy of the septum and perhaps also by the motion of the anterior leaflet of the mitral valve. See Fig. 20-9, which demonstrates this systolic anterior motion (SAM).

Prophylactic antibiotic therapy appears logical for patients with outflow tract obstruction because infective endocarditis does occur in a small proportion.[4] Pregnancy generally leads to a worsening of symptoms, a fact which may be related to the decreased peripheral arterial resistance.[15] There is generally no cause for termination of the pregnancy, however.

The clinical course of hypertrophic cardiomyopathy is quite variable. Many patients may remain relatively stable over a five-year period and a few may improve spontaneously. Many, however, have a slowly progressive deterioration with increased dyspnea during exertion.[1,12,13] Atrial arrhythmias are common and may be associated with any phase. They are particularly disturbing because of the importance of the atrial contribution to left ventricular filling. Atrial fibrillation can be catastrophic both because of the loss of the atrial "kick" and because of the tachycardia which further limits filling of the ventricle during diastole.

The average age of death is approximately 40, after 5–10 years of increasing symptoms. A particularly disturbing feature of this disease is that sudden cardiac death (due to ventricular fibrillation with or without preceding atrial dysrhythmias) may be the presenting problem. In 26 patients who had hypertrophic cardiomyopathy presenting with sudden cardiac death reviewed by Maron *et al*, 23/26 (88%) were less than 25 years of age (range from 8 to 49 years old).[18] Males outnumbered females by 2.7 to 1. Half of them died suddenly following moderate to severe physical exertion. Although the ventricular septum was moderately to severely thickened (17 mm or more) and the electrocardiogram was abnormal (typically showing left ventricular hypertrophy) in all patients, these features would not identify these asymptomatic patients who subsequently died suddenly.

The slowly progressive deterioration may not be altered by therapy. Propranolol may decrease left ventricular stiffness and does reduce the heart rate, both at rest and during exercise, permitting a greater time for ventricular filling. Lower doses of propranolol may not be sufficient. A reasonable starting dose is 40 mg., 4 times a day, which could be progressively increased until the resting pulse is 50–60 bpm. Although the symptom of dyspnea is frequently associated with congestive failure, the mechanism for dyspnea in this condition is typically improved by the administration of propranolol. Some patients may also have arrhythmias in spite of propranolol therapy. Although they are typically atrial, aggressive treatment is important. A good initial choice would be to prescribe quinidine as well. There is theoretical and some clinical justification for treatment with verapamil.[14,20,21] The hypercontractile state of the hypertrophic cardiomyopathies may be related in some way to calcium metabolism, and patients frequently feel better taking either verapamil or a placebo than while taking propranolol, because of fatigue. Following administration of verapamil, the heart rate is somewhat decreased (about 10 beats/minute). The PR interval measured from an ECG is usually prolonged relative to pretreatment levels and may lead to a reversible first-degree or even second-degree heart block. The systolic pressure is frequently reduced, some-

times dramatically, and may be associated with increased chest pain. Measures which increase contractility or reduce ventricular volume, such as digitalis or diuretic administration, may increase the outflow obstruction and should therefore be avoided.

Surgical removal of the focal hypertrophy in the septum typically leads to subjective patient improvement (75%), and may be of value if medical therapy has not been satisfactory.[17] The outflow gradient is reduced or abolished, but the elevated end diastolic pressure generally does not change. If mitral regurgitation was present, it usually resolves. There is no convincing evidence that the risk of sudden death is reduced. Patients would need to be treated medically for dyspnea or arrhythmias.

The etiology of hypertrophic cardiomyopathy is not known with any certainty. A familial (non-sex-linked autosomal dominant) form of inheritance has been recognized in about a third of these patients and may be associated with an increased frequency of sudden cardiac death. The most striking feature at the time of autopsy is not only the marked ventricular hypertrophy, frequently involving both ventricles but also, particularly, focal hypertrophy high in the ventricular septum. Because this septal dimension is typically greater than the free-wall thickness, some leading investigators call this disease "Asymmetric Septal Hypertrophy". Examination of the myocardial fibers, particularly from the hypertrophied septal region, shows a striking disarray in orientation. It is not established whether this disarray is a primary heart disease or secondary to some other problem.

Coronary artery stenosis demonstrated by coronary arteriography documents the presence of coronary artery disease, but there is no single test that defines the presence of alcoholic or peripartum cardiomyopathy. These cardiomyopathies, therefore, must be diagnoses of exclusion. The association of congestive heart failure in an alcoholic is not adequate to establish that alcohol caused the heart failure. The etiology for congestive heart failure in the alcoholic may still be ischemic heart disease, which may not have been obvious, particularly if anginal symptoms have been absent. Also, peripartum cardiomyopathy will be immediately considered when a young woman who has delivered a baby subsequently develops congestive heart failure. Other possible etiologies must also be considered, however, such as mitral valvular disease, which may not have been recognized previously.

During an acute episode, the diagnosis of viral myocarditis can be strongly supported by increasing viral antibody titers. At a later time, however, evaluating the etiology of focal contraction abnormalities observed with contrast or radionuclide angiography can be difficult. Focal contraction abnormalities are typically caused by prior myocardial infarction due to coronary artery disease. Other etiologies are usually not considered. Mitral valvular thickening noted echocardiographically is accepted as convincing evidence for rheumatic heart disease, even in the absence of a history for the acute episode. An unknown proportion of these patients have actually had viral myocarditis.

The person with no symptoms poses the greatest problem in the early recognition of both hypertrophic and alcoholic cardiomyopathies. A family history of sudden death in young individuals should lead to an evaluation for hypertrophic cardiomyopathy. Detection of a murmur is frequently the first indication in those who have outflow obstruction. A specific question about alcohol consumption can help avoid missing this condition at an early stage. Teaching asymptomatic patients about potentially life-threatening diseases which may need a change in life style is both important and challenging.[11]

In brief, asymptomatic individuals may have an important cardiomyopathy, and patients known to have a heart problem may be given common diagnoses incorrectly.

REFERENCES

1. Adelman AG, Wigle ED, Ranganathan N et al: The clinical course in muscular subaortic stenosis: A retrospective and prospective study of 60 human dynamically proven cases. Ann Intern Med 77:515–525, 1972
2. Alexander CS: Cobalt—Beer cardiomyopathy: A clinical and pathological study of twenty-eight cases. Am J Med 53:395–417, 1972
3. Asokan SK, Frank MJ, Witham AC: Cardiomyopathy without cardiomegaly in alcoholics. Am. Heart J 84:13–18, 1972
4. Braunwald E: Wolstenholne GEW, O'Connor M (eds): Natural history of idiopathic hypertrophic subaortic stenosis. In Hypertrophic Obstructive Cardiomyopathy, pp 30–39. Ciba Foundation Study Group 37, London, J & A Churchill, 1971
5. Burch GE, Sun SC, Colcolough HL et al: Coxsackie B viral myocarditis and valvulitis identified in routine autopsy specimens by immunofluorescent techniques. Am Heart J 74:13–23, 1967
6. Burch GE, Depasquale NP: Alcoholic cardiomyopathy. Am J Cardiol 23:723–731, 1969
7. Burch GE, Gilcs TD, Colcolouch HL: Pathogenesis of "rheumatic" heart disease: Critique and theory. Am Heart J 80:556–561, 1970
8. Burch GE, Shewey LL: Viral coronary arteritis and myocardial infarction. Am Heart J 92:11–14, 1976
9. Demakis JG, Rahimtoola SH: Peripartum cardiomyopathy. Circulation 44:964–968, 1971
10. Desa'neto A, Bullington JD, Bullington RH et al: Coxsackie B5 heart disease: Demonstration of inferiolateral wall myocardial necrosis. Am J Med 68:295–298, 1980
11. Dracup KA: Unraveling the mysteries of cardiomyopathy. Nursing 79. 9:84–87, 1979
12. Frank MJ, Abdulla AM, Canedo MI et al: Long-term medical management of hypertrophic obstructive cardiomyopathy. Am J Cardiol 42:993–1001, 1978
13. Frank S, Braunwald E: Idiopathic hypertrophic subaortic stenosis: Clinical analysis of 126 patients with emphasis on the natural history. Circulation 37:759–788, 1968
14. Kaltenbach M, Hopf R, Kober G et al: Treatment of hypertrophic obstructive cardiomyopathy with verapamil. Br Heart J 42:35–42, 1979
15. Kolibash AJ, Ruiz DE, Lewis RP: Idiopathic hypertrophic subaortic stenosis in pregnancy. Ann Intern Med 82:791–794, 1975
16. Lerner AM, Wilson FM, Reyes MP: Enteroviruses and the heart (with special emphasis of coxsackieviruses, group B, Types 1–5). I. Epidemiological and experimental studies. Mod Concepts Cardiovasc Dis 44:7–10, 1975
17. Maron BJ, Merrill WH, Freier PA et al: Long-term clinical course and symptomatic status of patients after operation for hypertrophic subaortic stenosis. Circulation 57:1205–1213, 1978
18. Maron BJ, Roberts WC, Edwards JE et al: Sudden death in patients with hypertrophic cardiomyopathy: Characterization of 26 patients without functional limitation. Am J Cardiol 41:803–810, 1978
19. McDonald CD, Burch GE, Walsh JJ: Alcoholic cardiomyopathy managed with prolonged bed rest. Ann Intern Med 74:681–691, 1971
20. Rosing DR, Kent KM, Borer JS et al: Verapamil therapy: A new approach to the pharmacologic treatment of hypertrophic cardiomyopathy. I. Hemodynamic effects. Circulation 60:1201–1207, 1979
21. Rosing DR, Kent KM, Maron BJ et al: Verapamil therapy: A new approach to to the pharmacologic treatment of hypertrophic cardiomyopathy. II. Effects on exercise capacity and symptomatic status. Circulation 60:1208–1213, 1979
22. Sutton MG, Tajik AJ, Gibson DG et al: Echocardiographic assessment of left ventricular filling and septal and posterior wall dynamics in idiopathic hypertrophic subaortic stenosis. Circulation 57:512–520, 1978
23. Woods JD, Nimmo MJ, Makay-Scollay EM: Acute transmural myocardial infarction associated with active Coxsackie virus B infection. Am Heart J 89:283–287, 1975

50

Infective Endocarditis

DIANNE J. CHRISTOPHERSON R.N., M.N.

and

ERIKA SEIBERLER SIVARAJAN, R.N., M.A.

Infective endocarditis is a bacterial, fungal, or rickettsial infection of the valves or endocardium usually occurring in a heart already damaged by congenital or acquired heart disease. The incidence of the disease is relatively rare, and it occurs more frequently in men than in women. The mean age of onset of the disease is increasing in relation to the incidence of the diseases predisposing to endocarditis.[4,8,13] The predisposing factors, symptoms and signs, and complications of endocarditis all vary according to the site of cardiac involvement (that is, right-sided versus left-sided lesions).

PATHOPHYSIOLOGY

Predisposing Causes

A combined list of the predisposing causes of endocarditis is given in Table 50-1. Frequent causes of endocarditis affecting the right side of the heart are parenteral drug abuse,[14] the insertion of intravenous catheters used for hyperalimentation, dialysis shunts, and cardiac pacemakers.[3] The predisposing factors associated with left-sided endocarditis are rheumatic and congenital heart disease.[3] About half of the patients who develop the disease have a history of rheumatic fever, but this percentage is declining because the incidence of rheumatic fever is declining. Patients who have cardiac surgery or who have foreign bodies permanently placed in their cardiovascular systems, for example, prosthetic heart valves, form an important subgroup. The congenital lesions most frequently associated with endocarditis are ventricular septal defects and bicuspic

aortic valves. Despite these numerous known predisposing factors of endocarditis, no underlying cardiac lesion can be found in 20%–40% of the cases.[13]

Etiology

The organisms causing endocarditis vary with the predisposing factor and with the patient population. Staphylococcus and streptococcus are the two most common organisms causing bacterial endocarditis. Staphylococcus bacteremias frequently occur with parenteral drug abuse and may also occur following cardiac surgery. Streptococcus bacteremias occur more commonly after dental work or upper respiratory procedures. Candida albicans and Aspergillis are the usual organisms causing fungal endocarditis.[3,18]

Mechanisms

Introduction of the offending organism into the blood stream can occur not only after a major traumatic procedure, such as heart surgery, but also from injury to mucous membranes after minor procedures. Bacteremia can occur from damage to gums after toothbrushing, use of water pressure cleaning devices in the mouth, after bronchoscopy, tonsillectomy, sigmoidoscopy, after transurethral resections or urinary catheterizations.[6] Only in a minority of patients, however, can the initiating incident for endocarditis be identified.

Prosthetic Valve Endocarditis

Endocarditis occurs 2–3 times more commonly after valve replacement using prosthetic valves than after other types

TABLE 50-1 CONDITIONS PREDISPOSING TO ENDOCARDITIS

Congenital heart disease
Rheumatic heart disease
Cardiac surgery
Parenteral drug abuse
Intravascular foreign bodies such as:
  Intravenous catheters
  Dialysis shunts
  Hyperalimentation catheters
  Pacemakers

of heart surgery.[5,16] Prosthetic valve endocarditis is classified by onset of symptoms into early-onset endocarditis with the infection occurring in the perioperative period, and late-onset (more than two months after surgery) due to a subsequent initiating event. Prolonged cardiopulmonary bypass, the intracardiac foreign body, and numerous invasive procedures in the immediate postoperative period predispose these patients to endocarditis.

Pathology

The characteristic pathologic feature of infective endocarditis is a vegetation growing on the leaflets of the valve or the endocardium.[1] These lesions are composed primarily of platelets.[3] Stress creates a site of damaged endothelium on the valve, to which platelets adhere. The inherent "stickiness" of the platelet, which serves so well in creating hemostasis at the site of a severed vessel, also leads to adherence of platelets at these sites of damaged endothelium.[3] Subsequent bacteremia may then lead to colonization of the platelet–fibrin mass and the establishment of an infection. The bacteria find a protective sanctuary in the platelet–fibrin vegetation, necessitating prolonged courses of antibiotic therapy.

The vegetations can be single or multiple, and vary in size and color.[1] They tend to occur where blood flows through a narrow orifice (for example, aortic stenosis) and usually grow on the low pressure side of a defect or injury (for example, in the aorta in cases of aortic stenosis). Both valves of the left side of the heart are involved more than those of the right. Of all lesions involving the valves, 37% involve the mitral valve, 27% involve the aortic valve, and 20% involve both valves.[1,16]

ASSESSMENT

Symptoms and Signs

Fever, splenomegaly, hematuria, petechiae, and cardiac murmurs are all common manifestations of infective endocarditis.[14] The fever course in endocarditis varies with the nature of the infection. In general, staphylococcus is associated with an acute fulminant infectious process and therefore causes temperature elevations, with spikes of higher temperature and shaking chills. Streptococcus usually produces a subacute infectious process with moderate temperature elevations (usually without chills), easy fatigability, splenomegaly, weight loss, anorexia, and night sweats.[7,14,16] Osler's nodes, petachiae, and emboli have been noted with both types. Osler's nodes are painful, red subcutaneous nodules that classically appear in the pads of the fingers.[16]

Other symptoms and signs associated with infective endocarditis are splinter hemorrhages in the nailbeds, clubbing of the nails and Roth's spots. Splinter hemorrhages of the nailbeds are single or multiple hemorrhages located in the distal one-third of the nail. The fingers may be clubbed in longstanding or prolonged endocarditis; however, underlying cyanotic congenital heart disease can be the cause. Roth's spots are retinal hemorrhages with a pale white center, located near the optic fundus.[16]

Cardiac Examination. Cardiac signs are related to the underlying cardiac disease and to the side of the heart involved. Cardiac failure may be present depending on the hemodynamic severity of the lesion. (See Chap. 27 for discussion of left-sided versus right-sided heart failure.) Tachycardia is common, often at a higher level than the patient's temperature would indicate, suggesting a compensatory mechanism for the cardiac failure. In left-sided endocarditis, the appearance of a new murmur (for example, systolic murmur of mitral insufficiency or early diastolic decrescendo murmur of aortic incompetence) in a person who has other symptoms of systemic infection is a cardinal sign of endocarditis.[16] If no murmur is present and other symptoms and signs indicate endocarditis, right-sided endocarditis should be suspected, and an assessment should be done with this in mind.[8]

Complications of Endocarditis

In addition to heart failure, other complications relate to embolization of parts of the vegetations to other organs with resultant infarctions. Some reports show that one-third of the patients diagnosed with endocarditis develop serious embolic complications. Right-sided endocarditis usually produces clots that travel to the lungs causing pulmonary infarction, which results in chest pain, and hemoptysis. These symptoms are difficult to distinguish from those of pneumonia. Left-sided emboli can travel to the brain, causing infarcts resulting in paralysis, sudden blindness, brain abscesses, or acute purulent meningitis. Emboli that move to the extremities usually provoke acute vascular insufficiency and pain. Emboli that move to the kidney produce hematuria, and emboli that move to the intestine cause acute abdominal pain with melena. Left-sided emboli can also cause myocardial or splenic infarction. The spleen is the most common site of embolic infarction in bacterial endocarditis. Splenic infarctions usually cause pain in the upper quadrant of the abdomen, which often radiates to the left shoulder.

Mycotic aneurysms are found in 10%–15% of endocarditis patients at autopsy.[7,16] These aneurysms are caused by direct bacterial invasion of the vessel wall, which leads to abscess formation and possible rupture of the vessel. They tend to occur at points of bifurcation in the arterial tree, most commonly in the cerebral artery (50%) and in the chest and abdomen (40%).[7,16]

Laboratory Values

The diagnosis of endocarditis is based primarily on positive culture of organisms present in the blood. The incidence of positive cultures is high (73%–93%) since the bacteremia of endocarditis is persistent.[2,7,15] Blood cultures in cases of fungal infection are, however, invariably negative. When unusual organisms are suspected, it is important to look specifically for fungi by using special culture techniques and for rickettsia by measuring antibody titers. The organisms grow as well from venous as from arterial specimens. The importance of using an aseptic technique for drawing the blood specimen is paramount, because contamination of the specimen at the time of venipuncture can cause erroneous results, may involve the patient in unnecessary treatment, and may also infect the patient.[7,8,14]

With endocarditis, few laboratory values appear consistently disrupted. A normochromic, normocytic anemia and an elevated sedimentation rate are the most consistent findings. The white blood count may be normal or may be elevated as high as 25,000 cells per cu mm. The differential white count may be normal or may show large numbers of immature granulocytes.

INTERVENTION

Medical Treatment

The plan for medical management of the patient with endocarditis consists of long-term parenteral administration of antibiotics against the causative organism. Guidelines for administration have been developed by the American Heart Association Committee on Prevention of Rheumatic Fever and Bacterial Endocarditis.[5,11,12] Treatment of the symptoms and signs associated with the underlying heart disease or heart failure is undertaken at the same time. The long duration of antibiotic therapy is important because the dense, avascular platelet–fibrin vegetation protects the microbes enmeshed within it from phagocytic cells and humoral agents. Parenteral administration of the antibiotics is considered essential in achieving effective concentrations of the drug in the serum. The concentration can be verified by assay. Valve replacement is recommended on the basis of the hemodynamic severity of the lesion produced by the endocarditis. Treatment of patients with infected prosthetic valves is more successful if the infected valve is replaced surgically and aggressive antibiotic therapy is maintained for 6–8 weeks after the replacement.[6,17]

Prognosis

Infective endocarditis has a 25%–35% mortality rate, even with treatment. Factors associated with a poor prognosis include involvement of the left side of the heart, especially the aortic valve; gram-negative bacteria and fungal infections; development of congestive heart failure (CHF) secondary to the incompetent valve, and endocarditis developing after replacement with a prosthetic valve.[7,15] The mortality rate for prosthetic valve endocarditis is significantly higher than with other forms of the disease (60%) because it is difficult to cure the infection without reoperating.[5,16]

Prophylaxis

For persons likely to contract endocarditis, the American Heart Association advocates use of antimicrobial therapy to prevent episodes of bacteremia before, during, and after invasive procedures; in most cases this includes parenteral antibiotics.[5] Procedures for which prophylaxis is recommended include dental curettage, because gingival bleeding may occur; surgical procedures or instrumentation of the upper respiratory tract, genitourinary tract or lower gastrointestinal tract. Procedures not requiring prophylaxis (unless the patient has a prosthetic heart valve) include normal vaginal delivery, upper gastrointestinal endoscopy, percutaneous liver biopsy, proctoscopy, barium enemas, insertion and removal of intrauterine devices (IUDs) and cardiac catheterizations. For the open heart surgery patient short-term antibiotic prophylaxis directed against staphylococcus is also recommended. Prophylactic administration of drugs for the prevention of rheumatic fever is ineffective in preventing endocarditis. For operative dental procedures the dosage is too small and the duration of prophylaxis too short; in the mouth the microorganisms will probably be resistant to penicillin.

Nursing Care

Nursing care of endocarditis may be considered in three areas:

1. Prevention of the disease through education of the population at risk
2. Prevention of the disease in the hospitalized population at risk
3. Care of the patient diagnosed as having endocarditis.

A nursing care plan for each of these patient situations is presented in Tables 50-2, 50-3, and 50-4.

Preventive Teaching

For the patient at risk, education is based on the premise that the individual with a clear understanding of the disease process will comply with therapy more readily and thus will be less likely to have a recurrence of the disease. It has been shown that the patients at highest risk have little awareness of the nature of their disease.[10] Teaching includes the parents of children with congenital heart disease, as well as adults at risk or diagnosed as having any predisposing heart disease. The teaching program should optimally begin in the pediatric cardiology clinic or outpatient setting at the time of the diagnosis of the primary heart lesion. From a public health perspective, aggressive follow-up of all streptococcal throat infections to ensure proper therapy is exceedingly important. This is aimed at reducing the number of cases of rheumatic fever, thus eliminating this disease as a predisposing factor of infective endocarditis.

A standard teaching plan for prevention of infective endocarditis should include cardiac anatomy and physiology,

(Text continues on page 662)

TABLE 50-2 NURSING CARE PLAN FOR PATIENT AT RISK FOR DEVELOPING ENDOCARDITIS

Potential Patient Problems	Nursing Goals	Nursing Actions	Rationale	Outcome Evaluation
Lack of knowledge about endocarditis among the population at risk	To instruct the patients at risk (or their parents) about the disease	Develop a comprehensive program for teaching about endocarditis, using basic written information, informal teaching settings, multiple small classes, and much reinforcement of the information	Providing information about the disease process using principles of adult education	
		Content should include knowledge of:		The patients (or their parents) will be able to describe:
		disease process; predisposing causes; indications for prophylactic antibiotic therapy;	Alerting medical and dental personnel to the need for proper prophylactic antibiotic therapy when needed	the nature of the disease; the major predisposing causes; the prophylactic antibiotic therapy and when it should be started.
		importance of understanding the difference between rheumatic fever and prophylaxis against endocarditis;	Recognizing the critical difference between them in duration and dosage	
		how to read a thermometer properly.	Detecting elevations in temperature promptly and seeking physician consultation when they are too high	The patients (or their parents) will: measure and record temperature accurately, and be aware that a spiking or a temperature above a given value requires physician consultation;
		importance of good daily oral hygiene, regular tooth brushing and flossing, avoiding the use of a water-pressure device;	Preventing endocarditis secondary to lesions of the gingiva	give evidence of knowing the importance of practicing good oral hygiene and making regular dental visits;
		importance of making known to dental and other health-care personnel the patient's history of congenital or rheumatic heart disease;		demonstrate that they know the reasons for keeping dental and medical personnel informed as to the course of the disease.
		importance of having emergency identification on the person at all times.	The American Heart Association has cards available for this identifying purpose for persons at risk. The use of emergency identifying cards saves lives.	The patients (or their parents) will demonstrate an awareness of the importance of wearing or carrying emergency identification at all times.
		Content for women in the childbearing years should include knowledge of:		
		Why intrauterine devices (IUDs) should be avoided	IUDs are a potential source of infection and provide an added risk for the patient with endocarditis.	The patients will demonstrate an understanding that IUDs are not a desirable form of contraception for a patient with heart disease.
		Why antibiotic therapy is no longer considered necessary for patients having a normal delivery	Antibiotics may be needed for more important reasons	The patients (or their parents) will demonstrate an awareness that normal vaginal deliveries do not require antibiotic prophylaxis.

TABLE 50-3   NURSING CARE PLAN FOR HOSPITALIZED PATIENT AT RISK FOR DEVELOPING ENDOCARDITIS

Potential Patient Problems	Nursing Goals	Nursing Actions	Rationale	Outcome Evaluation
Development of endocarditis in the hospitalized patient at risk	To prevent the hospitalized patient at risk from developing endocarditis by contracting nosocomial (hospital based) infections	Be aware of the population at risk: patients with a history of congenital or rheumatic heart disease; patients who have had cardiac surgery; parenteral drug abusers; patients with intravascular foreign bodies such as IV catheters, dialysis shunts, hyperalimentation catheters, or pacemakers.	Early detection and treatment of the disease may improve prognosis	Patients at risk remain free of endocarditis
		Graph temperature recordings daily; take temperature at least twice a day	Early detection of elevations and recognition of patterns	Vital signs are taken routinely, and charted with graphed temperatures
		Take vital signs accurately at least twice daily and note changes in cardiac auscultation, such as new or changed murmurs	A widened pulse pressure indicates increasing aortic incompetence. New or changed murmurs indicate a regurgitant heart valve.	Cardiac auscultation findings are charted routinely with vital signs and changes noted
		Observe basic general principles of asepsis and thorough handwashing when nursing the patient at risk	Handwashing is the simple most important infection control measure	Good handwashing technique is consistently practiced by all nursing personnel
		Maintain strict aseptic technique in the care and dressing changes of all intravascular catheters, pacemakers (wear mask, gown, gloves)	Airborne and contact organisms are prevented from entering sterile field	
		Develop protocols for aseptic technique such that, with change of the personnel, procedure is the same every day	Scientifically based protocol for procedures establish standards for nursing procedures, against which staff can be evaluated to ensure quality patient care.	Sterile technique is maintained during all dressing changes
		Plan staffing so that the procedure is performed by the same person, if possible, for continuity of observation	It is easier to note day to day changes if all personnel use the same techniques.	Same personnel do changes every day
		Develop policy for routine changes in peripheral intravenous sites	Prevent thrombophlebitis and allow the vein to be used more than once. Allows greater opportunity for isolation and growth of organisms.	Policies and procedures for consistent dressing changes are written and followed meticulously
		Recommended venipuncture technique for obtaining blood for cultures:		
		Prepare the skin with 2% iodine followed by 70% alcohol. Obtain at least three tubes of blood for culture, label them #1, #2, #3, according to the drawing order.	With the large numbers of bacteria residing on the skin, correct skin preparation to prevent contamination is crucial. If the organism is present in tube #1, skin contamination must be suspected. If present in all three, endocarditis is confirmed.	Aseptic technique is maintained throughout venipuncture for blood cultures
		Incubate the blood specimens in both aerobic and anaerobic media	Detection of both types of organisms	

TABLE 50-3 NURSING CARE PLAN FOR HOSPITALIZED PATIENT AT RISK FOR DEVELOPING ENDOCARDITIS (Cont.)

Potential Patient Problems	Nursing Goals	Nursing Actions	Rationale	Outcome Evaluation
		Monitor laboratory values: Watch for elevated white blood count, elevated sedimentation rates, and presence of normochromic, normocytic anemia	All indicate an inflammatory process and are signs of endocarditis	Laboratory values, symptoms and signs of embolization and the disease are assessed frequently and changes are noted in the chart
		Monitor the patient for: Malaise, weakness, easy fatiguability, and night sweats	All are indicative of a subacute infectious process. The patient may have these symptoms and signs on admission	
		Symptoms and signs of embolization: Cerebral: changes in level of consciousness, visual changes, blindness, headache Splenic: upper left abdominal pain radiating to the left shoulder Pulmonary: shortness of breath, chest pain with hemoptysis Renal: hematuria, reduced urine output, increased serum creatinine and blood urea nitrogen Cardiac: arrhythmias, complete heart block, pericarditis		

TABLE 50-4 NURSING CARE PLAN FOR PATIENT HOSPITALIZED WITH ENDOCARDITIS (SELECTED PROBLEMS)

Potential Patient Problems	Nursing Goals	Nursing Actions	Rationale	Outcome Evaluation
Difficulty maintaining effective antibiotic administration in the patient diagnosed as having infective endocarditis	To maintain muscle tissue and venous sites of entry in optimum condition for effective drug administration and patient comfort	Develop a chart for rotation of sites for intramuscular injections Maintain rotation schedule of intravenous site	Rotation of sites ensures that muscle is maintained in best condition for even drug absorption	Charts for intramuscular and intravenous injection made and used Muscle tissue and venous sites maintained in near-normal condition so that drug absorption is ensured
		Add small quantity of hydrocortisone to intravenous antibiotic and/or dilute the drug in a large quantity of diluent	Prevents thrombophlebitis and vein irritation: aids in conservation of veins	The patient's comfort is maintained at optimal level Intravenous sites are kept free of irritation from medications and from thrombophlebitis
Depression, social and financial problems associated with long hospitalization	To assist the patient to cope effectively with prolonged hospitalization	Foster the concept of primary nursing where possible, so that the patient benefits from long-term relationships with one or two staff members	This develops rapport between patient and nurse and communicates a sense of continuity and caring	Patient copes effectively with long hospitalization and remains optimistic about the outcome of the disease
		Encourage ventilation of feelings and concerns regarding hospitalization		Changes in the patient's mental outlook is noted in nursing notes and interventions are initiated if appropriate
		Assess the patient's anxiety, depression, and ability to solve social and financial problems and make use of their support systems		

(Table continues on page 662)

TABLE 50-4 NURSING CARE PLAN FOR PATIENT HOSPITALIZED WITH ENDOCARDITIS (SELECTED PROBLEMS) (Cont.)

Potential Patient Problems	Nursing Goals	Nursing Actions	Rationale	Outcome Evaluation
		Initiate referrals for occupational therapy and social services, as appropriate		Referrals are initiated, as appropriate
		Observe for side effects from long-term antibiotic therapy	To make early detection of side effects of antibiotics and to minimize complications from therapy	
		Monitor the patient for disturbances of balance, vertigo, and hearing loss	Ototoxicity and renal toxicity are both side effects of streptomycin and vancomycin. Hearing loss first occurs at the top and bottom of the hearing range, thus making the patient initially unaware of the loss	The patient is monitored for side effects of antibiotic therapy; prompt action is taken if symptoms and signs appear
		Obtain baseline audiograms before antibiotic therapy begins, and regularly throughout therapy		A baseline audiogram is obtained and evaluated for hearing loss before and during therapy.
		Monitor laboratory values for elevations in blood urea nitrogen and serum creatinine levels		Laboratory values are monitored and prompt action is taken if changes appear as described

predisposing factors, oral hygiene, birth control and pregnancy planning, information regarding recurrent symptoms, and knowledge of prophylaxis.[9] Cardiac anatomy and physiology can help the patient conceptualize the disease process and make it more graphic to him. The use of heart models, diagrams, and colored photographs will usually aid in his understanding. Identification of the valves or areas involved can be beneficial in individualizing a standard teaching plan. The long list of predisposing factors is best used when simplified and placed in written form to be kept as a reference by the patient. Generalized statements, such as a record of major dental work, all operations, any procedures for which a tube or object is placed inside the body, and any infections or lacerations for which antibiotic therapy was prescribed, should be included in this list.

The importance of good oral hygiene must be stressed. The patient must understand the importance of informing his dentist about his history of valvular or congenital heart disease. Recommended are regular dental visits every six months and regular brushing and flossing of the teeth, and avoiding the use of water-pressure cleaning devices because of the risk of bacteremia.

For women in the childbearing years, the patient's education should include facts concerning the use of IUDs. The IUD is not recommended, because it may provide a portal of entry for bacteria. Unless the patient has a prosthetic heart valve, the use of prophylactic antibiotics is usually not advised for normal vaginal deliveries.

A good understanding of the symptoms and signs of the disease will help ensure that the patient will seek prompt medical attention should they recur. Basic skills, such as reading a thermometer, should be taught and accuracy of the patient's skill verified. Individuals with a history of

rheumatic fever must be informed of the difference between prophylaxis for rheumatic fever and prophylaxis for endocarditis. Patients should be encouraged to carry an emergency medical identification card with them at all times. Wallet cards are available from the American Heart Association for this purpose.

Prevention in the Hospital

For the hospitalized patient, infection control is a primary nursing consideration which takes on added importance in the population exposed to the risk of developing endocarditis. Basic aseptic measures such as handwashing should be rigidly observed. The care of all intravascular catheters and devices must be meticulous and consistent to prevent them from becoming a source of infection. If temperature spikes occur, all intravascular catheters should be suspect and the sites of entry changed.

Patient Care

For the patient diagnosed as having infective endocarditis, frequent vital signs with graphed temperatures are indicated. Monitoring the blood pressure is important and a sudden widening between the systolic and diastolic pressure (pulse pressure) is important to note. A dramatic increase in pulse pressure may indicate a worsening of aortic regurgitation. Graphing temperatures makes peaks and patterns easier to detect. Frequent testing of the urine to detect occult hematuria is advised.

Once antimicrobial therapy has been instituted for the patient with endocarditis, maintenance of the sites for drug administration and observation for side-effects are important nursing concerns. The number of intramuscular and intravenous injections necessitates routine rotation of all parenteral sites. Assessment of the patient's hearing before starting therapy and throughout its course is advised to detect the presence of ototoxicity or any other side-effects of antimicrobial therapy. Renal toxicity can be assessed by monitoring the serum creatinine and the blood urea nitrogen.

The long duration of therapy necessitates an equally long hospitalization. The patient may develop feelings of depression and hopelessness about being out of the work force and away from his family, and financial and personal anxieties may surface. Occupational therapy can be beneficial as a diversion and can open up new opportunities for employment. Social services can assist in obtaining financial assistance and psychologic support for both the patient and the family. The patient with infective endocarditis who is of a different sociocultural background from that of the health care providers presents a particular challenge. For example, a former drug abuser may not be motivated to remain in the hospital for the full course of intravenous therapy. An approach that is sensitive to the needs and perception of the individual patient, while emphasizing the importance of therapy, is usually most productive in these situations.

In summary, infective endocarditis is a serious disease. Nursing care of the patient with infective endocarditis is a challenging and demanding task. Innovative and comprehensive care provided by the nurse contributes largely in assisting the patient to cope effectively with this potentially debilitating disease.

REFERENCES

1. Angrist A, Oka M, Nakao K: Vegetative endocarditis. Pathology Annual 2:155–212, 1967
2. Casey J, Miller M: Infective endocarditis: New diagnostic techniques. Am Heart J 96(1):123–127, 1978
3. Clawson CC: Role of platelets in the pathogenesis of endocarditis. In Kaplan E, Taranta A (eds): Infective Endocarditis, p 24. American Heart Association Monograph #52. Dallas, American Heart Association, 1977
4. Durack DT, Petersdorf RG: Changes in epidemiology of endocarditis. In Kaplan E, Taranta A (eds): Infective Endocarditis, p 3. American Heart Association Monograph #52. Dallas, American Heart Association, 1977
5. Committee on Prevention of Rheumatic Fever and Bacterial Endocarditis of the American Heart Association: Prevention of bacterial endocarditis. Circulation 56(1):139A–143A, 1977
6. Karchimer AW, Swartz MN: Infective endocarditis in patients with prosthetic heart valves. In Kaplan E, Taranta A (eds): Infective Endocarditis, p 58. American Heart Association Monograph #52. Dallas, American Heart Association, 1977
7. Kaye D: Infective Endocarditis. Baltimore, University Park Press, 1976
8. Lange M, Salaki J, Middleton J et al: Infective endocarditis in heroin addicts: Epidemiological observations and some unusual cases. Am Heart J 96(2):144–152, 1978
9. Mashak BJ: Patient education and prevention of endocarditis. Nurs Clin North Am 11(2):319–327, 1976
10. McGowan DS, Tuohy O: Dental treatment in patients with valvular heart disease. Br Med J 124:519–521, 1968
11. Miller M, Casey J: Infective endocarditis: Current therapy. Am Heart J 96(2):263–269, 1978
12. Pankey GA: The prevention and treatment of bacterial endocarditis. Am Heart J 98(1):102–118, 1979
13. Pazin G, Peterson KL, Griff FW et al: Determination of sites of infective endocarditis. Ann Intern Med 82:746–750, 1975
14. Pelletier LL, Petersdorf RG: Infective endocarditis. In Wintrobe MM, Thorn GW, Adams RD et al (eds): Harrison's Principles of Internal Medicine, 8th ed, p 797. New York, McGraw-Hill, 1977
15. Pelletier LL, Petersdorf RG: Infective endocarditis: A review of 125 cases from the University of Washington Hospitals 1963–1972. Medicine 56(4):287–313, 1977
16. Santoro J, Kaye D: Axioms on infective endocarditis. Hosp Med, February, 8–21, 1977
17. Wilson W, Haumin PM, Danielson GK et al: Prosthetic valve endocarditis. Ann Intern Med 82:751–756, 1975
18. Williams RC: Bacterial endocarditis: An analysis of immunopathology. In Kaplan E, Taranta A (eds): Infective Endocarditis, p 20. American Heart Association Monograph #52. Dallas, American Heart Association, 1977

51

Pulmonary Heart Disease

MARTHA TYLER, R.N., M.N.

The lungs, heart, and vascular system share a common physiologic goal—supplying the oxygen required for tissue metabolism and removing carbon dioxide, a waste product of metabolism. It is not surprising, therefore, that disease or dysfunction in one of the components of the system results in altered function or dysfunction in one or more of the other components. The effect of heart failure on the lung's ability to maintain normal gas exchange, particularly of oxygenation, is discussed in Chapter 27. This chapter describes the effect of dysfunction in the respiratory system on the pulmonary vascular bed and ultimately, the heart. The modern terminology for heart disease resulting from respiratory dysfunction is pulmonary heart disease (PHD). An older but still frequently used term for this condition is cor pulmonale.

DEFINITION

The accepted definition of pulmonary heart disease is:

An alteration in structure or function of the right ventricle resulting from disease affecting the structure or function of the lung or its vasculature, except when this alteration results from disease of the left side of the heart or congenital heart disease.[38]

This definition was the result of the deliberations of a committee of the World Health Organization which met in 1963. The definition was endorsed in 1970 by the Pulmonary Heart Disease Study Group of the Inter-Society Commission for Heart Disease Resources.[1] The possible changes in structure or function of the right ventricle (mentioned in the official definition) have been defined as "either hypertrophy or dilatation or failure or any combination detected clinically, radiologically, electrocardiographically, by cardiac catheterization, or by autopsy studies."[3]

In the clinical setting, PHD is often diagnosed only when signs of right ventricular failure, such as peripheral edema or distention of the jugular veins, are present. However, keeping the accepted definition in mind, it is obvious that PHD is often present long before the patient has overt signs of right heart failure. Since the cause of PHD is pulmonary artery hypertension, the increased use of the balloon-tipped flotation catheter and the availability of pulmonary artery pressure measurements (Chap. 21), should result in earlier and more accurate diagnosis and treatment of pulmonary heart disease.

NORMAL PULMONARY CIRCULATION

The arteries, capillaries, and veins of the lung form a low resistance system because there is very little muscular tissue in the arteries and arterioles of the lung. In addition, there is very little autonomic innervation in these vessels.[13] The result is a vascular bed that is capable, through recruitment and distention, of accepting large increases in cardiac output without an increase in intravascular pressure (see Chap. 5). Recruitment is the opening of previously closed capillaries. Distention is the dilation of already open capillaries. In the adult, the normal pulmonary artery pressure is 25 mm Hg systolic, 9 mm Hg diastolic, and 15 mm Hg mean. The upper limits of normal are 32 mm Hg systolic, 13 mm Hg diastolic, and 19 mm Hg mean.[40] During exercise, despite the accompanying large increases in cardiac output, pressures do not usually exceed 30 mm Hg systolic, 14 mm Hg diastolic, and 20 mm Hg mean.[12]

Normal and abnormal pulmonary arterial and left ventricular pressure contours are shown in Fig. 51-1. As revealed by the normal pressure contours in the left panel of the figure, when the lung and heart are normal the left ventricular end-diastolic pressure determines the pulmonary arterial diastolic pressure. In contrast to that of the systemic vascular system, the pulmonary arterial systolic pressure is due to volume distention of the pulmonary artery and is determined by the right ventricular stroke volume, the level of the diastolic pressure, and the compliance of the central pulmonary vessels.[15]

Pulmonary vascular resistance is determined by the pressure drop in the system from the pulmonary artery to the left atrium, and the cardiac output. Therefore, pulmonary vascular resistance equals input pressure minus outflow pressure divided by the blood flow. Substituting normal values (15 mm Hg minus 5 mm Hg divided by 6 l/min) the "usual" pulmonary vascular resistance is found to be 1.7 mm Hg/liter/minute, or approximately 100 dynes/sec/cm^{-5}.[36] The latter terms are those used most frequently by cardiologists, while the former are found more often in respiratory physiology texts.

PULMONARY HYPERTENSION

Pulmonary hypertension results when the normal determinants of vascular pressures in the lung are altered by disease or dysfunction. The three major causes of pulmonary hypertension are: (1) elevation of left atrial pressure; (2) massive increases in pulmonary blood flow; (3) an increase in pulmonary vascular resistance.

Increased left atrial pressure results in passive pulmonary hypertension. It is termed passive because it is secondary to congestion of the pulmonary veins due to failure of the left ventricle (Fig. 51-1, center panel, also Chap. 27).

Another cause of pulmonary hypertension, massive increases in pulmonary blood flow, occurs in congenital defects that result in left-to-right intracardiac shunts, such as most atrial and ventricular septal defects. With such defects, pulmonary artery pressures may equal or exceed systemic pressures.

The last and most common cause of pulmonary hypertension is increased pulmonary vascular resistance.[9] The pulmonary arterial pressure contours in increased pulmonary vascular resistance are illustrated on the right side of Fig. 51-1. Of the three causes of pulmonary hypertension listed, the first two are obviously due to diseases of structure and function of the *heart*. They are, therefore, by definition, eliminated as causes of pulmonary heart disease. Only increased pulmonary vascular resistance remains as a cause of pulmonary hypertension and, if changes in the structure or function of the right ventricle ensue, of pulmonary heart disease.

Increased Pulmonary Vascular Resistance

The mechanisms or causes of abnormally high pulmonary vascular resistance have been categorized as obstructive, obliterative, or vasoactive.[9]

An example of an obstructive mechanism is pulmonary embolism or thrombosis. Pulmonary vascular resistance increases when the vascular bed is obstructed by emboli. However, if the lung is normal, the emboli must be either massive or numerous and recurrent to cause pulmonary hypertension, because pulmonary artery pressures do not increase until approximately two-thirds of the lung vessels are obstructed. When underlying lung disease is present, this is a more important source of increased pulmonary vascular resistance.

Functional or anatomic obliteration of the pulmonary capillary bed also results in increased pulmonary vascular resistance. Included in this category are diffuse diseases causing arteritis of the pulmonary vessels, diseases which anatomically reduce the vascular bed, such as severe and far advanced emphysema, and rare pulmonary venous occlusive diseases.

Vasoactive causes of increased pulmonary vascular resistance include all substances or states known to

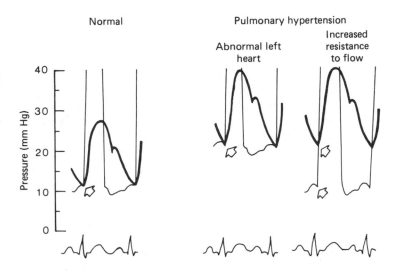

Fig. 51-1. Schematic representation of the relation between left ventricular (*thin line*) and pulmonary arterial (*thick line*) blood pressure contours. Peak left ventricular pressure lies off the diagram at this amplification. Under normal circumstances (*left*) end-diastolic pressure is identical at both sites (*single arrow*) and lies at the upper limit of normal values. In the presence of abnormal left heart function (*center panel*) left ventricular end-diastolic pressure is elevated above normal levels, and pulmonary arterial diastolic pressure rises passively to the same extent (*single arrow*). When pulmonary hypertension stems from abnormal structure or function of the pulmonary vessels (*right*) pressure in the pulmonary artery exceeds left ventricular pressure at the end of the diastole (*two arrows*). (Enson Y, Thomas HM III, Bosken CH, et al: Trans Assoc Am Phys 88:248–255, 1975)

have a *vasoconstrictive* effect on the precapillary pulmonary arterioles. The most important of these is alveolar hypoxia.[10,11,16,26,37] Others are increased hydrogen-ion concentration (usually due to hypercarbia), norepinephrine, and serotonin.[11,21,25] While there is very little smooth muscle in the pulmonary arteries, the vessels that have the most smooth muscle are in direct contact with the alveoli. Alveolar hypoxia and acidemia cause the pulmonary vessels to constrict by uncertain mechanisms. However, it has been shown that when the alveolar oxygen tension is low or the *p*H of blood perfusing the area falls, local arteriolar vasoconstriction results.[23] The vasoconstrictive response may be due to the release of vasoactive substances from mast cells, as a result of the direct effect of local hypoxia on the mast cell.[20] In 1974, Bergofsky reviewed other possible mechanisms of vasoconstriction and the status of research in this area.[2]

We have been discussing the effect of the vasoconstrictive response to alveolar hypoxia and acidemia in terms of its potential for increasing pulmonary vascular resistance and causing pulmonary artery hypertension. It should be recognized that ordinarily this is a beneficial response. For example, when areas of atelectasis or pulmonary consolidation cause localized hypoventilation and hypoxia, the resulting pulmonary artery vasoconstriction is also localized to the immediate area. Thus blood is directed from the hypoxic area to areas of the lung where alveolar ventilation is more normal, resulting overall in better matching of ventilation and perfusion, and subsequently in more efficient oxygenation and carbon dioxide excretion. However, when large areas of the lung are poorly ventilated, or when total alveolar ventilation is low (for example, in advanced obstructive lung diseases or diseases of the respiratory center or respiratory muscles) widespread hypoxic vasoconstriction results in a generalized increase in pulmonary vascular resistance, which in turn causes a marked increase in pulmonary artery pressure.

It is also important to remember that alterations of both structure and *function* of the respiratory system cause PHD. Therefore, diseases associated with PHD do not always directly involve the lung parenchyma or airways. For instance, dysfunction in the respiratory center or the respiratory muscles, or in the shape or mobility of the chest wall and diaphragm is associated with altered function of the lung, resulting in hypoxia, or alveolar hypoventilation, or both; this in turn leads to increased pulmonary vascular resistance, pulmonary hypertension and, ultimately, pulmonary heart disease.

Some examples of the wide variety of diseases associated with pulmonary heart disease can be seen in Table 51-1.

Anatomic Changes Due to Pulmonary Hypertension

Pulmonary Vessels. A sustained but modest increase in vascular resistance and pulmonary artery pressure results in medial hypertrophy of small pulmonary arteries. With higher elevations of resistance, intimal hyperplasia is seen. And, finally, when pulmonary hypertension is severe, intimal fibrosis occurs.[12] These changes are often seen in patients with diffuse interstitial lung disease.[13] They are seldom seen in patients with chronic obstructive pulmonary disease

---

TABLE 51-1 CAUSES OF PULMONARY HEART DISEASE

Chronic Obstructive Pulmonary Disease
Chronic bronchitis
Emphysema
Asthma

Other Abnormalities of Alveolar Ventilation
Kyphoscoliosis and other structural abnormalities of the thorax
Pleural disease
Neuromuscular disease
Alveolar hypoventilation associated with obesity
Abnormal ventilatory drive
Residence at high altitude
Airway obstruction due to hypertrophied tonsils and adenoids or prolapsed tongue (during sleep)

Pulmonary Vascular Obstruction or Disease
Systemic venous thrombosis or embolism
Idiopathic pulmonary thrombosis
Sickle cell anemia with pulmonary thrombosis
Malignant pulmonary emboli
Schistosomiasis

Infiltrative, Inflammatory, or Fibrotic Pulmonary Disease
Silicosis and other pneumoconioses
Tuberculosis
Sarcoidosis
Berylliosis
Idiopathic diffuse interstitial fibrosis
Collagen vascular disorders
Radiation damage
Idiopathic pulmonary hypertension

(Adapted from Behnke RH, Blount SG, Bristow JD et al: Circulation 41(A):17–23, 1970)

(COPD) because pulmonary hypertension is usually not sustained in the latter group.[22] If the patient has far advanced COPD with particularly low alveolar oxygen levels, medial hypertrophy with intimal proliferation may be seen. However, both medial hypertrophy and intimal proliferation can regress when the source(s) of pulmonary hypertension (usually alveolar hypoxia and increased hydrogen-ion concentration) are corrected. This is not true if intimal fibrosis has occurred, because it is a fixed anatomic change.

Right Ventricle. The speed with which pulmonary hypertension develops determines the nature of the response of the right ventricle (RV) to the hypertensive stress. With sustained and gradual worsening of gas exchange and slowly developing pulmonary hypertension, protein synthesis occurs and the right ventricle hypertrophies (or becomes hypertrophic).[27] However, when the increase in pulmonary artery pressure is sudden and severe, dilation of the right ventricle occurs immediately and is rapidly followed by failure. An example of this process can be seen in the patient with COPD who has a sudden worsening of gas exchange and respiratory failure, often due to infection. Rapid dilation of the right ventricle can occur; however, documentation of the dilated heart may be missed if initial treatment results in a prompt reversal of alveolar hypoxia and hypoventilation, because the right ventricular dilatation may have subsided before an electrocardiogram or chest radiograph can be obtained.

PULMONARY HEART DISEASE IN COPD

Chronic obstructive pulmonary disease is by far the most common cause of PHD. The incidence of PHD parallels COPD and is next only to coronary artery disease and hypertension among diseases of the heart in the population over 50 years.[14] The obstructive and obliterative pulmonary diseases listed earlier as possible causes of PHD have either been discussed elsewhere (for example, pulmonary emboli in Chap. 28), or are diseases or conditions of low incidence. The remainder of this chapter will deal with PHD as it will most frequently be encountered, a complication of chronic obstructive pulmonary disease.

Pathogenesis of PHD

The major mechanism of pulmonary heart disease in COPD is an increase in pulmonary artery pressure due to an increase in pulmonary vascular resistance. Pulmonary vascular resistance, in turn, is caused by the vasoconstrictive effects of generalized alveolar hypoxia and acidemia on the pulmonary arterioles. A secondary mechanism of PHD is also possible in COPD. Late in the course of COPD there may be sufficient loss of alveolar–capillary tissue to cause pulmonary hypertension on the basis of too much blood flow for the remaining pulmonary vascular bed. Pulmonary hypertension is fixed or irreversible in this case, but it must be stressed that significant anatomic reduction of lung tissue does not happen in all COPD patients, and when it does occur it is very late in the course of the disease. Therefore, patients with COPD may have repeated episodes of PHD due to the potentially reversible pulmonary hypertension associated with hypoxia and acidemia before (if ever) lung tissue destruction becomes a factor in the pathogenesis of PHD. This is important because therapy can potentially alter

the outcome of a functional (or physiologic) derangement, or alveolar hypoxia, but anatomic changes of the lung are not alterable. Figure 51-2 summarizes the mechanisms leading to PHD in the COPD patient.

Alveolar Hypoxia. The most frequent cause of alveolar hypoxia in COPD is multiple areas of poor ventilation, which also results in ventilation–perfusion ($\dot{V}/\dot{Q}$) mismatch.[14] The reduction in ventilation may be due to a variety of causes including retained secretions, hypertrophy and hyperplasia of bronchial mucous membranes, and bronchospasm. When perfusion continues to underventilated areas of the lung there is little, if any, gas exchange, and blood leaves these areas with essentially venous levels of oxygen and carbon dioxide. As mentioned before, blood is usually directed away from these areas by local vasoconstriction, but when the areas of poor ventilation are widespread, generalized vasoconstriction occurs throughout the lung, resulting in pulmonary hypertension. The outcome of the mismatch of ventilation and perfusion is arterial hypoxemia (and in certain situations, hypercarbia) because the blood perfusing normal areas of the lung is unable to make up for the desaturation in the blood coming from the poorly ventilated areas. During exacerbations of COPD, generalized alveolar hypoventilation (indicated by an elevated $PaCO_2$) and intrapulmonary shunting are additive mechanisms of alveolar hypoxia and acidemia.

Another factor in the genesis of PHD in COPD may be variations in respiratory drive. There is a wide variation in the ventilatory response to hypoxic and hypercarbic stimuli to respiration in the general population.[35] It is, therefore, possible that an abnormal response to hypoxemia or hypercarbia accounts for some of the variation in the levels of alveolar ventilation seen between patients with apparently equal amounts of obstruction to airflow.

In chronic alveolar hypoxia, muscularization of the precapillary pulmonary arterioles is seen. This appears to be

Fig. 51-2. The primary mechanism (*solid lines*) in the pathogenesis of pulmonary heart disease in chronic obstructive pulmonary disease is through the reversible effect of alveolar hypoxia and acidemia on pulmonary artery pressure. Late in the course (*dashed lines*) of COPD, particularly in patients with a significant component of emphysema, anatomic reduction of alveolar-capillary surface area can result in an additional, or rarely, single source of irreversible pulmonary hypertension. (Adapted from Ferrer MI: Cardiovasc Clin 8(3):216–217, 1977)

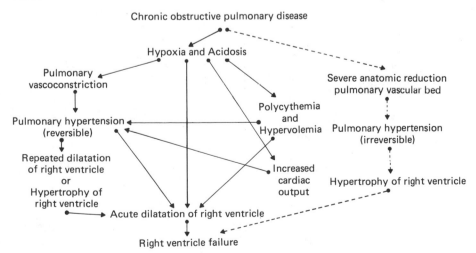

reversible in most patients with COPD if the hypoxia is corrected. If untreated, right ventricular dilation, hypertrophy, and failure appear at varying intervals after the onset of the pulmonary hypertension.

Acidemia. In addition to the precapillary vasoconstriction produced by alveolar hypoxia, vasoconstriction may be augmented[11,21] by the inability of the COPD patient to maintain homeostasis in acid–base balance, which results in increased hydrogen-ion concentration in the blood. The acidemia of COPD is usually produced by carbon dioxide retention due to alveolar hypoventilation, but lactic acid production due to anaerobic metabolism may be an additional source of excess acid.

NURSING CARE IN PULMONARY HEART DISEASE

From this discussion, it is apparent that the pulmonary hypertension associated with COPD is reversible in early stages in most patients. Therefore, nursing care based on an understanding of the pathophysiology of PHD can result in improved life style[32] and perhaps delayed mortality[28] for many patients with PHD.

The objective of both medical therapy and nursing care is to prevent pulmonary hypertension by assisting the patient in maximizing gas exchange and if, despite optimal therapy, hypoxia is still present, normalizing alveolar oxygen tension with oxygen therapy.

Prevention

Prevention of the majority of the cases of PHD requires the prevention of COPD. The etiology of COPD is almost always cigarette smoking.[17] Although many nurses may not realize it or perhaps agree, this is where nursing care should start. The nursing profession has the numbers to provide a widespread health exemplar of non-smoking. This does not seem to be the case, however, particularly when compared to the reduction in smoking by physicians in response to the first Surgeon General's Report.[33]

Patient Problems

The majority of the patient problems seen in PHD are associated with the underlying disease process, COPD, and its major pathophysiologic consequences; alveolar hypoxia and acidemia. Additional problems are also associated with the effects of hypoxia on the hemapoietic and circulatory systems. Recognition of hypoxia, assessment of its potential for causing PHD and definitive nursing interventions to correct or alleviate alveolar hypoxia are the core of the nursing process in treating PHD.

Abnormal Gas Exchange. Alveolar hypoxia is the actual causative factor in pulmonary vascular vasoconstriction, however, it is not an easily measured value. The arterial hypoxemia that results from widespread alveolar hypoxia is easily measured, so arterial blood gas values are the objective

criteria on which judgments regarding the likelihood of a patient with COPD developing PHD are made. Direct measurement of pulmonary artery pressures by pulmonary artery catheterization is, of course, possible. The graph shown in Figure 51-3 allows the prediction of levels of pulmonary artery mean pressure (and, therefore, of potential or actual PHD) from more easily determined arterial pH and oxygen saturation values.

The clinical signs of hypoxemia are those associated with tissue hypoxia in critical organ systems, particularly the brain and heart. Confusion, restlessness, headache (due to cerebrovascular dilatation), tachycardia, and tachyarrhythmias are cardinal signs and symptoms of hypoxemia and hypercarbia. Associated pulmonary symptoms are not prominent but may include increased dyspnea, cough, and sputum production. Both the acute and the chronic hypoxemia seen in COPD are usually associated with retained secretions.

The first step in secretion control is usually cessation of smoking. The nurse's role is to make sure that the patient has a clear idea of the benefits of stopping smoking entirely or at least of reducing the number of cigarettes smoked per day. There is a dramatic decrease in symptoms (cough and sputum production) and a modest improvement in pulmonary function (increased rate of airflow) in those who stop smoking completely and lesser, but still worthwhile changes if consumption is reduced by at least 25%.[4] In addition, Fletcher has shown that susceptible smokers who, at age 40, stop or cut cigarette consumption to less than 15 a day clearly have a greater chance of survival and freedom from disability.[17]

Improving the clearance of secretions is usually attempted through bronchial hygiene routines. Nurses should teach these routines to the COPD patient just as they teach insulin injections and urine testing to the diabetic patient. Bronchial hygiene starts with inhalation of a bronchodilator to open airways as much as possible so that secretions are easier to

Fig. 51-3. Graphic representation of the relationship between pulmonary artery mean pressure and blood pH, considering arterial oxygen saturation as a fixed parameter, in patients with chronic obstructive pulmonary disease. (Adapted from Ferrer MI: Bull NY Acad Med 41(9):948, 1964)

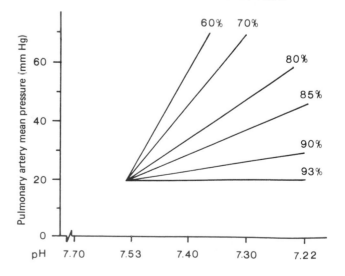

cough out. The effectiveness of bronchodilators should be assessed by auscultating the chest before and after administrating them, to see if there is evidence of a decrease in wheeze (if present) or an increase in breath sounds indicating improved airflow. Following the bronchodilator, steam (or, in the hospital, aerosol) is inhaled to loosen secretions. Although there is little scientific basis for this practice at present, many patients offer testimonials to its efficacy in raising secretions.

Once airways are opened and mucus is "loosened," secretions are cleared by postural drainage and coughing. The theoretic basis for postural drainage is that the flow of secretions toward the central airways will increase because of the effect of gravity on the secretions. An additional mechanism promoting the mobilization of secretions is the pressure change that occurs in the thorax when the body position is changed during postural drainage. The pressure relationships in the lungs are such that more airways and alveoli in the bases of the lung are open when the base of the lung temporarily becomes the "top of the lung" during postural drainage. Theoretically this should allow mucus trapped in airways in the base of the lung, which are usually closed in upright or lying positions, to flow centrally and be coughed out. If coughing is ineffective, suctioning is used to clear the mobilized secretions.

The desired outcome of teaching the patient bronchial hygiene is clearance of secretions and improved arterial oxygenation. Motivating the patient to change his daily routine to include these procedures is a major but not easily obtained goal of nursing intervention.

If severe hypoxemia (PaO_2 less than 50 mm Hg) is still present despite optimal bronchodilator and clearance therapy, the patient must start using supplementary oxygen. This is a stressful decision for most patients and for many physicians and nurses, too. The patient views oxygen therapy as a sign of impending death, and physicians and nurses see it as a failure of less expensive, conservative therapy. Actually, oxygen should be viewed simply as a medication which must, in most cases, be given continuously. The idea that oxygen must be taken continuously is a rather hard concept for patients to grasp, because most of them believe that oxygen can be stored up in the body. Also, there is often a feeling on the part of the family (and many professionals, too, unfortunately) that anybody who requires so little oxygen (1–2 liters is a usual dose) must not really "need" the oxygen and will become "dependent" on it. Patient, family, nurse, and physician must understand that it is the type of physiologic disturbance in gas exchange that determines the amount of oxygen supplementation required, and not the type of patient. The cause of hypoxemia most commonly present in COPD, $\dot{V}/\dot{Q}$ mismatch, requires only small increases in oxygen concentration to raise the alveolar oxygen tension to a level which brings the blood oxygen saturation to an acceptable level. Although ventilation may be poor, when oxygen is added to the inhaled air it eventually reaches the alveoli and raises the alveolar and ultimately the arterial oxygen level.

Long-term oxygen therapy is a major psychologic, social, and financial change in a patient's life. To promote adherence to this form of therapy, the patient must receive sound information about cost, convenience, risks and benefits.

Nurses should tell their patients that an improved lifestyle is an expected result of therapy, with increased ability to perform activities of daily living and reduction in hospital days the major benefits.[28,32]

Peripheral Edema. Caution is needed in assessing edema and related signs in patients with COPD[19]: (1) hyperinflation of the lungs may cause the diaphragm to partially obstruct the vena cava and lead to impaired inferior vena caval flow, resulting in leg edema despite a normal central venous pressure; (2) the depressed diaphragm may also result in a palpable liver edge without true engorgement; and (3) positive intrathoracic pressure generated during expiration through partially obstructed airways may cause distention of the jugular veins.

When edema is present in PHD, its usual cause is saline excess, due to renal sodium retention matched by water retention. The mechanism of why sodium is retained in PHD is not clearly understood but seems to be associated with redistribution of blood flow in the kidney due to hypoxemia.[29] Sodium retention is usually triggered by low cardiac output in congestive heart failure (CHF); however, in PHD, cardiac output often remains near normal, so the response in this case appears to be prompted by the low arterial oxygen tension (PaO_2) of the circulating blood. In PHD, it is theorized that blood flow is preferentially increased in the medulla of the kidney. This provides the oxygen needed for the aerobic demands of sodium reabsorption. While diuretics are sometimes used, simply correcting hypoxemia (by secretion clearance or oxygen therapy) is usually sufficient to cause diuresis in pulmonary heart disease.[7,39]

Nursing assessment includes accurate records of changes in weight and presence of leg edema. However, reliance on weight gain as a predictor of PHD has been questioned[8] and serial measurements of PaO_2 showing increasing hypoxemia may be more valuable in predicting impending right ventricular (RV) failure than weight gain or edema.

In selected cases, nursing intervention includes teaching the patient control of sodium balance through dietary restrictions of salt. This is often very trying for the patient and may add disinclination to eat tasteless food to the anorexia that is often already present. Anorexia is due to hepatic engorgement and poor circulation in the gastrointestinal tract as hypoxemia causes the shunting of blood from the gut to more vital organs.

Potassium Imbalance. Potassium and chloride depletion can easily occur in PHD when diuretics are given or diuresis is brisk in response to correction of hypoxemia. Potassium depletion is of concern in the PHD patient because digitalis therapy is sometimes used when RV failure is present and digitalis toxicity is increased in hypokalemia. The use of digitalis in PHD is controversial, with most authors saying it should not be used.[7,18,19,30,39] Since the pathogenesis of the congestive failure in PHD is pulmonary artery hypertension, which responds to correction of hypoxemia, it is difficult to develop a rationale for giving a cardiotonic drug in this setting (Chap. 34).

Nursing intervention includes dietary advice. Patients can replace some potassium by eating potassium-rich food, such as oranges and bananas, and should be encouraged to do so by nurses, because compliance with taking potassium supplements is poor. Adherence to medication regimes can be assessed by the frequency or infrequency with which refill prescriptions are requested.

Acid–Base Balance. Acidemia may be due to alveolar hypoventilation causing hypercarbia or to hypoxemia-induced lactic acidosis, or both. Acute respiratory failure (ARF) is a common complication in COPD. Acute respiratory failure is defined as a sudden fall in PaO_2 to less than 50 mm Hg with or without an acute rise in $PaCO_2$ to more than 50 mm Hg. A PaO_2 in this range will produce an oxygen saturation of less than 85% so (even without acidemia) one can expect the mean pulmonary artery pressure (PAP) to be 25 mm Hg or greater (see Fig. 51-3). The addition of acidemia, even a modest drop to a pH of 7.3, can be expected to raise the mean pulmonary artery pressure to approximately 35 mm Hg according to the graph. The vulnerability of the patient in acute respiratory failure to PHD is readily evident. Nursing interventions include prompt treatment of hypoxemia with oxygen therapy and, if there is also acidemia, bicarbonate administration may buy time until secretion clearance results in improved ventilation and $\dot{V}/\dot{Q}$ balance.

Cardiovascular Insufficiency. Left heart failure can, and often does, coexist with PHD when coronary heart disease (CHD) is also present.[6] It is not surprising that many patients have both conditions, since COPD—the main reservoir of PHD—has the same risk factors as CHD. Coexistence of COPD and CHD is a particularly serious situation. Many CHD patients in chronic left heart failure have "occult" pulmonary edema in the interstitium of the lung. This fluid tends to close small airways, worsening $\dot{V}/\dot{Q}$ relationships and increasing hypoxemia.[34]

There is no consistent type or pattern of cardiac arrhythmia seen in PHD. The arrhythmias seen in patients with PHD usually occur only when acute respiratory failure is also present. The incidence of arrhythmias varies indirectly with the PaO_2 and can be one of the earliest indications of a sudden deterioration of gas exchange.

Nursing intervention in cardiovascular insufficiency includes careful monitoring for signs of pulmonary edema, arrhythmias and worsening oxygenation. Placing patients with coexisting left heart failure in an upright position, seated or semi-Fowler, facilitates oxygenation.[5]

Sleep Disturbances. Normal persons are known to have increases in $PaCO_2$ and decreases in PaO_2 due to alveolar hypoventilation during sleep. The observed changes in PaO_2 and $PaCO_2$ in patients with COPD are of the same order[24,31] but because the patients start out with a lower PaO_2 when awake, the "normal" drop in PaO_2 during sleep may cause significant arterial desaturation, and pulmonary hypertension. Subjects often arouse when significant changes in gas exchange occur. This means that patients with COPD and PHD may have a significant disturbance in normal sleep patterns.

The nursing implications are clear. Hypoxemic patients must be assisted in keeping their oxygen on at night. Certain patients who have a reasonable oxygen saturation (greater than 85%) during the day will need to use oxygen only during the night to prevent pulmonary hypertension and PHD. Blood gas studies should be performed during sleep in patients with borderline daytime PaO_2 values.

Pain. Pain is not a prominent feature of PHD or the underlying hypoxemia of COPD. Occasionally pulmonary hypertension is associated with substernal, generalized but nonradiating pain[18] of mild degree. Sudden hepatomegaly in acute PHD can also cause pain by stretching the liver capsule. Overall, control of pain does not often present a problem in PHD. However, use of narcotics, sedatives, and tranquilizers for the control of pain from other sources would have to be carefully planned in a hypoxemic or a hypercarbic COPD patient because of their sedative effect on the respiratory center.

In summary, the nursing care and prevention of pulmonary heart disease is usually the prevention and care of persons with COPD and hypoxemia. Pulmonary heart disease is a preventable complication of COPD, if a close watch is kept on the patient's blood gas status, and appropriate therapy is promptly initiated.

REFERENCES

1. Behnke RH, Blount SG, Bristow JD et al: Primary prevention of pulmonary heart disease. Pulmonary heart disease study group. Circulation 41(A):17–23, 1970
2. Bergofsky EH: Mechanisms underlying vasomotor regulation of regional pulmonary blood flow in normal and disease states. Am J Med 57(3):378–394, 1974
3. Bhargava RK: Cor Pulmonale (Pulmonary Heart Disease). Mt. Kisco, Futura Publishing, 1973
4. Buist AS, Sexton GJ, Nagy JM et al: The effect of smoking cessation and modification on lung function. Am Rev Respir Dis 114(1):115–122, 1976
5. Bunke B: Respiratory function after acute MI: Implications for nursing. Cardiovasc Nurs 9(3):13–18, 1973
6. Burrows B, Kettel LJ, Niden AH et al: Patterns of cardiovascular dysfunction in chronic obstructive lung disease. N Engl J Med 286(17):912–918, 1972
7. Burrows B, Knudson RJ, Kettel LJ: Respiratory Insufficiency, pp 86–90. Chicago, Year Book Medical Publishers, 1975
8. Campbell RHA, Brand HL, Cox JR et al: Body weight and body water in chronic cor pulmonale. Clin Sci Mol Med 49(4):323–335, 1975
9. Crofton J, Douglas A: Respiratory Diseases, 2nd ed, pp 360–367. Oxford, Blackwell Scientific Publications, 1975
10. Doyle JT, Wilson JS, Warren JV: The pulmonary vascular responses to short-term hypoxia in human subjects. Circulation 5(2):263–270, 1952
11. Enson Y, Giuntini C, Lewis ML et al: The influence of hydrogen ion concentration and hypoxia on the pulmonary circulation. J Clin Invest 43(6):1146–1162, 1964
12. Enson Y: Pulmonary heart disease: Relation of pulmonary hypertension to abnormal lung structure and function. Bull NY Acad Med 53(6):551–566, 1977
13. Enson Y, Thomas HM III, Bosken CH et al: Pulmonary hypertension in interstitial lung disease: Relation of vascular resistance to abnormal lung structure. Trans Assoc Am Phys 88:248–255, 1975
14. Ferrer MI: Cor pulmonale (pulmonary heart disease): Present-day status. Am Heart J 89(5):657–664, 1975
15. Ferrer MI, Enson Y, Kilcoyne MM et al: Effects of isoproterenol on the pulmonary circulation in patients with chronic obstructive lung disease. Circulation 43(4):528–537, 1971

16. Fishman AP, McClement J, Himmelstein A et al: Effects of acute anoxia on circulation and respiration in patients with chronic pulmonary disease studied during "steady state." J Clin Invest 31(8):770–781, 1952

17. Fletcher C, Peto R, Tinker C et al: The Natural History of Chronic Bronchitis and Emphysema: An Eight-Year Study of Early Chronic Obstructive Lung Disease in Working Men in London, pp 129–132. Oxford, Oxford University Press, 1976

18. Fowler NO: Chronic cor pulmonale caused by lung disease. In Baum GL (ed): Textbook of Pulmonary Diseases. Boston, Little, Brown & Co, 1974

19. Guenter CA, Welch MH: Pulmonary Medicine, pp 587–591. Philadelphia, JB Lippincott, 1977

20. Haas F, Bergoffsky EH: Role of the mast cell in the pulmonary pressor response to hypoxia. J Clin Invest 51(12):3154–3162, 1972

21. Harvey RM, Enson Y, Betti R et al: Further observations on the effect of hydrogen ion on the pulmonary circulation. Circulation 35(6):1019–1027, 1967

22. Hasleton PS, Heath D, Brewer DB: Hypertensive pulmonary vascular disease in states of chronic hypoxia. J Pathol Bacteriol 95(2):431–440, 1968

23. Jameson AG: Diffusion of gases from alveolus to precapillary arteries. Science, 139(3557):826–828, 1963

24. Koo KW, Sox DS, Snider GL: Arterial blood gases and pH during sleep in chronic obstructive pulmonary disease. Am J Med 58(5):663–670, 1975

25. Liljestrand G: Chemical control of the distribution of pulmonary blood flow. Acta Physiol Scand 44:216–240, 1958

26. Lloyd TC Jr: Effect of alveolar hypoxia on pulmonary vascular resistance. J Appl Physiol 19(6):1086–1094, 1964

27. Morkin E: Activation of synthetic processes in cardiac hypertrophy. Circ Res (Suppl)35(8):37–48, 1974

28. Neff TA, Petty TL: Long-term continuous oxygen therapy in chronic airway obstruction: Mortality in relationship to cor pulmonale, hypoxia and hypercapnia. Ann Intern Med 72(5):621–626, 1970

29. Editorial: Oedemia in cor pulmonale. Lancet ii (7948): 1289–1290, 1975

30. Petty TL: Intensive and Rehabilitative Respiratory Care, 2nd ed, pp 35, 242. Philadelphia, Lea & Febiger, 1974

31. Pierce AK, Jarrett CE, Werkle G Jr et al: Respiratory function during sleep in patients with chronic obstructive disease. J Clin Invest 45(5):631–636, 1966

32. Stewart BN, Hood CI, Black AJ: Long-term results of continuous oxygen therapy at sea level. Chest 68(4):486–492, 1975

33. U.S. Department of Health, Eduction and Welfare. The Health Consequences of Smoking, A Report of the Surgeon General, Public Health Service. Washington, DC, U.S. Government Printing Office, 1971

34. Valencia A, Burgess JH: Arterial hypoxemia following acute myocardial infarction. Circulation 40(5):641–652, 1969

35. Weil JV, Bynne-Quinn E, Sodal IE et al: Hypoxic ventilatory drive in normal man. J Clin Invest 49:1061–1072, 1970

36. West JB: Respiratory Physiology—the Essentials. Baltimore, Williams & Wilkins, 1974

37. Westcott RN, Fowler NO, Scott RC et al: Anoxia and human pulmonary vascular resistance. J Clin Invest 30(9):957–970, 1951

38. World Health Organization. Chronic cor pulmonale: Report of an expert committee. Circulation 27(4):594–615, 1963

39. Wynne JW: The treatment of cor pulmonale. JAMA 239(21):2283, 1978

40. Yang SS, Bentivoglio LG, Maranhão V et al: From Cardiac Catheterization Data to Hemodynamic Parameters, 2nd ed, pp 90–91. Philadelphia, FA Davis, 1978

52

Cardiac Abnormalities Associated with Intracranial Events

WANDA ROBERTS, R.N. M.N.

and

SANDRA L. UNDERHILL, R.N., M.N.

Functional relationships between the heart and the brain are obvious. Stress and emotions can alter blood pressure, heart rate (HR), and cardiac contractility.[4,37] Conversely, a reduction in cardiac output below a critical level can lead to hemodynamic and metabolic disturbances in the brain. The adverse cardiac effects of intracranial lesions are less widely realized and appreciated. Patients with cerebrovascular accidents often manifest electrocardiographic changes[18] and are admitted to the Cardiac Care Unit to establish the presence or absence of myocardial infarction (MI). Once MI has been ruled out, these patients are transferred to general neurologic units without further cardiac monitoring. However, unrecognized cardiac damage can occur and can produce serious consequences. Neurologic patients often die unexpectedly of cardiac arrest, arrhythmias, or severe hypotension, without evidence of preexisting heart disease or blood loss.[5,25]

The earliest report associating cardiac abnormalities with intracranial disease was published in 1947.[3] An abnormal electrocardiogram (ECG) was noted in a patient with documented subarachnoid hemorrhage (SAH). Numerous clinical and experimental reports describing a variety of ECG abnormalities and myocardial lesions associated with intracranial disturbances have appeared since then. Many of the earliest notations were the result of incidental findings.[2,3,9,26,38] While ECG changes and myocardial lesions generally occur more frequently in patients with intracranial hemorrhages (ICH), they have also been found in patients with other intracranial disorders including meningitis, space-occupying lesions, head trauma, and cerebral thromboembolism.[10,21,25] Sixty-one percent–90% of all patients with acute strokes have demonstrated ECG abnormalities.[10,33]

ELECTROCARDIOGRAPHIC ABNORMALITIES

Table 52-1 lists the ECG morphologic changes and arrhythmias that have been documented in patients with intracranial disorders. These changes were seen in human subjects[19–21,23,31,35] and in experimental animals. The animals underwent electrical stimulation of selected brain areas or were subjected to various procedures that simulated intracranial lesions found in humans.[16,22,28,29,32] Many of the arrhythmias can be life-threatening. The morphologic changes in the electrocardiographic wave forms frequently mimic myocardial ischemia and infarction,[7,12,27] although hearts examined at autopsy often disclose no infarction.[10] The ECG changes can be transient or permanent.[25] They can appear at any time from the onset of the neurologic symptoms to several days afterwards.[12,34,35] The appearance of ECG changes in patients with ICH is associated with a poorer prognosis when these patients are compared with patients without ECG abnormalities. Such ECG changes may indicate the more severe brain lesions.[25]

SUGGESTED MECHANISMS OF ECG ALTERATIONS

Several explanations for the development of ECG changes with intracranial disorders have been put forward. These include electrolyte disturbances, arterial blood gas changes,

TABLE 52-1	ELECTROCARDIOGRAPHIC MANIFESTATIONS OF INTRACRANIAL EVENTS	
Morphologic Changes	**Arrhythmias**
Deeply inverted T waves	Sinus:
Flat T waves	bradycardia
Tall peaked T waves	tachycardia
Broad T-U fusion waves	arrhythmia
S-T segment depression or elevation	Atrial:
Prolonged U waves	fibrillation
Increased R wave voltage	flutter
Tall P waves	tachycardia
Notched or biphasic T waves	wandering pacemaker
	premature contractions
	paroxysmal tachycardia
	Junctional:
	bradycardia
	tachycardia
	Conduction disturbances:
	AV dissociation
	Mobitz II AV block
	Ventricular:
	premature beats (unifocal and multifocal)
	bigeminy and quadrigeminy
	tachycardia
	fibrillation

autonomic nervous system (ANS) dysfunction, and selective myocardial cell necrosis.[33] Neither electrolyte disturbances nor changes in arterial blood gases have been consistently correlated with ECG abnormalities.[14] The consensus is that the intracranial lesions (particularly SAH) produce an imbalance of autonomic outflow, resulting in an excess sympathetic and parasympathetic discharge. Early reports supported the belief that excess vagal activity was primarily responsible for the cardiac abnormalities, since stimulation of the main cortical representation of the parasympathetic nervous system* produced grossly abnormal electrocardiograms.[19,22,35,40] However, both sympathetic and parasympathetic discharge probably contribute to the overall disturbances in cardiac function.

It has been found that an excess of activity in one division of the ANS will produce an increase in the activity of the opposing division in an effort to maintain homeostasis.[15] Furthermore, electrical stimulation of hypothalamic nuclei have repeatedly been shown to produce strong systemic autonomic reactions. An abnormal hypothalamic response induced by spasms of small vessels supplying the hypothalamus may be a possible cause of autonomic overactivity associated with SAH, since hypothalamic and myocardial lesions have been found to coexist in patients with SAH.[11]

Excessive autonomic activity can produce focal myocardial cell necrosis. This lesion is believed to be partially responsible for the ECG abnormalities noted with intracranial disorders.[2,6,11,14,15,17,20,22,27] Focal myocardial cell necrosis is

characterized by patchy, diffuse areas of injury of myocardial cells interspersed between normal cells. Capillaries and blood flow remain intact. The areas of necrosis are randomly dispersed and, unlike MI, they do not follow the distribution of the coronary vasculature.[8,15,27] The histologic characteristics of this lesion are similar to those seen in sudden cardiac death and are described in detail in Chapter 13.

In several instances focal myocardial cell necrosis was found to be more extensive in areas immediately adjacent to adrenergic nerves throughout the myocardium and less severe in more distal areas.[14,15] This distribution factor supports the idea that these myocardial lesions are primarily neurogenic in origin and are caused by the metabolic effects of norepinephrine on the heart. Circulating catecholamines may also play a part in the genesis of myocardial lesions by increasing myocardial metabolism in the face of reduced coronary blood flow.[14,17]

In most instances, the neurogenically-induced ECG changes are believed to reflect impairment of myocardial repolarization.[32] Prolonged Q-T, S-T, and T-wave changes and ectopic arrhythmias have been associated with nonuniformity in the rates of repolarization of myocardial cells. Since sympathetic stimulation, catecholamine administration, and slow heart rates have been shown to increase nonuniformity of repolarization, it seems likely that sympathetic activity is the mechanism responsible for the ECG alterations demonstrated in patients with intracranial disorders, either alone or in conjunction with selective myocardial cell necrosis.[33,35]

INTERVENTION

Once the myocardium of patients with intracranial lesions has been damaged there is little evidence that therapy can alter the situation. Serious and life-threatening arrhythmias respond to conventional antiarrhythmic therapy and this should be instituted when necessary. Beyond this, therapy is primarily aimed at preventing cardiac complications. "Chemical denervation" of the heart by pharmacologic means has been recommended as a protective measure for patients who are likely to develop cardiac abnormalities. Therapy should begin as soon as possible after the onset of intracranial hemorrhage.[39]

Propranolol will block the sympathetic response of the beta adrenergic receptors in the myocardium and has experimentally demonstrated a protective effect on the hearts of animals with intracranial lesions.[17,20,27,34] Because of evidence suggesting the presence of alpha adrenergic receptors in the heart, alpha blockade with such drugs as phentolamine has now been recommended in conjunction with beta blockade.[13,36] To achieve parasympathetic or vagal blockade, atropine, an acetylcholine antagonist, can be administered.[15,33] Much experimental evidence advocating the usefulness of drug therapy exists; only recently has clinical evidence become available.[30] The true efficacy of pharmacologic autonomic blockade for preventing myocardial necrosis and arrhythmias and influencing mortality in patients with intracranial lesions requires further investigation.

* The main cortical representation of the parasympathetic nervous system is area 13, the Brodmann area, and is located on the orbital surface of the frontal lobes, with relay stations in the anterior hypothalamus and connections to the brainstem.

MEDICAL AND NURSING IMPLICATIONS

The transient nature of many of these ECG abnormalities makes them difficult to detect, unless patients undergo careful cardiac monitoring during the acute phase of their neurologic illness. Many patients are currently not monitored. Continuous cardiac monitoring can facilitate prompt recognition and treatment of these complications,[18] thereby preventing serious consequences to the patient, as well as adding significant information to the present body of knowledge about cardiac abnormalities of intracranial events.

Knowledge of the ECG changes associated with central nervous system disease is important for several other reasons. In patients with intracranial hemorrhage a misinterpretation of ECG changes as indicative of an MI may cause a delay in surgery or diagnostic testing, both of which may be necessary to prevent a second, often fatal, hemorrhage. The use of catecholamines in hypotensive neurologic patients may cause further myocardial damge and should be used with caution.[5,33] Patients who die from catastrophic intracranial events are often considered potential cardiac donors. Since both cardiac damage and ECG changes can occur, adrenergic blockade may be necessary to preserve the myocardium in these donors prior to transplantation.

Additional factors known to stress the heart and potentially compound myocardial damage should be carefully avoided. Hypoxemia, high intensity cardiac defibrillation, and hypokalemia have all been associated with myocardial damage. Nasal decongestants and bronchodilators have readily absorbable forms of catecholamines, nicotine causes catecholamine release from the adrenal medulla, and cyclic antidepressants prevent the inactivation of norepinephrine. The use of these latter agents in neurologic patients who risk having cardiac complications should be questioned. The contribution of severe emotional reactions to the development of cardiac abnormalities in neurologic patients has not been fully elucidated, but it seems logical that prevention of these stresses would be beneficial.

Many questions remain unanswered concerning the long-term effects of myocardial cell necrosis on overall cardiac function and on morbidity and mortality rates. Activity restrictions may be indicated for patients with intracranial events who manifest ECG changes. This may be accomplished by guidelines for progressive activity similar to those developed for patients after myocardial infarction. Close monitoring of these patients during activity would also be important in determining the exercise tolerance for individual patients.

Early recognition and prompt treatment are essential aspects of the management of cardiac complications of intracranial events. Continuous cardiac monitoring facilitates recognition of the abnormalities. Preventive drug therapy should also be considered.

REFERENCES

1. Bajusz E, Jasmin G: Influence of variations in electrolyte intake upon the development of cardiac necrosis produced by vasopressor amines. Lab Invest 13(7):757–66, 1964
2. Burch GE, Meyers R, Abildskov JA: A new electrocardiogram pattern observed in cerebrovascular accidents. Circulation 9(5):719–23, 1953
3. Byer E, Ashmen R, Toth L: Electrocardiograms with large upright T waves and long Q–T intervals. Am Heart J 33:796–806, 1947
4. Check W: Stress' route through brain to heart. JAMA 240(25):2712–14, 1978
5. Connor RC: Myocardial damage secondary to brain lesions. Am Heart J 78(2):145–48, 1969
6. Connor RC: Heart damage associated with intracranial lesions. Br Med J 3:29–31, 1968
7. Coodley E: The diagnosis of myocardial infarction by enzyme analysis. In Meltzer L, Dunning L (eds): Textbook of Coronary Care, pp 82–92. Philadelphia, Charles Press, 1972
8. Cowan MJ: Sudden cardiac death and selective myocardial cell necrosis. Heart Lung 8(3):559–63, 1979
9. Cropp GJ, Manning GW: Electrocardiographic changes simulating myocardial ischemia and infarction associated with spontaneous intracranial hemorrhage. Circulation 22:25–38, 1960
10. Dimant J, Grob D: Electrocardiographic changes and myocardial damage in patients with acute cerebrovascular accidents. Stroke 8(4):448–55, 1977
11. Doshi R, Neil-Dwyer G: Hypothalamic and myocardial lesions after subarachnoid hemorrhage. J Neurol, Neurosurg Psychiatry 40:821–26, 1977
12. Estanol B, Marin O: Cardiac arrhythmias and sudden death in subarachnoid hemorrhage. Stroke 6:382–86, 1975
13. Falk RH, Cassells W: Effect of drugs on myocardial necrosis after subarachnoid hemorrhage. Br Med J 2:1501, 1978
14. Greenhoot J, Reichenbach D: Cardiac injury and subarachnoid hemorrhage. J Neurosurg 30:521–31, 1969
15. Groover ME, Stout C: Neurogenic myocardial necrosis. Angiology 16:180–86, 1965
16. Gurdjian ES: Impact Head Injury, pp 192–202. Springfield, Charles C Thomas, 1975
17. Hawkins WE, Clower B: Myocardial damage after head trauma and simulated intracranial hemorrhage in mice: Role of the autonomic nervous system. Cardiovasc Res 5:524–29, 1971
18. Heaney LM: Cardiac and respiratory monitoring of acute stroke patients. Heart Lung 6(3):469–74, 1977
19. Hersch C: Electrocardiographic changes in subarachnoid hemorrhage, meningitis and intracranial space-occupying lesions. Br Heart J 26:785–93, 1964
20. Hunt D, McRae C, Zapf P: Electrocardiographic and serum enzyme changes in subarachnoid hemorrhage. Am Heart J 77(4):479–88, 1969
21. Jachuck SJ, Ramani PS, Clark P et al: Electrocardiographic abnormalities associated with raised intracranial pressure. Br Med J 1:242–44, 1975
22. Jacob WA, VanBogaert A, De Groodt-Lasseel M: Myocardial ultrastructure and hemodynamic reactions during experimental subarachnoid hemorrhage. J Mol Cell Cardiol 4:287–98, 1972
23. Korczyn AD: Respiratory and cardiac abnormalities in brain stem ischemia. J Neurol, Neurosurg Psychiatry 38:187–90, 1975
24. Koskelo P, Punsar S, Sipila W: Subendocardial hemorrhage and ECG changes in intracranial bleeding. Br Med J 1:1479–80, 1964
25. Lavy S, Yaar I, Melamed E et al: The effect of acute stroke on cardiac functioning as observed in an intensive stroke care unit. Stroke 5:775–79, 1974
26. Levine HD: Nonspecificity of the electrocardiogram associated with coronary heart disease. Am J Med 15(3):344–55, 1953
27. McNair J, Clower B, Sanford R: The effect of reserpine pretreatment on myocardial damage associated with simulated intracranial hemorrhage in mice. Eur J Pharmacol 9:1–6, 1970
28. Manning JW, Cotten M: Mechanisms of cardiac arrhythmias induced by diencephalic stimulation. Am J Physiol 203:1120–24, 1962
29. Mellville K, Blum B, Shister H et al: Cardiac ischemic changes and arrhythmias induced by hypothalamic stimulation. Am J Cardiol 12:781–91, 1963
30. Neil-Dwyer G, Walter P, Cruikshank J et al: Effect of propranolol and phentolamine on myocardial necrosis after subarachnoid hemorrhage. Br Med J 2:990–92, 1978

31. Parizel G: Life-threatening arrhythmias in subarachnoid hemorrhage. Angiology 24:17–21, 1973
32. Porter RW, Kamikawa K, Greenhoot J: Persistent electrocardiographic abnormalities experimentally induced by stimulation of the brain. Am Heart J 64(6):815–19, 1962
33. Reinstein L, Gracey J, Kline J et al: Cardiac monitoring of the acute stroke patient. Arch Phys Med Rehabil 53:311–14, 1972
34. Smith M, Rhorpe R: Cardiac arrhythmias, increased intracranial pressure, and the autonomic nervous system. Chest 61(2)125–33, 1972
35. Smith M, Rhorpe R: Ventricular bigeminy and quadrigeminy occurring in a case of subarachnoid hemorrhage. Journal of Electrocardiol 5(1):78–85, 1972
36. Van der Ark GD, Norton L, Pomerantz M: Cardiovascular effects of increased intracranial pressure. Surg Forum 23:409–11, 1972
37. Vaisrub S: Brain and heart—The autonomic connection. JAMA 234(9):959, 1975
38. Wasserman F, Choquelle G, Cassinelli R et al: Electrocardiographic observations in patients with cerebrovascular accidents: Report of 12 cases. Am J Med Sci 231(5):502–510, 1956
39. Weilder DJ: Myocardial damage and cardiac arrhythmias after intracranial hemorrhage. Stroke 5:759–64, 1974
40. Weintraub B, McHenry L: Cardiac abnormalities in subarachnoid hemorrhage: A resume. Stroke 5:384–91, 1974

53

Disorders of the Peripheral Vascular System

RUTH F. CRAVEN, R.N., M.N.

.and

MARY BOOZER, R.N., M.N.

Some of the common peripheral vascular diseases encountered in the care of the cardiac patient will be discussed in this chapter. Hypertension, discussed in Chapter 47, is implicated in many of the peripheral vascular diseases. Any circulatory disruption decreases the supply of oxygen and nutrients in the tissues, possibly resulting in anoxia, cell destruction, ulceration, and gangrene. Varicose veins are very common and increase the patient's susceptability to thrombophlebitis. Aneurysms sometimes occur, and are due to diseases of the blood vessel wall. Raynaud's disease, Raynaud's phenomenon, and thromboangitis obliterans may also be encountered in patients with cardiac disease. Arteriosclerosis obliterans is the leading cause of obstructive arterial disease of the extremities in the population seen in the intensive care units, and frequently occurs in conjunction with coronary artery disease.

ARTERIOSCLEROSIS OBLITERANS

Arteriosclerosis obliterans, resulting from atherosclerosis of the aorta and its branches to the extremities, is the most common chronic occlusive arterial disease of the extremities after the age of 50. This disorder involves the descending aorta, the common iliac, superficial femoral, popliteal, and the posterior and anterior tibial arteries. The intimal plaque which is the primary lesion of atherosclerosis causes progressive narrowing and, in many cases, complete occlusion of segments of these arteries.[6] The pathogenesis of atherosclerosis is discussed in depth in Chapter 10. Men are more commonly affected by arteriosclerosis obliterans than are women. Persons with diabetes mellitus are prone to develop

the disease and have greater frequency of vessel involvement distal to the knee.[1]

Pathophysiology

Arteriosclerosis obliterans is a slowly developing disease that manifests itself when an abnormally large pressure gradient develops across a stenosis or occlusion, and the distal flow is severely restricted. The decreased blood flow and pressure result in ischemic pain during exercise or rest. Persons who only develop ischemic symptoms during exercise may have normal blood flow while at rest. During exercise, the flow of blood may be so diminished that the contracting muscle obstructs the arterial flow markedly or completely, resulting in ischemic pain.[1] This type of cramping, ischemic pain brought on by exercise and relieved with rest, is *intermittent claudication,* the most common symptom of arteriosclerosis obliterans. The mechanisms by which the resulting tissue ischemia cause vasodilation or reactive hyperemia are described in Chapter 5.

Clinical Manifestations

Inadequate oxygenation of the tissues distal to the site of occlusion is the hallmark of arteriosclerosis obliterans. The most common symptoms are intermittent cramping pain, numbness, aching, and severe fatigue when ischemic muscles are active. These symptoms are relieved promptly by rest. This exercise-pain-rest cycle is constant from day to day, and is aggravated by walking up a hill or stairs. The amount of activity that produces intermittent claudication, for example, walking one flight of stairs or one-half to one block, is relatively constant and helps determine the severity of the problem. Since the major part of the work of walking is done by the calf muscles, they are the most common sites of claudication for occlusive lesions above the level of the knee.

Another important symptom of occlusive disease is the occurrence of pain at rest. Rest pain, which is worse at night, clearly indicates that the flow of blood to the area has been severely diminished and is inadequate to meet the oxygen demands of tissues at rest. The increasing occlusion, or the inadequacy of the collateral circulation, produces ischemia to the nerves as well as to the other tissues and produces lancinating, shooting pain which is most severe in the toes and foot, even at rest. Elevation of the limb always aggravates the pain because gravitational pull further decreases blood flow. Conversely, in the early stages, pain may be relieved by having the limb in a dependent position.

Other symptoms are secondary results of progressive ischemia distal to the occlusion or narrowing. The affected limb is cool compared with its counterpart or to the proximal part of the same limb. The involved extremity may show corresponding color changes, such as pallor due to the decreased blood flow; cyanosis due to diminished, inadequate blood flow; or reddish-blue discoloration due to capillary and venular responses to anoxia. In response to chronic, severe ischemia, the skin becomes dry, shiny, and devoid of hair, and the toenails become hard, brittle, thickened, and deformed. When the collateral blood flow to areas of the limb is no longer adequate, ischemic ulcerations and areas of gangrene may develop, often in the toes and sometimes on the anterior and lateral areas of the lower leg.[1]

Diagnosis

The most revealing function in diagnosing arteriosclerosis obliterans is careful palpation of the peripheral pulses. The pulses should be palpated at each of the sites shown in Figure 53-1, comparing them bilaterally for presence and strength. Palpation must be gentle over the dorsalis pedis and posterior tibial pulses, because a firm touch may compress an artery which has a minimally adequate blood flow and no pulsation will be felt. These two pulses may be difficult to palpate, or may be congenitally absent in some persons. This is when bilateral comparisons, changes in skin color and temperature, and the patient's history become important components in the assessment.

The Doppler ultrasound velocity detector helps to evaluate the presence of questionable pulses by amplifying sound (Chap. 28) and is used to measure the systolic pressure in the limb. Ankle pressures normally should be equal to or higher than the brachial artery pressures. Ankle pressure is reduced with disease. The magnitude of ankle pressure is related to the extent of the arterial occlusion. These ankle pressures and pulses may be present at rest. However, when a person with arteriosclerosis obliterans is asked to exercise to the point of claudication, the pressures fall markedly and are often unrecordable for a period of 30 seconds to several minutes.

In addition to ultrasound and plethysmography, physical examination and measurement of ankle pressure and adequacy of collateral circulation may be roughly estimated by

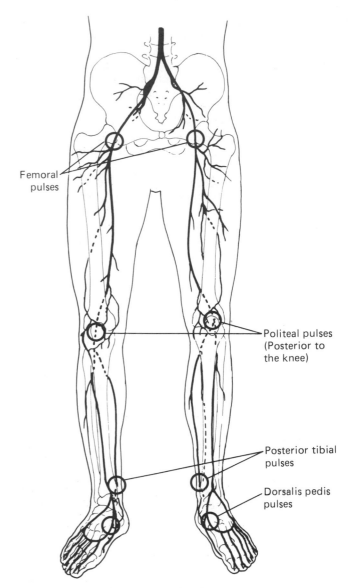

Fig. 53-1. Locations for palpating the peripheral arteries of the leg

elevating the legs. After the patient is placed in a flat position and his leg raised to a 45-degree angle, the plantar surface of the foot should remain pink. The appearance of pallor is indicative of inadequate blood flow. This test should be followed by having the patient sit up quickly, with the feet dependent, to assess the rate of filling. Normally the color should return to the foot within 10 seconds. Times in excess of 30 seconds denote severe ischemia with inadequate collateral blood flow.[1] Careful evaluation of case history, peripheral pulses and pressures are sufficient means to diagnose arteriosclerosis obliterans in most persons. Arteriography is used to localize the occlusion precisely in preparation for surgical intervention.

Medical Management

Early in the course of the disease, the person should establish measures to control and stabilize the disease for as long as possible. Losing excess weight in order to reduce the workload on the lower extremities, and restricting the use of tobacco which causes peripheral vasoconstriction, are two such measures. In conjunction, a daily exercise program in which the person walks on a flat surface for a distance short of the onset of claudication, followed by a rest period, is thought to help promote the development of collateral circulation.

If symptoms become progressively worse, as evidenced by paresthesias, unrelenting pain at rest, and advanced ischemic changes, surgery should be considered. Through arteriography it is possible to determine the exact location and extent of the occlusion, as well as the patency of the distal vessels. The type of surgery chosen is based on this information. Endarterectomy, sympathectomy, and bypass grafts have all been successful in improving blood flow, but bypass grafts are used most frequently. If surgery is not successful and gangrene occurs, then amputation of the limb becomes a necessity. This surgical procedure must be done at the level of patent flow and well-perfused tissue.

Nursing Management

The person with arteriosclerosis obliterans has a chronic progressive disease and needs understanding, supportive nursing care. Patient teaching is an important feature of nursing therapy. Reinforcing the need for weight reduction and for restricting the use of tobacco is an essential element in controlling the progress of the disease. In preventing excessive ischemia and tissue breakdown, instruction must include meticulous foot care; this means properly fitting shoes, immediate attention to blisters and cuts, and careful nail trimming. The person also should avoid such restrictive clothing as tight stockings or garters, and should not cross his legs. Both of these practices mechanically impede the blood flow in already compromised arteries. Encouraging adherence to a daily exercise program in an effort to stimulate the development of collateral circulation helps the person's mental outlook as well as his physical progress. For the person who has developed minor ulcerations or other tissue breakdown, a diet with adequate protein and vitamin C for wound healing and for re-establishing and maintaining integrity is needed.

While the person with arteriosclerosis obliterans soon learns that having his legs in a dependent position lower than the heart relieves some of his symptoms, keeping the legs hanging down increases the venous pressure and promotes dependent edema. The presence of edema further compromises tissue nutrition. The patient should be horizontal with the legs at the level of the heart or slightly lower in order to promote the most effective hemodynamics. The person with peripheral arterial insufficiency should *never* be positioned with the affected limb elevated above heart level.

The person with arteriosclerosis obliterans must be constantly alert to prevent tissue trauma and breakdown in the affected limb. As circulation becomes increasingly impaired, this problem becomes increasingly important. Patients with diabetes in particular may have a peripheral neuropathy. The result of this is a decreased sensitivity to thermal changes—heat and cold—and to pain. Heating pads and hot bath water may cause burns before the person is aware of it. Abrasions, bruises, and cuts may occur without the expected warning of pain. The neuropathy, particularly combined with poor tissue perfusion, will make even the smallest blister or ulcer the basis for infection and subsequent gangrene, and may tip the balance from a limb surviving on minimally adequate blood flow to one that must be amputated.

With severe ischemia, constant pain at rest often becomes a dominating factor. The unrelenting pain causes the person to experience sleeplessness, fatigue, and depression, which further stresses his reserves and his ability to cope with activities of daily living. Surgical intervention may be a necessity at this time. The procedure most frequently used is the implantation of a bypass graft to provide unobstructed flow around the area of occlusion.

The patient who has had bypass grafting requires consistent, continuous assessment of the peripheral circulation. The maintenance of normal systemic fluid volume for an adequate perfusion pressure helps prevent thrombus of the graft and can be monitored, as discussed in Chap. 28. The patency of the graft and the adequacy of the peripheral circulation is documented by assessing the peripheral pulsations distal to the graft. Two very common graft sites are the aortofemoral and the ileofemoral, as illustrated in Figure 53-2.

The popliteal, dorsalis pedis and posterior tibial pulses should be assessed every 15 minutes until stable and at least hourly after surgery, using a Doppler ultrasound velocity detector probe. Once the pulses are located, marking the skin with ink helps ensure consistent assessment. A difference in color and warmth of skin of the operated limb and the unoperated limb provides additional information on tissue perfusion. Other symptoms to watch for are numbness, tingling, weakness, severe pain, and pallor or cyanosis in the operated limb. These symptoms may occur at any time in the postoperative period. As soon as the patient is able, he should participate in the check and be taught how to monitor these changes. He should be told of the importance of any changes, and the need to report these changes to the physician. After vascular surgery, patients should also be monitored closely for bleeding, which is always a potential complication.

The patient should be positioned with continual consideration of the location of the graft. For example, a patient who has undergone bypass grafting as shown in Figure 53-2 should never be positioned with 90-degree hip flexion, because this would encourage pooling of blood in the pelvic region and promote thrombus formation in the graft. To avoid this, the patient should lie flat in bed or in a mild reclining position, avoiding pillows or other pressure sources under the knees. Patients should be reminded not to cross their legs at any time, but they should be encouraged to exercise the legs and feet during bed rest.

Ambulation can begin on the first postoperative day, provided that there are no other intervening problems. In addition to all the other well-known benefits of ambulation, it stimulates arterial circulation to the extremities, while the muscular action in the legs promotes venous return. Supporting devices such as crutches, a walker, and support hose may be necessary for the first few days or longer, depending upon the degree of disability.

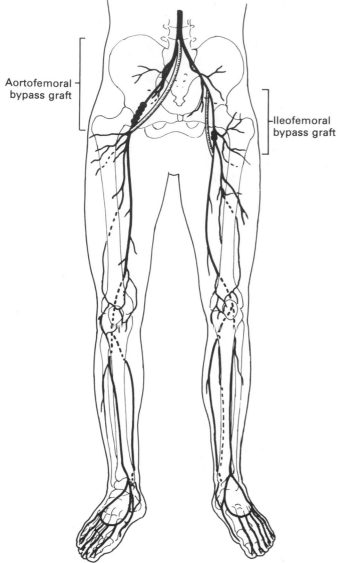

Aortofemoral
bypass graft

Ileofemoral
bypass graft

Fig. 53-2. Examples of common sites of peripheral bypass grafts

The goal of postoperative rehabilitation of the patient with a peripheral vascular graft is to maintain the improved blood flow and prevent further complications. Following the initial postoperative course, all patient teaching, discharge planning, and follow-up care should have that goal as the central focus.

ANEURYSMS

Pathophysiology

An aneurysm is a ballooning enlargement of any artery caused by weakening of the vessel wall. It may be small and localized or large and diffuse. The weakening of the vessel wall can be the end result of a variety of conditions. The large majority of aneurysms are due to the presence of arteriosclerosis in the aging person with hypertension

(Chap. 47). Some other conditions that may produce an aneurysm are syphilis, atherosclerosis (Chap. 10), congenital vascular defects, trauma, and infections in the vascular wall. The material presented in this section will be confined to discussion of aneurysms in the aorta, since aneurysms are more commonly seen at this site.

Regardless of the etiology of the aneurysm formation, the pathophysiologic changes are similar. The basic defect is in the walls of the blood vessels. The aorta, like all arterial vessels, is composed of three layers: the tunica intima, the tunica media and tunic adventitia. The intima is the innermost layer, consisting mainly of a single layer of endothelial cells. The media, or middle layer, of the aorta is thick and highly elastic. This elasticity is very important in circulatory dynamics, because it controls the necessary vasodilation and constriction of the vessel. The outer layer or adventitia is a cover of connective tissue which contains some elastic fibers (Fig. 5-5).

In an aortic aneurysm, all three layers of the vessel wall are involved, but the main defect is the destruction of the elastic fibers in the media. This defect allows the remaining fibrous tissue to stretch and increase the diameter of the aorta in the involved portion. Since the arteries are a closed conducting system filled with blood under high pressure, a weakness in the wall of a vessel will cause a distention of the blood vessel in the weakened area. If the pressure is great enough, the distention can lead to rupture of the aorta. Surgery is the treatment of choice, because of this ever-present possibility of rupture. Some patients are managed medically, and the treatment selected is based upon many considerations, including the condition of the patient and the size of the aneurysm.

Aneurysms are frequently classified as of a certain type. Some of the common classifications encountered will be discussed. The most common aneurysm is classified as fusiform and is one in which the wall of a whole segment of the artery is dilated (Fig. 53-3B). The saccular aneurysm is a ballooning outpouching of a portion of the wall (Fig. 53-3A). This type of aneurysm is more subject to rupture than is the fusiform. A dissecting aneurysm begins with a tear in the intimal wall, allowing blood under pressure to get between the layers in the vessel wall (Fig. 53-3C, and Fig. 53-3D.) In this way blood under pressure forms an extending hematoma and, as it increases in size, it further separates the layers of the vessel wall. The separating of the vessel layers can occur either forward from the intimal tear or backward toward the heart. (Further discussion of this will be found under thoracic aneurysm.)

Abdominal Aortic Aneurysm

Clinical Manifestations and Diagnosis. The most common site of an aneurysm, approximately 75%, is in the abdominal aorta just below the renal arteries (Fig. 53-4A). Frequently the patient is asymptomatic and the diagnosis is made during a physical examination. The majority of persons with abdominal aortic aneurysms are males over the age of 60 who have arteriosclerosis, hypertension, coronary artery disease (CAD) and respiratory disease. Careful abdominal palpation of persons with these criteria may reveal a pulsating

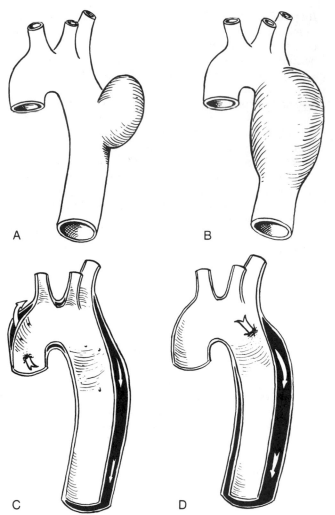

Fig. 53-3. Aneurysms of the thoracic aorta. **(A)** Saccular. **(B)** Fusiform. **(C)** Dissecting: typical site of tear in intima of proximal ascending aorta with dissection of the entire thoracic aorta. **(D)** Dissecting: dissection originating just distal to left subclavian artery. (From Phipps WJ, Long BC, Woods NF: Shafer's Medical—Surgical Nursing, 7th ed, pp 459—460. St. Louis, CV Mosby, 1980)

abdominal mass in the mid and upper abdomen. The majority of the diagnoses are made during a routine physical examination or using an abdominal radiographic film. Some patients may have low back pain radiating to the lumbar region, some may have abdominal pain and some may note the presence of a pulsating mass in the abdomen. A film of the abdomen may show wall calcification that would prompt further diagnostic tests. Aortography can be used in certain cases, but ultrasonography is the diagnostic method of choice. Ultrasonography is noninvasive and can be repeated to check on any changes in the size of the aneurysm, with little risk and without discomfort to the patient.

Medical Management

Surgery is the treatment of choice. The prognosis depends upon the size of the aneurysm and the overall condition of the patient. Elective surgery is advised for all abdominal aortic aneurysms 6 cm in diameter and larger, unless

contraindicated for reasons of other medical problems. For high-risk patients with aneurysms of 4–6 cm, close follow-up is advised, with immediate surgery if the aneurysm is expanding or shows signs of impending rupture.[5] If the aneurysm ruptures, the prognosis is grave, and surgery is done immediately.

Prior to elective surgery, a complete work-up is done to establish the patient's health status. The patient is brought up to his optimum state of health, while being observed for any signs and symptoms of an impending rupture. The success of the surgery varies with his overall physical condition and the size of the aneurysm. This analysis of the patient's health status is good routine preoperative care for surgery of the abdomen. In addition, the pedal pulse sites are identified and marked to assist in the postoperative location of both the posterior tibial and the dorsalis pedis pulses.

At the time of surgery, the aneurysm is clamped off, and it may or may not be removed (Fig. 53-4B and C). A Dacron or Teflon graft is anastomosed to the aorta and to the right and left common iliac arteries (Fig. 53-4D). This graft serves as the conduit for the blood in place of the disconnected section with the aneurysm.

Fig. 53-4. Fusiform aneurysm of abdominal aorta and surgical repair. **(A)** Usual location of aneurysm below renal arteries and involving bifurcation to a varying degree. **(B)**, **(C)** Proximal and distal control with clamps is followed by removal of the aneurysm. **(D)** Graft implantation. (Rhoads JE, Allen JG, Harkins, HN et al: Surgery: Principles and Practice, Philadelphia, JB Lippincott, 1970)

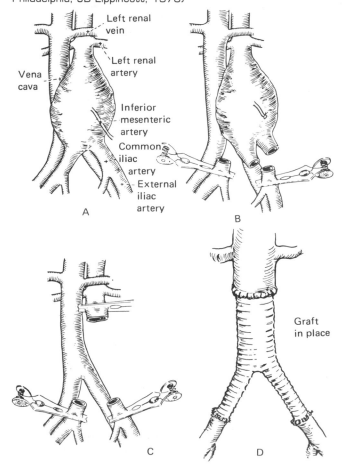

Nursing Management

The most common postoperative complications are hemorrhage and shock. Other complications that can occur in the postoperative period are occlusion at the site of the graft anastomosis, formation of a false aneurysm or of an enteric fistula, and infection.[5] On rare occasions, sacrifice of the inferior mesenteric artery may result in colonic ischemia (Fig. 53-4A). This ischemia can be prevented if the surgeon checks collateral blood flow to the colon at the time of surgery and reimplants the inferior mesenteric artery, if necessary.

Postoperatively, the patient is monitored very carefully for the first 24–48 hours in the same manner as is the cardiac surgery patient (see Chap. 24). Pedal pulses are evaluated as discussed in the section on postoperative care of arteriosclerosis obliterans. Likewise, assessment for possible destruction of the graft is the same, and patient teaching is important (p. 678, this chapter). These patients are often elderly and have other health problems which need to be identified and managed, in addition to the assessments that must be made relative to the surgery. This type of incision is frequently large and painful; the patient will require adequate medication to control the pain. Any effect on respiration and other vital signs is carefully noted and adjustments made in the dosage of medication.

Initially, the patient is placed in a flat position with his head turned to the side. As he recovers from surgery, the head of the bed can be raised to 30–45 degrees. Hip flexion should be avoided and, as the patient becomes ambulatory, he should *not* be allowed to sit up. Compression of the blood vessels must be avoided, but exercise of the legs and feet during bed rest is encouraged, and early ambulation is important to recovery.

Most patients will have a period of paralytic ileus after operation. Auscultation of the abdomen and assessment of bowel tones are an important part of the care. The close approximation of the graft to the renal arteries makes the observation of renal function very important. Intake and output are carefully monitored. Since these patients are subject to the usual postoperative complications, such as thrombophlebitis; the use of elastic stockings is often recommended. Coughing and deep breathing are important, as are other routine postoperative procedures.

Thoracic Aortic Aneurysms

Clinical Manifestations and Diagnosis. Thoracic aneurysms can also be caused by a variety of disease processes but the majority are caused by arteriosclerosis and syphilis. Aneurysms can occur anywhere along the course of the thoracic aorta: the ascending segment, the arch, or the descending segment. The descending aorta is the second most common site of aortic aneurysms and the majority are due to arteriosclerosis. Many patients with a thoracic aortic aneurysm are asymptomatic. Sometimes the diagnosis is first suspected from a routine chest film. If symptoms occur they are usually related to pressure on other structures. The patient may have symptoms of dysphagia, hoarseness, chest pain, dyspnea, cough, and hemoptysis. These symptoms are more common when the aneurysm is in the aortic arch, the least common site.

If an aneurysm is suspected, chest radiography and fluoroscopy can be helpful in confirming the diagnosis. Aortic angiography is the most definitive diagnostic tool.

Aneurysms due to syphilis occur in the tertiary stage of the disease, usually 20 to 30 years after the initial infection. These aneurysms may be saccular or fusiform. A course of penicillin therapy will be given if the person has not been previously treated. The treatment of choice in all thoracic aortic lesions is surgical repair if the patient can tolerate the surgical procedure.

A dissecting aneurysm of the thoracic aorta occurs because of a tear in the intima, allowing blood to enter and separate the blood vessel layers. The majority of these patients are males with arteriosclerosis who have a history of hypertension. A disorder of the media identified as idiopathic cystic medial necrosis associated with Marfan's syndrome has been associated with the stress of hypertension and medial destruction. Marfan's syndrome is characterized by defective formation of collagen and elastic fibers.

The most prominent symptom of a dissecting aortic aneurysm is sudden onset of severe pain in the anterior or posterior chest; it is sometimes confused with the pain of a myocardial infarction. The patient in some instances has identified the pain as a ripping, tearing pain. Dyspnea is usual and respiration is often rapid. Congestive heart failure may occur, usually related to severe aortic regurgitation, which frequently occurs in proximal dissection of the aorta. Cerebrovascular accidents, syncope, paraplegia, and pulse loss have all been described as symptoms of a dissecting aneurysm. The patient appears to be in shock, even though blood pressure is elevated.

Medical Management

Dissecting aortic aneurysms have a high mortality rate and constitute a medical emergency. Without treatment they are almost always fatal. Immediate intensive care treatments, aimed at controlling the pain and lowering the systolic blood pressure, should be instituted. Some controversy exists over how soon surgery should be performed, but surgery is the treatment of choice if the patient can tolerate it.

If time permits, the patient is brought to the optimum health status and prepared for surgical intervention. The patient is closely monitored in an intensive care unit. Preoperative preparation is the same as that for a patient being prepared for cardiac surgery (Chap. 24).

Surgery on the thoracic aorta may require that the patient be placed on the heart-lung bypass machine during surgery. This depends upon the size and location of the aneurysm. The aneurysm is located and a Dacron or Teflon graft is anastamosed to institute the repair. If the aneurysm is saccular, a patch-graft is used (Fig. 53-5A). If the aneurysm is fusiform or dissecting, a longer tubular graft is necessary (Fig. 53-5B).

Nursing Management

Postoperative nursing care is the same as that for the patient undergoing cardiac surgery (Chap. 24).

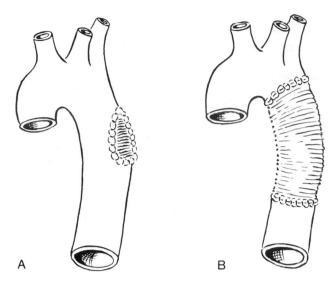

Fig. 53-5. (**A**) Patch graft repair of saccular aneurysm. (**B**) Replacement graft for fusiform aneurysm. (From Phipps WJ, Long BC, Woods NF: Shafer's Medical–Surgical Nursing, 7th ed, p 460. St. Louis, CV Mosby, 1980)

RAYNAUD'S DISEASE

Raynaud's disease is a functional peripheral arterial disease characterized by intermittent vasospasm, primarily in the fingers and toes, which results in pallor, coldness, tissue ischemia, and parasthesias. These attacks of intermittent vasospasm occur with varying frequency and severity, and are commonly precipitated by emotional stress or by exposure to cold. While the etiology is still unknown, recent evidence supports the theory that there may be a defect in basal heat production, limiting the ability to dilate cutaneous vessels. This is supported by the unusual sensitivity to cold and the tendency to shiver exhibited by those affected.[3]

Pathophysiology

The involved extremities undergo characteristic color changes during the vasospastic ischemic attack. Initially, they become blanched with a "dead white" appearance; they are cold, numb, painful, and may be damp with perspiration. The pallor indicates vasoconstriction of the small cutaneous vessels. Digits become cyanotic as the digital capillaries and venules dilate and the slowed blood flow allows the hemoglobin to release more of its oxygen. When the vasoconstriction is relieved, blood flow increases greatly, imparting a red color (rubor) to the previously ischemic digits.[1] The aching, throbbing pain in the digits which accompanies the change from cyanosis to rubor is believed to be the result of the accumulation and subsequent mobilization of abnormal metabolic products due to the ischemia. The length of the attack varies, depending on how soon the person is able to warm his body or hands or is able to relax and reduce the stress response.

Clinical Manifestations and Diagnosis

In general, the hands appear normal between attacks, depending on the severity and cause. Gradually, however, the cyanosis may persist and trophic skin changes may

begin. As a result of the tissue ischemia, fingers become thinner; the skin becomes white or discolored, shiny, taut, and smoother; and the nails may be deformed and clubbed. Diminished sensation in the fingers causes awkwardness with fine movements and increased potential of trauma and of thermal injury. There are no specific diagnostic tests for Raynaud's disease.

The terms *Raynaud's disease* and *Raynaud's phenomenon* are often used interchangeably. They do share many commonalities, such as coldness of involved extremities, color changes, pain, numbness and paresthesias but they also have certain distinctions. The medical diagnosis is based upon the history which is uniquely characteristic of Raynaud's syndrome.

Raynaud's disease (primary) occurs almost exclusively in young women between the ages of 18 and 40 years, with a gradual onset, most often in the late teens and in the twenties. The symptoms are bilaterally symmetrical in the fingers and, less often, in the toes. Raynaud's disease is usually defined as being a primary condition with no other evidence of occlusive peripheral vascular disease as in a primary systemic disease. It ranges from mild, causing little disability, to severe, with increasing pain and disability.

In contrast, Raynaud's phenomenon (secondary) occurs in persons of either sex, has a later onset, and is due to some underlying systemic disorder. The symptoms of Raynaud's phenomenon can be asymmetrical and may involve the thumbs as well as the fingers, with a thickening or tightening of the skin of the hands and possible ulceration of the fingertips. This phenomenon may occur with so-called collagen disorders, such as rheumatoid arthritis and scleroderma, and may precede their diagnosis by many years.[1] This may also occur in occupations where vibrating tools are used. Several years of follow-up examinations are important in patients who are over 30 when symptoms first develop, in order to differentiate between Raynaud's disease and Raynaud's phenomenon.

Medical Management

Pharmacotherapy is of some value in relieving vasoconstriction. Many patients find the side-effects of medications unpleasant, however, and would rather suffer with the symptoms of the disease. Oral doses of Rauwolfia alkaloids such as Reserpine (0.25–0.5 mg daily), are used to decrease peripheral vasoconstriction. Vasodilating drugs, such as Dibenamine (phenoxybenzamine), Priscoline hydrochloride (tolazoline hydrochloride), Roniacol (nicotinyl alcohol), Arlidin (nylidrin), and Cyclospasmol (cyclandelate) are also used for Raynaud patients. In some cases vasodilating drugs cause facial flushing and headaches. Several other drugs have been recommended, including triiodothyronine, guanethidine, and methyldopa, but these are still somewhat controversial.

For patients who have severe symptoms and have not obtained relief by any other method, a sympathectomy is often considered. Lumbar ganglion sympathectomy gives complete relief of symptoms in most cases where the feet are involved; however, with involvement of the arm, the results of a sympathetic ganglionectomy are much less predictable.

Biofeedback and progressive relaxation therapy are therapies that are gaining increasing attention as means for the individual to gain awareness of and control over the vasoconstriction process. These are discussed in Chapter 22.

Nursing Management

Relieving vasospasm and preventing its occurrence by avoiding exposure to cold and to stressful environments are the primary goals of management for the person with either Raynaud's disease or Raynaud's phenomenon. Reassurance that the symptoms are unlikely to result in serious disability is important to the psychologic and emotional well-being of the person.

Nurses can assist patients in identifying situations which tend to precipitate attacks, in order to cope with or eliminate them if possible. Occupational health nurses, in particular, can participate in the prevention of prolonged exposure of workers to conditions that may precipitate Raynaud's attacks, as well as in planning and implementing health education.

One very important area in nursing management is patient instruction to minimize exposure to cold to avoid precipitation of attacks. This is an area for nursing assessment and intervention, because the physician may not have the time or the background to explain practical pointers for avoiding cold exposure in everyday life. Although a move to a warmer climate may improve the symptoms, susceptible patients may have attacks in almost any climate; therefore, other measures should be emphasized. Smoking is definitely contraindicated because it causes vasoconstriction; nurses can reinforce the reasons for not smoking.

In order to keep the total body warm and thus prevent vasospasm in the digits, clothing should be of an insulative type which will retain body heat by trapping it in layers of air. Tightly and thickly woven arctic-type clothing, such as wool socks and mittens (not gloves) and fleece-lined footwear, should be worn in cold weather and can greatly decrease heat loss in the hands and feet. Recently inner soles for shoes made of reflective material have appeared on the market. These retain more of the body temperature that would normally be lost to the pavement or cold ground. Patients and medical literature agree that it is very important to have hands warm before putting mittens on, because once the fingers become cold they require an external source of warmth, such as water, to be rewarmed. Other suggestions to reduce discomfort include using mittens or gloves to remove cold items from the refrigerator or freezer, washing vegetables with tepid water, and using electric or thermal blankets on the bed. Activities which require a lot of pressure on the fingers such as typing, piano playing, sewing, and chopping foods by hand, may precipitate symptoms in some people with more advanced involvement.

Hikers and skiers use some specific techniques for keeping warm. Facing the sun rather than away from it helps to keep feet and hands warm. Holding the arms above the head to drain the venous blood from the hands, followed by circular whirling of the arms to drive arterial blood into the collapsed capillaries by centrifugal force is another physiologic technique for warming the hands. This process can be done repeatedly. It provides warmth and at the same time keeps the person moving and active. The more relaxed a person is when skiing or climbing, the less likelihood there is of a vasoconstrictive episode.[4]

Relief of vasoconstriction may be hastened by immersion of the hand or foot in warm water; however, the water should be no warmer than 90° F (32.2° C), in order to prevent adding thermal trauma to the already ischemic tissue. Relief may be obtained more quickly and satisfactorily by warming the backs of the hands first, or the backs of the shoulders and upper thoracic area where the sympathetic ganglia lie. The backs of the hands can be warmed by running warm water over them and the backs of the shoulders and upper thoracic region can be warmed by a heating pad, covered hot water bottle, a warm shower, or by getting into a warm tub and placing a warm washcloth over the area.

Patients of both sexes exposed to vibratory tools such as jackhammers, chain saws, and grinding wheels may manifest Raynaud's symptoms. Nurses in industrial settings may be called upon to recognize the symptoms, identify the predisposition to Raynaud's in pre-employment and follow-up physicals, refer the symptomatic person for further work-up, attempt to reduce that person's exposure to trauma, and aid in their transfer to a different work environment, if this is appropriate. Nurses in any setting may be involved in teaching patients about their therapy, in counseling patients, or in assisting them with day-to-day living with their symptoms.[2]

THROMBOANGIITIS OBLITERANS

Thromboangiitis obliterans (Buerger's disease) is an occlusive inflammatory disease of the small to medium peripheral arteries and veins. Whether this condition is a specific disease entity or a syndrome is still being argued. There is, however, agreement that its pathogenesis has a definite relationship to tobacco use.

Pathophysiology

The disease is characterized by inflammatory thrombus formation in segments of arteries and veins. Inflammatory cells extend through the vessel walls and into the thrombus. The presence of a thrombus and inflammation results in stenosis and occlusion of the vessel and in peripheral ischemia. The course of the disease is characterized by exacerbation and remission; however, the occlusive disease is progressive and often overtakes the development of collateral circulation. As the ischemia increases, non-healing ulcers and gangrene in the extremity may lead to the necessity for amputation.[1]

Clinical Manifestations

The person with Buerger's disease is typically a young male, 20–45 years old, who smokes cigarettes and complains of pain and coldness, most often of the upper extremities. Migratory thrombophlebitis as well as sensitivity to cold may occur early in the disease. Ischemic symptoms found in arteriosclerosis with obliterans, such as intermittent claudication of the instep of the foot, rest pain, and eventual tissue destruction and gangrene, are also indicators of Buerger's disease.

Diagnostic Tests

Diagnosis is based predominantly on the history and subsequent course of symptoms. Arteriography can be used to demonstrate the presence or absence of occlusion in the vessels.

Medical Management

The treatment of thromboangiitis obliterans is similar to that for arteriosclerosis obliterans, except that *total and permanent* abstinence from tobacco is imperative. While there is no specific evidence that tobacco causes Buerger's disease, nicotine does promote some vasoconstriction, which increases peripheral ischemia. If ischemia progresses to the point of ulcerations and gangrene, then amputation is almost always necessary.

Nursing Management

The goal in nursing care is to assist the patient with Buerger's disease to control the symptoms. The one known effective therapy for achieving this is the cessation of tobacco use. Long-term habits of smoking are difficult to interrupt and the patient will need consistent encouragement and reinforcement in this. As the disease progresses, the nursing care is the same as that described for arteriosclerosis obliterans.

VARICOSE VEINS

Varicose veins are dilated, distended tortuous veins, usually those in the lower extremities, which have incompetent valves. The hemodynamic disturbance present in varicosities is the result of the backflow and pooling of blood due to the valvular incompetency within the affected vein. Hereditary factors are considered important in the development of varicose veins. Other predisposing factors which increase venous pressure include pregnancy, obesity, ascites, tumors, and various occupations which require prolonged standing or sitting. More women are affected than men.

Pathophysiology

The affected veins no longer move the blood efficiently from the legs and feet, resulting in alterations of the hemodynamics which promote pooling and pain. The increased hydrostatic pressure within the varicosities exceeds the tissue pressure, results in dependent edema, and impedes tissue nutrition.

Manifestations

When the superficial veins are involved (primary varicose veins), the dilated, tortuous veins are visible superficially and may be accompanied by pedal edema. When the varicose veins are due to involvement of the deep venous system, they are referred to as secondary. While aching and fatigue may be experienced in the lower leg after a period of weight bearing, bed rest overnight usually relieves the edema and the discomfort. Hardened, fibrotic edema (brawny edema) may occur, together with a rash and changes in skin color and sensation in the affected extremity, particularly with secondary varicose veins.

Diagnosis

The history and clinical picture are usually sufficient for diagnosis. In addition, tests which demonstrate venous filling may be used for confirmation. Venography is useful to evaluate the deep venous system.

Medical Management

Support hose, elastic stockings, or elastic (ace) bandages are used to increase tissue hydrostatic pressure and thus venous pressure. The increased venous flow reduces the edema and improves tissue perfusion. For maximum support and benefit, these devices should be put on before the person arises, while the veins are minimally filled, as discussed in Chapter 28. Elastic garters, panty girdles, or other clothing causing constriction of the veins of the lower legs should be avoided (Chap. 38). Vein stripping is a surgical option if the conservative methods are inadequate, but this is rarely necessary unless other complications (for example, spontaneous rupture of the vein, stasis ulcers, or local infections) necessitate it.

Nursing Management

The focus of nursing care is teaching the patient how to fit the activities and demands of daily living with the discomfort imposed by varicose veins. Proper application of support stockings or bandages should be emphasized. Limiting long periods of standing or sitting and resting with the legs elevated above the level of the heart are actions which should be incorporated into daily living. Nursing care for the patient who develops thrombophlebitis and is on anticoagulant therapy is discussed in Chapter 28 and Chapter 38, respectively.

REFERENCES

1. Coffman JD: Diseases of the peripheral vessels. In Beeson P, McDermott W, Wyngaarden J (eds): Cecil's Textbook of Medicine, 15th ed. pp 1306–1307. Philadelphia, WB Saunders, 1979
2. Craven R, Curry T: When the diagnosis is Raynaud's. Am J Nurs 81(5):1007–1009, 1981
3. Frolich E: Pathophysiology, 2nd ed. p 37. Philadelphia, JB Lippincott, 1976
4. Leitch C, Tinker R: Primary Carc. Philadelphia, FA Davis, 1978
5. Slater EE, Desanctis RW: Diseases of the aorta. In Braunwald E (ed): Heart Disease: A Textbook of Cardiovascular Medicine. pp 1597–1629. Philadelphia, WB Saunders, 1980
6. Strandness DE: Vascular diseases of the extremities. In Isselbacher K et al (eds): Harrison's Principles of Internal Medicine, 9th ed. pp 1181–1188. New York, McGraw-Hill, 1980

ADDITIONAL READING

Atchinson JS, Murray J: Post vascular surgery. Nursing '78. 12:36–39, 1978
Bouhoutsos J, Morris T, Martin P: Unilateral Raynaud's phenomenon in the hand. Surgery 82(5):547–551, 1977

Brunner LR, Suddarth DS: Textbook of Medical–Surgical Nursing, 4th ed, pp 622–626. Philadelphia, JB Lippincott, 1980

Burgess EM, Marsden W: Major lower extremity amputations following arterial reconstruction. Arch Surg 108:655–660, 1974

Burrell ZL, Burrell LO: Critical Care, 3rd ed, pp 117–125. St. Louis, CV Mosby, 1977

Coffman JD: Intermittent claudication and rest pain: Physiologic concepts and therapeutic approaches. Progr Cardiovasc Dis 22(1):53–72, 1979

Dalen JE: Diseases of the aorta. In Isselbacher KJ et al (eds): Harrison's Principles of Internal Medicine, 9th ed, pp 1178–1181. New York, McGraw-Hill, 1980

Drain CB: The Recovery Room, pp 357–361. Philadelphia, WB Saunders, 1979

Eddy ME: Teaching patients with peripheral vascular disease. Nurs Clin North Am 12:151–160, 1977

Fronek A, Coel M, Bernstein EF: The importance of combined multisegmental pressure and Doppler flow velocity studies in the diagnosis of peripheral arterial occlusive disease. Surgery 84(6):840–847, 1978

Gardner E, Gray DJ, O'Rahilly R: Anatomy, 4th ed, pp 37–43. Philadelphia, WB Saunders, 1975

Halperin JL, Coffman JD: Pathophysiology of Raynaud's disease. Arch Intern Med 139:89–92, 1979

Hoffman GS: Raynaud's disease and phenomenon. Am Fam Physician 21(1):91–97, 1980

Imparato AM, Kim GE, Davidson T et al: Intermittent claudication: It's natural course. Surgery 78(6):795–799, 1975

Kessro B: Peripheral arterial insufficiency: Postoperative nursing care. Nurs Clin North Am 12:143–150, 1977

King OM: Care of the Cardiac Surgical Patient, pp 141–143. St. Louis, CV Mosby, 1975

Long GD: Managing the patient with abdominal aortic aneurysm. Nursing '78, 8:21–27, 1978

Miller K: Assessing peripheral perfusion. Am J Nurs 8:1673–1674, 1978

Phipps WJ, Long BC, Woods NF: Shafer's Medical-Surgical Nursing, 7th ed, pp 447–477. St. Louis, CV Mosby, 1980

Robbins SL, Angell M: Basic Pathology, 2nd ed, pp 145, 265–287. Philadelphia, WB Saunders, 1976

Roberts B: The acutely ischemic limb. Heart Lung 5:273–276, 1976

Robson AK: Aortofemoral graft. Nursing Times 75:18–22, 1979

Ryzewski J: Factors in the rehabilitation of patients with peripheral vascular disease. Nurs Clin North Am 12:161–168, 1977

Sexton DL: The patient with peripheral arterial occlusive disease. Nurs Clin North Am 12:89–100, 1977

Smith DW, Germain, CP: Care of the Adult Patient, pp 662–684. Philadelphia, JB Lippincott, 1975

Sodeman W Jr, Sodeman W: Pathologic Physiology, 6th ed. Philadelphia, WB Saunders, 1979

Sparks C: Peripheral pulses. Am J Nurs 75:1132–1133, 1975

Spencer FC, Imparato AM: Peripheral arterial disease. In Schwartz SI, et al (eds): Principles of Surgery, 2nd ed, pp 839–906. New York, McGraw-Hill, 1974

Spittell JA: Recognition and management of chronic atherosclerotic occlusive peripheral arterial disease. Mod Concepts Cardiovasc Dis 50(4):19–23, 1981

Taggart E: The physical assessment of the patient with arterial disease. Nurs Clin North Am 12:109–118, 1977

GLOSSARY

Activity. Refers to those movements that are accomplished in the course of meeting human physiological needs.

Afterload. The force opposing ventricular ejection (Fig. 2-7).

Ampere. The basic unit of electric current flow. The flow of a specific number of electrons past a point in 1 second.

Angina pectoris (angina). Chest discomfort, which is a symptom of myocardial ischemia; "strangling of the chest."

    classic angina. Angina that is typical in its onset, duration, location, radiation, and character.

    stable angina. Angina that has not changed in frequency, intensity, duration, or character for 60 days.

    unstable angina. Angina that has increased in frequency, intensity, duration, or character, heralding possible progression to infarction.

    variant angina (Printzmetal's angina). Chest discomfort similar in character but of longer duration than classic angina; usually not due to exertion; caused by spasm of the coronary arteries.

Angiocardiography, serial. Single or biplane serial x-ray films taken at filming rates of 4 to 12 frames per second. The advantages are high resolution, clear definition of anatomic detail, and large size, which permits filming of even grossly dilated ventricles for quantitative angiography. Disadvantages include relatively high x-ray exposure, blurring of moving structures due to long exposure times, and poor appreciation of dynamic events due to slow filming rates.

Angstrom (A or Å). 10^{-8} centimeter or $\frac{1}{100}$ millionth of a centimeter.

Arteriosclerosis. Hardening of the arteries; a general term describing atherosclerosis, medial calcific sclerosis, or arteriolar sclerosis.

Atherosclerosis. A type of arteriosclerosis with proliferation of smooth muscle cells and accumulation of lipids in the intima of large and middle-sized arteries; causes coronary artery disease.

Auscultatory gap. The period during which Korotkov sounds indicating true systolic pressure fade away and reappear at a lower pressure point; responsible for errors made in recording falsely low systolic BPs, especially in hypertensive patients, or up to 25 mm Hg; avoid by pumping cuff 30 mm Hg beyond palpable systolic pressure (Fig. 14-3).

Automaticity. Spontaneous impulse formation, a property of all pacemaker cells. A mechanism of abnormal impulse formation.

Biofeedback. During biological monitoring of a specific body function, the biological information that is returned, or "fed back," to the subject in order to facilitate the modification of that same function; examples include blood pressure biofeedback, heart rate biofeedback, and electromyogram biofeedback.

Blood flow rate (Q̇). The quantity of blood passing a given point in the circulation at a given point in time; volume/ unit of time; expressed as ml/min or cm³/sec; $\dot{Q} = \frac{\Delta P}{R}$ where $\dot{Q}$ = flow, ΔP is pressure difference along the length of a tube, and R = resistance (Fig. 5-3).

Cardiac Care Unit (CCU). An area equipped and staffed primarily to treat patients with suspected or definite myocardial infarction and patients with potentially lethal arrhythmias.

Cardiac index. Cardiac output per square meter of body surface area.

Cardiac output. Amount of blood ejected from the right or left ventricle per minute, expressed in liters per minute. Cardiac output is equal to the stroke volume multiplied by heart rate.

Cardiac rehabilitation. The process of actively assisting the known cardiac patient to achieve and maintain an optimal state of health.

Cardiac reserve. The extent to which cardiac output can be increased by an increase in heart rate or stroke volume. Heart rate is usually increased to a greater extent than is stroke volume (Fig. 6-5).

Cardiovascular collapse. A nonspecific term referring to functional failure of the heart or vasculature resulting in low tissue perfusion pressure and shock.

Cardioversion. Restoration of sinus rhythm. This is accomplished by vagal stimulation, drugs, and precordial synchronized shock.

Carotid sinus massage. Manual compression for 5 seconds of one carotid sinus, resulting in reflex vagal stimulation.

Cineangiocardiography. Single or biplane filming of the image on an image intensifier by a motion picture camera during cardiac catheterization. The advantages include clarity of movement and dynamic events of the cardiac cycle, television visualization, instant replay capability, and low x-ray exposure. The major disadvantage is limited field size.

Compensatory pause. With a complete compensatory pause, the combined R–R cycles of a normal and a premature beat together equal the time taken by two consecutive normal heart cycles. With an incomplete compensatory pause, the combined R–R cycles of a normal and a premature beat together do not equal the time taken by two consecutive normal heart cycles.

Compliance (C). The change in volume for a given change in pressure. $C = \dfrac{\Delta V}{\Delta P}$ where Δ = change, V = volume, and P = pressure.

Concealed conduction. If a stimulus reaches any part of the conducting system before it has finished repolarization, the conduction may be blocked or slowed. If it passes slowly, it is eventually blocked, resulting in tissue that is refractory. Refractory tissue either demonstrates an altered response or no response to a stimulus. This concealed conduction (no ECG change) affects transmission of the next impulse as it encounters the refractory tissue.

Conduction. Antegrade conduction is the normal direction of impulse propagation. In retrograde conduction, the impulse propagation is in the reverse direction.

Conduction velocity. Rate of rise of phase 0 of the action potential; speed at which the wave of depolarization is conducted through the myocardium.

Conductivity. Impulse propagation, which is dependent on membrane excitability, responsiveness, and refractoriness.

Cholesterol. A sterol found in animal tissue.

Chylomicron. A particle secreted by the intestinal wall lymph that transports fat; 90% of the chylomicron is triglyceride.

Contractility. Intrinsic ability of myocardial fibers to shorten, develop tension, or both, independent of variations induced by alterations in preload or afterload (Fig 2-8).

Coronary artery disease. Atherosclerosis of the coronary arteries, manifested by angina pectoris, myocardial infarction, or sudden cardiac death.

Crackles (formerly rales). Discontinuous sounds created by alveolar fluid or explosive reopening of closed alveoli; nonspecific, but may indicate atelectasis or congestive heart failure (Fig. 14-27 A).

Decremental conduction. Decay of action potential, leading to block.

Defibrillation. The use of asynchronized precordial electrical shock to depolarize the heart to terminate ventricular fibrillation.

dP/dt. Rate of rise of ventricular pressure per unit of time, an index of contractility. d = change, P = pressure, t = time.

Ectopic impulse. An electrical impulse from an area of the heart other than the sinus node.

Electrogram. A unipolar or bipolar record of electrical activity of the heart taken with the electrode(s) within a heart chamber or in contact with the myocardium.

Electrophoresis. The movement on various substrates of charged particles suspended in a liquid under the influence of an applied electric field; a qualitative test.

Escape impulse. One or two impulses (atrial, junctional, or ventricular) arising from delay in the formation or arrival of the prevailing pacemaker.

Escape interval. The time between the patient's own depolarization (ectopic or sinus-beat) and the initial pacemaker impulse (a preset interval in the circuitry). It can be either a shorter or a longer time period than the pulse interval.

Escape rhythm. Three or more consecutive impulses at a rate not exceeding the upper limit of the inherent pacemaker. Rate of impulse formation at the SA node is 60 to 100 impulses/minute; rate at the AV node is 40 to 60 impulses/minute; rate in the ventricular myocardium is 20 to 40 impulses/minute.

Excitability. Describes the ease with which a cardiac cell can be brought to threshold and made to fire either a normal or abnormal action potential. If it takes a large depolarizing current to make a cell reach threshold, excitability is low; if only a small depolarizing current is required, the cell is said to be highly excitable.

Exercise. Refers to physical exertion at prescribed intensity, duration, and frequency for improvement of health, prevention of deconditioning, or correction of a physical deformity or disability.

Fatty streak. Yellowish, smooth lesion protruding slightly into arterial lumen; controversy exists regarding its irreversibility and whether it is a precursor of the fibrous plaque.

Fibrillation threshold. Least intensity of an electrical stimulus that will initiate fibrillation.

Fibrous plaque. Characteristic lesion of atherosclerosis; yellow—gray elevation on surface of the artery.

Functional aerobic impairment (FAI). The degree of duration of the test observed and duration expected for a healthy person of the same age, sex, and habitual activity status as the patient, expressed as a percentage of the normal.

Half-life (plasma half-life, or t½). The amount of time needed for a drug concentration to change by 50%; used to describe the time course of disappearance of the drug from the plasma due to elimination of the drug from the body.

Hemiblock. Blockage of one of the two main divisions (left anterior or left posterior) of the left bundle branch.

Hyperlipidemia. An abnormal elevation of serum cholesterol, triglycerides, or both; may be primary, secondary, or familial.

heterozygous hyperlipoproteinemia. Familial lipid disorder transmitted to the child by only one parent.

homozygous hyperlipoproteinemia. Familial lipid disorder transmitted to the child by both parents.

Hyperlipoproteinemia. An abnormal elevation of serum lipoproteins.

J point. The junction between the QRS complex and the ST segment; the point at which the ST segment begins (Fig. 17-6).

Law of LaPlace. $P \propto T/r$, where P = distending pressure, T = wall tension, r = radius, $\propto$ = is proportional to. Also, $T = \dfrac{P \times r}{\text{wall thickness}}$. One implication of these relationships is that, at any given pressure, wall tension increases as the radius of the cylinder increases (Chaps. 2, 5, 27).

Leakage current. Current conveyed from accessible parts of an appliance to ground or to other accessible parts of an appliance.

Lipid. Naturally occurring organic substances, including triglycerides, phospholipids, and plant and animal sterols.

Lipoprotein. A combination of a lipid and a protein having the general properties of the protein, including that of solubility.

Maximum diastolic potential. The most negative voltage achieved across the membrane of a spontaneously depolarizing cell. This is achieved after repolarization, at the beginning of phase-4 depolarization.

Membrane responsiveness. The relationship between maximum velocity (V max) and the membrane potential at which the depolarizing stimulus was delivered. The more negative the potential difference across a membrane, the more rapid will be the V max.

Mole. The quantity of a chemical substance having a weight in grams equal to its molecular weight; one mole consists of 6.02257×10^{23} molecules.

Monosaturated fatty acid. Fatty acids that contain one double bond.

Nernst equation. Gives the equilibrium potential for each ion; the equilibrium potential is the point at which the forces promoting outward movement of an ion are balanced by the forces promoting inward movement (Chapter 3). For example, the equilibrium potential for potassium is:

$$E_k = \frac{RT}{FZ_k} \ln \frac{[K_o^+]}{[K_i^+]}$$

where E_k = equilibrium potential for K^+

$\quad$ R = gas constant

$\quad$ T = absolute temperature

$\quad$ F = the faraday (number of coulombs per mol of charge)

$\quad$ Z_k = the valence of K^+ (+1)

$\quad$ $[K_o^+]$ = K^+ concentration outside the cell (for example, 4mM)

$\quad$ $[K_i^+]$ = K^+ concentration inside the cell (for example, 155mM)

Converting from the natural log to the base 10 log and replacing the constants with numerical values, the equation becomes approximately

$$E_k = 61 \log_{10} \frac{[K_o^+]}{[K_i^+]} \text{ at } 37°C$$

$$E_k = 61 \log_{10} \frac{155}{4} = -97mv$$

Nursing diagnosis. A problem that can be treated by a nursing prescription; usually interferes with the patient's ability to perform ADLs, such as shortness of breath, or prevents the patient from coping adequately with any situation, such as denial of MI.

Nursing process. The basis of all nursing care, consisting of assessment, diagnosis, prescription, implementation, and evaluation.

Obesity. A body-mass index $\left(\frac{weight}{height}\right)^2$ or kg/m² greater than 20% above ideal values.

Ohm. The basic unit of electrical resistance against which a current of one ampere can be maintained by an electromotive force of one volt.

Ohm's law. Amperage (I) is equal to voltage (E) divided by the resistance (R) in ohms $\left(I = \frac{E}{R}\right)$.

Phlebostatic axis. The crossing of two reference lines: first, a line from the fourth intercostal space at the point where it joins the sternum drawn out to the side of body beneath the axilla; second, a line midpoint between the anterior and posterior surfaces of the chest (Fig. 21-1). The phlebostatic level is a horizontal line through the phlebostatic axis (Fig. 21-2).

Placebo. A simulated treatment given to improve symptoms but without the ability to act upon the underlying pathophysiologic process, as the real treatment would.

Placebo effect. The reaction of the patient to the placebo.

Plasma. The liquid phase of whole blood obtained by centrifuging or sedimenting out the solid phase (cells).

Polyunsaturated fatty acid. Fatty acids that contain two or more double bonds.

Poiseuille's law. Describes streamlined nonpulsitile flow of a substance with uniform viscosity: $\dot{Q} = \frac{\pi r^4 (P_i - P_0)}{8 \eta l}$ where $\dot{Q}$ = flow, $\frac{\pi}{8}$ = a constant, r = radius, $P_i - P_0$ = driving pressure, η = viscosity, and l = length. Thus, flow is proportional to the driving pressure, the fourth power of the radius, and a constant, and is inversely proportional to the viscosity of the liquid and the length of the tube (Fig. 5-3).

Preload. The distending force stretching the ventricular muscle (Fig. 2-6).

Pressure (P). Force (F) per unit area (P = F/A), for example, the force exerted by the blood in the heart or in a blood vessel. Pressure is exerted equally in all directions. In a liquid system, P = h.p.g., where h = height of volume of liquid, p = density of the liquid, and g = gravitational force; expressed as dyne/cm²; $\Delta P = \dot{Q} \times R$; also, $\Delta P = \frac{\Delta V}{C}$; also, BP = CO × SVR, where ΔP = change in pressure, $\dot{Q}$ = flow, R = resistance, ΔV = change in volume, C = compliance, BP = blood pressure, CO = cardiac output, and SVR = systemic vascular resistance.

pressure gradient. Difference in pressure from one point to another. A pressure gradient ($P_i - P_o$; P_i = pressure at inflow end, and P_o = pressure at outflow end) promotes flow. In the peripheral vascular system, this is the pressure difference between two points along a blood vessel, while, in the heart, it is the pressure difference between two adjacent cardiac chambers when the valve that separates them is open.

total pressure. In a vascular channel, the pressure of the kinetic energy of the flowing fluid plus the lateral pressure.

transmural pressure. Pressure on one side of a vessel wall minus pressure on the other side of the wall.

Pressure—rate product. The product of systolic blood pressure and heart rate divided by 100; highly correlated with myocardial oxygen consumption.

Pulse pressure. The difference between the systolic and

diastolic BP; reflects stroke volume, ejection velocity, and peripheral resistance (Fig. 14-4).

Reentry. When the impulse propagates along two different pathways and encounters a block along one of them (unidirectional block), the impulse traveling through the other pathway returns in a retrograde fashion through the blocked area and reenters the circuit, causing reexcitation of the myocardium. With unidirectional block, antegrade conduction is blocked because repolarization is retarded and retrograde conduction is slow, which allows the tissue to repolarize and to readmit an impulse (Figs. 26-1A and 26-1B).

Refractory period. The period in the cardiac cycle in which the excitability threshold is higher than normal and conduction is slower than normal.

> **absolute (effective) refractory period.** The period in the cardiac cycle when no action potential can be initiated by an electrical stimulus.

> **relative refractory period.** The period in the cardiac cycle in which the excitability threshold is higher and conduction is slower than normal.

Resistance. Opposition to force; factors that hinder or retard flow; in the vascular system, the hindrance provided by the vessels to the flow of viscous blood; $R = \frac{8\,\eta\,l}{\pi\,r^4}$ of Poiseuilles equation (see above); units are dyne sec/cm^{-5}. $R = \frac{\text{mean driving pressure }(\Delta P)}{\text{mean flow }\dot{Q}}$, so $R = \frac{\Delta P}{\dot{Q}}$; also, $SVR = \frac{BP}{CO}$ where SVR = systemic vascular resistance, BP = blood pressure, and CO = cardiac output.

> **peripheral resistance unit (PRU).** An expression of flow resistance useful in making comparisons in peripheral vascular beds, for example:
>
> $$\frac{1\ mm\ Hg}{1\,l\ min} = \frac{1333\ dynes/cm^2}{1000\ cm^3/60\ sec}$$
> $$= \frac{1333 \times 60\ dynes\ sec}{1000\ cm^5} = 80\ dynes\ sec\ cm^{-5}.$$
>
> PRUs are sometimes expressed per 100 g tissue.

> **pulmonary arteriolar resistance (PAR).** Resistance in pulmonary vascular beds. $PAR = \frac{PA - LA}{CO}$, where PA = mean pulmonary artery pressure, LA = mean left arterial pressure, and CO = cardiac output; approximately 67 dynes sec cm^{-5}.

> **systemic vascular resistance (SVR).** Resistance in systemic vascular beds; $SVR = \frac{MAP - PRA}{CO}$ where

MAP = mean systemic arterial pressure, PRA = mean right atrial pressure, and CO = cardiac output; approximately 1130 dynes sec cm^{-5}.

> **total pulmonary resistance (TPR).** Resistance in pulmonary vascular beds. $TPR = \frac{PA}{CO}$ where PA = mean pulmonary artery pressure, and CO = cardiac output; approximately 205 dynes sec cm^{-5}.

> **total systemic resistance (TSR).** Total resistance of systemic vascular beds; $TSR = \frac{MAP}{CO}$, where MAP = mean systemic arterial pressure, and CO = cardiac output.

Risk factors (of coronary artery disease). Characteristic findings associated with the presence of coronary artery disease; the three major risk factors are hyperlipoproteinemia, high blood pressure, and cigarette smoking.

Selective myocardial cell necrosis (myofibrillar degeneration). Small focal areas of myocardial cell death; the interstitial cells (capillaries, nerves, etc.) remain viable.

Sensitivity. The probability, usually expressed in percent, of classifying correctly a true positive test.

Serum. The liquid left after clotting of blood when fibrinogen has been removed.

Specificity. The probability, usually expressed in percent, of correctly classifying a negative test.

Tension. An elongating force that is exerted in the direction of pull; stress on a material produced by the pull of forces tending to cause extension. Like pressure, it may be expressed as force per unit area, but, unlike pressure, it is not equal in all directions. The term may be used to describe the force generated by a muscle or to describe the force within the wall of a cardiac chamber. It can be thought of as a force that would tend to pull apart the sides of an imagined slit in the myocardial wall.

Triglyceride. A compound consisting of three molecules of fatty acid esterified to glycerol; a neutral fat that is the usual storage form of lipids in animals.

Volt. Unit of electromotive force (pressure that causes current to flow).

Voltage. The driving force that causes current to flow.

Vulnerable period. A period during the cardiac action potential when a propagated impulse may result in a repetitive response or fibrillation.

Watt. The product of current pressure and current flow. One watt of power is equal to one ampere at the pressure of one volt.

INDEX

A

Q

R

W

X

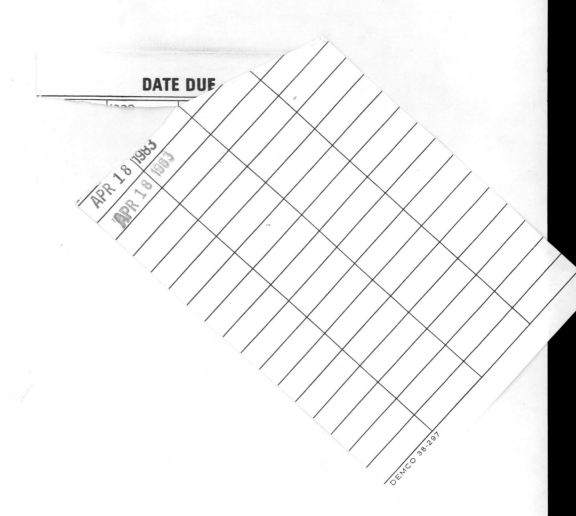